MASSACHUSETTS GENERAL HOSPITAL REVIEW OF CRITICAL CARE MEDICINE

SECOND EDITION

MASSACHUSETTS GENERAL HOSPITAL REVIEW OF CRITICAL CARE MEDICINE

SECOND EDITION

Editors

Marvin G. Chang, MD, PhD
Assistant Professor, Harvard Medical School
Associate Program Director, Critical Care-Anesthesiology Fellowship
Director, Perioperative Transthoracic Echocardiography (Point of Care Ultrasound)
Department of Anesthesia, Critical Care and Pain Medicine
Massachusetts General Hospital
Boston, Massachusetts

Casey M. Luckhurst, MD
Instructor in Surgery
Harvard Medical School
Division of Trauma, Emergency Surgery, and Surgical Critical Care
Department of Surgery
Massachusetts General Hospital
Boston, Massachusetts

Raghu R. Chivukula, MD, PhD
Assistant Professor of Medicine and Surgery
Harvard Medical School
Department of Medicine
Massachusetts General Hospital
Boston, Massachusetts

David M. Dudzinski, MD, JD
Associate Professor of Medicine
Harvard Medical School
Chief, Cardiac Critical Care Section
Director, Cardiac Intensive Care Unit
Program Director, Critical Care Cardiology Fellowship
Massachusetts General Hospital
Boston, Massachusetts

Saef Izzy, MD, MBChB, FNCS, FAAN
Associate Professor of Neurology
Division of Neurocritical Care and Cerebrovascular Diseases
Department of Neurology
Harvard Medical School
Mass General Brigham
Head of Immunology of CNS Injury Program
Ann Romney Center for Neurologic Diseases
Boston, Massachusetts

Edward A. Bittner, MD, PhD
Associate Professor of Anaesthesia
Department of Anaesthesia
Harvard Medical School
Program Director, Critical Care-Anesthesiology Fellowship
Associate Director, Surgical Intensive Care Unit
Massachusetts General Hospital
Boston, Massachusetts

Wolters Kluwer

Philadelphia • Baltimore • New York • London
Buenos Aires • Hong Kong • Sydney • Tokyo

Acquisitions Editor: Keith Donellan
Development Editor: Ashley Fischer
Editorial Coordinator: Sunmerrilika Baskar
Marketing Manager: Janet Feeney
Senior Production Specialist: Bridgett Dougherty
Manager, Graphic Arts & Design: Stephen Druding
Manufacturing Coordinator: Lisa Bowling
Prepress Vendor: S4Carlisle Publishing Services

2nd edition

9 8 7 6 5 4 3 2 1

Printed in The United States of America

Library of Congress Cataloging-in-Publication Data

ISBN-13: 978-1-975243-01-2

Library of Congress Control Number: 2026931608

shop.lww.com

MPP0326

To our teachers and fellows—past, present, and future.

Preface

Premise

Critical care medicine is one of the most dynamic fields in medicine, demanding both broad and deep clinical expertise. When we first created this resource more than a decade ago, there was a clear need for a comprehensive, high-quality critical care board review book. Since then, numerous advances in evidence-based medicine and multidisciplinary practices have significantly reshaped critical care medicine practiced today. This edition has been updated to reflect the major developments of the past decade. Our primary objective remains to provide a reliable resource for board certification and recertification, while also serving as a refresher and practical guide for rapid reference. We have continued to provide a concise, high-yield format that supports efficient study while still providing a comprehensive review of essential critical care topics. In addition, this new edition includes numerous questions and answers designed to reinforce key concepts and enhance retention of board-relevant material.

Requirements

At least one author must be a critical care attending/fellow either trained at Massachusetts General Hospital (MGH) or currently/previously practicing at MGH (to ensure consistency in terminology/approach and to provide the "MGH flavor of critical care"). Editors and contributors are drawn from the major specialty areas that encompass adult critical care medicine, including anesthesiology, surgery, emergency medicine, neurology, and medicine. The topic list for chapters was developed using the content outlines for the subspecialty critical care board examinations.

Contents

Contributors

Moustafa Abdalla, MD, DPhil
Resident
Department of Surgery
Massachusetts General Hospital
Boston, Massachusetts

Yasmin Aghajan, MD
Neurointensivist
Department of Neurology
Brigham and Women's Hospital
Boston, Massachusetts

Aaron D. Aguirre, MD, PhD
Cardiologist
Division of Cardiology
Department of Medicine
Massachusetts General Hospital
Boston, Massachusetts

Rashid A. Ahmed, MD
Fellow
Department of Neurology
Harvard Medical School
Massachusetts General Hospital
Brigham and Women's Hospital
Boston, Massachusetts

Katherine H. Albutt, MD, MPH
Attending Surgeon
Division of Trauma, Emergency Surgery, and Surgical Critical Care
Department of Surgery
Massachusetts General Hospital
Boston, Massachusetts

Glasiele C. Alcala, PhD
Research Fellow
Department of Anesthesiology, Critical Care and Pain Medicine
Massachusetts General Hospital
Boston, Massachusetts

Ali A. Alsarah, MD
Fellow
Department of Neurology
Harvard Medical School
Massachusetts General Hospital
Boston, Massachusetts

Andrea Ansari, MD
Fellow
Department of Anesthesiology, Critical Care and Pain Medicine
Massachusetts General Hospital
Boston, Massachusetts

Omar Arnaout, MD
Associate Professor of Neurosurgery
Department of Surgery
Harvard School of Medicine
Mass General Brigham
Boston, Massachusetts

Brandon J. Aubrey, MBBS, PhD
Fellow
Leukemia Service
Harvard Medical School
Massachusetts General Hospital
Boston, Massachusetts

Sharl Azar, MD
Medical Director
Department of Hematology
Massachusetts General Hospital
Boston, Massachusetts

Diana Barragan-Bradford, MD
Anesthesiologist and Critical Care Intensivist
Department of Anesthesia, Critical Care and Pain Medicine
Massachusetts General Hospital
Boston, Massachusetts

Matthew Bartek, MD, MPH
Instructor
Departments of Surgery and Medicine
Massachusetts General Hospital
Boston, Massachusetts

Lisa Bartucca, MD
Fellow
Pediatric Critical Care Medicine
Massachusetts General Hospital
Boston, Massachusetts

Lisa M. Bebell, MD, MSc
Assistant Professor
Department of Medicine
Harvard Medical School
Massachusetts General Hospital
Boston, Massachusetts

Sophia Bechek, MD
Anesthesiologist
Department of Anesthesia and Perioperative Medicine
Maine Medical Center
Spectrum HealthCare Partners
Portland, Maine

Emily Anne Smith Bergbower, MD, PhD
Fellow
Department of Anesthesiology
University of Maryland Medical Center
Baltimore, Maryland

Kristina Bermas, MD
Trauma Surgeon
Division of Trauma, Emergency Surgery, and Surgical Critical Care
Department of Surgery
Massachusetts General Hospital
Boston, Massachusetts

Samuel Bernard, MD
Assistant Professor of Medicine, Attending Cardiologist
Division of Cardiology
Department of Medicine
New York University Grossman School of Medicine
New York, New York

Lorenzo Berra, MD
Anesthesiologist and Critical Care Physician
Medical Director of Respiratory Care
Department of Anesthesia, Critical Care and Pain Medicine
Harvard Medical School
Massachusetts General Hospital
Mass General Brigham
Boston, Massachusetts

Edward A. Bittner, MD, PhD
Associate Professor of Anaesthesia
Department of Anaesthesia
Harvard Medical School
Program Director, Critical Care-Anesthesiology Fellowship
Associate Director, Surgical Intensive Care Unit
Massachusetts General Hospital
Boston, Massachusetts

Katharine Black, MD
Assistant Physician
Department of Medicine
Massachusetts General Hospital
Boston, Massachusetts

Eran Brauner, MD
Physician
Department of Surgery
Massachusetts General Hospital
Boston, Massachusetts

Kait Brennan, DO, MPH
Assistant Professor of Anesthesiology and Critical Care Medicine
Department of Anesthesiology
Vanderbilt University Medical Center
Nashville, Tennessee

Jason Brocker, MD
Chief of Trauma and Acute Care Surgery
Department of Surgery
Mass General Brigham—Salem
Swampscott, Massachusetts

Kemar J. Brown, MD
Cardiologist
Department of Medicine
Massachusetts General Hospital
Boston, Massachusetts

Patricia A.R. Brunker, MD, DPhil
Medical Director, Blood Transfusion Patient Services
Department of Pathology
Massachusetts General Hospital
Boston, Massachusetts

Andrew M. Brunner, MD
Associate Professor
Mass General Brigham Cancer Institute
Massachusetts General Hospital
Boston, Massachusetts

Giovanni Bruno, MD
Fellow
Department of Anesthesia, Critical Care and Pain Medicine
Massachusetts General Hospital
Boston, Massachusetts

John Bryant, MD
Assistant Professor
Department of Anesthesiology and Critical Care
Vanderbilt University Medical Center
Nashville, Tennessee

Jeffrey W. Cannon, MD
Anesthesiologist and Critical Care Physician
Winchester Anesthesia Associates
Winchester, Massachusetts

Sandra Carvajal-Raga, MD
Assistant Professor
Department of Anesthesiology
Keck Hospital of USC
Los Angeles, California

Gianna Lauren Casal, PharmD
Clinical Pharmacist
Pharmacy Department
Massachusetts General Hospital
Boston, Massachusetts

Maurizio Cereda, MD
Associate Professor
Department of Anesthesia, Critical Care and Pain Medicine
Massachusetts General Hospital
Boston, Massachusetts

Marvin G. Chang, MD, PhD
Assistant Professor, Harvard Medical School
Associate Program Director, Critical Care-Anesthesiology
Fellowship
Director, Perioperative Transthoracic Echocardiography (Point of Care Ultrasound)
Department of Anesthesia, Critical Care and Pain Medicine
Massachusetts General Hospital
Boston, Massachusetts

Safia Chatur, MD
Cardiologist and Instructor in Medicine
Department of Cardiology
Harvard Medical School
Massachusetts General Hospital
Boston, Massachusetts

Brian W. Chin, MD, MS
Attending Physician
Department of Emergency Medicine
Temecula Valley Hospital
Temecula, California

Raghu R. Chivukula, MD, PhD
Assistant Professor of Medicine and Surgery
Harvard Medical School
Department of Medicine
Massachusetts General Hospital
Boston, Massachusetts

Paul B. Comish, MD, MPH
Fellow
Department of Surgery
Massachusetts General Hospital
Boston, Massachusetts

Christopher V. Cosgriff, MD, MPH
Fellow
Department of Medicine
Massachusetts General Hospital
Boston, Massachusetts

Devan Cote, MD
Instructor in Anesthesia
Department of Anesthesia, Critical Care and Pain Medicine
Massachusetts General Hospital
Boston, Massachusetts

Leigh Anne Dageforde, MD, MPH
Assistant Professor of Surgery
Division of Transplantation, Department of Surgery
Massachusetts General Hospital
Boston, Massachusetts

Amory de Roulet, MD
Surgeon
Department of Surgery
Massachusetts General Hospital
Boston, Massachusetts

Michael P. DeWane, MD
Trauma and Acute Care Surgeon
Department of Surgery
Massachusetts General Hospital
Boston, Massachusetts

Anahat Dhillon, MD
Vice Chair of Critical Care
Department of Anesthesiology
Keck School of Medicine of USC
Los Angeles, California

Jose L. Diaz-Gomez, MD, MAS
Chair, Integrated Hospital Care Institute
Department of Critical Care Medicine
Cleveland Clinic
Abu Dhabi, United Arab Emirates

Ryan Dodge, III, MD
Anesthesiologist
Department of Anesthesia, Critical Care and Pain Medicine
Massachusetts General Hospital
Boston, Massachusetts

David M. Dudzinski, MD, JD
Associate Professor of Medicine
Harvard Medical School
Chief, Cardiac Critical Care Section
Director, Cardiac Intensive Care Unit
Program Director, Critical Care Cardiology Fellowship
Massachusetts General Hospital
Boston, Massachusetts

Jonathan A. Duskin, MD
Fellow
Division of Neurocritical Care
Department of Neurology
Mass General Brigham
Boston, Massachusetts

Kiran Dyamenahalli, MD, PhD
Fellow
Department of Anesthesia, Critical Care and Pain Medicine
Department of Surgery
Harvard Medical School
Massachusetts General Hospital
Boston, Massachusetts

Gamonmas Ekkapat, MD
Attending Anesthesiologist and Critical Care Physician
Department of Anesthesiology
Faculty of Medicine
Chulalongkorn University
King Chulalongkorn Memorial Hospital
Thai Red Cross Society
Bangkok, Thailand

Amjad Elmashala, MD
Fellow
Division of Neurocritical Care
Department of Neurology
Mass General Brigham
Boston, Massachusetts

Matthew Elson, MD
Fellow
Department of Surgery
Massachusetts General Hospital
Boston, Massachusetts

Logan Ernst, MD
Anesthesiologist/Intensivist
Department of Anesthesiology
Tufts Medical Center
Boston, Massachusetts

Bijan Safaee Fakhr, MD
Attending Physician
Department of Anesthesia, Critical Care and Pain Medicine
Massachusetts General Hospital
Boston, Massachusetts

David I. Feldman, MD, MPH
Fellow
Department of Medicine
Massachusetts General Hospital
Boston, Massachusetts

Karim Fikry, MD
Division Director, Anesthesia Critical Care
Department of Anesthesia
Lahey Hospital and Medical Center
Burlington, Massachusetts

Michael G. Fitzsimons, MD
Associate Professor, Section Head of Cardiac Anesthesia
Harvard Medical School
Vice Chair for Faculty Development
Department of Anesthesiology
Mass General Brigham
Boston, Massachusetts

Michael Flaherty, DO
Physician
Department of Pediatrics
Massachusetts General Hospital
Boston, Massachusetts

John Fountain, MD
Fellow
Division of Pulmonary and Critical Care Medicine
Department of Medicine
Massachusetts General Hospital
Boston, Massachusetts

Rachel C. Frank, MD
Staff Cardiologist and Program Director at Hopkins
Division of Cardiology, Department of Medicine
Massachusetts General Hospital
Boston, Massachusetts

Gabriel Fregoso, MD
Fellow
Department of Anesthesia, Critical Care and Pain Medicine
Massachusetts General Hospital
Boston, Massachusetts

Tiffany Gardner, MD
Fellow
Department of Medicine
Massachusetts General Hospital
Boston, Massachusetts

Timothy G. Gaulton, MD, MSc
Assistant Professor of Anesthesia
Department of Anesthesia, Critical Care and Pain Medicine
Massachusetts General Hospital
Boston, Massachusetts

Mina Ghobrial, MD
Physician
Department of Anesthesiology
UC San Diego School of Medicine
San Diego, California

Adam C. Glaser, MD
Resident
Department of Neurosurgery
Brigham and Women's Hospital
Boston Children's Hospital
Boston, Massachusetts

Rachel Goldberg, MD, MBA
Fellow
Division of Cardiovascular Medicine
Department of Medicine
Massachusetts General Hospital
Boston, Massachusetts

Jeremy Goverman, MD, FACS, FABA
Associate Professor
Department of Surgery
Massachusetts General Hospital
Boston, Massachusetts

Kylee Greider, MD
Assistant Professor
Department of Emergency Medicine and Critical Care
University of New Mexico School of Medicine
Albuquerque, New Mexico

Jason Griffith, MD, PhD
Assistant Physician in Medicine
Division of Pulmonary and Critical Care
Department of Medicine
Massachusetts General Hospital
Boston, Massachusetts

Esra Gumuser, MD
Fellow
Division of Cardiology
Department of Medicine
Massachusetts General Hospital
Boston, Massachusetts

Simran Gupta, MD
Fellow
Department of Infectious Diseases
Massachusetts General Hospital
Boston, Massachusetts

Samantha E. Halpern MD, MHS
Resident
Department of Surgery
Massachusetts General Hospital
Boston, Massachusetts

Dusan Hanidziar, MD, PhD
Assistant Professor of Anesthesia
Department of Anesthesiology
Massachusetts General Hospital
Boston, Massachusetts

Cara Hannigan, MD
Clinical Staff
Division of Trauma, Emergency Surgery, and Critical Care
Department of Surgery
Massachusetts General Hospital
Boston, Massachusetts

Daniel S. Harrison, MD
Assistant Professor
Department of Neurology
Boston University School of Medicine
Boston, Massachusetts

Scott A. Harvey, MD, MS, FACOG, FCCM
Associate Clinical Professor
Department of Obstetrics, Gynecology, and Reproductive Sciences
UC San Diego Health
La Jolla, California

John A. Helmstetter, MD
Physician
Department of Anesthesiology
University Medical Center New Orleans
New Orleans, Louisiana

Emma Huebner, MD
Critical Care Anesthesiologist
Anesthesiology
University of Washington
Seattle, Washington

Sean A. Hickey, MD
Associate Professor Surgery
Department of Surgery
UC San Diego School of Medicine
La Jolla, California

Karan S. Hingorani, MD, PhD
Fellow
Section of Neurocritical Care
Department of Neurology
Mass General Brigham
Boston, Massachusetts

Ryan J. Horvath, MD, PhD
Anesthesiologist and Critical Care Intensivist PACU Director
Department of Anesthesia, Critical Care and Pain Medicine
Massachusetts General Hospital
Boston, Massachusetts

William J. Hucker, MD, PhD
Cardiac Electrophysiologist
Division of Cardiology
Department of Medicine
Massachusetts General Hospital
Boston, Massachusetts

Olivia L. Hulme, MD
Fellow
Division of Cardiovascular Disease
Department of Medicine
Massachusetts General Hospital
Boston, Massachusetts

John O. Hwabejire, MD, MPH
Assistant Professor of Surgery
Department of Surgery
Massachusetts General Hospital
Boston, Massachusetts

Omar Hyder, MD
Attending Anesthesiologist
Department of Anesthesia, Critical Care and Pain Medicine
Massachusetts General Hospital
Boston, Massachusetts

Eric M. Isselbacher, MD, MSc
Associate Professor
Harvard Medical School
Edmund N. Ansin Endowed Chair in Healthcare Transformation
Director, Healthcare Transformation Lab
Co-Director, MGH Thoracic Aortic Center
Department of Cardiology
Massachusetts General Hospital
Boston, Massachusetts

Saef Izzy, MD, MBChB, FNCS, FAAN
Associate Professor of Neurology
Division of Neurocritical Care and Cerebrovascular Diseases
Department of Neurology
Harvard Medical School
Mass General Brigham
Head of Immunology of CNS Injury Program
Ann Romney Center for Neurologic Diseases
Boston, Massachusetts

Craig S. Jabaley, MD
Associate Professor
Department of Anesthesiology
Emory University School of Medicine
Atlanta, Georgia

Christina Anne Jelly, MD, MS
Assistant Professor
Department of Cardiothoracic Anesthesiology and Critical Care
Vanderbilt University Medical Center
Nashville, Tennessee

Caroline H. Jensen, MD
Fellow
Department of Anesthesia, Critical Care and Pain Medicine
Massachusetts General Hospital
Boston, Massachusetts

Debbie Jiang, MD
Instructor
Department of Internal Medicine
Massachusetts General Hospital
Boston, Massachusetts

Daniel W. Johnson, MD
Professor
Department Chief of Critical Care
Department of Anesthesiology
University of Nebraska Medical Center
Omaha, Nebraska

Q. Joyce Han, MD
Fellow
Division of Cardiology
Department of Medicine
Massachusetts General Hospital
Boston, Massachusetts

Usaamah Khan, MD
Fellow
Department of Neurology
Massachusetts General Hospital
Boston, Massachusetts

Fayez Kheir, MD, MSc
Physician
Division of Pulmonary and Critical Care Medicine
Department of Medicine
Massachusetts General Hospital
Boston, Massachusetts

Sumeet A. Khetarpal, MD, PhD
Fellow
Division of Cardiovascular Disease
Department of Medicine
Massachusetts General Hospital
Boston, Massachusetts

Emmett A. Kistler, MD, MHQS
Instructor in Medicine
Department of Medicine
Mount Auburn Hospital
Cambridge, Massachusetts

John Klick, MD, FCCP, FASE, FCCM
Critical Care Division Chief
Department of Anesthesiology
University of Vermont Medical Center
Burlington, Vermont

Davit Kocharyan, MD, MSc
Assistant Professor
Department of Anesthesiology and Critical Care
University of New Mexico Hospital
Albuquerque, New Mexico

Jean Kwo, MD
Assistant Professor of Anesthesia
Department of Anesthesia, Critical Care and Pain Medicine
Harvard Medical School
Massachusetts General Hospital
Boston, Massachusetts

Tenzing T. Lama, MD, MSc
Fellow
Department of Anesthesia, Critical Care and Pain Medicine
Massachusetts General Hospital
Boston, Massachusetts

Jacqueline Lange, PharmD, BCCP
Clinical Pharmacist
Department of Pharmacy
Massachusetts General Hospital
Boston, Massachusetts

Mariana L. Laporta Miranda, MD
Physician
Department of Anesthesiology and Critical Care
Mayo Clinic
Rochester, Minnesota

Danielle Leahy, MD.
Assistant Professor of Anesthesiology
Tufts University School of Medicine
Attending Physician
Department of Anesthesiology and Critical Care Medicine
Maine Medical Center
Portland, Maine

Grace C. Lee, MD
Surgeon
Department of Surgery
Massachusetts General Hospital
Boston, Massachusetts

Jarone Lee, MD, MPH, FCCM
Vice Chief, Critical Care
Medical Director, ICU
Division of Trauma, Emergency Surgery, and Surgical Critical Care
Department of Surgery
Massachusetts General Hospital
Boston, Massachusetts

Mary M. Leech, MD
Physician
Department of Surgery
Massachusetts General Hospital
Boston, Massachusetts

Srihari K. Lella, MD
Physician
Department of Surgery
Massachusetts General Hospital
Boston, Massachusetts

David Lewandowski, MD, MS
Clinical Instructor
Division of Emergency Critical Care Medicine
Brigham and Women's Hospital
Boston, Massachusetts

Worawan B. Limpitikul, MD, PhD
Fellow
Division of Cardiology
Department of Medicine
Massachusetts General Hospital
Boston, Massachusetts

Alban Longchamp, MD, PhD
Transplant Surgeon
Department of Surgery
Massachusetts General Hospital
Boston, Massachusetts

Natasha Lopez, PharmD
Critical Care Clinical Pharmacist
Pharmacy Department
Massachusetts General Hospital
Boston, Massachusetts

Spencer Lord, MD
Physician
Department of Surgery
Massachusetts General Hospital
Boston, Massachusetts

Casey M. Luckhurst, MD
Instructor in Surgery
Harvard Medical School
Division of Trauma, Emergency Surgery, and Surgical Critical Care
Department of Surgery
Massachusetts General Hospital
Boston, Massachusetts

John Luckoski, MD
Fellow
Department of Surgery
Massachusetts General Hospital
Boston, Massachusetts

Simona I. Lupu, MD
Instructor
Department of Anesthesia, Critical Care and Pain Medicine
Massachusetts General Hospital
Boston, Massachusetts

Jay Luther, MD
Director, Inpatient Gastroenterology and Hepatology
Department of Medicine
Massachusetts General Hospital
Boston, Massachusetts

Kyle A. Lyman, MD, PhD
Physician
Department of Neurology
Mass General Brigham
Boston, Massachusetts

Angela Ma, MD
Clinical Fellow in Medicine
Division of Pulmonary and Critical Care
Department of Medicine
Massachusetts General Hospital
Beth Israel Deaconess Medical Center
Boston, Massachusetts

Giovanna S. Manzano, MD
Neuroimmunologist
Department of Neurology
Harvard Medical School
Massachusetts General Hospital
Brigham and Women's Hospital
Boston, Massachusetts

Sandro Marini, MD
Fellow
Department of Neurology
Mass General Brigham
Boston, Massachusetts

Lukas H. Matern, MD
Staff Anesthesiologist and Intensivist
Department of Anesthesia, Critical Care and Pain Medicine
Massachusetts General Hospital
Boston, Massachusetts

Lydia Maurer, MD, MPH
Fellow
Department of Surgery
Perelman School of Medicine at the University of Pennsylvania
Philadelphia, Pennsylvania

James Tanner McMahon, MD
Physician
Department of Neurosurgery
Harvard Medical School
Brigham and Women's Hospital
Boston, Massachusetts

Nadia McMillan, MD, PhD
Fellow
Department of Neurology
Mass General Brigham
Boston, Massachusetts

Benjamin D. Medoff, MD
Associate Professor of Medicine
Division of Pulmonary and Critical Care Medicine
Department of Medicine
Massachusetts General Hospital
Boston, Massachusetts

Angela Meier, MD, PhD
Professor of Clinical Anesthesiology
Division of Critical Care, Department of Anesthesiology
UC San Diego School of Medicine
San Diego, California

Joseph Meyer, MD
Instructor in Medicine
Division of Cardiology
Department of Medicine
Massachusetts General Hospital
Boston, Massachusetts

Cristina Mietto, MD
Physician
Department of Anesthesia, Critical Care and Pain Medicine
Massachusetts General Hospital
Boston, Massachusetts

Ibrahim Migdady, MD
Assistant Professor of Neurosurgery
Division of Neurocritical Care
Department of Neurosurgery
McGovern Medical School—UTHealth Houston
Houston, Texas

Ilan Mizrahi, MD
Anesthesiologist
Department of Anesthesia, Critical Care and Pain Medicine
Massachusetts General Hospital
Boston, Massachusetts

Jahan Mohebali, MD MPH
Assistant Professor of Surgery
Division of Vascular and Endovascular Surgery
Department of Surgery
Harvard Medical School
Massachusetts General Hospital
Boston, Massachusetts

Philicia Moonsamy, MD, MPH
Surgeon
Department of Thoracic Surgery
Cedars Sinai Medical Center
Los Angeles, California

Scott Moses, MD, BCh, BAO
Fellow
Department of Anesthesia, Critical Care and Pain Medicine
Massachusetts General Hospital
Boston, Massachusetts

Matthew Mueller, DO, MPH
Assistant Professor
Critical Care Medicine, Emergency Medicine
MedStar Washington Hospital Center
Washington, DC

Christoph G.S. Nabzdyk, MD
Consultant and Associate Professor
Department of Critical Care and Cardiac Anesthesia
Department of Anesthesiology and Perioperative Medicine
Mayo Clinic
Rochester, Minnesota

Lakshmi Nemani, MD, MPH
Fellow
Department of Anesthesiology
Brigham and Women's Hospital
Boston, Massachusetts

Richard A. Newcomb, MD
Physician
Mass General Brigham Cancer Institute
Massachusetts General Hospital
Boston, Massachusetts

Joshua S. Ng-Kamstra, MDCM, MPH
Trauma and Acute Care Surgeon
Surgical Intensivist
Department of Surgery
Massachusetts General Hospital
Boston, Massachusetts

Crystal M. North, MD, MPH
Assistant Professor of Medicine
Division of Pulmonary and Critical Care Medicine
Department of Medicine
Harvard Medical School
Massachusetts General Hospital / Harvard Medical School
Boston, Massachusetts

Alice Nova, MD
Fellow
Department of Anesthesia, Critical Care and Pain Medicine
Anesthesia Center for Critical Care Research
Massachusetts General Hospital
Boston, Massachusetts

Michelle L. O'Donoghue, MD MPH
McGillycuddy-Logue Distinguished Chair in Cardiovascular Medicine
Heart Vascular Institute
Brigham and Women's Hospital
Boston, Massachusetts

Jamel Ortoleva, MD
Cardiothoracic Anesthesiologist and Intensivist
Department of Anesthesiology
Boston Medical Center
Boston, Massachusetts

Miriam A. Osei, MD, MPH
Fellow
Department of Hematology
Dana Farber Cancer Institute
Mass General Brigham
Boston, Massachusetts

Eduardo M.H. Padrao, MD
Fellow
Division of Pulmonary and Critical Care
Department of Medicine
Massachusetts General Hospital
Boston, Massachusetts

Nikhil Panda, MD, MPH
Physician
Division of Cardiothoracic Surgery
Department of Surgery
Massachusetts General Hospital
Boston, Massachusetts

Jun Soo Park, MD
Associate Physician
Cardiac Surgery Intensive Care Unit
Kaiser Permanente
Los Angeles, California

Jonathan Parks, MD
Instructor in Surgery
Division of Trauma, Emergency Surgery, and Surgical Critical Care
Department of Surgery
Harvard Medical School
Massachusetts General Hospital
Boston, Massachusetts

Raymond C. Parrish, MD
Fellow
Division of Pulmonary and Critical Care Medicine
Department of Medicine
Massachusetts General Hospital
Boston, Massachusetts

Naomi J. Patel, MD, MPH
Rheumatologist
Division of Rheumatology, Allergy and Immunology
Department of Medicine
Massachusetts General Hospital
Boston, Massachusetts

Nilay K. Patel, MD
Interventional and Structural Cardiologist
Division of Cardiology
Department of Medicine
Massachusetts General Hospital
Boston, Massachusetts

Parth N. Patel, MD
Fellow
Department of Medicine
Massachusetts General Hospital
Boston, Massachusetts

Thomas Peponis, MD
Assistant Professor of Surgery
Division of Colon and Rectal Surgery
Department of Surgery
UMass Chan Medical School
Worcester, Massachusetts

Christopher Piccuito, MSEd
Assistant Director
Respiratory Care Services
Massachusetts General Hospital
Boston, Massachusetts

Richard M. Pino, MD, PhD, FCCM
Professor and Head
Department of Anesthesiology
Louisiana State University Health Sciences Center
New Orleans, Louisiana

Will Pohlman, MD, MPH
Resident
Department of Medicine
Massachusetts General Hospital
Boston, Massachusetts

Avanthi Raghavan, MD
Cardiologist
Division of Cardiology
Department of Medicine
Massachusetts General Hospital
Boston, Massachusetts

Sean Rajnic, MD
Assistant Professor
Department of Anesthesiology
University of Nebraska Medical Center
Omaha, Nebraska

Spandan Rajuri, MBBS, DNB, FNB, EDAIC
Associate Staff Physician
Critical Care Department
Cleveland Clinic Abu Dhabi
Abu Dhabi, United Arab Emirates

Erika L. Rangel, MD, MS
Associate Professor of Surgery
Department of Surgery
Massachusetts General Hospital
Boston, Massachusetts

Pattara Rattanawong, MD
Cardiac Electrophysiologist
Sport and Genetic Electrophysiology Clinic
Pali Momi Heart Center
Pali Momi Medical Center
Aiea, Hawaii

Robert W. Regenhardt, MD, PhD
Staff Neurointerventionist
Departments of Neurosurgery and Neurology
Harvard Medical School
Massachusetts General Hospital
Boston, Massachusetts

Kerry Reynolds, MD
Clinical Director, Inpatient Oncology
Director, Severe Immunotherapy Complications Service
Department of Oncology
Massachusetts General Hospital
Boston, Massachusetts

Christopher Richards, MD
Associate Physician
Division of Pulmonary and Critical Care Medicine
Department of Medicine
Massachusetts General Hospital
Boston, Massachusetts

Juan G. Ripoll Sanz, MD
Cardiothoracic Anesthesiologist and Intensivist
Department of Anesthesiology and Perioperative Medicine
Mayo Clinic
Rochester, Minnesota

Guy A. Rordorf, MD
Associate Professor of Neurology
Department of Neurology
Harvard Medical School
Massachusetts General Hospital
Boston, Massachusetts

Jonathan Rosand, MD, MSc
Professor of Neurology
Department of Neurology
Harvard Medical School
Managing Director
Mass General Neuroscience Institute
Co-Founder and Co-Director
McCance Center for Brain Health
Chief
Division of Neurocritical Care and Emergency Neurology
Department of Neurology
Massachusetts General Hospital
Boston, Massachusetts

Eric S. Rosenthal, MD
Associate Professor
Director, MGH NeuroICU
Department of Neurology
Harvard Medical School
Mass General Brigham
Boston, Massachusetts

Daniel B. Rubin, MD, PhD
Assistant Professor of Neurology
Division of Pulmonary and Critical Care Medicine
Department of Medicine
Harvard Medical School
Massachusetts General Hospital
Boston, Massachusetts

Jonah Rubin, MD
Assistant Professor of Medicine
Pulmonary and Critical Care Medicine
Harvard Medical School
Massachusetts General Hospital
Boston, Massachusetts

Jay Saggu, MD
Fellow
Department of Anesthesia
Brigham and Women's Hospital
Boston, Massachusetts

Takashi Sakano, MD, PharmD
Anesthesiologist and Intensivist
Department of Anesthesia, Critical Care and Pain Medicine
Massachusetts General Hospital
Boston, Massachusetts

Jonathan R. Salik, MD, MS-HPEd
Cardiologist
Department of Medicine
Massachusetts General Hospital
Boston, Massachusetts

Michael Salt, DO
Physician
Department of Pediatrics
Mass General Brigham for Children
Boston, Massachusetts

Danielle L. Saly, MD, MPH
Nephrologist
Division of Nephrology
Department of Medicine
Massachusetts General Hospital
Boston, Massachusetts

Kyle Sanchez, MD†
Massachusetts General Hospital
Boston, Massachusetts

Roberta Ribeiro De Santis Santiago, MD, PhD, RRT
Instructor in Anaesthesia and Respiratory Therapist
Department of Anesthesia, Critical Care and Pain Medicine
Respiratory Care Services
Massachusetts General Hospital
Boston, Massachusetts

Minhazur Sarker, MD
Fellow
Department of Obstetrics and Gynecology
UC San Diego School of Medicine
San Diego, California

Ulrich H. Schmidt, MD, PhD, MBA
Vice Chair, Critical Care Medicine
Department of Anesthesiology
UC San Diego Health
San Diego, California

Kenneth Shelton, MD
Critical Care Division Chief
Department of Anesthesia, Critical Care and Pain Medicine
Massachusetts General Hospital
Boston, Massachusetts

† Deceased

Samer Shoshan, MBBS, MBA
Associate Staff Physician
Integrated Hospital Care Institute
Critical Care Division
Cleveland Clinic Abu Dhabi
Abu Dhabi, United Arab of Emirates

Matthew Sigakis, MD
Clinical Assistant Professor
Department of Anesthesiology and Critical Care Medicine
University of Michigan Medical School
Ann Arbor, Michigan

Robert D. Sinyard, MD, MBA
Fellow
Department of Acute Care Surgery
Vanderbilt University Medical Center
Nashville, Tennessee

Edmond Solomon, PharmD
Clinical Pharmacist
Pharmacy Department
Massachusetts General Hospital
Boston, Massachusetts

Phillip Song, MD
Associate Professor, Otolaryngology and Head and Neck Surgery
Department of Otolaryngology
Massachusetts Eye and Ear Infirmary
Boston, Massachusetts

Jamie L. Sparling, MD
Instructor of Anesthesia
Department of Anesthesia, Critical Care and Pain Medicine
Massachusetts General Hospital
Boston, Massachusetts

Stefano Spina, MD
Anesthesiologist and Intensivist
Department of Anesthesia, Critical Care and Pain Medicine
Massachusetts General Hospital
Boston, Massachusetts

Priya Srikanth, MD, PhD
Instructor
Department of Neurology
Mass General Brigham
Boston, Massachusetts

Ada C. Stefanescu Schmidt, MD, MSc
Cardiologist
Corrigan Minehan Heart Center
Massachusetts General Hospital
Boston, Massachusetts

Samantha J. Stein, MD
Clinical Fellow
Department of Anesthesia, Critical Care, and Pain Medicine
Massachusetts General Hospital
Boston, Massachusetts

Alexandra Steverson, MD, MPH
Fellow
Division of Cardiology
Department of Medicine
Massachusetts General Hospital
Boston, Massachusetts

Smrithi Sukumar, MD
Fellow
Division of Cardiology
Department of Medicine
Massachusetts General Hospital
Boston, Massachusetts

David B. Sykes, MD, PhD
Assistant Professor
Mass General Brigham Cancer Institute
Massachusetts General Hospital
Boston, Massachusetts

Christopher Tainter, MD
Attending Physician
Department of Medicine
Guam Regional Medical City
Dededo, Guam

Yasmine Tameze, MD
Instructor of Anesthesia
Department of Anesthesia, Critical Care and Pain Medicine
Massachusetts General Hospital
Boston, Massachusetts

Richard Teo, MD
Transplant Surgeon
Department of Surgery
Massachusetts General Hospital
Boston, Massachusetts

B. Taylor Thompson, MD
Professor of Medicine
Harvard Medical School
Physician
Division of Pulmonary and Critical Care Medicine
Department of Medicine
Massachusetts General Hospital
Boston, Massachusetts

Luke Tseng, MD
Fellow
Department of Anesthesia, Critical Care and Pain Medicine
Massachusetts General Hospital
Boston, Massachusetts

Matthew G. Tung, MD
Anesthesiologist
Department of Anesthesia, Critical Care and Pain Medicine
Massachusetts General Hospital
Boston, Massachusetts

Sarah M. Urbut, MD, PhD
Instructor
Cardiology, Heart Vascular Institute
Massachusetts General Hospital
Boston, Massachusetts

George Velmahos, MD, PhD, MSEd
John F. Burke Professor of Surgery
Harvard Medical School and Massachusetts General Hospital
Boston, Massachusetts

Maysa Vilbert, MD
Research Fellow
Division of Hematology/Oncology, Severe Immunotherapy Complications Program
Massachusetts General Hospital Cancer Center
Boston, Massachusetts

Elisa C. Walsh, MD
Anesthesiologist
Department of Anesthesia, Critical Care and Pain Medicine
Massachusetts General Hospital
Boston, Massachusetts

Annette A. Wang, MD
Resident
Department of Anesthesia, Critical Care, and Pain Medicine
Massachusetts General Hospital
Boston, Massachusetts

Danny Wang, MD
Resident
Department of Surgery
Cardiothoracic Surgery Fellow
Division of Thoracic Surgery
Massachusetts General Hospital
Boston, Massachusetts

Helen S. Wei, MD, PhD
Fellow
Division of Trauma, Emergency Surgery and Surgical Critical Care
Department of Surgery
Massachusetts General Hospital
Boston, Massachusetts

Elizabeth Cox Williams, MD
Assistant Professor
Department of Anesthesiology
University of Maryland School of Medicine
Baltimore, Maryland

Alison S. Witkin, MD
Assistant Professor of Medicine
Division of Pulmonary and Critical Care
Department of Medicine
Massachusetts General Hospital
Boston, Massachusetts

Michael Wolfe, MD
Anesthesiologist, Intensivist
Department of Anesthesia
David Geffen School of Medicine at UCLA
UCLA Health
Los Angeles, California

Christopher M. Worsham, MD, MPH
Assistant Professor of Medicine
Division of Pulmonary and Critical Care Medicine
Department of Medicine
Harvard Medical School
Massachusetts General Hospital
Boston, Massachusetts

Chia-Yun Wu, MD, PhD
Professor of Pathology
Harvard Medical School
Director, Genitourinary Pathology Services
Fellow
Division of Hematology/Oncology, Severe Immunotherapy Complications Program
Massachusetts General Hospital
Boston, Massachusetts

Tiffany Wu, PharmD
Infectious Diseases Clinical Pharmacist
Massachusetts General Hospital
Boston, Massachusetts

Amanda S. Xi, MD, MSE
Director, Pre-Procedure Evaluation, Critical Care
Anesthesiologist
Department of Anesthesia, Critical Care and Pain Medicine
Massachusetts General Hospital
Boston, Massachusetts

Nirupama Yechoor, MD, MSc
Instructor
Division of Neurocritical Care
Department of Neurology
Massachusetts General Hospital
Boston, Massachusetts

Laura J. Yockey, MD, PhD
Fellow
Rheumatology Unit
Department of General Internal Medicine
Massachusetts General Hospital
Boston, Massachusetts

Evin Yucel, MD, MSc
Cardiologist
Director of Interventional Cardiology
Department of General Internal Medicine
Massachusetts General Hospital
Boston, Massachusetts

Christine Zachek, MD, MPH
Fellow
Department of Anesthesia, Critical Care and Pain Medicine
Massachusetts General Hospital
Boston, Massachusetts

Sahar F. Zafar, MBBS, MSc
Associate Professor
Department of Neurology
Mass General Brigham
Boston, Massachusetts

Levi Zehr, MD, BSN
Assistant Professor
Department of Anesthesiology
University of Nebraska Medical Center
Omaha, Nebraska

Randall M. Zusman, MD
Associate Professor
Director, Hypertension Section
Division of Cardiology
Department of Medicine
Massachusetts General Hospital
Boston, Massachusetts

SECTION 1

Shock

Section Editors: Edward A. Bittner and David M. Dudzinski

1.1

Distributive Shock

Logan Ernst and Jean Kwo

- Also called vasodilatory shock, includes several phenotypes that cause systemic vasodilation leading to tissue hypoperfusion and organ dysfunction
  - Most common causes: sepsis and anaphylaxis
  - Less common: neurogenic shock, adrenal insufficiency, and drug overdose or toxicity

Septic Shock

- Septic shock and sepsis are significant causes of morbidity and mortality in the intensive care unit (ICU).
- Sepsis is one of the most common reasons for admission into the ICU.

Definitions

- Per the 2016 Sepsis-3 Guidelines, sepsis is defined as: life-threatening organ dysfunction caused by a dysregulated host response to infection.
- No longer defined with any specific criteria (eg, systemic inflammatory response syndrome [SIRS])
    - Can be identified with any of several verified scoring systems for organ dysfunction, including sequential organ failure assessment (SOFA) or Logistic Organ Dysfunction System Score
    - With SOFA: organ dysfunction defined by a change of >2 in total SOFA score
      - Baseline SOFA score of patients without organ dysfunction is 0.
      - Change in SOFA score >2 is associated with an overall mortality risk of 10% in a hospitalized population.
      - The quick SOFA (qSOFA) score was developed to quickly screen patients likely to have sepsis. This score includes:
        - Glasgow Coma Scale score ≤13
        - Systolic blood pressure (SBP) ≤100 mm Hg and/or
        - Respiratory rate >22/min
- Septic shock: a subset of sepsis in which underlying circulatory and cellular metabolism abnormalities are profound enough to substantially increase mortality.
  - Criteria for diagnosis:
    - Hypotension (mean arterial pressure [MAP] <65)
    - Elevated lactate level (>2 mmol/L [18 mg/dL])
      - If lactate level not available, other outward signs of tissue hypoperfusion, including delayed capillary refill or skin mottling
    - Sustained need for vasopressor therapy

Causes

- ANY infection can be complicated by sepsis!
  - Gram-positive bacteremia (ie, *Staphylococcus*, *Streptococcus*, *Clostridium*) via exposed peptidoglycan in their cell walls, exotoxins
  - Gram-negative bacteremia (*Escherichia coli*, *Pseudomonas*, *Acinetobacter*) via endotoxins (lipopolysaccharides)
  - Secondary bacterial infection after viral infection (eg, SARS-CoV-2, influenza)

Epidemiology

- Per the Centers for Disease Control and Prevention (CDC), 1.7 million people in the United States develop sepsis yearly.
- 28-Day mortality rate >25% for critically ill patients
- ~350,000 deaths per year in the United States
- Can occur at any age, but there is a correlation with advanced age of not only the incidence of septic shock but also increased mortality
- There are disparities in sepsis outcomes due to socioeconomic and racial factors. Black, Hispanic, and Native American populations in the United States have higher rates of sepsis-related complications and mortality compared to White populations.

Key Pathophysiology

- Sepsis results from the interaction of several factors, including the infectious agent, the patient's concomitant medical problems, and their immune system.
  - Immune response

- Proinflammatory response mediated by cytokines
  - Interleukin-1 (IL-1) and IL-6; tumor necrosis factor-alpha (TNF-α)
- Activated by antigen-antibody complexes
- Complement system activated by bacterial wall sugars and endotoxin
  - Activates neutrophils, lymphocytes, prostaglandins, and acute phase reactant proteins
- Proinflammatory mediators are counteracted by anti-inflammatory mediators.
  - IL-4 and IL-10
- Anti-inflammatory mediators can limit the effects of proinflammatory mediators, leading to a state of "relative" immunosuppression or immunoparalysis.
  - Leads to a reduction of human leukocyte antigen (HLA) proteins on monocytes
  - Contributes to increased morbidity and mortality

- Cellular dysfunction
  - Disturbance of mitochondrial oxygen utilization
  - Results in cytopathic hypoxia: low adenosine triphosphate (ATP) production in the setting of adequate oxygen delivery
  - Pathogenic activation of apoptosis
- Endothelial dysfunction and loss of hemostatic balance
  - Endothelial cells assist in the regulation of vascular tone and coagulation (via expression of heparin sulfate).
  - Inflammation is a known procoagulant state.
  - Nitric oxide (NO) is a potent vasodilator produced by NO synthase.
  - In sepsis, inducible NO synthase is stimulated by IL-6 and TNF-α, leading to an increased production of NO and subsequent profound vasodilation.
  - Endothelial surfaces normally have anticoagulant properties.
  - In sepsis, this anticoagulant balance is disturbed by procoagulant inducers (C-reactive protein, CRP), leading to intravascular thrombosis.
  - Tissue edema develops secondary to capillary leakage.
  - Fluids are subsequently shifted into the third space.
- Central nervous system dysfunction
  - Decreased oxygen delivery to the brain can lead to sepsis-induced encephalopathy (confusion, delirium, obtundation).
- Cardiac and circulatory dysfunction
  - Tachycardia compensates for severe systemic vasodilatation to maintain stroke volume.
  - Myocardial contractility eventually decreases and further contributes to the marked hypotension.
  - Impaired oxygen delivery combined with increased oxygen consumption and cardiac work leads to cardiac dysfunction.
- Respiratory dysfunction
  - Sepsis is accompanied by an increased work of breathing.
  - Capillary leak within the lungs leads to hypoxia.
  - Patients with severe sepsis can develop acute respiratory distress syndrome (ARDS).
- Renal dysfunction
  - Hypotension can lead to impaired perfusion, causing oliguria.
  - Acute tubular necrosis (ATN), which can further precipitate renal failure
  - In severe cases, patients may require renal replacement therapy.
- Hepatic dysfunction
  - Hypoperfusion can cause "shock liver," characterized by transaminitis.
  - Cholestasis and hyperbilirubinemia may be present.
- Endocrine dysfunction
  - Adrenal insufficiency
    - Sepsis can impair the normal stress response.
    - Results in an inadequate increase in serum cortisol levels
  - Insulin deficiency
    - Impaired function of pancreatic beta cells
    - Hyperglycemia is detrimental due to an increased frequency of infections, delayed wound healing, and reduced granulocyte function.
  - Vasopressin deficiency
    - Usually secreted in response to hypotension and hypovolemia
    - However, vasopressin levels are decreased in patients with septic shock.
    - Possible mechanisms include depletion of vasopressin stores, impaired baroreceptor-mediated vasopressin release, or desensitization of vasopressin receptors.

Differential Diagnosis

- The diagnosis of sepsis can be as straightforward as fulfilling the definitions of sepsis.
- However, there are patients with hypotension where the question of sepsis is less clear, and etiologies of hypotension overlap.
- Always try to rule out other causes of shock.
- The mainstay of diagnosing sepsis is the early identification of the etiology.
  - This begins by obtaining cultures: blood, urine, sputum, cerebrospinal fluid, and any other fluid sample (eg, abdominal drains) appropriate to the clinical situation.
  - Diagnostic imaging (plain films, ultrasound, and computed tomography [CT] scans) may also be helpful.

Management and Treatment

- The Surviving Sepsis Campaign is the result of the combined work of international groups to improve sepsis treatment and decrease mortality.
- This effort brought evidence-based guidelines to the treatment of sepsis.
- The most recent guidelines (2021) can be found at www.survivingsepsis.org

Hour-1 Bundle

- Emphasizes that sepsis is a medical emergency
- In the first hour
  - Obtain lactate levels and blood cultures.
  - Start broad-spectrum antibiotics after cultures are obtained.
  - Fluid resuscitation with crystalloid (30 mL/kg) for hypotension or lactate >4
  - Start vasopressor therapy if MAP <65.
    - Vasopressors can safely be administered peripherally with proper monitoring. Waiting for central line

placement is not necessary and presents potential harm to the patient.

Surviving Sepsis Guidelines

- Recognition of sepsis
  - Hospitals and health care systems should implement programs to screen for and treat sepsis.
  - The qSOFA should not be used as the single screening tool.
    - Sepsis scoring systems are not designed to screen for sepsis. Rather, they predict the risk of clinical deterioration and/or death.
- Source control is KEY!
  - Identification of the causative agent and controlling the infection
- Timely administration of antimicrobial therapy is a key component in treating sepsis.
  - The goal is to begin therapy within 1 hour of the presumptive diagnosis.
  - Ideally, obtain cultures prior to starting antimicrobial therapy.
  - Start broad-spectrum antibiotics based on the presumed source and narrow them once culture results are reported.
- Fluid resuscitation to ensure adequate intravascular volume and maintain perfusion
  - Fluid resuscitation after the initial 30 mL/kg bolus should be guided by dynamic measures (eg, stroke volume variation, echocardiography).
    - Over- and under-fluid resuscitation are both associated with harm.
  - Resuscitation should be guided by decreasing lactate levels, recognizing that lactate may not normalize in some patients.
  - Use balanced crystalloids with resuscitation. Avoid normal saline.
  - Can consider colloids (albumin) when the patient continues to require a significant amount of crystalloid to maintain MAP
  - Avoid hetastarch
- If MAP <65 mm Hg or SBP <90 mm Hg, initiate vasopressors:
  - Norepinephrine (NE) is the first drug of choice.
  - Start vasopressin when NE dose >0.25 to 5 μg/kg/min.
  - Add epinephrine if MAP remains <65 mm Hg on both NE and vasopressin.
  - Add dobutamine or epinephrine if there is evidence of myocardial dysfunction and persistent hypoperfusion.
  - If persistent hypotension despite fluid resuscitation and vasopressors, add corticosteroids
    - Dose: 200 mg hydrocortisone per day (50 mg every 6 hours)
- Ensure patients are well oxygenated and correct hypoxemia.
  - Hemodynamically unstable patients will often require endotracheal intubation.
  - 40% of patients with septic shock will develop ARDS. Use lung protective strategies including:
    - Low tidal volume ventilation (<6 mL/kg)
    - Plateau pressure <30 cm H_2O
    - Driving pressure <15 cm H_2O
- Glucose control
  - <180 mg/dL per NICE-SUGAR Trial findings
    - Tighter glucose control is not associated with better outcomes.
    - Avoid hypoglycemia.
- Ensure adequate nutritional support.
  - Enteral nutrition is preferred when there are no contraindications.
  - Initiate enteral nutrition early (within 72 hours).
  - Stress ulcer prophylaxis for patients at risk for gastrointestinal (GI) bleeding
- Therapies that are not recommended:
  - Intravenous (IV) Vitamin C
  - Bicarbonate for lactic acidemia
    - Bicarbonate should be administered to patients in shock with acute kidney injury and severe metabolic acidosis (pH ≤7.2).
- Goals of care
  - Discussion of prognosis and goals of care with patients and families should occur within 72 hours.
    - Sepsis is associated with multiorgan failure, poor functional recovery, and death. An understanding of what is acceptable to patients is crucial.

Outcomes

- Survivors of sepsis have a 1-year postdischarge mortality rate that ranges from 7% to 43%.
- They are also at increased risk of rehospitalization within 90 days.
- Survivors of sepsis report increased physical limitations, cognitive impairment, and psychological distress due to anxiety, depression, and posttraumatic stress disorder, and progression of preexisting medical conditions.
  - Surviving sepsis guidelines recommend assessment and follow-up for these issues.
  - Referral to a postcritical illness follow-up program, if available, is recommended.

Anaphylaxis

Definitions

- A serious and life-threatening hypersensitivity reaction that is usually rapid in onset and may cause death.
- Per the 2020 World Allergy Organization (WAO) definition, anaphylaxis is likely diagnosed when one of the following two criteria is met:
  - Acute onset of an illness (minutes to hours) with involvement of the skin, mucosal tissue, or both, and at least one of the following:
    - Respiratory compromise (dyspnea, bronchospasm, stridor, hypoxemia)
    - Reduced blood pressure (BP) or associated symptoms of end-organ dysfunction (hypotonia, syncope, incontinence)
    - Severe GI symptoms (severe abdominal pain, vomiting)
  - Acute onset of hypotension or bronchospasm or laryngeal involvement after exposure to a known or highly probable allergen for that patient, even in the absence of typical skin involvement
    - Excluding lower respiratory symptoms triggered by common inhalant allergens or food allergens perceived to cause "inhalational" reaction

- While the WAO recommends that anaphylaxis be divided into immunologic and nonimmunologic reactions (with elimination of the term "anaphylactoid"), the American Academy of Allergy, Asthma, and Immunology continues to use the term "anaphylactoid" to refer to non–immunoglobulin (Ig)E-mediated reactions that produce the same clinical response as anaphylaxis.

Common Causes to Remember

- Dependent on age and geographic areas
- Most common causes worldwide are food, venom (insect), and medications.

  (Table from Section 1.4: Obstructive Shock)

Epidemiology

- Global incidence ranges from 50 to 112 episodes per 100,000 person-years.
- Lifetime prevalence is 0.3% to 5.1%.
- Mortality is low: 0.21 to 0.56 per million per year in the United States.
- Perioperative anaphylaxis: occurs at a rate of 15.3 per 100,000 cases and is associated with increased health care costs, prolonged hospital stay, and a mortality of 2%.

Pathophysiology

- Immunologic anaphylaxis includes IgE-mediated reactions, IgG-mediated reactions, and immune complex/complement reactions.
- Nonimmunologic anaphylaxis includes reactions in which mast cells and basophils are activated without involvement of IgE or immune complexes.
- The "classic pathway" of anaphylaxis involves the production of allergen-specific IgE in peripheral lymphoid tissue following exposure to an allergen.
  - IgE binds to high-affinity IgE receptors on the surface of mast cells and basophils.
  - Subsequent exposure to the allergen allows surface-bound IgE to cross-link, leading to the activation and degranulation of mast cells and basophils.
  - Subsequent exposure to the allergen allows surface-bound IgE to cross-link, leading to the activation and degranulation of mast cells and basophils.
  - This results in the release of preformed chemical mediators of anaphylaxis (eg, histamine, tryptase, platelet-activating factor, prostaglandins, leukotrienes, cytokines, chemokines).
- Anaphylaxis is primarily categorized as a distributive shock syndrome characterized by profound vasodilation.
  - However, increased vascular permeability can cause massive amounts of fluid to move into the extravascular space, leading to concomitant hypovolemic shock.
  - Direct myocardial depression may also occur.

Differential Diagnosis

- Syndromes caused by excess endogenous production of histamine:
  - Systemic mastocytosis
  - Urticaria pigmentosa
  - Basophilic leukemia
- Vasovagal reactions
- Flushing disorders:
  - Carcinoid syndrome
  - Alcohol induced
  - Medullary carcinoma of the thyroid
  - Autonomic epilepsy
  - Vasointestinal peptide-secreting GI disorders
- Other forms of shock: hypovolemic, cardiogenic, obstructive
- Miscellaneous
  - C1 esterase deficiency syndromes
  - Pheochromocytoma
  - Capillary leak syndrome

Diagnosis and Treatment

- As anaphylaxis can be life-threatening, the diagnosis should be made by history and physical examination alone (see World Health Organization [WHO] criteria). However, laboratory studies may be helpful in confirming the diagnosis.
  - Plasma histamine levels peak 5 to 10 minutes after the onset of symptoms and remain elevated for 30 to 60 minutes.
  - Serum tryptase levels peak at 60 to 90 minutes after the onset of symptoms and persist for as long as 5 hours. However, serum tryptase levels should ideally be drawn between 30 minutes and 4 hours after symptom onset.
  - Serial histamine and tryptase measurements increase the sensitivity of tests to diagnose anaphylaxis.
  - A normal tryptase level, however, does not rule out anaphylaxis. For example, in food-induced anaphylaxis, basophil involvement may predominate over mast cell involvement; thus, an elevation in tryptase may not be seen.
- Skin tests or in vitro tests can determine the presence of specific IgE antibodies to foods, medications, or stinging insects. However, standardized skin testing is not available for the majority of allergens.
- Management of anaphylaxis:
  - Assess airway, breathing, and circulation. Remove offending allergen.
  - Epinephrine is the mainstay of management and should be administered as soon as possible.
    - Intramuscular (IM) administration is first-line in most situations. It is the fastest and most consistent administration method and is well tolerated.
    - IV route is not recommended initially due to risk of arrhythmias.
    - Dose: 0.01 mg/kg (up to max dose of 0.5 mg) IM every 5 to 15 minutes as necessary to control symptoms and increase BP
  - Clinicians should not wait for overt signs of shock to develop before administering epinephrine, as delays in epinephrine administration are associated with fatal anaphylaxis.
  - Epinephrine ameliorates the clinical symptoms of anaphylaxis via its action on adrenergic receptors: alpha-1 agonist effects include vasoconstriction and decreased mucosal edema. Beta-2 agonist effects include bronchodilation and decreased mediator release from mast cells and basophils.
  - In patients who remain hypotensive, IV epinephrine may be required.

- Continuous infusions of epinephrine are superior to bolus IV dosing.
- Infusion rates should be started at a rate of 0.1 to 1 μg/kg/min and titrated to hemodynamic data.

- Fluid management: large increases in vascular permeability can cause hypovolemia.
- Consider H1 blockers (eg, diphenhydramine) and H2 blockers (ranitidine or famotidine)
  - These agents treat the cutaneous manifestations of anaphylaxis and should never be used alone without epinephrine.
- Consider inhaled beta-agonists (albuterol) for bronchoconstriction resistant to epinephrine
- Glucocorticoid use is controversial. They were commonly given to prevent protracted symptoms or to prevent biphasic reactions. However, there is evidence that glucocorticoids may be of no benefit and can possibly cause harm.
- Other possible adjunctive therapies include glucagon (in patients treated with beta-blockers), vasopressin, methylene blue, and tranexamic acid.

Anaphylaxis Temporal Patterns

- Uniphasic: most common type. Symptoms peak within hours and resolve within a few hours with treatment.
- Persistent or protracted: symptoms present for >4 hours without clear resolution.
- Refractory anaphylaxis: continued symptoms despite adequate epinephrine dosing (at least three doses of epinephrine or initiation of epinephrine infusion) and medical management
- Biphasic anaphylaxis: when the patient develops anaphylaxis after initial signs and symptoms have completely resolved for at least 1 hour and a return of anaphylaxis within 48 hours without reexposure to the trigger
  - Incidence varies from 0.4% to 23% and varies with allergen.
  - Risk factors include:
    - Severe initial symptoms
    - Patients requiring >1 dose epinephrine
  - A period of subsequent observation is recommended following the initial episode.
  - There is no consensus on the optimal length of this observation period.

Outcomes

- Fortunately, mortality associated with anaphylaxis is low. However, the outcome/severity of reaction depends on the agent/dose that caused the anaphylaxis and cofactors (which can either mask initial symptoms or increase the risk of exposure to agents causing anaphylaxis).
  - Age (eg, adolescents/young adults may have increased risk-taking behaviors, older adults have increased risk from medication exposure)
  - Concomitant medical conditions (eg, asthma, atopic diseases, cardiovascular disease)
  - Concurrent medications (eg, beta-blockers, nonsteroidal anti-inflammatory drugs [NSAIDs])
  - Sedatives (eg, recreational drugs, ethyl alcohol [EtOH]) can mask recognition of symptoms.
  - Other factors: infection, sleep deprivation, emotional stress
- Upon discharge, patients should be educated on the avoidance of triggers and provided with an epinephrine autoinjector. A tailored individual anaphylaxis management plan and follow-up with allergy/immunology specialists to confirm anaphylaxis triggers should be in place.

Neurogenic Shock

Definitions

- Vasoplegic shock due to disruption of sympathetic control over vascular tone

Epidemiology

- In the United States, spinal cord injury (SCI) occurs at a rate of 55 new cases per million population per year.
- Early mortality with SCI is ~7%, and patients with tetraplegia have the highest risk.
- After the initial presentation, the mortality increases are almost double at 1 year.

Physiology and Treatment

- Autonomic function is transmitted in the anteromedial tract of the spinal cord, and its disruption leads to autonomic dysfunction.
- Sympathetic fibers exit at C7-T1 through T2, and parasympathetic fibers at S2-4.
- High-level spinal cord lesions are associated with the withdrawal of the sympathetic neural outflow (sympathectomy), leading to an unopposed parasympathetic neural output (mediated by the vagus nerve), resulting in bradycardia, vasodilation, and hypothermia.
- After complete cervical SCI, 60% to 70% of patients demonstrate neurogenic shock.
- Patients with traumatic SCI are at risk of developing other types of shock secondary to their other injuries and complications (eg, hypovolemia). These other causes must be identified and treated.
- Current trauma guidelines state to aim for a goal MAP of >85 to 90 mm Hg for 7 days after injury.
  - This recommendation is based on limited data, and the benefits should be weighed against the potential risks on a case-by-case basis.
  - After adequate volume resuscitation, vasopressors should be started to achieve goal MAP.
    - Vasopressors with both alpha- and beta-agonist properties (eg, NE, dopamine) are recommended.
      - There is some evidence that NE may decrease intrathecal cerebrospinal fluid pressure and improve spinal cord perfusion pressure.
    - Avoid vasopressors with solely alpha-1 agonist effect (eg, phenylephrine).
      - Can worsen bradycardia and possibly cause left ventricular failure and pulmonary edema
- Avoid hypotension. BP is correlated with spinal cord perfusion pressure. Secondary hypoperfusion can adversely affect the neurologic outcome.
- There is emerging evidence regarding the use of spinal cord perfusion pressure monitoring via lumbar intrathecal

pressure monitoring catheters, but the use of these has not yet shown benefit in large studies.

- Bradycardia can be treated with anticholinergic medications (eg, atropine, glycopyrrolate).
  - Temporary pacemakers are sometimes required in cases of prolonged or severe bradycardia.
    - Bradycardia associated with SCI often resolves within weeks to months; a permanent pacemaker is rarely required.
- Thermoregulation is disrupted with high SCI. Patients are unable to regulate core body temperature (in both heat and cold environments), and close monitoring is paramount.
- Glucocorticoids (methylprednisolone), if administered, should be given within 8 hours of injury. However, administration of glucocorticoids is not definitively recommended in SCI.
- Studies to enhance motor recovery with medications (eg, riluzole, glyburide, granulocyte colony-stimulating factor), cell-based therapies (eg, Schwann cells), and spinal scaffolds to guide nerve regrowth are currently under investigation.

SUGGESTED READINGS

Angus DC, van der Poll T. Severe sepsis and septic shock. *N Engl J Med*. 2013;369(9):840-851.

Annane D, Sébille V, Charpentier C, et al. Effect of treatment with low doses of hydrocortisone and fludrocortisone on mortality in patients with septic shock. *JAMA*. 2002;288(7):862-871.

Cardona V, Ansotegui IJ, Ebisawa M, et al. World Allergy Organization anaphylaxis guidance 2020. *World Allergy Organ J*. 2020;13(10):100472.

Dribin TE, Sampson HA, Camargo CA Jr, et al. Persistent, refractory, and biphasic anaphylaxis: a multidisciplinary Delphi study. *J Allergy Clin Immunol*. 2020;146:1089-1096.

Evans L, Rhodes A, Alhazzani W, et al. Surviving sepsis campaign: international guidelines for management of sepsis and septic shock 2021. *Crit Care Med*. 2021;49(11):e1063-e1143.

Golden DBK, Wang J, Waserman S, et al. Anaphylaxis: a 2023 practice parameter update. *Ann Allergy Asthma Immunol*. 2024;132(2):124-176.

Kemp SF, Lockey RF. Anaphylaxis: a review of causes and mechanisms. *Curr Rev Allergy Clin Immunol*. 2002;110:341-348.

Kumar A, Roberts D, Wood KE, et al. Duration of hypotension before initiation of effective antimicrobial therapy is the critical determinant of survival in human septic shock. *Crit Care Med*. 2006;34(6):1589-1596.

Lee YS, Kim KT, Kwon BK. Hemodynamic management of acute spinal cord injury: a literature review. *Neurospine*. 2021;18(1):7-14.

NICE-SUGAR Study Investigators; Finfer S, Chittock DR, Yu-Shuo Su S, et al. Intensive versus conventional glucose control in critically ill patients. *N Engl J Med*. 2009;360(13):1283-1297.

Paoli C, Reynolds MA, Sinha M, et al. Epidemiology and costs of sepsis in the United States—an analysis based on timing of diagnosis and severity level. *Crit Care Med*. 2018;46(12):1889-1897.

Prescott HC, Angus DC. Enhancing recovery from sepsis: a review. *JAMA*. 2018;319(1):62-75.

Rhee C, Jones TM, Hamad Y, et al. Prevalence, underlying causes, and preventability of sepsis-associated mortality in US acute care hospitals. *JAMA Netw Open*. 2019;2(2):e18757.

Singer M, Deutschman CS, Seymour CW, et al. The third international consensus definitions for sepsis and septic shock (Sepsis-3). *JAMA*. 2016;315(8):801-810.

Smith N, Lopez RA, Silberman M. Distributive Shock. [Updated 2023 Jul 24]. In: StatPearls [Internet]. Treasure Island (FL): StatPearls Publishing; 2025 Jan-. Available from: https://www.ncbi.nlm.nih.gov/books/NBK470316/.

1.2

Hypovolemic Shock

John Bryant and Christina Anne Jelly

Definitions

- Inadequate tissue oxygenation and end-organ hypoperfusion are seen as a result of a decrease and/or subsequent lack of circulating intravascular volume.
- Mean arterial pressure (MAP), cardiac output (CO), pulmonary artery wedge pressure (PAWP), and mixed venous oxygen saturation (Svo_2) will also be decreased, and systemic vascular resistance (SVR) will be increased in an attempt to maintain blood pressure. Compensatory mechanisms to maintain adequate end-organ perfusion may become overwhelmed and lead to multisystem organ dysfunction.
- The approach to any patient in shock is to first rule out hypovolemia as a potential cause.

Common Causes to Remember

- The most common causes of hypovolemic shock are identified in patients undergoing surgery, experiencing trauma, and with burns.
  - Hemorrhage (*Table 1.2.1*)
  - Dehydration (due to gastrointestinal [GI] losses)
  - Third spacing (due to burns)

Epidemiology

- Hypovolemia and hemorrhage are responsible for over half of deaths in acute trauma.
- Approximately one-third of these deaths occur out of the hospital.
- Hemorrhage and resulting hypovolemic shock are major causes of mortality within 4 hours of injury.
- The mechanism of injury and the immediate availability of a trauma center play a role in the mortality of these patients.

Key Pathophysiology

- Total body water (TBW) in the average adult male is equal to 60% of lean body weight (vs 50% in females).
- Two-thirds of the TBW is intracellular fluid (ICF).

TABLE 1.2.1 Causes of Traumatic and Nontraumatic Hemorrhagic Shock

Traumatic		Nontraumatic
Head and neck	Scalp lacerations Carotid injury	
Chest	Great vessel injury Cardiac rupture Hilar injury Hemothorax	Ventricular rupture status post MI Ruptured aneurysm (eg, TAAA)
Abdominal	Liver injury Spleen injury Renal laceration Visceral vessel injury (SMA, IMA, celiac) Great vessel injury (aorta, IVC)	Ruptured aneurysm —AAA —Visceral vessel Peptic ulcer disease Diverticulosis Colon cancer Intraabdominal cyst
Pelvic	Pelvic fracture Iliac vessel injury	Ruptured ovarian cyst Uterine rupture Postpartum bleeding Placental abruption and accreta
Orthopedic	Femur fracture Other long bone fractures	Severe hemarthrosis

AAA, abdominal aortic aneurysm; IMA, inferior mesenteric artery; IVC, inferior vena cava; MI, myocardial infarction; SMA, superior mesenteric artery; TAAA, thoracoabdominal aortic aneurysm.

- The remaining extracellular fluid (ECF) is further divided into interstitial fluid and plasma. Plasma volume is about 20% to 25% of ECF fluid volume. This distribution is important when evaluating the volume effects of sodium-based fluids. Sodium will equilibrate throughout the ECF, so on average, 75% of infused saline solutions will distribute in the interstitial fluid and 25% will distribute in the plasma.
- The average adult has ~5 to 6 L of blood, which is equivalent to about 8% of the TBW.
- An example of this calculation is shown in the following for an 80-kg male:

$$0.6 \times 80 \text{ kg} = 48 \text{ L of TBW}$$
$$2/3 \times 48 \text{ L} = 32 \text{ L ICF}$$
$$\text{TBW} - \text{ICF} = \text{ECF}$$
$$48 \text{ L} - 32 \text{ L} = 16 \text{ L ECF}$$
$$3/4 \times 16 \text{ L} = 12 \text{ L of interstitial fluid}$$
$$1/4 \times 16 = 4 \text{ L of plasma}$$

- When the body is hypovolemic, the earliest response is the movement of interstitial fluid into the capillaries.
- This transcapillary fluid shift is able to replace up to 15% of the intravascular volume, thus providing the mechanism for compensation in stage I shock.
- Acute blood loss results in the activation of the renin-angiotensin-aldosterone (RAA) system.

❑ ***Hypovolemic shock is classified into four stages based on the volume of blood loss and the patient's physiologic response.***

- Stage I shock results from a decrease of up to 15% of the circulating volume, or 750 to 1,000 mL.
  - Referred to as "compensated shock" because the body is able to physiologically adjust without showing clinical evidence of hypovolemia
  - Tachycardia, decreased systolic blood pressure, decreased pulse pressure, and decreased urine output do not occur.
  - Routine blood donation is an example of stage I shock.
- Stage II shock is associated with a 15% to 30% decrease in intravascular volume, or 1,000 to 1,500 mL.
  - Referred to as "mild shock"
  - The hallmark of this stage is mild tachycardia accompanied by normal systolic blood pressure and decreased pulse pressure.
- Stage III shock is characterized by decreased systolic blood pressure, decreased urine output, and mental status changes.
  - Referred to as "decompensated shock"
- Stage IV shock results from the loss of >2 L of circulating fluid.
  - Referred to as "severe shock"
  - Patients present with respiratory failure, anuria, and obtundation.
  - Patients with trauma that present in decompensated and severe shock have a markedly increased mortality.

Stage	I	II	III	IV
Blood loss (mL)	<15% (750-1,000)	15%-30% (1,000-1,500)	30%-40% (1,500-2,000)	>40% (>2,000)
HR (bpm)	<100	120	140	>140
SBP (mm Hg)	>100	>100	<100	<100
Pulse pressure	Normal	Decreased	Decreased	Decreased
RR (breaths/min)	12-20	20-30	30-40	>40
Urine output (mL/h)	>30	20-30	<20	None
Capillary refill	<2 s	>2 s; clammy skin	>3 s; cold pale skin	>4 s; cold mottled skin
Mental status	Normal	Anxious	Confusion, agitation	Obtunded

HR, heart rate; RR, respiratory rate; SBP, systolic blood pressure.

Differential Diagnosis

- Hypovolemic shock occurs after a loss of at least 20% of the body's intravascular volume.
  - The most dramatic cause of hypovolemia is rapid blood loss, referred to as hemorrhagic shock.
  - Liver and splenic injuries are the most common sources of hemorrhage following both penetrating and blunt abdominal trauma.
  - Orthopedic injuries such as pelvic and femur fractures can also be associated with massive blood loss.
  - The most common causes of nontraumatic hemorrhage include ruptured aneurysms and GI bleeds.
    - Peptic ulcers and diverticulosis are responsible for most cases of upper and lower GI bleeds, respectively.
- Hypovolemic shock also results from nonhemorrhagic intravascular volume loss.
  - Dehydration from poor oral intake, vomiting, or diarrhea can lead to hypovolemia.
  - Additional sources of GI fluid loss include high-output fistulas and stomas.
  - Insensible fluid losses also contribute to total body fluid balance.
  - Examples of increased insensible losses leading to hypovolemia include burns, open wounds, excessive sweating, and heat stroke.
  - The kidneys are another potential source of volume depletion: uncontrolled urine output, such as the recovery phase of acute tubular necrosis, or diabetic ketoacidosis can lead to hypovolemia.
- Rule out other causes of shock.

Evaluation of Volume Status

- When deciding whether to administer fluids, two key questions must be asked: (1) What is the patient's intravascular volume status? (2) Will fluid improve physiologic variables such as BP, urine output, and tissue perfusion? There is no gold standard assessment tool to determine volume status and fluid responsiveness, but several commonly used strategies to clinically assess volume status are as follows:
- Central venous pressure (CVP): commonly used. Studies have shown that CVP or changes in CVP do not reliably predict blood volume or change in stroke volume with volume challenge. Pulmonary artery occlusion pressure is proportional to left ventricular end diastolic volume and may be a better predictor, but its use is limited as it requires placement of a pulmonary artery catheter.
- Straight leg raise: Transition patient from 45-degree head-up position to flat with maximal effect in 30 to 90 seconds. Assess for increase in stroke volume (carbon monoxide monitor or pulse pressure). An increase of 10% is often used as a cutoff for fluid responsiveness. This is a reversible, noninvasive easy-to-perform test that studies have shown to correlate well with volume responsiveness. It can be unreliable in patients with severe hypovolemia, and positional changes may be challenging in the acutely ill patient.
- Pulse pressure variation (PPV): Changes in intrathoracic pressure will alter left and right ventricular preload and afterload. Changes are dependent on whether the patient is spontaneously ventilating versus being mechanically ventilated with positive pressure. PPV has been validated in patients who are mechanically ventilated and not breathing spontaneously. PPV is increased in patients with hypovolemia, but may also increase in patients with tamponade, constrictive pericarditis, bronchospasm, and increased intraabdominal or intrathoracic pressure.
- Point-of-care ultrasound: Often performed with evaluation of IVC size and collapsibility in patients who are spontaneously ventilating or with the IVC distensibility index in patients who are being mechanically ventilated. IVC assessment to determine volume status and fluid responsiveness are limited by operator experience, probe placement, patient positioning, and patient ultrasound windows. Stroke volume assessment via left ventricular outflow tract velocity time integral (LVOT VTI) and CO estimates has also been utilized to determine fluid responsiveness.

Management and Treatment

> *Resuscitation is complete when the oxygen debt has been repaid, tissue acidosis eliminated, and normal aerobic metabolism restored in all tissue beds.*
>
> —*EAST Practice Management Guideline Committee*

- The treatment of hypovolemic shock centers on rapid hemostasis and fluid resuscitation.
- In order to maintain end-organ function, oxygen delivery and consumption must be optimized.
- Traditional end points of resuscitation include the restoration of blood pressure and pulse, as well as urine output and CVP.
- However, the normalization of these parameters does not necessarily indicate that tissue hypoperfusion has ceased.
- For this reason, additional end points must be utilized.
- Biochemical measures of resuscitation include arterial pH, base deficit, lactate, serum bicarbonate, and central venous oxygen saturation.
- The time to normalization of pH, lactate, and base deficit has prognostic ramifications. In the trauma population, patients whose pH and lactate levels have returned to baseline within 24 hours have markedly improved survival rate.

SUGGESTED READINGS

Bradley CA, Ma C, Hollon M. Perioperative point of care ultrasound for hemodynamic assessment: a narrative review. *Semin Cardiothorac Vasc Anesth*. 2023;27(3):208-222.

Cannon JW. Hemorrhagic shock. *N Engl J Med*. 2018;378(4):370-379.

Kalantari K, Chang JN, Ronco C, Rosner MH. Assessment of intravascular volume status and volume responsiveness in critically ill patients. *Kidney Int*. 2013;83(6):1017-1028.

Murphy JT, Gentilello LM. Shock. In: *Greenfield's Surgery: Scientific Principles and Practice*. 4th ed. Editors for the 4th Edition: by M.W. Mulholland, Keith D. Lillemoe, Gerard M. Doherty, Ronald V. Maier, Gilbert R. Upchurch. Lippincott Williams & Wilkins; 2006:179-182.

Suresh MR, Chung KK, Convertino VA. Unmasking the hypovolemic shock continuum: the compensatory reserve. *J Intensive Care Med*. 2019; 34(9):696-706.

Tisherman SA, Barie P, Bokhari F, et al. Resuscitation endpoints. The Eastern Association for the Surgery of Trauma practice management guidelines. *J Trauma*. 2004;57(4):898-912. chrome-extension://efaidnbmnnnibpcajpcglclefindmkaj/https://www.east.org/Content/documents/practicemanagementguidelines/resuscitation-endpoints_JTACS_Publication.pdf

1.3

Cardiogenic Shock

Rachel C. Frank and Samuel Bernard

Definition

- Low cardiac output state resulting in life-threatening end-organ hypoperfusion and hypoxia
  - Systolic blood pressure (SBP) <90 mm Hg for ≥30 minutes or vasopressors required to achieve SBP ≥90 mm Hg
  - End-organ hypoperfusion
    - Altered mental status
    - Cold/clammy skin and extremities
    - Urine output <30 mL/h
    - Acute kidney or liver injury
    - Lactate >2.0 mmol/L

Hemodynamic Definitions (Table 1.3.1)

- Cardiac index ≤2.2 L/min/m^2
- Narrow pulse pressure (<25 mm Hg)
- Elevated systemic vascular resistance (SVR >1,200 dynes·s/cm^5)
  - 80·(Mean arterial pressure [MAP] [mm Hg] − Central venous pressure [CVP] [mm Hg])/Cardiac output [L/min]
- *Left-sided heart failure*
  - Pulmonary capillary wedge pressure (PCWP) ≥18 mm Hg
  - Normal (or low) CVP
- *Right-sided heart failure*
  - CVP >15 mm Hg
  - CVP/PCWP >0.63

TABLE 1.3.1 Clinical and Hemodynamic Definitions for Different Phenotypes of Cardiogenic Shock

Left-Sided	Right-Sided	Biven-tricular	Obstructive
SBP <90 mm Hg for >30 min OR addition of vasopressors for SBP ≥90 **End-organ hypoperfusion** **Cardiac index ≤2.2 L/min/m^2** **AND**			
• CVP ↓ • PCWP ↑ • CVP/PCWP normal (<0.63) • PAPi normal (>1.0)	• CVP ↑ • PCWP ↓ • CVP/PCWP ↑ (>0.63) • PAPi ↓ (<1.0)	• CVP ↑ • PCWP ↑ • PAPi ↓ (<1.0)	• Equalization of diastolic pressures

CVP, central venous pressure; PAPi, Pulmonary artery pulsatility index; PCWP, pulmonary capillary wedge pressure; SBP, systolic blood pressure.

  - Pulmonary artery pulsatility index (PAPi) <1.0
    - (Pulmonary artery systolic pressure − pulmonary artery diastolic pressure)/CVP
  - Normal (or low) PCWP
- *Biventricular failure*
  - Combination of left- and right-sided heart failure
- *Obstructive*
  - Tamponade—"equalization" of pressures (CVP = pulmonary artery diastolic pressure = PCWP)

Differential Diagnosis (Table 1.3.2)

- Broadly grouped into left-sided, right-sided, biventricular, or obstructive shock
- Can occur concomitantly with other types of shock (eg, septic, anaphylactic, hemorrhagic)—known as mixed shock state
- May require a pulmonary artery catheter (PAC) to delineate the hemodynamic profile

General Management Strategies

- Optimize volume status: diuretics for volume overload (cardiogenic shock)
- Optimize contractility: inotropic therapy (ie, inodilators dobutamine, milrinone; inoconstrictor epinephrine)
  - Milrinone is associated with greatest reductions in SVR and pulmonary vascular resistance (PVR)
  - Epinephrine is associated with higher rates of refractory shock compared to dobutamine.
  - However, may need to choose an agent depending on MAP and SVR goals, and whether the inotrope vasodilates or vasoconstricts
  - All of these agents can increase heart rate or cause tachyarrhythmia
- Optimize MAP and SVR: vasopressor therapy for goal MAP ≥65 mm Hg in general, but may need to adjust based on patient's baseline blood pressure and end-organ needs
  - Norepinephrine generally preferred as first-line therapy overall
  - Vasopressin also used as a first-line agent, may also result in decreased PVR
  - Dopamine associated with increased tachyarrhythmia and may have higher mortality in cardiogenic shock (SOAP II trial)
  - Phenylephrine is preferred in patients with left ventricular (LV) outflow tract obstruction, but is otherwise generally avoided due to its pure increase in SVR and PVR
- Afterload reduction (if hypertensive) for goal MAP 65-70 mm Hg
- Decrease PVR in right-sided heart failure using inhaled nitric oxide or inhaled prostacyclin
- Invasive or noninvasive ventilator management
  - Positive end-expiratory pressure (PEEP) is *beneficial* in left-sided heart failure due to decreased LV preload, decreased LV afterload, and hydrostatic displacement of pulmonary edema
  - Suboptimal PEEP is *detrimental* in right-sided heart failure, due to increased right ventricular (RV) afterload.
    - If too low, PVR increases from atelectasis and collapsed alveolar-pulmonary capillary units

TABLE 1.3.2 Differential Diagnosis for Different Phenotypes of Cardiogenic Shock

Left-Sided *Only*	Left-Sided *or* Biventricular	Right-Sided *Only*	Obstructive
• Acute myocardial infarction (MI) • Left-sided valvular disease • Left ventricular outflow tract obstruction • Post-MI papillary muscle rupture • Post-MI pseudoaneurysm	• Nonischemic dilated cardiomyopathy • Acute myocarditis • Tachyarrhythmia-induced cardiomyopathy • Post-MI ventricular septal rupture • Takotsubo cardiomyopathy • Infiltrative cardiomyopathy (eg, amyloidosis, sarcoidosis) • Restrictive cardiomyopathy • Drugs (eg, alcohol, cocaine) • Chemotherapy (eg, anthracyclines) • Immunotherapy (eg, checkpoint inhibitors) • Peripartum cardiomyopathy • Septic cardiomyopathy • Thyrotoxicosis • Allograft rejection (after heart transplant)	• Right ventricular MI • Arrhythmogenic right ventricular cardiomyopathy (ARVC) • Right-sided valvular disease (eg, severe tricuspid regurgitation) • Pulmonary hypertension • Acute hypoxemia/hypercarbia	• Tamponade • Pulmonary embolism • Amniotic fluid/fat embolus • Tension pneumothorax

    - If too high, PVR increases from alveolar overdistension and compressed pulmonary vasculature
  - Maintain normoxia and normocarbia to avoid adverse effects on PVR
- Optimize rhythm: low threshold for cardioversion of arrhythmia if thought to be a significant contributor to shock (as per Advanced Cardiac Life Support [ACLS] protocol, but also consider noncompliant ventricles where atrial "kick" is required for stroke volume)

Specific Disease Management Strategies

- Acute myocardial infarction–related cardiogenic shock (AMI-CS)
  - AMI causes ~80% of cardiogenic shock
  - Dual antiplatelet therapy (aspirin with clopidogrel, prasugrel, or ticagrelor) + heparin
  - Mortality benefit of early revascularization (SHOCK trial)
- Left ventricular outflow tract obstruction
  - Due to systolic anterior motion (SAM) of the mitral valve with hypercontractile basal LV segments
  - Significant concomitant mitral regurgitation (MR) is common
  - Associated with hypertrophic cardiomyopathy, Takotsubo cardiomyopathy, and large anterior infarction
  - Treatment with beta-blockade (or non-dihydropyridine calcium channel blocker), fluids, and phenylephrine (or vasopressin)
  - AVOID afterload reducing agents and insults to preload, which can worsen cavitary obstruction.
- Left-sided valvular disease
  - Surgical evaluation/heart team meeting for all patients
  - Acute MR
    - *Etiologies*: Prolapse/flail, endocarditis, papillary muscle rupture, trauma/deceleration injury, acute rheumatic fever
    - *Surgical emergency*, however, may be bridged with mechanical circulatory support (MCS)
    - Can be considered for transcatheter edge-to-edge repair in certain select cases
  - Acute aortic regurgitation (AR)
    - *Etiologies*: Endocarditis, aortic dissection, prolapse/flail, trauma/deceleration injury, procedural complication
    - Maintain high heart rate (with isoproterenol or transvenous pacing) to maintain shorter times in diastole
    - Surgical emergency and with few available MCS options
    - Very limited percutaneous options
  - Acute decompensation of chronic severe aortic stenosis (AS)
    - Most frequently calcific AS
    - May be treated with percutaneous balloon aortic valvuloplasty (PBAV) as a bridge to surgery
    - Surgery is *definitive* therapy, but is rarely emergent.
  - Acute decompensation of chronic severe mitral stenosis (MS)
    - May be rheumatic or calcific
    - Decrease heart rate (with beta-blockers or nondihydropyridine calcium channel blockers) to prolong diastole and decrease mean mitral valve gradient
    - *Rheumatic* MS may be treated *definitively* with percutaneous balloon mitral valvuloplasty (PBMV)
    - Surgery is *definitive* therapy, but is rarely emergent.
- Acute/fulminant myocarditis
  - *Etiologies*: Giant cell, eosinophilic, lymphocytic, viral, idiopathic, drug-induced (eg, checkpoint inhibitors, clozapine)
  - May present with ventricular arrhythmias or complete heart block
  - Empiric intravenous (IV) glucocorticoids (only some myocarditis etiologies are steroid responsive, including

giant cell, eosinophilic, and checkpoint inhibitor myocarditis)
            - Long-term immunosuppression (eg, cyclosporine, azathioprine) may be appropriate in some cases
    - May need MCS to await recovery versus need for advanced therapies (eg, left ventricular assist device [LVAD] or transplant)
- Cardiac tamponade
    - Support with IV fluid
    - Pericardiocentesis

Mechanical Circulatory Support

- Temporary forms of cardiac support while awaiting recovery, or as bridge to LVAD or heart transplant
- Choice of temporary MCS is determined by shock hemodynamic profile and needs
- Intraaortic balloon pump (IABP)
    - Inflation during diastole, deflation during systole
    - Improves coronary perfusion, decreases LV afterload
    - Provides ~ 0.5 to 1.0 L/min of cardiac output
    - Can be placed via femoral or axillary artery
    - Cannot be used with severe AR or aortic dissection
    - No clear benefit of medical therapy in patients with AMI-CS (IABP-SHOCK II trial). Thus, current intensive care unit (ICU) use can be for procedural support for coronary revascularization, MCS bridge to surgery in acute MR, left heart failure in patients without AMI-CS, and as an LV "vent" in patients on venoarterial extracorporeal membrane oxygenation (VA-ECMO)
- Microaxial flow pump (percutaneous ventricular assist device, eg, Impella)
    - Provides 2.5 to 5.5 L/min of cardiac output depending on specific device
    - Placed via femoral or axillary artery and sits across the aortic valve
    - Unloads the LV and provides forward systemic flow
    - Cannot be used with severe AR, mechanical aortic prosthesis, aortic dissection, left ventricular thrombus
    - Recent data suggesting benefit compared to medical therapy in patients with cardiogenic shock due to myocardial infarction (MI; DanGer trial)
    - Right-sided assist devices available to support postprocedure left-sided cardiogenic shock
- VA-ECMO
    - Complete bypass of the heart and lungs
    - Can provide up to 6 L/min of cardiac output
    - MCS of choice for severe biventricular failure, and cardiogenic shock combined with respiratory failure (eg, severe pulmonary embolism)
    - Drainage cannula (central venous system) circulates blood through a pump and oxygenator, wherein blood is delivered to the femoral artery via the return cannula.
    - Aortic return reaches the heart in retrograde fashion. VA-ECMO *increases* the afterload on the LV, and so may be paired with another form of MCS (eg, IABP or microaxial flow pump) for LV unloading or "venting." Marked aortic insufficiency is a contraindication
    - Major risks include bleeding, stroke, or vascular complications
- The intensivist must proactively consider available durable heart replacement strategies when evaluating a patient for MCS, so there is a destination or "exit" option in case the heart does not recover so as to liberate from the MCS.

SUGGESTED READINGS

Al-Khatib SM, Stevenson WG, Ackerman MJ, et al. 2017 AHA/ACC/HRS guideline for management of patients with ventricular arrhythmias and the prevention of sudden cardiac death: a report of the American College of Cardiology/American Heart Association Task Force on Clinical Practice Guidelines and the Heart Rhythm Society. *J Am Coll Cardiol*. 2018;72(14):e91-e220.

Alviar CL, Miller PE, McAreavey D, et al; ACC Critical Care Cardiology Working Group. Positive pressure ventilation in the cardiac intensive care unit. *J Am Coll Cardiol*. 2018;72(13):1532-1553.

Basso C. Myocarditis. *N Engl J Med*. 2022;387(16):1488-1500.

Davis MB, Arany Z, McNamara DM, Goland S, Elkayam U. Peripartum cardiomyopathy: JACC state-of-the-art review. *J Am Coll Cardiol*. 2020;75(2):207-221.

De Backer D, Biston P, Devriendt J, et al; SOAP II Investigators. Comparison of dopamine and norepinephrine in the treatment of shock. *N Engl J Med*. 2010;362(9):779-789.

Geller BJ, Sinha SS, Kapur NK, et al; American Heart Association Acute Cardiac Care and General Cardiology Committee of the Council on Clinical Cardiology; Council on Cardiopulmonary, Critical Care, Perioperative and Resuscitation; Council on Cardiovascular Radiology and Intervention; Council on Cardiovascular and Stroke Nursing; Council on Peripheral Vascular Disease; and Council on Cardiovascular Surgery and Anesthesia. Escalating and de-escalating temporary mechanical circulatory support in cardiogenic shock: a scientific statement from the American Heart Association. *Circulation*. 2022;146(6):e50-e68.

Heidenreich PA, Bozkurt B, Aguilar D, et al. 2022 AHA/ACC/HFSA guideline for the management of heart failure: a report of the American College of Cardiology/American Heart Association Joint Committee on Clinical Practice Guidelines. *Circulation*. 2022;145(18):e895-e1032.

Hochman JS, Sleeper LA, Webb JG, et al; SHOCK Investigators (Should We Emergently Revascularize Occluded Coronaries for Cardiogenic Shock). Early revascularization in acute myocardial infarction complicated by cardiogenic shock. *N Engl J Med*. 1999;341(9):625-634.

Møller JE, Engstrøm T, Jensen LO, et al; DanGer Shock Investigators. Microaxial flow pump or standard care in infarct-related cardiogenic shock. *N Engl J Med*. 2024;390(15):1382-1393.

Naidu SS, Baran DA, Jentzer JC, et al. SCAI SHOCK stage classification expert consensus update: a review and incorporation of validation studies: this statement was endorsed by the American College of Cardiology (ACC), American College of Emergency Physicians (ACEP), American Heart Association (AHA), European Society of Cardiology (ESC) Association for Acute Cardiovascular Care (ACVC), International Society for Heart and Lung Transplantation (ISHLT), Society of Critical Care Medicine (SCCM), and Society of Thoracic Surgeons (STS) in December 2021. *J Am Coll Cardiol*. 2022;79(9):933-946.

Thiele H, Zeymer U, Neumann FJ, et al; IABP-SHOCK II Trial Investigators. Intraaortic balloon support for myocardial infarction with cardiogenic shock. *N Engl J Med*. 2012;367(14):1287-1296.

Vahdatpour C, Collins D, Goldberg S. Cardiogenic shock. *J Am Heart Assoc*. 2019;8(8):e011991.

van Diepen S, Katz JN, Albert NM, et al; American Heart Association Council on Clinical Cardiology; Council on Cardiovascular and Stroke Nursing; Council on Quality of Care and Outcomes Research; and Mission: Lifeline. Contemporary management of cardiogenic shock: a scientific statement from the American Heart Association. *Circulation*. 2017;136(16):e232-e268.

1.4

Obstructive Shock

Lukas H. Matern

Overview of Obstructive Shock

- Obstructive shock occurs when a mechanical impediment to flow within the cardiovascular system results in inadequate end-organ perfusion.
- Major etiologies of obstructive shock include tension pneumothorax, cardiac tamponade, pulmonary embolism (PE), and central vascular compression (see *Table 1.4.1*).
    - Physiologically, these conditions may reduce preload, increase afterload, and/or reduce cardiac contractility to produce shock.
    - In most cases of obstructive shock, diastolic filling of the right or left ventricle is impaired and may be considered the primary hemodynamic problem.
    - Acute aortic dissection, particularly with ascending aortic (ie, type A) involvement, may sufficiently increase left ventricular afterload to precipitate obstructive shock, though this type of shock will not be covered in detail here.
- Key examination findings in obstructive shock may resemble cardiogenic shock.
    - The pulse pressure is typically narrow.
    - The extremities are cool or mottled.
    - Jugular venous distension may be present.
- In general, effective treatment of obstructive shock depends on timely relief of the mechanical obstruction in addition to aggressive supportive care until this occurs.

TABLE 1.4.1 Summary of Selected Causes of Obstructive Shock

Cause of Shock	Pathophysiology	Treatment
Tension pneumothorax	Reduced preload due to accumulation of pressurized air within the pleural space	Needle decompression with thoracostomy tube placement
Cardiac tamponade	Right ventricular diastolic failure due to compression by fluid within the pericardium	Pericardiocentesis followed by continuous pericardial drainage
Pulmonary embolism	Right ventricular dysfunction due to obstructing debris within the pulmonary arteries	Systemic anticoagulation with thrombolysis and/or embolectomy (for thromboembolism)
Caval obstruction or compression	Preload reduction due to compression or blockage of the superior and/or inferior venae cavae	Volume administration with prompt removal of the obstruction

- While pharmacotherapies such as thrombolysis may be effective in treating disorders such as PE and caval thrombosis, most causes of mechanical obstruction require urgent mechanical interventions (eg, needle or tube drainage).

Tension Pneumothorax

- Under normal circumstances, the pleural cavity is a negative pressure space, with tight pleural apposition permitting lung expansion during spontaneous ventilation.
- A pneumothorax is present when air accumulates in the pleural space, which may compromise ventilation as well as perfusion.
    - A simple pneumothorax may present without hemodynamic or respiratory consequences and may not require intervention (when <2-3 cm in size).
    - Additional material, such as blood, chyle, or exudate, may accumulate within a pneumothorax (resulting in a concomitant hemothorax, chylothorax, or pleural effusion, respectively).
- A tension pneumothorax develops when sufficient air has accumulated in the pleural space to compromise the circulation.
    - A pneumothorax may expand as gas enters from injured lung parenchyma (eg, in the setting of a ruptured bulla) or from the atmosphere (eg, in the presence of a sucking chest wound).
    - Without a route for escape, pleural air accumulates under positive pressure, producing mediastinal shift, reducing venous return, and lowering cardiac output to cause obstructive shock.
- Signs and symptoms of tension pneumothorax include an absence of lung sounds and hyperresonance to percussion of the affected hemothorax, jugular venous distension, hypotension, and respiratory distress.
    - Chest radiography may demonstrate an area of radiolucency without visible lung markings, reduced lung volumes, and contralateral shift of the mediastinum.
    - Bedside ultrasonography will reveal an absence of lung sliding and may demonstrate lung points, a highly specific finding of pneumothorax.
    - Ultimately, tension pneumothorax requires a rapid clinical diagnosis with swift intervention, and treatment should not be delayed for any specific study.
- Management of the tension pneumothorax requires emergent release of trapped air from the pleural cavity.
    - Needle decompression may be performed by inserting a 5-cm large-bore needle at the second intercostal space at the midclavicular line or around the fifth intercostal space at the midaxillary line.
    - While needle decompression may be immediately lifesaving, insertion of a chest tube (thoracostomy tube) is also required to allow ongoing drainage of air from the pleural space and prevent recurrence of the pneumothorax.
        - Depending on clinician experience and resource availability, emergent tube thoracostomy may also be performed for primary decompression.
        - Guidelines recommend insertion of chest tubes over the rib within the "triangle of safety," which is bounded by the lateral border of the pectoralis major muscle, the anterior edge of the latissimus dorsi muscle, the axilla, and the nipple line.

   - If an open or "sucking" chest wound is present, a semi-occlusive dressing may be placed to create a one-way escape valve and reduce air entry.
- When intubation and mechanical ventilation are otherwise indicated, these interventions should be delayed until after decompression of the tension pneumothorax.
  - Positive pressure ventilation may directly increase the size of a pneumothorax and compromise venous return, accelerating hemodynamic collapse.

Cardiac Tamponade

- In many cases, a pericardial effusion may be present without tamponade.
  - Fluid may accumulate within the pericardium due to fluid transudation, inflammatory exudation, or bleeding (ie, hemopericardium).
  - Chronic accumulation of pericardial fluid may be hemodynamically tolerated due to gradual increases in pericardial compliance, which results in a low-pressure pericardial effusion without significant cardiac compression.
- Cardiac tamponade develops when fluid within the pericardium accumulates too rapidly or in volumes too high to allow for pericardial compensation, which results in extrinsic compression of the cardiac chambers and reduced cardiac output.
  - The atria, which function as low-pressure collecting systems for blood, are the first to experience compression or inversion.
  - Compression of the right ventricle with impaired diastolic filling ultimately causes cardiovascular collapse as tamponade progresses.
- Signs and symptoms of tamponade include hypotension, jugular venous distension, and distant or muffled heart sounds (the Beck triad), though these "classic" findings are not always present.
  - Pulsus paradoxus, an exaggerated decrease in systolic blood pressure on inspiration ($\geq$10 mm Hg), is associated with, but not specific for, tamponade.
  - An electrocardiogram may show a decreased amplitude of the QRS complex or, in the presence of a large effusion, an electrical alternans pattern.
  - Chest radiographs may demonstrate enlargement of the cardiac silhouette but are often normal in acute tamponade.
  - As intrapericardial pressure builds, equalization of filling pressures between the cardiac chambers may be measured via placement of a pulmonary artery catheter.
  - Echocardiography allows for definitive diagnosis and reveals a pericardial effusion with atrial inversion, collapse of the right ventricle, and a hyperkinetic and underfilled left ventricle.
- Management of tamponade centers on the expeditious drainage of pericardial fluid.
  - Bedside needle pericardiocentesis may be performed under ultrasound guidance via subxiphoid or parasternal approaches.
  - Subsequent pericardial drainage via an indwelling catheter or surgical subxiphoid window is needed to prevent reaccumulation of fluid.
  - Until drainage can be achieved, a patient's hemodynamics may be managed supportively with volume resuscitation and vasopressor administration.
- Further interventions may be required to address complex precipitating causes, especially if tamponade occurs secondary to conditions such as aortic dissection or trauma.

Pulmonary Embolism

- PE occurs when intravascular debris, such as a migratory thrombus from a deep vein, embolizes into the pulmonary arterial tree and produces obstruction with increased right ventricular afterload.
  - Other types of emboli may also occlude pulmonary blood flow, including tumor cells, fat, air, and amniotic fluid or fetoplacental material.
- PE due to venous thromboembolism may be classified as low, intermediate, or high risk (generally preferred over qualifiers such as "submassive" and "massive").
  - Intermediate-risk PE arises when evidence of right ventricular dysfunction or strain appears without overt hemodynamic compromise.
  - High-risk PE is accompanied by hypotension, signaling true obstructive shock.
- Signs and symptoms of high-risk PE include dyspnea, tachycardia, pleuritic chest pain, hypoxia, hemoptysis, and hypotension.
  - Radiographs are most often normal, though a minority of patients with PE may present with a pleural-based opacity (Hampton hump) or a focus of peripheral lung radiolucency (Westermark sign).
  - Electrocardiographic findings are nonspecific and may include tachycardia or, in some cases, ST depression in lead I, deep Q waves in lead III, and inverted T waves in lead III (the "$S_1Q_3T_3$" pattern of right ventricular or inferior wall strain).
  - In the setting of a thromboembolic PE, a diagnosis may also be supported by evidence of a thrombus in a deep venous structure (eg, a femoral vein).
  - Echocardiography may aid in the diagnosis, demonstrating right ventricular dilation, bowing or flattening of the interventricular septum, right ventricular free wall hypokinesis with apical sparing (the McConnell sign), a small and hyperkinetic left ventricle, or a thrombus within the heart or pulmonary arteries.
  - Definitive diagnosis requires computed tomographic (CT) pulmonary angiography or, in select cases, a nuclear ventilation-perfusion scan or invasive angiogram.
- High-risk PE from thromboembolism requires prompt administration of systemic anticoagulation, usually with a bolus and infusion of unfractionated heparin, in addition to systemic thrombolytics to break down the obstructing clot.
  - In select cases, catheter-directed interventions or surgical pulmonary embolectomy may also be indicated, especially if systemic thrombolytic therapy is ineffective or contraindicated.
  - Patients with high-risk PE may require volume administration, vasopressors or inotropes, and/or mechanical circulatory support as a bridge to definitive intervention.
  - The decision to administer thrombolytics—as well as the optimal dose—in intermediate-risk PE remains an area of study, and patients are often evaluated for candidacy by multidisciplinary response teams.

- Other embolic phenomena producing obstructive shock require different management strategies.
  - For example, air embolism may arise from venous air entry during invasive procedures (eg, intracranial neurosurgery or central venous catheterization), rapid changes in ambient pressure, or aggressive mechanical ventilation.
  - Acute embolism of ≥200 mL air in the average adult (~3 mL/kg) may produce a right ventricular "air lock" with flow obstruction.
    - Treatment includes head-down positioning, administration of 100% inspired oxygen, and hemodynamic support with fluids and vasopressors.
- A cornerstone of PE management lies in diligent prevention.
  - Immobilized patients, especially those with systemic inflammatory or hypercoagulable states, are at high risk for venous thromboembolism and PE.
  - Barring contraindications, most critically ill patients should receive chemical and/or mechanical prophylaxis against venous thromboembolic disease.
  - Patients at high risk of venous air entrainment, such as neurosurgical patients requiring dissection around the venous sinuses, should be monitored closely with appropriate modalities (eg, precordial Doppler ultrasound) with measures taken to reduce the risk of air entry.

Caval Obstruction

- Occlusion or compression of the great veins, especially the superior vena cava (SVC) and inferior vena cava (IVC), may result in hemodynamic consequences sufficient to precipitate obstructive shock.
  - The mechanism of shock in the setting of major venous compression is almost universally a decrease in right ventricular preload.
- While major caval obstruction is relatively uncommon, this condition may result from tumor embolism or caval extension (eg, hematogenous spread of renal cell carcinoma), caval thrombosis, mediastinal tumor mass effect, or late-trimester pregnancy.
  - Thrombosis of the IVC, while rare, requires aggressive intervention with thrombolytics and/or systemic anticoagulation.
  - Aortocaval compression by the gravid uterus, particularly with IVC obstruction, may occur in patients in the third trimester of pregnancy when lying supine.
    - Complete caval collapse has been noted to occur in a large proportion of parturients in a fully supine position at term.
    - Hypotension thought to be due to caval compression in pregnancy may be treated with leftward uterine displacement or lateral decubitus positioning in addition to volume and vasopressor administration.
    - Manual leftward uterine displacement continues to be recommended as a component of maternal advanced cardiac life support protocols to improve venous return.

SUGGESTED READINGS

Grocott HP, Gulati H, Srinathan S, Mackensen GB. Anesthesia and the patient with pericardial disease. *Can J Anaesth*. 2011;58(10):952-966.

Konstantinides SV, Meyer G, Becattini C, et al. 2019 ESC guidelines for the diagnosis and management of acute pulmonary embolism developed in collaboration with the European Respiratory Society (ERS). *Eur Heart J*. 2020;41(4):543-603.

Meyer G, Vicaut E, Danays T, et al. Fibrinolysis for patients with intermediate-risk pulmonary embolism. *N Engl J Med*. 2014;370(15):1402-1411.

Zotzmann V, Rottmann FA, Katharina Müller-Pelzer K, et al. Obstructive shock, from diagnosis to treatment. *Rev Cardiovasc Med*. 2022;23(7):248.

SECTION 2

Cardiovascular

Section Editors: David M. Dudzinski and Marvin G. Chang

2.1

Coronary Artery Disease, Myocardial Ischemia, and Infarction

Parth N. Patel, Sarah M. Urbut, Michelle L. O'Donoghue, and Nilay K. Patel

Definitions

- Coronary artery disease (CAD) refers to atherosclerotic narrowing of the epicardial coronary arteries that supply the myocardium with oxygen and nutrients.
- Acute coronary syndromes (ACSs) occur when there is newly partial or complete obstruction of the coronary artery lumen, leading to myocardial ischemia. ACS typically indicates rupture (or erosion) of a coronary atherosclerotic plaque.
- Myocardial injury is defined as an elevation in cardiac troponin values with at least one value above the 99th percentile of the upper reference limit. Myocardial injury is acute when there is a sudden rise (or fall) of troponin values. Several conditions commonly seen in intensive care unit (ICU) settings, such as hypotension, hypoxemia, anemia, arrhythmias, heart failure, and renal dysfunction, can cause myocardial injury (and which are not necessarily ACS).
- Myocardial infarction (MI) is diagnosed in the presence of acute myocardial injury with clinical evidence of myocardial ischemia. Supporting clinical evidence can include patient-reported symptoms, new ischemic changes on electrocardiogram (ECG), development of pathologic Q waves, or imaging demonstrating new loss of viable myocardium.

Epidemiology

- Ischemic heart disease is the #1 leading cause of death worldwide, accounting for 15% of all deaths globally each year.
- > 9 million deaths were attributable to ischemic heart disease in 2021.
- CAD affects some 300 million individuals worldwide.
- The prevalence of ischemic heart disease tends to increase with age.

Pathophysiology

- CAD has been linked to a combination of modifiable and nonmodifiable risk factors—most notably high levels of low-density lipoprotein cholesterol (LDL-C), hypertension, diabetes mellitus (DM), tobacco use, and family history.
- Additionally, high levels of lipoprotein(a) and vascular inflammation are recognized contributors to the initiation and propagation of atherosclerosis.
- Mature atherosclerotic plaques are composed of a lipid core that is separated from the vessel lumen by a fibrous cap made of collagen. Plaques that contain a thin fibrous cap overlying the lipid core are less stable and thus more prone to spontaneously rupture.

Type 1 Versus Type 2 Myocardial Infarction

- Type 1 MI describes the instance in which atherosclerotic plaque disruption leads to acute exposure of the prothrombotic lipid core to the bloodstream, leading to rapid platelet aggregation and thrombus formation in the coronary artery lumen.
- Type 2 MI occurs if there is inadequate myocardial oxygen supply to meet myocardial oxygen demand, coupled with clinical evidence of myocardial ischemia, in the absence of coronary atherothrombosis.
  - Some specific examples of inadequate coronary blood and myocardial oxygen supply (though not due to plaque rupture) include coronary artery spasm, spontaneous coronary artery dissection, severe anemia, tamponade, acute cor pulmonale (cf pulmonary embolism, with reduced right to left blood flow), hypoxemic respiratory failure, severe bradyarrhythmia, or cardiogenic shock.
  - Some specific examples of increased myocardial oxygen demand include left ventricular (LV) distention or pressurization, sustained tachyarrhythmia, severe anemia (heart will compensate by trying to increase cardiac output), fever, elevated sympathetic tone, hyperthyroidism, surgery, shock, vasopressors or inotropes, withdrawal

of negative chronotropic agents, or certain mechanical circulatory support devices like peripheral venoarterial extracorporeal membrane oxygenation (VA ECMO). Any factor that increases myocardial intrinsic contractility, the heart rate, or systolic wall tension will increase demand.
   - In the ICU settings, fixed coronary atherosclerotic obstruction, combined with acute stressor or with increase in physiologic demands, can cause type 2 MI.

Coronary Anatomy

- The left main coronary artery normally arises from the left sinus of Valsalva within the aortic root and divides into the left anterior descending (LAD) and left circumflex (LCX) arteries.
   - The LAD courses along the anterior interventricular groove (between the right ventricle and LV) toward the apex of the heart. The LAD gives origin to diagonal arteries, which supply blood to the anterolateral aspect of the myocardium, as well as septal perforators that provide blood to the anterior 2/3 of the interventricular septum (Figure 2.1.1).
   - The LCX courses along the left AV groove (between the left atrium [LA] and LV) toward the posterior aspect of the heart. The LCX gives origin to obtuse marginal arteries that supply blood to the lateral wall of the heart.
- The right coronary artery (RCA) normally arises from the right sinus of Valsalva within the aortic root.
   - The RCA travels in the right AV groove (between the right atrium and the right ventricle) toward the posterior aspect of the heart. The RCA provides blood supply to the sinus node and later provides acute marginal arteries that supply the free wall of the right ventricle.
- The dominance of the coronary circulation is determined by which blood vessel supplies the posterior descending artery (PDA), which runs along the inferior interventricular groove (between the right ventricle and LV). The PDA gives origin to septal perforators that supply blood to the inferior 1/3 of the interventricular septum.
   - Estimates suggest 70% of the population is right dominant (RCA provides PDA), 10% is left dominant (LCX provides PDA), and 20% is codominant.
   - Small branches from the dominant artery provide blood supply to the AV node. Ischemia to this territory may result in AV blocks in certain ischemic syndromes.
   - The dominant artery is usually the only blood supply to the posterior papillary muscle, placing it at risk for rupture in the setting of an inferior MI.
- Correlation of ischemic ECG changes, wall motion abnormalities on echocardiography, or new electrical or mechanical disturbances with knowledge of coronary anatomy can help localize the affected territory in the setting of coronary ischemia. Nevertheless, the intensivist should be prepared to consider that there can be variability among patients in exact distributions of anatomy, including anomalous coronary origins and trajectories, as well as artery-to-artery collateralization.

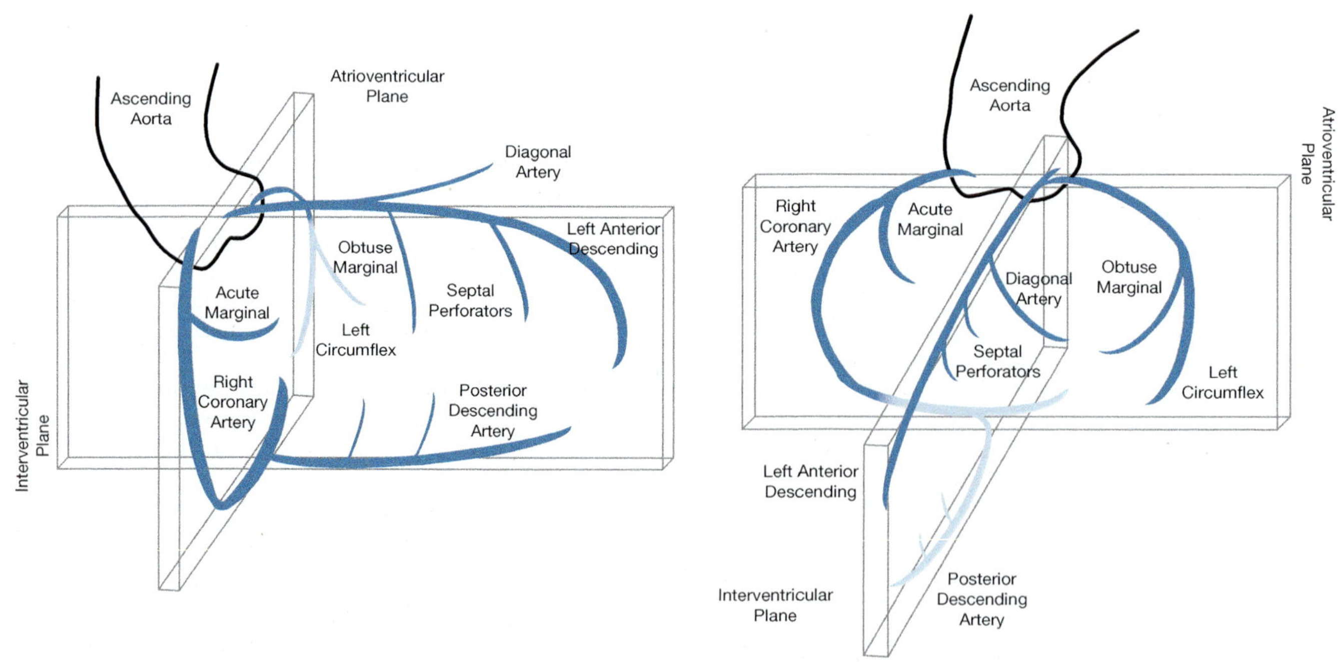

FIGURE 2.1.1 Schematic of coronary artery anatomy and distribution. The major coronary arteries are defined by their course along two distinct orthogonal planes. The left anterior descending artery and posterior descending artery course along the interventricular plane on the anterior and posterior aspects of the heart, respectively. The left circumflex coronary artery and right coronary artery traverse the atrioventricular plane on the left and right sides of the heart, respectively. Branches of these major coronary arteries supply blood flow to all myocardial segments.

Acute Management of Coronary Ischemia

- Acute MI is recognized and diagnosed by laboratory evidence of myocardial injury and supporting evidence of myocardial ischemia.
- Treatment should be aimed at reducing further injury and working to reperfuse the injured myocardium.

Key Subtypes

- Complete occlusion of an epicardial coronary artery leads to transmural myocardial ischemia, biomarker release, myocardial necrosis, and manifests as an ST-elevation myocardial infarction (STEMI).
  - Reperfusion should be offered to all patients with STEMI within 12 hours of symptom onset and who have no contraindications. Faster time to reperfusion confers increased benefit.
  - The benefit appears to attenuate after 12 hours, though restoration of flow in the infarct-related artery may improve clinical outcomes up to 24 hours after symptom onset.
  - Primary percutaneous coronary intervention (PCI) has been shown to reduce major adverse cardiovascular events when compared to fibrinolysis.
  - Primary PCI remains superior to fibrinolysis even when it requires transfer to the PCI-capable hospital, as long as the transfer-related delay to receive PCI is $<$120 minutes.
- Partial occlusion of an epicardial coronary artery with downstream myocardial ischemia manifests as either unstable angina (UA) if there is no detectable release of cardiac biomarkers or non–ST-elevation myocardial infarction (NSTEMI) if there is evidence of myocardial necrosis.
  - In the majority of patients, the decision to proceed with and optimal timing for catheterization is determined on a case-by-case basis after considering patient stability, clinical comorbidities, and risk for recurrent ischemic events.
  - In select patients with electrical instability, cardiogenic shock complicating MI, or with ongoing anginal symptoms despite maximal medical therapy, urgent cardiac catheterization and revascularization is recommended.

Medical Management

- Aspirin should be considered and given as soon as possible, since it has a demonstrable benefit in patients presenting with suspected MI, with a number needed to treat of 42 to prevent one death at 35 days.
  - All patients should be given a loading dose $\geq$300 mg to initiate treatment.
  - Following loading, higher dose aspirin (300-325 mg) does not reduce ischemic events compared to lower dose aspirin (75-100 mg) but is associated with a higher risk of bleeding.
- Nitroglycerin may provide relief of chest pain through dilation of the capacitance vessels (venodilatation) and reducing ventricular wall tension.
  - Dosing can be provided through sublingual administration or through intravenous infusion.
  - Use is contraindicated in patients on phosphodiesterase inhibitors (sildenafil, vardenafil, tadalafil) and in patients with suspected right ventricular infarction, as these patients are preload dependent and administration causing venodilatation may precipitate hypotension or shock.
- Beta-blockade reduces myocardial oxygen demand and decreases rates of ventricular arrhythmias but, in large trials, has been shown to increase the risk of cardiogenic shock.
  - Oral beta-blockade should be initiated within 24 hours of acute MI as long as there is no evidence of AV block, heart failure, or low output state.
  - Beta-blockers can cause harm in patients with increased time since symptom onset, elevated heart rate, low pulse pressure, and cool extremities. These features can be risk factors and signs of evolving cardiogenic shock.
- $P2Y_{12}$ inhibitors (clopidogrel, ticagrelor, prasugrel) improve outcomes in patients with ACS; however, treatment with these medications increases rates of major bleeding.
  - Loading generally occurs once coronary anatomy has been defined and a decision has been made whether the patient will receive PCI, coronary artery bypass grafting (CABG), or medical therapy.
- Anticoagulation is believed to slow propagation of thrombus, stabilize vulnerable plaques, and restore vessel patency in patients with a suspected atherothrombotic mechanism of infarction (type 1 MI).
  - If clinical suspicion for type 1 MI is high, and anticoagulation is reasonably safe, treatment with unfractionated heparin, low-molecular-weight heparin, or bivalirudin should be initiated in the acute setting.
- Statins reduce LDL-C levels and are believed to have pleotropic effects along many pathogenic pathways, including reducing inflammation, oxidative stress, and endothelial dysfunction.
  - High-intensity statin therapy in the acute setting may stabilize both culprit and other at-risk coronary plaques and should be started as soon as ACS is suspected.
  - Furthermore, reduction of LDL-C levels leads to dose-dependent reduction in the risk of recurrent major atherosclerotic events in follow-up that is proportional to the absolute magnitude of the reduction in achieved LDL-C.
- Following the acute ischemic event, several proven secondary prevention measures should be initiated prior to discharge, including additional LDL-C lowering, glycemic control, and smoking cessation.
- In patients with signs or symptoms of heart failure and low LV ejection fraction following ACS, angiotensin-converting enzyme inhibitors (ACEi), angiotensin receptor blockers (ARBs), and mineralocorticoid receptor antagonists (MRAs) have all been shown to improve long-term survival (these agents may not be able to be initiated immediately after ACS).

Myocardial Revascularization

- Optimal timing of coronary revascularization depends on the acuity and severity of the myocardial insult, as described earlier.

- The preferred strategy for revascularization depends on several factors, including clinical characteristics, anatomic features, technical aspects, and supportive long-term data.
  - PCI is generally preferred to CABG in patients requiring urgent revascularization or in cases of low-complexity, single- or two-vessel CAD.
    - While "complete revascularization" (cf culprit lesion and nonculprit lesions) has emerged as the default strategy in ACS, in patients with cardiogenic shock, culprit vessel–only PCI is performed (higher risks periprocedurally were observed in cardiogenic shock patients, including renal dysfunction).
  - CABG is generally favored over PCI in patients with left main or high-complexity CAD, multivessel CAD with DM, and multivessel CAD with low LV ejection fraction.
  - Other factors that often affect the decision for PCI versus CABG include the presence of adequate bypass grafts and targets, clinical comorbidities (eg, aortic disease, which could affect cannulation needed for CABG; or severe lung disease, which affects post-CABG recovery), hemodynamic status, ability to tolerate dual-antiplatelet therapy, patient frailty, and rehabilitation potential.

Complications of Myocardial Infarction

- Prompt recognition of complications of MI requires integration of examination findings, hemodynamics, coronary anatomy, cardiac physiology, and clinical knowledge of the time elapsed since the MI occurred. Complications of MI can lead to cardiogenic shock and be fatal if left untreated.
- Cardiac arrhythmias such as heart block, atrial fibrillation, and ventricular arrhythmias are most common in the first few days after MI.
  - Polymorphic ventricular tachycardia or ventricular fibrillation can be caused by acute myocardial ischemia and occur within 4 hours of MI.
  - Monomorphic ventricular tachycardia is more frequently seen > 48 hours after MI due to the development of myocardial scar and cardiac remodeling.
  - Sinus node dysfunction is usually caused by RCA infarct.
  - Heart block (AV nodal dysfunction) can be observed when there is infarction of the dominant artery that supplies the PDA.
  - Bundle branch blocks can also result from ischemia (eg, left bundle branch block [LBBB] from proximal left coronary occlusion). Severe heart blocks may be an indication for temporary pacing post-MI.
- Mechanical complications such as papillary muscle rupture, ventricular septal rupture, and free wall rupture are most likely between 3 and 14 days of MI, especially in cases of inadequate coronary revascularization.
  - Papillary muscle rupture presents as acute severe mitral regurgitation, pulmonary edema (may be unilateral), hypoxemia, and cardiogenic shock. The posteromedial papillary muscle has a single blood supply from the dominant coronary artery and is particularly prone to injury in inferior MI. High index of suspicion is required as the murmur may be minimal as there is rapid equilibration of regurgitant flow from LV to LA.
  - Ventricular septal rupture can occur in infarctions that involve the LAD (which provides blood to the anterior 2/3 of septum) or PDA (inferior 1/3 of the septum). Ventricular septal rupture leads to significant left-to-right blood shunting and should be suspected in cases with new murmur (holosystolic, left sternal border) and pulmonary edema. Left-to-right shunting can be detected as an increase in oxygen saturation from the level at the right atrium to the right ventricle. Right heart failure may occur.
  - Free wall rupture can occur if there is transmural infarction in any myocardial location abutting the pericardial space. Myocardial free wall rupture presents as cardiac tamponade and sudden obstructive shock. A rupture of the ventricular free wall that is contained by overlying, adherent pericardium is called a pseudoaneurysm. Pseudoaneurysms and free wall ruptures are both cardiac surgical emergencies.
- Cerebral and systemic embolization can be seen with infarctions that lead to akinetic or aneurysmal myocardial segments, as these provide a nidus for ventricular thrombus formation.
- Pericardial inflammation (Dressler syndrome) can be seen in large transmural infarcts several weeks after MI.

Mimickers of ST-Segment Myocardial Infarction

- In the ICU setting, differentiating true STEMI from its mimics is essential to avoid inappropriate treatments and to ensure optimal patient care.
- A thorough recognition of the potential mimics (Table 2.1.1) and a systematic approach can aid in accurate diagnosis and management.

Diagnostic Approach to Coronary Artery Disease and Myocardial Ischemia in the Intensive Care Unit

- Clinical correlation
  - Assess patient's history, symptoms, and risk factors.
  - Construct differential diagnosis based on presenting signs and symptoms.
- ECG monitoring
  - Obtain serial ECGs to monitor changes over time.
  - When ACS is suspected, several repeat ECGs will be needed in the first 10 minutes.
  - Look for evolving patterns consistent with MI.
- Cardiac biomarkers
  - Measure troponin levels to assess for myocardial injury.
  - Interpret in conjunction with clinical and ECG findings.
- Imaging studies
  - Perform echocardiogram to evaluate wall motion abnormalities.
  - Consider cardiac magnetic resonance imaging (MRI) for detailed assessment if diagnosis remains uncertain.
- Consultation
  - Consider consulting a cardiologist for protean or complex cases.
  - Utilize a multidisciplinary approach for comprehensive management.

TABLE 2.1.1 STEMI Mimics

Condition	Supportive ECG Criteria	Clinical Pearls
Pericarditis	Widespread diffuse concave ST-segment elevation PR depression in majority of limb and precordial leads PR elevation in aVR	Inflammation of the pericardium leads to pleuritic chest discomfort. Pericardial friction rub or effusion may be seen.
Left ventricular hypertrophy	Increased R-wave amplitude in leads I, aVL, and V4-V6 Increased S-wave amplitude in V1-V3 Discordant ST elevation can be seen in V1-V3 due to repolarization abnormalities.	Patients will have increased left ventricular wall thickness due to chronic pressure overload conditions such as hypertension or aortic stenosis. ECG changes due to repolarization are not dynamic.
Benign early repolarization	Elevation of the J-point between the end of the QRS complex and beginning of the ST segment Concave ST elevation, usually most prominent V2-V5 No reciprocal ST depression	Most commonly seen in young, healthy patients <50 y of age
Left ventricular aneurysm	Deep Q waves with ST elevation in territory of prior infarct	Seen in patients with previous MI. Often related to incomplete reperfusion and transmural scar
RV-paced rhythm or left bundle branch block	Ventricular pacing or QRS duration >120 ms Dominant S wave in V1 Broad monophasic R wave in leads I, aVL, V5-V6 Discordant ST elevation can be seen in V1-V3 due to repolarization abnormalities.	Concordant or excessively discordant ST-segment deviations can help diagnose MI in the setting of ventricular pacing or left bundle branch block (Sgarbossa criteria).
Brugada syndrome	Characteristic appearance of coved ST elevation followed by a negative T wave in leads V1-V3 (type 1)	Diagnosis of Brugada syndrome requires characteristic ECG findings with supportive clinical history of syncope, ventricular arrhythmia, or sudden cardiac death. ECG findings can be elicited by drugs, illness, or fever.
Coronary spasm	Localized ST elevation in pattern identical to acute STEMI Reciprocal ST depressions present	Coronary spasm is unable to be differentiated from STEMI by ECG alone. Changes are transient and reversible with vasodilators.

ECG, electrocardiogram; MI, myocardial infarction; RV, right ventricle; STEMI, ST-elevation myocardial infarction.

SUGGESTED READINGS

Amsterdam EA, Wenger NK, Brindis RG, et al. 2014 AHA/ACC guideline for the management of patients with non-ST-elevation acute coronary syndromes. *Circulation*. 2014;130(25):e344-e426.

Martin SS, Aday AW, Almarzooq ZI, et al. 2024 heart disease and stroke statistics: a report of US and global data from the American Heart Association. *Circulation*. 2024;149(8):e347-e913.

Reed GW, Rossi JE, Cannon CP. Acute myocardial infarction. *Lancet*. 2017;389(10065):197-210.

Thygesen K, Alpert JS, Jaffe AS, et al. Fourth universal definition of myocardial infarction (2018). *J Am Coll Cardiol*. 2018;72(18):2231-2264.

Vaduganathan M, Mensah GA, Turco JV, et al. The global burden of cardiovascular diseases and risk: a compass for future health. *J Am Coll Cardiol*. 2022;80(25):2361-2371.

2.2

Heart Failure

Kemar J. Brown, Safia Chatur, and David M. Dudzinski

Myocardial Pathology—Heart Failure

- Heart failure (HF) is a clinical syndrome that is characterized by the mismatch between the ability to generate cardiac output (CO) versus metabolic tissue demands (or the ability to meet metabolic tissue demands but only at abnormally elevated cardiac filling pressures).
- Impairment in effective stroke volume (SV) may be driven by systolic dysfunction (as in HF with reduced ejection fraction [HFrEF]), poor compliance and impaired diastolic filling (as in HF with preserved ejection fraction [HFpEF]), inadequate left ventricular (LV) preload (right ventricular [RV] failure) or, more rarely, insufficient heart rate (HR) in cases of inappropriate bradycardia.
- Patients with HF typically present with signs of congestion and/or low output (cardiac index <2.2 L/min/m^2). General management of acute decompensation, irrespective of etiology, hinges on relieving congestion (diuresis) and on hemodynamic support (eg, inotropes or mechanical support).

TABLE 2.2.1 Classifications

Category	Name	Properties
HFrEF	HF with reduced EF	EF ≤40% Often accompanied by LV dilatation and myocardial fibrosis
HFmrEF	HF with mildly reduced EF or midrange EF	EF 41%-49%
HFimpEF	HF with improved EF	EF >40% following previously documented EF ≤40%
HFpEF	HF with preserved EF	EF >50% and evidence of HF (elevated biomarkers or elevated filling pressures)

EF, ejection fraction; HF, heart failure; LV, left ventricle.

Echocardiographic Classification of Heart Failure

- Classification is typically dependent on the LV ejection fraction (EF) assessed via transthoracic echocardiography (Table 2.2.1).
- Functional classifications are shown in Table 2.2.2.

Key Heart Failure Pathophysiology

- Increase in cardiac filling pressures in an attempt to preserve SV
- Decreased SV causes an increase in HR to maintain CO.
- Later decrease in CO heralds decompensated HF.
- Upregulated renin-angiotensin system activation results from decreased CO.

TABLE 2.2.2 NYHA and AHA/ACC Classifications and Stages

NYHA Class	AHA/ACC Stage	Comments
(I) Asymptomatic, no physical limitation	(A) At risk,[a] but neither signs nor symptoms of HF, structural heart disease, or cardiac biomarkers	Stages A and B correlate with NYHA I-II.
(II) Mild symptoms	(B) Asymptomatic with evidence of structural heart disease, increased filling pressures, or abnormal cardiac biomarkers	
(III) Significant symptoms	(C) Structural heart disease, with symptoms (current or prior)	Stage C can have range of NYHA I-III.
(IV) Symptoms at rest	(D) Refractory HF[b]	Stage D correlates with class IV symptoms.

ACC, American College of Cardiology; AHA, American Heart Association; HF, heart failure; NYHA, New York Heart Association; VE, ventilatory efficiency.

[a]Patients with hypertension, atherosclerosis, diabetes, metabolic syndrome and obesity, exposure to cardiotoxic agents, genetic variant for cardiomyopathy, or positive family history of cardiomyopathy.

[b]Cardiopulmonary exercise testing (CPET) is important for risk stratification and planning for advanced therapies. High-risk features on CPET at maximal effort (respiratory exchange ratio ≥1.1) include peak Vo_2 <14 mL/kg/min (12 mL/kg/min with beta-blocker) or peak Vo_2 <50% of predicted, VE/Vco_2 slope >36, and exercise oscillatory respiration.

- In diastolic HF, impairments in isovolumic relaxation or compliance during LV filling

Epidemiology

- Though the landscape of medical therapy for HF continues to widen, about 26 million people are afflicted worldwide (6 million people in the United States, or 2% of the US population).
- Acute decompensation, refractory congestion, and recurrent hospitalizations (over 1 million HF hospitalizations in the United States annually) become more problematic as the HF stage progresses.
- Acute HF = leading cause of admissions in people older than 65 years.
- Large disparities in HF incidence and prevalence are seen primarily among Black individuals.
- Lifetime risk of HF through age 75 is 21.3% for Black men compared to 19.1% for White men, 23.9% for Black women compared to 13.4% for White women.

Common Heart Failure Causes to Remember

- The etiologies of HF are quite broad, and these are also associated with echocardiographic classification into HFrEF versus HFpEF (see Table 2.2.3).

Differential Diagnosis of Heart Failure

- Cardiac (pericardial effusion and tamponade, constrictive pericarditis, acute/severe primary valvular disease)
- Noncardiac (volume overload, hypertension, anemia, sepsis, renal failure, cirrhosis, superior vena cava [SVC] syndrome)
- Pulmonary (acute respiratory distress syndrome [ARDS], pneumothorax, chronic obstructive pulmonary disease [COPD], emphysema, pneumonia, pulmonary embolus [PE], pulmonary fibrosis)

Common Heart Failure Triggers to Remember

- Patients are counseled on the need to avoid common triggers, including dietary indiscretions (high sodium and fluid intake) and medication nonadherence.

TABLE 2.2.3 Etiologies of Heart Failure

Systolic Dysfunction Etiologies	Diastolic Dysfunction Etiologies
Coronary artery disease	Metabolic/endocrine (diabetes, obesity, thyroid)
Hypertension	Hypertension
Cardiomyopathy (CM) (ischemic, dilated, peripartum)	Cardiomyopathy (hypertrophic, restrictive, sarcoid, amyloidosis, hemochromatosis)
Other cardiac (arrhythmia, valvular)	Other cardiac (valvular)
Inflammation (infection, sepsis, myocarditis) Drugs (alcohol, cocaine, doxorubicin)	

- HF exacerbations can also be precipitated by ischemia and infarction; excessive use of cardioinhibitory medications that decrease chronotropy, inotropy, or both, such as beta-blockers, calcium channel antagonists, and sodium channel blockers; worsening valve disease; tachyarrhythmias, bradyarrhythmias; pacemaker related; comorbid renal or liver failure; and medications like nonsteroidal antiinflammatory drugs (NSAIDs).

Diagnostic Evaluation of Heart Failure

- History and physical examination are the foundation, with a specific focus on volume examination and peripheral perfusion.
- Laboratory testing for volume overload and end-organ perfusion: NT-proBNP, troponin, basic metabolic panel, liver function tests (LFTs), lactate
- Pulmonary artery catheter placement for tailoring of therapies (LV and RV filling pressures, CO, mixed venous O_2 saturation, etc) (see Table 2.2.4)
- Repeat transthoracic echocardiogram (TTE) to reassess for new structural or valvular changes.
- Cardiac magnetic resonance imaging (cMRI) and endomyocardial biopsy must be considered if there is heightened concern for giant cell myocarditis and/or eosinophilic myocarditis, which have distinct histopathologic findings that can aid in diagnosis and which may have distinct therapeutic imperatives.
- Coronary angiogram is necessary with overt ischemic changes on electrocardiogram (ECG), wall motion abnormalities on TTE, frequent ventricular ectopy (especially if polymorphic), recurrent angina with rising cardiac troponin, and otherwise unexplained acute or subacute new or worsening systolic dysfunction.

Goals and Management of Acute Heart Failure Care (Tailored Therapy)

- *Acute HF goals include hemodynamic and respiratory support and symptomatic relief.*
- Clinically (or hemodynamically) determine volume status (for pulmonary capillary wedge pressure) and systemic perfusion (for CO). This matrix can be used for clinical assessment of acute and chronic HF by grouping patients based on *hemodynamic profile* (warm vs cold) and *congestion* (wet vs dry) (see Table 2.2.5).
  - These classifications can also help guide management and predict outcomes. Profile C has the highest mortality as these patients are in cardiogenic shock. Acute care is needed in the intensive care unit (ICU) setting with inotropes, diuretics, intravenous (IV) afterload reduction, and ± temporary mechanical circulatory supports as a bridge-to-recovery or to more durable heart replacement therapy.
  - Type L patients require pharmacologic and mechanical support.
- Address *precipitating factors* (eg, coronary angiogram if indicated to rule out myocardial ischemia).
- Optimize *volume status* (preload): IV diuretics targeting filling pressure goals, urine output, pulmonary edema on chest radiograph, weight, and clinical signs of congestion on physical examination.
- Adjust *afterload*: especially essential in low output states or in aortic or mitral regurgitation to reduce regurgitant volume.
- Adjust *contractility* with inotropes in low output states. Composite hemodynamic goals:
  - *Cardiac index* >*2.2 L/min/m*^{2}
  - *Mean arterial pressure (MAP)* >*65 mm Hg* (can individualize to try to support organ dysfunction, eg, renal; if carotid or other stenosis; if baseline hypertension, or baseline hypotension, eg, cirrhosis)
  - *Central venous pressure (CVP)* <*10 mm Hg* (can individualize if RV dysfunction or marked tricuspid regurgitation [TR])
  - *Pulmonary capillary wedge pressure (PCWP)* 12 to 14 mm Hg (possibly higher in patients with acute myocardial infarction [MI] or restrictive cardiomyopathy [CM] that have impaired LV compliance). In some patients, the pulmonary artery diastolic pressure (*PADP*) is used as a surrogate for PCWP; however, there can be differences between these two values if there is pulmonary vascular remodeling.
  - *Systemic vascular resistance (SVR) reduction*: this reduces LV afterload and may facilitate ejection.
- Avoid offending agents like beta-blockers and calcium channel blockers that provide negative inotropy. Attempt to reverse the inciting cause if one is identified.
- Noninvasive positive pressure ventilation (NIPPV) in acute HF decreases the need for intubation by 50% and reduces hospital mortality by 40%.
- Consider roles for interventional therapies (coronary artery bypass grafting/percutaneous coronary intervention [CABG/PCI], valve replacement), device therapies (cardiac resynchronization), and bridge-to-heart transplant with mechanical circulatory support if refractory HF syndrome.
- Acute diastolic HF care based on volume optimization and treating underlying triggers (atrial fibrillation with rapid ventricular response, infection, dietary indiscretions)
  - Lusitropic agents might help ventricular relaxation, but none are in contemporary clinical use.

TABLE 2.2.4 Therapies

Blood Pressure	PCWP	CO	Therapy
High	High	Low	Vasodilator, diuresis
Normal	High	Low	Inodilator vs vasodilator, diuresis
Low	High	Low	Inotrope, mechanical assist devices, diuresis

Early consult to advanced heart failure service for supportive management of vasoactive therapy, consideration for temporary mechanical circulatory support, and assessment of candidacy for heart replacement therapy (LVAD and heart transplantation). CO, cardiac output; LVAD, left ventricular assist device; PCWP, pulmonary capillary wedge pressure.

TABLE 2.2.5 Hemodynamic Profile

	Congestion (–)	Congestion (+)
Malperfusion (–)	Warm and dry *Type A*	Warm and wet *Type B*
Malperfusion (+)	Cold and dry *Type L*	Cold and wet *Type C*

Right Ventricular Failure

- RV predominant failure can also be seen in the ICU and can be difficult to manage in the acute setting. Etiologies of isolated acute RV dysfunction may include acute pulmonary embolism, RV ischemia/infarction, acute respiratory failure/ARDS, acute increases in RV afterload, or RV dysfunction following placement of left-sided mechanical supports (either percutaneous or durable left ventricular assist device [LVAD]). Arrhythmogenic RV CM is rarely seen.
- Management hinges on inotropic support, RV afterload reduction, optimization of RV preload (shock secondary to acutely increased RV afterload or reduction in contractility [as in RV infarct] may benefit from volume loading to increase RV SV as well as transpulmonary blood transit), increased chronotropy (to augment CO since LV preload will be relatively fixed in severe RV impairment), maintenance of atrioventricular synchrony, and reducing the risk of tachyarrhythmias. Digoxin should be considered for rate control (if needed) and may afford more inotropy.
- If a transvenous pacer is in place, higher pacing rate may provide benefit. This is important in the ICU immediately post-heart transplant when there is often postbypass and posttransplant RV dysfunction, and augmenting HR is a method to augment CO.
- Generally, seek to avoid RV-only pacing since this may result in ventricular dyssynchrony in the short-term and longer term myocardial dysfunction. In those cases, also consider upgrading to dual-chamber device or cardiac resynchronization therapy with defibrillator (CRT-D).

Durable Heart Replacement Therapies

- Heart replacement therapy (HRT) becomes necessary in most patients with end-stage HF with New York Heart Association (NYHA) IV symptoms, American Heart Association/American College of Cardiology (AHA/ACC) stage D that become refractory to medical management.
- Advanced HF specialists need to be consulted to assess candidacy for durable LVAD and heart transplantation.
- Contraindications for heart transplant include recent smoking (within 6 months), active substance use, untreated malignancy, treated malignancy (in remission for <5 years), uncontrolled diabetes, body mass index (BMI) >35, severe peripheral artery disease, pulmonary vascular resistance (PVR) >3.5 Wood units (because this increases risk of allograft RV failure), severe systemic illnesses, and irreversible multiorgan dysfunction.
- Pretransplant optimization may depend on United Network for Organ Sharing (UNOS) status:
  - Status 1: venoarterial extracorporeal membrane oxygenation (VA ECMO), nondischargeable biventricular assist device (BiVAD), mechanical circulatory support (MCS) with life-threatening arrhythmias
  - Status 2: intra-aortic balloon pump, sustained ventricular tachycardia/ventricular fibrillation (VT/VF), nondischargeable LVAD, MCS with malfunction, percutaneous MCS
  - Status 3: dischargeable LVAD (has 30 days at status 3 time), MCS with complication, intravenous inotrope with hemodynamic monitoring
  - Status 4: inotropes without hemodynamic monitoring, stable LVAD, ischemia with intractable angina, congenital heart disease, hypertrophic CM, restrictive CM, re-do transplant
  - Status 5: combined organ transplant
  - Status 6: remaining active transplant
  - Status 7: inactivated
- A large focus, including in the ICU, is placed on physical and nutritional optimization before and after heart transplant.
- Recipient may receive organ from DBD (donor after brain death) or DCD (donor after circulatory death). DCD organs are more susceptible to RV dysfunction in the immediate posttransplant period, especially if pulmonary pressures are on the higher end of acceptable, if donor is very young, or prolonged organ transit time in OCS (organ care system). RV dysfunction post-heart transplant can be isolated with normal graft LV function. In these cases, SV may be fixed due to ongoing myocardial edema and/or perfusion injury. Exposures to negative inotropes such as amiodarone or sotalol pretransplant may also increase the risk of primary graft dysfunction (PGD).
- Post-heart transplant management is focused on:
  - Preload optimization to optimize RV function
  - RV afterload reduction (inhaled nitric oxide, milrinone)
  - Atrial pacing 100 to 110 bpm to maintain CO is the setting of transiently impaired SV
  - Inotropic support (epinephrine, milrinone, dobutamine); dual inotropes used immediately posttransplant and weaned within 72 hours to 5 days posttransplant
  - Early detection of severe RV dysfunction and PGD may require evaluation for early mechanical support if needed.
  - Early endotracheal extubation is prioritized.
  - Early initiation of posttransplant immunosuppression and opportunistic infection prophylaxis
- Immunosuppression:
  - Induction often with antithymocyte antibodies if recipient is highly sensitized pretransplant
  - Maintenance with high-dose corticosteroids (tapered over time), calcineurin inhibitor (tacrolimus), and an antiproliferative agent (mycophenolate mofetil). Care is given to balancing rejection, infection, malignancy, drug toxicity, and side effects over time.
  - Prophylactic agents are used to minimize the risks of cytomegalovirus (CMV), *Pneumocystis jirovecii* pneumonia (PJP), herpes simplex virus (HSV), and *Candida* infections over the first 3 to 12 months after transplant.
  - If hepatitis C virus (HCV)-positive organ is utilized, anti-HCV therapy will be required.
  - Coronary artery vasculopathy is addressed with aspirin, statin, and risk factor control.
  - Additional prophylaxis measures are taken to maintain bone health and minimize gastric ulcers, given exposure to high-dose corticosteroids.
- Patients deemed less than ideal candidates for HRT may be considered for palliative inotropes. These patients are followed longitudinally by the HF team.
- Average life expectancy after LVAD ~5 years, after transplant ~10 to 15 years

Outcomes

- Mortality following hospitalization with HF is 10% at 30 days, 42% at 5 years.
- Mortality >50% for NYHA class IV, ACC/AHA stage D HF.
- Inpatient mortality is 20% to 40% if HF with acute MI, 80% if also hypotensive.
- Hyponatremia is an independent predictor of poor outcomes.

Management of Chronic Heart Failure

- Cornerstone of chronic HFrEF management is initiation and titration of guideline-directed medical therapy (GDMT):
  - Beta-blocker
  - Renin-angiotensin-aldosterone system inhibitor (RAASi) ± neprilysin inhibitor
  - Mineralocorticoid receptor antagonist (MRA)
  - Sodium-glucose cotransporter-2 inhibitor (SGLT2i)
- These represent the "four pillars" of contemporary chronic HFrEF treatment and, when used together, confer synergistic benefit toward positive remodeling of the heart, reduced frequent hospitalization, and improved mortality.
- Peripartum CM, typically occurring during the last month of pregnancy or within 5 months of delivery (in the absence of other causes), is treated similarly. Risk of LV thrombus is elevated due to systolic dysfunction and hypercoagulable state, so TTE is necessary to screen for thrombus formation. When still pregnant, RAASi and MRA should be avoided. Multidisciplinary management is required with HF, maternal-fetal-medicine, and cardio-obstetrics teams.
- Iron panels: patients should be screened for iron deficiency, and IV iron (eg, iron sucrose or ferric carboxymaltose) should be given if necessary (ferritin <100 or ferritin 100-299 if transferrin saturation <20%). Oral iron supplementation is not effective.

SUGGESTED READINGS

Bozkurt B, Ahmad T, Alexander K, et al. HF STATS 2024: heart failure epidemiology and outcomes statistics an updated 2024 report from The Heart Failure Society of America. *J Card Fail*. 2025;31(1):66-116.

Bozkurt B, Coats AJ, Tsutsui H, et al. Universal definition and classification of heart failure: a report of the Heart Failure Society of America, Heart Failure Association of the European Society of Cardiology, Japanese Heart Failure Society and Writing Committee of the Universal Definition of Heart Failure. *J Card Fail*. 2021;27(4):387-413.

Crespo-Leiro MG, Costanzo MR, Gustafsson F, et al. Heart transplantation: focus on donor recovery strategies, left ventricular assist devices, and novel therapies. *Eur Heart J*. 2022;43(23):2237-2246.

Guglin M, Zucker MJ, Borlaug BA, et al. Evaluation for heart transplantation and LVAD implantation. *J Am Coll Cardiol*. 2020;75(12):1471-1487.

Lam CSP, Docherty KF, Ho JE, McMurray JJV, Myhre PL, Omland T. Recent successes in heart failure treatment. *Nat Med*. 2023;29(10):2424-2437.

Lindenfeld J, Miller GG, Shakar SF, et al. Drug therapy in the heart transplant recipient. *Circulation*. 2004;110(24):3734-3740.

Maddox TM, Januzzi JL, Allen LA, et al. 2024 ACC expert consensus decision pathway for treatment of heart failure with reduced ejection fraction. *J Am Coll Cardiol*. 2024;83(15):1444-1488.

Maitra NS, Dugger SJ, Balachandran IC, Civitello AB, Khazanie P, Rogers JG. Impact of the 2018 UNOS heart transplant policy changes on patient outcomes. *JACC Heart Fail*. 2023;11(5):491-503.

Miller L, Birks E, Guglin M, Lamba H, Frazier OH. Use of ventricular assist devices and heart transplantation for advanced heart failure. *Circ Res*. 2019;124(11):1658-1678.

Murphy SP, Ibrahim NE, Januzzi JL Jr. Heart failure with reduced ejection fraction: a review. *JAMA*. 2020;324(5):488-504.

Ommen SR, Ho CY, Asif IM, et al. 2024 AHA/ACC/AMSSM/HRS/PACES/SCMR guideline for the management of hypertrophic cardiomyopathy: a report of the American Heart Association/American College of Cardiology Joint Committee on Clinical Practice Guidelines. *Circulation*. 2024;149(23):e1239-e1311.

Sharma A, Verma S, Bhatt DL, et al. Optimizing foundational therapies in patients with HFrEF: how do we translate these findings into clinical care? *JACC Basic Transl Sci*. 2022;7(5):504-517.

Simonenko M, Hansen D, Niebauer J, et al. Prevention and rehabilitation after heart transplantation: a clinical consensus statement of the European Association of Preventive Cardiology, Heart Failure Association of the ESC, and the European Cardio Thoracic Transplant Association, a section of ESOT. *Eur J Prev Cardiol*. 2024;31(11):1385-1399.

Velleca A, Shullo MA, Dhital K, et al. The International Society for Heart and Lung Transplantation (ISHLT) guidelines for the care of heart transplant recipients. *J Heart Lung Transplant*. 2023;42(5):e1-e141.

2.3

Rhythm Disturbances

Worawan B. Limpitikul, Pattara Rattanawong, and William J. Hucker

Key Points

- The first decision point is patient's hemodynamic stability. For unstable patients, follow Advanced Cardiovascular Life Support (ACLS) algorithms. For stable patients, treat underlying causes.
- Identify the rhythms and treat accordingly.

Definitions

- Cardiac arrhythmias are relatively common in the intensive care unit (ICU).
- Proper and timely care depends on the rapid identification of life-threatening rhythms.

Epidemiology

- Cardiac dysrhythmias are common in the ICU, with an incidence of between 12% and 31%.
- Atrial fibrillation in postcardiac surgery patients has the highest incidence.
- Acute left ventricular dysfunction, a major contributor to cardiac dysrhythmias, occurs in approximately one-third of critically ill patients.
- New-onset cardiac arrhythmias are associated with poorer outcomes in critically ill patients.

Key Pathophysiology

- Cardiac rhythm and function are affected by several factors, both structural (intrinsic) and exogenous in origin.
- Ischemia, electrolyte imbalances, volume status (particularly hypervolemia), shock of any kind (cardiogenic, obstructive [including tamponade, tension pneumothorax], distributive [sepsis], hypovolemic), and pain/anxiety are among the precipitating factors in new-onset cardiac dysrhythmias.
- Preexisting risk factors include scarred myocardium (previous myocardial infarction [MI]), cardiomyopathies, and valvular disturbances (eg, mitral regurgitation), hypertension (HTN), diabetes mellitus (DM), thyroid disease, and smoking or drug history.

Common Approaches to Dysrhythmia

- Immediate goal: determine hemodynamic stability.
  - If unstable/life-threatening, follow ACLS guidelines for resuscitation.
- Is the rhythm a *perfusing* one?
  - Hint: look at arterial line tracing (or SpO_2 tracing if no arterial line) in concert with electrocardiogram (ECG) rhythm on monitor.
  - If nonperfusing, cardiovert/shock based on ACLS guidelines.
- If a perfusing rhythm, obtain 12-lead ECG and/or rhythm strip for closer inspection, treating cardiovascular instability as necessary.
- Identify and treat underlying causes.
  - Obtain full chemistry panel (especially look at Mg^{2+}, K^+, and ionized Ca^{2+}) and complete blood count (CBC) to check for anemia and correct as necessary.
  - Assess fluid status (central venous pressure [CVP] or noninvasive monitor). Diurese or replete as necessary.
  - Address oxygenation, pain, and other issues as needed.

Bradycardia

- Definition: heart rate (HR) <50 bpm
- Common causes:
  - Medications: calcium channel and beta-blockers (causing sinus node and atrioventricular [AV] nodal inhibition), cholinergic agents, sedating medications (dexmedetomidine)
  - Metabolic: hyperkalemia, hypermagnesemia, hypocalcemia, hypothyroid
  - Ischemic heart disease: inferior MI
  - Increased vagal tone: sleep
  - Hypothermia: temperature management postcardiac arrest
  - Others: myocarditis, aortic valve endocarditis, infiltrative diseases, congenital heart disease, postcardiac surgery/post-transcatheter aortic valve replacement (TAVR)
- Management:
  - First, assess patient's hemodynamic stability and for evidence of inadequate end-organ perfusion.
  - If unstable bradycardia,
    - give intravenous (IV) atropine 1 mg every 3 to 5 minutes, up to 3 mg total.
      - be cautious with atropine use in Mobitz II and third-degree heart block (atropine will increase the sinoatrial node rate; but the AV block degree may worsen if the AV node is "stressed" by higher HR input).
    - then, start dopamine gtt 5 to 20 μg/kg/min, isoproterenol gtt 1 to 20 μg/min, or epinephrine gtt 2 to 10 μg/min (can choose in part based on blood pressure, as dopamine and epinephrine are vasoconstrictors while isoproterenol is a vasodilator).
  - Identify and treat reversible causes. Stop offending medications.
  - Identify the level of lesion (sinoatrial [SA] nodal dysfunction, AV nodal block, infranodal block) and the origin of the escape rhythms (in part based on QRS width). A wide escape rhythm from outside the conduction system should not be considered stable.
    - Sinus node dysfunction may respond to pharmacotherapy. Long pauses refractory to medical management may sometimes require temporary pacing.
    - AV nodal block: first-degree, second-degree type I (Wenckebach) can be monitored if the patient is hemodynamically stable, and these will likely respond to pharmacotherapy.
    - Infranodal block: likely will not respond to pharmacotherapy. Mobitz II can be monitored if hemodynamically stable. Third-degree block requires immediate intervention.
  - Consider transcutaneous/transvenous temporary pacing if unable to treat underlying causes. Transcutaneous pacing can be used in an emergency, but will cause pain to an awake patient from electrical discharges.

Tachycardia

- Definition: HR ≥150 bpm
- DDx: see Figure 2.3.1
- Management:
  - First, assess patients' hemodynamic stability and identify rhythm. If unstable, follow ACLS.
  - In stable patients, identify rhythm (Figure 2.3.1) and treat accordingly.
  - Sinus tachycardia usually represents a body's compensatory effort to underlying pathologies. Identify and treat these underlying reversible causes rather than treating the HR. In some cases, however, a primary treatment goal will be reduction of the HR (eg, acute MI, to reduce myocardial oxygen demand; or aortic dissection, to reduce shear stress on the aorta).
  - Supraventricular tachycardia (SVT): vagal maneuvers, give adenosine 6 mg peripheral IV push followed by 12 mg peripheral IV push as needed (if using central line access, halve these doses); ensure patient is on telemetry monitor and pacing is available. For SVT, can also trial beta-blockers/calcium channel blockers.
  - New-onset atrial fibrillation or atrial flutter:
    - Calcium channel blockers/beta-blockers for rate control in the setting of preserved ventricular function

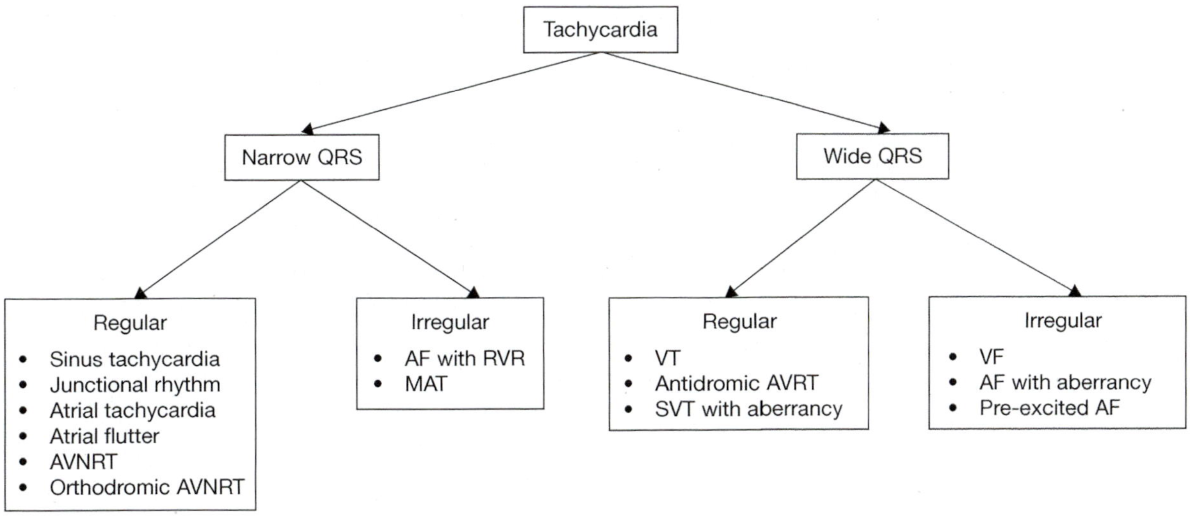

FIGURE 2.3.1 **Differential diagnosis for tachycardia.** AF, atrial fibrillation; AVNRT, atrioventricular nodal reentrant tachycardia; AVRT, atrioventricular reentrant tachycardia; MAT, multifocal atrial tachycardia; SVT, supraventricular tachycardia; VF, ventricular fibrillation; VT, ventricular tachycardia.

    - Amiodarone (rate and rhythm control) or digoxin (rate control) in the setting of poor ventricular function
    - Note that digoxin does not reliably terminate atrial fibrillation and its time of onset may be rather slow, especially in emergent situations.
  - Wolff-Parkinson-White (WPW) with atrial fibrillation/SVT:
    - Direct cardioversion is recommended for all hemodynamically unstable patients. In WPW, the very fast atrial rate can be conducted directly to the ventricle via a bypass tract, which is why this is a medical emergency.
    - Nodal blockades (IV beta-blockers, digitalis, adenosine, lidocaine, and nondihydropyridine calcium channel antagonists) are contraindicated with atrial fibrillation in WPW.
    - In the absence of experience with procainamide or ibutilide (for wide-complex atrial fibrillation) or flecainide for rapid ventricular response (RVR), amiodarone can be useful.
  - Monomorphic ventricular tachycardia (VT)
    - Consider myocardial scar. Follow ACLS.
  - Polymorphic VT
    - Generally a reflection of myocardial ischemia. Follow ACLS and evaluate for coronary ischemia and reperfusion.
  - Torsade de Pointes (TdP), a form of polymorphic VT with "twisting" of the QRS axis
    - This rhythm occurs in the setting of prolonged QTc in baseline ECG, with rhythm triggered by early afterdepolarizations occurring during the prolonged repolarization.
    - TdP is called "pause dependent," often occurring following long-short R-R intervals.
    - Give magnesium: slow 2 g IV push.
    - Consider isoproterenol or temporary pacing to increase HR and shorten QTc.

Electrical Storm

- Definition: ≥3 episodes of VT/VF (ventricular fibrillation) in 24 hours
- Common causes:
  - Myocardial scar: ischemic, intrinsic cardiomyopathy
  - Acute myocardial ischemia
  - Electrolyte disturbances
  - QTc prolonging medications
- Management:
  - See Figure 2.3.2
  - IV antiarrhythmics: see Table 2.3.1 for commonly used IV antiarrhythmics
  - For recalcitrant VT/VF,
    - Consider sedation (reduce sympathetic tone) and intubation.
    - Seek expert consultation for further management.
      - Stellate ganglion block
      - VT/VF ablation
      - Mechanical circulatory support

Outcomes

- Patients with new-onset dysrhythmias have poorer outcomes.
- Atrial fibrillation is associated with a 2-fold increase in in-hospital mortality.
- However, almost 90% of patients with postoperative atrial fibrillation return to sinus rhythm by 2 months after surgery.

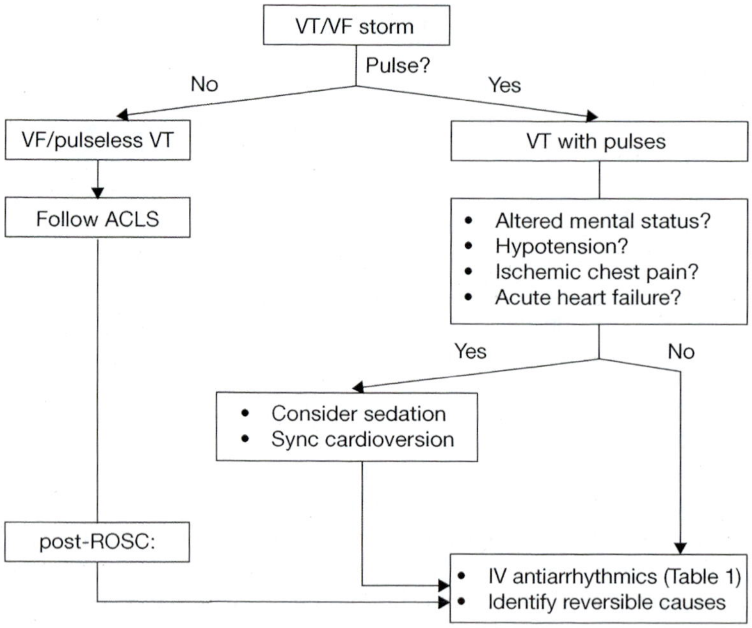

FIGURE 2.3.2 **Management of electrical storm.** ACLS, Advanced Cardiovascular Life Support; mono VT, monomorphic ventricular tachycardia; poly VT, polymorphic ventricular tachycardia; ROSC, return of spontaneous circulation; VF, ventricular fibrillation; VT, ventricular tachycardia.

TABLE 2.3.1 Commonly Used IV Antiarrhythmics

Antiarrhythmics	Dose	Monitoring	Adverse Effects
Metoprolol	IV 5 mg q5 min up to 3 doses		Bradycardia, hypotension, AVB
Esmolol	IV bolus 0.5 mg/kg → then gtt at 0.05 mg/kg/min		Bradycardia, hypotension, AVB
Amiodarone	IV bolus 150 mg → then gtt at 1 mg/min × 6 h → then 0.5 mg/min × 18 h	↑ QTc ↑ DFT	Acute: hypotension, TdP, AVB Chronic: pulmonary fibrosis, pneumonitis, thyroid abnormalities
Lidocaine (ischemic VT/VF)	IV bolus 1 mg/kg (can repeat with 0.5-0.75 mg/kg every 5-10 min, up to max of 3 mg/kg) → then gtt at 1-4 mg/min	↓ QTc Check lidocaine level (reaches steady state in 18-24 h)	Tinnitus, visual changes, seizure, tremor, delirium, psychosis, bradycardia, nausea/vomiting
Procainamide	IV bolus 10 mg/kg over 20 min → gtt at 1-4 mg/min for up to 12-24 h	↑ QTc ↑ DFT Check procainamide and NAPA levels (reaches steady state depending on renal and hepatic function)	TdP, AVB, HF exacerbation Lupus-like syndrome

AVB, atrioventricular block; DFT, defibrillation threshold; HF, heart failure; IV, intravenous; NAPA, *N*-acetyl procainamide; q, every; TdP, torsades de pointes; VF, ventricular fibrillation; VT, ventricular tachycardia.

SUGGESTED READINGS

Annane D, Sébille V, Duboc D, et al. Incidence and prognosis of sustained arrhythmias in critically ill patients. *Am J Respir Crit Care Med*. 2008;178(1):20-25.

Crawford TC, Oral H. Cardiac arrhythmias: management of atrial fibrillation in the critically ill patient. *Crit Care Clin*. 2007;23(4):855-872.

Falk RH, Knowlton AA, Bernard SA, et al. Digoxin for converting recent-onset atrial fibrillation to sinus rhythm: a randomized, double-blinded trial. *Ann Intern Med*. 1987;106:503-506.

Joglar JA, Chung MK, Armbruster AL, et al. 2023 ACC/AHA/ACCP/HRS guideline for the diagnosis and management of atrial fibrillation: a report of the American College of Cardiology/American Heart Association Joint Committee on Clinical Practice Guidelines. *Circulation*. 2024;149(1):e1-e156.

Kowlgi G, Cha Y. Management of ventricular electrical storm: a contemporary appraisal. *Europace*. 2020;22:1768-1780.

Reinelt P, Karth GD, Geppert A, Heinz G. Incidence and type of cardiac arrhythmias in critically ill patients: a single center experience in a medical-cardiological ICU. *Intensive Care Med*. 2001;27(9):1466-1473.

Roy D, Talajic M, Nattel S, et al. Atrial fibrillation and congestive heart failure investigators. rhythm control versus rate control for atrial fibrillation and heart failure. *N Engl J Med*. 2008;358(25):2667-2677.

Tsadok MA, Jackevicius CA, Essebag V, et al. Rhythm versus rate control therapy and subsequent stroke or transient ischemic attack in patients with atrial fibrillation. *Circulation*. 2012;126(23):2680-2687.

2.4

Valvular Disorders

David I. Feldman, Olivia L. Hulme, and Evin Yucel

Definition

- Valvular heart disease (VHD) includes a myriad of diseases with different pathophysiology, valve hemodynamics, clinical presentation, impact on cardiac structure and function, and clinical outcomes.
- Types of VHD include aortic stenosis (AS), aortic regurgitation (AR), mitral stenosis (MS), mitral regurgitation (MR), tricuspid stenosis (TS), tricuspid regurgitation (TR), pulmonic stenosis (PS), and pulmonic regurgitation (PR).
- Echocardiography is the first-line noninvasive diagnostic test for evaluating VHD.
- Depending on the severity of VHD, intervention with valve repair or replacement may be needed, with pharmacologic or mechanical circulatory support as a bridge to definitive treatment, all of which should involve a multidisciplinary heart team discussion.

Aortic Stenosis

Etiologies

- Calcific degeneration is the most common cause of AS (in Western nations). Other causes include congenital bicuspid or unicuspid aortic valve (AV), rheumatic heart disease, and radiation.

Epidemiology

- Prevalence increases with age, 1% to 2% and 12% of people >65 and >75 years of age have calcific AS, respectively.
- Congenital bicuspid valve is found in ~1% to 2% live births, with 3:1 male predominance.
- Rheumatic AS, characterized by nodular thickening of the valve leaflets, is invariably associated with concurrent rheumatic changes of the mitral valve (MV).

Pathophysiology

- Regardless of the initial cause, the progressive pathophysiology of AS is similar.
- Gradual worsening of obstruction leads to compensatory left ventricular hypertrophy (LVH) that reduces ventricular wall stress and preserves ejection fraction (EF).
- The changes in the structure and function of the LV result in myocardial fibrosis, myocardial ischemia, LV diastolic dysfunction, and eventually LV systolic dysfunction.
- Additionally, the resultant LV hypertrophy and pressure overload from AS results in increased pressure transmitted to the left atrium (LA), causing pulmonary congestion, as well as the pulmonary vasculature causing pulmonary hypertension.
- Decompensation occurs under several possible conditions.
    - Depressed LV contractility occurs, independent of AS sequelae.
    - Rising LV afterload that outpaces compensatory LVH leads to a critical decrease in EF, and exertional syncope ensues.
    - Atrial fibrillation (AF) prevents adequate LV preload.
    - An increased oxygen demand (eg, exercise, tachyarrhythmia) leads to subendocardial ischemia because hypertrophied heart muscle requires more oxygen than its vasculature can support under stress, and angina ensues.
    - Reduced systemic vascular resistance (eg, systemic inflammatory response syndrome, heavy analgesia, or sedation) leads to hypotension as the stroke volume (SV) cannot be raised by the LV against a fixed stenotic AV.

Symptoms, Physical Examination, and Differential Diagnosis

- Symptoms: dyspnea, angina, syncope/presyncope, heart failure symptoms (orthopnea, paroxysmal nocturnal dyspnea [PND], edema)
- Physical examination findings: low amplitude and slow rise of arterial pulse (pulsus parvus et tardus), reduced pulse pressure, crescendo-decrescendo systolic murmur (severe when S2 is absent)
- Diagnostic testing:
    - electrocardiogram (ECG)—LVH;
    - chest x-ray (CXR)—AV calcification;
    - cardiac computed tomography (CT)—AV calcium score >1,200 Agatston Units (AU) and >2,000 AU for females and males, respectively;
    - TTE—severe high-gradient AS: mean gradient >40 mm Hg, peak velocity >4 m/s, and AV area (AVA) <1 cm^2.
- Severe low-flow, low-gradient AS: AVA ≤ 1 cm^2 with resting aortic V_{max} <4 m/s or mean gradient <40 mm Hg due to low left ventricular ejection fraction (LVEF) (low flow: indicated by stroke volume index [SVi] on echocardiogram <35 mL/m^2); consider dobutamine stress echocardiogram to see if increased cardiac output (CO) generates mean gradient or peak velocity consistent with severe AS. Severe paradoxical low-flow, low gradient AS: AVA ≤1 cm^2 with resting aortic V_{max} <4 m/s or mean gradient <40 mm Hg and SVi <35 mL/m^2 despite normal LVEF (EF ≥50%). Aortic sclerosis: focal thickening and calcification of AV leaflets, no AV obstruction to flow, ejection murmur that mimics that of AS, differentiated on echo by jet velocity <2.5 m/s in aortic sclerosis and higher in AS.
- AS must also be differentiated from supravalvular stenosis, subvalvular stenosis, and hypertrophic obstructive cardiomyopathy (HOCM).

Management and Treatment

- There is no medical management for progressive AS.
- Statins have not been shown to slow the rate of AS progression. Sodium-glucose cotransporter-2 (SGLT2) inhibitors are being investigated to slow the rate of AS progression.
- For patients with rheumatic AS, antibiotics are indicated for the prevention of recurrent rheumatic fever until the age of 40 years.
- Treatment of acutely decompensated AS (LV dysfunction, shock): invasive hemodynamic monitoring with pulmonary artery catheter (PAC), prompt inotropic support, and, rarely, percutaneous aortic balloon valvuloplasty (PABV) as

a bridge to valve replacement (c.f. transcatheter aortic valve replacement [TAVR]) in patients with cardiogenic shock.

- Hemodynamic goals during acute management: preload augmentation, heart rate (HR) <90, maintain sinus rhythm, maintain contractility (avoid beta-blockade), maintain or augment systemic vascular resistance (vasopressors norepinephrine, phenylephrine)
- Aortic valve replacement (AVR) indications: symptomatic severe AS, asymptomatic severe AS with LVEF <50%, moderate AS in patients undergoing coronary artery bypass grafting or aortic aneurysm repair
- Post-AVR care: expect SV to increase and LV end-diastolic pressure (LVEDP) to decrease, LVH persists for an extended period and may require preload augmentation, especially in the cases of "suicide LV," which is characterized by a dynamic intraventricular gradient after the abrupt decrease in systemic afterload in the setting of a hypercontractile LV, leading to circulatory collapse. Treatment depends on increasing preload and afterload (ideally pure vasoconstrictors without inotropic effect to avoid worsening the outflow gradient).

Outcomes

- Once moderate stenosis has developed, further progression is almost certain.
- Without intervention, survival is 2 to 3 years after the onset of symptoms.
- PABV has no long-term benefit in acutely decompensated AS and is primarily reserved as a short-term bridge to definitive valve replacement.
- TAVR versus surgical AVR should be decided in the context of a heart team discussion, which is based on a combination of individual risk (ie, comorbidities, frailty, age etc), technical factors, and patient preference.
- AVR improves symptoms and survival.
- TAVR perioperative mortality is <1%, rates of permanent pacemaker are up to 7% post-TAVR and higher in individuals with baseline conduction abnormalities (bundle branch blocks: 30%-50%).
- Surgical AVR perioperative mortality is estimated using the Society of Thoracic Surgeons (STS) risk scoring; risk is higher when combined with bypass grafting.

Aortic Regurgitation

Common Causes to Remember

- Causes of acute AR: infective endocarditis (IE), aortic dissection, blunt chest trauma, acute-on-chronic decompensation of AR
- Many causes of chronic AR: bicuspid valve, calcific degeneration, rheumatic heart disease, aortic aneurysm, degenerative aortic dilation
- Etiology of AR can be characterized by leaflet abnormalities, aortic root abnormalities, or combined valve and aortic root abnormalities.

Epidemiology

- AR occurs in young (20-40 years of age) and older adults (>60 years of age) in the setting of bicuspid AV and calcific AV disease, respectively.
- Aortic root disease is the most common cause of isolated AR, accounting for >50% of patients with isolated AR who undergo AVR.

Key Pathophysiology

Acute Aortic Regurgitation

- Sudden regurgitant retrograde flow through the aortic orifice causes an abrupt rise in LV diastolic pressure, and subsequent elevation of LA pressure (LAP) and pulmonary vascular pressure, resulting in pulmonary edema and dyspnea. Acute AR is often associated with tachycardia.
- Forward SV drops as the LV cannot undergo immediate compensatory dilation to maintain SV, resulting in hypotension and, in some cases, cardiogenic shock.

Chronic Aortic Regurgitation

- Regurgitant flow through the aortic orifice over a prolonged period leads to LV compensatory dilation and eccentric hypertrophy to maintain LV systolic function. The large regurgitant volume increases SV, resulting in elevated systolic blood pressure (SBP) while lowering diastolic blood pressure (DBP).
- Reduced DBP lowers coronary perfusion pressure, LV dilation increases wall tension, and oxygen demand can outstrip supply.
- Over time, the LV remodels, preload reserve is exhausted, systolic performance declines, pulmonary vascular pressures rise, and congestive heart failure (HF) symptoms appear.

Symptoms, Physical Examination, and Findings

- Acute severe AR: sudden onset, weakness, dyspnea, presyncope, hypotension, tachycardia, bounding pulse, early and short diastolic murmur, possible pulmonary edema on CXR
  - Use multiple echo parameters to evaluate the regurgitant AV jet and severity.
- Chronic AR: symptoms may be absent/mild/severe, elevated SBP and low DBP, bounding pulse (several eponymous signs), long diastolic murmur, LVH on ECG, cardiomegaly, and, possibly, pulmonary edema on CXR.
- Nocturnal angina can occur late in the course, result of decreased HR, and subsequent decline in arterial diastolic pressure.

Management and Treatment

Acute Hemodynamic Management of Mild/Moderate Aortic Regurgitation

- Increase LV preload, increase HR, maintain contractility, decrease systemic vascular resistance (SVR), and maintain pulmonary vascular resistance (PVR).

Acute Severe Aortic Regurgitation

- Surgical intervention (AVR) takes precedence over medical management in acute severe AR.
- Consideration can also be given to valve-in-valve TAVR for acute prosthetic valve AR when surgical risk is prohibitive.

- HF and cardiogenic shock therapies: vasodilation and diuresis as tolerated, inotropes as needed; note intra-aortic balloon pump (IABP) contraindicated as it will worsen AR
- Antibiotics for IE, and assess the need for definitive surgery.
- Type A acute aortic dissection: beta-blockade for impulse control with caution (compensatory tachycardia should not be prevented), emergency repair surgery
- Post-AVR care: LVEDP decreases while LVH and LV dilation persist, may require augmentation of LV preload; if LV function declines, inotropes or IABP may be necessary.

Outcomes

- Acute severe AR leads to death without rapid intervention.
- AVR perioperative mortality is 3% to 4%, higher when combined with bypass grafting.
- TAVR has not yet been approved as a treatment for either acute or chronic AR; JenaValve is being studied as a transcatheter option for the treatment of severe AR.

Mitral Stenosis

Common Causes to Remember

- Rheumatic heart disease is the most common cause.
- Other nonrheumatic causes are degenerative due to annular calcification, leaflet calcification, radiation, congenital disease, autoimmune (systemic lupus erythematosus and rheumatoid arthritis), postintervention (secondary to surgical or transcatheter MV interventions).

Epidemiology

- 40% of patients with rheumatic heart disease have isolated MS. The male-to-female ratio of rheumatic MS is 1:2.
- Degenerative MS is most common in the Western world and is primarily related to mitral annular calcification (MAC) (1%-2% of patients with MAC).

Key Pathophysiology

- Severe MS may take 20 to 40 years to develop following acute rheumatic fever in rheumatic MS; degenerative MS due to MAC usually develops later in life.
- Significant hemodynamic changes and symptoms occur when the MV area decreases to <1.5 cm^2 and the gradient exceeds 10 mm Hg.
- Incomplete LA emptying leads to increased LAP and reactive pulmonary hypertension; HF symptoms can follow if reactive pulmonary hypertension fails to adequately compensate for elevated LAP. LAP is variable, though, and depends on HR (tachycardia reduces filling time) and CO (gradient across the MV increases as a square of flow [CO]).
- AF can result from chronic enlargement of LA from sustained elevated LAP.
- Low flow in the LA predisposes to thrombus formation, while turbulent flow across the MV increases the risk for IE.
- Right ventricular (RV) dysfunction occurs later in the disease course because of pulmonary arterial hypertrophy (PAH). LV function is usually spared unless affected by similar mechanisms, resulting in MS (ie, degenerative MS due to existing comorbidities).

Symptoms, Physical Examination, and Differential Diagnosis

- Mild-to-moderate MS is typically asymptomatic at rest (MV area >1.5 cm^2 with gradient <10 mm Hg; normal MV area >4 cm^2).
- Severe MS: AF commonly leads to acute decompensation; presents with dyspnea, orthopnea, PND, fatigue; examination shows signs of HF, loud S1 and opening snap in rheumatic MS, low-pitch diastolic "rumbling" murmur is a classic finding but may be absent in AF or low-output states, presystolic accentuation due to atrial contraction (absent in AF); LA enlargement ± right ventricular hypertrophy (RVH) on ECG and CXR, pulmonary edema on CXR in advanced disease; on echo valve area <1 cm^2 is critical. Transthoracic echocardiogram is first-line testing for diagnosis and is also used for percutaneous balloon mitral valvuloplasty (PBMV); transesophageal echocardiogram is needed to exonerate LA appendage prior to the procedure.
- Asymptomatic MS usually progresses to symptomatic MS in 10 years, with most being symptomatic within 20 years of the development of MS.
- Known MS without typical pulmonary congestion symptoms should raise concern for concomitant TS.

Management and Treatment

- Acute management: address precipitating factor(s), increase LV preload, decrease HR, maintain contractility, maintain SVR, decrease PVR
- Anticoagulation for MS with AF, or MS with prior embolic event
- Surgical treatment
  - PBMV—for severe MS with certain valve anatomy and absence of both LA thrombus and > moderate MR
  - MV commissurotomy—for severe, symptomatic MS when valve anatomy not acceptable for PBMV
  - MV replacement (MVR)—for moderate-to-severe MS with abnormal valve anatomy
  - Intervention of coexisting valvular or coronary disease should be considered at time of MV operation.
  - Transcatheter options include valve-in-MAC, or valve in ring or valve in valve for those with prior surgical interventions leading to MS; valve anatomy and neo-left ventricular outflow tract size must be considered to determine eligibility of transcatheter options.
- Management after surgical intervention: The chronically deprived LV may fail in the setting of acute increase in volume across the now open MV, inotropic support may be necessary, maintaining preload and reducing SVR may also be beneficial.

Outcomes

- Asymptomatic patients with MS have >80% 10-year survival.
- Symptomatic severe MS results in a mortality rate of 8% to 13% per year in the first 5 years without intervention.
- Natural history of untreated MS is death by heart failure, systemic or pulmonary embolism, or infection.
- Outcomes for surgical intervention are dependent on institutional experience, patient comorbidities, and valve morphology.
- Perioperative mortality for MVR and MV repair is estimated using STS risk scoring; mortality increases for both when combined with bypass grafting.

Mitral Regurgitation

Common Causes to Remember

- Acute MR can result from a rapid precipitating factor affecting an otherwise normal valve.
- Etiologies of acute MR can be divided into primary or secondary. Most common cause of primary MR is myxomatous degeneration of the MV leaflets leading to MV prolapse. Other less common causes include leaflet perforation, cleft leaflets, radiation, and rheumatic and connective tissue disease. Most common causes of secondary MR include annular dilation and leaflet tethering from a ventricular disease.
- Most common causes of acute MR include MV flail, acute myocardial infarction leading to papillary muscle rupture or dysfunction, rheumatic heart disease, IE, and trauma.

Epidemiology

- Exact incidence and prevalence are unknown; however, MR is among the most common VHD in the United States.

Key Pathophysiology

Acute Mitral Regurgitation

- Sudden regurgitation of LV SV into the LA decreases forward CO, raises LA volume, and increases the LV end-diastolic volume (LVEDV) as regurgitant and normal pulmonic blood both enter the LV during diastole.
- Decreased forward CO leads to systemic hypotension.
- The LA in acute MR cannot adapt its compliance to sudden increased volume, leading to increased LAP, pulmonary congestion, and subsequent dyspnea and pulmonary edema.
- Initially, the LV systolic function will increase in the setting of acute MR. Eventually, increased LVEDV may stretch the myocardium beyond optimal place on the Starling curve, reducing contractility and further impairing forward CO.

Chronic Mitral Regurgitation

- Gradually worsening regurgitation causes chronic stretching and compensatory increased compliance of the LA, which abrogates pulmonary congestion.
- As the LA dilates with time, the LAP drops and an increasing portion of the LV SV becomes regurgitant, leading to diminishing forward CO and ultimately symptoms of low CO.
- Chronically increased LVEDV leads to LV dilation and eventual poor contractility, contributing to low CO.
- Chronically dilated LA predisposes to AF.

Symptoms, Physical Examination, and Differential Diagnosis

- Acute severe MR: dyspnea, cough, chest pain, ± hypotension, tachycardia, tachypnea, rales, variable holosystolic murmur (acute MR—lower pitch and softer than chronic MR murmur; sometimes a murmur is not heart in acute severe MR due to rapid equilibration between LA and LV), S4 common, early closure of P2, paradoxical splitting of S2 when PAH present, possible AF or atrial flutter, pulmonary edema on CXR; echo can identify specific mechanistic abnormality, regurgitant jet, and severity (qualitative vs quantitative). Acute severe MR, especially following papillary muscle rupture, can be difficult to identify on physical examination and transthoracic echocardiogram due to rapid and very short jet of MR.
- Decompensated chronic MR: symptoms of HF, early soft systolic murmur, cardiomegaly on ECG and CXR, pulmonary edema on CXR; echocardiogram can show LA and LV dilation, identify specific mechanistic abnormality, regurgitant jet, and severity (qualitative vs quantitative).
- Consider unilateral pulmonary edema as caused by acute flail or papillary muscle rupture.

Management and Treatment

Mild/Moderate Mitral Regurgitation

- Preload based on clinical response, maintain or increase HR, maintain contractility, decrease SVR, decrease PVR; guideline-directed medical therapy when MR is functional (goal-directed medical therapy for heart failure with reduced ejection fraction [HFrEF]).

Acute Severe Mitral Regurgitation

- Medical management of HF and cardiogenic shock: vasodilation and diuresis as tolerated, inotropes, IABP as needed; antibiotics for IE
- It is possible to medically stabilize a patient with acute severe MR prior to operative intervention (unlike acute severe AR); however, mechanical circulatory support may be needed (IABP, percutaneous left ventricular assist device [LVAD], and/or venoarterial extracorporeal membrane oxygenation [VA ECMO]).
- MV repair preferred if technically feasible
- MVR if native tissue is inadequate for repair (bioprosthetic vs mechanical)
- Management after surgical intervention: Inotropic support or IABP may be needed as LV contracts against a new elevated afterload, and the LV has less preload than before. AF must be aggressively treated.
- Transcatheter options for the treatment of acute MR are often limited to those with surgical valve interventions where repeat surgical intervention poses prohibitive surgical risk (ie, valve-in-valve, valve-in-ring). Percutaneous treatment options, such as transcatheter edge-to-edge repair (TEER), are most often reserved for chronic MR.

Outcomes

- Without surgical intervention, prognosis for patients with MR and heart failure is poor.
- TEER is only approved for patients at high surgical risk; transcatheter mitral valve replacement (TMVR) is currently investigational and is not yet approved, with only high and prohibitively high surgical risk patients being enrolled in trials.

Pulmonic Stenosis

Common Causes to Remember

- Almost always congenital (ie, Noonan syndrome, tetralogy of Fallot, Williams syndrome), rarely carcinoid or rheumatic related

Epidemiology

- 0.5/1,000 live births worldwide
- Coexisting valvular disease common when carcinoid or rheumatic cause

Key Pathophysiology

- With progression of PS, compensatory RVH occurs, increasing the risk of RV ischemia and eventual RV failure.

Differential Diagnosis

- Mild and moderate PS are typically asymptomatic.
- Severe PS: fatigue, dyspnea, presyncope, syncope, and symptoms of RV failure (abdominal distension/bloating, edema); central venous a-wave, systolic murmur (increases with inspiration), ejection click moves closer to S1 (absent when severe), RV heave, ECG may show right atrial (RA) enlargement, RVH, RV strain; RVH, pulmonary artery dilation on CXR; echo shows thick pulmonic cusps and systolic doming, severity can be graded by peak gradient.
- Other causes of right heart failure must be considered in workup of PS.

Management and Treatment

- Acute management: increase RV preload, increase HR, maintain contractility, maintain SVR, maintain or moderately decrease PVR.
- Moderate PS progresses to the point of requiring intervention in 25% of cases.
- Percutaneous pulmonary balloon valvuloplasty (PBV) for peak gradient ≥50 mm Hg is preferred; beta-blockade should precede PBV to prevent postprocedural acute outflow tract obstruction from RVH.
- Surgical valvotomy or valve replacement is indicated following poor result with PBV, unfavorable valve morphology, severe PR, and fixed subvalvular or supravalvular PS.
- Transcatheter valve replacement is becoming increasingly more common for PS with excellent outcomes.

Outcomes

- Normal life expectancy following successful surgical relief of moderate or severe PS; repeat procedures are often required.
- Mild PS has minimal progression and excellent outcome.

Pulmonic Regurgitation

Common Causes to Remember

- Prior intervention for congenital heart disease (eg, valvotomy for PS, tetralogy of Fallot repair)
- Rheumatic heart disease, carcinoid heart disease, endocarditis, pulmonary hypertension (dilation of the valve ring or pulmonary artery)

Key Pathophysiology

- PR leads to progressive RV dilation; the dilated RV predisposes to low CO, HF, QRS prolongation, and arrhythmias.

Symptoms, Physical Examination, and Differential Diagnosis

- Mild PR is marked by a benign course.
- Severe or long-standing PR: exercise intolerance, diastolic decrescendo low-pitched murmur (increases with inspiration) ± pulmonic systolic ejection murmur, palpable RV heave, wide splitting of S2, RV S3, and/or S4, signs of HF, prolonged QRS with rSR pattern and/or RVH on ECG, RV prominence on CXR; echo shows continuous wave Doppler profile with short pressure half-time that ends prior to end of diastole, severity can be graded by assessing pressure half-time (reduced) and flow reversal in the pulmonary artery (severe when present).
- Other causes of right heart failure and diastolic murmurs must be considered in the workup of PR.

Management and Treatment

- No proven medical therapies
- Cardiac magnetic resonance imaging (MRI): used to assess right-sided size and function to plan the timing of valve replacement
- Pulmonary valve (PV) replacement indicated for severe PR with symptoms (including arrhythmias and diminished exercise tolerance), RV ejection fraction (RVEF) <40%, progressive RV dilation, moderate or worse TR, prolonged or increasing QRS, and severe PR in a patient undergoing a cardiac operation for another indication

Outcomes

- Mild PR typically a benign course
- Chronic severe PR usually well tolerated for many years
- Sudden death can occur as a result of arrhythmias in severe RV dilation.
- Improved exercise tolerance following PV replacement with good long-term outcomes if intervened upon prior to irreversible RV dysfunction

Tricuspid Stenosis

Common Causes to Remember

- Rare; nearly always rheumatic (more commonly affects left-sided valves and so expect concurrent mitral > aortic rheumatic valvulopathy)
- Less common causes: congenital (tricuspid atresia), carcinoid heart disease, endomyocardial fibrosis, vegetations; functional stenosis from RA tumor or extrinsic compression (extracardiac tumors)

Epidemiology

- Exceedingly rare in developed countries
- More common in females
- Patients with rheumatic TS almost always have coexisting MV disease.
- Clinically significant TS present in about 5% of patients with rheumatic heart disease.

Key Pathophysiology

- Following a prolonged asymptomatic period, worsening TS causes RA enlargement that predisposes to atrial arrhythmias.

- Inspiration or exercise causes an increase in the gradient across the tricuspid valve (TV).
- RA dilation also predisposes to RA thrombus formation with the risk for pulmonary embolus.

Symptoms, Physical Examination, and Differential Diagnosis

- TS: fatigue, dyspnea, ascites, peripheral edema; increased venous pressure, difficult to distinguish from MS with auscultation (opening snap, rumbling diastolic murmur [often inaudible]), presystolic hepatic pulsation may be present, clear lung fields despite distended neck veins; AF or RA enlargement on ECG, elevated central venous a-wave, increased central venous pressure; RA enlargement on CXR; echo shows commissural fusion, diastolic leaflet doming, mean gradient >10 mm Hg, pressure half-time >190 ms, enlarged RA and dilated inferior vena cava (IVC)
- TR: rheumatic tricuspid disease usually presents with TR or a combination of TR and TS.
- Symptoms of MS may be masked by TS, especially when due to rheumatic disease.

Management and Treatment

- Medical therapy is frequently ineffective: rate control for AF; sodium restriction and diuresis may optimize preoperative hepatic function.
- Acute management: increase RV preload, slow or maintain HR, maintain contractility, increase SVR, and maintain PVR.
- Tricuspid balloon valvotomy for some patients, TR is a common complication.
- TV replacement is preferred treatment; surgical versus transcatheter based on heart team discussion.
- In patients with concomitant MS, TS correction alone is contraindicated as this can lead to pulmonary congestion.
- Postoperative management: If a PAC is required, it should be placed across a prosthetic valve intraoperatively under direct vision; RV dysfunction from increased load after TV replacement can be offset by afterload reduction (ie, reduction in pulmonary artery pressure) and positive inotropy.

Tricuspid Regurgitation

Common Causes to Remember

- Most commonly due to any process causing annular (atrial functional) and/or RV failure and dilation (ie, pulmonary hypertension, chronic obstructive pulmonary disease [COPD], chronic thromboembolic pulmonary hypertension [CTEPH], atrial septal defect [ASD], anomalous pulmonary venous return)
- Congenital TV abnormalities: Ebstein anomaly, AV canal defects
- Primary TV abnormalities: prolapse
- Acquired TV abnormalities: endocarditis, trauma, rheumatic heart disease, carcinoid heart disease, myxomatous change, device related (ie, PPM, ICD), radiation or drug exposure

Key Pathophysiology

- After an extended latency, progressive RV and RA volume overload leads to right heart failure, RA dilation predisposes to atrial arrhythmias.

Symptoms, Physical Examination, and Differential Diagnosis

- Often asymptomatic until RV failure or pulmonary hypertension develop, nonspecific symptoms are present, such as fatigue, exercise intolerance, anorexia; signs of right heart failure with long-standing severe TR (ascites, edema, cardiac cirrhosis), central venous v-wave; atrial arrhythmias on ECG due to atrial dilation
- Other valvular diseases should be investigated as MS or AS can lead to TR.
- An investigation for an underlying etiology of annular dilation should be performed, for example, pulmonary hypertension, ASD, anomalous pulmonary venous return, and LV dysfunction.

Management and Treatment

- Volume overload management: diuretics, sodium restriction, fluid restriction
- TV repair or replacement for symptomatic severe TR, progressive RV enlargement, severe TR resulting from blunt chest trauma, severe TR in a patient undergoing a cardiac operation for another indication
- Acute management: reduce RV preload, increase or maintain HR, maintain contractility, maintain SVR, decrease PVR.
- In addition to surgical repair and replacement, tricuspid TEER and/or transcatheter tricuspid valve replacement (TTVR) are now options for patients requiring TV intervention with prohibitive surgical risk.
- Postoperative management: after TV repair or replacement, the increased RV pressure can lead to RV dysfunction requiring inotropic support.

Outcomes

- Right-sided chamber enlargement increases morbidity even in asymptomatic patients.
- Severe TR reduces long-term survival either alone and in combination with other valvular abnormalities.
- Symptomatic improvement and a reduction in mortality result from surgical intervention; TV repair for organic disease tends to have better outcome than TV replacement. Further studies are needed to better understand the long-term outcomes associated with transcatheter options.

SUGGESTED READINGS

Bonow RO, Carabello BA, Chatterjee K, et al. 2008 focused update incorporated into the ACC/AHA 2006 guidelines for the management of patients with valvular heart disease: a report of the American College of Cardiology/American Heart Association Task Force on Practice Guidelines (Writing Committee to develop guidelines for the management of patients with valvular heart disease). *J Am Coll Cardiol*. 2008;52:e1-e142.

Bruce CJ, Connolly HM. Right-sided valve disease deserves a little more respect. *Circulation*. 2009;119:2726.

Carabello BA. Modern management of mitral stenosis. *Circulation*. 2005;112(3):432-437.

Chan KL, Teo K, Dumesnil JG, et al. Effect of lipid lowering with rosuvastatin on progression of aortic stenosis: results of the Aortic Stenosis Progression Observation: Measuring Effects of Rosuvastatin (ASTRONOMER) trial. *Circulation*. 2010;121:306.

Chiang CW, Lo SK, Ko YS, et al. Predictors of systemic embolism in patients with mitral stenosis: a prospective study. *Ann Intern Med*. 1998;128:885-889.

Freeman RV, Otto CM. Spectrum of calcific aortic valve disease: pathogenesis, disease progression, and treatment strategies. *Circulation*. 2005; 111(24):3316-3326.

Hayes C, Gersony W, Driscoll D, et al. Second natural history study of congenital heart defects: results of treatment of patients with pulmonary valvar stenosis. *Circulation*. 1993;87(suppl):I28-I37.

Hoffman JIE, Kaplan S. The incidence of congenital heart disease. *J Am Coll Cardiol*. 2002;39(12):1890-1900.

Maron BJ. Hypertrophic cardiomyopathy. In: Bonow RO, Mann DL, Zipes DP, Libby P, eds. *Bonow: Braunwald's Heart Disease*. 9th ed. Elsevier Saunders; 2011:1582-1594.

Maron BJ, Gardin JM, Flack JM, et al. Assessment of the prevalence of hypertrophic cardiomyopathy in a general population of young adults: echocardiographic analysis of 4111 subjects in the CARDIA study. *Circulation*. 1995;92:785.

Maron BJ, McKenna WJ, Danielson GK, et al. American College of Cardiology/European Society of Cardiology clinical expert consensus document on hypertrophic cardiomyopathy. *J Am Coll Cardiol*. 2003;42:1687.

Maron MS, Olivotto I, Zenovich AG, et al. Hypertrophic cardiomyopathy is predominantly a disease of left ventricular outflow tract obstruction. *Circulation*. 2006;114:216.

Moore RA, Martin DE. Anesthetic management for the treatment of valvular heart disease. In: Hensley FA, Martin DE, Gravlee GP, eds. *A Practical Approach to Cardiac Anesthesia*. 3rd ed. Lippincott, Williams, and Wilkins; 2003:302-335.

O'Brien SM, Shahian DM, Filardo G, et al. The Society of Thoracic Surgeons 2008 cardiac surgery risk models: part 2—isolated valve surgery. *Ann Thorac Surg*. 2009;88:S23.

Oh JK, Seward JB, Tajik AJ, eds. Cardiomyopathies. In: *The Echo Manual*. 3rd ed. Lippincott, Williams, and Wilkins; 2007:251-273.

Otto CM, Bonow R: Valvular heart disease. In: Bonow RO, Mann DL, Zipes DP, Libby P, eds. *Bonow: Braunwald's Heart Disease*. 9th ed. Elsevier Saunders; 2011:1582-1594.

Otto CM, Lind BK, Kitzman DW, et al. Association of aortic-valve sclerosis with cardiovascular mortality and morbidity in the elderly. *N Engl J Med*. 1999;341:142-147.

Rossebo AB, Pedersen TR, Boman K, et al. Intensive lipid lowering with simvastatin and ezetimibe in aortic stenosis. *N Engl J Med*. 2008;359:1343.

Safian RD, Berman AD, Diver DJ, et al. Balloon aortic valvuloplasty in 170 consecutive patients. *N Engl J Med*. 1988;319:125-130.

Selzer A, Cohn KE. Natural history of mitral stenosis: a review. *Circulation*. 1972;45:878-890.

Shahian DM, O'Brien SM, Filardo G, et al. The Society of Thoracic Surgeons 2008 cardiac surgery risk models: part 3—valve plus coronary artery bypass grafting surgery. *Ann Thorac Surg*. 2009;88:S43.

Smith CR, Leon MB, Mack MJ. Transcatheter versus surgical aortic-valve replacement in high-risk patients. *N Engl J Med*. 2011;364:2187-2198.

Sorajja P, Valeti U, Nishimura RA, et al. Outcome of alcohol septal ablation for obstructive hypertrophic cardiomyopathy. *Circulation*. 2008;118:131.

Waller BF, Howard J, Fess S. Pathology of mitral valve stenosis and pure mitral regurgitation—part I. *Clin Cardiol*. 1994;17(6):330-336.

Whitlow PL, Feldman T, Pedersen WR, et al. Acute and 12-month results with catheter-based mitral valve leaflet repair. *J Am Coll Cardiol*. 2012; 59:130-139.

Wood P. An appreciation of mitral stenosis, I: clinical features. *Br Med J*. 1954;4870:1051-1063.

Wood P. An appreciation of mitral stenosis, II: investigations and results. *Br Med J*. 1954;4871:1113-1124.

2.5

Pericardial Disease

Esra Gumuser and Jonathan R. Salik

Anatomy, Structure, and Function

- The pericardium surrounds the heart and the roots of the great vessels.
- Consists of an outer dense fibrous pericardium and inner serous pericardium separated by a "pericardial space" containing 15 to 50 mL of plasma ultrafiltrate. Serous layer contains a parietal (outer) and visceral (inner) layer.
- Serves multiple functions:
  - Mechanical: prevents chamber dilation, enhances ventricular compliance
  - Membranous: prevents infection, provides lubrication, minimizes friction between the heart and the surrounding structures
  - Ligamentous: promotes stability within the thorax
- The phrenic, vagus, and sympathetic trunks innervate the parietal serous layer; visceral serous layer is insensate.
- Blood supply is via the pericardio-phrenic branches of the internal thoracic artery (internal mammary artery).
- Common forms of pericardial disease include:
  - Acute and recurrent pericarditis
  - Pericardial effusion ± cardiac tamponade
  - Constrictive pericarditis (CP)
  - Effusive CP

Pericarditis

Background

- Most common form of pericardial disease; accounts for 5% of emergency department (ED) visits for non-acute coronary syndrome (ACS) chest pain
- Common causes
  - Idiopathic (viral): most common cause in developed world (>80%).
  - Postcardiac injury syndrome: post-myocardial infarction (MI) (early vs late/Dressler syndrome), postpericardiotomy, posttraumatic, postablation
  - Autoimmune: systemic lupus erythematosus (SLE), rheumatoid arthritis, scleroderma, adult-onset Still disease, vasculitis
  - Malignancy
    - Usually secondary malignancy (lung most common, followed by breast, mediastinal lymphomas, and hematologic malignancies)
    - Rarely primary pericardial malignancy (mesothelioma, teratoma, sarcoma)
  - Tuberculosis: most common cause of pericarditis in developing world
  - Purulent
  - Metabolic: uremia, ovarian hyperstimulation syndrome, hypothyroidism

  - Drugs/toxins
  - Aortic dissection
- Complications: recurrent pericarditis (15%-30%), tamponade (3%), CP (1%-2%)
- Definitions
  - Recurrent pericarditis: pericarditis that occurs after a previously documented episode, following a symptom-free interval of at least 4 to 6 weeks
  - Incessant pericarditis: episode of pericarditis lasting >4 to 6 weeks (but ≤3 months) without remission
  - Chronic pericarditis: pericarditis lasting for >3 months

Diagnosis

- Acute pericarditis
  - Defined as: pleuritic, positional (worse supine, relieved by sitting forward) chest pain with 2 or more of the following:
    - Pericardial friction rub: three components (two systolic and one diastolic), best heard at the left lower sternal border with patient leaning forward
    - Typical electrocardiogram (ECG) changes: diffuse STE/PR depressions in nonvascular distribution (with STD and PR elevations in leads aVR/V1); as pericarditis evolves, T waves invert before normalizing
    - Elevated inflammatory markers (CRP, ESR)
    - New or worsening pericardial effusion
    - Pericardial inflammation on cardiac MRI
  - Initial testing: all patients should receive complete blood count (CBC) with differential, basic metabolic panel (BMP), troponin, erythrocyte sedimentation rate (ESR), C-reactive protein (CRP), thyroid-stimulating hormone (TSH), transthoracic echocardiogram (TTE), and chest x-ray.
    - Additional tests to consider based on clinical presentation: antinuclear antibody (ANA), cyclic citrullinated peptide/rheumatoid factor (CCP/RF), T-spot, blood cultures, viral studies (eg, human immunodeficiency virus [HIV], hepatitis C virus [HCV], viral respiratory panel), Lyme testing, computed tomography (CT) of the chest/anterior/posterior (A/P) for malignancy
- Recurrent pericarditis: often presents with pericardial chest pain in the absence of other typical signs/symptoms of pericarditis → advanced imaging may help make the diagnosis
  - Cardiac magnetic resonance imaging (cMRI): helps differentiate between active inflammation (late gadolinium enhancement [LGE] + pericardial edema on T2 short-tau inversion recovery time [STIR]), chronic inflammation (LGE without pericardial edema), and fibrosis (pericardial thickening without significant LGE). Can also quantify the degree of pericardial thickening and assess for hemodynamic effects (eg, constriction)
  - CT scan: quantifies the degree of calcification and pericardial thickening; does not readily assess for extent of inflammation nor hemodynamic effects

Management

- Acute pericarditis: first-line therapy is nonsteroidal antiinflammatory drugs (NSAIDs) + colchicine.
  - NSAIDs: wean once patient is asymptomatic ± CRP normalization; start proton pump inhibitor (PPI) if on antiplatelet or anticoagulation, history of peptic ulcer disease (PUD), or age ≥65
    - Ibuprofen: 600 to 800 mg 3 times daily (tid) (wean by 200 mg/dose q1-2 weeks)
    - Aspirin: 650 to 975 mg tid (wean by 162-324 mg/dose q1-2 weeks)
      - Preferred if post-MI, stage 4 to 5 chronic kidney disease (CKD) (glomerular filtration rate [GFR] <30), concomitant myocarditis (HF) or concurrent atrial fibrillation (AF)
  - Colchicine: 0.6 mg 2 times daily (bid) for 3 months (dose reduction with CKD, weight <70 kg, or concurrent P-glycoprotein inhibitor [macrolides, verapamil] or CYP 3A4 inhibitor)
  - Prednisone: should be avoided whenever possible because ↑ risk of rebound pericarditis, ↑ adverse effects; consider if uremic pericarditis, stage 4 to 5 CKD, pregnancy ≥20 weeks, connective tissue disease, pain refractory to NSAIDs/colchicine, or contraindication to NSAIDs
    - Starting dose: prednisone 0.25 to 0.5 mg/kg—taper very slowly (guided by CRP)
  - Exercise restriction until resolution of symptoms/CRP, minimum 1 month
- Recurrent pericarditis:
  - First recurrence: NSAIDs + colchicine
    - NSAIDs: wean guided by both symptoms *and* CRP
    - Colchicine: extend the duration to 6 months
  - Multiple recurrences: treatment guided by underlying phenotype
    - Auto-inflammatory: (+) ESR/CRP, (+) cMRI LGE, (−) antibodies
      - Interleukin-1 (IL-1) inhibitors (injectable) have become the standard of care versus prednisone.
        - Anakinra (daily), rilonacept (weekly)
        - Contraindications: active malignancy or infection, pregnancy, concomitant CYP450 inhibitor, immunosuppressed
      - Radical pericardiectomy: reserved for refractory cases
    - Autoimmune phenotype: (+) ESR/CRP, (+) cMRI LGE, (±) antibodies
      - Treatment directed at the underlying disease; consider IL-1 inhibitors for refractory symptoms.
    - Noninflammatory phenotype: (−) ESR/CRP, (−) cMRI, (−) antibodies
      - Alternative pain agents (acetaminophen, tricyclic antidepressants (TCAs), serotonin-norepinephrine reuptake inhibitor (SNRI), gabapentin/pregabalin)
      - Avoid steroids

Pericardial Effusion and Tamponade

Background

- Etiology: pericarditis (most common cause), malignancy, uremia, tuberculosis, autoimmune disease, iatrogenic (post-percutaneous coronary intervention [PCI]/ablation), hypothyroidism, drug/toxin, pulmonary hypertension, acute MI, aortic dissection
- Hemodynamic significance depends on the speed of accumulation—slow accumulation may be accommodated without symptoms, whereas rapid accumulation may present as tamponade with obstructive shock.

- Tamponade: occurs when intrapericardial pressure exceeds intracardiac pressure, causing chamber collapse, compromised venous return, and obstructive shock

Pathophysiology

- In tamponade, the primary hemodynamic consequence is interventricular interdependence (one ventricle fills at the expense of the other) due to the presence of tense pericardial fluid that causes a fixed total volume for ventricular filling.
  - In tamponade, the inspiratory drop in intrathoracic pressure is still able to be transmitted across the cardiac chambers, which can be accommodated to some extent by the pericardium, which remains un-thickened and elastic (unlike in constriction) → Kussmaul sign is thus typically absent in tamponade.
- As intrapericardial pressure begins to exceed intracardiac pressure, right-sided chamber collapse occurs, markedly impeding right-sided filling and thus left-sided filling, causing circulatory collapse and obstructive shock.

Physical Examination

- Findings consistent with cardiac tamponade include:
  - Pulsus paradoxus: systolic blood pressure reduction of >10 mm Hg during inspiration (reflective of interventricular interdependence)
  - Beck's triad: hypotension, muffled heart sounds, elevated jugular venous pressure (JVP). Beck's triad is insensitive, but more specific, for acute tamponade (note, there is a Beck triad for chronic tamponade: muffled heart sounds, elevated JVP, and ascites).

Diagnostic Studies

- Tamponade is a clinical diagnosis.
- ECG: sinus tachycardia, electrical alternans, low QRS voltage, ± signs of pericarditis (eg, diffuse STE/PR depressions)
- TTE
  - Pericardial effusion (measured in diastole)—trivial (only seen in systole), small (<10 mm), moderate (10-20 mm), large (>20 mm)
  - Dilated inferior vena cava (IVC) with reduced respiratory collapse ("IVC plethora")
  - Mitral/tricuspid inflow velocity: exaggerated respiratory variation (indicative of interventricular interdependence)
    - Tricuspid valve (TV): increase in flow during inspiration by ≥60%
    - Mitral valve (MV): increase in flow during expiration by ≥30%
  - Right atrial (RA) collapse > occurring 1/3 cardiac cycle
  - Right ventricular (RV) diastolic collapse
- Right heart catheterization (RHC)
  - Diastolic pressure equalization in all four chambers
  - Central venous pressure (CVP)/RA tracing: blunted Y-descent (due to decreased filling throughout the entirety of diastole)

Management

- Medical stabilization: intravenous fluids, discontinue beta-blockers (to promote higher heart rates), vasopressors (norepinephrine first line)
- Urgent needle pericardiocentesis via fluoroscopic/TTE guidance
  - Can consider up-front cardiac surgery if purulent effusion or hemopericardium (eg, aortic dissection)
- For pericardial effusions likely to reaccumulate (eg, malignant effusions), pericardial window (usually performed by cardiac or thoracic surgery) may be necessary to drain the pericardium into the pleural (or peritoneal) space.
- For patients with pericarditis, concurrent management of pericarditis should also be pursued (eg, NSAIDs, colchicine).
- In patients with malignant, noninflammatory effusions, colchicine has been shown to improve clinical outcomes.

Pericardial Constriction (Also Known as Constrictive Pericarditis)

Overview

- Insult that causes fibrosis of the pericardium, resulting in rigid, noncompliant pericardium encasing the heart. This restricts mid- and later-diastolic ventricular filling (most filling will occur in early diastole).
- Pericardial constriction is a heart failure preserved ejection fraction (HFpEF) mimic.
- Suspect in patients with right-sided heart failure (↑JVP, edema, hepatomegaly, ascites) with normal right ventricular systolic pressure/mean pulmonary arterial pressure (RVSP/mPAP), especially if history of chest radiation, cardiac surgery, tuberculosis, or prior idiopathic pericarditis
- Etiology: idiopathic/viral (~50%), cardiac surgery, radiation therapy, autoimmune disease, tuberculosis, purulent pericarditis

Pathophysiology

- Primary hemodynamic consequence is interventricular interdependence, which arises from two interrelated phenomena:
  - Dissociation of intrathoracic and intracardiac pressure:
    - In constriction, cardiac chambers are "shielded" from intrathoracic respiratory pressure variations due to encasement by the rigid pericardium (unlike in tamponade).
    - As a result, during inspiration, pulmonary capillary wedge pressure (PCWP) falls (because the pulmonary veins are entirely intrathoracic), but the left atrial/left ventricular (LA/LV) pressures remain elevated → results in decreased LV filling during inspiration, causing septum to shift toward the left, which increases right-sided filling and creates interventricular interdependence.
  - Limitation of the total volume of blood:
    - The rigid pericardium limits the total volume of blood that can fill the heart, which causes the septum to bow even more to the left during inspiration as the RV is unable to expand outward in response to the respirophasic increase in right-sided filling, further creating interventricular interdependence.

Physical Examination

- Right-sided heart failure symptoms (hepatic congestion, peripheral edema, ascites, elevated JVP)
- Kussmaul sign—paradoxical rise in JVP during inspiration due to the inability of the noncomplaint pericardium to accommodate superior vena cava (SVC) flow into the RA
- Pericardial "knock"—diastolic extra heart sound, often confused with S3; due to abrupt cessation of filling during early diastole
- Pulsus paradoxus (only seen in ~1/3 of patients)

Diagnosis

- TTE
  - Septal bounce: abrupt, paradoxical movement of the interventricular septum toward the LV in early diastole during inspiration
  - Septal shift: respirophasic change in septal position (indicates ventricular interdependence)
  - Dilated IVC with reduced respiratory collapse ("IVC plethora")
  - Mitral/tricuspid inflow: exaggerated respiratory variation (indicative of interventricular interdependence)
    - TV: increase in flow during inspiration by ≥40%
    - MV: increase in flow during expiration by ≥25%
  - Diastolic expiratory hepatic vein flow reversal
  - Mitral inflow typically shows restrictive filling (*E/A* >2).
  - Preserved (exaggerated) medial (septal) mitral annulus early diastolic velocity (*e′*) ≥8 cm/s (this is distinct from restrictive cardiomyopathies [RCMs], which as a myocardial disease will have lower *e′* values)
    - Annulus reversus: septal *e′* > lateral *e′* (due to tethering of lateral LV wall by the rigid pericardium) (this is opposite normal physiology, where lateral *e′* is usually higher)
    - Annulus paradoxus: as left ventricular end-diastolic pressure (LVEDP) rises, *E/e′* ratio remains low (<15) due to preserved *e′* velocity (this is "paradoxical" because typically higher *E/e′* ratio suggests higher LVEDP).
- RHC
  - CVP/RA tracing: prominent X-descent (due to preserved atrial relaxation), prominent Y-descent (due to enhanced, rapid early ventricular diastolic filling)
  - RV tracing: square root ("dip and plateau") sign → due to rapid RV filling during early diastole (dip) followed by abrupt cessation during mid-to-late diastole (plateau)
  - Hemodynamic criteria for CP are shown in Table 2.5.1.

Constrictive Pericarditis Versus Restrictive Cardiomyopathy

- Why is this important? Both CP and RCM are HFpEF mimics, and both manifest as biventricular diastolic dysfunction with elevated CVP and pulmonary venous pressures and possible negative impact on cardiac output. However, the similarities end at clinical presentation: the etiologies are very different, and the treatments are distinct (surgical pericardiectomy for CP, which may be curative, while RCM has limited treatment options).
- Key difference is the presence of interventricular interdependence, which is present in constriction but *not* in restriction.
- TTE
  - Findings favoring restriction: biatrial dilation, elevated RVSP, LV wall thickening, diastolic inspiratory hepatic vein flow reversal
  - Findings favoring constriction: septal bounce/shift, exaggerated respiratory variation across MV/TV, annulus reversus, diastolic expiratory hepatic vein flow reversal
- Labs
  - Normal NT-proBNP favors constriction (reduced distensibility of the cardiac chambers limits natriuretic peptide secretion).
- Invasive hemodynamics: simultaneous LV/RV pressure assessment is gold standard.
  - Restriction: ventricular concordance during inspiration and expiration (ie, LV/RV pressures rise and fall together)
  - Constriction: ventricular discordance during inspiration and expiration (ie, RV pressure increases during inspiration while LV pressure decreases during inspiration; this is due to interventricular interdependence)

Management

- Transient CP may be seen with acute pericarditis or after cardiac surgery → treat with antiinflammatory therapy (eg, NSAIDs/colchicine).

TABLE 2.5.1 Hemodynamic Criteria for Constrictive Pericarditis

Criterion	Sensitivity (%)	Specificity (%)	Positive Predictive Accuracy (%)	Negative Predictive Accuracy (%)
LVEDP—RVEDP ≤5 mm Hg	46	54	58	40
PASP <55 mm Hg	90	29	73	66
RVEDP/RVSP >1/3	93	46	71	79
LVRFW >7 mm Hg	45	44	62	42
Inspiratory decrease in RAP <5 mm Hg	71	37	62	39
Systolic area index >1.1	97	100	100	95

In general, these factors help separate restrictive myopathic disease from constrictive pericarditis. LVRFW, height of left ventricular rapid filling wave (effectively height from the dip to the plateau). Systolic area index is the ratio of the area of the RV systolic tracing to the area of the LV systolic tracing in inspiration versus expiration; an increase indicates increased ventricular interdependence (effectively the ratio of stroke volumes).

LV, left ventricular; LVEDP, left ventricular end-diastolic pressure; PASP, pulmonary artery systolic pressure; RAP, right atrial pressure; RVEDP, right ventricular end-diastolic pressure; RVSP, right ventricular systolic pressure.

From Talreja DR, Nishimura RA, Oh JK, Holmes DR. Constrictive pericarditis in the modern era: novel criteria for diagnosis in the cardiac catheterization laboratory. *J Am Coll Cardiol*. 2008;51(3):315-319.

- For chronic constriction without pericardial inflammation, preferred management is with radical pericardiectomy (complete removal of the pericardium via sternotomy).
  - Indications
    - Persistent symptoms despite IL-1 inhibitor treatment
    - New York Heart Association (NHYA) III/IV symptoms
    - Absence of end-stage symptoms (eg, cardiac cachexia, reduced cardiac output, hypoalbuminemia, cardiac cirrhosis)
    - Lack of co-occurring RCM
    - No other surgical contraindications

Effusive-Constrictive Pericarditis

Overview/Diagnosis

- Condition characterized by concurrent pericardial effusion (often with tamponade) and pericardial constriction
- Diagnosis: simultaneous pericardiocentesis and RHC demonstrate persistent elevation of RA pressure despite normalization of intrapericardial pressure.
  - Criteria: failure of RA pressure to decrease by >50% *or* to a level <10 mm Hg after pericardiocentesis

Pathophysiology

- Rigid parietal pericardium increases intrapericardial pressure, leading to increased tension on the pericardial effusion, often causing tamponade.
- Similarly, rigid visceral pericardium constricts ventricular filling and causes concomitant pericardial constriction that persists despite fluid drainage.

Management

- If acute (ie, due to transient inflammation), treat as acute pericarditis (eg, NSAIDs/colchicine).
- If chronic (ie, inflammation absent), treat as CP with radical pericardiectomy.

SUGGESTED READINGS

Adler Y, Charron P, Imazio M, et al. 2015 ESC guidelines for the diagnosis and management of pericardial diseases: the task force for the diagnosis and management of pericardial diseases of the European Society of Cardiology (ESC). *Eur Heart J*. 2015;36(42):2921-2964.

Garcia MJ. Constrictive pericarditis versus restrictive cardiomyopathy. *JACC*. 2016;67(17):2061-2076.

Geske JB, Anavekar NS, Nishimura R, Oh JK, Gersh BJ. Differentiation of constriction and restriction: complex cardiovascular hemodynamics. *JACC*. 2016;68(21):2329-2347.

Imazio M, Bobbio M, Cecchi E, et al. Colchicine in addition to conventional therapy for acute pericarditis: results of the colchicine for acute pericarditis (COPE) trial. *Circulation*. 2005;112(13):2012-2016.

Little WC, Freeman GL. Pericardial disease. *Circulation*. 2006;113(12):1622-1632.

Talreja DR, Nishimura RA, Oh JK, Holmes DR. Constrictive pericarditis in the modern era: novel criteria for diagnosis in the cardiac catheterization laboratory. *JACC*. 2008;51(3):315-319.

2.6

Myocardial Disorders

Kemar J. Brown, Safia Chatur, and David M. Dudzinski

Myocardial Pathology—Cardiomyopathy

- Heterogeneous group of myocardial disorders associated with structural abnormalities, mechanical impairment, and often accompanied by electrical disturbances
- Some definitions require the absence of coronary artery disease, hypertension, valvular, or congenital disease as alternative etiologies for myocardial dysfunction.

Dilated Cardiomyopathy

Definitions

- Characterized by eccentric ventricular remodeling with impaired systolic and diastolic function
- Older definition requires left ventricular ejection fraction (LVEF) <40% or fractional shortening <25%.

Common Dilated Cardiomyopathy Causes to Remember

- Idiopathic (50%)
- Genetic/familial (20%-30%) including inherited or de novo mutations. Common mutations include titin (TTN), lamin (LMNA), RBM20, and BAG3.
- Cardiac (ischemic heart disease, congenital heart disease, valvular diseases, high output states)
- Deposition/infiltrative (amyloidosis, hemochromatosis)
- Inflammatory or autoimmune (sarcoidosis, scleroderma, giant cell arteritis, eosinophilic, idiopathic myocarditis)
- Chemical/toxic exposures (alcohol, cocaine, amphetamines, chemotherapy, immune checkpoint inhibitors, hydroxychloroquine)
- Infectious (viral, protozoa, Chagas)
- Tachyarrhythmias, pacemaker mediated
- Peripartum cardiomyopathy (CM)

Epidemiology

- Incidence in the United States is 5 to 8 out of 100,000 people, mostly 20 to 60 years old, and more common in men than in women.
- Bimodal age presentation, with large number of patients having long latent period
- Most common indication for heart transplant

Key Pathophysiology

- Reduced sarcomere contractility, eccentric hypertrophy, myocardial fibrosis resulting from insult to myocardium or underlying genetic abnormality, together causes low cardiac output (CO) and electrophysiologic disturbances
- Renin-angiotensin axis compensates for low CO, increased vasoconstriction (vasopressin), and volume expansion (aldosterone and atrial natriuretic peptide)
- Dilated cardiomyopathy (DCM) can present in decompensated heart failure (HF), malignant arrhythmias, thromboembolic events, or sudden death.

Differential Diagnosis

- Acute coronary syndrome (ACS)
- Valvular disease
- Restrictive (RCM)
- Hypertrophic CM (HCM)
- Acute endocarditis
- Cardiac tamponade

Management and Treatment

- Hallmarks of chronic DCM management include prescription of maximum tolerated guideline-directed medical therapy (GDMT), volume management with loop diuretics, afterload reduction, implantable cardioverter-defibrillator/cardiac resynchronization therapy with a defibrillator (ICD/CRT-D) if indicated, referral to advanced HF specialist for consideration of advanced therapies (LV assist device [LVAD] and cardiac transplantation). Cardiopulmonary exercise test is used to predict mortality and determine candidacy for heart replacement therapy.
- Acute decompensation
  - Intravenous administration of loop diuretics for preload optimization with or without inotropic support, aggressive afterload optimization to augment CO by facilitating LVEF, and tailoring with pulmonary artery catheter if needed.
  - Noninvasive positive pressure ventilation (NIPPV) may avoid intubation.
  - Adequate control of ventricular and supraventricular arrhythmias
  - Temporary mechanical circulatory support if needed—consult advanced HF specialist.

Outcomes

- 5-year survival after initial HF presentation ~50%
- 60-day mortality from HF exacerbation admission 8% to 20%
- Durability of remission on GDMT is highly dependent on underlying cause and presence of extracardiac comorbidities.

Hypertrophic Cardiomyopathy

Definitions

- Autosomal dominant cardiac myocyte disease resulting from mutations in sarcomere genes, resulting in cardiomyocyte hypertrophy, increased ventricular wall thickness, excessive extracellular matrix deposition, and myofibrillar disarray
- Increased LV wall thickness results in clinically significant diastolic dysfunction, myocardial ischemia, arrhythmias, and, sometimes, dynamic LV outflow tract obstruction (LVOTO).

Epidemiology

- The most common cause of sudden death in individuals <35 years of age. More common in males and usually presents in the third decade of life
- 1:500 prevalence worldwide
- 25% of first-degree relatives affected with proven morphologic abnormalities on multimodality imaging.

Key Pathophysiology

- 60% of patients harbor known pathogenic gene mutation of sarcomere or sarcomere-related genes inherited in a Mendelian pattern with incomplete penetrance and variable expression.
- Gene mutations in MYH7 and MYBPC3 account for 75% of cases. Additional mutations include TNNT2, TNNI3, TPMP1, and MYL2.
- Wall thickening most commonly affects the interventricular septum, although any region of LV myocardium can be affected. Septal and posterior wall thickness is >13 mm (normotensive) or >15 mm (hypertensive).
- Wall thickening is associated with significant diastolic dysfunction with delayed inactivation from abnormal calcium reuptake as well as mismatch between myocardial oxygen supply and demand, chronic myocardial ischemia, and fibrosis. Furthermore, inappropriate firing of stress-sensitive mechanoreceptors in the hypertrophic myocardium results in dysautonomia.
- Although atrial fibrillation is a common arrhythmia (25%), fibrosis and myocardial disarray are main drivers of ventricular tachycardia (20%-30%) in HCM. Tachyarrhythmias in general are poorly tolerated since >35% of LV preload in HCM is dependent on atrial kick.
- LVOTO can result from either (1) septal hypertrophy causing systolic anterior motion (SAM) of the mitral valve or (2) structural dysmorphology of the mitral valve and displacement of the papillary muscles and valve apparatus anteriorly.

Differential Diagnosis

- Severe aortic stenosis
- Hypertensive heart disease
- RCM
- Fabry disease
- Noonan syndrome
- Athlete's heart

Management and Treatment

- Detailed personal, family history, genetic testing for risk stratification of proband and biologic relatives
- LVOTO with gradient ≥30 mm Hg is considered hemodynamically significant and associated with death and HF. Gradient ≥50 mm Hg is threshold for surgical/percutaneous intervention. (See Table 2.6.1.)
- Cardiac magnetic resonance imaging (MRI) indicated in cases of high clinical suspicion and if transthoracic echocardiogram (TTE) is inconclusive. Cardiac MRI also helps to

TABLE 2.6.1 Risk Factors for Sudden Cardiac Death in HCM[a]
Unexplained syncope
SCD in relative (HCM related)
LV apical aneurysm
NSVT (≥3 beats at ≥120 bpm)
LVEF ≤50%
Wall thickness >30 mm
Extensive LGE on CMR imaging (≥15% of LV mass)

[a]At least one of the above.
CMR, cardiac magnetic resonance; HCM, hypertrophic cardiomyopathy; LGE, late gadolinium enhancement; LV, left ventricle; LVEF, left ventricular ejection fraction; NSVT, nonsustained ventricular tachycardia; SCD, sudden cardiac death.

assess burden of late gadolinium enhancement (LGE). LGE >15% and/or nonsustained ventricular tachycardia (NSVT) meet Class IIb criteria for ICD placement.
- Beta-blockers are the first line of management. Use of calcium channel blockers may be limited by their vasodilatory properties. Disopyramide is used off-label to reduce outflow tract obstruction. Mavacamten is a selective, allosteric, reversible small-molecule adenosine triphosphatase inhibitor of cardiac myosin that blocks actin-myosin interaction and augment lusitropy; currently recommended for New York Heart Association (NYHA) II and III symptoms. Diuretics and vasodilators must be used with caution to avoid intravascular depletion and reduced preload. Use of inotropes and vasopressors should be cautioned to avoid tachyarrhythmias, and inotropes can worsen or provoke LVOTO.
- Heart transplant for failed medical/surgical interventions

Outcomes

- Women diagnosed later and have worse prognosis.
- Mortality 0.5% to 4%, ICD placement has been attributed to improved mortality.
- Left atrial enlargement (volume >118 mL) is associated with increased risk, HF, and atrial fibrillation.

Restrictive Cardiomyopathy

Definitions

- Characterized by impaired ventricular relaxation, reduced diastolic ventricle volume, and impaired CO (fixed stroke volume, so patient is heart rate [HR] dependent).
- Typical hemodynamic signs include "dip and plateau"/"square root sign," elevated and rapid equalization of filling pressures in all chambers during diastole.
- Structurally, findings for RCM on TTE include normal or mildly reduced LV and right ventricular (RV) function, nondilated ventricles, biatrial enlargement, tissue Doppler with elevated *E/e′* ratio, and other indicia of diastolic impairment.

Common Causes to Remember

- Deposition/infiltrative/inflammatory (amyloidosis, sarcoidosis)
- Storage diseases (hemochromatosis, Fabry, Gaucher, Hurler, Danon, Niemann-Pick, Friedrich ataxia)
- Noninfiltrative (idiopathic, familial)
- Radiation therapy
- Endomyocardial disease
- Metastatic disease
- Carcinoid
- Post-heart transplant

Epidemiology

- 5% of primary heart muscle disease
- Most common in the United States is amyloidosis and idiopathic RCM, while globally is Loeffler endocarditis and chronic endomyocardial fibrosis. Sarcoidosis more common in African American women, with highest incidence in Japan.

Key Pathophysiology

- Majority of RCM cases are due to abnormal deposition of intercellular or intracellular material or dysregulated fibroblast activity within the pericardial or endocardium, all resulting in reduced ventricular compliance. Decreased stroke volume and CO leads to symptomatic HF, and increased filling pressures lead to pulmonary and systemic congestion.
- CO will be HR dependent, as stroke volume is generally fixed. This has implications for therapy with beta-blockers, as more diastolic time will not improve filling but will contribute to overall CO reduction.
- Microarchitectural disruption often involves the atrioventricular (AV) node and results in complete heart block.
- Atrial fibrosis and enlargement increase the susceptibility to atrial fibrillation/atrial flutter development.
- One-third of patients also have deep venous thrombosis (DVT) and thromboembolic disease.

Differential Diagnosis

- Pericarditis (constrictive, acute)
- Aortic stenosis
- Cardiac tamponade
- HCM and DCM
- Hypertensive heart disease
- Sarcoidosis

Management and Treatment

- Hemodynamic/respiratory support, optimize pulmonary/systemic volume status
- Volume status tenuous as high filling pressures needed to maintain CO, but diuresis may be indicated.
- Agents that induce vasodilation and negative chronotropy should be used with caution. Excessive preload reduction may compromise LV filling and result in decreased CO. Afterload reducing agents (angiotensin-converting enzyme inhibitor [ACEi], angiotensin receptor blocker [ARB], angiotensin receptor-neprilysin inhibitor [ARNI], nitrates) should be titrated carefully to avoid hypotension and low CO. Similarly, CO in RCM is dependent on higher HR due to relatively fixed and reduced stroke volume. Prolonged diastole at low HR may exacerbate pulmonary congestion. Consequently, calcium channel blockers and beta-blockade should also be administered with caution.

- AV synchrony is essential and may require dual-chamber pacemaker.
- Anticoagulation and rate control for atrial fibrillation if not otherwise contraindicated
- Cardiac transplantation considered if intractable HF and irreversible etiology

Outcomes

- Variable with 2- to 5-year survival of 64% and 10-year survival 37%, with two-thirds being cardiovascular deaths. Of survivors, 10% had cardiac transplant, 63% being moderately symptomatic.

Myocarditis

Definition

- Inflammation/necrosis of myocytes causing cardiac dysfunction

Common Causes to Remember

- Viral most common worldwide (HIV, Lyme, coxsackie B)
- Toxins (medication, environment)
- Immunologic/autoimmune (rheumatoid, sarcoidosis)

Epidemiology

- Asymptomatic to sudden death (up to 1.3%)
- Seen in up to 20% of young patients with sudden cardiac death
- Average age 42 years, with slightly higher incidence in males

Key Pathophysiology

- Impaired myocardial function with anemia, fever, and tachycardia
- Some patients have rapid cell death without interstitial infiltrate, leading to ventricular dysfunction and cardiovascular collapse.
- Typically, a week after viral infection, proinflammatory cells target myocardium expressing viral RNA.
  - Attack results in negative inotropic effects and acute HF.
  - Chronically, this causes DCM and HF.

Differential Diagnosis

- Cardiac (ACS, HF)
- Aortic dissection
- Pulmonary (pulmonary edema, pneumonia, asthma, pulmonary emboli)
- Esophageal perforation

Management and Treatment

- Most have mild viral symptoms and recover with outpatient care.
- If severe disease, focus on respiratory/hemodynamic support, including temporary pacemakers for high-grade conduction blocks.
- Bridge to heart transplant with mechanical circulatory support may be required.
- Workup includes cardiac troponin I (positive in 35% patients), antinuclear antibody (ANA), viral polymerase chain reaction (PCR), electrocardiogram (ECG), and TTE.
  - MRI can be helpful.
  - Endocardial biopsy is the gold standard.
- LV dysfunction is treated as acute HF exacerbation.
- Beta-blockers are useful in reducing myocardial damage in recovery phase.
- Immunosuppressant therapy benefit is seen in patients with cardiac sarcoidosis, hypersensitivity, or giant cell myocarditis.

Outcomes

- Mortality varies with presentation (4%-25%).
- Most are undiagnosed and resolve.
- Fulminant myocarditis is severe but typically has complete recovery.
- In contrast, subacute myocarditis presentations may have continued cardiac dysfunction.

Cardiac Contusions

Definitions

- Complication of blunt thoracic trauma
- Definitive diagnosis by histopathology, but clinical diagnosis with cardiac biomarkers, ECG, and TTE

Common Causes to Remember

- Cardiopulmonary resuscitation
- Trauma (fall >20 ft, motor vehicle accident, low-velocity trauma not excluded)

Epidemiology

- True incidence unknown
- Present in 14% of immediate fatalities from blunt injury, ranges from 0% to 76% depending on clinical or postmortem diagnosis

Key Pathophysiology

- Deceleration force causes direct pressure on myocardium, with increased intrathoracic pressure and shear forces.
- RV commonly injured (it is the most anterior cardiac structure, located immediately retrosternal). RV injury reduces preload to LV, with resultant decreased CO.
- Intraventricular septum can shift, reducing LV compliance with 40% decrease in CO that can persist for weeks.
- Damaged valves, chordae tendineae, papillary muscles, and interventricular septum can compromise cardiac function.
- Thrombosis, vasospasm, and interruption of myocardial blood supply may occur.
- Presentation ranges widely (asymptomatic to arrhythmias, HF, ventricular aneurysm, pericardial effusion with tamponade, cardiac rupture).

Differential Diagnosis

- Cardiac (tamponade, injury to aorta, intrathoracic vessels)
- Pulmonary (contusions, pneumothorax, hemothorax, diaphragm rupture)
- Musculoskeletal (rib fractures, flail chest, sternal fractures)

Management and Treatment

- Respiratory and hemodynamic support (judicious volume, medications, procedural interventions)

- Consider myocardial injury if persistent hypotension with no source of bleed.
- Cautious inotropic support as injured myocardium sensitive to inotropic effects and prone to arrhythmias
- TTE helpful for volume status and cardiac function while ruling out tamponade
- ECG abnormalities probably warrant telemetry for 24 hours with electrolyte disturbance correction.
- Cardiac biomarkers suggest the presence and degree of injury.
- Nuclear imaging studies can provide imaging evidence of cardiac contusion.

Outcome

- Most recover fully as bruised part of the heart regains function.

Catecholamine-Induced Cardiomyopathy

Definitions

- Often transient injury to the myocardium that results from states of catecholamine excess, resulting from a significant antecedent emotional or physical stressor, thereby causing myocardial necrosis. Given the high degree of overlap with ACS, stress CM is often deemed a diagnosis of exclusion. In some cases, there is no clear stress trigger.
- Characterized by regional wall motion abnormalities most classically of the LV mid and apical segment, with apical ballooning ("takotsubo CM," the pattern seen in 80%); the basal segment can be hyperkinetic. This classic pattern can mimic a left coronary artery injury distribution. As such, coronary angiogram should demonstrate nonobstructive epicardial coronary disease or coronary disease that does not explain the extent of myocardial dysfunction.
- Other variants include midcavitary variant (with the apex and basal segments hyperdynamic), reverse takotsubo (apical hyperkinesis with basal hypokinesis), and isolated RV-predominant variant.

Common Causes to Remember

- Takotsubo (stress CM)
- Pheochromocytoma
- Paraganglioma
- Critical illness
- Physical trauma
- Cerebrovascular events/seizures
- Postcardiac surgery/reperfusion
- Emotional stress/trauma
- Multivessel coronary vasospasm
- Impaired microvascular function and endothelial dysfunction

Epidemiology

- Mean age 67. Takotsubo CM most common in female, 90% predominance. Most common in Asian (57%) and White (40%) individuals. Approximately 2% of suspected ACS represents patients subsequently diagnosed with takotsubo CM.

Key Pathophysiology

- Hyperkinetic basal segments cause LV narrowing and increased intraventricular pressure gradient, with possible systolic collapse of RV, and also cause LVOTO.
- Preserved myocardial perfusion and metabolism means cardiac dysfunction responds to inotropes.
- In cases of myocardial stunning, transient ischemia glucose utilization > fatty acid metabolism, which results in impaired cardiac function. Glucose utilization becomes the main energy source in stress CM as well. Repeated stunning leads to "hibernating myocardium," characterized by impaired myocardial function of limited duration, tissue ischemia without necrosis, and recovery of function after revascularization.
- Classic histologic findings include focal myocytolysis, mononuclear infiltrates, and contraction band necrosis.

Differential Diagnosis

- Myocardial infarction/ACS
- DCM
- Postpartum CM
- Alcoholic CM

Management and Treatment

- Respiratory/hemodynamic support (address tachyarrhythmias, administer inotropes and vasodilators as needed)
- TTE may show apical ballooning, dyskinesia, and dilatation of apex and mid segment; cardiac catheterization to exclude coronary pathology.
- Dobutamine stress echocardiography or positron emission tomography/single-photon emission computed tomography (PET/SPECT) imaging has been used to characterize myocardial contractility.
- Early initiation and uptitration of GDMT. Referral to advanced HF

Outcome

Most patients recover fully within days to weeks.

SUGGESTED READINGS

Ammirati E, Moslehi JJ. Diagnosis and treatment of acute myocarditis: a review. *JAMA*. 2023;329(13):1098-1113.

Bansal MK, Maraj S, Chewaproug D, Amanullah A. Myocardial contusion injury: redefining the diagnostic algorithm. *Emerg Med J*. 2005;22(7):465.

Basso C. Myocarditis. *N Engl J Med*. 2022;387(16):1488-1500.

Braunwald E. Cardiomyopathies. *Circ Res*. 2017;121(7):711-721.

Cooper LT. Myocarditis. *N Engl J Med*. 2009;360(15):1526-1538.

de Miguel V, Arias A, Paissan A, et al. Catecholamine-induced myocarditis in pheochromocytoma. *Circulation*. 2014;129(12):1348-1349.

Dec GW, Fuster V. Idiopathic dilated cardiomyopathy. *N Engl J Med*. 1994;331(23):1564-1575.

Ellis CR, Di Salvo T. Myocarditis: basic and clinical aspects. *Cardiol Rev*. 2007;15(4):170-177.

Frank RC, Yunis AA, Dudzinski DM. Heart failure. In: Bittner EA, Berra L, Lee J, Kwo J, Fagenholz P, Sonny A, eds. *Critical Care Handbook of the Massachusetts General Hospital*. 7th ed. Lippincott Williams & Wilkins; 2024:252-266.

Gigli M, Stolfo D, Merlo M, Sinagra G, Taylor MRG, Mestroni L. Pathophysiology of dilated cardiomyopathy: from mechanisms to precision medicine. *Nat Rev Cardiol*. 2025;22(3):183-198.

Kassim TA, Clarke DD, Mai VQ, Clyde PW, Shakir KMM. Catecholamine-induced cardiomyopathy. *Endocr Pract*. 2008;14(9):1137-1149.

Marian AJ, Braunwald E. Hypertrophic cardiomyopathy. *Circ Res*. 2017;121(7):749-770.

Maron BJ, Desai MY, Nishimura RA, et al. Diagnosis and evaluation of hypertrophic cardiomyopathy. *J Am Coll Cardiol*. 2022;79(4):372-389.

McNally EM, Mestroni L. Dilated cardiomyopathy. *Circ Res*. 2017;121(7):731-748.
Muchtar E, Blauwet LA, Gertz MA. Restrictive cardiomyopathy. *Circ Res*. 2017;121(7):819-837.
Nair L, Winkle B, Senanayake E. Managing blunt cardiac injury. *J Cardiothorac Surg*. 2023;18(1):71.
Pabba K, Widmer RJ, Nguyen V, Martinez MW. Cardiac contusion complicated by heart failure in a young athlete. *JACC Case Rep*. 2022;4(17):1124-1128.
Pereira NL, Grogan M, Dec GW. Spectrum of restrictive and infiltrative cardiomyopathies. *J Am Coll Cardiol*. 2018;71(10):1130-1148.
Pereira N, Grogan M, Dec GW. Spectrum of restrictive and infiltrative cardiomyopathies. *J Am Coll Cardiol*. 2018;71(10):1149-1166.
Rapezzi C, Aimo A, Barison A, et al. Restrictive cardiomyopathy: definition and diagnosis. *Eur Heart J*. 2022;43(45):4679-4693.
Reisinger J, Dubrey SW, Falk RH. Restrictive cardiomyopathy. *N Engl J Med*. 1997;336(26):1917-1918.
Scagliola R, Seitun S, Balbi M. Cardiac contusions in the acute care setting: historical background, evaluation and management. *Am J Emerg Med*. 2022;61:152-157.
Schultheiss HP, Fairweather D, Caforio ALP, et al. Dilated cardiomyopathy. *Nat Rev Dis Primer*. 2019;5(1):32.
Seidman CE, Seidman JG, Robbins J, Watkins H. Identifying sarcomere gene mutations in hypertrophic cardiomyopathy. *Circ Res*. 2011;108(6):743-750.
Tenzer ML. The spectrum of myocardial contusion: a review. *J Trauma Acute Care Surg*. 1985;25(7):620-627.
Thevathasan T, Kenny MA, Gaul AL, et al. Sex and age characteristics in acute or chronic myocarditis. *JACC Adv*. 2024;3(4):100857.
Tschöpe C, Ammirati E, Bozkurt B, et al. Myocarditis and inflammatory cardiomyopathy: current evidence and future directions. *Nat Rev Cardiol*. 2021;18(3):169-193.

2.7

Congenital Heart Disease in Adults

Q. Joyce Han, and Ada C. Stefanescu Schmidt

- There is a rapidly growing number of adult patients with congenital heart disease (CHD), due to improved surgical and medical therapies and increased survival and longevity of children with CHD.
- Caring for patients with CHD relies on understanding their cardiac anatomy, prior interventions, and any associated lesions and complications.
- The care for patients with adult congenital heart disease (ACHD) requires an interdisciplinary approach, including congenital cardiologists and cardiac surgeons.
- The complexity and significant heterogeneity of this population are associated with a lack of large clinical trials, but registry data are increasingly robust; interinstitutional collaboration is especially important for rare circumstances.

Hemodynamic Monitoring and Testing Considerations in Population With Congenital Heart Disease

Blood Pressure Monitoring

- Always check bilateral arm pressures and four extremity blood pressures (BPs) when possible; the higher arm BP is correct (ie, reflective of central aorta pressure), while lower pressures may be falsely low due to prior surgeries.
- Classic Blalock-Taussig-Thomas (BTT) shunt (*direct anastomosis* between the transected subclavian artery and the pulmonary artery [PA]) will lead to underestimation of ipsilateral arm BP.
- Modified BT shunt (*synthetic graft* between the subclavian artery and the PA) does not significantly affect the BP measurement.
- Subclavian flap for coarctation repair: falsely low BP on the surgical side

Oxygen Saturation Monitoring

Always check for baseline saturation on room air at prior visits, especially for patients with known right-to-left shunts. Patients with chronic cyanosis will tolerate saturations of 80% (or sometimes 70%) at rest.

Vascular Access

- Ultrasound is recommended for line insertion as veins might be occluded or fibrosed. Review prior access and pacemaker insertion records if possible. Note cut-down scars over peripheral arteries.
- Consider abnormal venous anatomy: persistent left superior vena cava (SVC), baffle leaks or obstruction, and Fontan physiology (wherein catheters should be situated in the SVC proximal to the SVC-to-PA anastomosis)
- Filter all intravenous (IV) lines in patients with right-to-left shunt.
- In particular, due to fibrosis at sites of prior procedures, access may be particularly painful, and in some patients, associated with posttraumatic stress disorder. Adequate sedation prior to and during procedures is important.

Imaging

- Echocardiogram can be technically challenging and requires special expertise.
- Echocardiographic estimates of RV systolic pressure are unreliable in the presence of RV outflow tract obstruction.
- Computed tomography (CT) angiograms in Fontan patients are challenging: contrast injected in the upper extremity during a CT scan will stream preferentially into one of the PAs, unless the scan is protocolled to provide adequate opacification, and may falsely suspect a pulmonary embolus.

Common Adult Congenital Heart Disease–Related Critical Care Scenarios by Organ System

Cardiac

- Acute decompensated heart failure (HF)
  - Pressors and inotropes. *Note that increasing cardiac contractility with pharmacologic agents may result in the poorly tolerated increase in myocardial oxygen demand and impairment of diastolic function.*
    - At low doses, vasopressin acts through a nitric oxide–dependent mechanism to vasodilate the pulmonary circulation and has demonstrated safety in patients with pulmonary hypertension.
    - Milrinone, compared to dobutamine, produces more pulmonary and systemic vasodilation, less tachycardia and myocardial oxygen consumption, and an increased rate of myocardial relaxation.
  - Mechanical circulatory support (MCS)
    - Utilized significantly less in patients with ACHD due to the inherent anatomic and physiologic variations
    - Commonly used in decompensated HF and the postoperative period after reoperation
    - Indications include left-sided HF, right-sided HF, biventricular HF, persistent arrhythmia, and significant hypoxemia.
    - The INTERMACS scale is a helpful tool to stratify patients with HF with ACHD requiring MCS.
  - Long-term therapies
    - Cardiac transplantation is the most definitive long-term treatment.
    - Ventricular assist device (VAD), biventricular assist device (BiVAD), and total artificial heart (TAH) can improve survival as a bridge to transplantation, though increased adverse events have been found in patients with ACHD.
- Arrhythmia and conduction disturbances
  - Up to 50% of post-Fontan patients will develop atrial tachyarrhythmias, which are often associated with hemodynamic instability; rhythm control is preferred in all patients if possible.
  - Intra-atrial reentrant tachycardia (IART), or atypical flutter, is particularly common among surgically repaired ACHD. It may be harder to detect on an electrocardiogram (ECG) and requires a high level of suspicion: Any regular tachycardia with a constant rate should be considered IART until proven otherwise (rather than a sinus tachycardia, for instance).
    - In particular seen in patients with Fontan, Mustard, Senning, and tetralogy of Fallot (TOF)
    - Vagal maneuvers can be attempted, followed by IV beta-blockers, diltiazem, or verapamil. Cardioversion is indicated in the presence of hemodynamic instability.
    - Catheter ablation is generally considered the preferred strategy for long-term management. Sotalol is frequently used; amiodarone may be used in the short term.
- Sinus node dysfunction is common in atrially repaired D-transposition, patch-repaired superior sinus venosus arterial septal defect (ASD), and the Fontan procedure.
- Atrioventricular (AV) nodal block is commonly associated with L-transposition of the great arteries and primum ASD.

Pulmonary

- Airway management and mechanical ventilation
  - Assess for increased risk for cervical instability (atlantoaxial instability) in Down syndrome.
  - In patients without a subpulmonic ventricle (Fontan), intubation increases intrathoracic pressure, which can raise PVR and reduce LV preload, leading to shock.
  - Dexmedetomidine and propofol are safe in patients with CHD and pulmonary hypertension as they do not increase PVR. For pain management, fentanyl does not impact pulmonary vascular tone. Early extubation is a priority in all patients with pulmonary hypertension or Fontan.
  - Abnormal lung mechanics (such as restrictive lung disease) is common.
  - In Fontan, systemic venous return is dependent on negative intrathoracic pressure during inspiration; thus, positive end-expiratory pressure (PEEP) should be minimized when possible.
- Pulmonary hypertension
  - PA hypertension, occurring in 30% of uncorrected and 15% of corrected CHD, with RV failure being one of the most common causes of morbidity and early mortality.
  - In patients with right-to-left shunt, avoid increasing PVR or decreasing systemic vascular resistance (SVR), both of which will lead to increased right-to-left shunting and subsequent worsening hypoxemia.
    - Conditions that increase PVR include hypoxemia, hypercapnia, positive pressure ventilation, hypothermia, metabolic acidosis, alpha-adrenergic stimulation, and high hematocrit.
    - Pulmonary vasodilators such as nitric oxide may be used to decrease PVR.
    - Conditions that decrease SVR include vasodilators, spinal or epidural anesthesia, hyperthermia, infection/distributive insult, heavy sedation, and excessive narcotic administration.
- Restrictive lung disease
  - Occurs in up to half of adults with CHD, especially in Fontan and TOF patients

Nephrology

- Acute kidney injury
- Cyanotic CHD has the highest risk for *chronic kidney disease* due to chronic hyperviscosity and hypoxia; creatinine often overestimates glomerular filtration, cystatin C is more accurate.

Hepatology/Gastroenteropathy

- High-filling pressures are required to drive forward flow through the pulmonary vasculature in the absence of a subpulmonic ventricle → portal hypertension and hepatic congestion → liver cirrhosis and hepatocellular carcinoma. MELD-XI is a significant predictor of major adverse *cardiac* events.
- 10% of Fontan patients may present with protein-losing enteropathy.

Hematology

- Anemia. Independently associated with increased mortality in CHD. Iron deficiency is the most common etiology.

- Bleeding and thrombosis
  - Common due to platelet dysfunction and increased red blood cell production
  - Fontan patients are at particularly high risk for systemic and pulmonary thromboembolic events, partly because of the low-flow circuit. Warfarin is the anticoagulant of choice in patients with a Fontan and a newly diagnosed thrombus.

Infectious Disease

- Patients with heterotaxy syndrome may have ciliary dysmotility, leading to an increased risk for pneumonia.
- Consider hepatitis C in adults who underwent surgery before 1991.

Neurology/Psychiatry

- Acknowledge anticipated anxiety and review coping strategies.
- Assess for learning disabilities.
- Important to contact and include their social support system in discussions and plans

Review of Congenital Heart Conditions

There are many other CHDs that impact the care of adult patients. However, the basic principles of understanding the anatomy, the relative pressures for blood flow, and the coexisting diseases can be followed in the management of all these patients.

Fontan Procedure

- Used in *functional single-ventricle physiology* (tricuspid atresia, pulmonary atresia, hypoplastic left heart syndrome, double-inlet LV)
- Pulmonary blood flow is driven by venous pressure, augmented by intrathoracic pressure swings during inspiration, relaxation of the systemic ventricle, and peripheral skeletal muscles. Therefore, Fontan patients are particularly sensitive to hemodynamic and respiratory shifts. Small increases in PVR can significantly decrease cardiac output.
- Very important to know the anatomy:
  - *Classic Fontan*: the right atrial (RA) appendage is connected to the PA.
  - *Lateral tunnel Fontan*: a synthetic baffle is inserted in the RA connecting the SVC to the PA.
  - *Extracardiac Fontan*: a synthetic tube connecting the inferior vena cava (IVC) to the PAs
  - A *fenestration* is often performed at the time of surgery as a "pop-off" right-to-left shunt to preserve cardiac output in the initial postoperative period when the PVR might be elevated. The fenestration is often closed later in childhood.
- Not cyanotic at baseline, but arterial oxygen saturation on room air rarely >95% for numerous reasons. Consider the following conditions if arterial oxygen saturation fails to correct with supplemental oxygen: systemic venous-to-pulmonary venous connections (via development of collateral vessels, also called "venovenous collaterals" [VVCs]), pulmonary arteriovenous malformations (AVMs), obstruction along the Fontan pathway (IVC-to-PA, SVC-to-PA, and PAs), and fenestrations.
- If a patient presents with a resistant arrhythmia, the patency of the Fontan circuit needs to be evaluated for obstruction.

Atrial Level Shunt

- Leads to RV volume overload
- Hemodynamic significance depends on the side of the defect and the left-to-right shunt.
- Pulmonary hypertension is common.
- ASD closure is indicated in patients with (Qp: pulmonary blood flow; Qs: systemic blood flow) → 1.5 with RV enlargement and without evidence of resting or exertional cyanosis. Contraindicated if mean pulmonary artery pressure (mPAP) >2/3 MAP (mean arterial pressure), PVR >2/3 SVR (either suggesting "irreversible pulmonary hypertension"), or primarily right-to-left shunt (ie, Eisenmenger syndrome).

Ventricular Level Shunt

- Leads to PA, left atrial (LA), and LV dilation
- Small ventricular septal defects (VSDs) usually have no clinical significance. Large VSDs may lead to pulmonary vascular disease and Eisenmenger syndrome.
- Associated with an increased risk of endocarditis

Eisenmenger Syndrome

- Most common causes of cyanotic CHDs in adults
- Eisenmenger syndrome refers to the process by which a congenital heart defect causes left-to-right shunting that leads to progressive right heart and pulmonary vascular hypertension, which eventually leads to right-to-left reversal of the shunt and cyanosis.

Tetralogy of Fallot

- The most common cyanotic congenital heart defect
- Four anatomic heart abnormalities: VSD, pulmonic stenosis, overriding aorta, and RV hypertrophy
- Presently, full repair of TOF is performed before 6 months of age with a low mortality (<2%). Complete surgical repair of TOF involves a VSD patch, RV outflow tract patch, and infundibular resection and/or pulmonic valvular repair.
- Common complications postrepair: pulmonary insufficiency leads to RV overload and dysfunction

Ebstein Anomaly

- An abnormality of the tricuspid valve in which the leaflets are apically displaced into the RV, with a malformed anterior leaflet abnormally attached to the RV free wall associated with atrialization of the RV
- 80% of patients with Ebstein have an intra-atrial communication through which right-to-left shunting may occur.
- Children may present as severely cyanotic with decompensated failure.
- Adults may present later in life with arrhythmia (Wolff-Parkinson-White [WPW] is common), dyspnea, or paradoxical embolization.
- Pathophysiology is determined by the degree of tricuspid involvement, the amount of right-to-left shunting, ventricular dysfunction, and the occurrence of tachyarrhythmias.

SUGGESTED READINGS

Baumgartner H, De Backer J, Babu-Narayan SV, et al. 2020 ESC guidelines for the management of adult congenital heart disease. *Eur Heart J*. 2021;42:563-645.

Buber J, Valle C, Valente AM. Common congenital heart problems in acute and intensive care. *Eur Heart J Acute Cardiovasc Care*. 2023;12:267-279.

Das T, Rampersad P, Ghobrial J. Caring for the critically ill adult congenital heart disease patient. *Curr Cardiol Rep*. 2024;26:283-291.

Gilboa SM, Salemi JL, Nembhard WN, Fixler DE, Correa A. Mortality resulting from congenital heart disease among children and adults in the United States, 1999 to 2006. *Circulation*. 2010;122:2254-2263.

Kendsersky P, Krasuski RA. Intensive care unit management of the adult with congenital heart disease. *Curr Cardiol Rep*. 2020;22:136.

Ramlakhan KP, van der Bie M, den Uil CA, Dubois EA, Roos-Hesselink JW. Adult patients with congenital heart disease in the intensive care unit. *Heart*. 2022;108:1452-1460.

Stout KK, Daniels CJ, Aboulhosn JA, et al. 2018 AHA/ACC guideline for the management of adults with congenital heart disease: a report of the American College of Cardiology/American Heart Association Task Force on Clinical Practice Guidelines. *Circulation*. 2019;139:e698-e800.

2.8

Cardiogenic Pulmonary Edema versus Noncardiogenic Pulmonary Edema

Roberta Ribeiro De Santis Santiago

Definition

- Pulmonary edema is the accumulation of fluids in the alveolar and/or interstitial spaces. The fluid (extravascular lung water—EVLW) can have a transudative or exudative composition depending on the concentration of protein/cells. It is etiologically classified as cardiogenic and noncardiogenic pulmonary edema.
- Pulmonary edema results from disturbances of the fluid net flow through the membrane between the vascular bed and alveolar/interstitial spaces (ie, hydrostatic pressure, oncotic pressure, vascular permeability, and surface area available for fluid movement) originally described as Starling forces.
- The pulmonary edema progression can be divided into:
- Stage 1 (*compensated*): the lymphatic drainage can counteract the fluid accumulation and keep the fluid net at zero.
- Stage 2 (*perihilar edema*): the lymphatic drainage can no longer compensate for the fluid accumulation. Edema is identified around bronchioles and lung vasculature and is represented radiologically by findings such as the Kerley B lines and peribronchial cuffing.
- Stage 3 (*alveolar edema*): initially around the alveolar membrane (stage 3a), evolving to the alveolar membrane rupture and flood (stage 3b).
- Etiology
    - *Cardiogenic pulmonary edema*: the fluid accumulation is generally due to increased left atrial pressures, resulting in relatively higher hydrostatic pressures of the pulmonary capillary bed in comparison to the hydrostatic pressures of the pulmonary interstitium and demonstrated by increased pulmonary artery wedge pressures (>18 mmHg). Conditions other than left cardiac dysfunction that can increase cardiac filling pressures include primary fluid overload, severe hypertension, and severe renal disease (Table 2.8.1).
- *Noncardiogenic pulmonary edema*: the fluid accumulation is due to injury or increased pulmonary capillary permeability demonstrated by a pulmonary artery wedge pressure <18 mmHg (Table 2.8.1).
- At the bedside, the distinction between cardiogenic and noncardiogenic pulmonary edema often cannot be made clinically. The pulmonary edema presentations frequently overlap, especially in patients with multiple comorbidities (Figure 2.8.1). When the underlying etiology of pulmonary edema is unclear, a pulmonary artery catheter can be placed, and the measurement of pulmonary artery wedge pressure helps differentiate between cardiogenic and noncardiogenic pulmonary edema (Table 2.8.2).

TABLE 2.8.1 Causes of Pulmonary Edema

Cardiogenic Pulmonary Edema
Acute myocardial ischemia/infarction
Systolic heart failure
Diastolic heart failure
Arrhythmias
Valvular dysfunction (aortic insufficiency, mitral regurgitation)
Cardiomyopathy (myocarditis, Takotsubo syndrome)
Cardiac tamponade
Other forms of "volume overload" (intake/output imbalances, renal failure, transfusion-associated circulatory overload [TACO])
Toxic/metabolic (scorpion venom, pheochromocytoma, β-blocker or calcium channel antagonist overdose)
Swimming induced (swimmers and divers)
Noncardiogenic Pulmonary Edema
ARDS
Pulmonary embolism
Transfusion-related acute lung injury (TRALI)
Drug toxicity (opioid, aspirin, tocolytic agents, chemotherapeutic agents, aerolized/inhaled agent)
Neurogenic
High altitude
Fat embolism syndrome
Amniotic fluid embolism
Engraftment syndrome (following stem cell transplant)
Ovarian hyperstimulation syndrome
Reexpansion

ARDS, acute respiratory distress syndrome.

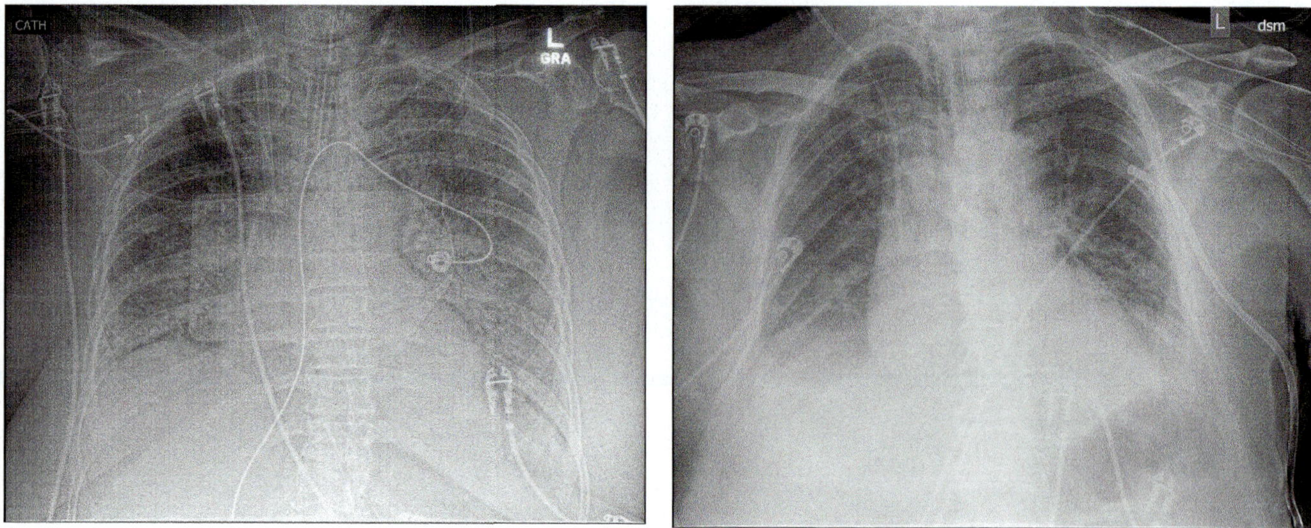

A B

FIGURE 2.8.1 **Two patients with multiple comorbidities and overlapping cardiogenic and noncardiogenic pulmonary edema. (A)** 51 y.o., female, underlying interstitial lung disease due to Sjögren syndrome. Acute respiratory failure secondary to acute respiratory failure secondary to pneumonia complicated with acute respiratory distress syndrome (ARDS) and cardiogenic component of pulmonary edema. **(B)** 71 y.o., male, underlying heart failure (ejection fraction of 30%) and pulmonary embolism. Acute respiratory failure secondary to angioedema complicated with ARDS.

Causes of Pulmonary Edema

See Table 2.8.1.

Epidemiology

Overall, true prevalence and incidence vary with underlying etiology. Regarding cardiogenic pulmonary edema, evidence shows an in-hospital mortality rate of 15% to 20%, 50% survival after 1 year, and 15% survival after 6 years.

Differential Diagnosis

TABLE 2.8.2 Differential Diagnosis

Cardiogenic Pulmonary Edema	Noncardiogenic Pulmonary Edema
Clinical presentation: • Setting of acute coronary syndrome • Patient with established heart failure noncompliant to medication and/or diet • Chest pain, orthopnea • Prolonged hospital stay with positive fluid net balance • Setting of multiple transfusions	Clinical presentation: • Setting of sepsis, pancreatitis • Medication overdose • Settings of multiple transfusions
Physical examination: • Lungs auscultation → bilateral crackles, abolished • Lungs percussion → dullness at pulmonary bases • Cardiac auscultation → S3 • Jugular vein dilation, positive hepatojugular reflex • Lower extremities edema	Physical examination: • Lungs auscultation → crackles • No signs of volume overload
Laboratory examinations: • Elevated plasma levels of BNP (brain natriuretic peptide) • Hemodilution • Elevated liver function markers (hepatic congestion) • Acute ST changes in the ECG	Laboratory examinations: • Normal plasma levels of BNP • No hemodilution • Unaltered liver function markers
Chest radiography: • Bilateral pleural effusion • Enlarged cardiac silhouette • Vascular cephalization ("bat wings") • Kerley B lines	Chest radiography: • Diffuse, bilateral infiltration • Regular cardiac silhouette • Lack of vascular cephalization ("bat wings") • Lack of Kerley B lines
Lung ultrasound: • Normal lung sliding • Ground glass rocket • Thin even pleural line • Homogeneous lung tissue • Transudative pleural effusion	Lung ultrasound: • Ground glass rocket • Thick/uneven pleural line • Inhomogeneous lung tissue • Lung tissue consolidation/air bronchogram • Transudative pleural effusion
Transpulmonary thermodilution • Elevated EVLW with increased cardiac preload	Transpulmonary thermodilution • Elevated EVLW with decreased cardiac preload

ECG, electrocardiogram; EVLW, extravascular lung water.

Management and Treatment

Cardiogenic Pulmonary Edema

Ultimately, all treatment options will address the underlying etiology of the exacerbation of left-sided heart disease.

- Appropriate supplemental oxygen. Oxygen therapy should be adjusted to treat hypoxemia and avoided if SpO2> 90%.
- *Assisted ventilation.* In the onset of respiratory distress with hypoxemia and/or acidosis, noninvasive positive

pressure should be considered (continuous or bilevel positive pressure ventilation). Studies have demonstrated multiple benefits (reduced mortality, reduced cost, reduced intubation rates) for the use of noninvasive positive pressure noninvasive positive pressure ventilation in managing cardiogenic pulmonary edema.
- *Diuretics.* The primary treatment is the intravenous administration of loop diuretics (eg, furosemide). Early initiation improves symptoms and may reduce mortality.
- *Vasodilators.* In patients not responding to diuretics, nitroglycerin may be added to the treatment to reduce preload and improve symptoms. In patients with increased afterload, nitroprusside can help reduce arterial tone.
- *Ultrafiltration.* Intervention may be considered in patients with volume overload who are resistant to diuretics and have renal dysfunction.
- Emergent cardiac catheterization, mitral or aortic valve repair/replacement

These interventions may be essential to addressing the primary cause of cardiogenic pulmonary edema.

Noncardiogenic Pulmonary Edema

- Evidence-based treatment options are limited, and supportive care (maintaining hemodynamics and optimizing respiratory function) is the mainstay.
- Treatment strategies are similar to those employed in the management of acute respiratory distress syndrome (ARDS).

SUGGESTED READINGS

Assaad S, Shelley B, Perrino A. Transpulmonary thermodilution: its role in assessment of lung water and pulmonary edema. *J Cardiothorac Vasc Anesth*. 2017;31(4):1471-1480.

Bello G, De Santis P, Antonelli M. Non-invasive ventilation in cardiogenic pulmonary edema. *Ann Transl Med*. 2018;6(18):355.

Briasoulis E, Pavlidis N. Noncardiogenic pulmonary edema: an unusual and serious complication of anticancer therapy. *Oncologist*. 2001;6(2):153-161.

Budev MM, Arroliga AC, Falcone T. Ovarian hyperstimulation syndrome. *Crit Care Med*. 2005;33(10 suppl):S301-S306.

Busl KM, Bleck TP. Neurogenic pulmonary edema. *Crit Care Med*. 2015;43(8):1710-1715.

Chadda K, Annane D, Hart N, Gajdos P, Raphaël JC, Lofaso F. Cardiac and respiratory effects of continuous positive airway pressure and noninvasive ventilation in acute cardiac pulmonary edema. *Crit Care Med*. 2002;30(11):2457-2461.

Crane SD. Epidemiology, treatment and outcome of acidotic, acute, cardiogenic pulmonary oedema presenting to an emergency department. *Eur J Emerg Med*. 2002;9(4):320-324.

De Backer D, Aissaoui N, Cecconi M, et al. How can assessing hemodynamics help to assess volume status? *Intensive Care Med*. 2022;48(10):1482-1494.

Ingbar DH. Cardiogenic pulmonary edema: mechanisms and treatment—an intensivist's view. *Curr Opin Crit Care*. 2019;25(4):371-378.

Lee-Chiong T, Matthay RA. Drug-induced pulmonary edema and acute respiratory distress syndrome. *Clin Chest Med*. 2004;25(1):95-104.

Lichtenstein DA, Mezière GA. Relevance of lung ultrasound in the diagnosis of acute respiratory failure: the blue protocol. *Chest*. 2008;134(1):117-125.

Semple JW, Rebetz J, Kapur R. Transfusion-associated circulatory overload and transfusion-related acute lung injury. *Blood*. 2019;133(17):1840-1853.

Spitzer TR. Engraftment syndrome following hematopoietic stem cell transplantation. *Bone Marrow Transplant*. 2001;27(9):893-898.

Ware LB, Matthay MA. Clinical practice. Acute pulmonary edema. *N Engl J Med*. 2005;353(26):2788-2796.

2.9

Systemic Hypertension

Sumeet A. Khetarpal and Randall M. Zusman

Definitions (American College of Cardiology/American Heart Association 2025 guidelines)

- Normal blood pressure (BP)—systolic BP (SBP) <120 mm Hg and diastolic BP (DBP) <80 mm Hg
- Elevated BP—SBP 120 to 129 mm Hg and DBP <80
- Stage 1 hypertension (HTN): SBP 130 to 139 mm Hg or DBP 80 to 89 mm Hg
- Stage 2 HTN: SBP ≥140 mm Hg or DBP ≥90 mm Hg
- Severe HTN: SBP ≥180 mm Hg and/or DBP ≥120 mm Hg
  - Hypertensive urgency: severe HTN in an asymptomatic patient or associated with mild headache but *no* symptoms or evidence of acute end-organ malperfusion
  - Hypertensive emergency: severe HTN and concomitant end-organ malperfusion

Additional Hypertensive Conditions

- Postoperative HTN: SBP >190 mm Hg and/or DBP >110 mm Hg on two consecutive measurements following surgery; usually begins 30 minutes after the operation and lasts 2 hours
  - *Risk factors:* chronic baseline HTN, pain, delirium with agitation, hypothermia with shivering, distended bladder, nausea and vomiting, withdrawal from opioids or alcohol, unrecognized baseline obstructive sleep apnea contributing to hypercarbia and hypoxemia
- Hypertensive disorders in pregnancy:
  - Gestational HTN: new onset SBP ≥140 mm Hg and/or DBP ≥90 mm Hg on at least two occasions separated by 4 hours after 20 weeks of gestation in an individual who was previously normotensive prior to pregnancy AND no proteinuria or signs/symptoms of preeclampsia associated with end-organ malperfusion
  - Preeclampsia: BP criteria of gestational HTN along with proteinuria ≥300 mg per 24-hour collection or urine protein:creatinine ratio ≥0.3 or urine dipstick ≥2+ protein

- Preeclampsia with severe features: preeclampsia with SBP ≥160 mm Hg and/or DBP ≥110 mm Hg (two separate occasions separated by 4 hours), or preeclampsia with signs/symptoms of end-organ malperfusion
  - Thrombocytopenia (platelet count <100,000/μL)
  - Transaminase elevation ≥2× upper limit of normal and/or severe persistent right upper quadrant pain not accounted for by other etiologies
  - Acute kidney injury (serum creatinine >1.1 mg/dL)
  - Pulmonary edema
  - Persistent cerebral or visual disturbances
- Eclampsia: preeclampsia accompanied by generalized seizure not attributable to other diagnoses
- HELLP syndrome: *H*emolysis, *E*levated *L*iver enzymes, and *L*ow *P*latelets: features identified in patient with preeclampsia indicate increased rates of maternal and neonatal morbidity and mortality

Epidemiology

- HTN affects ~30% of the US population.
- Increased prevalence among males, Black adults, old age, obesity, chronic kidney disease, diabetes, excessive alcohol consumption
- Hypertensive crisis is seen in only 1% of all hypertensive cases.
- Incidence of postoperative HTN varies from 4% to 35%.
- Preeclampsia is seen in 5% of pregnancies.

Pathophysiology

- Perfusion of the brain, heart, and kidney remains relatively constant in the setting of normally fluctuating BP due to vascular autoregulation.
- With prolonged severe HTN, autoregulatory vasoconstriction protects the vital organs from excessive pressure and creates a new homeostatic set point.
- End-organ malperfusion associated with hypertensive emergency reflects failure of normal autoregulation along with abrupt changes in systemic vascular resistance.
- Concurrent endovascular injury with fibrinoid necrosis of arterioles results in vascular occlusion and ischemia, platelet dysfunction, as well as production of vasoactive intermediates results in further disruption of autoregulation.

Differential Diagnosis

- Primary (essential) HTN
  - Most common cause of hypertensive urgency or emergency due to the prevalence of primary HTN in the population
- Secondary HTN
  - Renal etiologies: (account for 80% of secondary HTN): renovascular disease (renal artery stenosis), parenchymal disease (glomerulonephritis)
  - Neurologic etiologies: central nervous system (CNS) trauma, cerebrovascular accident (CVA), autonomic hyperreactivity, spinal cord injury, Guillain-Barré syndrome (GBS)
  - Endocrine etiologies: renin- or aldosterone-secreting tumors, pheochromocytoma, hypothyroidism or hyperthyroidism, Cushing syndrome
  - Autoimmune etiologies: vasculitis, collagen vascular disorders (eg, scleroderma)
  - Medication/toxin-mediated etiologies: neuroleptic malignant syndrome, serotonin syndrome, cocaine and amphetamines, alcohol withdrawal
  - Pregnancy-related etiologies: (see earlier)
  - Anatomic causes: coarctation of the aorta

Clinical Features

- Major organs affected include brain, eyes, heart, great vessels, kidneys, and gravid uterus.
- Single-organ involvement in 83% cases, two organs in 14% cases, and three or more organs in only 3%
- Common features
  - Cerebral infarction (24.5%)
  - Intracerebral (ICH) or subarachnoid hemorrhage (4.5%)
  - Hypertensive encephalopathy (16.3%)
  - Acute congestive heart failure (14.3%)
  - Left ventricular hypertrophy (6.3%-18.3%)
  - Acute myocardial infarction or unstable angina (12.0%)
  - Aortic dissection (2%)
  - Acute pulmonary edema (22.4%)
  - Eclampsia (2%)
  - Retinopathy marked by papilledema, retinal hemorrhages, and exudates

Evaluation

- Initial evaluation includes clinical examination and measurement of chemistries (particularly K^+ and Ca^{2+}), renal function, urinalysis, electrocardiogram (ECG), and chest x-ray (CXR).
- Signs and symptoms concerning for aortic dissection (severe, sharp, ripping or tearing chest, abdominal, or back pain or pain radiating to the back) require emergent imaging.

Management of Hypertensive Emergencies

- *Overall:* avoid rapid swings in BP and hypoperfusion of already damaged end organs.
  - For most cases, mean arterial pressure (MAP) should be reduced by no >10% to 20% in the first hour and subsequently by 5% to 15% over the initial 24-hour period. This usually achieves the target BP of <180/<120 mm Hg for the first hour and <160/<110 mm Hg by 24 hours.
- Verify accuracy of BP result: appropriately sized cuff with manual sphygmomanometry
- Consider the need for continuous intra-arterial BP monitoring (particularly necessary if considering bolus or continuous intravenous vasoactive medication administration).
- Assess for etiologies for reactive HTN: pain, anxiety, urinary retention, sympathomimetics, or drug or alcohol withdrawal.
- *Management goals* depend on involved end organs and underlying etiology.
  - Hypertensive encephalopathy, CVA, ICH: avoid hypoperfusion; do not decrease BP >20%; no clear benefit of BP reduction in ischemic stroke.

- Agents of choice: nicardipine decreases cerebral ischemia; favor ultrashort-acting therapies given the consequences of hypoperfusion (esmolol, nitroprusside).
- Acute congestive heart failure or pulmonary edema: reduce BP via vasodilation and diuresis
  - Agents of choice: intravenous (IV) nitrates (low doses dilate capacitance vessels, higher doses dilate arterioles and lower BP), morphine, IV angiotensin-converting enzyme inhibitor (ACE-I), IV diuretics
- Acute coronary syndrome: reduce BP (decreases afterload and myocardial oxygen demand)
  - Agents of choice: IV nitrates and IV beta-blockers
- Aortic dissection: reduce BP and shear force (decrease heart rate [HR])
  - Agents of choice: (initially) IV beta-blocker to decrease shear force; other antihypertensives (IV nitroprusside); avoid reflex tachycardia by starting beta-blocker first.
  - Continuous intra-arterial BP monitoring is necessary.
- Sympathomimetic intoxication: reduce sympathomimetic drive with benzodiazepines, IV nitroglycerin, IV hydralazine; avoid isolated beta-blockade resulting in unopposed alpha receptor activity, particularly with cocaine

Selected Antihypertensive Agents

- Labetalol: combination alpha-1 blocker and nonselective beta-blocker; onset 2 to 5 minutes and duration of action 2 to 4 hours; metabolized by liver; IV load with 20 mg, then infusion at 1 to 2 mg/min
- Esmolol: ultrashort-acting beta-blocker; onset 60 seconds, duration of action 10 to 20 minutes; IV 0.5 to 1 mg/kg load over 1 minute, then infusion at 50 g/kg/min up to 300 g/kg/min
- Nicardipine: dihydropyridine-derived calcium channel blocker, onset of action in 5 to 15 minutes with duration of action 4 to 6 hours; crosses blood blood-brain barrier; dosing independent of weight, starting at 5 mg/h IV infusion
- Nitroprusside: arterial and venous vasodilator; impairs cerebral and cardiac blood flow and increases intracranial pressure (ICP); onset within seconds; duration of action 1 to 2 minutes; can result in cyanide toxicity
- Hydralazine: direct vasodilator, onset of 5 to 15 minutes, can last for 12 hours
- Fenoldopam: short-acting dopamine (D1) agonist that increases renal perfusion and sodium excretion; onset 5 minutes with maximal effect at 15 minutes and duration of action between 30 to 60 minutes; 0.1 g/kg/min to start; particularly useful for HTN emergencies primarily presenting with acute renal failure (acute hypertensive nephrosclerosis)

Outcomes

- Long-term risk of cardiovascular disease begins at BP 115/75 and doubles with each increment of 20/10 mm Hg.
- Despite effective therapy, most patients with a history of hypertensive emergency have moderate-to-severe chronic vascular damage with associated risk for coronary, renal, and cerebrovascular disease.
- First large natural history study of hypertensive emergency in the era prior to widespread antihypertensive use demonstrated a 1-year mortality of 79% and median survival of 10.5 months.
- More recent data demonstrate 70% survival at 5 years, lower survival with chronic kidney disease.

SUGGESTED READINGS

Ault MJ, Ellrodt AG. Pathophysiological events leading to the end-organ effects of acute hypertension. *Am J Emerg Med*. 1985;3:10-15.

Carey RM, Moran AE, Whelton PK. Treatment of hypertension: a review. *JAMA*. 2022;328:1849.

Flanigan JS, Vitberg D. Hypertensive emergency and severe hypertension: what to treat, who to treat, and how to treat. *Med Clin North Am*. 2006;90:439-451.

Flint AC, Conell C, Ren X, et al. Effect of systolic and diastolic blood pressure on cardiovascular outcomes. *N Engl J Med*. 2019;381:243.

Fuchs FD, Maestri MK, Bredemeier M, et al. Study of the usefulness of optic fundi examination of patients with hypertension in a clinical setting. *J Hum Hypertens*. 1995;9:547-551.

Gal TJ, Cooperman LH. Hypertension in the immediate postoperative period. *Br J Anaesth*. 1975;47:70-74.

James PA, Oparil S, Carter BL, et al. 2014 evidence-based guideline for the management of high blood pressure in adults: report from the panel members appointed to the Eighth Joint National Committee (JNC 8). *JAMA*. 2014;311:507.

Levy D, Larson MG, Vasan RS, et al. The progression from hypertension to congestive heart failure. *JAMA*. 1996;275:1557.

Rodriguez MA, Kumar SK, De Caro M. Hypertensive crisis. *Cardiol Rev*. 2010;18:102-107.

Slama M, Modeliar SS. Hypertension in the intensive care unit. *Curr Opin Cardiol*. 2006;21:279-287.

Staessen JA, Wang J, Bianchi G, Birkenhäger WH. Essential hypertension. *Lancet*. 2003;361:1629.

Vakili BA, Okin PM, Devereux RB. Prognostic implications of left ventricular hypertrophy. *Am Heart J*. 2001;141:334.

Whelton PK, Carey RM, Aronow WS, et al. 2025 ACC/AHA/AAPA/ABC/ACPM/AGS/APhA/ASH/ASPC/NMA/PCNA guideline for the prevention, detection, evaluation, and management of high blood pressure in adults: a report of the American College of Cardiology/American Heart Association task force on clinical practice guidelines. *https://www.ahajournals.org/doi/10.1161/HYP.0000000000000249*

2.10

Pulmonary Hypertension

Gabriel Fregoso and Marvin G. Chang

Definition

- Pulmonary hypertension (PH): mean pulmonary arterial pressure (mPAP) of >20 mm Hg (previously ≥25 mm Hg), measured at rest by right heart catheterization
- PH can be classified into five groups based on etiology and hemodynamics (pre- and postcapillary PH).
- In PH, right ventricular (RV) afterload is increased due to elevated pulmonary pressures, which can lead to RV dysfunction and ultimately RV failure.
- Long-term treatment of PH is group specific, aimed at addressing the underlying condition while improving pulmonary vascular resistance (PVR) and RV function.

Diagnostics and Differential Diagnosis

- The gold standard for the diagnosis of PH is invasive hemodynamics with right heart catheterization and can help distinguish precapillary from postcapillary etiologies of PH.
- Echocardiography is useful for screening and identifying possible PH and can be used to estimate PAPs and assess RV function.
  - Precapillary PH: mPAP >20 mm Hg, pulmonary capillary wedge pressure (PCWP) ≤15 mm Hg, and PVR >2 Woods Units (WU); World Health Organization (WHO) groups I, III, and IV
  - Postcapillary PH: mPAP >20 mm Hg, PCWP >15 mm Hg, and PVR <2 WU; WHO group II and pulmonary veno-occlusive disease (PVOD)
  - High cardiac output associated PH: mPAP >20 mm Hg, low PCWP <15 mm Hg, low PVR ≤2 WU; typically secondary to systemic conditions such as hyperthyroidism, anemia, pregnancy, liver failure, or sepsis, where increased cardiac output leads to elevated pulmonary pressures without significant increases in PVR
- PH encompasses heterogeneous diseases that cause elevations in PAPs that are classified into the five WHO groups based on underlying etiology (Table 2.10.1).
- WHO classification
- Additional clinical data that can aid in the diagnosis of PH prior to diagnosis with right heart catheterization include the following:
  - Symptoms
    - Dyspnea, fatigue, syncope or presyncope, chest pain, palpitations, or edema
    - Syncope/presyncope is particularly concerning.
  - Physical examination findings
    - Related to elevated pulmonary pressures
      - Loud P2, tricuspid regurgitation and pulmonic regurgitation murmur, RV S4

TABLE 2.10.1 WHO Classification

Group	Description	Treatment
Group I Pulmonary arterial hypertension, PVOD, and pulmonary capillary hemangiomatosis (PCH)	Pulmonary arterial hypertensions: idiopathic, familiar, or "associated." The latter includes collagen vascular diseases, portal hypertension, HIV, congenital left-to-right shunt, drugs and toxins, PVOD, and PCH.	PAH-specific treatments
Group II Left-sided heart disease	LV systolic failure (HFrEF), diastolic dysfunction (HFpEF), and valvular disease (ie, mitral or aortic valve disease)	Treatment of underlying heart disease
Group III Primary lung disease or hypoxemia	COPD, ILDs, sleep-disordered breathing, exposure to high altitudes	Treatment of underlying lung disease
Group IV Embolic	Thromboembolic (PE or chronic PE) as well as nonthrombotic (tumor, parasites)	Anticoagulation, balloon pulmonary angioplasty, surgical intervention
Group V "Others"	Includes sarcoidosis, lymphangiomatosis	Dependent on specific condition

COPD, chronic obstructive pulmonary disorder; HFrEF, heart failure with reduced ejection fraction; HIV, human immunodeficiency virus; ILD, interstitial lung disease; LV, left ventricle; PAH, pulmonary arterial hypertension; PE, pulmonary embolism; PVOD, pulmonary veno-occlusive disorder; WHO, World Health Organization.

    - Related to RV failure: jugular vein distention (JVD), ascites, hepatomegaly, edema
  - Electrocardiogram (ECG) findings
    - RV hypertrophy: right atrial (RA) dilation, RV hypertrophy, and dilation, RV strain
      - S1Q3T3 pattern: S-wave in lead I, Q-wave and inverted T-wave in lead III
  - Imaging findings
    - Chest x-ray (CXR): RV enlargement, proximal vascular enlargement, peripheral hypovascularity
    - Computed tomography (CT) findings: RV enlargement, PA enlargement (PA should not be larger than the aorta)
  - NT-BNP can be used to track disease progression and has prognostic value in determining disease severity.
  - Findings on echocardiogram
    - RV pressures (RV systolic pressure or RVSP) are estimated based on tricuspid regurgitation jet velocity and central venous pressure (CVP), which can be used to estimate the pressure difference between the RA and RV, and reflect the pulmonary artery systolic pressure (PASP), provided there is no pulmonary valve (PV) disease or RV outflow obstruction.
    - RV hypertrophy is often present in chronic PH.
    - RV hypokinesis, RV dilation, and RA dilation may suggest advanced disease or acute decompensation.
    - Left atrial (LA) enlargement may suggest elevated left-sided etiology contributing to PH.

        - Reduced PV velocity-time integral (VTI) and pulmonary acceleration time (PAT) suggest RV dysfunction and increased pulmonary pressures, respectively. The PV VTI waveform with significant notching (W wave) may also indicate significantly elevated pulmonary pressures.
        - D-shaped septum during systole suggests RV pressure overload, while during diastole suggests RV volume overload. Both impair left ventricular (LV) filling, reflecting ventricular interdependence, which may be due to PH.
        - Tricuspid Annular Plane Systolic Excursion (TAPSE), RV systolic velocity (RV S′), and RV strain are important echocardiographic markers of RV function in PH. A reduced TAPSE, decreased RV S′ velocity, and impaired RV strain suggest RV dysfunction, which may be secondary to increased RV afterload from elevated pulmonary pressures. These measurements may provide valuable insights into the severity of RV impairment and prognosis in these patients.
        - Examine for anatomic causes, including shunts (ie, patent foramen ovale) and valvular abnormalities (ie, tricuspid regurgitation, PV insufficiency, and mitral/aortic valve disease), which can impact RV afterload and volume overload, potentially contributing to PH.
- Standard workup is aimed at classification, assessing underlying etiology, and establishing a baseline disease severity. This typically includes ECG, CXR, echocardiogram, CT angiography, $\dot{V}/\dot{Q}$ scan, pulmonary function tests (PFTs), sleep studies, human immunodeficiency virus (HIV), antinuclear antibody (ANA), and liver function tests (LFTs).
- CT angiography is generally preferred to $\dot{V}/\dot{Q}$ scans for diagnosing chronic thromboembolic disease (CTED) due to its higher sensitivity in detecting thromboembolic obstructions and detailed anatomic information. However, $\dot{V}/\dot{Q}$ scans are still used in certain situations, such as when CT imaging may be less feasible (eg, contrast allergy, renal failure, and pregnancy, considering the associated risks and benefits) or when CT angiography is inconclusive.

Epidemiology

- Global prevalence of PH is 1%.
    - Most common etiologies include WHO groups II and III.
    - Groups I, IV, and V are rare causes of PH.
    - Group I is more common in women. Many subtypes of pulmonary arterial hypertension (PAH) have significant family associations.
    - Many patients have a concomitant presence of connective tissue diseases, HIV, interstitial lung disease, thromboembolic disease, and liver disease.
- Mortality is worsened in PH with increasing mPAP and WU, independent of WHO group subtype.
    - Multiple calculators have been developed for disease severity classification based on symptoms, functional status, and other clinical data. Worsening disease severity calculation predicts increased mortality, with <50% of patients with high disease severity classification having 5-year transplant-free survival.
    - Poor prognostic indicators include high New York Heart Association (NYHA) functional class, low 6-mile walking distance, low exercise oxygen consumption, tachycardia, low systolic blood pressure (SBP), increasing mPAP or mean right atrial pressure (RAP), decreased cardiac index, presence of ANY pericardial effusion, RA/RV enlargement, renal failure, and high NT-BNP.
    - Prognosis is dependent on the etiology of PH.

Key Pathophysiology

- PAH
    - Pathophysiology involves vascular remodeling leading to decreased luminal cross-section.
    - Vasoconstriction can play a role in ~20% of patients.
- Precapillary PH
    - Similar to PAH, but the underlying etiology of increased PVR due to decreased cross-sectional area is secondary to disease-specific processes seen in WHO group III (chronic lung disease or sleep apnea) and group IV (chronic thromboembolic pulmonary hypertension, or CTEPH), where the increased resistance results from vascular obstruction (as seen in CTEPH) or hypoxia-induced vascular remodeling (as seen in chronic lung disease or sleep apnea).
- Postcapillary PH
    - Most often secondary to elevated LA pressures
- RV response and decompensation to PH
    - While the disease is often diagnosed and monitored in terms of elevated PAPs, it is usually the eventual decompensation of the RV that leads to symptoms. Thus, if the rise in pressure is gradual, patients can often tolerate much higher pressures with less symptoms.
    - RV decompensation can occur with both volume overload and insufficient preload.
    - In cases of fluid overload and acute decompensation due to a sudden increase in PAP, the RV dilates. This leads to decreased RV output, impaired coronary perfusion (due to RV dilation), potential ischemic injury, and decreased LV output due to interventricular septal bowing of the RV into the LV chamber.
- Falling cardiac output suggests advanced disease or acute decompensation.
- Increased cardiac output, particularly when coupled with normal/decreased PVR and normal PCWP, suggests a physiologic response to a systemic condition (sepsis, anemia, liver failure, thyrotoxicosis, pregnancy).

Management and Treatment

- PAH-specific therapies: three classes of drugs aimed at treating pathophysiology associated with PAH. Although approved mostly for group I disease, their applications outside this have been expanding, particularly for diseases that include crossover between classes.
    - Calcium channel blockers, though not PAH specific, can help control mild-to-moderate PH in patients with a positive vasodilatory challenge.
        - Improved survival for responders
        - Vasodilatory challenge
            - Can use inhaled nitric oxide (iNO), epoprostenol, or adenosine during right heart catheterization
            - A positive response is a 20% fall in PAP/PVR.

- Prostacyclin analogs
  - Include epoprostenol (infusion), treprostinil (infusion, subcutaneous, inhaled, and oral), iloprost (inhaled), and oral selexipag
  - Continuous intravenous epoprostenol (Flolan) is the oldest of the PAH-specific medications and has been shown to improve hemodynamics, 6-minute walk test, and survival in severe PAH (idiopathic PAH/familial).
  - Epoprostenol is the only drug that has directly shown improved survival. Other PAH-specific medications have trials that have shown improvement in surrogate measures, such as symptoms, 6-minute walk test, and improved hemodynamics.
- NO-soluble guanylate cyclase-cGMP pathway
  - Phosphodiesterase 5 (PDE5) inhibitors include sildenafil and tadalafil.
  - Soluble guanylate cyclase analogs include riociguat.
  - Have been shown to improve symptoms, exercise tolerance, hemodynamics
- Endothelin receptor antagonists bosentan, ambrisentan, and macitentan
  - Have been shown to improve symptoms, exercise tolerance, hemodynamics
- Sotatercept: new antiproliferative specifically targeting pulmonary vasculature by modulating the activin receptor signaling pathway, which plays a role in vascular remodeling
- Approved 2024 for the treatment of PAH; significant improvements in hemodynamics, functional status, and event-free survival

- Combination therapy in PAH leads to improved functional and mortality outcomes compared to monotherapy. Initial combination therapy, particularly with endothelin receptor antagonists and PDE5 inhibitors, is now recommended for most patients with PAH.
- Treatment of non-group I disease
  - Group II disease: if secondary to left-sided heart disease, treatment involves correcting it (diuresis, surgery to correct valves, reducing left-sided afterload).
  - Group III disease: treat underlying lung disease, optimize oxygenation, and consider pulmonary rehabilitation. Supplemental oxygen therapy can improve exercise capacity and symptoms and may also improve survival in chronic hypoxemic lung disease–associated PH.
  - Group IV disease: for thromboembolic disease, anticoagulation should be considered. For CTEPH, a multidisciplinary approach is recommended and may also involve consideration of balloon angioplasty (BPA) or pulmonary endarterectomy, depending on operability. Pulmonary endarterectomy has shown particularly favorable results when performed at specialized centers.
- Atrial septotomy: creates a shunt between the right and left circulation, which improves cardiac output but worsens systemic oxygenation. High morbidity
- Organ transplant
  - Lung transplants have been shown to be helpful in some subgroups of end-stage PAH, PVOD, and group III disease and can be considered in many other subgroups as well.
  - Liver transplantation is often helpful in portopulmonary disease.
  - PH is no longer an absolute contraindication to liver transplant.
- Monitoring
  - Periodic assessment of functional class and 6-minute walk test, and echocardiogram
  - The 6-minute walk test measures the "unencouraged" distance walked in 6 minutes as well as oxygen saturation during the test. It is the standard metric for assessing the functional status of patients with PH and correlates with disease severity and prognosis.
- PH and intensive care unit (ICU)
  - Very challenging because fluid overload and mechanical ventilation both worsen RV failure
  - The RV (particularly in PH) cannot accommodate sudden increases in higher pressures and dilates.
  - RV dilation also leads to RV ischemia (and thus further dysfunction), LV dysfunction through septal bowing, and exacerbation of right-to-left shunts that may contribute to hypoxemia.
  - This ultimately leads to circulatory failure.
  - General approach is based on the type of insult as well as etiology of PH.
  - Expert consultation is recommended.
  - Specifics to keep in mind
    - Mechanical ventilation: high positive end-expiratory pressure (PEEP) and large tidal volumes both can lead to increased PVR and decreased RV function in already decompensated patients. Hypoxemia should be minimized as hypoxic vasoconstriction increases PVR. Additionally, permissive hypercapnia can further increase PVR and worsen RV function.
    - Choice of pressors in right heart failure:
      - Milrinone not only reduces PVR but also decreases systemic vascular resistance (SVR), which can improve RV function in PH, although it may lead to systemic hypotension.
      - Dobutamine and epinephrine provide RV inotropic support to improve RV output.
      - Vasopressin increases SVR without directly affecting PVR, helping to maintain systemic pressures higher than pulmonary pressures, thus preventing cardiovascular collapse.
    - Volume status and management: careful fluid resuscitation is necessary to avoid RV volume overload.
    - iNO, inhaled epoprostenol, and intravenous (IV) epoprostenol can be considered to lower PVR acutely.
    - Acute RV failure in the ICU requires prompt recognition and management, as delays can lead to irreversible circulatory collapse. Mechanical circulatory support may be considered in refractory cases.

SUGGESTED READINGS

Andreassen AK, Ragnhild W, Svein S, et al. N-terminal pro-B-type natriuretic peptide as an indicator of disease severity in a heterogeneous group of patients with chronic precapillary pulmonary hypertension. *Am J Cardiol*. 2006;98(4):525-529.

Badesch DB, Champion HC, Sanchez MA, et al. Diagnosis and assessment of pulmonary arterial hypertension. *J Am Coll Cardiol*. 2009;54(1 suppl):S55-S66.

Barnett CF, O'Brien C, De Marco T. Critical care management of the patient with pulmonary hypertension. *Eur Heart J Acute Cardiovasc Care*. 2022;11(1):77-83.

Barst RJ, Gibbs JS, Ghofrani HA, et al. Updated evidence-based treatment algorithm in pulmonary arterial hypertension. *J Am Coll Cardiol*. 2009;54(1 suppl):S78-S84.

Barst RJ, McGoon M, Torbicki A, et al. Diagnosis and differential assessment of pulmonary arterial hypertension. *J Am Coll Cardiol*. 2004;43 (12 suppl):40S-47S.

Benza RL, Miller DP, Gomberg-Maitland M, et al. Predicting survival in pulmonary arterial hypertension: insights from the registry to evaluate early and long-term pulmonary arterial hypertension disease management (REVEAL). *Circulation*. 2010;122(2):164-172.

Chang KY, Duval S, Badesch DB, et al. Mortality in pulmonary arterial hypertension in the modern era: early insights from the Pulmonary Hypertension Association Registry. *J Am Heart Assoc*. 2022;11(9):e024969.

Condliffe R, Kiely DG. Critical care management of pulmonary hypertension. *BJA Educ*. 2017;17(7):228-234.

Galiè N, Barberà JA, Frost AE, et al. Initial use of ambrisentan plus tadalafil in pulmonary arterial hypertension. *N Eng J Med*. 2015;373(9):834-844.

Humbert M, Kovacs G, Hoeper MM, et al. 2022 ESC/ERS guidelines for the diagnosis and treatment of pulmonary hypertension. *Eur Respir J*. 2023;61(1):2200879.

Marius HM, Badesch DB, Ghofrani H, et al. Phase 3 trial of sotatercept for treatment of pulmonary arterial hypertension. *N Engl J Med*. 2023; 388(16):1478-1490.

Maron BA. Revised definition of pulmonary hypertension and approach to management: a clinical primer. *J Am Heart Assoc*. 2023;12(8):e029024.

Maron BA, Brittain EL, Hess E, et al. Pulmonary vascular resistance and clinical outcomes in patients with pulmonary hypertension: a retrospective cohort study. *Lancet Respir Med*. 2020;8(9):873-884.

Maron BA, Hess E, Maddox TM, et al. Association of borderline pulmonary hypertension with mortality and hospitalization in a large patient cohort: insights from the Veterans Affairs Clinical Assessment, Reporting, and Tracking Program. *Circulation*. 2016;133(13):1240-1248.

McGoon M, Gutterman D, Steen V, et al. Screening, early detection, and diagnosis of pulmonary arterial hypertension: ACCP evidence-based clinical practice guidelines. *Chest*. 2004;126:14S-34S.

McLaughlin VV, Archer SL, Badesch DB, et al. ACCF/AHA 2009 expert consensus document on pulmonary hypertension a report of the American College of Cardiology foundation task force on expert consensus documents and the American Heart Association developed in collaboration with the American College of Chest Physicians; American Thoracic Society, Inc.; and the Pulmonary Hypertension Association. *J Am Coll Cardiol*. 2009;53:1573-1619.

McLaughlin VV, Presberg KW, Doyle RL, et al. Prognosis of pulmonary arterial hypertension: ACCP evidence-based clinical practice guidelines. *Chest*. 2004;126:78S-92S.

Rich S, Dantzker DR, Ayres SM, et al. Primary pulmonary hypertension: a national prospective study. *Ann Intern Med*. 1987;107:216-223.

Stringham R, Shah NR. Pulmonary arterial hypertension: an update on diagnosis and treatment. *Am Fam Phys*. 2010;82(4):370-377.

Tapson VF, Humbert M. Incidence and prevalence of chronic thromboembolic pulmonary hypertension: from acute to chronic pulmonary embolism. *Proc Am Thorac Soc*. 2006;3(7):564-567.

Zamanian RT, Haddad F, Doyle RL, Weinacker AB. Management strategies for patients with pulmonary hypertension in the intensive care unit. *Crit Care Med*. 2007;35(9):2037-2050.

2.11

Aneurysms and Dissections

Avanthi Raghavan and Eric M. Isselbacher

Aortic Aneurysms

- Conventional definition of an aneurysm is abnormal dilation of an artery to >50% of its expected diameter.
  - This definition is most applicable to the descending thoracic and abdominal aorta.
  - For the ascending aorta, aneurysm is more accurately defined as a diameter ≥4.5 cm.
- The risk of acute aortic syndromes increases with increasing diameter.
- The anatomic site of an aneurysm provides clues about the underlying etiology (Table 2.11.1).
- Aneurysm can also be described according to morphology:
  - Symmetric, circumferential dilation: *fusiform*
  - Localized outpouching of a portion of the wall: *saccular*

TABLE 2.11.1 Etiology: Aneurysm

Anatomic Site	Common Causes

Ascending thoracic aortic aneurysm (TAA)
• Includes aortic root and ascending aortic aneurysms up to the innominate artery
	• Typically due to a heritable or congenital etiology:
	  • Heritable cases can be syndromic (associated with a connective tissue disorder, such as Marfan or Loeys-Dietz syndrome) or nonsyndromic
	  • Congenital: bicuspid aortic valve (most common), coarctation, Turner syndrome
	• Inflammation (Takayasu arteritis, giant cell arteritis)
	• Infection
	• Thoracic trauma
	• Previous aortic dissection
	• Hypertension, atherosclerosis, and degenerative disease less common

Descending TAA • Arises distal to the left subclavian artery, to the diaphragm	• Typically due to degenerative disease and atherosclerosis
Abdominal aortic aneurysm (AAA) • Below the diaphragm, generally infrarenal (75%)	• Typically occurs in the context of atherosclerosis; smoking is an important risk factor.

Epidemiology

- Thoracic aortic aneurysm (TAA) has a prevalence of <1%, compared to 3% to 8% for abdominal aortic aneurysm (AAA).
- Both TAA and AAA occur disproportionately in men compared to women.
- Ascending TAA is generally diagnosed at an earlier age compared to descending TAA.

Key Pathophysiology

- Most cases of aneurysm are slowly progressive and result from gradual expansion of the aorta over an individual's lifetime.
  - Exception is certain acquired etiologies (infection, trauma, and inflammatory conditions).
- Cystic medial necrosis is the classic pathologic finding in aneurysm and results from smooth muscle dysfunction and extracellular matrix breakdown.

Presenting Symptoms and Diagnosis

- Most cases are clinically silent.
- Aortic root or ascending aortic aneurysms may be complicated by aortic regurgitation.
  - In these cases, clinical presentation may include congestive heart failure.
- Large TAA may cause symptoms related to mass effect or compression of adjacent structures.
  - Chest pain
  - Hoarseness due to stretching of the recurrent laryngeal nerve
  - Dysphagia due to esophageal compression
  - Stridor and dyspnea due to pressure on the left main bronchus
- TAA, however, is typically an incidental finding on imaging performed for another purpose.
  - Chest radiograph
    - Prominent right aortic border on the anteroposterior view in cases of ascending aortic aneurysm
    - Mediastinal widening
    - Enlarged descending aorta in the lateral view in cases of descending aortic aneurysm
  - Echocardiography
    - Transthoracic echocardiography for measurement of the aortic root and ascending aorta, aortic valve anatomy, aortic regurgitation, ventricular function
    - Limited visualization of the aortic arch and descending aorta
  - Axial imaging, including computed tomography (CT) and magnetic resonance imaging (MRI) with three-dimensional reconstruction:
    - Both modalities allow imaging of the entire aorta and its branches.
    - Advantage of CT is fast acquisition time; disadvantages are radiation exposure and need for iodinated contrast for optimal visualization of the vessel lumen.
- AAA may rarely present as a pulsatile mass on abdominal examination.
- AAA is more commonly detected via screening ultrasonography of at-risk individuals (older age, male, smoking history, and family history).

Management and Treatment

- Management includes strict blood pressure control and periodic surveillance imaging until the aortic size reaches prophylactic repair thresholds, or the patient has an acute aortic syndrome.
  - Elective repair thresholds depend on a complex interplay of factors, but generally range from 5.0 to 5.5 cm, and may be even lower in certain cases of inherited aortic aneurysm.
- TAA
  - Ascending TAA is managed with an open surgical approach.
    - Aneurysmal aortic segment is excised and replaced with a graft.
      - Choose aortic valve–sparing root replacement procedure versus composite graft (ie, graft that includes a prosthetic aortic valve), depending on the presence and severity of native valve disease.
      - Aortic root replacement requires coronary reimplantation.
  - Aortic arch aneurysm is managed with an open surgical approach.
    - Hemiarch replacement does not involve arch vessels; total arch replacement requires concomitant branch vessel replacement.
    - "Elephant trunk" operation extends the aortic arch graft into the descending thoracic aorta, creating a landing zone for future operation.
  - Descending TAA is managed with an open surgical or endovascular approach.
    - Open repair performed via left thoracotomy; maintenance of spinal perfusion is critical.
      - Preferred for patients with underlying connective tissue disease
    - Thoracic endovascular aortic repair (TEVAR) is associated with less perioperative morbidity compared to open repair but requires more frequent postoperative surveillance and higher need for reinterventions.
  - AAA is managed with an open surgical or endovascular approach.
    - Endovascular aneurysm repair (EVAR) preferred for high-risk patients and is associated with less morbidity, but requires more frequent postoperative surveillance.
  - Postoperative complications
    - Open repair
      - Immediate complications
        - Hemodynamic instability
        - Coagulopathy
        - Respiratory failure
        - Renal failure
        - Mesenteric, cerebral, or spinal cord ischemia
      - Delayed complications
        - Graft infection
        - Anastomotic pseudoaneurysm
    - Endovascular repair
      - Immediate complications
        - Renal failure
        - Bowel ischemia: CT or MRI scan indicated in any case of severe abdominal pain

- Paraplegia: increased risk in cases of long or multiple stent grafts, especially in the T8-L2 segments, or concomitant AAA repair
  - Preoperative cerebrospinal fluid (CSF) drainage advised in these cases
  - Emergency drainage in new-onset paraparesis in the intensive care unit (ICU)
- Stroke
- Endoleak is persistent blood flow into the aneurysm sac that is outside the lumen of the repair graft. Endoleak may cause pain due to expansion or remain asymptomatic.
  - Type I: occurs at the proximal/distal attachment site
  - Type II: retrograde via side branches
  - Type III: ineffective sealing of overlapping graft joints
  - Type IV: due to the porosity of the graft fabric
  - Type I and III endoleaks should be treated without delay due to the increased rate of open conversion or aneurysm rupture.
- Myocardial infarction
- Vascular access complications: hematoma, distal ischemia

- Delayed complications
  - Endoleak (type I, II, III, IV)
  - Stent-graft migration or embolization, infection, fracture/collapse, or erosion into esophagus
  - Bowel or lower limb ischemia

Outcomes

- Outcomes for prophylactic open surgical and endovascular repair are generally excellent when performed by experienced cardiac and vascular surgeons as part of a multidisciplinary aortic team.
- Endovascular repair is associated with lower perioperative morbidity compared to open repair and favorable short- and intermediate-term outcomes, but no clear long-term mortality benefit.

Acute Aortic Syndromes

The most common acute aortic syndromes are aortic dissection, intramural hematoma (IMH), and penetrating atherosclerotic ulcer (PAU); all can culminate in aortic rupture.

Aortic Dissection

Tear in the intima and delamination of the aortic wall characterized by:

- Blood entering the aortic intima creating a blood-filled space: *false lumen*
- Proximal or distal spread of the intimal flap that can involve the branches of the aorta
- Classified according to the anatomic site of involvement is shown in Table 2.11.2

TABLE 2.11.2 Anatomic Site Classifications

Stanford classification	Type A: all dissections involving the ascending aorta (regardless of the site of origin)
	Type B: all dissections that do not involve the ascending aorta
DeBakey classification	Type I: dissection originates in ascending aorta and extends distally to involve the arch and descending aorta.
	Type II: dissection only involves the ascending aorta.
	Type III: dissection originates in descending aorta.

Epidemiology

- 5 to 30 cases per million people per year
- Most common in the fifth to seventh decades of life; male > female predominance
- Younger patients (<40 years of age): connective tissue disorder, bicuspid aortic valve, coarctation of aorta, pregnancy (third trimester)

Presenting Symptoms

- Abrupt, severe sharp or stabbing chest or back pain that is worst at onset and occasionally radiates
- Additional symptoms depend on the extent of the dissection and/or involvement of branch vessels (Table 2.11.3).

Differential Diagnosis

- IMH: absence of intimal flap and false lumen, crescentic shape
- Penetrating atherosclerotic ulcer: older hypertensive male, crater-like lesion with evidence of atherosclerotic disease
- Aortic mural thrombus
- Symptomatic aortic aneurysm

TABLE 2.11.3 Clinical Presentation: Dissection

Clinical Presentation	Pathophysiology
Pulse deficit (>20 mm Hg BP differential between limbs)	Dissection extends into the branch vessels.
Chest pain due to myocardial ischemia	Dissection extends into the coronary artery (commonly right coronary artery).
Heart failure with new diastolic murmur	Incomplete aortic valve closure due to leaflet tethering or prolapse from aortic root dissection
Hypotension/shock	Cardiac tamponade, acute severe aortic regurgitation, hemothorax, aortic rupture
Stroke	Dissection extends into the carotid or vertebral arteries.
Paraplegia	Dissection extends into the intercostal arteries, causing spinal ischemia.
Hematuria/oliguria	Dissection extends into the renal arteries.
Abdominal pain, bowel ischemia, and/or gastrointestinal bleeding	Dissection extends into the celiac or superior mesenteric artery.
Lower extremity ischemia	Dissection extends into the iliac artery.
Syncope	Transient occlusion of the carotid artery, cardiac tamponade

BP, blood pressure.

Diagnosis

- CT is the preferred imaging modality due to its accuracy, availability, noninvasive nature, and rapid acquisition time.
  - Can identify the location of intimal tear and assess the extent of aortic involvement, branch vessel involvement, radiographic evidence of malperfusion, hemopericardium, and pleural effusion
  - Can assess for concomitant IMH, PAU
  - Can identify periaortic hematoma, which suggests contained rupture
  - Disadvantages: requires iodinated contrast, patient must be stable enough to travel
- Echocardiography
  - Transthoracic echocardiography
    - Rapid acquisition and can be performed at bedside
    - Can assess for complications of aortic dissection, including aortic regurgitation and pericardial effusion/tamponade
    - Disadvantages: limited ability to visualize distal dissection flaps
  - Transesophageal echocardiography
    - Improved anatomic resolution and sensitivity compared to transthoracic echocardiography
    - Can be performed for bedside diagnosis; more frequently done in the operating room (OR) after the diagnosis of dissection is confirmed by CT
- Chest radiography
  - May demonstrate mediastinal widening and/or pleural effusions, but nonspecific
- MRI
  - Limited utility in the diagnosis of acute aortic dissection due to prolonged acquisition times; more useful for stable patients with contrast allergy or for longitudinal follow-up

Management and Treatment

- Type A dissection
  - Surgical emergency: surgery is the definitive therapy.
    - Goals of open surgical repair:
      - Prevent retrograde propagation of dissection flap into the aortic root
      - Prevent antegrade propagation of dissection flap into the distal aorta
      - Prevent or repair aortic rupture
      - Address branch occlusion, leading to malperfusion syndromes
    - If cardiac tamponade is documented, it should only be evacuated in the OR (not percutaneously).
  - While awaiting surgical correction, medical management with antiimpulse therapy (need to decrease d*P*/d*t*)
    - Intravenous beta-blockers to achieve target heart rate of 60 to 80 bpm
    - If patient remains hypertensive after intravenous beta-blockers, then initiate intravenous vasodilator therapy (ie, sodium nitroprusside) to achieve systolic blood pressure <120 mm Hg.
      - Avoid as initial treatment, due to the risk of compensatory tachycardia.
    - Invasive blood pressure monitoring with arterial line is recommended.
      - Be aware of pseudohypotension due to branch occlusion by dissection flap.
- Type B dissection
  - Medical management is the cornerstone of treatment for uncomplicated cases.
    - First-line treatment is the utilization of beta-blockers, such as labetalol.
  - Target systolic blood pressure <120 mm Hg
  - Surgical management:
    - In the acute setting, surgical management is associated with increased mortality and paraplegia.
    - Surgery reserved for patients who develop complications:
      - Free or contained rupture (periaortic hematoma, hemothorax, mediastinal hematoma)
      - Malperfusion syndromes (renal, mesenteric, or peripheral ischemia)
      - Retrograde dissection
      - Progressive aortic enlargement
      - Refractory pain
    - Endovascular stent grafting, percutaneous fenestration of a dissection flap, or both can be used in complicated cases.

Outcomes

- Type A dissections portend a mortality rate of 1% to 2% per hour after symptom onset.
- Prompt intervention leads to good outcomes, particularly in patients treated at high-volume aortic centers.

Intramural Hematoma

Hemorrhage into the medial layer of the aortic wall due to spontaneous rupture of the vasa vasorum, without an intimal tear

- Classification scheme is identical to aortic dissection.

Epidemiology

- IMH comprises 5% to 25% of acute aortic syndromes.
- Higher incidence in individuals of Asian descent

Presenting Symptoms and Diagnosis

- Symptoms are similar to acute aortic dissection.
- CT is the diagnostic imaging modality of choice.
  - On noncontrast imaging, there is focal, high-attenuation crescentic thickening of the aortic wall; intimal calcium may be displaced inward (in contrast to mural thrombus).
  - On contrast imaging, no intimal flap or false lumen is observed.
- Transesophageal echocardiography demonstrates eccentric wall thickening with mixed echogenicity.

Management and Treatment

- Acute type A IMH and complicated type B IMH are surgical emergencies.
  - May progress to dissection or rupture
  - Complicated IMH: malperfusion, periaortic hematoma, pericardial effusion with tamponade, refractory pain, rupture
- Uncomplicated type B IMH can be managed medically.

Penetrating Atherosclerotic Ulcer

Ulcerated aortic plaque penetrates into the aortic wall, leading to medial hemorrhage.

Epidemiology

- Most commonly seen in older patients with extensive atherosclerotic disease

Presenting Symptoms and Diagnosis

- Symptoms are similar to acute aortic dissection.
- Diagnosis by CT; concomitant vascular disease is often seen.

Management and Treatment

- Typically occur in the descending aorta; can be managed medically in the absence of high-risk features
- Urgent surgical repair is recommended for PAU with rupture or PAU with associated IMH of the ascending aorta.
- PAU involving the ascending aorta can be treated with open surgical repair; PAU involving the descending aorta may be amenable to endovascular repair.

SUGGESTED READINGS

Braverman AC. Acute aortic dissection: clinician update. *Circulation*. 2010; 122:184-188.

Braverman AC, Schermerhorn M. Diseases of the aorta. In: Libby P, Bonow RO, Mann DL, Tomaselli GF, Bhatt DL, Solomon SD, eds. *Braunwald's Heart Disease*. 12th ed. Elsevier; 2021:806-836.

Elkouri S, Gloviezky P, McKusic MA, et al. Perioperative complications and early outcome after endovascular and open surgical repair of abdominal aortic aneurysms. *J Vasc Surg*. 2004;39:497-505.

Evangelista A, Mukherjee D, Mehta RH, et al. Acute intramural hematoma of the aorta. *Circulation*. 2005;111:1063-1070.

Flachskampf FA, Banbury M, Smedira N, Thomas JD, Garcia M. Transesophageal echocardiography diagnosis of intramural hematoma of the ascending aorta: a word of caution. *J Am Soc Echocardiogr*. 1999; 12(10):866-870.

Gaul C, Dietrich W, Erbguth FJ. Neurological symptoms in acute aortic dissection: a challenge for neurologists. *Cerebrovasc Dis*. 2008;26:1-8.

Golledge J, Norman P. Pathophysiology of abdominal aortic aneurysm relevant to improvements in patients' management. *Curr Opin Cardiol*. 2009;24:532-538.

Greeven AP, Bouwman LH, Smeets HJ, van Baalen JM, Hamming JF. Outcome of patients with ruptured abdominal aortic aneurysm after cardiopulmonary resuscitation. *Acta Chir Bel*. 2011;111(2):78-82.

Hagan PG, Nienaber CA, Isselbacher EM, et al. International Registry of Acute Aortic Dissection (IRAD): new insights from an old disease. *JAMA*. 2000;283:897-903.

Harkin DW, Dillon M, Blair PH, Ellis PK, Kee F. Endovascular ruptured abdominal aortic aneurysm repair (EVRAR): a systematic review. *Eur J Vasc Endovasc Surg*. 2007;34(6):673-681.

Hiratzka LF, Bakris GL, Beckman JA, et al. American College of Cardiology Foundation/American Heart Association task force on practice guidelines; American Association for Thoracic Surgery; American College of Radiology; American Stroke Association; Society of Cardiovascular Anesthesiologists; Society for Cardiovascular Angiography and Interventions; Society of Interventional Radiology; Society of Thoracic Surgeons; Society for Vascular Medicine: guidelines for the diagnosis and management of patients with thoracic aortic disease. *Circulation*. 2010; 121:e266-e3369.

Isselbacher EM, Cigarroa JE, Eagle KA. Cardiac tamponade complicating proximal aortic dissection. Is percardiocentesis harmful? *Circulation*. 1994;90(5):2375-2378.

Isselbacher EM, Preventza O, Hamilton Black J, et al. 2022 ACC/AHA guideline for the diagnosis and management of aortic disease: a report of the American Heart Association/American College of Cardiology Joint Committee on Clinical Practice Guidelines. *Circulation*. 2022; 146:e334-e482.

Lall P, Gloviczki P, Agarwal G, et al. Comparison of EVAR and open repair in patients with small aortic aneurysms: can we predict results of the PIVOTAL trial. *J Vasc Surg*. 2009;49(1):52-59.

Hoyert DL, Arias E, Smith BL, Murphy SL, Kochanek MA. *Deaths: final data for 1999. National Vital Statistics Reports*. National Center for Health Statistics. Accessed October 13, 2025. https://www.cdc.gov/nchs/data/nvsr/nvsr49/nvsr49_08.pdf

Miraude A, Bosch JL, Halpern EF, et al. Elective endovascular versus open surgical repair of abdominal aortic aneurysms: systematic review of short-term results. *Radiology*. 2002;224:739-747.

Noorani A, Page A, Walsh SR, Varty K, Hayes PD, Boyle JR. Mid-term outcomes following emergency endovascular aortic aneurysm repair for ruptured abdominal aortic aneurysms. *Eur J Vasc Endovasc Surg*. 2012;43(4):382-385.

O'Connor CJ. Abdominal aortic aneurysm repair. In: Atlee JL, ed. *Complications in Anesthesia*. 2nd ed. Saunders Elsevier; 2007:390-394.

Rogers AM, Herman LK, Booher AM, et al. Sensitivity of the aortic dissection risk score, a novel guideline based tool for identification of acute aortic dissection at initial presentation: results from the International Registry of Acute Aortic Dissection. *Circulation*. 2011;123:2213-2228.

Spoerke N, Michalek J, Schreiber M, et al. Crystalloid resuscitation improves survival in trauma patients receiving low ratios of fresh frozen plasma to packed red blood cells. *J Trauma*. 2011;71(2):S380-S383.

Upchuch GR, Nienaber C, Fattori R, et al. Acute aortic dissection presenting primarily abdominal pain: a rare manifestation of a deadly disease. *Ann Vasc Surg*. 2005;19:367-373.

2.12

Cardiovascular Infections

Olivia L. Hulme, Simran Gupta, and Lisa M. Bebell

Infective Endocarditis

- *Infective endocarditis* (IE) should be considered a systemic disease, involving multiple organs, and embolic phenomena may be the first sign of this disease (brain, lung, spleen, kidney, skin).
- Mortality in native valve endocarditis ranges from 16% to 25%, though varies by pathogen and comorbidities.
- With a decline in rheumatic fever prevalence and an increase in cardiac device and transcatheter heart valve implantations, the demographics of patients with IE have changed over the last 20 years.
- In developed countries, the presence of intracardiac devices and degenerative valve disease has also shifted incidence and prevalence to an older age (mean age 61 years with >50% of patients older than 50 years), though the mean age of patients with injection drug use (IDU)-associated IE is ~36 to 41 years.
- A multidisciplinary team composed of infectious disease specialists, cardiologists, cardiac surgeons, neurologists, radiologists, and other specialists should be involved in the care of patients with IE to shorten the time to diagnosis and improve survival. Depending on the situation and the patient, intensivists, addiction specialists, oral surgeons, and psychiatrists may be important as well.

Epidemiology

- Incidence ~3 to 7/100,000 person-years and increasing
- Incidence higher in men (male:female ≥2:1) but women have worse prognosis.
- Prevalence of IDU-associated IE has risen in the past decade, with affected individuals more likely to be younger, on Medicaid and in the lowest quartile of median household income, and more likely to have hepatitis C and HIV.
- Risk factors include:
  - IDU
  - Prosthetic valves or other intracardiac prosthetic material (including devices)
  - Prior history of IE
  - Age-related degenerative valve disease
  - Poor dentition, periodontal disease, and other dental infections
  - Immunosuppression and immunodeficiency
  - Chronic hemodialysis
  - Cyanotic congenital heart disease that has either not been repaired or incompletely repaired with residual intracardiac shunting

Pathophysiology

- Staphylococci, streptococci, and enterococci spp. account for 70% to 80% of all cases of endocarditis: staphylococci (40%-45%, mainly *Staphylococcus aureus*), streptococci (35%-40%, mainly viridans group), and enterococci (10%).
- With the highest risk population changing over the last 20 years, the microbiology of IE has also changed. Viridans group streptococci were once most common, now *S. aureus* is predominant, postulated to be due to increases in IDU and intracardiac device–related IE.
- *Enterococcus* spp. IE is often associated with prior transcatheter aortic valve replacement (TAVR) or mitral valve replacement.
- Fungal IE is most associated with cardiac implantable electronic devices (CIEDs), prosthetic valves, and IDU.
  - *Candida* and *Aspergillus* spp. most common
  - High mortality rate (up to 70%), more likely to need surgery
- Right-sided IE more commonly associated with IDU, CIED, and central venous catheters. In addition to staphylococcal and streptococcal infections, *Pseudomonas aeruginosa,* and other Gram-negative bacteria are more prevalent in right-sided IE.

Prosthetic Valve Infective Endocarditis

- Low overall incidence of prosthetic valve endocarditis (PVE) post-TAVR (0.3-2 per 100 person-years), but PVE represents 20% of all IE cases.
- Early infection common (<2 months post-surgery), prosthetic material is not yet endothelialized, giving organisms direct access to prosthetic-annulus interface and perivalvular tissue.
- Perivalvular abscesses more common with PVE than native valve IE (NVE) since the annulus is the primary site of infection.
- Staphylococci (32%), streptococci (25%), and enterococci (16%) are the main causes.
- For early or periprocedural (during the initial 2 months after valve replacement) TAVR-related IE, *Enterococcus* is the primary cause.
- PVE should be considered in patients with a history of valve replacement and:
  - Bacteremia with an organism commonly causing IE
  - Persistent constitutional symptoms
  - New prosthetic valve dysfunction
  - Unexplained stroke or septic emboli
- Transesophageal echocardiogram (TEE) has higher sensitivity than transthoracic echocardiogram (TTE) for detecting vegetations and complications like abscess or fistulae.
- Cardiac computed tomography (Cardiac CT) or fluorodeoxyglucose (18F) (^{18}F-FDG) positron emission tomography (PET)/CT may be used if the presence of artifact and shadowing from the prosthetic valve limits echocardiographic evaluation.

Cardiac Implantable Electronic Device Infective Endocarditis

- ~10% of IE cases worldwide
- CIED infection is defined in an expert consensus statement as:
  - *Definite* lead or valvular infection:
    - Pre-extraction: ≥2 positive blood cultures for *S. aureus* or identical species of coagulase-negative staphylococci with no alternative source *and* TEE findings consistent with vegetation *or* ^{18}F-FDG PET/CT with metabolic activity along leads or valves

- Post-extraction: device, tissue, or fluid culture growth of identical organisms isolated from blood cultures
  - *Possible* lead or valvular infection:
    - Persistent (>72 hours) bacteremia due to nonstaphylococcal organisms despite adequate pathogen-directed therapy with no alternative source
- Primarily caused by *S. aureus,* with other Gram-positive cocci (streptococci and enterococci) also implicated
- ^{18}F-FDG PET/CT is useful for identifying pocket infections and lead-associated IE.
- Definite CIED infection requires complete device removal, given a high rate of relapse with device retention.
- Reimplantation should be delayed until local and systemic infection has resolved (and up to 14 days if evidence of valvular IE).

Diagnosis (Tables 2.12.1 and 2.12.2)

- Initial evaluation includes electrocardiogram (ECG) and chest x-ray (CXR):
  - Heart block or conduction delay may indicate aortic paravalvular extension.
  - Myocardial ischemia may indicate coronary artery septic embolism.
  - CXR may demonstrate septic pulmonary emboli.
  - TTE to evaluate for vegetations, valvular dysfunction, left ventricular (LV) function, abscess, leaflet perforation, aortic pseudoaneurysm, and fistula
  - If clinical suspicion still high after negative TTE, pursue TEE.
- Cardiac CT (CCT) can be used if TEE contraindicated, or images are suboptimal.
  - Less sensitive for vegetations (64% vs 94%)
  - More sensitive for pseudoaneurysm or abscess (78% vs 69%)

Management and Treatment

- Antibiotic therapy is the mainstay, and surgery can be important, especially for complications.
- *Antimicrobial therapy*
  - Target antimicrobials to isolated organism.
  - Duration should be calculated from the first day of negative blood cultures, or date of surgery if intraoperative tissue cultures are positive for the causative organism.
- *Empiric therapy*
  - Regimen should cover most common pathogens, including staphylococci (methicillin sensitive and resistant), streptococci, and enterococci.
  - Reasonable empiric regimen for suspected NVE is vancomycin plus ceftriaxone.
    - If risk for oral or gastrointestinal (GI) source, consider ampicillin/sulbactam in lieu of ceftriaxone.
    - In patients at risk of nosocomial *Pseudomonas* infection, could substitute cefepime or piperacillin/tazobactam for ceftriaxone.
  - Tailoring therapy to specific pathogens
    - Consult your ID colleague!
    - Methicillin-sensitive *Staphylococcus aureus* (MSSA)
      - Intravenous (IV) oxacillin/nafcillin or cefazolin
        - Use oxacillin or nafcillin for patients with central nervous system (CNS) involvement for better penetration.

TABLE 2.12.1 2023 Duke-International Society for Cardiovascular Infectious Diseases Criteria for the Diagnosis of IE

Major	
Microbiologic	1. *Positive blood cultures*
	a. Microorganisms that commonly cause IE isolated from ≥2 separate blood culture sets *or*
	b. Microorganisms that occasionally or rarely cause IE isolated from ≥3 separate blood culture sets
	2. *Positive laboratory tests*
	a. Positive PCR or other nucleic acid–based technique for *Coxiella burnetii, Bartonella* spp., or *Tropheryma whipplei* from blood *or*
	b. *C. burnetii* phase 1 IgG titer >1:800, or isolated from a single blood culture
	c. Indirect immunofluorescence assay with positive IgM and IgG to *Bartonella henselae* or *Bartonella quintana* with IgG titer ≥1:800
Imaging	1. *Echocardiography and/or CT*
	a. TTE, TEE, and/or CT with vegetation, valvular/leaflet perforation, aneurysm, abscess, pseudoaneurysm, or intracardiac fistula *or*
	b. Significant new valvular regurgitation *or*
	c. New-partial prosthetic valve dehiscence
	2. ^{18}*F-FDG PET/CT* with abnormal metabolic activity involving native or prosthetic valve, ascending aortic graft, CIED leads, or other prosthetic material
Surgical	Evidence of IE on intraoperative direct inspection
Minor	
Predisposition	Prior history of IE, prosthetic valve or valve repair, CIED, IDU, HOCM, congenital heart disease, more than mild regurgitation or stenosis
Fever	Documented fever >38.0 °C/100.4 °F
Vascular phenomena	Arterial emboli, septic pulmonary infarcts, cerebral or splenic abscess, mycotic aneurysm, intracranial hemorrhage, conjunctival hemorrhage, Janeway lesions, purulent purpura
Immunologic phenomena	Immune complex–mediated glomerulonephritis, Roth spots, Osler nodes, positive rheumatoid factor
Microbiologic (not meeting major criterion)	1. Positive blood culture for organisms consistent with IE but not meeting major criterion *or* 2. Positive culture, PCR, or nucleic acid test for IE organism from a sterile body site or a single PCR positive for a skin bacterium on a valve/wire without other supportive evidence
Imaging	Abnormal ^{18}F-FDG PET/CT metabolic activity within 3 mo of implantation of prosthetic valve, ascending aortic graft (with concomitant evidence of valve involvement), CIED leads, or other prosthetic material
Physical examination	New regurgitation on auscultation when TTE/TEE is not available

CIED, cardiac implantable electronic device; CT, computed tomography; HOCM, hypertrophic obstructive cardiomyopathy; IDU, injection drug use; IE, infective endocarditis; IgG, immunoglobulin G; PCR, polymerase chain reaction; PET, positron emission tomography; TEE, transesophageal echocardiogram; TTE, transthoracic echocardiogram; FDG, fluorodeoxyglucose.

TABLE 2.12.2 Identifying Definite and Possible Endocarditis With Major and Minor Criteria

Definite endocarditis	*Pathologic criteria*	Microorganisms or active IE identified in a vegetation from cardiac tissue, explanted prosthetic valve or sewing ring, ascending aortic graft, CIED, or arterial embolus with clinical signs of IE
	Clinical criteria	2 major
		1 major + 3 minor
		5 minor
Possible endocarditis	*Clinical criteria*	1 major + 1 minor
		3 minor

CIED, cardiac implantable electronic device; IE, infective endocarditis.

- Methicillin-resistant *Staphylococcus aureus* (MRSA)
  - IV vancomycin is first line.
  - Daptomycin is an alternative.
- Streptococci
  - Viridans group
    - IV penicillin G or ceftriaxone, depending on the penicillin minimum inhibitory concentration (MIC)
  - Groups A, B, C, F, and G
    - IV penicillin G is typically first line.
- Enterococci
  - IV ceftriaxone plus IV ampicillin *or* IV penicillin, G *or* IV ampicillin plus IV gentamicin
  - Depends on susceptibility testing
- HACEK organisms
  - *Haemophilus/Aggregatibacter aphrophilus, Actinobacillus/Aggregatibacter actinomycetemcomitans, Cardiobacterium hominis, Eikenella corrodens, Kingella kingae*
  - Nearly all are highly susceptible to third-generation cephalosporins (eg, ceftriaxone).
- *Candida*
  - Typically fluconazole (IV → oral [PO]) or IV micafungin depending on species and susceptibility testing

- Duration of therapy
  - Generally, 6 weeks for uncomplicated left-sided NVE with MSSA, 4 to 6 weeks for enterococci, 4 weeks for highly penicillin-susceptible streptococci
  - For uncomplicated right-sided MSSA NVE and all IE due to HACEK organisms, 4 weeks may be considered.
  - For PVE, >6 weeks, IV with possible oral tail if needed for suppression
  - IV antibiotics historically used for the entire duration of therapy though now more data support a switch to PO toward the end of the course in certain situations (but should be guided by ID consultation)

Surgical Treatment

- May be needed in up to 50%, though high surgical risk may preclude surgery
- Goal of surgery is to remove infected or damaged valve tissue, abscesses, repair fistula/aneurysm, and replace valves as needed (repair preferred, if possible).
- American College of Cardiology/American Heart Association/European Society of Cardiology (ACC/AHA/ESC) guidelines for surgical indications:
  - Acute heart failure, cardiogenic shock, or severe valvular regurgitation
  - Uncontrolled infection (local, fungal or resistant organisms, failure to clear blood cultures, sepsis)
  - Embolic risk reduction—early surgery for mobile left-sided vegetations >10 mm
  - PVE—early surgery for PVE with relapsing infection (recurrent bacteremia posttreatment)

Percutaneous Aspiration

- Large-bore aspiration device approved in 2023 for nonsurgical removal of right heart vegetations in nonsurgical candidates without complete valve destruction

Complications and Outcomes

Complications

- Cardiac complications are most common, in up to 50%.
  - Heart failure is most common cause of death.
  - Perivalvular abscess (30%-40%), usually aortic valve and annulus
    - Can lead to heart block; PR interval prolongation seen with an enlarging abscess
  - Pericarditis
  - Intracardiac fistula
- Metastatic infection, including embolization, mycotic aneurysm, and noncardiac abscess
  - Septic embolization in up to 45%—highest incidence with anterior mitral valve leaflet involvement, PVE, *S. aureus, Candida,* HACEK
    - Left-sided IE → systemic embolization (or via intracardiac shunt)
    - Cerebrovascular accident (CVA), myocardial infarction (MI), paralysis, splenic/renal infarction, limb ischemia, osteomyelitis, and septic arthritis possible
    - Right-sided IE → pulmonary embolization (bacterial pneumonia, lung abscess, pleural effusion)
- Cerebrovascular complications in up to 35% (embolic or hemorrhagic stroke, brain abscess, meningitis, seizure)

Outcomes

- In-hospital mortality up to 25%—intracardiac abscess and LV ejection fraction (EF) <40% are independent predictors.
- Higher mortality with *S. aureus*, heart failure, embolization, perivalvular abscess, larger vegetation, persistent bacteremia, positive valve culture, poor surgical candidacy, female sex, and concomitant diabetes mellitus

SUGGESTED READINGS

Baddour LM, Esquer Garrigos Z, Rizwan Sohail M, et al. Update on cardiovascular implantable electronic device infections and their prevention, diagnosis, and management: a scientific statement from the American Heart Association. *Circulation*. 2024;149(2):e201-e216.

Cimmino G, Bottino R, Formisano T, et al. Current views on infective endocarditis: changing epidemiology, improving diagnostic tools and centering the patient for up-to-date management. *Life (Basel)*. 2023;13(2):377.

Farina JM, Liblik K, Iomini P, et al. Infections and cardiovascular disease. *J Am Coll Cardiol*. 2023;81(1):71-80.
Fong IW. New perspectives of infections in cardiovascular disease. *Curr Cardiol Rev*. 2009;5(2):87-104.
Fowler VG, Durack DT, Selton-Suty C, et al. The 2023 Duke-International Society for cardiovascular infectious diseases criteria for infective endocarditis: updating the modified Duke criteria. *Clin Infect Dis*. 2023;77(4):518-526.
Kirkbride RR, Rawal B, Mirsadraee S, et al. Imaging of cardiac infections: a comprehensive review and investigation flowchart for diagnostic workup. *J Thorac Imaging*. 2021;36(5):W70.
Yucel E, Bearnot B, Paras ML, et al. Diagnosis and management of infective endocarditis in people who inject drugs: JACC state-of-the-art review. *J Am Coll Cardiol*. 2022;79:2037-2057.

2.13

Implantable Cardiac Devices

Will Pohlman, Smrithi Sukumar, and David M. Dudzinski

Implanted Cardiovascular Electronic Pulse Generators

Permanent Pacemakers and Implantable Cardioverter-Defibrillators

- >80% of pacemakers implanted are in older patients, with average age of pacemaker recipients 75 ± 10 years.
- It is important to determine the type of device in any patient who has a device.
- In patients who are unable to explain why their device was implanted, radiographic findings on chest x-ray (CXR) may provide clues about the device type:
  - Identifying the number and position of leads
  - Identifying one or two large shocking coils on CXR indicates the device is an implantable cardioverter-defibrillator (ICD).
  - Commercially available applications that use a cell phone camera to analyze CXR can be useful in identifying the device manufacturer.
- Dual-chamber right atrial and right ventricular permanent pacemaker (PPM) contributes to atrioventricular (AV) synchrony. However, in permanent atrial fibrillation (AF), for example, atrial lead is not often placed as it will not contribute to AV synchrony.
- Leadless pacemakers are placed directly in the right ventricle and do not require a separate generator in the pectoral position. However, they can only provide ventricular pacing. Leadless pacemakers are gaining the capability to sense the atrial activity and attempt synchrony, but overall outcome studies are needed in comparison to the traditional transvenous approach.
- The practitioner should observe that not all electronic generators implanted in the chest are cardiac devices, despite being located in the pectoral position, which is the usual location for cardiac generators.
  - Electronic devices placed for other disorders (eg, nerve stimulators for diaphragmatic stimulation, vagus nerve simulators for epilepsy) may occupy this location in the chest as well.
  - Additionally, subcutaneously placed ICD (S-ICD) may avoid some lead complications (infection, tricuspid regurgitation); consider if issues with infection risk or venous access, noting antitachycardic pacing is not available.

Cardiac Resynchronization Therapy

- Provides synchronized right and left ventricular (LV) pacing ("biventricular pacing") in patient with heart failure with reduced ejection fraction (HFrEF), to reduce electrical dyssynchrony and thus mechanical dyssynchrony, resulting in improved ejection fraction (EF)
  - Cardiac resynchronization therapy with a pacemaker (CRT-P): biventricular ± right atrial pacing
  - Cardiac resynchronization therapy defibrillator (CRT-D): CRT-P with addition of ICD functions
- CRT is typically achieved with a lead that reaches the LV via the coronary sinus.
- The biventricular pacing rate should be as high as possible (close to 100%) to obtain benefit from CRT.

Indications for Device Implantation

- The indications for PPM include the following:
  - Symptomatic disease of impulse formation (sinus node disease, eg, symptomatic bradycardia, iatrogenic bradycardia due to necessary medications)
  - Symptomatic disease of impulse conduction (higher grade disease of the AV node)
  - Long QT syndrome (though most of these patients receive ICD in current practice)
  - Hypertrophic obstructive cardiomyopathy (HOCM) (infrequently done for symptom relief)
- The indications for ICD placement include the following:
  - Hemodynamically significant or sustained ventricular tachycardia (VT); ventricular fibrillation (VF); high risk of lethal VT/VF; resuscitated sudden cardiac death (SCD)
  - Patients awaiting heart transplant
  - Long QT syndrome
  - Arrhythmogenic right ventricular cardiomyopathy, cardiac sarcoidosis
  - Brugada syndrome (right bundle branch block [RBBB], ST-segment elevation in leads V1-V3) and other channelopathies

- Symptomatic heart failure (New York Heart Association [NYHA] II, III), with EF ≤35% despite ≥3 months of guideline-directed medical therapy
- Primary prevention in HOCM (e.g. unexplained syncope, massive LVH, family history SCD)
- Post-myocardial infarction (>40 days) with EF ≤30%, or EF ≤40% and nonsustained VT

- The indications for CRT placement include the following:
  - Symptomatic heart failure (NYHA II, III, and ambulatory class IV), with left ventricular ejection fraction (LVEF) ≤35%, QRS ≥150 ms, and left bundle branch block (LBBB)
  - Consider if LVEF ≤35% and QRS 130 to 149 ms with LBBB or QRS ≥150 ms with non-LBBB
  - Also consider if EF 36% to 50% and indication for PPM and there is expected high-pacing burden—however, "conduction area pacing" either His bundle or left bundle branch pacing wire positions are becoming alternative options
- The vast majority (>90%) of the indications for pacemaker implantation is composed of patients suffering from sick sinus syndrome and AV block.

Pacemaker Operating Modes

- The pacemaker mode classification consists of a five-letter system designed to indicate the chamber location for sensed, response, programmability, and multisite pacing function. (See Table 2.13.1 for additional details.)
  - Position IV refers to the device programmability with regard to rate modulation to ensure heart rate response matches oxygen demand or consumption by the body.
    - The purpose of this setting is to ensure an increase in heart rate in response to an increase in oxygen demand in those patients who are unable to do so on their own.
    - Two common rate response sensors exist:
      - Accelerometers, which operate based on the movements of the patient
      - Transthoracic impedance monitors that are triggered by the patient's ventilation
      - The rate response is a programmable feature.
    - Typically, the accelerated heart rate will persist for several minutes following cessation of the activity that led to the required increase in heart rate.
      - Should not cause concern to the practitioner as this will eventually cease
    - The rate response mode should be disabled while a patient is in the hospital as this function can be triggered by other medical devices such as ventilators, respiratory rate monitors, and electrocautery.

TABLE 2.13.1 Pacemaker Mode Classifications

Character Position	Letter Codes
I—Chamber(s) paced	O = none, A = atrium, V = ventricle, D = dual (A+V)
II—Chamber(s) sensed	O = none, A = atrium, V = ventricle, D = dual (A+V)
III—Response to sensing	O = no response, I = inhibited, T = triggered, D = dual (T+I)
IV—Rate modulation	O = none, R = rate modulation
V—Multisite pacing	O = none, A = atrium, V = ventricle, D = dual (A+V)

Understanding the Function of Implantable Cardioverter-Defibrillators

- These devices serve to terminate ventricular tachydysrhythmias (ie, VT and VF).
- They function by routinely monitoring the R-R interval.
- If a certain number of short R-R intervals are detected, the antitachycardia event counter begins, and the device charges in preparation to deliver a defibrillatory shock. Antitachycardia pacing attempts to pace at a high rate to disrupt a tachycardic episode.
- Most devices have a reconfirmation period at which point the presence of a dysrhythmia is reestablished before a shock is delivered by the device.
- Regardless of whether a shock is delivered, the battery stores will be depleted each time the device is charged.

Altering Pacemaker Function With the Application of a Magnet

- It is important to be aware that NOT all pacemakers will convert to a continuous asynchronous mode with the application of a magnet.
- In some devices, the effect of placing a magnet can be changed with programming, or it can be completely removed.
- Response to the magnet will be dictated by the device make/model and especially by the manufacturer.
- Although manufacturers may publish reference guidelines for their devices, some devices with programmable magnet behavior will require interrogation to determine their current settings.
- Similarly, magnet behavior in ICDs can be changed with reprogramming:
  - Suspension of tachyarrhythmia detection is the typical mode ICD devices assume when a magnet is applied.
  - It is important that the practitioner remain vigilant in determining what effect placing a magnet over the device will have *prior* to applying it.
  - This may even involve calling the manufacturer of the device to verify these settings.

Device Dysfunction

- General causes of device dysfunction include lead failure, failure to capture, or generator failure.
- Lead failure tends to be uncommon, with lead perforation occurring in ~1% of patients and can present as either undersensing (undetected intrinsic activity), oversensing, or inadequate delivery of energy from the device.
- There is a reduced risk of lead fracture in older adults.
- Generator failure is rare, especially in devices that are not near the end of their battery life.

- The strongest determinant of increased generator longevity is larger battery capacity.
- In the event of device failure, rule out electrolyte abnormalities, acid-base disturbances, antiarrhythmic drugs, or new myocardial damage when trying to determine the potential cause.
- In unstable patients experiencing device dysfunction, certain maneuvers may be initiated as temporizing measures for hemodynamic stability including the following:
- Apply a magnet if the device's default mode is asynchronous pacing.
  - This eliminates sensing of intrinsic activity by the device.
- Alternative means of temporary pacing should be considered (ie, transvenous, transthoracic, or transesophageal pacing).
  - Transesophageal pacing requires both functioning atria and AV node and is generally contraindicated when a permanent implanted cardiovascular electronic pulse generator is present.
- Sympathomimetic drugs (ie, epinephrine, dopamine, isoproterenol) may be administered as these drugs decrease the depolarization threshold, increase chronotropy, or do both.
- Complications following device implantation should be high on the physician's differential in instances of pacemaker dysfunction in patients with recently placed devices, with the understanding that older patients (>75 years of age) are at increased risk for these complications.
- Early postimplant complications may include lead dislodgement or loss of capture, cardiac perforation, pneumothorax, hematoma, infection, and death.
- Complication rates following pacemaker implantation have varied between 3.3% and 3.8% in different large clinical trials.

Other Device Parameters

- Most contemporary device generators are "magnetic resonance imaging (MRI) conditional." Electrophysiology consultant is typically needed to safely undergo an MRI. Some older devices (and some intensive care unit [ICU] devices) preclude MRI.
- If patients with an implanted PPM or ICD present with a systemic infection syndrome, or bacteremia, consider device endovascular infection.

Other Implantable Devices That May Be Encountered

- Implantable loop recorder (ILR)
  - Small device placed subcutaneously in the left chest that provides continuous rhythm monitoring up to 3 years (eg, palpitations or syncope evaluation)
- Pulmonary artery pressure monitors (eg, CardioMEMS)
  - Device the size of a paperclip and implanted in a pulmonary artery (PA) that provides wireless measurements of PA pressures to assist in longitudinal diuretic management.
  - Pressures can be monitored remotely or interrogated in the clinic or while hospitalized.
- Baroreflex activation therapy (BAT) (eg, Barostim)
  - Lead placed over the carotid sinus, subcutaneously tunneled to implantable pulse generator in the pectoral position
  - Electrical stimulation of the carotid sinus augments parasympathetic outflow and inhibits sympathetic activity.
  - Used in patients with heart failure to reduce symptoms. Studies are ongoing, assessing impacts on morbidity and mortality.
- Durable implanted mechanical circulatory support devices (ventricular assist device [VAD]) are covered in Section 2.18: Hemodynamic and Mechanical Circulatory Support.

SUGGESTED READINGS

Al-Khatib SM. Cardiac implantable electronic devices. *N Engl J Med*. 2024;390(5):442-454.

Armaganijan LV, Toff WD, Nielson JC, et al. Are elderly patients at increased risk of complications following pacemaker implantation? A meta-analysis of randomized trials. *Pacing Clin Electrophysiol*. 2012;35:131-134.

Chauhan A, Grace AA, Newell SA, et al. Early complications after dual chamber versus single chamber pacemaker implantation. *Pacing Clin Electrophysiol*. 1994;17:2012-2015.

Crossley GH, Poole JE, Rozner MA, et al. Heart Rhythm Society/American Society of Anesthesiologists Expert Consensus Statement on the perioperative management of patients with implantable defibrillators, pacemakers and arrhythmia monitors: facilities and patient management. *Heart Rhythm*. 2011;8(7):1114-1152.

Healey J, Connolly SJ, Morillo CA. The management of patients with carotid sinus syndrome: is pacing the answer? *Clin Auton Res*. 2004;14(suppl 1):80-86.

Healey JS, Toff WD, Lamas GA, et al. Cardiovascular outcomes with atrial-based pacing compared with ventricular pacing: meta-analysis of randomized trails, using individual patient data. *Circulation*. 2006;114:11-17.

Lamas GA, Orav EJ, Stambler BS, et al. Quality of life and clinical outcomes in elderly patients treated with ventricular pacing as compared with dual-chamber pacing. Pacemaker Selection in the Elderly Investigators. *N Eng J Med*. 1998;338:1097-1104.

Lattell J, Upadhyay GA. Bradyarrhythmias and physiologic pacing in the ICU. *J Intensive Care Med*. 2022:37(5):595-610.

Miller RD, Eriksson LI, Fleisher LA, Wiener-Kronish JP, Young WL. *Miller's Anesthesia*. 6th ed. Churchill Livingstone; 2010.

Nakai T, Ikeya Y, Kogawa R, Okumura Y. Cardiac resynchronization therapy: current status and near-future prospects. *J Cardiol*. 2022;79(3):352-357.

Rosenthal LS, Mester S, Rakovec P, et al. Factors influencing pacemaker generator longevity: results from the complete automatic pacing threshold utilization recorded in the CAPTURE trial. *Pacing Clin Electrophysiol*. 2010;33:1020-1030.

Zaidan JR, Apfelbaum JL, Belott P, Connis RT, Nickinovich DG, Rozner MA. Practice advisory for the peri-operative management of patients with cardiac implantable electronic devices: pacemakers and implantable cardioverter-defibrillators. *Anesthesiology*. 2011;114(2):247-261.

2.14

Hemodynamic Monitoring and Bioengineering

Q. Joyce Han and Aaron D. Aguirre

Background

- Hemodynamic monitoring is defined as the measurement and interpretation of biologic signals about cardiac physiology and blood flows that describe the overall performance of the cardiovascular system.
- Hemodynamic monitoring does not serve a direct therapeutic purpose.
- When data derived from monitors are accurately interpreted by the clinician, appropriate therapeutic interventions may be employed to improve patient outcomes.
- Advances in hemodynamic monitoring have introduced noninvasive and minimally invasive technologies that provide continuous, real-time cardiovascular data.
- It is important to realize the strengths and weaknesses of each individual monitor and stream of data when guiding patient care.

Electrocardiogram Monitoring/Telemetry

- Continuous assessment of cardiac rhythms and electrical activity, allowing real-time detection of arrhythmias and ischemic events
- Used for high-risk patients, postoperative cardiac care, heart failure, and arrhythmia monitoring
- The telemetry system wirelessly transmits electrocardiogram (ECG) data to a central station, allowing remote monitoring of multiple patients simultaneously.
- Real-time ECG waveforms on standard limb leads and precordial leads are recorded (usually two leads are displayed), with alarms for arrhythmias or abnormal cardiac activity.
    - Lead II often serves as the primary lead for rhythm monitoring as it is aligned with the electrical axis of the atria.
    - Detection of ischemia in lead V5 has a sensitivity of 75%. When combining multiple leads, the sensitivity goes up to 98%.
- Challenges: sensitive to electrode misplacement, skin issues, and signal interference. Regular checks and proper placement of electrodes are crucial for accuracy.
- New systems are integrating artificial intelligence (AI)-based algorithms to analyze ECG data and detect subtle abnormalities real time, to identify ischemia, estimate cardiac output (CO), and predict clinical deterioration. Examples include:
    - GE Healthcare MUSE System: uses AI to detect subtle changes in ECG waveforms, aiding in early detection of ischemia, myocardial infarction, and other cardiac events
    - Philips IntelliVue Guardian: incorporates AI for early detection of patient deterioration based on ECG and vital sign trends
- New analytical techniques and developments using ECG signals: esCCO (Nihon Kohden)
    - esCCO uses pulse-wave transit time and ECG signals to estimate CO noninvasively, offering continuous hemodynamic monitoring.
    - *Devices needed:* ECG, pulse oximeter, esCCO system
    - *Input:* ECG and pulse-wave transit time
    - *Output:* CO, heart rate, and stroke volume
    - *Limitations:* may not be as accurate as invasive methods, particularly in patients with arrhythmias

Noninvasive Blood Pressure

- Oscillometric and auscultatory measurements are widely available.
    - Oscillometric method: most commonly used in automatic blood pressure (BP) cuffs; measures the oscillations in arterial wall pressure caused by blood flow and computes systolic and diastolic pressures
    - Auscultatory method: uses a stethoscope and manual sphygmomanometer to detect Korotkoff sounds, providing accurate systolic and diastolic pressure readings
- Cuffs must be properly fitted
    - Cuff too large: artificially low reading
    - Cuff too small: artificially high readings
- The location of the cuff relative to the right atrium (RA) will affect the measured pressure.
- BP might be different between arms due to peripheral artery disease (subclavian stenosis etc).
- Limitations in critically ill patients
    - In critically unstable patients, continuous and highly accurate BP readings are often required, necessitating the use of invasive arterial lines instead.

New Developments Using Noninvasive Blood Pressure Measurements

- ClearSight (Edwards Lifesciences)
    - ClearSight uses finger arterial pressure waveforms to provide continuous noninvasive BP and hemodynamic parameters such as CO.
    - *Devices needed:* finger cuff, ClearSight system
    - *Input:* finger arterial pressure
    - *Output:* continuous noninvasive BP, CO, and stroke volume
    - *Limitations:* sensitive to patient movement and improper cuff placement
- CNAP (CNSystems)
    - CNAP uses finger sensors to capture arterial pressure waveforms for continuous noninvasive BP monitoring.
    - *Devices needed:* finger cuff, CNAP monitor
    - *Input:* finger arterial pressure
    - *Output:* continuous noninvasive BP, stroke volume, and CO
    - *Limitations:* susceptible to noise from movement and improper calibration
- T-line system (Tensys Medical)
    - T-line system uses a sensor placed over the radial artery to capture continuous arterial waveforms, allowing real-time noninvasive BP measurements.

- *Devices needed:* radial artery sensor, T-line monitor
- *Input:* radial artery pressure waveform
- *Output:* continuous noninvasive arterial pressure, CO
- *Limitations:* sensitive to sensor placement and patient movement

Direct Arterial Pressure Monitoring

- Direct arterial pressure monitoring is primarily performed using a catheter inserted into the radial artery, although other sites such as the brachial, femoral, axillary, and dorsalis pedis arteries can also be utilized. This method provides real-time BP readings and is an essential practice in critically ill patients.
- Indications: hemodynamic instability, continuous BP monitoring, respiratory failure (monitor $PaCO_2$), need for frequent blood samples
- The arterial pressure wave is transmitted through the tubing to a transducer, which converts the pressure wave into an electrical signal.
  - Various physiologic factors can affect the characteristics of the arterial pressure waveform, including changes in vascular compliance due to age, the presence of valvular abnormalities, and peripheral vascular disease.
  - Mechanical factors that may affect accuracy include tubing length, stiffness, or compliance, and the presence of air in the line.
- Complications: limb ischemia, bleeding, vascular injury, nerve injury

New Developments Using Direct Arterial Pressure Measurements

- FloTrac (Edwards Lifesciences)
  - FloTrac uses arterial waveform analysis from a standard arterial line to provide continuous CO and stroke volume without external calibration.
  - *Devices needed:* arterial catheter, FloTrac sensor, FloTrac monitor
  - *Input:* arterial waveform
  - *Output:* continuous CO, stroke volume variation, and BP
  - *Limitations:* accuracy can vary with vascular tone changes and requires an arterial line.
- ProAQT (Getinge)
  - ProAQT utilizes pulse contour analysis through an existing arterial line to measure CO and stroke volume continuously.
  - *Devices needed:* arterial catheter, ProAQT system
  - *Input:* arterial pressure waveform
  - *Output:* continuous CO, stroke volume, and dynamic parameters
  - *Limitations:* dependent on arterial line quality and calibration
- Argos (Retia Medical)
  - Argos uses advanced arterial waveform analysis for real-time monitoring of CO and hemodynamic parameters.
  - *Devices needed:* arterial catheter, Argos system
  - *Input:* arterial waveform
  - *Output:* continuous CO, stroke volume, and pulse pressure variation
  - *Limitations*: accuracy may be influenced by vasomotor tone and requires an arterial line.
- LidCO rapid system (Masimo)
  - LidCO rapid uses pulse contour analysis of arterial pressure to provide real-time continuous CO and stroke volume.
  - *Devices needed:* arterial catheter, LidCO monitor
  - *Input:* arterial pressure waveform
  - *Output:* continuous CO, stroke volume, and stroke volume variation
  - *Limitations:* accuracy can be affected by vascular tone and arterial waveform quality.

Central Venous Pressure

- Central venous pressure (CVP) refers to the pressure in the thoracic vena cava near the RA, reflecting RA pressure (RAP). It provides valuable insights into a patient's fluid status (right heart filling pressures), cardiac function, and overall hemodynamics, making it crucial for managing critically ill patients.
- Performed via catheterization of a central vein, most often the internal jugular, subclavian, femoral, or antecubital vein
- The 2011 Centers for Disease Control and Prevention (CDC) guidelines recommend subclavian vein placement as the preferred site to reduce the incidence of central line–associated bloodstream infections (CLABSIs). However, clinician expertise plays a significant role in minimizing the risk of CLABSI.
- The internal jugular vein may be preferred in patients at risk of bleeding as direct vascular pressure can be easily applied to this site while the subclavian site is relatively noncompressible.
- Indications for central catheter placement:
  - Central administrations of medications
  - CVP monitoring, central oximetry monitoring
  - Venous access for large-volume resuscitation or when peripheral access is poor
  - Pulmonary artery (PA) catheterization or transvenous pacing
  - Hemodialysis, noting that subclavian placement should be avoided in patients with advanced kidney disease to prevent subclavian vein stenosis
- Both the measured pressure and waveform provide useful clinical information, though care must be taken in the interpretation of the CVP; the complete clinical picture must be assessed. The CVP waves are divided by elements of the cardiac cycle.
  - a wave: <u>a</u>trial contraction; occurs in end diastole, just after the ECG P wave; this correlates with the echocardiographic A wave.
    - "Cannon A waves" indicate atrioventricular (AV) dissociation (atrial contraction against a closed tricuspid valve [TV], such as ventricular tachycardia [VT], AV blocks).
    - Absent a waves in atrial fibrillation/flutter
    - Large a wave with slow y-descent in TV stenosis, or pulmonic valve stenosis or right ventricular (RV) failure
  - c wave: bowing of TV into RA during ventricular <u>c</u>ontraction; follows the R wave on ECG
  - x-descent: atrial rela<u>x</u>ation (early x-descent), downward movement of TV (late x-descent)

- Steep x-descent in constriction: due to exaggerated ventricular longitudinal contraction and preserved atrial relaxation (thus it will be lost in atrial fibrillation)
- x-descent can be decreased in RV dysfunction (due to reduced ventricular longitudinal contraction).

  - v wave: passive atrial filling (venous return) when TV closed; coincides with T wave
    - Prominent v waves seen in TR
  - y-descent: early diastolic ventricular filling, from rapid atrial emptying following opening of the TV (ventricular diastole) as RAP drives blood into the RV. This correlates with the echocardiographic E wave.
    - Prominent x and y descents seen in pericardial constriction
    - Prominent y-descent in restriction as well (high atrial pressures), but there will also be a blunted x-descent. (As regard a noncompliant RV, rapid inflow of blood will lead to a rapid rise in pressure—the "square root" sign.)
    - Blunted y-descent seen in tamponade because the intrapericardial pressure reduces the RA-RV gradient (equalization of diastolic pressures).
- Complications primarily from central venous catheter placement may include vascular injury, cardiac tamponade, bleeding, infection, pneumothorax, venous thrombosis, and thromboembolism.

New Developments Using Direct Arterial Pressure Measurements

- PiCCO (Getinge)
  - PiCCO uses thermodilution (TD) and pulse contour analysis to provide comprehensive hemodynamic monitoring, including CO, preload, and extravascular lung water.
  - *Devices needed:* arterial catheter, central venous catheter, PiCCO monitor
  - *Input:* arterial pressure waveform, TD bolus
  - *Output:* CO, preload parameters, extravascular lung water
  - *Limitations:* requires both arterial and central venous lines, and TD can be cumbersome.

Pulmonary Arterial Catheter

- The PA catheter (or Swan-Ganz catheter, or right heart catheter) is advanced through the RA and RV into the PA.
- Indication: tailored therapy; diagnose (1) etiology of shock (eg, cardiogenic vs distributive); (2) cardiogenic versus noncardiogenic pulmonary edema; (3) left ventricular (LV) versus RV failure; (4) etiology of pulmonary hypertension; (5) L → R shunting; (6) valve disease; (7) pericardial disease
- Waveforms and tracings
  - Pulmonary capillary wedge pressure (PCWP) waveform: obtained by advancing the catheter into a small PA branch and inflating the balloon, providing an indirect estimate of left atrial (LA) pressure.
  - The waveforms for the LA in the PCWP tracing follow those of the RA in the CVP tracing.
  - Used for assessing LV preload and differentiating cardiogenic from noncardiogenic pulmonary edema
- CO measurement techniques
  - Fick principle: estimates CO using oxygen consumption (Vo_2) and arterial-venous oxygen difference
    - Equation: $CO = Vo_2/(13.4 \times Hgb \times [Spo_2 - Mvo_2])$.
    - Limitations: Vo_2 is often estimated, which may not reflect the true metabolic state, especially in critically ill patients.
  - TD
    - Involves injecting a bolus of cold crystalloid into the RA and measuring the downstream temperature change in the PA
    - Uses the Stewart-Hamilton formula to calculate CO
    - Limitations: inaccurate in the presence of significant tricuspid regurgitation or intracardiac shunts
- Hemodynamic calculations
  - Cardiac index (CI) = CO/BSA (accounts for body size), where BSA is body surface area
  - Systemic vascular resistance (SVR) = (MAP − CVP)/CO, where MAP is mean arterial pressure.
  - Pulmonary vascular resistance (PVR) = (mPAP − PCWP)/CO, mPAP is mean pulmonary artery pressure.
  - Pulmonary arterial pulsatility index (PAPi) = (SPAP − DPAP)/RAP, an indicator of RV function (where SPAP is systolic pulmonary artery pressure, and DPAP is diastolic pulmonary artery pressure)
    - Lower values (especially <2) indicate poor RV function and may predict adverse outcomes in patients with RV failure, postcardiac surgery, post-LV assist device, and those with acute myocardial infarction.
- Troubleshooting
  - Catheter motion artifacts: may cause sharp pressure waveforms at the beginning of systole
  - Underdamping and overdamping: can lead to over- or underestimation of PA pulse pressures
- Complications
  - Risks associated with PA catheter placement include accidental PA puncture, air embolism, pneumothorax, ventricular arrhythmias, and the development of right bundle branch block (RBBB).
  - Infection risk: prolonged use can increase the risk of catheter-associated bloodstream infections.
  - PA injury: "overwedging" (line tip too distal, or balloon overinflated) or improper placement can cause PA perforation or rupture, especially in fragile vessels.

Additional Developments for Continuous Hemodynamic Monitoring

- Esophageal Doppler (Deltex Medical)
  - The esophageal Doppler measures blood flow velocity in the descending aorta via a probe inserted into the esophagus, providing real-time CO and stroke volume.
  - *Devices needed:* esophageal Doppler probe, Doppler monitor
  - *Input:* Doppler ultrasound of the descending aorta
  - *Output:* stroke volume, CO
  - *Limitations:* invasive due to probe placement in the esophagus, requires precise positioning

SUGGESTED READINGS

Bootsma IT, Boerma EC, de Lange F, Scheeren TWL. The contemporary pulmonary artery catheter. Part 1: placement and waveform analysis. *J Clin Monit Comput*. 2022;36(1):5-15.

Bootsma IT, Boerma EC, Scheeren TWL, de Lange F. The contemporary pulmonary artery catheter. Part 2: measurements, limitations, and clinical applications. *J Clin Monit Comput*. 2022;36(1):17-31.

Cecconi M, De Backer D, Antonelli M, et al. Consensus on circulatory shock and hemodynamic monitoring. Task force of the European Society of Intensive Care Medicine. *Intensive Care Med*. 2014;40(12):1795-1815.

Couture EJ, Laferrière-Langlois P, Denault A. New developments in continuous hemodynamic monitoring of the critically ill patient. *Can J Cardiol*. 2023;39(4):432-443.

Garland A, Arbour R. Pulmonary artery catheter use in critical care: a review of the evidence and a look to the future. *Crit Care Med*. 2014;42(7):1701-1711.

Kulkarni AP, Govil D, Samavedam S, et al. ISCCM guidelines for hemodynamic monitoring in the critically ill. *Indian J Crit Care Med*. 2022;26(suppl 2):S66.

Landesberg G, Mosseri M, Wolf Y, Vesselov Y, Weissman C. Perioperative myocardial ischemia and infarction: identification by continuous 12-lead electrocardiogram with online ST-segment monitoring. *Anesthesiology*. 2002;96(2):264-270.

Vincent J-L, Pinsky MR. Understanding cardiac output monitoring: a practical guide. *J Crit Care*. 2018;48:1-6.

2.15

Cardiac Imaging

Alexandra Steverson, Rachel Goldberg, Joseph Meyer, and David M. Dudzinski

Transthoracic Echocardiogram

- Standard windows (Figure 2.15.1)
  - Optimization of views using probe manipulation: rocking, sliding, rotation
- Common echocardiogram imaging modes
  - Color Doppler: applies color to area of interest to evaluate timing, velocity, direction, and turbulence of flow
  - M-mode: displays motion over time occurring along a single scanning "line" through the heart and offers high temporal resolution
  - Pulse-wave (PW) Doppler: displays blood flow velocities from a specific cardiac location over time
  - Continuous wave (CW) Doppler: displays all blood flow velocities recorded along a scanning line continuously

STAT Echocardiography Indications

- Tamponade
  - Right atrial (RA) collapse (>⅓ cardiac cycle) and right ventricular (RV) diastolic inversion
    - Less sensitive in patients with elevated right-sided filling pressures
  - Left-sided chamber collapse (more specific, less sensitive)
  - Respiratory inflow variation across the mitral valve (MV) (>25%) and tricuspid (>40%)
  - Inferior vena cava (IVC) plethora is a sensitive (not specific) marker.
  - Tamponade can be regional (especially in postoperative patients), so need to visualize pericardial space in multiple views.
- Acute RV strain/dysfunction
  - Reduced RV free wall motion with hyperdynamic RV apex (McConnell sign)
  - Seen in: pulmonary embolism, RV myocardial infarction (MI)
  - Need to include direction of effect: dilated RV, reduced indicators of annular function (tricuspid annular plane systolic excursion [TAPSE], S')
  - In the case of pulmonary embolism, should evaluate for clot-in-transit
- New cardiomyopathy/acute decompensated heart failure/cardiogenic shock
  - Assess biventricular function (assess univentricular vs biventricular), wall thickness (to assess for myocardial edema/infiltration), chamber size (nondilated may suggest acute process), valvular dysfunction, shunts, and wall motion abnormalities (WMAs) to construct differential diagnosis
  - Echo parameters may also bear on possible mechanical circulatory support modalities (assess aortic regurgitation, chamber sizes, RV function, and exclude left ventricular [LV] thrombus)
- Post-MI mechanical complications
  - Ventricular septal rupture (VSR)
    - Color Doppler through the septum with PW/CW to evaluate the degree of left-to-right shunting; look for "drop-out" on two-dimensional (2D) echo and regional WMA.
    - Anterior MI usually leads to apical VSR (check subcostal and apical view); inferior MI leads to basal VSR, which can be more serpiginous (check parasternal long-axis or subcostal view).
  - Ischemic mitral regurgitation (MR)
    - Identify mechanism: ischemic (leaflet tethering), functional (LV dilatation), papillary muscle dysfunction or rupture
  - Other: free wall rupture, pericardial effusion, LV thrombus, LV aneurysm
- Postcardiac surgery
  - Complications: identify effusion/tamponade, hematoma, new WMA (coronary entrapment, kinking, or air embolism). Left circumflex can be damaged during MV surgeries. RCA can be damaged during TV surgeries.
  - Post-heart transplant: identify caval, pulmonary artery (PA), left atrial, and aortic anastomoses; assess RV dysfunction.

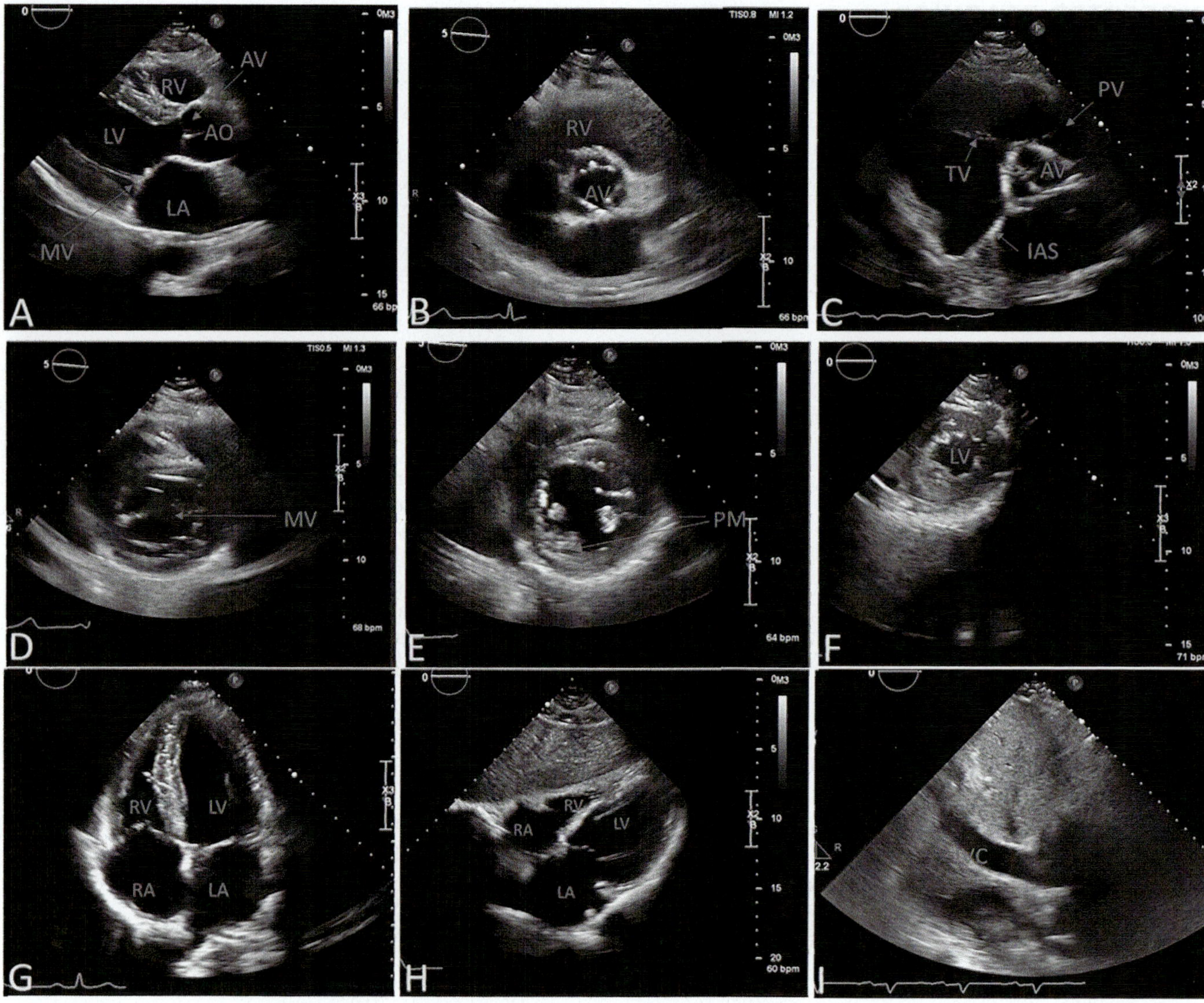

FIGURE 2.15.1 Standard echocardiogram views. A. Parasternal long-axis view. **B** and **C.** Parasternal short-axis (PSAX) view, in systole (B) and diastole (C). **D.** PSAX view, mitral valve/basal LV level. **E.** PSAX view, papillary muscle/mid LV level. **F.** PSAX view, apical level. **G.** Apical four-chamber view. **H.** Subcostal view. **I.** Subcostal view—IVC. AO, aorta; AV, aortic valve; IVC, inferior vena cava; LA, left atrium; LV, left ventricle; MV, mitral valve; PM, papillary muscle; PV, pulmonic valve; RA, right atrium; RV, right ventricle; TV, tricuspid valve.

Other Common Clinical Scenarios in the Intensive Care Unit

- Aortic stenosis (AS)
  - Valvular obstruction of the LV outflow tract (LVOT), often due to leaflet degeneration and calcification, or congenital valvulopathy
  - 2D transthoracic echocardiogram (TTE) is used for assessing valve morphology (eg, tricuspid, congenital bicuspid), leaflet motion and thickening (often restricted and thickened), and quantitative measures of severity. Do not forget to assess for aortopathy if a bicuspid valve is identified.
    - Use parasternal long-axis and short-axis views, zoomed on the aortic valve, for qualitative assessment.
    - Severe AS is defined as: peak velocity>4 m/s and mean gradient >40 mm Hg obtained by CW Doppler (typically from apical five- and three-chamber views), and an aortic valve area <1.0 cm^2.
    - Special circumstances: low-flow low-gradient AS occurs most often in the setting of LV dysfunction and manifests as low stroke volume (SV) (indexed SV <35 mL/m^2), low mean gradient, aortic valve area (AVA) <1.0 cm^2.
- Mitral stenosis (MS)
  - Valvular obstruction at the level of the MV, often due to rheumatic or degenerative calcific disease (most common in the United States)
  - 2D TTE is used for assessing valve morphology, leaflet motion and thickening, and quantitative measures of severity.
    - Rheumatic MS is characterized by commissural and chordal fusion, causing the leaflets to open with a "doming" motion ("hockey stick" appearance in diastole). Degenerative MS is age related and often associated with annular and eventual leaflet calcification.

    - Severe MS is defined as: mitral valve area (MVA) <1.5 cm^2 by planimetry (by 2D parasternal short axis), continuity equation, or diastolic pressure half-time obtained by CW Doppler (apical four- or two-chamber).
    - Other hemodynamic features: mean gradient by CW Doppler often 10 mm Hg when severe (note: mean gradient is very heart rate [HR] dependent and can be elevated in high flow states), LA enlargement, and elevated right ventricular systolic pressure (RVSP).
    - Remember in significant MS, there will be underfilling of the LV, with the LA pressure (or pulmonary capillary wedge pressure [PCWP]) higher than LV end-diastolic pressure (LVEDP).
- Obstructive hypertrophic cardiomyopathy (HCM) (Figure 2.15.2)
  - Often asymmetric LV hypertrophy (LVH) of the septum ≥15 mm without other risk factors for hypertrophy (note: other forms of HCM exist, such as apical) associated with LVOT obstruction (gradient ≥30 mm Hg) due to systolic anterior motion (SAM) of the anterior leaflet of the MV
  - 2D TTE used for assessing the location and degree of hypertrophy, LV wall thickness (in parasternal long-axis and short-axis views), associated MV pathology (parasternal or apical), CW/PW Doppler to assess for LVOT obstruction (apical views)
    - MV SAM results in posteriorly directed eccentric MR and LVOT obstruction if ≥40% of the cardiac cycle.
    - Dynamic outflow obstruction seen with late-peaking systolic gradient, described as "dagger shaped," as seen in Figure 2.15.2. Can be exacerbated with Valsalva, exercise, inotropes, or distributive or hypovolemic physiology
- MR
  - Often caused by primary lesions of the valve apparatus (leaflets, chords, and papillary muscles) or secondary to annular dilation (functional)
  - 2D TTE used to assess etiology by assessing valve motion in parasternal and apical views (prolapse, flail, thickening, or vegetation)
  - Severity assessed using CW and PW Doppler to determine vena contracta width (≥0.7 cm for severe), evidence of flail or perforation, and advanced quantitation
- LV thrombus (Figure 2.15.3)
  - Typically seen after transmural MI with apical regional WMA (akinesis or dyskinesis) resulting in stagnant blood flow
  - Assess on TTE using off-axis views (as shown in Figure 2.15.3) and using color Doppler and contrast imaging
  - Pedunculated, mobile thrombus is at the highest risk of embolism.

Other Structures/Procedures

- Assessing the location of cardiac devices (mechanical circulatory support [MCS] positioning, PA line, extracorporeal membrane oxygenation[ECMO] cannulae) (Figure 2.15.4)
- TTE can also be used in ventilator adjustments to optimize RV and LV interactions.
- Ramp echo studies are performed using TTE to optimize MCS and determine the need for escalation or weaning of support.

Transesophageal Echocardiogram

- Indications: evaluation of cardiac structures and function where findings will alter management, intraoperative guidance, guidance of transcatheter procedures, and critically ill patients
- Contraindications
  - Absolute: perforated viscus, esophageal stricture, esophageal tumor, esophageal perforation or laceration, esophageal diverticulum, or active upper gastrointestinal (GI) bleed
  - Relative: history of radiation to neck and mediastinum, restriction of neck mobility (severe cervical arthritis, atlantoaxial joint disease, cervical spinal abscess); Barrett's esophagus, dysphagia, esophageal varices, active esophagitis; history of GI surgery (such as gastric bypass), recent upper GI bleed, active peptic ulcer disease, symptomatic hiatal hernia; coagulopathy, (<50)
- Common clinical scenarios
  - Endocarditis evaluation typically performed with a moderate or high pretest probability (eg, staphylococcal > streptococcal bacteremia, fungemia, prosthetic heart valve, or intracardiac device)
    - Involves assessment of all four cardiac valves for evidence of vegetation, valve regurgitation or stenosis (flail or perforated leaflets), sequelae such as perivalvular abscess
    - Prosthetic valves also need to be assessed for paravalvular leak, dehiscence.
  - Left atrial appendage (LAA) assessment for cardioversion performed at multiple angles (minimum at 0, 45, 90, and 135 degrees)
    - Organized thrombus is well circumscribed and may appear mobile.
    - Spontaneous echocardiographic contrast (slow blood flow) may appear "smoke-like" due to its slow motion and lack of definition.
    - LAA-emptying velocities of by PW <20 cm/s are associated with thrombus formation and embolic events.
  - Aortic dissection: can visualize the aortic root, ascending thoracic aorta (120-140 degrees), arch and descending aorta (0 or 90 degrees)
    - Assess with color Doppler to identify and assess dissection flap (such as fenestration in the flap, identify true versus false lumen and false-lumen thrombosis)
    - For proximal dissection, also evaluate the aortic valve and for aortic regurgitation; dissection flap can impact leaflet geometry or impair.
    - Note: transesophageal echocardiogram cannot visualize the entire thoracic aorta due to the interposition of airways between the probe and the aorta; may not see parts of the distal ascending aorta or arch.
  - Critically ill patients with poor TTE windows

Point-of-Care Ultrasound

- Indications: qualitative but interactive assessment of effusion, biventricular function, basic valvular assessment, IVC evaluation
- Not validated for use in more complex cases, such as evaluation of endocarditis, WMA, severity of stenotic or regurgitant lesions, where high resolution and Doppler are required

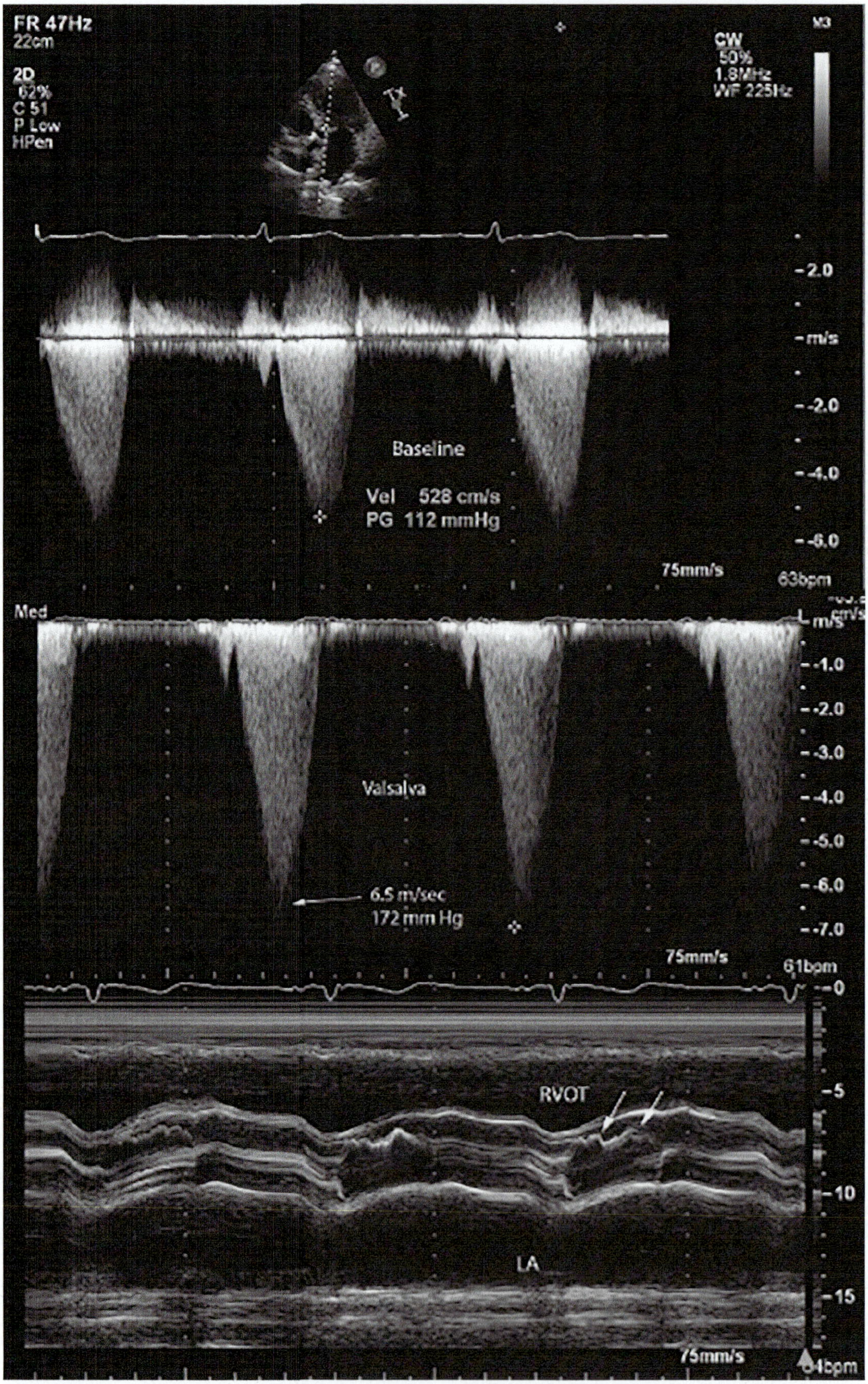

FIGURE 2.15.2 Continuous wave Doppler demonstrating LVOT obstruction at rest, which worsened with the Valsalva maneuver. M-mode demonstrating late-systolic systolic anterior motion of the mitral valve (arrows), which leads to dynamic LVOT obstruction. LA, left atrium; LVOT, left ventricular outflow tract; RVOT, right ventricular outflow tract.

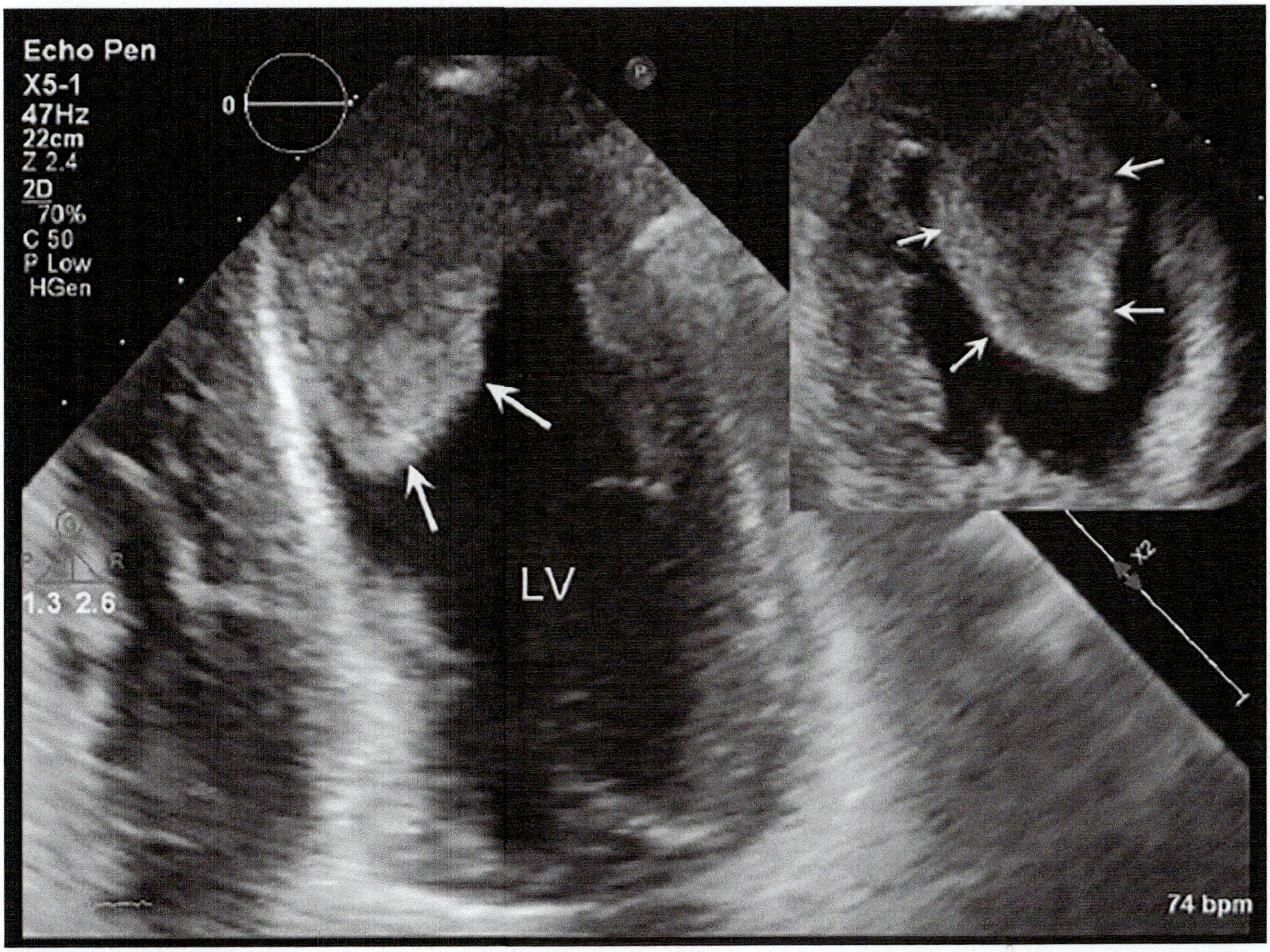

FIGURE 2.15.3 **Apical four-chamber view demonstrating left ventricular (LV), indicated by arrows.**

- IVC evaluation in the subcostal window 0.5 to 3 cm from the RA
  - IVC diameter ≤2.1 cm and collapses >50% with inspiration (or a sniff) = RA pressure (RAP) of 3 mm Hg
  - IVC diameter >2.1 cm that collapses <50% with inspiration (or sniff) = RAP of 15 mm Hg
  - If one of the criteria is present, RAP is intermediate (RAP of 8 mm Hg).
  - Intubated patients on positive pressure ventilation, IVC is commonly dilated and not an accurate estimate of RAP.
- Lung ultrasound can be used to assess B-lines (pulmonary edema), pneumothorax, and pleural effusion.

Chest X-Ray

- Evidence of volume overload/pulmonary edema: Kerley B-lines, peribronchial cuffing, pulmonary venous congestion, fissure thickening/fluid, air space opacification, pleural/pericardial effusions
- Widened mediastinum: differential diagnosis includes aortic dilatation or injury, venous anomalies, mediastinal mass, enlarged PA, postcardiac surgery
- Lines and cardiac device positioning
  - Sternal wires—indicate prior cardiac surgeries
  - Identify valve prostheses and pacing/defibrillator leads
  - PA catheter positioning: tip within the middle third of chest x-ray (CXR) ideally
  - Intra-aortic balloon placement: ideally distal tip within the aorto-pulmonary window
  - Endotracheal tube placement: ideally tip 2 to 4 cm above the carina

Cardiac Computed Tomography

- Coronary evaluation, including fractional flow reserve, to evaluate the hemodynamic significance of coronary vessel lesions
- Aortic calcium score to help determine the severity of AS when there are discordant data
- Access/device planning for percutaneous/surgical interventions
- May also be useful in evaluating LAA, and in endocarditis evaluations (eg, perivalvular abscess), cardiac masses (including thrombus)

Cardiac Magnetic Resonance Imaging

- Diagnosis: myocarditis, infiltrative processes (amyloidosis, sarcoidosis), pericardial processes (pericarditis, constriction, malignancy), viability, and scar
- Typically requires prolonged imaging and thus less available in critically ill patients

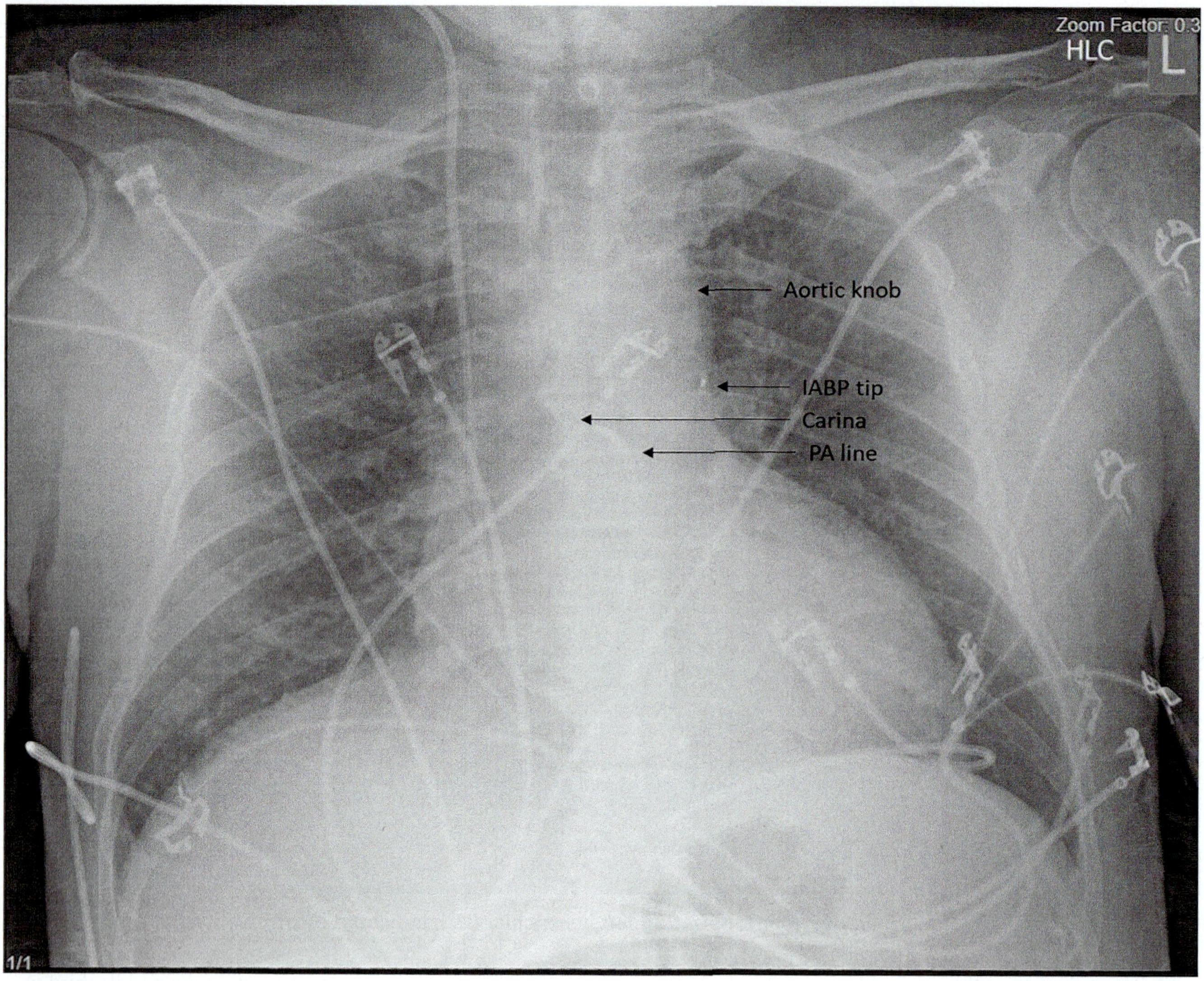

FIGURE 2.15.4 Chest x-ray with demonstrative anatomy/devices identified. IABP, intra-aortic balloon pump; PA line, pulmonary arterial line.

SUGGESTED READINGS

Armstrong WF, Ryan T. *Feigenbaum's Echocardiography: Ebook Without Multimedia*. 8th ed. Wolters Kluwer; 2018.

Baumgartner H, Hung J, Bermejo J, et al. Echocardiographic assessment of valve stenosis: EAE/ASE recommendations for clinical practice. *Eur J Echocardiogr*. 2009;10(1):1-25.

Hahn, RT, Abraham T, Adams MS, et al. Guidelines for performing a comprehensive transesophageal echocardiographic examination. *J Am Soc Echocardiogr*. 2013;26:921-964.

Kirkpatrick JN, Grimm R, Johri AM, et al. Recommendations for echocardiography laboratories participating in cardiac point of care cardiac ultrasound (POCUS) and critical care echocardiography training: report from the American Society of Echocardiography. *J Am Soc Echocardiogr*. 2020;33(4):409-422.

Klein AL, Asher CR, eds. *Clinical Echocardiography Review: A Self-Assessment Tool*. Lippincott Williams & Wilkins; 2011.

Mitchell C, Rahko PS, Blauwet LA, et al. Guidelines for performing a comprehensive transthoracic echocardiographic examination in adults: recommendations from the American Society of Echocardiography. *J Am Soc Echocardiogr*. 2019;32(1):1-64.

Nagueh SF, Phelan D, Abraham T, et al. Recommendations for multimodality cardiovascular imaging of patients with hypertrophic cardiomyopathy: an update from the American Society of Echocardiography, in collaboration with the American Society of Nuclear Cardiology, the Society for Cardiovascular Magnetic Resonance, and the Society of Cardiovascular Computed Tomography. *J Am Soc Echocardiogr*. 2022;35(6):533-569.

Otto CM, Nishimura RA, Bonow RO, et al. 2020 ACC/AHA guideline for the management of patients with valvular heart disease: a report of the American College of Cardiology/American Heart Association Joint Committee on Clinical Practice Guidelines. *Circulation*. 2021;143:e72-e227.

Volpicelli G, Elbarbary M, Blaivas M, et al. International evidence-based recommendations for point-of-care lung ultrasound. *Intensive Care Med*. 2012;38:577-591.

Zoghbi WA, Adams D, Bonow RO, et al. Recommendations for noninvasive evaluation of native valvular regurgitation: a report from the American Society of Echocardiography developed in collaboration with the Society for Cardiovascular Magnetic Resonance. *J Am Soc Echocardiogr*. 2017;30(4):303-371.

2.16

Pharmacologic Therapies for Cardiac Disorders

Edmond Solomon and David M. Dudzinski

Antiarrhythmics and Nodal Agents

Sodium Channel Blockers

Lidocaine (Intravenous)

- Indications: ventricular tachycardia/fibrillation (VT/VF) (enhanced efficacy in ischemic tissue; local anaerobic metabolism → intracellular acidosis → potassium efflux → increased affinity of lidocaine to sodium channels)
- Dosing: bolus 1 to 1.5 mg/kg ×1 (~100 mg), may repeat 0.75 mg/kg every 5 minutes (max cumulative dose 3 mg/kg), followed by infusion at 1 to 4 mg/min
- Adverse drug reactions (ADRs) (increased risk if hepatic/renal dysfunction) are related to sodium channel antagonism: local anesthetic toxicity (confusion, somnolence tremors, seizures, hallucination), QRS prolongation, bradycardia, nausea
- Therapeutic drug monitoring (TDM): consider monitoring if infusion > 24 hours. Therapeutic levels: 1.5 to 5 µg/mL, toxic >5 µg/mL (may have symptoms of toxicity at levels <5 µg/mL)

Procainamide (Intravenous)

- Indications: atrial fibrillation (AF)/flutter, supraventricular tachycardia (SVT), Wolff-Parkinson-White (WPW), VT/VF
- Dosing: load/bolus 10 to 17 mg/kg ×1 or 100 mg q5min until arrhythmia controlled, hypotension, or QRS widens by 50%, followed by infusion at 1 to 4 mg/min if needed
- ADRs (increased risk if hepatic/renal dysfunction): PR/QRS/QTc prolongation, bradycardia, positive antinuclear antibody (ANA), lupus-like drug reaction, cytopenia, local anesthetic toxicity (see earlier)
- TDM: consider monitoring if infusion >24 hours. Therapeutic: procainamide 4 to 10 µg/mL, NAPA (N-acetylprocainamide) 15 to 25 µg/mL

Mexiletine (Oral)

- Indications: VT/VF
- Dosing: 100 to 200 mg q8-12h (max 1.2 g/d)
- ADRs: nausea, vomiting (taking with food limits gastrointestinal [GI] upset)
- Notes: Oral option for patients on lidocaine infusions, give the first dose when lidocaine stopped, prolonged half-life in hepatic dysfunction

Quinidine (Oral)

- Indications: AF/flutter, VT, Brugada syndrome
- Dosing: 200 to 400 mg q6h (sulfate), 324 to 648 mg q8 (gluconate)
- ADRs: QRS/QTc prolongation, diarrhea, nausea, hepatotoxicity, hemolysis (if G6PD deficient)
- Notes: Oral option for patients on procainamide infusions, give the first dose when procainamide stopped. Prolonged half-life in patients with heart failure (HF), renal/hepatic dose adjustments needed

Potassium Channel Blockers

Amiodarone (Intravenous/Oral)

- Indications: AF/flutter, SVT, VT/VF
- Dosing: VT/VF arrest: 300 mg rapid bolus, second dose 150 mg rapid bolus if needed. AF/SVT/VT: 150 mg intravenous (IV) followed by 1 mg/min 6 hours, then 0.5 mg/min for 18 hours. After IV, complete oral (PO) 400 mg q8-12h for a total load of 6 g (atrial) or 10 g (ventricular). Maintenance dose 100 to 400 mg daily
- ADRs: QTc prolongation, bradycardia, hypotension; chronic use can cause pulmonary/thyroid/liver/ocular toxicity (iodine-containing medication) and requires surveillance.

Beta-Blockers

Esmolol (Intravenous)

- Indications: AF/flutter, acute aortic syndromes, VT
- Dosing: 500 to 1,000 µg/kg bolus (optional), continuous infusion 25 to 300 µ/kg/min
- ADRs: bradycardia, hypotension, negative inotropy (avoid in acute decompensated heart failure [ADHF])
- Notes: Beta-2 selective, first-line therapy in acute aortic syndromes for rate and impulse control. High doses = high fluid intake and high cost

Labetalol (Intravenous/Oral)

- Indications: AF/flutter, acute aortic syndromes, hypertension
- Dosing: (PO) 200 to 800 mg q8-12h (max 2,400 mg/d), (IV) 5 to 20 mg q10m as needed, continuous infusion 0.5 to 4 mg/min
- ADRs: bradycardia, hypotension, negative inotropy (avoid in ADHF)
- Notes: Beta:alpha receptor activity ratio 3:1 for PO and 7:1 for IV

Metoprolol (Intravenous/Oral)

- Indications: AF/flutter, SVT, VT, acute coronary syndrome (ACS), chronic HF
- Dosing: (PO) IR 25 to 200 mg/d divided into q6-12h, ER 50 to 400 mg/d divided q12-24hr, (IV) 2.5 to 10 mg q10-15 min as needed
- ADRs: bradycardia, hypotension, negative inotropy (avoid in ADHF)
- Notes: IV to PO 2.5:1 (5 mg IV = 12.5 mg PO), beta-1 selective

Calcium Channel Blockers

Diltiazem (Intravenous/Oral)

- Indications: AF/flutter, angina, coronary vasospasm, SVT
- Dosing: (PO) IR 30 to 90 mg q6h (max 480 mg/d), ER 120 to 480 mg q24h/d, (IV) 0.25 mg/kg IV (10-20 mg),

may repeat 0.35 mg/kg q10-15m as needed or continuous infusion 5 to 15 mg/h

- ADRs: bradycardia, hypotension, negative inotropy (avoid in ADHF)
- Notes: Nondihydropyridine calcium channel blocker (CCB). Half-life prolonged with continuous infusion

Verapamil (Intravenous/Oral)

- Indications: AF/flutter, angina, coronary vasospasm, SVT
- Dosing: (PO) IR 40 mg q8h (max 480 mg/d), ER 120 to 480 mg divided q12-24h (IV) 5 to 10 mg q10-15min as needed
- ADRs: bradycardia, hypotension, negative inotropy (avoid in ADHF), constipation
- Notes: Nondihydropyridine CCB

Miscellaneous

Adenosine (Intravenous)

- Indications: SVT (also in Advanced Cardiac Life Support [ACLS] algorithm for regular wide-complex tachycardia as there are adenosine-sensitive VT)
- Dosing: 6 mg rapid IV bolus followed by 12 mg ×2 (if needed). Central line administration or heart transplant patients reduce these doses by 50% (3 mg/6 mg/6 mg).
- ADRs: transient atrioventricular (AV) block, flushing, headache, dyspnea
- Notes: Avoid in polymorphic wide-complex tachycardia, short half-life so administer 10 mL flush immediately after dose given and can raise arm where infused.

Digoxin (Intravenous/Oral)

- Indications: AF/flutter, SVT, HF
- Dosing: loading dose 8 to 12 μg/kg (ideal body weight), 50% as first dose followed by 25% q6h × 2 doses. No loading doses needed for HF. Maintenance dose 62.5 to 250 μg/d based on renal function. Use extreme caution in end-stage renal disease (ESRD) (not dialyzable).
- ADRs: bradycardia, nausea/vomiting, vision disturbances, ventricular arrhythmias
- TDM: trough levels 0.5 to 0.9 for HF, <2 for atrial arrhythmias
- Notes: Antidote = digoxin immune Fab, each 40 mg vial reverses ~0.5 mg digoxin, indications for reversal: life-threatening arrhythmias, acute ingestion >10 mg or trough level >10 ng/mL (acute ingestion) or >6 ng/mL (chronic ingestion), K^+ >5.5 mEq/L with worsening symptoms

Vasoactive Agents

Vasopressors

Norepinephrine (Intravenous)

- Indications: vasodilatory shock, mixed shock
- Dosing: 1 to 30 μg/min (0.02-0.3 μg/kg/min)
- Receptor activation: $\alpha1 = \beta1 > \beta2$
- ADRs: arrhythmias, coronary/limb ischemia
- Notes: Caution in left ventricular (LV) outflow tract obstruction due to β1 agonism, first-line vasopressor in septic shock

Phenylephrine (Intravenous)

- Indications: vasodilatory shock, hypotension from atrial/ventricular arrhythmias, cardiogenic shock due to aortic/mitral stenosis or LV outflow tract obstruction
- Dosing: 10 to 400 μg/min (0.1-5 μg/kg/min)
- Receptor activation: α1 only
- ADRs: reflex bradycardia, limb ischemia
- Notes: First-line vasopressor for hypotension due to LV outflow tract obstruction (hypertrophic obstructive cardiomyopathy [HOCM]/stress cardiomyopathy) or mitral/aortic stenosis. Avoid in cardiogenic shock due to other causes, may be useful in hypotension with rapid atrial arrhythmias.

Vasopressin (Intravenous)

- Indications: vasodilatory shock, diabetes insipidus
- Dosing: 0.03 to 0.04 units/min IV (shock), 5 to 10 units subcutaneously (SC) 2 to 3×'s daily (diabetes insipidus)
- Receptor activation: V1 and V2 (nonnoradrenergic receptors)
- ADRs: mesenteric/digital ischemia, reflex bradycardia, hyponatremia
- Notes: Second-line vasopressor for septic shock after norepinephrine, limited effect on pulmonary vascular resistance (so may be advantageous in pulmonary arterial hypertension [PAH] or right ventricular [RV] failure)

Methylene Blue (Intravenous)

- Indications: refractory vasodilatory shock, vasoplegia postcardiac surgery, methemoglobinemia
- Dosing: shock 1 to 2 mg/kg bolus followed by infusion (if needed) 0.25 to 1 mg/kg/h, methemoglobinemia 1 mg/kg bolus may repeat 1 hour later if methemoglobin remains >30% or if symptoms persist
- Pharmacology: nitric oxide synthase inhibitor to limit its vasodilatory effect in shock
- ADRs: serotonin syndrome (monoamine oxidase inhibitor [MAOI]), methemoglobinemia (high doses or in renal failure with prolonged infusion), blue/green discoloration of body fluids, increased pulmonary vascular resistance (PVR), hemolytic anemia (if G6PD deficient)
- Notes: May cause pulse oximetry inaccuracy, hold serotonergic medications if administered, avoid in known G6PD deficiency.

Hydroxocobalamin (Intravenous)

- Indications: refractory vasodilatory shock (off-label); cyanide poisoning
- Dosing: 5 to 10 g IV over 10 to 15 minutes for shock; or continuous infusion 250 to 500 mg/h after 125 to 250 mg bolus
- Mechanism: inhibits nitric oxide–mediated vasodilatation and binds H_2S as well (latter may be produced by bacteria in septic shock)
- ADRs: red chromaturia, elevated blood pressure (BP), photosensitivity, renal injury
- Notes: Consult Poison Control Center if using for cyanide poisoning. May interfere with intensive care unit (ICU) devices that employ colorimetric technologies

Angiotensin II (Intravenous)

- Indications: refractory vasodilatory shock
- Dosing: 1.25 to 80 ng/kg/min (max 80 ng/kg/min for 3 hours, then 40 ng/kg/min)
- Receptor activation: angiotensin II
- ADRs: arterial/venous thromboembolism, mesenteric/peripheral ischemia, acidosis, thrombocytopenia
- Notes: Last line after failure of other vasopressors, costly

Inotropes

Epinephrine (Intravenous, Subcutaneous, Intramuscular)

- Indications: cardiogenic or vasodilatory shock, symptomatic bradycardia, anaphylaxis, cardiac arrest
- Dosing: 1 to 20 μg/min (0.01-0.2 μg/kg/min) for shock/bradycardia, 1 mg IV bolus every 3 to 5 minutes for cardiac arrest, 0.3 to 0.5 mg intramuscularly (IM) for anaphylaxis
- Receptor activation: α1, β1, and β2
- ADRs: arrhythmias, coronary/limb ischemia; can increase lactate levels
- Notes: Caution in LV outflow tract obstruction and unrevascularized coronary disease due to β1 agonism, first-line vasopressor in anaphylactic shock, first-line inotrope in ADHF with significant hypotension

Dobutamine (Intravenous)

- Indications: ADHF, cardiogenic shock
- Dosing: starting dose 2.5 to 5 μg/kg/min, titrated to effect (max 10 μg/kg/min)
- Receptor activation: β1>β2
- ADRs: tachycardia, arrhythmias, reduced BP
- Notes: Usually mean arterial pressure (MAP) neutral (β2-induced vasodilation offset by β1-induced increase in stroke volume), fast onset/offset (~10-20 minutes)

Milrinone (Intravenous)

- Indications: ADHF, cardiogenic shock (especially RV dysfunction)
- Dosing: starting dose 0.125 to 0.25 μg/kg/min titrated to effect (max 0.75 μg/kg/min)
- Pharmacology: PDE3 inhibitor
- ADRs: tachycardia, arrhythmias, hypotension
- Notes: Arterial/venous/pulmonary vasodilation = reduction in MAP/PVR, bolus doses cause significant hypotension, long half-life, which is further prolonged in renal failure, slow titrations and weaning, therefore, required

Chronotropes

Dopamine (Intravenous)

- Indications: symptomatic bradycardia, ADHF (rarely)
- Dosing: 5 to 20 μg/kg/min
- Receptor activation: D1 and D2> β1> β2> α1 (only at higher doses ~10 μg/kg/min)
- ADRs: tachyarrhythmias, peripheral ischemia
- Notes: Used first line in the treatment of symptomatic bradycardia, rarely used as an inotrope

Isoproterenol (Intravenous)

- Indications: symptomatic bradycardia, bradycardia-induced torsade de pointes
- Dosing: 1 to 20 μg/min
- Receptor activation: β1 and β2 agonists
- ADRs: angina, coronary vasospasm, arrhythmias
- Notes: Doses >10 μg/min have a limited effect on heart rate (HR), alternative agent for symptomatic bradycardia if hypertension associated with dopamine or epinephrine, may consider first line for rate-dependent torsade de pointes.

Atropine (Intravenous)

- Indication: symptomatic bradycardia
- Dosing: 0.5 to 1 mg q3-5min (max total dose 3 mg)
- Pharmacology: muscarinic (M2) receptor antagonist
- ADRs: arrhythmias, paradoxical bradycardia
- Notes: Do not administer doses <0.5 mg (paradoxical bradycardia), ineffective in heart transplant recipients due to denervation.

Vasodilators

Nitroglycerin (Intravenous, and Also Oral, Sublingual, Transdermal)

- Indications: ACS, angina, hypertension, pulmonary decongestion and preload modulation in HF
- Mechanism: nitrate donor (causes venodilatation > arterial vasodilatation)
- Dosing: 5 to 400 μg/min (higher doses needed for arterial dilation, tachyphylaxis can occur after 24-48 hour). Onset (immediate), duration of action (minutes) independent of renal/hepatic function
- ADRs: reflex tachycardia, headache
- Notes: Venous >>> arterial dilation, first line for angina and acute cardiogenic pulmonary edema, use caution in inferior myocardial infarction (MI)/RV MI (preload sensitive states) or if phosphodiesterase-5 inhibitor (PDE5-I) use within last 24 hours

Nitroprusside (Intravenous)

- Indications: acute aortic dissection, ADHF, hypertension
- Mechanism: nitrate donor
- Dosing: 0.2 to 0.5 μg/kg/min (max of 10 μg/kg/min × 10 min then 5 μg/kg/min); onset (minutes), duration of action (<10 min) independent of renal/hepatic function
- ADRs: cyanide/thiocyanate toxicity if hepatic/renal impairment or with higher doses (>3 μg/kg/min) or long duration (>3 day), methemoglobinemia with high doses
- Notes: Venous = arterial dilation effect; avoid in acute ACS or unrevascularized coronary artery disease (CAD) due to the risk of "coronary steal syndrome," avoid if PDE5-I use within last 24 hours.

Nicardipine (Intravenous)

- Indications: acute aortic dissection, hypertension (including pregnancy-induced), BP management in ischemic stroke
- Mechanism: dihydropyridine CCB
- Dosing: 2.5 to 15 mg/h, onset (<5 minute), duration of action (0.5-2 hour) prolonged in hepatic dysfunction

- ADRs: potential pulmonary shunting, headache
- Notes: Arterial dilation only, hepatic impairment will increase duration of action, first-line agent for hypertension.

Clevidipine (Intravenous)

- Indications: acute aortic dissection, hypertension, BP management in ischemic stroke
- Mechanism: dihydropyridine CCB
- Dosing: 1 to 21 mg/h; onset (<5 minute), duration (5-15 minute) independent of renal/hepatic function
- ADRs: potential pulmonary shunting, headache, increased triglycerides
- Notes: Arterial dilation only, fat emulsion (0.2 g/mL) so monitor triglycerides with prolonged use, use with caution in egg/soy allergy

Hydralazine (Intravenous/Oral)

- Indications: hypertension, chronic HF management (usually combined with isosorbide)
- Mechanism: direct arterial vasodilator via smooth muscle relaxation
- Dosing: 5 to 20 mg q4-6h (IV), 12.5 to 100 mg q6-8h, max 300 mg/d (PO)
- ADRs: hypotension, headache, reflex tachycardia
- Notes: Rare risk of systemic lupus erythematosus (SLE)-like reaction

SUGGESTED READINGS

Al-Khatib SM, Stevenson WG, Ackerman MJ, et al. 2017 AHA/ACC/HRS Guideline for management of patients with ventricular arrhythmias and the prevention of sudden cardiac death: a report of the American College of Cardiology/American Heart Association Task Force on Clinical Practice Guidelines and the Heart Rhythm Society [published correction appears in *J Am Coll Cardiol*. 2018;72(14):1760.]. *J Am Coll Cardiol*. 2018; 72(14):e91-e220.

Aranda JM Jr, Schofield RS, Pauly DF, et al. Comparison of dobutamine versus milrinone therapy in hospitalized patients awaiting cardiac transplantation: a prospective, randomized trial. *Am Heart J*. 2003;145(2): 324-329.

Bress AP, Anderson TS, Flack JM, et al. The management of elevated blood pressure in the acute care setting: a scientific statement from the American Heart Association. *Hypertension*. 2024;81(8):e94-e106.

Dan GA, Martinez-Rubio A, Agewall S, et al. Antiarrhythmic drugs-clinical use and clinical decision making: a consensus document from the European Heart Rhythm Association (EHRA) and European Society of Cardiology (ESC) Working Group on Cardiovascular Pharmacology, endorsed by the Heart Rhythm Society (HRS), Asia-Pacific Heart Rhythm Society (APHRS) and International Society of Cardiovascular Pharmacotherapy (ISCP) [published correction appears in *Europace*. 2018;20(5):738.]. *Europace*. 2018;20(5):731-732.

Mathew R, Di Santo P, Jung RG, et al. Milrinone as compared with dobutamine in the treatment of cardiogenic shock. *N Engl J Med*. 2021;385:516.

Shankar A, Gurumurthy G, Sridharan L, et al. A clinical update on vasoactive medication in the management of cardiogenic shock. *Clin Med Insights Cardiol*. 2022;16:11795468221075064.

2.17

Cardiac Arrest and Resuscitation

David Lewandowski and Jarone Lee

The critical care physician is often called upon to assist in cardiopulmonary resuscitation (CPR) in the intensive care unit (ICU) as well as throughout the hospital. Cardiopulmonary arrest in the hospitalized patient often has a specific cause, and, as time to resuscitation is strongly linked to outcome, resuscitative efforts should be individualized.

Common Causes to Remember

- Myocardial infarction
- Pericardial tamponade
- Pulmonary embolus
- Tension pneumothorax
- Hypoxemia
- Acid-base derangements
- Hypovolemia
- Hemorrhage
- Hypothermia
- Electrolyte abnormalities

Epidemiology

- There are ~300,000 cardiac arrests among hospitalized patients in the United States annually.
- Less than half of the patients who undergo CPR will be resuscitated, and less than one half of those initially resuscitated will live until hospital discharge.
- As few as 5% of CPR recipients return to baseline functional status post arrest.
- The probability of successful resuscitation exponentially declines after 6 to 10 minutes of arrest.

Key Pathophysiology

- In-hospital cardiac arrest may be due to a variety of pathophysiologic insults.
- Respiratory failure leads to more than half of the cardiac arrest events in hospitalized patients, and it may be due to aspiration, excessive sedation, pulmonary embolism, airway obstruction, muscle weakness, and other causes.
  - Failure to rapidly restore oxygenation results in hypoxemia, which initially enhances the peripheral chemical drive to breathe and stimulates the heart rate.
  - However, profound hypoxemia depresses neural function and produces refractory bradycardia.
- Primary cardiovascular events can lead to cardiac arrest via an abrupt decrease in cardiac output due to arrhythmia or decreased pump function resulting from the following factors:
  - Decrease in preload
    - Venodilation
    - Hemorrhage

- Cardiac tamponade
- Tension pneumothorax
- Increase in afterload
  - Obstructive shock
  - Specifically increases in right ventricular (RV) afterload, such as pulmonary embolism
- Acute decreases in contractility via cardiac muscle fiber dysfunction
  - Drugs
  - Acidosis
  - Electrolyte disturbances

- Ultimately, a cascade of events leads to systemic hypoperfusion.
- Tissue hypoxemia leads to anaerobic metabolism and acidosis, which leads to systemic vasodilation, pulmonary vasoconstriction, reduced myocardial contractility, insensitivity to catecholamines, and eventual circulatory collapse.

Differential Diagnosis

- During in-hospital arrest, it is important that the team quickly consider the circumstances and incorporate appropriate treatment into the resuscitation to maintain perfusion and address the underlying cause.
- Depending on the clinical situation, a broad differential diagnosis for the cause of cardiac arrest may exist:
  - *Mechanical ventilation*: misplaced endotracheal (ET) tube, auto-positive end-expiratory pressure (PEEP), mucus plug, etc
  - *During or post central line placement*: tension pneumothorax, tachyarrhythmia, heart block/bradycardia, air embolism, tamponade, etc
  - *Acute head injury*: increased intracranial pressure (ICP), diabetes insipidus (DI)-induced hypovolemia, etc
  - *Recent myocardial infarction*: arrhythmia, cardiac rupture or tamponade, papillary muscle rupture, atrioventricular (AV) block, etc
  - *Renal insufficiency*: hyperkalemia, acidosis, hypoglycemia
  - *Pancreatitis*: hypovolemia, hypocalcemia, abdominal compartment syndrome, etc
  - *Medication error or overdose*: opioid, local anesthesia, insulin, beta-blocker, calcium channel blocker, digoxin, tricyclic antidepressant (TCA), monoamine oxidase inhibitor (MAOI), etc
  - *Trauma*: hemorrhage, tension pneumothorax, tamponade, etc
  - *Burns*: airway obstruction, carbon monoxide, cyanide toxicity, etc
  - *During patient transport*: displaced ET tube, interruption of vasoactive medications, etc

Management and Treatment

- CPR was initially conceived for otherwise healthy patients who suffer from sudden cardiac death from arrhythmia or myocardial infarction.
- The likelihood of successful CPR, meaning hospital discharge without neurologic impairment, depends on patient characteristics and time until return of circulation.
- Promptly instituted CPR in sudden cardiac arrest is highly successful, whereas CPR in patients with multiple organ failure and critical illness is very unlikely to be beneficial.
- Published guidelines for Basic Life Support (BLS) and Advanced Cardiac Life Support (ACLS) are updated regularly and provide a framework for resuscitation.
- A high-quality, organized, resuscitative effort is fundamental to success.
  - Establishing a *team leader* and *roles* early is important to ensure a coordinated and effective resuscitative effort.
  - High-quality *chest compressions* should be of adequate rate (100-120/min) and depth (5-6 cm) and allow for complete chest recoil after each compression.
  - Interruption of chest compressions should be limited, aiming for a chest compression fraction >80%.
  - End-tidal CO_2 ($ETCO_2$) correlates with cardiac output and cerebral and coronary perfusion pressure during CPR:
    - Quantitative waveform capnography should be monitored with bag-valve mask to monitor CPR quality and adjust chest compressions to improve $ETCO_2$.
    - In intubated patients, $ETCO_2$ <10 mm Hg during CPR suggests return of spontaneous circulation (ROSC) is unlikely.
    - An initial $ETCO_2$ or 20-minute $ETCO_2$ >20 is a strong predictor of ROSC.
    - It is reasonable to consider an abrupt increase in $ETCO_2$ as indicative of ROSC.
    - Diastolic blood pressure can be used as a surrogate for coronary perfusion pressure during CPR.
  - Initially, effective *ventilation* can usually be established with a bag-valve mask.
    - Consider head tilt, jaw thrust, nasopharyngeal airway or oropharyngeal airway, and two-operator bag-valve mask technique to improve ventilation.
  - CPR should be performed with cycles of 30 compressions and 2 breaths prior to placement of an advanced airway.
  - Advanced airway placement should be performed by an experienced operator and should not interfere with ongoing resuscitative efforts.
    - Supraglottic device insertion or ET intubation may be utilized as both demonstrate similar survival to discharge and neurologic outcome in cardiac arrest.
  - After the placement of an advanced airway, ventilation may be provided at 10 breaths per minute while performing continuous chest compressions.
    - Excessive ventilation impairs venous return and makes achieving ROSC more challenging.
  - For patients with ventricular fibrillation (VF) or pulseless ventricular tachycardia (VT), an unsynchronized shock should be delivered as quickly as possible.
  - Early intravenous or intraosseous access is important but should not interrupt ongoing CPR.
  - The ET route may be used for certain medications commonly remembered using the acronym NAVEL (naloxone, atropine, vasopressin, epinephrine, lidocaine) but is not a preferred route due to variable drug uptake.
  - ACLS drug therapy leads to increased rates of ROSC, though there are insufficient data to show that this translates into long-term survival benefit with good neurologic outcome.
    - Epinephrine should be administered every 3 to 5 minutes.

- Amiodarone or lidocaine may be considered for shockable rhythms.
- Magnesium sulfate is recommended only in torsades de pointes.

- Drugs NOT recommended for routine use during cardiac arrest include atropine, sodium bicarbonate, and calcium.
- Point-of-care ultrasound (POCUS) can help identify reversible causes of cardiac arrest (pneumothorax, cardiac tamponade, clot-in-transit, deep venous thrombosis, etc) and identification of ROSC, but the team must be mindful to minimize interruptions in chest compressions if performing cardiac ultrasound.
- Extracorporeal CPR (E-CPR) with venoarterial extracorporeal membrane oxygenation (VA ECMO) may be considered for both out-of-hospital (OHCA) and in-hospital (IHCA) cardiac arrest in select patients:
  - Witnessed cardiac arrest with initiation of CPR within 10 minutes (including bystander CPR)
  - Initial shockable rhythm
  - $ETCO_2$ >10 mm Hg during CPR
  - Intermittent ROSC or refractory VF
  - Those with signs of life (extremity movement, pupillary response, agonal respirations, etc)
  - No known end-stage organ disease (heart failure, end-stage renal disease [ESRD], chronic obstructive pulmonary disease [COPD], liver failure, or terminal illness)
  - Absence of significant aortic valve insufficiency
  - Prompt activation of the ECMO team so patient arrives at the ECMO capability facility within 30 minutes of cardiac arrest and ECMO cannulation achieved within 60 minutes of cardiac arrest.
  - May be considered for patients suffering cardiac arrest from toxidrome
- Time dedicated to identifying a pulse during rhythm checks must be limited to under 10 seconds to maintain a high chest compression fraction.
- After ROSC, efforts should be made to stabilize and reevaluate the patient.
  - This includes optimizing cardiopulmonary function and vital organ perfusion, transporting the patient to the appropriate critical care setting, as well as identifying and treating the precipitating cause of the arrest and taking measures to prevent recurrence.

- Postcardiac arrest care
  - Systematic postcardiac arrest care after ROSC can improve the likelihood of survival and quality of life.
  - After reevaluating and stabilizing the patient and transporting them to the appropriate critical care setting, subsequent objectives include:
    - Controlling the body temperature to optimize neurologic recovery
    - Optimizing mechanical ventilation
    - Identifying and treating acute coronary syndromes
    - Reducing the risk of multiorgan injury
    - Objectively assessing prognosis and recovery
  - Targeted temperature management (TTM) should be considered in any patient who is unable to follow commands after ROSC.
    - Hypothermia has multifactorial effects that ultimately reduce cell death, including inhibition of damaging neurotransmitters, preserving the blood-brain barrier, protecting adenosine triphosphate (ATP) stores, and decreasing ICP.
    - In a Cochrane meta-analysis, conventional hypothermia after ROSC resulted in improved neurologic outcome and survival in patients compared to standard treatment.
      - There is no difference found between therapeutic hypothermia and TTM at 36 °C.
      - Those undergoing therapeutic hypothermia experienced increased incidences of severe arrhythmia, hypokalemia, and pneumonia.
    - Any adult patient with OHCA or IHCA who remains comatose after ROSC should be managed with a deliberate target temperature strategy (32 °C to) ≤37.5 °C, regardless of initial rhythm (2023 American Heart Association [AHA] Class I recommendation).
    - Based on prior trial data suggesting neurologic benefit, it remains uncertain whether there are subpopulations of comatose arrest survivors who may benefit from hypothermia (eg, 32-34 °C) (2023 AHA Class IIb recommendation).
    - TTM for fever prevention should continue at least 24 hours (2023 AHA Class IIa recommendation); consider up to 72 hours if comatose. Fever after ROSC is associated with poor outcomes and should actively be prevented after initial TTM (2023 AHA Class IIb recommendation).
    - Potential complications associated with cooling include:
      - Coagulopathy
      - Arrhythmia
      - Hyperglycemia
      - Immune dysfunction
      - Electrolyte disarray
      - Shivering
    - The ongoing TTM3 and ICECAP trials will provide additional evidence to determine optimal targeted temperature and duration of management, respectively.
  - Optimizing mechanical ventilation includes adjusting FIO_2 to the minimum concentration needed to achieve arterial oxyhemoglobin saturation 92% to 98%, with a goal of avoiding hyperoxia while ensuring adequate oxygen delivery and avoiding hyperventilation as hypocapnia-induced vasoconstriction may worsen global brain ischemia.
  - Because of the high incidence of acute coronary ischemia as a cause of cardiac arrest, emergent coronary angiography should be undertaken in patients with evidence of ST-segment elevation myocardial infarction (STEMI) (2023 AHA Class I recommendation) or high risk of coronary artery disease and shock, electrical instability, or ongoing ischemia for which revascularization may benefit (2023 AHA Class IIa recommendation).
  - Seizures occur in 5% to 20% of patients after ROSC and may even be higher as the clinical diagnosis of seizures,

especially in sedated or paralyzed patients, may not be readily apparent.

- An electroencephalogram (EEG) should be performed and monitored frequently and continuously in comatose patients.
- Clinically evident seizures must be treated promptly. Nonconvulsive seizures, diagnosed by EEG, are reasonable to treat.

- As the goal of postcardiac arrest management is to return patients to their prearrest functional level, prognostication of neurologic outcome is important.
- There is no physical finding or diagnostic study that is reliable in predicting outcome in comatose survivors during the first 24 hours after arrest.
- A multimodal and multidisciplinary approach to neuroprognostication after at least 72 hours of normothermia is recommended.
  - In the era of modern ICU care and TTM, no single sign or combination of signs or symptoms predicts poor neurologic outcome within the first 72 hours of postarrest care.
  - Observation for >72 hours after ROSC and achieving normothermia should be considered before predicting poor outcome in these patients.
  - Minimizing sedation and the exclusion of other cofounders (acid-base disorders, electrolyte abnormalities, metabolic derangements, infections, etc) are important for neuroprognostication.
  - After 72 hours of ROSC, the absence of bilateral pupillary response and bilateral absence of N20 somatosensory evoked potentials (SSEP) on EEG are reliable predictors of poor neurological outcome.
  - Status myoclonus early in admission, elevated neuron-specific enolase at 48 to 72 hours, and unreactive or malignant EEG patterns after rewarming have a moderate predictive value of poor neurologic outcome.
  - Repeat advanced imaging (computed tomography [CT] or magnetic resonance imaging [MRI]) after the initial 72-hour period may provide some additional prognostic value.
  - For patients with indeterminate neuroprognosis, a longer period of observation is recommended if this aligns with their goals of care.
- Despite maximal efforts, some patients will remain brain dead after ROSC from cardiac arrest.
- If appropriate, these patients may be considered for organ donation as there is no difference in the functional outcome of organs transplanted from patients who are brain dead after cardiac arrest compared to those who are brain dead from other causes.
- Losing a patient after cardiac arrest can be traumatic for both the patient's loved ones and medical staff.
  - Survivors postarrest should be supported with appropriate rehabilitation services, such as social work and clergy.
- Medical team debriefing and feedback can improve resuscitation quality and performance.

SUGGESTED READINGS

Arrich J, Schütz N, Oppenauer J, et al. Hypothermia for neuroprotection in adults after cardiac arrest. *Cochrane Database Syst Rev*. 2023; 5(5):CD004128.

Belur AD, Sedhai YR, Truesdell AG, et al. Targeted temperature management in cardiac arrest: an updated narrative review. *Cardiol Ther*. 2023; 12(1):65-84.

Dankiewicz J, Cronberg T, Lilja G, et al. Hypothermia versus normothermia after out-of-hospital cardiac arrest. *N Engl J Med*. 2021;384(24): 2283-2294.

Dine CJ, Gersh RE, Leary M, Riegel BJ, Bellini LM, Abella BS. Improving cardiopulmonary resuscitation quality and resuscitation training by combining audiovisual feedback and debriefing. *Crit Care Med*. 2008; 36(10):2817-2822.

Holmberg MJ, Ross CE, Fitzmaurice GM, et al. Annual incidence of adult and pediatric in-hospital cardiac arrest in the United States. *Circ Cardiovasc Qual Outcomes*. 2019;12(7):e005580.

Paiva EF, Paxton JH, O'Neil BJ. The use of end-tidal carbon dioxide (ETCO2) measurement to guide management of cardiac arrest: a systematic review. *Resuscitation*. 2018;123:1-7.

Panchal AR, Bartos JA, Cabañas JG, et al. Part 3: adult basic and advanced life support: 2020 American Heart Association guidelines for cardiopulmonary resuscitation and emergency cardiovascular care. *Circulation*. 2020;142(16_suppl_2):S366-S468.

Perman SM, Elmer J, Maciel CB, et al. 2023 American Heart Association focused update on adult advanced cardiovascular life support: an update to the American Heart Association guidelines for cardiopulmonary resuscitation and emergency cardiovascular care. *Circulation*. 2024; 149(5):e254-e273.

Rajajee V, Muehlschlegel S, Wartenberg KE, et al. Guidelines for neuroprognostication in comatose adult survivors of cardiac arrest. *Neurocrit Care*. 2023;38(3):533-563.

Richardson ASC, Tonna JE, Nanjayya V, et al. Extracorporeal cardiopulmonary resuscitation in adults. Interim guideline consensus statement from the Extracorporeal Life Support Organization. *ASAIO J*. 2021; 67(3):221-228.

Sandroni C, Cariou A, Cavallaro F, et al. Prognostication in comatose survivors of cardiac arrest: an advisory statement from the European Resuscitation Council and the European Society of Intensive Care Medicine. *Resuscitation*. 2014;85(12):1779-1789.

Schmicker RH, Nichol G, Kudenchuk P, et al. CPR compression strategy 30:2 is difficult to adhere to, but has better survival than continuous chest compressions when done correctly. *Resuscitation*. 2021;165:31-37.

Vincent JL, Moore FA, Bellomo R, Marini J. *Textbook of Critical Care*. 8th ed. Elsevier; 2024.

2.18

Hemodynamic and Mechanical Circulatory Support

Jamel Ortoleva

Hemodynamic and mechanical circulatory support (MCS) is most commonly used in patients with cardiac or combined cardiopulmonary compromise refractory to conventional measures, such as inotropic support, diuresis, mechanical ventilation, and intravenous vasoactive support.

Indications

- Refractory heart or combined heart and lung compromise despite maximal conventional measures, such as diuresis, inotropic support, mechanical ventilation, and intravenous afterload
- Refractory arrhythmia (typically ventricular) that cannot be addressed with medications, defibrillation, and cardioversion, and sympathetic blockade such as stellate ganglion blockade
- Cardiac arrest (most commonly, extracorporeal cardiopulmonary resuscitation or eCPR)
- Planned and unplanned periprocedural support
- MCS is most effective in cardiogenic shock or pulmonary embolism (a type of obstructive shock).
- Patients with mixed shock can also benefit as long as cardiogenic shock is a major component (eg, sepsis with both distributive and cardiogenic components may still have acceptable outcomes with MCS).

Contraindications

- Pure distributive shock as MCS does not directly address the underlying pathology (ie, inflammation and cytokines, capillary leak)
- Patients with or without a pathway to recovery or durable therapy (durable left ventricular assist device [LVAD] or heart transplantation)
- Patients with no vascular access options due to peripheral vascular disease or vessel size

Mechanical Circulatory Support Types

Biventricular Support Types

- Currently available methods of biventricular support are venoarterial extracorporeal membrane oxygenation (VA ECMO) and the use of two devices to form biventricular assist devices (BiVADs).

Venoarterial Extracorporeal Membrane Oxygenation

Indications

- Need for rapid deployment (instability resulting in the inability to mobilize to an area with imaging), cardiac arrest, arrhythmia, periprocedural support, metabolic acidosis, and metabolic disarray (such as significant electrolyte abnormalities in addition to myocardial compromise) as the cause of cardiovascular decline, combined pulmonary and cardiac failure

Contraindications

- Moderate or worse aortic insufficiency (due to retroaortic blood flow in peripheral VA ECMO causing left ventricular [LV] distention, pulmonary edema, and ventricular arrhythmias that can cause significant lung injury)
- Inability to safely obtain vascular access due to significant peripheral vascular disease, aortic dissection, or high burden of deep venous thrombosis
- Unrecoverable heart or lung function without the possibility of transplant or other durable therapy
- Uncontrolled hemorrhage
- Distributive shock with no cardiogenic component
- Poor functional status at baseline
- Unrecoverable neurologic status and not an organ donor
- Patient or health care proxy refusal
- Do not resuscitate/do not intubate status

Survival Statistics

- The SAVE (Survival after Venoarterial ECMO) score is one method of approximating survival in patients undergoing VA ECMO cannulation when not performed for eCPR.
- Survival to hospital discharge of VA ECMO when not used in the setting of refractory cardiac arrest is ~40%.
- VA ECMO cannulation in the setting of an inability to achieve sustained return of spontaneous circulation carries a survival to hospital discharge of ~30%.

What Is Venoarterial Extracorporeal Membrane Oxygenation and How Is It Managed?

- VA ECMO is a method of continuous blood flow that provides both hemodynamic (via a centrifugal flow pump) and respiratory support via the presence of an oxygenator that directly adds oxygen and removes carbon dioxide from the blood.
- The oxygenator adds oxygen and removes carbon dioxide to and from the blood, respectively.
- The fraction of delivered oxygen (Fdo_2) and sweep gas flow rate control the percentage of oxygen and amount of carbon dioxide added to and removed from the blood flowing through the oxygenator.
- Higher sweep gas flow rates will remove more carbon dioxide but without an effect on oxygenation.
- VA ECMO blood flow rate is titrated to provide both hemodynamic support and oxygen delivery.

- Pressure lines connected to transducers just before the oxygenator (premembrane) and just after the oxygenator (postmembrane) assist in monitoring oxygenator function. This pressure difference is often referred to as the "delta P." Different oxygenators will have different acceptable delta P levels. This number is affected by blood flow rate as well (increased blood flow rates will increase delta P).
- Blood gas analysis from sites before and after the oxygenator is performed several times daily to assess oxygenator function (both oxygenation and carbon dioxide removal).
- Peripheral VA ECMO configurations with left femoral or left axillary arterial access will have a "mixing point" or "mixing cloud," which is the location in the aorta that blood coming from the LV (either by native contractility or through additional ventricular assist devices) meets blood flow from the VA ECMO circuit.
- If the lungs are not appropriately oxygenating blood, then relatively deoxygenated blood is proceeding through the heart and will be the blood supply proximal to the mixing point (or the point where native cardiac output meets VA ECMO blood flow). This could mean that the coronary arteries and brain could be receiving deoxygenated blood. While the blood flow to the coronary arteries cannot be readily sampled, brain oxygenation can be inferred from arterial blood gas analysis drawn from right upper extremity arterial lines. Thus, right radial arterial line oximetry must be monitored in peripheral VA ECMO to assess brain oxygenation, unless the arterial cannula is in the right axillary or right subclavian position.

Left Ventricular Distention and Left Ventricular Venting

- Peripheral VA ECMO increases LV afterload, which can reduce aortic valve opening and cause LV distention.
- While afterload may be increased with peripheral VA ECMO, a recent study in patients supported by VA ECMO and intra-aortic balloon pump found that increasing VA ECMO flows usually results in a reduction or no difference in pulmonary capillary wedge pressure.
- Some intrinsic myocardial function is necessary to avoid clotting in the right ventricle, pulmonary arteries (PAs), pulmonary veins, left atrium, LV, and aortic root. Generally, at least 5 mm Hg of PA pulsatility and 10 mm Hg of arterial line pulsatility (<10 points between systolic and diastolic pressure) should be maintained.
- High afterload on the LV also causes distention, which results in complications including pulmonary edema, pulmonary hemorrhage, and ventricular arrhythmias.
- Patients supported by VA ECMO require pulsatility or invasive methods of LV venting in order to prevent LV distention. Multiple methods are available to reduce the degree of LV distention.
- "LV venting" describes maneuvers that reduce LV distention and include diuresis, increased positive end-expiratory pressure, afterload reduction (pharmacologically or by reducing ECMO blood flow rates), and inotropic support.
- More invasive methods of LV venting include the use of an intra-aortic balloon pump, atrial septostomy, transvalvular catheterization, and suction of blood from the LV, transvalvular microaxial flow pumps, and surgical venting (such as with a drain via right upper pulmonary vein).
- It is currently unknown which method of LV venting is superior, and data to support indiscriminate LV venting are generally retrospective without significant granularity.
- Clinical triggers for immediate LV venting include ventricular arrhythmias due to ventricular distention, clinical evidence of pulmonary edema such as frothy secretions in the endotracheal tube, and a lack of pulsatility despite noninvasive maneuvers.
- At the current time, invasive methods of LV venting should be performed on a case-by-case basis, taking into account invasive hemodynamic assessment (via PA catheter monitoring), individual patient characteristics, and the overall goal after VA ECMO (eg, myocardial recovery vs plan for heart replacement therapy with LVAD or heart transplantation).

Venoarterial Extracorporeal Membrane Oxygenation Configurations

- Peripheral
  - *Femoral-femoral*
    - Femoral-femoral VA ECMO is by far the most straightforward, rapidly deployable method of support and may be performed outside a hospital setting, in the emergency department, in a general hospital ward, in the intensive care unit, in a procedural suite, or operating room.
    - This cannulation strategy may be performed using percutaneous or surgical access (via cut-down).
    - Venous drainage (21F-25F) and retrograde (directed toward the aorta) arterial access (15F-19F)
    - It is very rare that a patient will require a larger arterial cannula size than 17F because total VA ECMO flow targets need not achieve total body flow goals (a cardiac index <2.2 is acceptable in most cases, given the presence of some intrinsic cardiac function, unlike in cardiopulmonary bypass).
    - Larger arterial cannulas are also associated with more complications.
    - For distal limb perfusion and to reduce the risk of lower extremity ischemia, a third access point to direct blood flow in antegrade manner in the superficial femoral artery is placed on the extremity with the arterial cannula. This third access point is much smaller than either of the two main cannulas (5F-8F, metal reinforced sheaths are generally used).
    - Femoral-femoral VA ECMO can provide partial or complete hemodynamic support depending on blood flow rate, which is determined by cannula size and systemic vascular resistance.
    - Occasionally, myocardial recovery precedes pulmonary recovery. In this case, the heart may eject deoxygenated blood. In circuit configurations with femoral or left axillary arterial access, the mixing point will be more distal in the aorta, resulting in differential oxygenation, which has previously been referred to as "differential hypoxia", "north-south syndrome" or "harlequin syndrome. This can also occur in patients undergoing LV unloading with transvalvular microaxial flow pumps.
    - One example of differential oxygenation is when hypoxic blood enters the coronary arteries and the brain, which may limit myocardial recovery and cause neurologic complications.

- Significant north-south syndrome causes hypoxic blood to enter the coronary arteries and the brain, which may limit myocardial recovery and cause neurologic complications.
- Monitoring for differential oxygenation includes a pulse oximetry probe on the right upper extremity or right ear, and drawing all arterial blood gases from an arterial line in the right upper extremity (radial, brachial, or axillary).
- There is no widely available method to evaluate the oxygen saturation of blood entering the coronary arteries.

- *Axillary ECMO*
  - In patients with significant peripheral vascular disease, the left or right axillary artery is occasional used as a reinfusion cannula. If a cannula is used to access the vessel instead of a graft, a reperfusion sheath is still important, but given the relative rarity of this cannulation strategy, a definitive recommendation on distal reperfusion sheaths cannot be made.
  - Right axillary arterial cannulation prevents differential oxygenation, but left axillary arterial cannulation does not.

Central Venoarterial Extracorporeal Membrane Oxygenation Cannulation

- Central cannulation involves drainage from the right atrium (RA) and reinfusion to the aorta. Hybrid central cannulation can include peripheral venous cannulation with aortic reinfusion.
- Central cannulation provides the highest blood flow rates, obviates the need for reperfusion sheaths, and prevents the occurrence of differential oxygenation.
- Central cannulation is most frequently utilized in the case of the inability to separate from cardiopulmonary bypass due to postcardiotomy shock, because the cannulas are already in place in the operating room.
- Central cannulation is also used in cases of small blood vessels and significant peripheral vascular disease that prevents safe peripheral vascular access.
- Except in rare circumstances (such as eCPR in postcardiotomy patients), central cannulation generally requires an operating room and cannot be deployed as rapidly as peripheral cannulation.
- Central cannulation carries the disadvantage of increased bleeding and the possibility of mediastinitis.

Extracorporeal Membrane Oxygenation Complications

- Hemolysis, thrombosis, LV distention, limb ischemia if placed via a cannula in the axillary or femoral artery, stroke, seizure, worsening aortic insufficiency, aortic dissection, cannula site bleeding, vascular injury, cardiac injury, thrombocytopenia, von Willebrand factor deficiency, and infection.

Nondischargeable, percutaneous, and surgical BiVADs

- BiVADs represent a combination of left and right heart support devices, which are discussed later.
- BiVADs are utilized in patients as a method of recovery from refractory cardiac compromise that would not be possible on a shorter time scale with VA ECMO.
- BiVADs are also utilized in patients as a bridge to heart transplantation.
- BiVADs are helpful for patients with no meaningful biventricular function (either due to persistent arrhythmia or due to poor contractility) as a means of preventing thrombus formation in the heart and lungs while awaiting recovery, LVAD (should right heart function improve), or transplantation.
- BiVADs are contraindicated in patients who do not have an "exit strategy" (meaning a means to recovery or durable therapy such as heart transplant).
- Types of BiVADs:
- Percutaneous configurations
  - Transvalvular microaxial flow right ventricular assist device (RVAD) and LVAD
  - Dual-lumen single cannula RVAD and transvalvular microaxial flow LVAD
- Surgical BiVADs (consider if axillary arteries too small or cannot deploy peripheral RVAD due to vascular access issues or tricuspid/pulmonic valve pathology)

Right Ventricular Assist Devices

- RVADs are used in patients with predominant right heart failure and the absence of significant metabolic derangement that could subsequently result in LV failure.
- Percutaneous and surgical approaches are available.
- Percutaneous RVADs can be deployed in cardiac catheterization labs and are less invasive than surgically placed devices, but generate lower blood flow rates than surgical RVADs (typical maximum flow approximately 4 to 4.5 L/min).
- Importantly, all RVAD patients should at least initially be monitored with a PA catheter and an arterial line.
- PA catheters in RVAD patients will show reduced PA pulsatility due to the continuous flow mechanism of these devices.
- PA catheterization and monitoring of LV function are very important in this patient population because acute LV failure in patients with RVADs can result in ongoing forward flow from the RVAD, acute increases in left atrial pressure, and pulmonary edema as well as potentially fatal pulmonary hemorrhage.
- A brief description of available percutaneous devices is provided later. Devices are differentiated by the presence or absence of blood flow outside the body (extracorporeal support), which allows for the addition of an oxygenator for oxygenation and carbon dioxide removal. A description of surgical devices follows.

Percutaneous With Extracorporeal Blood Flow

- Some similarities to venovenous ECMO, except that oxygenated blood is directly infused into the PA and proper nomenclature is "VP ECMO".
  - Percutaneous single cannula dual-lumen strategies:
    - These devices are generally placed from the right internal jugular vein and terminate in the main PA.
    - Two percutaneous cannulas are currently available, both of which can be part of a configuration with an oxygenator:

- A dual-lumen single cannula (ProtekDuo, LivaNova) with drainage ports designed to be in the RA and right ventricle, with reinfusion ports at the distal tip, which terminates in the main PA
- A dual-lumen single cannula (Dual Lumen Cannula, Spectrum Medical, Gloucester) with drainage ports designed to be in the superior vena cava and RA with reinfusion ports at the distal tip, which terminates in the main PA
- Device flows can be up to ~4.5 L/min and can be controlled by modifying the revolutions per minute on the extracorporeal pump console.

Percutaneous With No Extracorporeal Blood Flow

- Transvalvular microaxial flow pumps (Impella RP or Impella RP Flex, Abiomed, Danvers, MA) that originate from either the right internal jugular vein or a femoral vein
  - These devices require either heparin or sodium bicarbonate infusion in a dedicated line connected to the device known as "the purge line." Infusion into this line functions to prevent thrombus in the pump. Purge line heparin can impact the partial thromboplastin time (PTT) because it is infused systemically.
  - Blood flow rates are determined by the selected "performance level" or P level, which ranges from P1 to P9 (least to most flow). Clinically, P8 is typically the maximum performance level that is used.
  - The axial flow nature of these pumps allows for the smaller pump size at the potential expense of a higher risk of hemolysis than centrifugal pumps used for VA ECMO and surgically placed ventricular assist devices.
  - For the device deployed from the femoral vein, an inlet port in the inferior vena cava allows blood entry through the device to the outflow port in the PA.
  - For the device deployed from the right internal jugular vein, an inlet port in the superior vena cava or the RA allows blood entry through the device to the outflow port in the PA.
  - Percutaneous RVADs are contraindicated in multiple conditions including:
    - Vascular anatomy, or devices such as inferior vena cava filters, which cannot accommodate the passage of the device or cannula
    - Severe insufficiency or stenosis of tricuspid or pulmonary valves
    - Thrombus in the RA, right ventricle, or main PA
    - The right internal jugular approach is contraindicated in patients with superior vena cava clot, and the femoral approach is contraindicated in patients with inferior vena cava clot.

Surgical Extracorporeal Right Ventricular Assist Device

- A large cannula is placed in the RA bringing blood outside the body to a pump, which is then attached to another cannula in the PA to reinfuse blood back to the patient.
- An oxygenator can be added to the circuit (after the pump) to a surgically placed RVAD to provide oxygenation and carbon dioxide removal (VP ECMO).

Left-Sided Support Devices

- Left-sided support devices are generally placed in patients with refractory LV failure without significant metabolic derangement. Invasive hemodynamic monitoring with the use of a PA catheter to identify right heart failure, at least for a period of time after initial implantation, is necessary. Additionally, in patients with left heart failure as the primary cause of decompensation, patients with signs of right heart failure due to left heart failure can receive these devices.
- Configurations With Extracorporeal Blood Flow:
  - Left atrial to femoral arterial support (TandemHeart, LivaNova) involves placing a cannula from the femoral vein, across the interatrial septum into the left atrium to drain blood and return it to the femoral artery.
    - An oxygenator may be added to this configuration.
    - If an oxygenator is not added to this configuration, care teams must be aware that if the cannula inlet migrates from the left atrium into the RA, a shunt of venous blood to the femoral artery will result.
    - This support type can provide significant left heart decompression (flows of up to ~5 L/min) but requires vigilance to ensure adequate cannula positioning. Additionally, given the presence of a peripheral arterial cannula, limb ischemia can result if a distal perfusion catheter is not in place.
    - Contraindications to this device type include:
      - Lack of vascular access points, significant peripheral vascular disease, left atrial thrombus, severe aortic insufficiency (relative, reports of this support platform in patients with this pathology exist), and certain inferior vena cava filters that cannot accommodate the passage of a cannula.
    - Complications
      - Hemolysis, limb ischemia, stroke, cannula site bleeding, vascular injury, RA or left atrial perforation, infection, right heart failure
- Surgical temporary extracorporeal LVAD
  - Indications
    - Surgical temporary extracorporeal LVADs are most frequently placed in patients who qualify for LV mechanical support but either do not have the anatomy or vasculature to accommodate a less invasive LVAD, or require flows higher than can be delivered by other devices.
  - Contraindications
    - Nonrecoverable cardiac pathology and not a candidate for durable therapy, nonrecoverable organ failure and not a candidate for multiorgan transplant, significant aortic disease and no other large-vessel cannulation options, patients with LV abnormalities, such as pseudoaneurysm, can be difficult to support with this method.
  - Surgical temporary extracorporeal LVADs are placed via sternotomy or thoracotomy and involve either cannulation of the LV apex or the left atrium for blood drainage with reinfusion to the aorta.
  - An oxygenator may be added to the circuit of these devices, but due to the reinfusion cannula in the ascending aorta, vigilance for thrombus burden on the post-oxygenator side is critical.
  - Support types without extracorporeal blood flow
    - Transvalvular microaxial flow pumps

- Transvalvular microaxial flow LVADs (Impella CP, Impella 5.5, Abiomed, Danvers, MA) can be deployed from femoral or axillary vessels as well as the innominate artery or aorta.
- Blood flow rates are determined by the selected "performance level" or P level, which ranges from P1 to P9 (least to most flow). Clinically, P8 is typically the maximum performance level that is used.
- The axial flow nature of these pumps allows for the smaller pump size at the potential expense of a higher risk of hemolysis than centrifugal pumps used for VA-ECMO and surgically placed ventricular assist devices.
- Larger transvalvular microaxial flow LVADs can provide adequate blood flow for full LV support in the absence of LV contractility, but require surgical cut- down and graft placement in the axillary artery, the subclavian artery, the innominate artery, or the aorta.
- These devices require either heparin or sodium bicarbonate infusion in a dedicated line known as "the purge line". Purge line heparin can impact the PTT because it is infused systemically.
- These devices can be used for isolated left heart support, part of a BiVAD configuration, or for LV venting in the VA ECMO population.
- The console for these devices contains a "placement signal" waveform that allows for rapid confirmation of correct device placement (with inlet in the LV and outlet in the aorta). In patients with minimal or no intrinsic LV function, the LV and aortic waveforms will appear nonpulsatile.
- Contraindications
  - These devices are contraindicated in patients with atrial or ventricular septal defects, aortic dissection, mechanical aortic valves, LV thrombus, moderate or worse aortic insufficiency, aortic stenosis with a valve area of ≤0.6 cm^2, and vascular anatomy that precludes placement.
- Complications
  - Hemolysis, thrombosis, aortic valve leaflet injury, entanglement in the mitral subvalvular apparatus with regurgitation, arrhythmias, and limb ischemia if placed via a sheath in the femoral artery.

- Intra-aortic balloon pump (IABP) counterpulsation is the oldest form of temporary MCS. IABP involves placing an inflatable balloon in the aorta that is triggered by either electrocardiogram (ECG) or pressure sensing. IABP may also be set to a specific rate in patients undergoing cardiopulmonary bypass.
  - IABP inflates at the time of the aortic blood pressure dicrotic notch and deflates at the end of diastole just before aortic valve opening.
  - IABP can also be set to inflate at the middle of the T wave and deflate at the peak of the R wave.
  - IABP is used in the treatment of left heart failure, for coronary artery disease and ischemia, and for LV venting.
  - IABP functions by reducing LV afterload and increasing coronary perfusion pressure. If functioning properly, the IABP should reduce LV end-diastolic pressure and decrease pulmonary capillary wedge pressure.
  - IABP may be deployed via a femoral artery, the axillary artery, or the aorta.
  - IABP is the smallest of the left heart assist devices and provides the least support.
  - IABP may be set to inflate and deflate with every heartbeat (1:1), with every other heartbeat (1:2), and even as infrequently as 1:4 or 1:8. Practice varies among centers but also by indication for the IABP and severity of cardiac disease and shock.
  - Anticoagulation is preferable with IABP but is not required if left at 1:1.
  - Contraindicated
    - Aortic dissection, moderate or worse aortic insufficiency, peripheral vascular disease that precludes placement
  - Complications
    - Vascular injury at the access site, dissection, stroke, occlusion of abdominal vessels (including the renal arteries with organ dysfunction), thrombocytopenia, anemia, and thrombus formation on the device with distal embolism.

Weaning From Mechanical Circulatory Support

- Weaning from isolated left or right heart support involves reducing device settings and collecting information, including cardiac output, changes in vasoactive medication requirement, changes in invasively measured filling pressures (central venous pressure, PA pressures, and pulmonary capillary wedge pressure), echocardiographic analysis of myocardial and valve dysfunction, and ECG assessment of ischemia.
- Patients should not be weaned if they require high-dose vasoactive agents to support hemodynamics during device turn-downs.
- Weaning from biventricular support is generally performed sequentially based on which ventricle recovers first.
- Weaning from VA ECMO is more complicated as it supports both cardiac and lung function.
  - Weaning can be performed when patients have sufficient lung recovery to maintain safe ventilator settings with minimal sweep gas flow (1 L/min) and have acceptable hemodynamics with low to moderate doses of vasoactive agents.
  - After institutional protocols for adequate anticoagulation are followed, VA ECMO circuit blood flows can be turned down to 0.5 to 1 L/min for brief periods (<10 minutes), hemodynamics and arterial blood gas analysis measured, and turned back up to higher flows to prevent thrombosis.
  - VA ECMO decannulation can be performed surgically via cut-down and direct arterial repair, or percutaneously either with a closure device placed at the time of cannulation or by directly accessing the cannula lumen and placing a closure device after wire exchange.

Ethical Issues With Mechanical Circulatory Support

- Patients undergoing MCS are often not intubated or sedated and thus can participate in care decisions.
- It can be very challenging for patients, families, and care teams to navigate situations in which patients are conscious (and even ambulatory) while supported by temporary MCS, but are not recoverable and have no exit strategy to durable therapy.

- Ideally, just before MCS initiation or shortly thereafter, family members are provided a realistic explanation of the high mortality rate, high inherent complication rates of MCS, and potential for very difficult decisions during the course of MCS runs.
- Early involvement of ethics teams, palliative care, and other support systems is of paramount importance in this clinical scenario.

Conclusions and Summary Points

- MCS allows support for patients with refractory shock due to cardiac causes (or pulmonary embolism) and cardiac arrest.
- The decision of when to initiate MCS can be complex as premature initiation will result in complications in patients who did not require it.
- Late initiation of MCS will result in organ failure that is not recoverable.
- Signs of malperfusion, such as mild organ dysfunction and elevated blood lactate despite optimization of volume status, or increasing doses of vasoactives, should prompt immediate communication with shock teams to decide whether to initiate MCS and which configuration is best suited for the patient.
- Systemic anticoagulation is recommended for patients undergoing MCS, but consensus guidelines do not exist. There is significant institutional variability in anticoagulation protocols. Importantly, patients with bleeding can have anticoagulation withheld (particularly patients supported by VA ECMO) for long periods of time (days) so long as device flows are kept high. In the case of transvalvular microaxial flow pumps, sodium bicarbonate can be used instead of heparin in the purge flow solution.
- MCS is not a cure for the underlying illness, but rather allows for support of organ function while the heart recovers, or allows for a bridge to durable therapy, such as heart transplant or dischargeable LVAD.
- Patients undergoing VA ECMO support, particularly non-central, non-right axillary ECMO configurations, must always be ventilated with a mechanical ventilator if intubated to avoid differential oxygenation and potential coronary and brain hypoxia.
- Stroke, cardiac injury, vascular injury, bleeding, hemolysis, platelet dysfunction, infection, failure of the nonsupported ventricle, and many other complications accompany patients undergoing MCS.
- Small teams with experience and expertise in the management of the MCS population are crucial to optimize outcomes and maintain a high standard for the care of these patients.

SUGGESTED READINGS

Calhoun A, Lee MH, Pisano DV, Karavas A, Ortoleva J. Variability in triggers for mechanical left ventricular unloading in VA-ECMO: A literature search. J Extra Corpor Technol. 2025 Mar;57(1):24-31.

Carey MR, Tong W, Godfrey S, Takeda K, Nakagawa S. Withdrawal of temporary mechanical circulatory support in patients with capacity. *J Pain Symptom Manage*. 2022;63(3):387-394.

Combes A, Price S, Slutsky AS, Brodie D. Temporary circulatory support for cardiogenic shock. *Lancet*. 2020;396(10245):199-212.

Eckman PM, Katz JN, El Banayosy A, Bohula EA, Sun B, van Diepen S. Veno-arterial extracorporeal membrane oxygenation for cardiogenic shock: an introduction for the busy clinician. *Circulation*. 2019;140(24):2019-2037.

Esper SA, Welsby IJ, Subramaniam K, et al. Adult extracorporeal membrane oxygenation: an international survey of transfusion and anticoagulation techniques. *Vox Sang*. 2017;112(5):443-452.

Ezad SM, Ryan M, Donker DW, et al. Unloading the left ventricle in venoarterial ECMO: in whom, when, and how? *Circulation*. 2023;147(16):1237-1250.

Gandhi KD, Moras EC, Niroula S, et al. Left ventricular unloading with Impella versus IABP in patients with VA-ECMO: a systematic review and meta-analysis. *Am J Cardiol*. 2023;208:53-59.

Garan AR, Takeda K, Salna M, et al. Prospective comparison of a percutaneous ventricular assist device and venoarterial extracorporeal membrane oxygenation for patients with cardiogenic shock following acute myocardial infarction. *J Am Heart Assoc*. 2019;8(9):e012171.

Gillespie LE, Lane BH, Shaw CR, et al. The intra-aortic balloon pump: a focused review of physiology, transport logistics, mechanics, and complications. *J Soc Cardiovasc Angiogr Interv*. 2024;3(5):101337.

Kar B, Adkins LE, Civitello AB, et al. Clinical experience with the TandemHeart percutaneous ventricular assist device. *Tex Heart Inst J*. 2006;33(2):111-115.

Lorusso R, Shekar K, MacLaren G, et al. ELSO interim guidelines for veno-arterial extracorporeal membrane oxygenation in adult cardiac patients [published correction appears in *ASAIO J*. 2022;68(7):e133]. *ASAIO J*. 2021;67(8):827-844.

Makdisi G, Wang IW. Extra corporeal membrane oxygenation (ECMO) review of a lifesaving technology. *J Thorac Dis*. 2015;7(7):E166-E176.

Moghaddam N, van Diepen S, So D, Lawler PR, Fordyce CB. Cardiogenic shock teams and centres: a contemporary review of multidisciplinary care for cardiogenic shock. *ESC Heart Fail*. 2021;8(2):988-998.

Ortoleva JP, Alfadhel A, Dalia AA. Invasive hemodynamic and physiologic considerations in patients undergoing extracorporeal membrane oxygenation. *J Cardiothorac Vasc Anesth*. 2021;35(9):2549-2551.

Panda K, Glance LG, Mazzeffi M, et al. Perioperative extracorporeal cardiopulmonary resuscitation in adult patients: a review for the perioperative physician. *Anesthesiology*. 2024;140(5):1026-1042.

Richardson ASC, Tonna JE, Nanjayya V, et al. Extracorporeal cardiopulmonary resuscitation in adults. Interim guideline consensus statement from the Extracorporeal Life Support Organization. *ASAIO J*. 2021;67(3):221-228.

Salter BS, Gross CR, Weiner MM, et al. Temporary mechanical circulatory support devices: practical considerations for all stakeholders. *Nat Rev Cardiol*. 2023;20(4):263-277.

Santana JM, Dalia AA, Newton M, et al. Mechanical circulatory support options in patients with aortic valve pathology. *J Cardiothorac Vasc Anesth*. 2022;36(8 Pt B):3318-3326.

Saura O, Hékimian G, Del Marmol G, Lucenteforte M, Pineton de Chambrun M, Chommeloux J, Assouline B, Petit M, Juvin C, Gautier M, Moyon Q, Visinoni N, Luyt CE, Leprince P, Lebreton G, Schmidt M, Combes A, Levy D; PAPO-Flow Study Investigators. Effect of ECMO Flow Variations on Pulmonary Capillary Wedge Pressure in Patients With Cardiogenic Shock. J Am Coll Cardiol. 2025 Sep 16;86(11):768-778. doi: 10.1016/j.jacc.2025.06.048. PMID: 40930613.

Schmidt M, Burrell A, Roberts L, et al. Predicting survival after ECMO for refractory cardiogenic shock: the survival after veno-arterial-ECMO (SAVE)-score. *Eur Heart J*. 2015;36(33):2246-2256.

Takayama H, Soni L, Kalesan B, et al. Bridge-to-decision therapy with a continuous-flow external ventricular assist device in refractory cardiogenic shock of various causes. *Circ Heart Fail*. 2014;7(5):799-806.

Tonna JE, Boonstra PS, MacLaren G, et al. Extracorporeal Life Support Organization registry international report 2022: 100,000 survivors. *ASAIO J*. 2024;70(2):131-143.

Wu IY, Wyrobek JA, Naka Y, Dickstein ML, Glance LG. Perioperative management of patients receiving short-term mechanical circulatory support with the transvalvular heart pump. *Anesthesiology*. 2022;136(5):829-842.

2.19

Cardiac and Vascular Surgery Postoperative Management and Perioperative Complications

Caroline H. Jensen and Kenneth Shelton

Physiologic Consequences of Cardiac Surgery

- Much of early postoperative care relates to the use and consequences of the cardiopulmonary bypass (CPB) machine and cardioplegia intraoperatively.
  - The systemic inflammatory response after CPB is attributed to the interaction between the blood and the artificial surface of the bypass circuit, which can lead to the release of inflammatory cytokines.
  - Coagulopathy is commonly seen postoperatively, with a multifactorial etiology relating to residual systemic heparin, consumptive coagulopathy secondary to the systemic inflammatory response, hypothermia, and dilutional effect of crystalloid administration.
- Myocardial protection during open cardiac surgery is most often achieved using cardioplegia, which arrests the heart after cross-clamp placement. The successful use of cardioplegia reduces myocardial metabolism and oxygen demand.
  - Cardioplegia solution can be administered antegrade via the aortic root and retrograde via the coronary sinus.
  - Failure in myocardial protection with cardioplegia can occur with the introduction of air, severe coronary artery stenosis, or poor collateral flow. Evidence of poor myocardial protection is seen with postoperative echocardiographic wall motion abnormalities and electrocardiogram (ECG) changes.
  - Inadequate myocardial protection can manifest as transient myocardial depression, persistent myocardial injury and dysfunction, or arrhythmias.

Basics of Postoperative Cardiac Surgery Management

- Cardiac surgical patients typically arrive to the intensive care unit (ICU) with an arterial catheter, central venous catheter, possibly a pulmonary artery catheter (PAC), chest tubes, and a Foley catheter.
  - Continuous ECG, pulse oximetry, arterial blood pressure, invasive hemodynamic measurements, cardiac output (CO) calculated by thermodilution, pulse pressure variation, chest tube output, and urine output are monitored postoperatively.
  - On arrival, the patient should have a 12-lead ECG, chest radiograph, a physical examination, and laboratory studies.
    - The 12-lead ECG should be evaluated for ST-segment changes, new Q waves, interval development of a bundle branch block, and new arrhythmias (atrioventricular blocks).
    - The chest radiograph should verify correct placement of all existing tubes, including endotracheal tube, central venous catheter, PAC, pleural drains, and pericardial drains. Pneumothorax, hemothorax, pulmonary edema, and pleural effusions can also be identified on postoperative chest radiograph.
    - Physical examination should be done to evaluate the sternotomy and ensure warm extremities, strong pulses, nondistended stomach, equal pupils, and clear breath sounds.
- Hemodynamic management postoperatively can be challenging in the setting of myocardial depression, vasoplegia, and hypovolemia.
  - Blood pressure, filling pressures (central venous pressure [CVP] as surrogate for right atrial pressure; pulmonary artery diastolic pressure as a surrogate for left atrial pressure), and routine measurement of CO and cardiac index can guide hemodynamic management.
    - Cardiac index should be maintained >2.0 L/min/m^2.
    - Blood pressure should be maintained with a mean arterial pressure >70 mm Hg.
    - Pulmonary artery diastolic pressure should be maintained between 14 and 18 mm Hg, though patients with a dilated or scarred left ventricle may require higher pressures.
  - Markers of perfusion indicate how successful the hemodynamic management is. Typically, lactate, mixed venous oxygen saturation, and urine output are considered in the evaluation of perfusion.
    - Goal Lactate <2 mmol/L
    - Mixed venous saturation, measured from the pulmonary artery port of the Swan Ganz catheter, >65%
    - Urine output >0.5 mL/kg/h
  - Thermodilution and Fick equation can both be used to monitor CO.
    - The thermodilution method involves flushing a defined amount of saline at a set temperature and monitoring the temperature change in the blood. The saline will be injected into the right atrium, and the temperature change will be detected in the pulmonary artery by the PAC. The resultant thermodilution curve is indicative of the patient's CO.
    - By Fick's equation: CO = $Vo_2/(C_a - C_v)$, where Vo_2 is oxygen consumption, C_a is oxygen content of arterial blood, and C_v is oxygen content of mixed venous blood. The Vo_2 is often an estimated number based on population nomograms in healthy patients and so may not apply to critically ill patients. C_a and C_v can both be calculated using the patient's laboratory values, including hemoglobin, oxygen saturation on arterial blood gas (ABG), and mixed venous saturation from PAC.
  - Vasopressors and inotropes are likely to be required to achieve hemodynamic and perfusion goals.
    - Choice of vasopressor or inotrope is variable and often institution or practitioner dependent. Epinephrine is a common inotropic agent that

also has vasopressor activity. Norepinephrine and vasopressin are commonly used vasopressor agents. Inodilators (milrinone and dobutamine) are often used in conjunction with vasopressor agents to maintain blood pressure.
    - Inotropes increase myocardial oxygen demand and can be harmful in ischemic cardiac disease.
    - Inotropes are also proarrhythmogenic.
  - Afterload reduction plays an important role in optimizing cardiac function and increasing CO by facilitating ejection of the ventricle.
    - In addition, hypertension can exacerbate bleeding and stress at surgical anastomosis sites.
    - Sodium nitroprusside, nitroglycerin, clevidipine, and nicardipine are all appropriate agents in cardiac surgery patients.

Respiratory Management

- Patients typically arrive intubated to the ICU after cardiac surgery.
- Patients without significant complications and comorbidities are often placed on a "fast-track" protocol after arrival to the ICU, and they are extubated within 6 hours.
  - Cardiac surgery is a risk factor for acute respiratory distress syndrome (ARDS).
  - Hypercarbia can be a unique challenge in cardiac patients, as increased right ventricular (RV) afterload and respiratory acidosis may disproportionately affect patients with reduced RV function or existing pulmonary hypertension.

Fluid Management

- Resuscitation is classically the first phase of postoperative management in the setting of intravascular hypovolemia and relative vasoplegia.
- Typically, patients require up to 3 L of crystalloid in the first 12 hours postoperatively.
- Lactated Ringer solution or a balanced electrolyte solution is preferred to normal saline (0.9% sodium chloride), which is associated with increased incidence of metabolic acidosis and acute kidney injury (AKI). Albumin is acceptable in postoperative cardiac patients, though there is no evidence to suggest it is superior to crystalloid.
- Excessive resuscitation requirements should raise concern for other issues related to coagulopathy, bleeding, or cardiac dysfunction. Additionally, excessive fluid administration may worsen the patient's clinical condition by causing heart failure, pulmonary edema, dilutional coagulopathy, and intestinal edema and dysfunction.

Sedation

- Propofol is a favored agent for its short-acting sedation, with additional narcotic agents for analgesia as needed.
- Dexmedetomidine can be used as an alternative for "fast-track" patients for less sedation while maintaining anxiolysis.

Temperature

- Patients are cooled in the operating room, and they often require additional warming in the ICU prior to weaning sedation and extubation.
- If neuromuscular blocking agents are reversed prematurely, shivering occurs and increases oxygen consumption.
- Patients with temperatures <35 °C will peripherally vasoconstrict to augment their core body temperature; improvement in hypothermia may help hemodynamic management.
- Hypothermia can also negatively impact coagulation and wound healing.

Perioperative Complications

Bleeding

- Chest tube output is monitored continuously in the ICU, and chest tube output exceeding 300 to 400 mL in the first 1 to 2 hours or >200 mL/h for several hours is highly concerning for coagulopathy or mediastinal bleeding requiring surgical repair.
- Cardiac tamponade should be suspected after cardiac surgery in the setting of elevated filling pressures, hypotension, tachycardia, and low CO.
  - Suspicion should be high if chest tube output suddenly stops.
  - Arterial line tracing can show increased respiratory variation (pulsus paradoxus) and narrowing of the pulse pressure.
  - Chest x-ray (CXR) can show enlarged cardiac silhouette or widened mediastinum.
  - ECG often has decreased QRS voltage.
  - Echocardiographic findings for cardiac tamponade may not be impressive, as small posterior pericardial fluid pockets can still cause chamber or vessel compression and manifest significant hemodynamic effects.

Atrial Fibrillation

- Atrial fibrillation is a very common complication after cardiac surgery, occurring in about 25% of coronary artery bypass grafting (CABG) patients.
- For high-risk patients and procedures, amiodarone is started as a prophylactic agent on postoperative day 1; beta-blocker can be considered based on hemodynamic profile as in the previous section.

Myocardial Infarction

- Ischemia on ECG should be closely monitored postoperatively, as the patient may have incomplete revascularization, poor myocardial protection, anastomotic stenosis, or graft occlusion, kinking, or compression.
  - If concern for ischemia, nitroglycerin can be initiated for augmented coronary perfusion.
  - If there is concern for coronary spasm, calcium channel blockers can be considered.
  - Cardiac surgery and interventional cardiology should be involved for emergency angiography, followed by reexploration versus percutaneous coronary intervention.
  - Diffuse ST elevation with PR depressions often represents acute pericarditis.

Cardiac Biomarkers

- The utility of cardiac biomarkers after cardiac surgery is unclear, as they will be elevated in most patients.

- Troponin and CK-MB >5× the upper limit with ECG changes is cause for concern, and immediate angiography or echocardiography is warranted. Troponin is regarded as the most sensitive biomarker as it is cardiac specific.
  - Note that troponin clearance is reduced in the setting of kidney disease and is less reliable as a cardiac marker.

Cardiac Arrest

- Cardiac arrest should be managed with standard Advanced Cardiac Life Support (ACLS) protocols, though with some notable exceptions for postoperative cardiac patients in an ICU with continuous monitoring.
- If it is feasible to defibrillate or pace within 1 minute of witnessed arrest in the ICU, those actions should occur prior to cardiopulmonary resuscitation (CPR), as there is a heightened risk in poststernotomy patients; chest compressions may disrupt fresh suture lines or cause sternal injury to myocardium.
  - In case of pulseless ventricular tachycardia and ventricular fibrillation, defibrillation should be attempted 3 times within the first minute. A bolus of code-dose epinephrine should also be administered.
  - In case of asystole, external pacing (ideally using pacer wires) and atropine should be attempted.
  - Chest compressions have tremendous risk in patients with left ventricular assist device (LVAD) or extracorporeal membrane oxygenation (ECMO), as cannulae can be dislodged.
    - If defibrillation or pacing is not possible within 1 minute of arrest, chest compressions should be started.
    - If early CPR is not successful, early resternotomy with open chest massage should be attempted.
    - The likelihood of survival is related to the etiology of the arrest.
      - Etiologies to be explored and ruled out include hypovolemia, hypoxia, severe acidosis, electrolyte derangements including hyperkalemia and hypokalemia, tamponade, tension pneumothorax, thrombosis, pulmonary embolism, and iatrogenic drug administration.
- Mechanical circulatory support (MCS) is a relatively new form of support for patients in obstructive or cardiogenic shock manifesting signs of end-organ malperfusion. Specifically, in low CO states secondary to ischemia, LV failure, or RV failure, MCS can be a vital intervention and serve as a bridge to further intervention or overall hemometabolic recovery.
- Venoarterial (VA) ECMO is a cardiopulmonary support strategy that provides biventricular support. It also aids in appropriate ABG exchange, adding oxygenation and removing carbon dioxide. VA ECMO can be initiated with multiple configurations, including peripheral and central cannulation.
- Venovenous (VV) ECMO is a form of pulmonary support providing oxygenation and carbon dioxide removal, without cardiac support. Similar to VA ECMO, multiple configurations exist to provide VV-ECMO both peripherally and centrally.
- Durable LVAD support is generally reserved for patients as a bridge to heart transplantation or for durable support in patients with end-stage isolated LV failure. LVADs do not offer oxygenation or carbon dioxide removal and do not provide RV support.
- Percutaneous temporary LVAD (Impella) support has been used for periprocedural percutaneous coronary interventions or for isolated LV failure. This form of support may be used temporarily when inotropic therapy is insufficient to support organ perfusion. Impella devices may be placed percutaneously and offer significant antegrade flow, which minimizes LV distension, decreases LV wall tension, and lowers myocardial oxygen consumption.
- Intra-aortic balloon pump (IABP) support is largely reserved for refractory angina, acute mitral regurgitation, or ventricular septal defect as a mechanical complication of a myocardial infarction (MI). IABP support has not been shown in large, randomized trials to decrease the mortality of patients with acute MI cardiogenic shock.

Neurologic Injury

- Stroke after cardiac surgery ranges from 4% to 10%.
  - The etiology of stroke varies and can be attributed to mobilization of atherosclerotic emboli after aortic cross-clamping, air emboli, thrombi, and prolonged hypoperfusion after cardiac bypass.

Acute Kidney Injury

- AKI is a common problem after both cardiac surgery, and it is associated with higher rates of renal replacement therapy (RRT), longer ICU admissions, and higher mortality.
- The etiology of postoperative AKI is unclear, but it is likely related to sustained periods of hypoperfusion, increased inflammation and circulating cytokines, and hemolysis.

Considerations in Postoperative Vascular Surgery Patients

Overview of Vascular Surgery and Specific Considerations

- Vascular surgery patients have higher American Society of Anesthesiologists (ASA) scores, with higher rates of diabetes, chronic kidney disease, heart disease, and lung pathology.
- Vascular surgery encompasses a broad range of procedures, both surgical and endovascular, that implicate multiple organ systems: aortic aneurysm and dissection repair, carotid endarterectomy, and limb revascularization.
- In open thoracic or abdominal aneurysm repair, there are periods of cross-clamping and unclamping that predispose the patient to complications related to hypoperfusion and ischemia-reperfusion injury.
- Endovascular aneurysm repair (EVAR) and thoracic endovascular aneurysm repair (TEVAR) are becoming increasingly more popular as alternatives to open surgical repair. Endografts are deployed for thoracic and abdominal aneurysms and aortic dissections under fluoroscopic guidance.
- Fenestrated endovascular aortic repair (FEVAR) involves fenestrated grafts from the aortic graft that provide perfusion to the visceral arteries, which would otherwise be covered by the aortic graft.

- Landing zones are assessed prior to the deployment of grafts in TEVAR surgery. If there is a risk of the graft obstructing flow to the left subclavian artery, the patient will undergo a two-part staged procedure, starting with an open left carotid-subclavian bypass to ensure adequate flow in preparation for the second stage graft deployment.

Neurologic Injury

- Spinal cord ischemia, most often from anterior spinal arteries, is a tragic complication after vascular repair of thoracoabdominal aortic aneurysms (TAAAs). Typically, it is diagnosed with motor weakness, as well as loss of pain and temperature sensation.
  - The spinal cord perfusion pressure should be increased in the setting of motor weakness, which is often achieved through increasing blood pressure (mean arterial pressure [MAP] >90 mm Hg) and manipulating cerebrospinal fluid (CSF) pressure via a spinal drain.
    - Spinal drains work by draining CSF and reducing the CSF pressure, which enhances the spinal cord perfusion pressure by the following equation:
      a. Spinal cord perfusion pressure = MAP − CSF pressure (or CVP)
    - CSF drainage should be monitored hourly by the ICU and should not exceed 20 mL/h.
    - Excessive CSF drainage can adversely change the pressure differential in the brain vasculature, predisposing patients to a higher risk of subdural hematoma and subarachnoid hemorrhage.
    - Excessive and sustained blood pressure increases can predispose patient to hemorrhagic stroke.

Stroke

- Vascular surgery patient characteristics predispose this population to a higher risk of stroke.
- Typically, strokes in this population are secondary to ischemia from hypoperfusion or embolic phenomenon.
- Diagnosis: noncontrast computed tomography (CT) of the head (rule out hemorrhagic stroke) followed by magnetic resonance imaging (MRI) is appropriate for diagnosis.

Cardiovascular Complications

- Myocardial ischemia is of particular concern given the vascular surgery patient population, which exhibits higher rates of atherosclerosis, conduction abnormalities, and heart failure. Postoperative MI may be secondary to coronary thrombosis or low-flow across existing coronary artery lesions.
  - Workup of suspected coronary events should include an ECG, cardiac biomarkers (troponin), and transthoracic echocardiography to evaluate wall motion changes.
  - Management should include consultation with a cardiologist to determine if coronary angiography and revascularization are warranted.
- Unique to the carotid endarterectomy (CEA) procedure, postoperative bradycardia and hypotension can occur with increased arterial pressure on the carotid baroreceptors, causing a reflex response.
  - Reflex bradycardia and hypotension after CEA require vasopressor and chronotropic support.

Respiratory

- Most patients are extubated in the operating room after vascular surgery.
- The patients who remain intubated likely have significant comorbidities or underwent significant resuscitation and fluid shifts during the surgical course.
- Volume status is important to understand prior to extubation, and diuresis may be required to help mobilize third-spacing fluids in the postoperative period.

Mesenteric Ischemia

- Mesenteric ischemia is a dreaded complication of vascular surgery that can result from mechanical obstruction during surgery or embolic/thrombotic events postoperatively.
- Mesenteric ischemia should be suspected in the setting of persistent lactic acidosis, ongoing shock state, and abdominal pain out of proportion to physical examination. CT of the abdomen and pelvis may be obtained to help guide diagnosis.
- Clinical suspicion should prompt surgical consultation.
- Definitive treatment in the case of bowel necrosis is exploratory laparotomy with bowel resection. In the absence of frank necrosis, medical management with bowel rest and antibiotics may be deemed appropriate.

Acute Kidney Injury

- AKI is a common complication after vascular surgery that worsens outcomes; risk is heightened with preexisting renal dysfunction, intraoperative hypotension, suprarenal cross-clamping, and sustained periods of hypoperfusion.
- In open TAAA repair cases, there is a 20% to 30% incidence of postoperative renal injury, with 3% to 6% of patients requiring dialysis.
- For open TAAA repair, several intraoperative strategies exist to protect the kidneys until normal aortic flow is restored.
  - Cold crystalloid renal perfusion is the preferred option, which offers excellent protection to the kidneys.
  - Passive shunts, bypass grafts, and left heart bypass circuits are also technical strategies to maintain antegrade flow to the kidneys during cross-clamp time.
- Once AKI has occurred, careful attention to adequate intravascular volume and avoidance of nephrotoxic drugs is of the utmost importance.

Bleeding and Thrombosis

- Vascular surgery often involves heparinization, large volume resuscitation, and hypothermia, which all predispose the patient to coagulation derangements.
- Hemoglobin goal >7 g/dL should be targeted, but if there are concerns for spinal cord ischemia, a higher threshold may be warranted.
- Patients with catheter-assisted lysis after thrombectomy should be monitored in the ICU postoperatively.
  - Fibrinogen is monitored (maintained >150 mg/dL) as a marker for the risk of bleeding, though there is a paucity of evidence to support this practice.
- Depending on the vascular procedure and the corresponding concern for graft thrombosis, Doppler signals and pulse checks are performed hourly and require ICU monitoring.

Other Vascular Surgery Complications

- There can be direct injury at the site of vascular access/puncture, ranging from the development of a pseudoaneurysm to complete rupture requiring surgical repair.
- In cases with reperfusion, signs of compartment syndrome should be closely monitored by physical examination and CPK levels. Treatment is urgent fasciotomy.
- Retroperitoneal hematomas should be considered in the case of refractory hypotension and hemoglobin drop.
- Large sheaths placed in the femoral artery can compromise flow to the distal extremity and cause ischemic injury.
- Endoleaks and stent graft infections are typically late complications of vascular surgery.

SUGGESTED READINGS

Bhamidipati CM, Coselli JS, LeMaire SA. Perfusion techniques for renal protection during thoracoabdominal aortic surgery. *J Extra Corpor Technol*. 2012;44(1):P31-P37.

Bojar RM. *Manual of Perioperative Care in Adult Cardiac Surgery*. Wiley-Blackwell, John Wiley & Sons, Inc; 2021.

Chatterjee S, Preventza O, Orozco-Sevilla V, et al. Critical care management after open thoracoabdominal aortic aneurysm repair. *J Cardiovasc Surg (Torino)*. 2021;62(3):220-229.

Coselli JS, LeMaire SA, Köksoy C, et al. Cerebrospinal fluid drainage reduces paraplegia after thoracoabdominal aortic aneurysm repair: results of a randomized clinical trial. *J Vasc Surg*. 2002;35(4):631-639.

Crimi E, Hill CC. Postoperative ICU management of vascular surgery patients. *Anesthesiol Clin*. 2014;32(3):735-757.

Dunning J, Fabbri A, Kolh PH, et al; EACTS Clinical Guidelines Committee. Guideline for resuscitation in cardiac arrest after cardiac surgery. *Eur J Cardiothorac Surg*. 2009;36:3-28.

Herrmann C. Cardiac advanced life support-surgical guideline: overview and implementation. *AACN Adv Crit Care*. 2014;25:123-129.

Kaufman C, Kinney T, Quencer K. Practice trends of fibrinogen monitoring in thrombolysis. *J Clin Med*. 2018;7(5):111.

Mebazaa A, Pitsis AA, Rudiger A, et al. Clinical review: practical recommendations on the management of perioperative heart failure in cardiac surgery. *Crit Care*. 2010;14:201.

Ramsay JG, Shelton KT, Cudemus G. Extracorporeal membrane oxygenation and cardiac devices. In: Gropper M, ed. *Miller's Anesthesia*. 9th ed. Elsevier; 2019:2694-2712.

Sharifpour M, Bittner EA. Critical care of the vascular surgery patient. *Anesthesiol Clin*. 2022;40(4):775-790.

Singh S, Maldonado Y, Taylor MA. Optimal perioperative medical management of the vascular surgery patient. *Anesthesiol Clin*. 2014;32(3): 615-637.

Stephens RS, Shah AS, Whitman GJ. Lung injury and acute respiratory distress syndrome after cardiac surgery. *Ann Thorac Surg*. 2013;95:1122-1129.

Stephens RS, Whitman GJ. Postoperative critical care of the adult cardiac surgical patient. Part I: routine postoperative care. *Crit Care Med*. 2015; 43(7):1477-1497.

Stephens RS, Whitman GJ. Postoperative critical care of the adult cardiac surgical patient: part II: procedure-specific considerations, management of complications, and quality improvement. *Crit Care Med*. 2015;43(9): 1995-2014.

Thiele H, Zeymer U, Neumann FJ, et al. Intraaortic balloon support for myocardial infarction with cardiogenic shock. *N Engl J Med*. 2012; 367(14):1287-1296.

Werdan K, Gielen S, Ebelt H, et al. Mechanical circulatory support in cardiogenic shock. *Eur Heart J*. 2014;35:156-167.

SECTION 3

Pulmonary

Section Editors: Raghu R. Chivukula, Edward A. Bittner, and Casey M. Luckhurst

3.1

Pulmonary Mechanics

Raghu R. Chivukula

Definitions and Formulas

- Airway pressures: measured at proximal airways during mechanical ventilation (if intubated, this pressure reflects tracheal pressure)
  - Peak inspiratory pressure (PIP)
    - Maximal pressure measured at end inspiration
    - Determined *by both the elastic and resistive properties* of the respiratory system
  - Plateau pressure (P_{plat})
    - Estimation of peak alveolar pressure at a state of zero flow
    - Determined solely by tidal volume and compliance of respiratory system (*no contribution of airways resistance*)
    - Measured by applying an end-inspiratory breath-hold for 0.5 to 2 seconds (zero flow)
    - Measurement only valid during passive inflation (use assist control mode, not pressure support ventilation)
  - Compliance
    - Distensibility of system; inverse of elastance
    - Change in volume divided by the pressure required to produce that volume
    - Respiratory system compliance (compliance of chest wall + lung)
      - $C_{RS} = \Delta V/\Delta P = V_T/(P_{plat} - \text{PEEP})$
      - Normal value for mechanically ventilated patient is 50 to100 mL/cm H_2O.
    - Chest wall compliance: reflects all contributions to respiratory compliance other than from the lungs (includes chest, spine, abdomen, musculature)
      - Calculated using esophageal pressure (P_{ES}) as a surrogate for pleural pressure (P_{PL})
      - $C_{CW} = \Delta V/\Delta P = V_T/\Delta P_{PL}$
      - Normal value = 200 mL/cm H_2O
      - Causes of increased chest wall compliance: paralysis, flail chest
      - Causes of decreased chest wall compliance: obesity, abdominal distension, thoracic deformities, chest wall burns/edema, increased muscle tone
    - Lung compliance
      - Calculated using transpulmonary pressure, typically not possible directly unless pleural pressure is known
      - $C_L = \Delta V/\Delta P = V_T/((P_{plat} - \text{PEEP}) - \Delta P_{PL})$
      - Normal value = 200 mL/cm H_2O
      - Causes of increased lung compliance: emphysema
      - Causes of decreased lung compliance: consolidation, atelectasis, pulmonary edema, pulmonary fibrosis, pneumonectomy, mainstem intubation
  - Resistance
    - Opposition to air flow within airways
    - Change in pressure divided by flow
    - Inspiratory resistance:
      - $R_I = (\text{PIP} - P_{plat})/\dot{V}$
      - Set ventilator for constant inspiratory flow
    - Normal value for intubated and mechanically ventilated patients <10 cm H_2O/L/s at a flow of 1 L/s
    - Causes of increased resistance: bronchospasm, secretions, small endotracheal tube

Pressure-Volume Curves (Figure 3.1.1)

- Depict the static relationship between pressure and volume of respiratory system

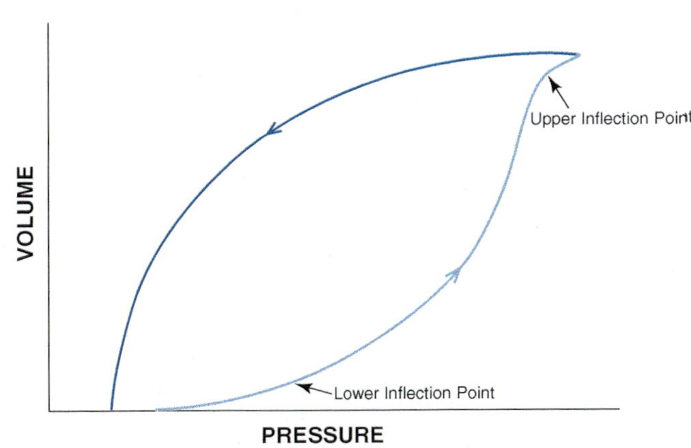

FIGURE 3.1.1 **Pressure-volume curves.**

- Constructed by measuring pressure as lungs are inflated or deflated (different curves due to hysteresis); accurate measurements require sedation and often paralysis.
- Normal shape is sigmoidal with lower and upper inflection points.
- Lower inflection point may represent the closing volume of the alveoli. Similarly, the upper inflection point may represent overdistension of the alveoli.
- Clinical utility of adjusting ventilator to avoid alveolar collapse and overdistension based on the pressure-volume curve is not clear.

SUGGESTED READINGS

Bigatello LM, Davignon KR, Stelfox HT. Respiratory mechanics and ventilator waveforms in the patient with acute lung injury. *Respir Care.* 2005;50(2):235-245.

Hess DR, Bigatello LM. The chest wall in acute lung injury/acute respiratory distress syndrome. *Curr Opin Crit Care.* 2008;14(1):94-102.

Hess DR, Medoff BD, Fessler MB. Pulmonary mechanics and graphics during positive pressure ventilation. *Int Anesthesiol Clin.* 1999;37(3):15-34.

Jubran A, Tobin MJ. Monitoring during mechanical ventilation. *Clin Chest Med.* 1996;17(3):453-473.

Lucangelo U, Bernabé F, Blanch L. Respiratory mechanics derived from signals in the ventilator circuit. *Respir Care.* 2005;50(1):55-65.

Lucangelo U, Bernabè F, Blanch L. Lung mechanics at the bedside: make it simple. *Curr Opin Crit Care.* 2007;13(1):64-72.

3.2

Respiratory Failure, Mechanical Ventilation, and Weaning

Raghu R. Chivukula

Definitions

- *Respiratory failure:* inability of the lungs to perform their basic task of gas exchange: the transfer of oxygen from inhaled air into the blood and the transfer of carbon dioxide from the blood into exhaled air
- *Hypoxemic respiratory failure* reflects inability to oxygenate (Pao_2 <60 mm Hg).
  - Classically, five potential physiologic causes:
    - Shunt: regions of lung with perfusion but zero ventilation
    - $\dot{V}/\dot{Q}$ mismatch: regions of lung with mismatched perfusion and ventilation
    - Hypoventilation: reduced minute ventilation causing elevated alveolar CO_2
    - Diffusion defect: impairment of oxygen movement across the alveolar and capillary basement membranes
    - Reduced Fio_2: either due to reduced oxygen fraction (rare) or due to reduced total barometric pressure (eg, at altitude)
- Hypercapnic respiratory failure reflects inability to clear CO_2 ($Paco_2$ >45 mm Hg).
  - Classically, two potential physiologic causes:
    - Reduced alveolar ventilation
      - Mechanical limitation: airway obstruction, neuromuscular weakness, chest wall stiffness
      - Loss of central respiratory drive: brain injury, narcotics
    - Increased CO_2 production (though rarely sufficient to manifest as hypercapnia on its own)

Common Causes to Remember (Table 3.2.1)

Key Pathophysiology

- Acute respiratory failure can result from pathology affecting any component of the respiratory pathway, from the central nervous system (CNS) control centers, to the spinal cord, to the muscles of respiration, to the lungs and their vasculature.
- Causes are often multifactorial.
- Understanding the cause of the acute respiratory failure is key to treating and reversing it.

Differential Diagnosis

- CNS: drugs, sedatives, central sleep apnea, encephalopathy
- Spinal cord: trauma, transverse myelitis
- Neuromuscular system: polio, Guillain-Barré syndrome, critical care/steroid myopathy
- Chest wall/pleural space: kyphosis, obesity, pleural effusion, pneumothorax, hemothorax
- Upper airways: obstructive sleep apnea, vocal cord paralysis, tracheomalacia

TABLE 3.2.1 Indications for Mechanical Ventilation

Hypoxemia	Hypoxemia (Spo_2 <90%) unresponsive to conservative measures (supplemental O_2, high-flow nasal cannula) OR concern for ongoing lung injury
Hypercapnia	No strict arterial pH cutoff; pH <7.3 with evidence of respiratory distress or somnolence is typical
Respiratory fatigue	Signs: tachypnea, dyspnea, use of accessory muscles, diaphoresis, tachycardia
Airway protection	Decreased mental status, increased aspiration risk

- Lower airways: bronchospasm, chronic obstructive disease, infection, congestive heart failure (CHF)
- Lung parenchyma: aspiration, infection, interstitial lung disease
- Pulmonary vasculature: pulmonary embolism, pulmonary hypertension

Management and Treatment

- Mechanical ventilation may be needed to treat hypoxemia, hypercarbia, and/or respiratory fatigue.
  - Ventilator settings should be chosen not only to provide adequate oxygenation and ventilation but also to promote patient-ventilator synchrony, maintain alveolar recruitment while avoiding alveolar overdistention, and avoid auto-positive end-expiratory pressure (PEEP) and ventilator-induced lung injury.
- Understanding the variables that determine how a ventilator breath is delivered, how to set the ventilator, and ventilator modes is essential to avoid the harmful effects of mechanical ventilation (Table 3.2.2).
- Ventilator settings
  - Should be tailored to the underlying condition resulting in respiratory failure
  - Tidal volume
    - Target tidal volume of 4 to 8 mL/kg predicted body a weight
    - Should use predicted body weight (based on gender and height of patient) to determine tidal volume:
      - Males: predicted body weight (PBW) = 50 + 2.3 × (height [inches] − 60)
      - Females: PBW = 45.5 + 2.3 × (height [inches] − 60)
    - In patients with acute respiratory distress syndrome (ARDS) or any form of acute lung injury (ALI), low tidal volume ventilation (4-8 mL/kg, frequently targeted to <6 mL/kg in practice) has been established as superior to high tidal volume ventilation.

TABLE 3.2.2 Ventilator Variables

Variable	Definition	Considerations
Trigger	Starts the inspiratory phase	Ventilator initiated: • Trigger is time (determined by set respiratory rate). Patient initiated: • Trigger is either change in pressure (pressure trigger), change in flow (flow trigger), or electrical activity of the diaphragm (Ead). • Trigger sensitivity that is set too high will require excessive patient effort to initiate a breath. • Trigger sensitivity that is set too low may result in auto-triggering of the ventilator by cardiac oscillations or other artifacts.
Control	Constant during inspiration	Volume (flow) or pressure
Cycle	Terminates inspiration	• Time for volume- or pressure-controlled ventilation • Flow for pressure support ventilation

    - Patients with neuromuscular disease may need higher tidal volumes (8-10 mL/kg) to prevent atelectasis.
    - Evidence for overdistension potentially requiring further reduction in tidal volumes includes P_{plat} >30 cm H_2O or driving pressure (DP, P_{plat} − PEEP) >15 cm H_2O.
  - Inspiratory time
    - Set directly in pressure-controlled ventilation
    - Determined by tidal volume, flow rate, and flow pattern in volume-controlled ventilation
    - Determined by cycle off (flow deceleration) sensitivity in pressure support ventilation
    - If set incorrectly (too long or too short), may result in patient/ventilator asynchrony
    - Should be set shorter than expiratory time to prevent inverse I:E ratio
  - Respiratory rate(s) can be shown in Table 3.2.3.
    - Minute ventilation is determined by tidal volume and respiratory rate.
    - Minute ventilation of 6 to 12 L/min is typical (higher with increased CO_2 production and/or dead space, body weight).
    - Adjust rate to achieve the desired pH and pco_2.
    - High respiratory rates can be associated with air trapping and auto-PEEP.
  - I:E ratio
    - Set directly in pressure-controlled ventilation
    - Determined by tidal volume, respiratory rate, and flow pattern in volume-controlled ventilation
    - Longer inspiratory time can result in improved oxygenation but is also associated with auto-PEEP and hemodynamic instability.
    - Expiratory time should be longer than inspiratory time and is determined by inspiratory time and respiratory rate.
  - PEEP
    - Increases functional residual capacity (FRC), decreases intrapulmonary shunt, can improve pulmonary compliance through recruitment of atelectatic units
    - Can produce hemodynamic instability through effects on venous return; can contribute to overdistension
    - PEEP can be titrated by:
      - Clinical parameters (oxygenation, hemodynamics, body habitus, radiograph)
      - PEEP tables (eg, ARDSnet tables)
      - Pressure-volume curves (see previous chapter), with PEEP titrated to approximate that pressure at which the lower inflection point occurs
      - "Best PEEP trial" to determine the best respiratory system compliance directly by assaying compliance at multiple tidal volumes
      - Esophageal pressure transduction, aiming to maintain end-expiratory transpulmonary pressure >0 cm H_2O
      - Electrical impedance tomography, an emerging technique
    - No clinical trial evidence supports a single method of PEEP titration as superior to others in all circumstances.

TABLE 3.2.3 Respiratory Rates

Mode	Control Variable	Tidal Volume	Respiratory Rate	I:E ratio
Volume control	Volume (flow)	Delivered tidal volume is set and constant regardless of airways resistance or respiratory system compliance.	Set: patient can trigger a rate greater than that set on ventilator but always receives the set rate.	Inspiratory time is determined by inspiratory flow and pattern, and tidal volume.
Pressure control	Pressure	Determined by pressure setting, airways resistance, respiratory system compliance, patient's inspiratory effort	Set: patient can trigger a rate greater than that set on ventilator but always receives the set rate.	I:E ratio can be set on the ventilator.
Pressure support	Pressure	Determined by pressure setting, airways resistance, respiratory system compliance, patient's inspiratory effort	All breaths are triggered by patient.	Ventilator cycles to expiratory phase when flow decreases to a preset level. Some ventilators have a backup time cycle to terminate inspiration.
Continuous positive airway pressure (CPAP)	Pressure	Determined by patient: ventilator does not provide inspiratory assistance.	All breaths are triggered by patient.	Determined by patient

Common Modes of Mechanical Ventilation

- Noninvasive ventilation (NIV), specifically continuous positive airway pressure (CPAP) and bilevel positive airway pressure (BiPAP). High-flow nasal cannula is sometimes considered NIV but is not discussed here as it does not provide significant mechanical support.
  - Indications include:
    - Cardiogenic pulmonary edema
    - Acute chronic obstructive pulmonary disease (COPD) exacerbation
    - Acute asthma exacerbation
    - Obstructive sleep apnea/obesity hypoventilation syndrome
    - Postextubation, specifically in patients intubated for hypercapnic respiratory failure (Note: neither routine extubation to NIV nor "rescue" BiPAP is well supported by available evidence.)
  - Contraindications
    - Cardiac or respiratory arrest
    - ARDS
    - Severe encephalopathy (eg, Glasgow Coma Scale [GCS] <10)
    - Severe upper gastrointestinal bleeding/gastric or esophageal surgery
    - Hemodynamic instability or unstable cardiac arrhythmia
    - Facial surgery, trauma, or deformity
    - Inability to cooperate/protect the airway
    - Inability to clear respiratory secretions
    - High risk for aspiration
  - Use of NIV requires frequent reassessment for success or failure. Delay in intubation may result in increased mortality. Consider prompt intubation if there is:
    - Increased accessory muscle use
    - Increased respiratory rate
    - Worsening arterial blood gas
    - Increased dyspnea
    - Increased heart rate
- Discontinuation of mechanical ventilation
  - Assessment of potential for ventilator discontinuation
    - Is there evidence of resolution of underlying disease that led to respiratory failure and need for mechanical ventilation?
    - Is gas exchange adequate?
      - Oxygenation: $Pao_2 > 60$, PEEP <8 cm H_2O, and $Fio_2 < 40\%$ to 50%
      - Ventilation: pH ≥ 7.25
    - Is the patient hemodynamically stable (no active myocardial ischemia or clinically important hypotension requiring vasoactive drug therapy)?
    - Can the patient initiate an inspiratory effort?
      - Sedation should be adjusted so patient can cooperate with weaning process.
- *The spontaneous breathing trial (SBT) is the best predictor of successful ventilation discontinuation.*
    - SBT is typically performed with minimal ventilator settings pressure support (PS) 0 to 5 + PEEP 0 to 5.
    - A successful SBT reflects >30 minutes of adequate gas exchange, respiratory effort, and hemodynamic stability. Longer SBT durations have not been demonstrated to increase the positive predictive value of SBT.
  - Criteria to determine tolerance of an SBT is shown in Table 3.2.4.

TABLE 3.2.4 Criteria for Successful SBT

Gas exchange	pH >7.32; $\uparrow Paco_2 \leq 10$ mm Hg; $Pao_2 \geq 50$-60 mm Hg; $Spo_2 \geq 88\%$
Hemodynamics	HR <120-140 bpm or Δ <20%; SBP <180-200 mm Hg and >90 mm Hg or Δ <20%
Respiratory rate	RR ≤30-35 breaths/min or Δ <50%
Subjective criteria	
Mental status	No new or excessive somnolence, anxiety, agitation
Discomfort/diaphoresis	No new or worsened
Work of breathing	No use of accessory respiratory muscles or thoracoabdominal paradoxical breathing pattern

HR, heart rate; RR, respiratory rate; SBP, systolic blood pressure.

- If patient fails SBT:
  - Set ventilator to comfortable, nonfatiguing mode for patient.
  - Look for cause of failed SBT.
    - Most common cause is need for further resolution of underlying disease.
    - Other contributory causes include dynamic hyperinflation, myocardial ischemia and cardiac disease, and critical illness neuropathy/myopathy.
    - Tracheostomy tube malposition should be considered if patient fails to wean off a low level of PS or develops respiratory distress quickly after removal of positive pressure ventilation.
- For example, bronchoscopic examination might reveal occlusion of airway device by the posterior membrane of the trachea.
  - SBT should be repeated once the cause for failed SBT is corrected.
- Use of weaning protocols is associated with reductions in weaning duration, total duration of mechanical ventilation, and intensive care unit (ICU) length of stay.
- Eligible patients should undergo daily, scheduled SBTs, and spontaneous awakening trials (SATs).

- Criteria for extubation
  - Successful completion of SBT
  - Ability to protect airway and clear secretions
    - Quality of cough
    - Quantity of secretions
    - Frequency of suctioning
  - Absence of upper airway edema
    - Can occur with prolonged mechanical ventilation, smaller airways (women, children), trauma, repeated or traumatic intubations
    - May be diagnosed with a leak test and/or direct visualization of airway with laryngoscopy or fiberoptic examination of glottis
      - Cuff leak test is indicated in patients at high risk for postextubation laryngeal edema: traumatic or difficult intubation, prolonged intubation (typically >6 days), use of a large endotracheal tube, female sex, or prior reintubation after unplanned extubation.
      - Leak test is performed with patient breathing spontaneously, off positive pressure ventilation, and endotracheal tube cuff deflated. A positive leak test is often defined as >100 mL or >15% of tidal volume loss due to leak.
      - Presence of a leak suggests the absence of significant airway swelling.
    - Absence of a cuff leak indicates the possibility of airway edema.
    - Guidelines suggest a single dose of intravenous (IV) methylprednisolone (~60 mg) in the event of no leak, followed by extubation >4 hours later. Repeat testing for cuff leak is not supported by evidence, nor are prolonged steroid administration regimens.
  - Patient cooperation
    - Patient should be awake, alert, comfortable, and able to follow instructions to cough.
      - Anxiolytics and pain medications may be titrated to achieve above goal.

Outcomes

- Mortality associated with mechanical ventilation: 30% to 60% depending on patient population studied
- Predictors of mortality include advanced age, a medical admitting diagnosis (vs surgical), respiratory failure due to primarily a pulmonary cause, and the inability to wean from mechanical ventilation.
- Predictors of failure to discontinue mechanical ventilation include a medical admitting diagnosis (vs surgical) and history of underlying respiratory disease.
- One study using ICD-9 codes to identify patients receiving mechanical ventilation found that only 30.8% of patients were discharged home from the hospital; 28.2% of patients were discharged to a nursing facility.
- In another study of Medicare beneficiaries aged ≥65, mechanical ventilation during hospitalization was associated with a 1-year mortality of 72% and significant disability.
- Estimated costs were $27 billion nationally or 12% of all hospital costs.

SUGGESTED READINGS

Barnato A, Albert S, Angus D, et al. Disability among elderly survivors of mechanical ventilation. *Am J Respir Crit Care Med.* 2011;183:1037-1042.

Bigatello L, Stelfox H, Berra L, et al. Outcome of patients undergoing prolonged mechanical ventilation after critical illness. *Crit Care Med.* 2007;35:2491-2249.

Blackwood B, Alderdice F, Burns K, et al. Use of weaning protocols for reducing duration of mechanical ventilation in critically ill adult patients: Cochrane systematic review and meta-analysis. *BMJ.* 2011;342:c7237.

Esan A, Hess D, Raoof S, et al. Severe hypoxemic respiratory failure: ventilation strategies. *Chest.* 2010;137:1203-1216.

Esteban A, Frutos F, Ferguson ND, et al. Noninvasive positive pressure ventilation for respiratory failure after extubation. *N Engl J Med.* 2004;350:2452-2460.

Esteban A, Frutos F, Tobin MJ, et al. A comparison of four methods of weaning patients from mechanical ventilation. *N Engl J Med.* 1995;332:345-350.

MacIntyre N. Current issues in mechanical ventilation for respiratory failure. *Chest.* 2005;128:561S-567S.

Mercat A, Richard J, Vielle B, et al. Positive end-expiratory pressure setting in adults with acute lung injury and acute respiratory distress syndrome: a randomized controlled trial. *JAMA.* 2008;200:637-645.

NIH/NHLBI ARDS Network. Ventilation with lower tidal volumes as compared with traditional tidal volumes for acute long injury and acute respiratory distress syndrome. *N Engl J Med.* 2000;342:1301-1308.

Schmidt GA, Girard TD, Kress JP, et al. Liberation from mechanical ventilation in critically ill adults: executive summary of an Official American College of Chest Physicians/American Thoracic Society Clinical Practice Guideline. *Chest.* 2017;151(1):160-165.

Wunsch H, Linde-Zwirble W, Angus D, et al. Epidemiology of mechanical ventilation use in the United States. *Crit Care Med.* 2010;38:1947-1953.

3.3

Acute Respiratory Distress Syndrome

Christopher V. Cosgriff and B. Taylor Thompson

Acute respiratory distress syndrome (ARDS) is fundamentally characterized by hypoxemia in the setting of bilateral pulmonary opacities representative of an exudative alveolar filling process caused by increased epithelial and endothelial permeability. Previously, definitionally limited to patients receiving positive pressure ventilation, attention to resource-limited settings and the extensive use of high-flow nasal cannula (HFNC) during the COVID-19 pandemic have yielded a new global definition with four criteria required to make the diagnosis:

- Precipitating factor and origin of alveolar edema: the process occurred following an acute risk factor (eg, pneumonia, aspiration, trauma), and the pulmonary edema and concomitant hypoxemia are not primarily or exclusively explained by cardiogenic pulmonary edema.
- Temporality: occurring within 7 days of the purported risk factor
- Chest imaging: bilateral opacities on chest radiography or computed tomography not fully explained by effusions, atelectasis, or nodules/masses, or ultrasonographic evidence such as bilateral B lines and/or consolidations
- Oxygenation
  - Nonintubated ARDS: Pao_2:Fio_2 ≤300 mm Hg or Spo_2:Fio_2 ≤315 (if Spo_2 ≤97%) on HFNC ≥30 L/min or noninvasive ventilation with at least 5 cm H_2O of end-expiratory pressure
  - Intubated ARDS:
    - Mild: 200< Pao_2:Fio_2 <=300 mm Hg or 235< Spo_2:Fio_2 <=315 (if Spo_2 ≤97%)
    - Moderate: 100< Pao_2:Fio_2 <=200 mm Hg or 148< Spo_2:Fio_2 <=235 (if Spo_2 ≤97%)
    - Severe: Pao_2:Fio_2 ≤100 mm Hg or Spo_2:Fio_2 ≤148 (if Spo_2 ≤97%)
  - Modified definition for resource-limited settings: Spo_2:Fio_2 ≤315 (if Spo_2 ≤97%), requiring neither positive end-expiratory pressure (PEEP) nor a minimum flow rate

Common Causes to Remember (Table 3.3.1)

TABLE 3.3.1 Common Causes of Pulmonary Injury and Remote Injury

Pulmonary Injury (Direct)	Remote Injury (Indirect)
• Pneumonia (pulmonary sepsis) • Infectious or chemical pneumonitis • Pulmonary contusion (think trauma) • Fat or amniotic fluid embolus • Near drowning	• Nonpulmonary sepsis • Severe burns • Pancreatitis • Severe trauma • Ischemia-reperfusion injury • Drug overdose • Transfusion-related acute lung injury (TRALI)

Epidemiology

- Pre–COVID-19 pandemic studies suggested 10% of all intensive care unit (ICU) patients and 23% of all mechanically ventilated patients met the previous definition for ARDS (now subsumed into intubated ARDS).
- Mortality for the syndrome is estimated at 35% to 45%, but heavily influenced by age and comorbidity burden.

Pathophysiology

Multiple mechanisms contribute to the development of alveolar filling with noncardiogenic pulmonary edema:

- Direct and indirect injuries, dysregulated inflammation, and recruitment of a cellular inflammatory response result in increased vascular and epithelial permeability to protein and solutes.
- Neutrophils are recruited as a central element of the innate immune response. Neutrophil extracellular traps (NETs) have been identified as a key driver of ongoing epithelial damage.
- Biomechanical propagation: because there is heterogeneity in the distribution of alveolar consolidations, areas of lung with greater consolidation become stiffer and can experience higher local transmural pressures, therefore causing them to act as local *stress raisers*—particularly at the interface between consolidated and nonconsolidated regions of the lung.

Syndrome Heterogeneity

Recent evidence suggests at least two biologically distinct subtypes of ARDS, referred to as endotypes:

- Hyperinflammatory: characterized by higher levels of serum cytokines (eg, interleukin-6 [IL-6], tumor necrosis factor-alpha [TNFα]), higher levels of multiorgan dysfunction, and higher mortality. Recent work has demonstrated that the primary cause of death in the majority of these patients is circulatory failure (shock).
- Hypoinflammatory: characterized by lower levels of inflammatory serum cytokines than the hyperinflammatory subtype, though still elevated over normal. The lungs remain the primary organ injured. Recent work has demonstrated that the primary cause of death in the majority of these patients is respiratory failure (failure to wean from the ventilator as opposed to refractory hypoxemia).

Retrospective analyses of randomized trials have suggested differential responses to various treatments and management strategies between these endotypes that may guide future targeted therapies.

Differential Diagnosis

A central tenet of treating ARDS is to identify the underlying cause. Many causes of ARDS require specific treatment in addition to supportive ICU care for optimal outcomes. After exonerating cardiogenic pulmonary edema as the primary cause, the differential diagnosis for bilateral opacities with hypoxemia includes:

- Organizing pneumonia (secondary or cryptogenic)
- Diffuse alveolar hemorrhage (bland or inflammatory)
- Vasculitis
- Acute eosinophilic pneumonia
- Acute hypersensitivity pneumonitis

- Drug-induced pneumonitis
- Acute exacerbation of interstitial lung disease
- Acute chest syndrome

However, aside from targeting the therapeutic strategy toward these underlying causes, the tenets of supportive care in terms of ventilator and fluid management remain largely the same with these diagnoses and ARDS.

Management and Treatment

The major goal of supportive care for ARDS supportive care is to limit ventilator-induced lung injury. This requires lower tidal volumes, higher inspiratory flow, end-expiratory pressure, and respiratory rates to ventilate a gently opened lung while limiting patient ventilator dyssynchrony.

In the patient with nonintubated ARDS, there remains equipoise between strategies that prioritize early intubation in an attempt to avoid the potential for patient self-induced lung injury (P-SILI) and strategies that attempt to judiciously stave off intubation when it is considered safe to continue support with HFNC or noninvasive positive pressure ventilation. Increased work of breathing and worsening hypoxemia are recommended triggers for intubation, and the Respiratory rate-OXygenation (ROX) index may help inform these decisions. Tidal volumes should be monitored on noninvasive ventilation as the combination of high respiratory drive and noninvasive inspiratory assist may result in very large tidal volumes, lung injury, and worse outcomes.

All intubated patients with suspected or confirmed ARDS should be initiated on *lung-protective ventilation*:

- Tidal volumes should be set (on volume control) or targeted at (on pressure control) *≤4 to 8 mL/kg of ideal body weight*.
- There remains a lack of certainty in the selection of the level of PEEP with previously explored strategies that include empiric selection based on hypoxemia, or selection tailored to driving pressure, imaging-based assessments of recruitability, esophageal balloon manometry–based estimation of transpulmonary pressure, and recruitability assessed by electrical impedance tomography. Current data support a recommendation of a higher PEEP strategy coupled with close monitoring of respiratory mechanics and hemodynamics in patients with moderate-to-severe ARDS.
    - Society guidelines recommend against recruitment maneuvers, which may be harmful.
    - Plateau pressures should be targeted at <30 cm H_2O and driving pressure should ideally be targeted at <15 cm H_2O, although the current randomized data support prioritization of plateau pressure as a target over driving pressure.
    - Sedation should be applied judiciously to ensure ventilator synchrony and should be weaned as aggressively as able, considering the known long-term sequelae of prolonged sedation. The addition of neuromuscular blockade may be needed for control of dyssynchrony.
    - There is discordance in existing data and society-derived recommendations on the use of neuromuscular blockade. We advise neuromuscular blockade for treating dyssynchrony that persists on optimal sedation and analgesia to maintain lung-protective ventilation, and meta-analysis supports its empiric use in severe ARDS.
    - The primary form of neuromuscular blockade studied is cisatracurium, and its purported benefits may be due to its role in reducing breath-stacking dyssynchrony, double triggering, and P-SILI.
    - Protracted exposure to neuromuscular blockade, particularly if a patient is also receiving steroids, is associated with the risk of critical illness myopathy. The need for neuromuscular blockade should be reevaluated daily.
    - In patients whose Pao_2:Fio_2 ratio is <150 while on PEEP >=5 and Fio_2 >=0.6, prone positioning is an evidence-based intervention that reduces mortality.
    - Prone positioning is a fundamentally lung-protective maneuver, and its benefit is independent of its effect on gas exchange.
- As with the decision to intubate the patient, there is a dearth of guidance on when it is safe to wean sedation and support toward a spontaneous breathing trial. However, current practice follows the original ARDSnet protocol in which the spontaneous breathing trial is attempted when the patient is on an Fio_2 ≤40% and PEEP ≤8 or an Fio_2 ≤50% and PEEP ≤5.

Beyond lung-protective ventilation, pharmacotherapeutic considerations include:

- Systemic corticosteroids: while prior studies suggested harm from high-dose steroids, particularly when administered late in the course of ARDS, recent data informed by the COVID-19 pandemic and studies on the management of severe pneumonia have led to a conditional recommendation to administer steroids in all patients with ARDS who do not have a contraindication. At present, there is no guidance on the selection of agent, dose, or duration, but reasonable options include hydrocortisone started at 200 mg/d and tapered according to clinical course as described in the CAPE COD study as well as dexamethasone started at 6 mg/d and applied as it was used in COVID-19 based on the RECOVERY study.
- Inhaled pulmonary vasodilators: Outside of indications for the reduction of right heart strain, inhaled pulmonary vasodilators such as nitric oxide and epoprostenol may improve $\dot{V}/\dot{Q}$ matching and thus reduce hypoxemia, but these therapies have not been shown to improve mortality, and their effect on hypoxemia should not result in a decision to forgo proning in a patient initially meeting the aforementioned criteria.
- Diuretics: conservative fluid management targeting a central venous pressure (CVP) <4 has been shown to reduce the duration of mechanical ventilation and intensive care without worsening nonpulmonary organ failures.

With respect to salvage therapy in patients failing conventional support:

- Inverse ratio ventilation, which increases the average mean airway pressure, may temporarily improve hypoxemia but at the cost of exacerbating lung injury, and with the potential for worsened auto-PEEP and hemodynamic compromise.
- Venovenous extracorporeal membranous oxygenation (ECMO): based on a small number of studies, ECMO is thought to be a lifesaving intervention in a select group of patients when applied judiciously and early to patients who have failed conventional management.
    - In patients with severe ARDS, there should be early consideration of transfer to an ECMO-capable center.

- Transfer to such centers is associated with better outcomes for patients who do not go on to ECMO, and patients who have spent a protracted period on HFNC and/or mechanical ventilation are less likely to benefit from initiation of ECMO.

Outcomes

- Morbidity and mortality for patients with ARDS remain high, although progress has been made with the introduction of lung-protective ventilation, proning, and protocolized nursing care.
- As described earlier, many patients with ARDS do not die from overwhelming hypoxemia, but rather from progressive nonpulmonary organ dysfunction.
  - The hyperinflammatory subtype of ARDS, which is associated with an increased incidence of shock, carries a higher mortality.
  - Long-term morbidity in many survivors is driven by muscle weakness and cognitive dysfunction, requiring protracted rehabilitation. Prevention involves shortening the duration of ventilation, sedation, and limiting the use of neuromuscular blockade.
  - Total lung capacity and vital capacity may return to the lower bounds of normal after ARDS, DLCO (diffusing capacity of the lungs for carbon monoxide) is reduced, and some patients will have persistent restrictive or mixed obstructive-restrictive deficits. The majority of survivors do not need long-term oxygen supplementation, and many return to active lives.

SUGGESTED READINGS

Evrard B, Sinha P, Delucchi K, et al. Causes and attributable fraction of death from ARDS in inflammatory phenotypes of sepsis. *Crit Care*. 2024;28(1):164.

Herridge M, Cheung A, Tansey C, et al. One-year outcomes in survivors of the acute respiratory distress syndrome. *N Engl J Med*. 2003;348:683-693.

Hopkins R, Weaver LK, Pope D, et al. Neuropsychological sequelae and impaired health status in survivors of severe acute respiratory distress syndrome. *Am J Respir Crit Care Med*. 1999;160:50-56.

Matthay MA, Arabi Y, Arroliga AC, et al. A new global definition of acute respiratory distress syndrome. *Am J Respir Crit Care Med*. 2024;209(1):37-47.

Meade M, Cook D, Guyatt G, et al. Ventilation strategy using low tidal volumes, recruitment maneuvers, and high positive end-expiratory pressure for acute lung injury and acute respiratory distress syndrome, a randomized controlled trial. *JAMA*. 2008;299(6):637-645.

Meyer NJ, Gattinoni L, Calfee CS. Acute respiratory distress syndrome. *Lancet*. 2021;398(10300):622-637.

Papazian L, Forel J, Gacouin A, et al. Neuromuscular blockers in early acute respiratory distress syndrome. *N Engl J Med*. 2010;363:1107-1116.

Qadir N, Sahetya S, Munshi L, et al. An update on management of adult patients with acute respiratory distress syndrome: an official American Thoracic Society clinical practice guideline. *Am J Respir Crit Care Med*. 2024;209(1):24-36.

Rizzo AN, Aggarwal NR, Thompson BT, Schmidt EP. Advancing precision medicine for the diagnosis and treatment of acute respiratory distress syndrome. *J Clin Med*. 2023;12(4):1563.

Rubenfeld GD, Caldwell E, Peabody E, et al. Incidence and outcomes of acute lung injury. *New Engl J Med*. 2005;353:1685-1693.

Santiago VR, Rzezinski AF, Nardelli LM, et al. Recruitment maneuver in experimental acute lung injury: the role of alveolar collapse and edema. *Crit Care Med*. 2010;38:2207-2214.

Sinha P, Neyton L, Sarma A, et al. Molecular phenotypes of acute respiratory distress syndrome in the ROSE trial have differential outcomes and gene expression patterns that differ at baseline and longitudinally over time. *Am J Respir Crit Care Med*. 2024;209(7):816-828.

Slutsky AS. Lung injury caused by mechanical ventilation. *Chest*. 1999;116(1 suppl):9S-15S.

Sud S, Friedrich JO, Taccone P, et al. Prone ventilation reduces mortality in patients with acute respiratory failure and severe hypoxemia: systematic review and metaanalysis. *Intensive Care Med*. 2010;36:585-599.

Talmor D, Sarge T, Malhotra A, et al. Mechanical ventilation guided by esophageal pressure in acute lung injury. *N Engl J Med*. 2008;359:2095-2104.

The Acute Respiratory Distress Syndrome Network. Ventilation with lower tidal volumes as compare with traditional tidal volumes for acute lung injury and the acute respiratory distress syndrome. *N Engl J Med*. 2000;342(18):1334-1349.

The National Heart, Lung, and Blood Institute ARDS Clinical Trials Network. Higher versus lower positive end-expiratory pressures in patients with the acute respiratory distress syndrome. *N Engl J Med*. 2004;351:327-336.

The National Heart, Lung, and Blood Institute ARDS Clinical Trials Network. Efficacy and safety of corticosteroids for persistent acute respiratory distress syndrome. *N Engl J Med*. 2006;354:1671-1684.

The National Heart, Lung, and Blood Institute ARDS Clinical Trials Network. Pulmonary-artery versus central venous catheter to guide treatment of acute lung injury. *N Engl J Med*. 2006;354:2213-2224.

The National Heart, Lung, and Blood Institute ARDS Clinical Trials Network. Comparison of two fluid-management strategies in acute lung injury. *N Engl J Med*. 2006;354:2564-2575.

Thompson BT, Chambers RC, Liu KD. Acute respiratory distress syndrome. *N Engl J Med*. 2017;377(6):562-572.

Tomashefski JF Jr. Pulmonary pathology of acute respiratory distress syndrome. *Clin Chest Med*. 2000;21(3):435-466.

Tremblay LN, Slutsky AS. Ventilator-induced lung injury: from the bench to the bedside. *Intensive Care Med*. 2006;32:24-33.

Wheeler AP, Bernard GR. Acute lung injury and the acute respiratory distress syndrome: a clinical review. *Lancet*. 2007;369:1553-1565.

3.4

Ventilator-Induced Lung Injury and Ventilator-Associated Lung Injury

Maurizio Cereda, Stefano Spina, and Glasiele C. Alcala

- Ventilator-induced lung injury (VILI): an acute inflammatory process resulting from the mechanical stress and strain placed on the lung during mechanical ventilation. Patients with acute respiratory distress syndrome (ARDS) are typically at high risk of excessive strain due to the dramatic reduction in end-expiratory lung volume and inhomogeneous inflation.
- Patient self-inflicted lung injury (P-SILI) arises when a patient's high respiratory drive leads to vigorous inspiratory efforts, which, in turn, increase transpulmonary pressure swings. The mechanical stress and strain from these efforts result in the cyclic opening and closing of alveoli, producing shear forces that further damage the delicate lung structure.

Common Causes to Remember

- *Barotrauma*: damage to the lung tissues due to high airway pressures, leading to alveolar overdistension and rupture
- *Volutrauma*: lung injury caused by excessive tidal volumes, which can lead to alveolar overinflation and shear stress
    - *Atelectrauma*: injury caused by repetitive opening and closing of alveoli (atelectasis), especially at lower lung volumes, leading to mechanical stress and strain on the alveolar walls
    - *Biotrauma*: release of inflammatory mediators and cytokines due to mechanical ventilation, contributing to lung inflammation and injury
    - *Oxygen toxicity*: lung injury caused by exposure to high concentrations of oxygen, which can lead to oxidative stress and damage to lung tissues
    - *Ventilator-associated pneumonia (VAP)*: infection of the lungs due to invasive mechanical ventilation, which can exacerbate lung injury and inflammation
    - Effective management and prevention of VILI require careful monitoring of ventilator settings, such as tidal volume, airway pressures, and oxygen levels, as well as strategies to minimize lung injury while maintaining adequate gas exchange and patient comfort.

Epidemiology

VILI occurs in a subset of patients undergoing mechanical ventilation, especially those with preexisting lung injury or acute respiratory failure causing altered lung mechanics. However, it is difficult to discriminate between secondary VILI and primary lung injury in individual patients. VILI is a significant concern in critical care settings, particularly among patients receiving mechanical ventilation for ARDS and other conditions, but it might also affect patients with noninjured lungs, for example, in the perioperative setting. The epidemiology of VILI highlights its impact and incidence:

1. *Prevalence*: VILI occurs in a subset of patients undergoing mechanical ventilation, especially those with preexisting lung injury and abnormal regional lung mechanics. The exact prevalence is unclear and probably varies depending on patient population, ventilation practices, and underlying conditions.
2. *Risk factors*: Patients at higher risk for VILI include those with severe ARDS, acute lung injury, or those requiring prolonged mechanical ventilation. Factors such as high tidal volumes, high airway pressures, inhomogeneous lung inflation, and inappropriate ventilator settings increase the risk.
3. *Consequences*: VILI can lead to worsened lung function, prolonged ventilator dependence, increased mortality rates, and longer intensive care unit (ICU) stays. It contributes to the morbidity and mortality associated with critical illness.
4. *Prevention strategies*: Guidelines and protocols emphasize protective ventilation strategies (eg, low tidal volumes, moderate positive end-expiratory pressure) to mitigate the risk of VILI. Monitoring and adjusting ventilator parameters based on patient response are critical in preventing lung injury.
5. *Research and advances*: Ongoing research focuses on refining ventilator management strategies to minimize VILI while optimizing respiratory support. This includes advancements in ventilator technology, understanding the pathophysiology of lung injury during mechanical ventilation, and identifying patients with risk factors for VILI.

Key Pathophysiology

- VILI involves several interconnected mechanisms that contribute to lung damage during mechanical ventilation.
- *Barotrauma:* which occurs when high airway pressures lead to the overdistension of alveoli. This overdistension can cause the alveolar walls to rupture, releasing air into surrounding tissues and resulting in complications such as pneumothorax, pneumomediastinum, and subcutaneous emphysema.
- *Volutrauma:* the use of excessive tidal volumes results in overinflation of the alveoli. This causes mechanical stress and strain on the alveolar-capillary membrane, leading to alveolar damage, increased permeability, and pulmonary edema.
- *Atelectrauma:* during the respiratory cycle, the repetitive opening and closing (atelectasis) of unstable airspaces generate shear forces that damage the alveolar walls. This cyclic recruitment and derecruitment of alveoli can lead to inflammation, surfactant dysfunction, and further lung injury. Atelectasis can be macroscopic (eg, lobar, segmental) or microscopic, where interspersed open and collapsed airspaces result in localized concentration of mechanical stress.
- *Biotrauma:* mechanical ventilation can trigger a local and systemic inflammatory response due to the release of pro-inflammatory cytokines and mediators from the injured lung tissue. This inflammatory response can exacerbate lung injury and contribute to multiple organ dysfunction syndrome.

- *Oxygen toxicity:* prolonged exposure to high concentrations of oxygen can generate reactive oxygen species, leading to oxidative stress, inflammation, alveolar-capillary membrane damage, and impaired gas exchange. Ideal target oxygen concentrations in ICU patients are, however, poorly defined.
- Multiple mechanisms can coexist, resulting in stress and strain to lung tissues during ventilation and causing cellular injury and disruption of the extracellular matrix.

Differential Diagnosis

- VILI should be considered in the differential diagnosis of any mechanically ventilated patient who experiences worsening respiratory status, need for increasing ventilator support, or worsening pulmonary infiltrates. However, susceptible patients can develop P-SILI before being intubated.
- As VILI is a diagnosis of exclusion that involves nonspecific clinical and radiographic changes, a thorough evaluation and investigation into alternative etiologies for respiratory decompensation should be undertaken before VILI/VALI (ventilator-associated lung injury) is considered a diagnosis.
- The skilled clinician will use all available clinical data to arrive at a convincing diagnosis and should take into account the following clinical conditions when composing a differential diagnosis:
  - Respiratory infection: suspected with new lobular pulmonary infiltrates, change in sputum production, fever, and new/worsening leukocytosis
  - Left-sided heart failure/cardiogenic shock: suspected with new, bilateral pulmonary infiltrates, known heart failure, elevated brain natriuretic peptide, electrocardiogram (ECG) changes, pink/frothy endotracheal tube secretions
  - Transfusion-related acute lung injury: suspected with rapid onset of clinical changes, bilateral infiltrates, recent transfusion of blood products
  - Pneumothorax: suspected with acute decompensation, loss of breath sounds in an isolated lung field, acutely elevated airway pressures
  - Diffuse alveolar hemorrhage: suspected with the development of bilateral infiltrates, ± changes in hematocrit, overt blood in endotracheal tube, underlying collagen vascular disease

Management and Treatment

- Given the subclinical nature of VILI and its close association with other lung pathologies, prevention is the best, and perhaps the only, treatment for VILI/VALI.
- Monitor lung mechanics to keep driving pressure <15 cm H_2O and plateau pressure <30 cm H_2O. The overarching objective of lung-protective ventilation strategies is to reduce the strain and stress caused by mechanical ventilation on the lungs, thereby minimizing VILI.
- All bedside decisions regarding ventilator management should respect the potential development of VILI in any patient.
- Monitor total driving pressure when patients transition to assisted or spontaneous ventilation. This can be obtained in two ways. (A) by performing an end-inspiratory pause to allow time for the inspiratory muscles to relax and obtain stable plateau pressures. Driving pressure is computed as the plateau pressure minus positive end-expiratory pressure (PEEP). (B) By performing an end-expiratory pause to estimate inspiratory pressure (occlusion pressure, Pocc). With this method, driving pressure is then estimated as 0.75 × Pocc + pressure support.
- PEEP: choose PEEP to improve hypoxemia while reducing lung collapse and consequently improving respiratory system compliance and lung strain. However, the value of more aggressive delivery of PEEP and recruitment maneuvers and the optimal strategies to recruit lung remain undefined.
- Decisions to prevent VILI mirror treatment goals in ARDS; prevention of VILI is generally achieved through the following treatment philosophies:
  - Protect the ventilated "baby" lung: VILI is a heterogeneous disease likely reflecting the fact that only a small portion of the lung participates in gas exchange.
    - Reduce cyclic atelectasis (opening and closing of lungs) by utilizing low tidal volume strategies (6 mL/kg of ideal body weight) and applying PEEP to maintain mean airway pressures below 30 cm H_2O.
  - Accept elevated arterial CO_2 values ("permissive hypercapnia") when not contraindicated (eg, in intracranial hypertension) as a trade-off for minimization of lung strain over normalization of gas analysis.
  - Several lines of evidence support the benefit of conservative versus liberal fluid administration in the management of ARDS ("A dry lung is a happy lung").

Outcomes

ARDS mortality remains elevated despite progress in medical care, reaching >40% death rates in patients who are more severely hypoxemic. However, outcomes vary greatly depending on coexisting conditions and the underlying pathophysiology responsible for mechanical ventilation.

SUGGESTED READINGS

Amato MB, Meade MO, Slutsky AS, et al. Driving pressure and survival in the acute respiratory distress syndrome. *N Engl J Med*. 2015;372(8):747-755.

Costa ELV, Alcala GC, Tucci MR, et al. Impact of extended lung protection during mechanical ventilation on lung recovery in patients with COVID-19 ARDS: a phase II randomized controlled trial. *Ann Intensive Care*. 2024;14(1):85.

Dianti J, Matelski J, Tisminetzky M, et al. Comparing the effects of tidal volume, driving pressure, and mechanical power on mortality in trials of lung-protective mechanical ventilation. *Respir Care*. 2021;66(2): 221-227.

Dreyfuss D, Sumon G. Ventilator-induced lung injury. *Am J Respir Crit Care Med*. 1998;157:294.

Gajic O, Dara SI, Mendez JL, et al. Ventilator-associated lung injury in patients without acute lung injury at the onset of mechanical ventilation. *Crit Care Med*. 2004;32(9):1817.

Gattinoni L, Pesenti A. The concept of "baby lung." *Intensive Care Med*. 2005;31:776.

Gattinoni L, Protti A, Caironi P, et al. Ventilator-induced lung injury: the anatomical and physiological framework. *Crit Care Med*. 2010; 38(10):S539.

National Heart, Lung, and Blood Institute Acute Respiratory Distress Syndrome (ARDS) Clinical Trials Network, Wheeler AP, Bernard GR, et al. Pulmonary-artery versus central venous catheter to guide treatment of acute lung injury. *N Engl J Med*. 2006;354:2213.

3.5

Pulmonary Embolic Disorders

Tiffany Gardner and Alison S. Witkin

Definition, Epidemiology, and Presentation

Definition

- Pulmonary embolism (PE) reflects the blockage of one of the pulmonary arteries caused by material having traveled through the bloodstream.
- Often caused by a deep venous thrombosis (DVT) of the lower extremities or pelvic vasculature that breaks off and travels (embolizes) to the lungs. Can also be caused by fat, air, or amniotic fluid

Predisposing Conditions

- Pregnancy, obesity, smoking, advanced age
- Immobility, particularly acute (eg, recent long travel)
- Cancer, heart failure, previous DVT or PE
- Kidney problems, nephritic syndrome
- Hormone replacement therapy, erythropoietin, tamoxifen
- Surgery, particularly involving hip, pelvis, or knee
- Fractures of long bones
- Inherited thrombophilia, polycythemia vera, antiphospholipid antibodies

Key Elements of History

- Shortness of breath
- Sharp chest pain, particularly with deep breath (pleuritic)
- Anxiety, cough, hemoptysis

Physical Examination Findings

- Vital signs: tachypnea, tachycardia, fevers
- Auscultation: crackles, prominent S2
- Peripheral edema

Diagnosis

Risk Assessment Prior to Dedicated Testing

- Wells proposed criteria for creating a score that would predict whether a PE was likely or not (Table 3.5.1).
- There are multiple other criteria that have been studied, including the PERC rule, Geneva Scoring System, Modified Geneva Scoring System, and YEARS algorithm (Table 3.5.1).
- These scoring criteria are primarily used to determine patients who are at a high enough risk of PE to obtain additional testing to confirm or rule out the diagnosis.

TABLE 3.5.1 Modified Wells Criteria

Criteria	Points
Clinical symptoms of DVT	3
No other diagnosis MORE likely	3
HR >100	1.5
Multiple days of immobilization or surgery in the past 4 wk	1.5
Previous DVT/PE	1.5
Hemoptysis	1
Malignancy	1

DVT, deep vein thrombosis; HR, heart rate; PE, pulmonary embolism.
PE Unlikely < or = to 4 points
PE likely > 4 points

Laboratory Findings

- Normal D-dimer can be used to exclude a PE in low probability cases but is often positive, limiting its utility. There is increasing evidence that D-dimer should be adjusted for age and that it may be appropriate to use an age-adjusted D-dimer.
- Troponins can be elevated and are associated with poor prognosis, but are not useful in excluding the diagnosis.
- Hypercapnia (due to increased dead space) and hypoxemia may be present but have limited negative predictive value.

Electrocardiographic Findings

- Electrocardiographic (ECG) findings suggestive of right ventricular (RV) strain (for acute PE) and right ventricular hypertrophy (RVH) (for chronic PE) should arouse suspicion but are often not present and are not specific.
  - Classic S1Q3T3 (large S in lead I, large Q and flipped T in lead III)
  - New right bundle branch block (RBBB) (often incomplete)
  - New ST-segment and T-wave abnormalities (particularly in inferior leads)
  - Late R/S transition

Chest X-ray Findings

- Common findings include cardiomegaly, pleural effusions, and atelectasis.
- No finding is sensitive or specific for PE.

Echocardiographic and Ultrasonographic Findings

- Transthoracic echocardiogram
  - Echocardiographic evidence of RV dysfunction can be suggestive of a PE but is not sensitive and not specific.
  - Findings of RV dysfunction include elevated RV systolic pressure, RV dilation, tricuspid regurgitation, and RV dysfunction.
  - In the presence of RV dysfunction, sparing of the apex of the RV is 94% specific for PE (McConnell sign) but can be seen in other forms of acute RV dysfunction (eg, in acute hypoxemic respiratory failure from acute respiratory distress syndrome [ARDS]).

- Lower extremity, upper extremity venous ultrasound
    - High suspicion of PE combined with finding DVT is diagnostic.
    - A negative DVT study does not exclude PE.

Pulmonary Artery Computed Tomographic Angiogram

- PIOPED II study found a sensitivity of 83% and specificity of 96% in a population in which reference studies and computed tomography (CT) scans were both performed.
- When risk stratified by Wells criteria, negative predictive value (NPV) at a low pretest probability was 96% and positive predictive value (PPV) at high pretest probability was 96%.

Ventilation-Perfusion Scan

- Difficulty with interpretation, especially when the patient has coexisting lung disease
- PIOPED I study showed the utility of ventilation-perfusion ($\dot{V}/\dot{Q}$) scan for the diagnosis of PE.
- Particularly useful with clear chest x-ray (CXR) and contraindication to obtaining a computed tomographic angiography (CTA)
- A completely normal $\dot{V}/\dot{Q}$ scan rules out PE.
- Very low probability and high probability $\dot{V}/\dot{Q}$ scans are useful if they are concordant with the clinical picture, for example, when the $\dot{V}/\dot{Q}$ shows a high probability of PE with a clinical picture that suggests a high probability of PE. Otherwise, further testing is needed.
- Low and intermediate probability readings do not rule in or rule out PE.
- $\dot{V}/\dot{Q}$ scans can often detect chronic clots that are no longer creating an obstructive lumen. Also, they are useful in diagnosing chronic thromboembolic disease.

Pulmonary Angiography

- Gold standard involves injection of dye by right heart catheterization.
- Requires invasive, right heart catheterization and its associated risks

Diagnostic Algorithm Based on the PIOPED II Study

- Low clinical suspicion: obtain D-dimer. If negative, PE is unlikely. If positive, perform CTA.
- Intermediate clinical suspicion: obtain D-dimer and DVT ultrasound. If D-dimer is positive, then CTA.
- High clinical suspicion: obtain CTA.

Management and Treatment

Initial Stabilization

- Aimed at preventing cardiovascular collapse
- Patients decompensate because of RV failure.
- Limited data on the optimal method of resuscitation
- Treat as standard therapy for acute RV failure (see Section 2.10: Pulmonary Hypertension).
- This includes ensuring adequate oxygenation, optimization of fluid status, and usage of inotropes.

Risk Stratification

- Approach to therapy in PE is guided by risk classification. Risk stratification comprises two components:
    - Hemodynamic instability or new hypotension
    - Right heart strain
        - With stable hemodynamics, right heart strain is the next best accepted prognostic indicator for poor outcome.
        - On echocardiogram, often a composite criterion of RV dysfunction (eg, hypokinesis) and RV dilation, especially when compared to the left ventricular (LV) in end-diastole
        - On CTA, RV dilation: measured by the ratio of RV to LV in end-diastole
        - Elevations in B-type natriuretic peptide (BNP), NT-proBNP, and troponin are all associated with death or hemodynamic decompensation, although the PPV of these is low.
- Risk classification
    - High risk: patients with shock and hemodynamic instability due to PE
    - High-intermediate risk: hemodynamically stable patients with RV strain by both imaging AND biomarkers
    - Low-intermediate risk: hemodynamically stable patients with RV strain by imaging OR biomarkers
    - Low risk: hemodynamically stable without RV strain and lack of other risk factors for progression or bad outcome

Anticoagulation

- Mainstay of therapy
- Immediate anticoagulation is recommended. This should not be delayed for diagnostic verification in cases of high suspicion, where there are no contraindications to anticoagulation.
- Given difficulties in achieving therapeutic levels, unfractionated heparin should only be used if there is a contraindication to another agent, such as low-molecular-weight heparin (LMWH) or a direct oral anticoagulant (DOAC). DOACs are often avoided in critically ill patients due to their long half-life.
- Even cases with low-to-moderate suspicion can be considered for empiric anticoagulation when there is a delay in definitive diagnosis.
- Contraindications to anticoagulation
    - Ongoing or recent major bleeding that cannot be easily treated
    - Any intracranial bleeding in the past 5 days
    - Severe thrombocytopenia
    - *Duration of therapy:* at least 3 months of anticoagulation is recommended for patients with a transient major provoking factor. Extended or indefinite therapy is often advised for unprovoked or persistent risk factors, especially if bleeding risk is low.

Thrombolysis

- While there are no large, randomized studies, systemic thrombolysis is considered first line for patients with shock and without contraindication.
- Criteria for thrombolysis

- Most sources consider hemodynamic instability as a criterion for considering thrombolysis.
- Other factors to consider include RV dysfunction, impending RV dysfunction, hypoxemia, and large clot burden.
- Assess the risks and benefits on a case-by-case basis.

- Contraindications for thrombolysis
  - *Absolute:* brain pathology suspicious for arteriovenous malformation (AVM), aneurysms, neoplasms, history of hemorrhagic stroke, recent head/spine surgery, recent stroke, uncontrolled hypertension with systolic blood pressure (SBP) >200 mm Hg, active internal bleeding, and bleeding diathesis
  - *Relative:* previous and remote history of the abovementioned events, pregnancy, age, recent trauma, recent surgery, and recent bleeding

Catheter-Based Interventions

- Catheter-directed thrombolysis
  - Minimally invasive procedure in which a thrombolytic drug is administered directly into the pulmonary arteries at the site of the thrombus via a catheter.
  - Ultrasound-enhanced catheters may disrupt fibrin-fibrin cross-links, increasing local delivery of drug.
- Catheter-based embolectomy:
  - percutaneous, minimally invasive procedure that mechanically removes thrombus from the pulmonary arteries using specialized catheters, without the use of systemic or local thrombolytic agents

Surgical Embolectomy

- In the acute setting, a pulmonary thromboembolectomy can restore hemodynamics.
- Indication: severe hemodynamic compromise, with an expected high mortality, and conservative measures are expected to fail or have failed.
- In chronic thromboembolic disease, pulmonary thromboendarterectomies (PTEs) are associated with significant reversal of hemodynamic compromise and functional improvement when performed in experienced centers.

Inferior Vena Cava (Greenfield) Filter Placement

- Can be placed in the inferior vena cava (IVC), superior vena cava (SVC), or large veins to prevent large clots from traveling to the right heart and the lung
- Indications
  - Prevention of PE in those who cannot be adequately anticoagulated
  - Presence of large DVTs or in patients with a low cardiopulmonary reserve with high potential for a fatal outcome if clot travels despite anticoagulation (more controversial indication)
- Contraindications:
  - Bacteremia
  - Thrombus that would prevent filter placement
  - Severe coagulopathy
- Efficacy
  - Rate of PE after placement of an IVC filter as low as 1.7%
  - Should be removed when no longer needed to reduce the risk of filter thrombus and DVT

Follow-Up

- Follow-up visit within 3 months of the acute PE event to assess for recurrent symptoms, anticoagulation adherence, and bleeding risk and to reevaluate the need for continued therapy. Consider referral to a PE clinic or specialist if available.

Outcomes

- High-risk PE (>50% occlusion) has a mortality as high as 70% within the first hour.
- ICOPER registry from 52 centers and seven countries suggests 17.4% 90-day mortality among all patients with PEs.

Resolution and Recurrence Risk

- Chronic thromboembolic pulmonary hypertension (CTEPH) complicates up to 3.8% of PE events.
- Pulmonary hypertension often results from a chronic clot burden. If persisting and progressive, may need pulmonary endarterectomy (see Section 2.10: Pulmonary Hypertension).
- Recurrence is an issue when the underlying cause of the initial clot is not resolved.
- In one study, there was a 3% recurrence in 3 months.
- The following factors increase the risk of recurrence: immobilization, hospitalization, increased age, chronic obstructive pulmonary disease (COPD), and malignancies.

SUGGESTED READINGS

Gibson NS, Sohne M, Kruip MJ, et al. Further validation and simplification of the Wells clinical decision rule in pulmonary embolism. Thromb Haemost. 2008;99(1):229-234. doi:10.1160/TH07-05-0321

Giri J, Sista AK, Weinberg I, et al. Interventional therapies for acute pulmonary embolism: current status and principles for the development of novel evidence: a scientific statement from the American Heart Association. *Circulation*. 2019;140(20):e774-e801.

Kahn SR, de Wit K. Pulmonary embolism. *N Engl J Med*. 2022;387(1):45-57.

Klok FA, Ageno W, Ay C, et al. Optimal follow-up after acute pulmonary embolism: a position paper of the European Society of Cardiology Working Group on pulmonary circulation and right ventricular function, in collaboration with the European Society of Cardiology Working Group on atherosclerosis and vascular biology. *Eur Heart J*. 2022;43(3):183-189.

Ortel TL, Neumann I, Ageno W, et al. American Society of Hematology 2020 guidelines for management of venous thromboembolism: treatment of deep vein thrombosis and pulmonary embolism. *Blood Adv*. 2020;4(19):4693-4738.

Stevens SM, Woller SC, Kreuziger LB, et al. Antithrombotic therapy for VTE disease: second update of the CHEST guideline and expert panel report. *Chest*. 2021;160(6):e545-e608.

van der Hulle T, Cheung WY, Kooij S, et al. Simplified diagnostic management of suspected pulmonary embolism (the YEARS study): a prospective, multicentre, cohort study [published correction appears in *Lancet*. 2017;390(10091):230]. *Lancet*. 2017;390(10091):289-297.

3.6

Severe and Life-Threatening Asthma Exacerbation

Eduardo M. H. Padrao and Benjamin D. Medoff

Evaluating the Severity of an Asthma Exacerbation

- A severe asthma exacerbation is a clinical diagnosis based on signs and symptoms, although many patients (up to 50%) may not manifest any of the following abnormalities:
  - Tachycardia >120 bpm
  - Tachypnea >30 ipm
  - Use of accessory muscles
  - Orthopnea
  - Pulsus paradoxus (may be absent in very severe disease as they develop respiratory muscle fatigue)
  - Inability to talk in full sentences without taking breaths
  - Diaphoresis
  - Tripod position
  - Spo_2 <90% on room air
  - Peak expiratory flow <50% (although recommended by most societies, the use of peak flow in severe cases can be inaccurate and delay treatment—it should be used as an adjunct data point)
- The evaluation should also include asking about risk factors for fatal asthma, such as:
  - Previous history of intubation due to asthma exacerbation
  - Hospitalization or visit to the emergency department (ED) in the past year for an asthma exacerbation
  - Severe exacerbation in patients using oral steroids
  - Poor adherence to inhaled corticosteroids
  - Utilization of >1 canister of albuterol per month
  - History of psychiatric comorbidities or psychosocial problems
  - History of severe food allergy

Initial Management for Severe or Life-threatening Asthma

- Inhaled beta-2 agonists
  - Nebulization of albuterol 2.5 mg every 20 minutes for 3 doses
  - If no improvement, can switch to *continuous albuterol nebulization* (10-15 mg over 1 hour)
  - Be aware that beta-2 agonists can cause worsening of oxygenation initially due to dilation of the pulmonary vasculature, reducing ventilation-perfusion matching. Other side effects include tachycardia, arrhythmias, tremors, anxiety, insomnia, paradoxical bronchospasm (4% of population—hypersensitivity to components), hypokalemia, and lactic acidosis.
- Inhaled muscarinic antagonists
  - Nebulization of *ipratropium* 0.5 mg in addition to albuterol
  - Evidence: ipratropium was shown in trials to improve FEV_1 and decrease hospitalization. The use in critically ill patients admitted to the intensive care unit (ICU) is recommended but extrapolated from these trials.
  - Side effects include dry mouth and dry secretions, paradoxical bronchospasm, dizziness, and blurry vision.
- Systemic glucocorticoids
  - Oral therapy if patients can take oral, or intravenous (IV) for those who are not able to take oral or at high risk for intubation
  - Usual dose *40 to 60 mg of prednisone or equivalent*. However, based on expert opinion, severe cases may require higher doses (commonly 80-125 mg of IV methylprednisolone every 6-8 hours based on clinical judgment). No role for inhaled glucocorticoids in patients with severe asthma exacerbation.
  - Side effects include hyperglycemia, hypertension, anxiety, agitation, and insomnia.
- Magnesium sulfate
  - IV *magnesium sulfate* 2 g over 20 minutes
  - Evidence: can improve FEV_1 and may be beneficial in severe patients, decreasing hospitalization. The use in critically ill patients admitted to the ICU is extrapolated.
  - Use with caution in patients with acute or chronic kidney injury and neuromuscular disease; side effects include bradycardia, flushing, and hypotension.

Patients That Do Not Respond to Initial Management

- Parenteral beta-2 agonists
  - Intramuscular *epinephrine* 0.3 to 0.5 mg (can be repeated every 5 minutes up to 3 doses) if asthma exacerbation concomitant with anaphylaxis, or 0.3 mg if life-threatening asthma (can be repeated every 20 minutes up to 3 doses)
  - Alternative: terbutaline subcutaneous 0.25 mg (can be repeated every 20 minutes up to 3 doses)
  - IV epinephrine 1 to 15 mg/min. Caution in patients with coronary artery disease.
  - Evidence is controversial, but most recent meta-analysis did not show benefit for the addition of IV or intramuscular beta-2 agonists to inhaled therapy in severe asthma, with a risk of increasing cardiovascular events.
- Helium-oxygen ("HeliOx")
  - Oxygen 20% to 30% and helium 70% to 80%. Works by reducing the density of inhaled gas, reducing the Reynolds number, and *restoring laminar flow* in the airways (vs turbulent flow). Functionally, this reduces resistance to airflow.
  - Most effective for patients with large or upper airway obstruction, such as inducible laryngeal obstruction. No randomized trials, based on anecdotal case reports and small studies.
- IV leukotriene receptor antagonists (LTRAs)
  - IV LTRAs have been studied in randomized clinical trials for acute asthma exacerbation. The evidence suggests that leukotriene antagonists do improve FEV_1.
  - Most guidelines do not recommend the routine use of IV LTRA. However, this can be considered in life-threatening asthma exacerbations.
  - Patients with nonsteroidal antiinflammatory drugs (NSAIDs) or aspirin-exacerbated respiratory disease may benefit from IV LTRA.
- Noninvasive Ventilation (NIV)
  - Trial of 1 to 2 hours, but should not delay intubation

- Evidence extrapolated from patients with chronic obstructive pulmonary disease (COPD) and small asthma trials showing benefit in improvement in gas exchange and obstruction
- Initial setup: Fio_2 titration for Spo_2 goal of 88% to 92% (except for pregnant women, for which the goal is >94%), titration of inspiratory positive airway pressure (IPAP) to a peak inspiratory pressure <20 cm H_2O, titration of expiratory positive airway pressure (EPAP) to avoid ineffective triggering

Intubation

The Decision to Intubate

- There are no studies or consensus on when to intubate patients with severe asthma. Patients with significant respiratory distress, impending extreme fatigue, altered mental status, lack of airway protection, and/or hemodynamic instability should be intubated.
- The decision to intubate should weigh the risks and benefits of the impending respiratory failure, the complications of mechanical ventilation, and a prolonged ICU stay.
- Arterial blood gas analysis can be used to aid with the decision but should not be used as the only determining factor. A normal but rising $Paco_2$ may be a sign of impending respiratory arrest.

Intubation Procedure

- Patients with severe asthma should be considered to have a physiologically difficult airway.
- Patients should be intubated with *rapid sequence intubation (RSI)* with a *large lumen endotracheal tube* by an *experienced operator*.
- Preoxygenation should maintain Spo_2 at least ≥94% to maximize apnea tolerance. This can be performed with spontaneous breathing with a bag valve mask, high-flow nasal cannula, or NIV.
- Premedication: albuterol if not used prior. Lidocaine can be used to suppress bronchospasm during laryngoscopy but is not recommended if the patient has already received beta-2 agonists.
- Ketamine and propofol are first-line agents for induction due to bronchodilatory effects. Ketamine can lead to increased oral secretions, and propofol can also be used but can cause peri-intubation hypotension.
- Patients with asthma are at risk for postintubation hypotension, acidosis, and barotrauma. Prolonged apnea time during intubation can lead to cardiac arrest or shock. Patients may require deep sedation and a period of paralysis after intubation.
- If there is immediate improvement in the patient's respiratory failure and normal lung mechanics (low airway resistance) after intubation, upper airway obstruction (such as vocal cord dysfunction) should be suspected as an alternative diagnosis.

Mechanical Ventilation

Mechanical Ventilation Goals

- Oxygenation: Sao_2 88% to 92% is appropriate other than in pregnancy, where the goal is >94%.
- Ventilation: pH >7.20 is typically targeted, though there are numerous cases of patients tolerating very low pH during mechanical ventilation for prolonged periods.
- Avoidance of dynamic hyperinflation: limiting minute ventilation and increasing inspiratory flow to improve expiration time are recommended. Ideally, one should target an auto-positive end-expiratory pressure (PEEP) <5 cm H_2O and plateau pressure <30 cm H_2O.
- Frequent reevaluations: patients with asthma have dynamic obstruction of the airways, and their physiology may change quickly.

Ventilator Settings and Monitoring

- Mode
  - Pressure-controlled modes are preferred, as they limit inspiratory pressure and hyperinflation, especially in patients with dynamic changes in airway resistance. However, it is often difficult to maintain adequate minute ventilation due to high airway resistance.
  - Volume-controlled ventilation will more reliably provide an appropriate tidal volume at the cost of an increased risk of high pressures and hyperinflation. Volume-controlled ventilation also provides fixed tidal volumes, which can allow appropriate delivery of inhaled therapy to the airways.
- Tidal volume
  - 6 to 10 mL/kg of ideal body weight is usually recommended. A more conservative approach should be used (4-8 mL/kg) if there is suspicion of concomitant acute respiratory distress syndrome (ARDS).
- Respiratory rate
  - Low respiratory rate between 10 and 12 breaths/min
- Fio_2
  - Titrated to achieve Spo_2 (88%-92%). Severe hypoxemia should prompt consideration of an alternative or superimposed etiology.
- Inspiratory flow and inspiratory time
  - High inspiratory flows (60-80 L/min) allow longer expiratory time. If the inspiratory time can be set, an appropriate initial time ranges between 0.8 and 1.2 seconds (*I:E* ratio ranging from 1:3 to 1:5).
  - High inspiratory flow against high airway resistance will result in high peak inspiratory pressures. Ventilator cutoff values may need to be set high (>50 cmH_2O).
- PEEP
  - The effects of PEEP in asthmatics may be variable and, in most patients, may drive hyperinflation by decreasing the expiratory driving pressure and increasing the time of expiration. There is often no expiratory dynamic airway closure in asthma.
  - Auto-PEEP and plateau pressures should be surveilled for with expiratory and inspiratory pauses, respectively.
  - Start with a PEEP of 0 and then carefully titrate the PEEP higher while monitoring plateau pressure and auto-PEEP. Choose a PEEP that limits auto-PEEP to <5 cm H_2O and plateau pressure <30 cm H_2O. Nonobese patients with no dynamic hyperinflation should have a PEEP of ~5 cm H_2O.
- Trigger:
  - Flow trigger may avoid ineffective triggering due to auto-PEEP when allowing spontaneous respiration. The flow sensitivity can be set at −2 L/min.

Complications of Mechanical Ventilation

- Patients with life-threatening asthma may develop complications from mechanical ventilation that should be

monitored. They are usually adverse effects from dynamic hyperinflation and/or respiratory acidosis.
    - Barotrauma
    - May lead to pneumothorax, subcutaneous emphysema, and/or pneumomediastinum. In most cases of pneumothorax, patients will require chest tube placement.
- Hemodynamic instability
  - Hemodynamic instability in the setting of increasing thoracic pressure (due to the hemodynamic effects of dynamic hyperinflation or pneumothorax). Ventilator should be adjusted with an increase in expiratory time.
  - Hemodynamic instability can happen in the setting of severe acidosis.
- Ineffective efforts
  - Hyperinflation can cause ineffective triggering when spontaneously breathing. More common in patients with COPD and asthma overlap. This is not an issue during controlled mechanical ventilation.
  - Switching trigger mode to flow and improving dynamic hyperinflation

Asthma Therapy While Mechanically Ventilated

- Continuation of inhaled beta-2 agonists, antimuscarinic, parenteral glucocorticoids
- Magnesium sulfate, parenteral beta-2 agonists, and HeliOx can be continued on a case-by-case basis. The use of parenteral beta-2 agonists may be required, especially in patients in whom low tidal volumes are needed to limit hyperinflation, thus limiting aerosol delivery to the airways. Note that many modern ventilators are not able to utilize HeliOx.

Sedation and Paralysis

- Propofol and/or ketamine as first-line sedative agents
- A paralytic agent can be considered in patients who are dyssynchronous with the ventilator.
- Due to the high risk of neuromuscular weakness, prolonged courses of paralytics should be avoided, ideally no >24 to 48 hours. An as-needed bolus strategy can be used.

Volatile Anesthetics

- Inhaled anesthetics such as halothane, isoflurane, and sevoflurane have bronchodilatory effects.
- Use requires the availability of an anesthesiologist, operating room–style ventilator.
- Risks include hypotension, myocardial depression, arrhythmias, and the risk of secondhand inhalation by ICU staff not accustomed to volatile anesthetics

Extracorporeal Membrane Oxygenation and Extracorporeal CO_2 Removal

- There are no randomized trials of extracorporeal membrane oxygenation (ECMO) on patients with life-threatening asthma.
- By reducing hypercapnia and improving pH, ECMO can allow ventilation with a lower minute ventilation, reducing the risk of dynamic hyperinflation and barotrauma. Survival rates of patients with severe asthma requiring ECMO range from 85% to 95%.
- Extracorporeal CO_2 removal (ECO_2R) cannulation is simpler than ECMO and requires significantly lower blood flow rates.
- Can help clear carbon dioxide while allowing ventilation strategy to avoid dynamic hyperinflation
- No studies on patients with life-threatening asthma

SUGGESTED READINGS

Baggott C, Hardy JK, Sparks J, et al. Epinephrine (adrenaline) compared to selective beta-2-agonist in adults or children with acute asthma: a systematic review and meta-analysis. *Thorax*. 2022;77(6):563-572.

Darioli R, Perret C. Mechanical controlled hypoventilation in status asthmaticus. *Am Rev Respir Dis*. 1984;129(3):385-387.

Davis DP, Hwang JQ, Dunford JV. Rate of decline in oxygen saturation at various pulse oximetry values with prehospital rapid sequence intubation. *Prehosp Emerg Care*. 2008;12(1):46-51.

Garner O, Ramey JS, Hanania NA. Management of life-threatening asthma: severe asthma series. *Chest*. 2022;162(4):747-756.

Goodacre S, Cohen J, Bradburn M, et al. The 3Mg trial: a randomised controlled trial of intravenous or nebulised magnesium sulphate versus placebo in adults with acute severe asthma. *Health Technol Assess*. 2014;18(22):1-168.

Homer-Bouthiette C, Shen BH, Dobie AC, et al. Practice patterns for acute asthma exacerbation in adult patients admitted to US intensive care units. *Ann Am Thorac Soc*. 2024;21(10):1441-1448.

Idris AH, McDermott MF, Raucci JC, Morrabel A, McGorray S, Hendeles L. Emergency department treatment of severe asthma. Metered-dose inhaler plus holding chamber is equivalent in effectiveness to nebulizer. *Chest*. 1993;103(3):665-672.

Kew KM, Kirtchuk L, Michell CI. Intravenous magnesium sulfate for treating adults with acute asthma in the emergency department. *Cochrane Database Syst Rev*. 2014;2014(5):CD010909.

Leatherman JW, McArthur C, Shapiro RS. Effect of prolongation of expiratory time on dynamic hyperinflation in mechanically ventilated patients with severe asthma. *Crit Care Med*. 2004;32(7):1542-1545.

Leatherman JW, Ravenscraft SA. Low measured auto-positive end-expiratory pressure during mechanical ventilation of patients with severe asthma: hidden auto-positive end-expiratory pressure. *Crit Care Med*. 1996;24(3):541-546.

Lozano-Espinosa M, Antolín-Amérigo D, Riera J, Gordo Vidal F, Quirce S, Álvarez Rodríguez J. Extracorporeal membrane oxygenation (ECMO) and beyond in near fatal asthma: a comprehensive review. *Respir Med*. 2023;215:107246.

Lugogo NL, MacIntyre NR. Life-threatening asthma: pathophysiology and management. *Respir Care*. 2008;53(6):726-739.

Medoff BD. Invasive and noninvasive ventilation in patients with asthma. *Respir Care*. 2008;53(6):740-750.

Normansell R, Kew KM, Mansour G. Different oral corticosteroid regimens for acute asthma. *Cochrane Database Syst Rev*. 2016;2016(5):CD011801.

Ranieri VM, Grasso S, Fiore T, Giuliani R. Auto-positive end-expiratory pressure and dynamic hyperinflation. *Clin Chest Med*. 1996;17(3):379-394.

Rodrigo GJ, Rodrigo C. First-line therapy for adult patients with acute asthma receiving a multiple-dose protocol of ipratropium bromide plus albuterol in the emergency department. *Am J Respir Crit Care Med*. 2000;161(6):1862-1868.

Tuxen DV, Williams TJ, Scheinkestel CD, Czarny D, Bowes G. Use of a measurement of pulmonary hyperinflation to control the level of mechanical ventilation in patients with acute severe asthma. *Am Rev Respir Dis*. 1992;146(5 pt 1):1136-1142.

Venkatesan P. 2023 GINA report for asthma. *Lancet Respir Med*. 2023;11(7):589.

3.7

Chronic Obstructive Pulmonary Disease

Katharine Black

Definition

- Chronic obstructive pulmonary disease (COPD) is characterized by:
  - *Epidemiology:* nearly all patients have a history of cigarette smoking; less commonly other inhaled environmental exposures; rarely genetic.
  - *Clinical presentation:*
    - Chronic cough, dyspnea (usually worse with exertion), and sputum production
    - Severity of dyspnea and frequency of exacerbations categorize patients.
    - Periodic exacerbations with increased dyspnea and increased production of more purulent sputum
  - *Physical examination:* rhonchi, wheezing, decreased intensity of breath sounds, and prolonged expiration; stigmata of hyperinflation (barrel chest) or of chronically elevated work of breathing (cachexia) may be present.
  - Pulmonary function testing: airflow limitation, not fully reversible, usually progressive

Common Causes to Remember

- Smoking is the most important contributor to COPD in the United States and Europe.
  - Tobacco smoking history is associated with 70% of all patients with COPD, though only about half of heavy smokers develop COPD.
- Other causes include hereditary deficiency of alpha-1 anti-trypsin (A1AT) and other genetic factors, premature birth or other abnormal lung development, airway infections, exposures to biomass, or household pollution and allergy.

Epidemiology

- It is estimated that 10 million Americans have been diagnosed with COPD, but up to 24 million have airflow limitation.
- An equal number is believed to be affected but undiagnosed. Global prevalence estimated at about 10%; estimated 3.5 million annual deaths. When combined, COPD is the fourth leading cause of death in the United States, with over 190,000 annual deaths.

Key Pathophysiology

- Patients with COPD can have features of emphysema (a pathologic diagnosis), chronic bronchitis (a clinical diagnosis), or both.
  - Emphysema is abnormal permanent enlargement of air spaces distal to the terminal bronchioles, with destruction of their walls and without obvious fibrosis.
    - Defined by radiology or pathology
  - Chronic bronchitis is excessive inflammation and secretion of bronchial mucus.
    - Defined clinically: daily productive cough for ≥3 months in at least 2 consecutive years
- About 30% of patients with COPD and about 25% of patients with asthma are thought to meet criteria for Asthma-COPD Overlap.

Clinical Presentation

- Emphysema-predominant patients often present with dyspnea as their primary complaint.
- Symptoms worsen with exertion and may be out of proportion to changes in oxygen. Bronchitis-predominant patients may present primarily with chronic productive cough.
- Uncomfortable, with accessory muscle use, may have audible wheezing.
- Blood gas can be normal or shows reduced Pao_2 and elevated $Paco_2$.
- Chemistries may show elevated bicarbonate as compensation for chronic CO_2 retention.
  - *Chest radiograph:* hyperinflation with flattened diaphragms, or bronchial wall thickening, increased interstitial markings especially at the bases
  - *Computed tomography (CT) scan findings:*
    - Upper lobe–predominant loss of alveolar septation in smoking-related emphysema
    - Panlobular in A1AT-related emphysema
    - Bronchitis may manifest as thickened bronchial walls, visible luminal secretions.

Pulmonary Function Tests

FEV_1	FVC	FEV_1/FVC	TLC	FRC	RV	DLCO
↓	↓	↓	↑	↑	↑	Normal or ↓

DLCO, diffusion lung capacity for carbon monoxide; FEV_1, forced expiratory volume in 1 second; FRC, forced residual capacity; FVC, forced vital capacity; RV, residual volume; TLC: total lung capacity.

- Airway obstruction is defined by postbronchodilator FEV_1/FVC <0.7 (GOLD criteria).
- ATS/ERS definition: FEV_1/FVC less than lower limit of normal/5th percentile predicted
- Severity of airflow obstruction is based on percent of predicted FEV_1:

	Mild	Moderate	Severe	Very Severe
GOLD: % predicted FEV_1	≥80%	50%-80%	30%-59%	<30%
ATS/ERS: Z-score	−1.65 to −2.5	−2.51 to −4	<−4	

- Bronchodilator response
  - *GOLD criteria:* do not formally recommend
  - *ATS/ERS:* increase in FEV_1 or FVC of over >10% relative to *predicted* FEV_1 or FVC
  - *Prior definition:* increase in FEV_1 or FVC of over >200 mL AND ≥12%

Differential Diagnosis

- Bronchial asthma: characterized by reversible airway obstruction, often associated with allergies; patients may be asymptomatic between exacerbations.

- Bronchiectasis: usually associated with chronic purulent sputum, recurrent pneumonia, hemoptysis, and digital clubbing. Chest imaging shows airway dilation and distortion.
- Cystic fibrosis: typically in childhood and early adulthood; variants increasingly being identified in late adulthood
- Central airflow obstruction (eg, by tumor): should usually be seen on imaging and will have a distinct appearance on flow-volume loops
- Congestive heart failure: physical examination, radiology, and lab findings such as brain natriuretic peptide (BNP)/pro-BNP can distinguish. May overlap with COPD
- Interstitial lung disease: restrictive pattern on spirometry, distinct CT scan findings

Management and Treatment

Ambulatory Patients

- *Smoking cessation:* by far the most important intervention
- *Oxygen therapy*: the only drug approved to change the natural history of patients with COPD with resting hypoxemia (Pao_2<55 mm Hg or Sao_2 <89%)
- *Pulmonary rehabilitation:* including graded aerobic physical exercise and patient education
- *Inhaled bronchodilators:* do not change, improve, or halt the decline in lung function, but provide symptomatic improvement for patients
  - Inhaled medications
    - Long-acting muscarinic antagonists (LAMAs) are first-line therapy for mild stable COPD.
    - Long-acting beta-2 agonists (LABAs) (eg, formoterol and salmeterol)
    - Inhaled corticosteroids
    - Combination beta agonist, LAMAs, inhaled steroid ("triple therapy")
  - Chronic azithromycin may reduce the rate of exacerbations through an immunomodulatory effect.
  - If peripheral eosinophil (absolute eosinophil count ≥300/μL), evidence-based guidelines suggest dupilumab or mepolizumab for patients with COPD.
  - Short-acting bronchodilators can be added during exacerbations: initial therapy includes short-acting bronchodilators and anticholinergics.
- *Corticosteroids:* systemic glucocorticoids reduce the frequency of COPD exacerbations and improve self-reported functional status, but come with significant long-term toxicities. Steroids should be used in combination with inhaled bronchodilators and should not be considered a first-line treatment modality.
- Antibiotics are used to (1) treat acute exacerbation; (2) treat acute bronchitis; and (3) prevent acute exacerbation.

Hospitalized Patients

- *Bronchodilator therapy:* typically nebulized short-acting bronchodilator preparations
- *Systemic glucocorticoids:* 40 mg prednisone (or equivalent) × 5 days is guideline therapy. However, recent evidence suggests that the benefits of steroids in acute exacerbations of COPD may be limited to those with peripheral blood eosinophilia.
- *Antibiotics:* decrease mortality and treatment failure in patients hospitalized for COPD. Doxycycline and/or azithromycin are reasonable for patients without risk factors for *Pseudomonas*.
- *Supplemental oxygen:* to maintain Sao_2 between 88% and 92% or Pao_2 of ~60 mm Hg. Higher oxygen targets may be associated with exacerbated $\dot{V}/\dot{Q}$ mismatch.
- Noninvasive ventilation has been shown to reduce the need for invasive ventilation and concomitant comorbidities and to be superior to high-flow nasal cannula (HFNC) for acute exacerbations of COPD.
- *Mechanical ventilation*
  - Indications: intractable hypercarbia, respiratory acidosis, work of breathing
  - 1% to 2% of patients hospitalized for COPD will require invasive ventilation.
  - Ventilator settings should avoid hyperinflation/worsening air trapping while maintaining lung protection. Moderate hypercapnia can be permitted (pH 7.25-7.30), requiring attention to airway resistance and intrinsic positive end-expiratory pressure (PEEP). Ensure adequate expiratory time to prevent auto-PEEP.
  - Patients with risk factors for *Pseudomonas* should receive either Zosyn (piperacillin and tazobactam) or cefepime, with attention to local antibiogram and relevant patient history.

Surgery for Chronic Obstructive Pulmonary Disease

- *Lung transplantation:* remains the only cure for severe COPD but has significant morbidity and limited long-term survival. Ongoing tobacco use always precludes lung transplant evaluation. Medical comorbidities, extremes of body mass index (BMI) (<16 or >35), and lack of psychosocial support can also be prohibitive barriers.
- *Lung volume reduction surgery (LVRS):* is a bilateral resection of overinflated lung volume in select patients; attempts to relieve dyspnea and improve exercise tolerance in patients with advanced lung hyperinflation and diffuse emphysema
- Bronchoscopic lung volume reduction may be considered for symptomatic improvement in selected patients but has no demonstrated mortality benefit.
- *Bullectomy:* this is a more historical procedure that is losing popularity in the management of COPD. It was most commonly performed when a single bulla occupied 30% to 50% of the hemithorax.

Outcomes

- The most important predictor is the degree of pulmonary function at the time of initial diagnosis.
- The median survival of patients with FEV_1<1 L is about 4 years.
- Other prognostic factors include BMI, dyspnea, and exercise capacity.
- Biomarkers

SUGGESTED READINGS

Ferrera MC, Labaki WW, Han MK. Advances in chronic obstructive pulmonary disease. *Annu Rev Med*. 2021;72:119-134.

Mein SA, Ferrera MC. Management of asthma and COPD exacerbations in adults in the ICU. *CHEST Crit Care*. 2025;3(1):100107.

Ramakrishnan S, Jeffers H, Langford-Wiley B, et al. Blood eosinophil-guided oral prednisolone for COPD exacerbations in primary care in the UK (STARR2): a non-inferiority, multicentre, double-blind, placebo-controlled, randomised controlled trial. *Lancet Respir Med*. 2024;12(1):67-77.

3.8

Restrictive Lung Diseases

Angela Ma and Crystal M. North

Diagnosis of a restrictive ventilatory defect requires (a) forced expiratory volume in 1 second (FEV_1) to forced vital capacity (FVC) ratio greater than the lower limit of normal and (b) total lung capacity (TLC) lower than the lower limit of normal. Reduced residual volume (RV) with normal TLC or reduced diffusing capacity for carbon monoxide (DLCO) with normal spirometry/lung volumes can indicate early/subclinical interstitial lung disease (ILD).

FEV_1	FVC	FEV_1/FVC	TLC	FRC	RV	DLCO
↓	↓	Normal/↑	↓	↓	↓	↓

The severity of restriction is determined by TLC.

Normal	Mild	Moderate	Severe
≥80% predicted	60%-79% predicted	40%-59% predicted	<40% predicted

Although this chapter focuses on ILDs, it is important to recognize that restrictive ventilatory deficits can also be caused by nonpulmonary etiologies, which include:

- Pleural disease (eg, large pleural effusion, pleural scarring/plaque)
- Chest wall/bony deformity (eg, ankylosing spondylitis, scoliosis/kyphosis, large bony resections, pectus excavatum, morbid obesity)
- Neuromuscular weakness (eg, amyotrophic lateral sclerosis [ALS], myasthenia gravis, Guillain-Barré, critical illness myopathy, diaphragmatic weakness/paralysis, paraplegia/quadriplegia)

General Principles in Interstitial Lung Disease

ILDs represent a large and etiologically diverse group of pulmonary disorders that share some common clinical features. This section focuses on general principles, while the following sections detail specific presentations, radiographic patterns, and treatment within each subgroup. Unfortunately, when advanced ILD culminates in intensive care unit (ICU) admission for respiratory failure, there are only rarely effective targeted therapies to offer (exceptions are noted later), highlighting the importance of early recognition and management. A pulmonologist with expertise in ILD should be involved in the care of critically ill patients with significant fibrotic lung disease.

Classification by Etiology

- Idiopathic
- Exposure related
- Autoimmune
- Genetic/other

Diagnostic Approach

- Presentation
  - Often insidious and progressive dyspnea and/or dry cough
  - Physical examination: inspiratory crackles (*"Velcro-like" with alveolar involvement*), inspiratory "squeaks" (more common in airway-centered etiologies), digital clubbing, evidence of concomitant connective tissue disease (CTD), hypoxemia
  - Radiographic abnormalities often incidentally noted on imaging performed for other reasons
- Beyond history and physical examination, initial workup should include:
  - Laboratory evaluation of erythrocyte sedimentation rate/c-reactive protein (ESR/CRP), antinuclear antibody (ANA), antineutrophil cytoplasmic antibody (ANCA), Scl-70, rheumatoid factor/cyclic citrullinated peptide (RF/CCP), Ro/La, U1-RNP, hypersensitivity pneumonitis (HP) antibody panel, myositis autoantibody panel
  - Pulmonary function testing (PFT) (including spirometry, lung volumes, DLCO) if possible (critically ill patients typically cannot have PFTs performed)
  - "ILD protocol" HRCT (high-resolution computed tomography) of the chest, which includes inspiratory and expiratory phases to assess for mosaic attenuation and air trapping as well as prone imaging to assess for atelectasis. In critically ill patients, standard chest CT is typically adequate to establish a diagnosis of ILD.
  - Consideration of bronchoscopy ± bronchoalveolar lavage (BAL), most helpful in evaluating eosinophilic pneumonia, HP, sarcoidosis, and diffuse alveolar hemorrhage (DAH)
  - Consideration of echocardiogram and right heart catheterization in patients with DLCO reduced out of proportion to radiographic findings, or CT evidence of possible pulmonary hypertension (PH). Patients with ILD and confirmed PH may benefit from inhaled treprostinil (INCREASE, *NEJM* 2021).
- Lung biopsy should be considered when clinical presentation, imaging, and laboratory studies do not establish a specific diagnosis. Relative contraindications include significant PH or hypoxemia, and it is important to recognize that lung biopsy can trigger ILD exacerbations. Biopsy can be obtained via multiple approaches:
  - *Transbronchial biopsy* (TBBx) is the least invasive and most helpful in airway-centered disease (sarcoidosis, HP).
  - *Cryobiopsy* has generally increased yield in comparison to TBBx, with lower risk and reasonable diagnostic agreement with surgical lung biopsy.
  - *Surgical lung biopsy* is the most invasive and highest yield and may be preferred in more peripheral disease, but requires multidisciplinary input of radiology and thoracic surgery to determine optimal biopsy site(s) and risk/benefit ratio.

Specific Radiographic Patterns and Disease Associations

Specific chest CT abnormalities can point to various etiologies of ILD and are, therefore, important to distinguish in consultation with thoracic radiology.

- Usual interstitial pneumonia (UIP)
  - CT findings: subpleural reticulations, honeycombing, and traction bronchiectasis typically *in a basilar-predominant distribution*
  - Most frequently seen in idiopathic pulmonary fibrosis (IPF) but also associated with rheumatoid arthritis (RA)-ILD, systemic sclerosis (SSc)-ILD, fibrotic HP, sarcoidosis, and pneumoconiosis. The presence of a UIP pattern in non-IPF etiologies portends a worse prognosis.
- Nonspecific interstitial pneumonia (NSIP)
  - CT findings: ground-glass opacities (GGOs—hazy areas of increased attenuation with preservation of airway and vascular markings) + subpleural sparing
  - Can be seen in idiopathic NSIP, CTD-ILD, drug-induced ILD
- Mosaic attenuation
  - CT findings: "patchwork" appearance with regions of differing attenuation, which reflects gas-trapping and/or pulmonary vascular disease
  - Can be seen in HP, sarcoidosis
- Consolidation
  - CT findings: dense areas of increased attenuation characterized by loss of airway and vascular markings
  - Can be seen in organizing pneumonia (OP), idiopathic inflammatory myopathy (IIM)-associated ILD, acute interstitial pneumonia (AIP), in addition to more common ICU pulmonary disorders
- Septal thickening
  - CT findings: thickening of the walls (septa) between the pulmonary lobules
  - Can be seen in acute eosinophilic pneumonia (AEP), pulmonary alveolar proteinosis (PAP), DAH
- Nodules
  - CT findings: small, dense/solid-appearing opacities
  - Centrilobular distribution can be suggestive of smoking-related ILDs, HP, and AEP. Perilymphatic or peribronchovascular distribution can be suggestive of sarcoidosis.
- Cysts
  - CT findings: well-circumscribed pockets of air within the lung tissue, differentiated from emphysema by the presence of a thin (or thick) wall and lack of central vessel
  - Can be seen in lymphangioleiomyomatosis (LAM), Langerhans cell histiocytosis (LCH), lymphoid interstitial pneumonia (LIP)

Specific Interstitial Lung Diseases: Presentation, Workup, and Management

Idiopathic Interstitial Pneumonias

The idiopathic interstitial pneumonias (IIPs) constitute a heterogeneous group of primary pulmonary disorders *not known to be caused by some other systemic illness*. Importantly, and confusingly, the same radiographic and clinical findings can also represent secondary effects of a variety of diseases, emphasizing that IIPs represent diagnoses of exclusion following exoneration of other causes.

Nonspecific Interstitial Pneumonia

- Epidemiology/clinical presentation: *most common IIP*, male > female, typically older adults (>50), often smokers. Systemic symptoms are rare in IPF, so premature graying, cytopenias, and/or concomitant liver disease should raise suspicion for familial and/or telomeropathy-associated disease.
  - Patients with low telomere length (<10th percentile) may have worse outcomes (FVC decline, lung transplant, death) with immunosuppression (PANTHER-IPF cohort post-hoc analysis, *AJRCCM* 2018).
- Diagnostics: UIP pattern on chest CT
- Management/prognosis: antifibrotics (nintedanib and pirfenidone) can slow disease progression but are not effective acutely. Acute exacerbations (AEs) are managed with corticosteroids (limited data), supportive care, consideration of palliative care, and/or transplant consultation, as *AE-IPF portends very poor prognosis*.

Nonspecific Interstitial Pneumonia

- Epidemiology/clinical presentation: more commonly associated with CTD or systemic disease, can be idiopathic
- Diagnostics: NSIP pattern on chest CT
- Management/prognosis: *generally responsive to immunosuppression*. Initial therapy typically corticosteroids, with steroid-sparing agents generally administered concomitantly in severe initial presentation and/or incomplete response to corticosteroids: azathioprine, mycophenolate mofetil (MMF). Refractory disease: rituximab, calcineurin inhibitors, intravenous immunoglobulin (IVIG). Outcome varies with underlying cause (if known), generally better than IPF.

Acute Interstitial Pneumonia

- Epidemiology/clinical presentation: previously healthy patients, prodrome of nonspecific constitutional and respiratory symptoms with subsequent rapid progression and fulminant respiratory failure ("*idiopathic acute respiratory distress syndrome [ARDS]*")
- Diagnostics: early exudative phase with bilateral GGOs and dense, dependent consolidative opacities followed by organizing phase with architectural distortion and traction bronchiectasis
- Management/prognosis: generally high-dose corticosteroids and supportive care. Consider extracorporeal membrane oxygenation (ECMO) ± lung transplant evaluation in select patients with severe, poorly responsive disease. *Mortality generally >50%.*

Acute Eosinophilic Pneumonia

- Epidemiology/clinical presentation: rare, men > women, younger age (<40); subacute cough, dyspnea, ± fever/systemic symptoms. Risk factors: tobacco use, inhalational drug use, medications (nonsteroidal antiinflammatory drugs [NSAIDs], antibiotics, selective serotonin reuptake inhibitors [SSRIs]), infections (fungal, parasitic)

- Diagnostics: early phase with septal thickening/reticular markings with progression to GGOs, poorly defined centrilobular nodules, denser consolidations. *>25% eosinophils on BAL* or eosinophilic pneumonia on lung biopsy (important to obtain prior to steroid exposure, if possible)
- Management/prognosis: *very steroid responsive* (higher doses in those with fulminant respiratory failure), tapered over 2 to 4 weeks. *Relapse is rare.*

Chronic Eosinophilic Pneumonia

- Epidemiology/clinical presentation: rare, women > men with underlying atopy; gradual onset of dyspnea, cough, fever, unintentional weight loss; less likely to cause fulminant respiratory failure versus AEP
- Diagnostics: GGOs and consolidative opacities with upper lobe and peripheral predominance. *Peripheral eosinophilia (can be absent), BAL with >25% eosinophils (commonly >40%).*
    - Extrapulmonary manifestations should prompt evaluation for eosinophilic granulomatosis with polyangiitis (EGPA), as these are rare in chronic eosinophilic pneumonia (CEP).
- Management/prognosis: *responsive to steroids*, taper over 3 to 6 months pending clinical response; *relapse fairly common*, though usually rapidly responsive to steroids. Off-label use of biologics (primarily mepolizumab and benralizumab; case reports of CEP precipitated by dupilumab)

Cryptogenic Organizing Pneumonia

- Epidemiology/clinical presentation: rare, more common in older patients (>50); typically insidious onset of cough, dyspnea, malaise, fatigue, weight loss usually <2 months prior to presentation; rapidly progressive respiratory failure (less frequent)
    - Note: OP can also arise in the setting of drug toxicity, autoimmune disease (notably RA, IIM, SSc), or infection (eg, nonresolving pneumonia, post–COVID-19).
- Diagnostics: migratory consolidative opacities, often peripheral. *"Reverse-halo" or "atoll" sign: GGO with rim of denser consolidation.* BAL may be helpful to rule out eosinophilic pneumonia.
- Management/prognosis: *typically steroid responsive*, variable taper depending on clinical response (typically ~6 months). Relapses are common and typically occur when the prednisone dose is <20 mg daily (or equivalent) and are usually responsive to increased dosing and/or steroid-sparing agents (eg, MMF, azathioprine).

Exposure-Related Interstitial Lung Diseases

Hypersensitivity Pneumonitis

- Epidemiology/clinical presentation: often >50 yo, *history reveals exposure to trigger (birds, feathers, farming, etc).* Examination with crackles and, classically, inspiratory squeaks
- Diagnostics: GGOs, mosaic attenuation, centrilobular nodules; fibrosis (random or mid-lung); "head cheese sign" (areas of mosaic attenuation, normal lung, and GGOs) is highly specific. HP panel (serologic immunoglobulin G [IgG] antibody panel) can be informative, BAL: lymphocytosis. Consider lung biopsy (TBBx vs cryobiopsy), in consultation with pulmonary specialists, to assist in diagnosis.
- Management/prognosis: *antigen avoidance is key*. Steroids more helpful in nonfibrotic > fibrotic HP (with consideration of steroid-sparing agents). Antifibrotic therapy in progressive disease. Outcome favorable in nonfibrotic HP if offending exposure is identified and removed; worse in patients with fibrotic HP.

Drug-Induced Lung Injury

- Epidemiology/clinical presentation: exposure to amiodarone, chemotherapy (eg, busulfan, bleomycin), immune checkpoint inhibitors (ICI), methotrexate, nitrofurantoin, among others. No specific CT pattern is required. *Pneumotox.com is an excellent resource for documented toxicities.*
- Diagnostics: careful search of drug exposure is critical.
- Management/prognosis: outcomes depend upon the specific agent, which should be discontinued, if possible. ICI pneumonitis is a commonly encountered immune-related adverse event (irAE) among inpatients who are receiving or have recently received ICI therapy and is discussed in detail elsewhere in this book.

Radiation-Induced Lung Injury

- Epidemiology/clinical presentation: >20 Gy cumulative radiation exposure, preceding/concurrent chemotherapy. Cough, dyspnea, fever, chest pain, and malaise that present weeks to months after radiation
- Diagnostics:
    - Acute phase: 3 to 12 weeks after radiation therapy (XRT); GGOs or consolidation within the radiation field. May resolve or may progress
    - Fibrotic phase: 6 to 12 months after XRT (can progress for up to 2 years); scarring, volume loss, and traction bronchiectasis; typically sharp delineation between damaged and normal lung not conforming to anatomic boundaries
    - Secondary OP: 3 to 17 months after XRT; involvement of lung outside areas of irradiated lung, contralateral lung
- Management/prognosis: *supportive/symptomatic management + steroids* in patients who have moderate/severe symptoms (tapered over 1-3 months), no evidence for antifibrotics. Improvement is not expected in the fibrotic phase.

Smoking-Related Interstitial Lung Diseases: Desquamative Interstitial Pneumonia and Respiratory Bronchiolitis-Interstitial Lung Disease

- Epidemiology/clinical presentation: respiratory bronchiolitis-ILD (RB-ILD, milder) and desquamative interstitial pneumonia (DIP, more severe) represent a continuum of smoking-related disorders that present nearly exclusively in active smokers >40 yo.
- Diagnostics: CT findings of GGOs (both DIP and RB-ILD), centrilobular nodules (RB-ILD). Often diagnoses of exclusion without histopathology
- Management/prognosis: *smoking cessation* (primary) with consideration of steroids in refractory/progressive cases. DIP more frequently requires treatment with steroids and occasionally antibiotics (macrolides) and steroid-sparing agents (azathioprine, cyclophosphamide) as second-line agents.

Pneumoconiosis

- Epidemiology/clinical presentation: caused by inhalation of inorganic/mineral dust (eg, construction, mining, welding, stone cutting); symptoms include dyspnea, dry cough, and chest tightness but may be asymptomatic in earlier stages.
- Diagnostics: radiographic findings depend upon the inhaled material. Examples include:
  - Asbestos: *pleural thickening*, lower lobe predominant parenchymal involvement with reticular opacities
  - Silica: nodules with progression to fibrosis/coalescing masses, punctate *"eggshell" calcifications* in the lymph nodes, upper lung zone predominance
- Management/prognosis: generally *supportive care, consideration of lung transplantation*; steroids (systemic or inhaled) may be used in chronic beryllium disease.

Autoimmune Interstitial Lung Diseases

General Considerations

- Epidemiology: ILD most commonly complicates SSc, RA, IIMs (myositis), mixed connective tissue disease (MCTD), and Sjögren disease. Typically women > men, except in RA-ILD
- Diagnostics: *NSIP most common*. UIP common in RA-ILD. OP common in myositis-associated ILD. Diagnosis often requires clinical, serologic, and radiographic data ± biopsy.
- Management/prognosis: treatment of the underlying autoimmune disorder, as noted later

Systemic Sclerosis-Interstitial Lung Disease

- Epidemiology/clinical presentation: high prevalence and leading cause of mortality in SSc; more common in diffuse cutaneous SSc; associated with anti–Scl-70
- Diagnostics: NSIP > UIP on CT; anti–Scl-70 antibody
- Management/prognosis: caution with corticosteroids due to the risk of precipitating scleroderma renal crisis (lower risk with daily prednisone equivalent <15 mg). The first-line steroid-sparing agent is MMF, followed by tocilizumab or rituximab.

Rheumatoid Arthritis-Interstitial Lung Disease

- Epidemiology/clinical presentation: pulmonary involvement can precede joint disease; the presence of ILD portends higher morbidity and mortality.
- Diagnostics: UIP > NSIP on CT; CCP/RF positivity
- Management/prognosis: immunosuppression ± disease-modifying antirheumatic drugs (DMARDs); active joint disease is associated with increased pulmonary mortality.

Myositis-Associated Interstitial Lung Disease

- Epidemiology/clinical presentation: high prevalence, *leading cause of mortality/morbidity in IIMs*, and ILD may be the first manifestation of IIM. *Patients can present critically ill with rapidly progressive disease, even without clinical myositis.*
- Diagnostics: NSIP, OP on CT. Thigh magnetic resonance imaging (MRI) can reveal active myositis. Associated with several myositis-associated autoantibodies (eg, Jo-1, MDA5, PL-7, PL-12). Elevated serum aldolase, creatine kinase
- Management/prognosis: limited data for immunosuppressive agents of choice, often multidrug regimen (steroids, cyclophosphamide, rituximab intravenous immunoglobulin [IVIG]) given the high risk of fulminant disease

Sarcoidosis

- Epidemiology/clinical presentation: female > male, increased lifetime risk in Black patients in the United States; clinical presentation is variable depending on which organ systems are involved (eg, cardiac, cutaneous, ocular).
  - Pulmonary symptoms include dry cough, dyspnea, fatigue, and weight loss.
- Diagnostics: CT with *peribronchovascular thickening*, perilymphatic/subpleural nodules, GGOs, mediastinal/hilar lymphadenopathy; four stages from just lymphadenopathy (stage I) to extensive parenchymal involvement/architectural distortion (stage IV). Biopsy with noncaseating granulomas
- Management/prognosis: low-moderate dose steroids (typically for >1 year) in symptomatic patients

SUGGESTED READINGS

Adegunsoye A, Ryerson CJ. Diagnostic classification of interstitial lung disease in clinical practice. *Clin Chest Med.* 2021;42(2):251-261.

Cottin V. Eosinophilic lung diseases. *Immunol Allergy Clin North Am.* 2023;43(2):289-322.

Crouser ED, Maier LA, Wilson KC, et al. Diagnosis and detection of sarcoidosis. An official American Thoracic Society clinical practice guideline. *Am J Respir Crit Care Med.* 2020;201(8):e26-e51.

De Giacomi F, Vassallo R, Yi ES, Ryu JH. Acute eosinophilic pneumonia. Causes, diagnosis, and management. *Am J Respir Crit Care Med.* 2018;197(6):728-736.

Hallowell RW, Danoff SK. Diagnosis and management of myositis-associated lung disease. *Chest.* 2023;163(6):1476-1491.

Lee AS, Scofield RH, Hammitt KM, et al. Consensus guidelines for evaluation and management of pulmonary disease in Sjögren's. *Chest.* 2021;159(2):683-698.

Levesque MH, Montesi SB, Sharma A. Diffuse parenchymal abnormalities in acutely dyspneic patients: a pattern-based approach. *J Thorac Imaging.* 2015;30(4):220.

Maher TM. Interstitial lung disease: a review. *JAMA.* 2024;331(19):1655.

Newton CA, Zhang D, Oldham JM, et al. Telomere length and use of immunosuppressive medications in idiopathic pulmonary fibrosis. *Am J Respir Crit Care Med.* 2019;200(3):336-347.

Podolanczuk AJ, Wong AW, Saito S, Lasky JA, Ryerson CJ, Eickelberg O. Update in interstitial lung disease 2020. *Am J Respir Crit Care Med.* 2021;203(11):1343-1352.

Raghu G, Remy-Jardin M, Richeldi L, et al. Idiopathic pulmonary fibrosis (an update) and progressive pulmonary fibrosis in adults: an official ATS/ERS/JRS/ALAT clinical practice guideline. *Am J Respir Crit Care Med.* 2022;205(9):e18-e47.

Raghu G, Remy-Jardin M, Ryerson CJ, et al. Diagnosis of hypersensitivity pneumonitis in adults: an official ATS/JRS/ALAT clinical practice guideline. *Am J Respir Crit Care Med.* 2020;202(3):e36-e69.

Waxman A, Restrepo-Jaramillo R, Thenappan T, et al. Inhaled treprostinil in pulmonary hypertension due to interstitial lung disease. *N Engl J Med.* 2021;384(4):325-334.

Wijsenbeek M, Suzuki A, Maher TM. Interstitial lung diseases. *Lancet.* 2022;400(10354):769-786.

3.9

Aspiration Syndromes

Giovanni Bruno and Cristina Mietto

Definition

Aspiration is defined as the abnormal entry of fluid, particulate exogenous substances, or endogenous secretions into the lower airways.

- Two main factors facilitate aspiration.
  - Compromised protection of lower airways, with microaspiration or macroaspiration passing through the trachea and larynx from oropharynx, stomach, duodenum, and exogenous sources
  - Pro-inflammatory aspirated material, which can include microbes, bile, pepsin, and particulates
- Based on the time of onset, aspiration syndromes can be divided into acute and chronic.
  - Acute: bronchospasm, asthma, acute bronchitis, chronic obstructive pulmonary disorder (COPD) exacerbation, pneumonia, pneumonitis, foreign body obstruction, acute respiratory distress syndrome (ARDS)
  - Chronic: bronchiectasis, chronic bronchitis, exogenous lipoid pneumonia, interstitial lung disease, organizing pneumonia, diffuse aspiration bronchiolitis
- Aspiration syndromes can also be divided into those affecting the airways or the lung parenchyma (Table 3.9.1).

Risk Factors for Aspiration

- Upper gastrointestinal (GI) disease (eg, gastroesophageal reflux disease [GERD], gastroparesis)
- Decreased level of consciousness
- Dysphagia
- Pharyngeal anesthesia
- Compromised airway defenses (eg, impaired cough reflex)

Epidemiology

- In patients younger than 80 years, pneumonia develops as a consequence of an aspiration event in 5% of cases. The incidence increases to >10% in patients older than 80 years.

TABLE 3.9.1 Classification of Aspiration Syndromes by Affected Area

Airways	Lung Parenchyma
Vocal cord dysfunction	Aspiration pneumonitis
Foreign body aspiration (mechanical obstruction)	Aspiration pneumonia
Bronchiectasis	Organizing pneumonia
Bronchoconstriction (eg, exacerbation of asthma)	Interstitial lung disease
Diffuse aspiration bronchiolitis/ bronchiolitis obliterans syndrome	Exogenous lipoid pneumonia

- Silent aspiration occurs in 40% to 70% of cases after cerebrovascular events.
- Silent aspiration is observed in >50% of hospitalized patients aged 70 years or above.
- Aspiration events are responsible for 18% to 30% of pneumonia occurring among nursing home residents.

Key Pathophysiology

- The pathophysiology depends on the type and volume of aspirated material, as well as the clinical condition of the individual, whether they are healthy or have multiple risk factors for severe disease.
- Aspiration can be divided into three forms:
  - Chemical
  - Bacterial
  - Fluids and particulate matter
- Chemical pneumonitis
  - Aspiration of substances toxic to the lower airways, mostly due to the aspiration of gastric secretions
  - Chemical pneumonitis is commonly caused by aspiration of a large volume of gastric contents with a low pH (usually <2.5).
    - Mendelson syndrome is a form of chemical pneumonitis occurring particularly during anesthesia, more commonly during emergency surgeries with "full stomach" patients.
  - Frequent microaspiration, such as those occurring during sleep, can lead to chronic lung injuries.
  - Macroaspiration can cause acute lung injury and diffuse alveolar damage.
  - In patients with GERD, direct exposure to refluxed gastroduodenal contents, which include acid, pepsin, and bile acid, can lead to laryngeal injury and mucosal damage.
  - Clinical features: depend on the amount of the inoculum and host factors
    - Usually, dyspnea with abrupt onset, low-grade fever, cyanosis, crackles, and severe hypoxemia
  - Infiltrates on chest x-ray (CXR): lower lobes in upright patients but superior segments of lower lobes and posterior segments of the upper lobes in the recumbent patient
- Diagnosis: based on clinical features and CXR findings, usually occurs within 2 hours. In patients with aspiration during anesthesia, clinical or radiographic abnormalities may not be immediately evident.
- Bacterial pneumonia
  - Bacterial pneumonia often results from aspiration due to impaired swallowing, leading to oropharyngeal or gastric contents entering the lungs, especially in those with a weak cough reflex.
  - Multiple risk factors increase the likelihood of aspiration pneumonia and mortality. Having multiple risk factors significantly raises 30-day and 6-month mortality rates.
  - Clinical features: indolent symptoms, predisposing conditions for aspiration, absence of rigors, failure to grow out typical pulmonary pathogens on sputum, putrid sputum, evidence of periodontal disease, CXR showing necrotic pneumonia, abscess, or empyema
  - Microbiology: recent studies on older patients have shown a shift in the pathogens responsible for pneumonia, likely due to demographic changes and

early sampling. Gram-negative bacteria account for 49% of cases, anaerobes for 16%, and *Staphylococcus aureus* for 12%. Community-acquired pneumonia primarily involves *Streptococcus pneumoniae*, *S. aureus*, *Haemophilus influenzae*, and Enterobacteriaceae, while hospital-acquired cases are dominated by Gram-negative bacilli, including *Pseudomonas aeruginosa*.
    - Diagnosis: although some studies have proposed using quantitative lung-lavage cultures to distinguish bacterial from noninfectious pneumonitis, and others suggest the use of procalcitonin, diagnosis remains primarily clinical. The initial CXR may appear negative in some cases of aspiration pneumonia.
- Fluids and particulate matter
    - Aspiration of fluids or particulate matter that are not toxic to the lungs but can cause mechanical obstruction or reflexive airway closure
    - The severity of respiratory obstruction depends on the object's size relative to airway caliber.
    - This is found more commonly in children from objects such as peanuts.
    - Large objects can lodge in the larynx or trachea and cause acute distress and should be treated with abdominal thrusts as per basic life support.
    - Smaller objects may cause an irritating cough, and there may be evidence of atelectasis or obstructive emphysema on CXR, while chest computed tomography (CT scan) can reveal intrabronchial masses and air trapping. The foreign body aspiration is often confirmed by bronchoscopy.

Treatment and Management

- Treatment of all three syndromes is mainly supportive.
- Prevention measures are strongly recommended (eg, antibiotic therapy may be considered for 24 hours in comatose patients after emergency intubation).
- Appropriate fasting time reduces the risk of postoperative chemical pneumonitis; the patient should fast for at least 8 hours and refrain from clear liquids for at least 2 hours before surgery.
- Patients require close respiratory monitoring, pulmonary toilet, and supportive treatment as needed, including intubation and mechanical ventilation.
- As with any critically ill patient, ventilator settings should be tailored to the patient's condition.
- Low-tidal volume ventilation is recommended for patients with ARDS or at risk for ARDS (see the section on ARDS and definition).
- Rigid bronchoscopic removal is typically required if the patient aspirated an object that requires removal (eg, a peanut).
    - To reduce the risk of postoperative chemical pneumonitis, the patient should fast for at least 8 hours and refrain from clear liquids for at least 2 hours before surgery.
    - If there is concern for infection, antibiotics should be given.
    - The site of infection acquisition and the risk factors for multidrug-resistant pathogens drive the appropriate antibiotic choice.
    - Antibiotics should appropriately cover the patient for pneumonia (eg, community-acquired pneumonia or health care–acquired pneumonia).
    - In patients with most community-acquired pneumonia, ampicillin-sulbactam, carbapenem, and fluoroquinolones are effective treatments.
    - Clindamycin can be added for high-risk anaerobic infections as severe periodontal disease, necrotizing pneumonia, or lung abscesses.
    - Patients showing a good clinical response without extrapulmonary infection are recommended 5 to 7 days of treatment.
    - Longer treatment is recommended for those with necrotizing pneumonia, lung abscess, or empyema.
- There is no established role for corticosteroids.
- Prevention of aspiration in the intensive care unit (ICU):
    - Minimize sedation to allow cough.
    - Consider aspiration of subglottic secretions with specialized endotracheal tubes.
    - Elevation of the head of the bed: studies found that raising the head of the bed 30 to 45 degree leads to a 3-fold reduction in hospital-acquired pneumonia.
    - Early versus late feeding:
        - Although early feeding increases aspiration versus no feeding, feeding is still recommended for its multiple benefits.
        - Interestingly, postpyloric feeding has not shown any benefit in reducing the risk of aspiration.
    - Oral antiseptics and mouthwash: decrease infection in the setting of post-coronary artery bypass grafting
    - Selective decontamination of the GI tract refers to a strategy used to prevent aspiration pneumonia by reducing the amount of potentially harmful bacteria in a patient's mouth and stomach through the application of topical antibiotics.

Outcomes

- Most patients recover, with 62% having a rapid clinical recovery.
- 12% of patients develop a fulminant course, characterized by ARDS and death.
- 26% of patients initially improve but then develop bacterial infection or ARDS.

SUGGESTED READINGS

Lee AS, Ryu JH. Aspiration pneumonia and related syndromes. *Mayo Clin Proc*. 2018;93:752-762.

Mandell LA, Niederman MS. Aspiration pneumonia. *N Engl J Med*. 2019;380:651-663.

Simpson AJ, Allen JL, Chatwin M, et al. BTS clinical statement on aspiration pneumonia. *Thorax*. 2023;78(suppl 1):s3-s21.

3.10

Pneumonia

Christopher Richards

- *Definition*
  - Pneumonia in the intensive care unit (ICU) falls into three categories based on the risk profiles of the patient and where they were likely to have acquired the infection.
    - Community-acquired pneumonia (CAP)
    - Hospital-acquired pneumonia (HAP)
    - Ventilator-associated pneumonia (VAP)
  - The American Thoracic Society (ATS) and the Infectious Disease Society of America (IDSA) provide guidelines in two areas: CAP published in 2019 and HAP/VAP published in 2016.
  - The 2016 update for HAP and VAP removed the designation of "Healthcare Associated Pneumonia."
  - These guidelines are broadly applicable but do not directly address immunocompromised patients and do not provide information on fungal pneumonias, nor COVID-19.
- *Burden of disease*
  - In high-income countries the monthly death rate from severe pneumonia is 10% to 12% and rises to 30% if patients receive any form of mechanical ventilation.
  - Pneumonia accounts for 50% of antibiotics prescribed in the ICU.
  - Pneumonia is the second most common nosocomial infection (after urinary tract infection [UTI]).
  - The diagnosis of pneumonia increases hospital stay by 7 to 9 days and adds $40,000 per patient to the cost of admission.
  - Intubation increases the risk of pneumonia by 6- to 20-fold.
  - HAP and CAP requiring ICU admission are associated with an attributable mortality of 33% to 50%.
- *Diagnosis*
  - The diagnosis of pneumonia requires clinical discretion, considering symptoms, imaging, and laboratory/microbiologic testing.
  - Differential diagnosis (in the ICU, any of these can occur concurrently with pneumonia):
    - Congestive heart failure
    - Atelectasis
    - Pulmonary embolism/infarction
    - Drug reaction/pneumonitis
    - Aspiration pneumonitis
    - Pulmonary hemorrhage
    - Acute respiratory distress syndrome (ARDS)
    - Transfusion-related complications
      - Transfusion-associated circulatory overload (TACO)
      - Transfusion-related acute lung injury (TRALI)
  - Sputum culture
    - Should be obtained in all patients with severe CAP in the ICU
      - Methods include:
        - Expectorated sputum
        - Induced sputa
        - Bronchoscopic airway lavage (BAL)
        - In line suctioning/mini-BAL through an established airway
  - Blood cultures
    - Should be obtained in all patients with severe CAP in the ICU
  - Procalcitonin (PCT)
    - PCT levels are highest among patients with bacterial infections.
    - High PCT levels are associated with increased risk of ICU transfer and mortality.
    - Role for PCT is best suited for discontinuation of antibiotics after 48 hours of treatment.
  - Viral swabs
    - Should be obtained in all patients with severe CAP in the ICU
    - A positive viral swab with a PCT ≤0.25 can be used to defer antibiotic treatment.
  - Methicillin-resistant *Staphylococcus aureus* (MRSA) nasal swabs
    - In culture-negative pneumonia, a negative MRSA nasal swab can reliably be used to de-escalate anti-MRSA antibiotics.
  - *Streptococcus pneumoniae* and *Legionella* urinary antigen testing
    - These tests can be considered in cases of severe CAP, but outside known high-risk exposures and epidemiologic outbreaks, they may be insensitive and lead to premature changes in antibiotic selection.
- *Management*
  - *CAP*
    - Overall, up to 10% of all patients admitted with CAP are admitted to the ICU.
    - Severity of CAP can be estimated using the criteria in Table 3.10.1.

TABLE 3.10.1 Severe CAP Requires One Major Criterion or Three or More Minor Criteria

Minor Criteria	Major Criteria
Respiratory rate ≥30 breaths/min	Septic shock requiring vasopressors
Pa_{O_2}/F_{IO_2} ratio ≤250	Respiratory failure requiring mechanical ventilation
Multilobar infiltrates	
Confusion/disorientation	
Uremia (blood urea nitrogen ≥20 mg/dL)	
Leukopenia (white blood cell count <4,000 cells/μL)	
Thrombocytopenia (platelet count <100,000/μL)	
Hypothermia (core temperature <36 °C)	
Hypotension requiring aggressive fluid resuscitation	

CAP, community-acquired pneumonia.

TABLE 3.10.2 CURB-65 Score

Confusion	1 point	Score 1: Low risk, consider outpatient treatment
BUN >19 mg/dL	1 point	
Respiratory rate ≥30	1 point	Score 2: Moderate risk, inpatient treatment, or outpatient treatment with close follow-up
Systolic BP <90 mm Hg or Diastolic BP ≤60 mm Hg	1 point	
Age ≥65	1 point	Score 3-5: High risk, inpatient treatment with possible ICU admission

The CURB-65 score is one of multiple predictive tools that can be used to triage patients who are presenting to the hospital with pneumonia. This tool is helpful in determining when a patient can be managed as an outpatient or admitted the hospital and can be calculated rather quickly.

BP, blood pressure; BUN, blood urea nitrogen; ICU, intensive care unit.

Triage decisions for admission to the hospital versus ICU can be informed using the CURB-65 score (Table 3.10.2) or pneumonia severity index (Table 3.10.3).

- Direct admission from the emergency department to the ICU is associated with decreased mortality compared to transfer from the hospital ward to the ICU.
  - Physician determination aided by a prognostic tool is the best method to triage patients.
- For patients with severe CAP, empiric therapy is recommended, based on the guidelines below, and should be given as soon as possible after admission (Table 3.10.4).
- A large Medicare study showed that 30-day CAP mortality was increased when administration of the first dose of antibiotic was delayed by >8 hours from the time of arrival to the hospital.

- *HAP/VAP*
  - HAP refers to pneumonia not associated with mechanical ventilation.
  - VAP refers to pneumonia associated with mechanical ventilation.
  - Risk factors include:
    - Intravenous (IV) antibiotic use in the 90 days prior
    - Septic shock at the time of HAP/VAP
    - ARDS preceding HAP/VAP
    - ≥5 days of hospitalization prior to HAP/VAP
    - Acute renal replacement therapy prior to HAP/VAP
  - Patients with HAP or VAP should receive empiric therapy based on the guidelines in Table 3.10.5.
    - Additional considerations to antibiotic selection should be made based on local resistance patterns and epidemiology.
  - Duration of therapy can be informed by:
    - Clinical improvement
    - PCT <0.25 at 48 hours
    - 7 days is generally sufficient for HAP and VAP, including infections caused by *Pseudomonas* and MRSA infections, but can be extended pending response.
  - Response to therapy is expected within 72 hours. Reasons for a lack of response include:

TABLE 3.10.3 Pneumonia Severity Index

		Classification	Risk	Point Value
Age	(Points = age)	I	Low	None
Sex	Female −10 Male 0	II	Low	≤70
Nursing home resident	+10	III	Low	71-90
Neoplastic disease history	+30	IV	Moderate	91-130
Liver disease history	+20	V	High	>130
Congestive heart failure history	+10			
Cerebrovascular history	+10			
Renal disease history	+10			
Altered mental status	+20			
Respiratory rate ≥30	+20			
Systolic blood pressure <90 mm Hg	+20			
Temperature <35 °C (95 °F) or >39.9 °C (103.8 °F)	+15			
Pulse ≥125 beats/min	+10			
pH <7.35	+30			
BUN ≥30 mg/dL or ≥11 mmol/L	+20			
Sodium <130 mmol/L	+20			
Glucose ≥250 mg/dL or ≥14 mmol/L	+10			
Hematocrit <30%	+10			
Partial pressure of oxygen <60 mm Hg or <8 kPa	+10			
Pleural effusion on x-ray	+10			

The pneumonia severity index is a risk assessment tool that can be used to stratify patients presenting with pneumonia to the appropriate level of care. Pitfalls include the emphasis on age that can understate severe disease in younger patients, and the number of entries make it less practical than the CURB-65 score.

BUN, blood urea nitrogen.

TABLE 3.10.4 Empiric Treatment for Severe CAP

Organism	Therapy
Group 1: no risks for *Pseudomonas aeruginosa* • Streptococcal pneumonia (including DRSP) • *Legionella* spp. • *Haemophilus influenza* • Enteric Gram-negative bacilli • *Staphylococcus aureus* • *Mycoplasma pneumonia* • Respiratory viruses • Miscellaneous: *Chlamydia pneumonia*, *Mycobacterium tuberculosis*, endemic fungi	Intravenous β-lactam (cefotaxime, ceftriaxone) Plus either Intravenous macrolide (azithromycin) Or Intravenous fluoroquinolone
Group 2: risks for *P. aeruginosa* (Structural lung disease, bronchiectasis, cystic fibrosis, tracheostomy, steroid therapy, broad-spectrum antibiotics in the last month, malnutrition, leukopenic immunosuppression) • All of the Group 1 pathogens plus *P. aeruginosa*	Selected intravenous antipseudomonal β-lactam (cefepime, imipenem, meropenem, piperacillin/tazobactam) Plus intravenous antipseudomonal quinoline (ciprofloxacin) Or Selected intravenous antipseudomonal β-lactam (cefepime, imipenem, meropenem, piperacillin/tazobactam) Plus Intravenous aminoglycoside plus either intravenous macrolide (azithromycin) Or Intravenous nonpseudomonal fluoroquinolone

Group 1, no risk of *P. aeruginosa*. Group 2, risk of *P. aeruginosa*.
CAP, community-acquired pneumonia; DRSP, drug-resistant *Streptococcus pneumoniae*.

- Inadequate antimicrobial selection or dosing
- Unusual pathogen
  - The list of unusual pathogens is broad. A pertinent history including occupational and travel histories, exposure to livestock, tick bites, endemic fungal exposures, and reasons for immune suppression should be explored.
- Complications of pneumonia (empyema or parapneumonic effusion)
  - Risk factors for empyema include patients under the age of 60, a history of alcohol misuse, seizure, loss of consciousness, diabetes, and poor dentition.
  - Common organisms include *S. pneumoniae, S. agalactiae, MRSA, Klebsiella,* and *Pseudomonas.*
- Noninfectious illness
  - These would include, among others, organizing pneumonia, acute eosinophilic pneumonia, drug reaction, drug pneumonitis from cancer immunotherapies, and complications of blood product transfusion.

○ *Steroids for pneumonia in the ICU*
- Community-Acquired Pneumonia: Evaluation of Corticosteroids (CAPE COD)

TABLE 3.10.5 Empiric Treatment for HAP/VAP

Potential Pathogen	Recommended Antibiotic
Streptococcal pneumonia *Haemophilus influenza* Methicillin-sensitive *Staphylococcus aureus* Antibiotic-sensitive enteric Gram-negative bacilli • *Escherichia coli* • *Klebsiella pneumoniae* • *Enterobacter* species • *Proteus* species *Serratia marcescens*	Ceftriaxone Or Levofloxacin, moxifloxacin, or ciprofloxacin Or Ampicillin/sulbactam Or Ertapenem
Pathogens as above plus MDR pathogens • *Pseudomonas aeruginosa* • *Klebsiella pneumoniae* (ESBL) • *Acinetobacter* species Methicillin-resistant *Staphylococcus aureus* (MRSA) *Legionella pneumonia*	Antipseudomonal cephalosporin (cefepime, ceftazidime) Or Antipseudomonal carbapenem (imipenem or meropenem) Or β-lactam/β-lactamase inhibitor (piperacillin-tazobactam) Plus Antipseudomonal fluoroquinolone (ciprofloxacin or levofloxacin) Or Aminoglycoside (amikacin, gentamicin, or tobramycin) Plus Linezolid or vancomycin

Sensitive pathogens as well as multidrug-resistant (MDR) organisms.
ESBL, extended-spectrum beta-lactamase; HAP, hospital-acquired pneumonia; VAP, ventilator-associated pneumonia.

- For patients with severe CAP (high-flow oxygen, mechanical ventilation, pneumonia severity index >130)
- Treat with 200 mg hydrocortisone IV daily for 4 days, then determine if there has been clinical improvement.
- Pending clinical improvement can decide to continue steroids for 8 or 14 days following a prescribed taper.
- Reduces 30-day mortality, intubation, use of vasopressors
- Did not include patients with influenza or COVID-19

● *Prevention of pneumonia in the ICU*

○ Common strategies include:
- Avoiding intubation
- Minimizing sedation
- Early extubating practices
- Early mobilization

○ Other commonly performed initiatives without clear benefit include:
- Head of bed elevation protocols are based on little data.
- Stress ulcer prophylaxis can increase risk of pneumonia.
- Chlorhexidine rinses may increase mortality risk.

● *Viral pneumonia in the ICU*

○ Respiratory viruses are found in 18% to 49% of patients in the ICU with severe respiratory tract infections.
- Influenza, COVID-19, and respiratory syncytial virus (RSV) are common actionable infections.

- Rhinovirus, enterovirus, parainfluenza, adenovirus, and human metapneumovirus are common infections with no specific therapy.
- *Influenza*
  - All patients presenting during "flu season" with severe acute respiratory illness or an acute worsening of a chronic respiratory illness should be tested for influenza.
  - The neuraminidase inhibitor oseltamivir is preferred and has similar enteral and IV absorption.
  - Benefits of oseltamivir are greatest within 48 hours of symptom onset.
  - There may be prolonged viral shedding in critically ill patients, extending treatment beyond 5 days can be made on a case-by-case basis.
- *COVID-19*
  - Treatments for COVID-19 are evolving, the recommendations here are derived from the 2023 IDSA COVID treatment guidelines.
  - Severe COVID-19: Spo_2 ≤94% on room air.
  - Critical illness COVID-19: mechanical ventilation or extracorporeal membrane oxygenation (ECMO) with other end-organ damage
  - Antiviral therapies:
    - Remdesivir is recommended for hospitalized patients with progressive, severe, or critically ill COVID-19.
    - Lopinavir/ritonavir is not recommended for severe or critically ill patients with COVID-19.
  - Antiinflammatory therapy is considered for patients with COVID-19 as many have a hyperinflammatory syndrome that leads to multisystem failure.
    - Dexamethasone (6 mg IV or orally [PO] for 10 days, or until discharged) is recommended for severely and critically ill patients with COVID-19.
    - For severe progressive or critically severe COVID-19, add tocilizumab (anti–IL-6) to standard of care.
    - Anakinra (anti–IL-1) is not recommended as the group most likely to benefit has not been identified.

SUGGESTED READINGS

Bhimraj A, Morgan RL, Shumaker AH, et al. Infectious Diseases Society of America guidelines on the treatment and management of patients with COVID-19. *Clin Infect Dis.* 2024;78:e250-e349.

Dequin PF, Meziani F, Quenot JP, et al. Hydrocortisone in severe community-acquired pneumonia. *N Engl J Med.* 2023;388(21):1931-1941.

Fine MJ, Auble TE, Yealy DM, et al. A prediction rule to identify low-risk patients with community-acquired pneumonia. *N Engl J Med.* 1997;336(4):243-250.

Huang HB, Peng JM, Weng L, Wang CY, Jiang W, Du B. Procalcitonin-guided antibiotic therapy in intensive care unit patients: a systematic review and meta-analysis. *Ann Intensive Care.* 2017;7(1):114.

Kalil AC, Metersky ML, Klompas M, et al. Management of adults with hospital-acquired and ventilator-associated pneumonia: 2016 clinical practice guidelines by the Infectious Diseases Society of America and the American Thoracic Society. *Clin Infect Dis.* 2016;63(5):e61-e111.

Klompas M. Prevention of intensive care unit-acquired pneumonia. *Semin Respir Crit Care Med.* 2019;40(4):548-557.

Metlay JP, Waterer GW, Long AC, et al. Diagnosis and treatment of adults with community-acquired pneumonia. An official clinical practice guideline of the American Thoracic Society and Infectious Diseases Society of America. *Am J Respir Crit Care Med.* 2019;200(7):e45-e67.

3.11

COVID-19

Jason Griffith

Since emerging in December 2019, severe acute respiratory syndrome coronavirus-2 (SARS-CoV-2), the virus responsible for COVID-19, has caused a global pandemic, resulting in millions of deaths and a profound impact on our society.

SARS-CoV-2 Biology

- SARS-CoV-2 virus is a member of the Coronavirus family, a positive-sense, single-stranded RNA virus and is the third highly pathogenic coronavirus to emerge from zoonotic sources within the past two decades.
- Structural proteins include the membrane-bound spike (S), envelope (E), membrane proteins (M), and the RNA-binding nucleocapsid (N) protein.
- Viral entry is mediated by S glycoprotein binding to the angiotensin-converting enzyme 2 (ACE2) and furin-mediated cleavage. ACE2 receptor distribution predominantly determines viral host cell infectivity. The N-terminal domain and the receptor-binding domain of the S glycoprotein are targeted by neutralizing antibodies and are the site of ongoing variation due to evolution.
- Variants continue to evolve from the original Wuhan-Hu-1 strain and are characterized by increased transmission advantages compared to prior variants. These variants include alpha (PANGO lineage B.1.1.7), beta (B1.351), gamma (P.1), delta (B.1.617.2/AY), and omicron (B.1.1.529). Omicron includes various sublineages such as BA.1, BA.2, BA.5, and JN.1 and its descendants KP.2 and KP.3.
- Early alpha and beta variants demonstrated optimized furin cleavage, thus enhancing transmissibility, while later variants demonstrate more immune escape.

Clinical Manifestations of COVID-19

- COVID-19 illness in most immunocompetent patients is characterized by an asymptomatic incubation period, a symptomatic period lasting a mean of 6 to 9 days and a recovery period. Viral rebound may occur in both treated and untreated patients. Additionally, a subset of individuals experience persistent symptoms postinfection, which is referred to as long COVID or post–acute sequelae of SARS-CoV-2 infection.

- Viral replication in immunocompromised patients (including patients with B- and T-cell deficiency, hematologic malignancy, solid-organ transplant, human immunodeficiency virus [HIV]) may be persistent with prolonged positive polymerase reaction chain (PCR) tests and symptoms.
- Up to 20% of infections may be asymptomatic. In the remainder of patients, respiratory viral infection symptoms are common and include fever, myalgia, sore throat, and runny nose.
- Severe COVID-19 requiring hospitalization generally occurs after a median of 6 days after symptom onset, and a viral pneumonia picture emerges with cough, fever, hypoxemia, and opacities on chest imaging.
- Lab values associated with severe COVID-19 include lymphopenia, as well as an elevated troponin, D-dimer, C-reactive protein (CRP), lactate dehydrogenase (LDH), ferritin, and creatine kinase.
- Multiorgan failure is a common feature in severe COVID-19 illness. Cardiac manifestations, including myocarditis, arrhythmias, and myocardial infarction, have all been reported. Acute kidney injury is common as are neurologic sequelae, including syncope and stroke. Skin lesions include "COVID toes," which are swollen erythematous digits with discoloration consistent with pernio. An elevated risk of arterial and venous thrombi occurs in the first 7 days of infection and may last up to a year postinfection.

Risk Factors for Severe COVID-19

- The strongest association with severity remains age, and age >65 vaccinated or >50 unvaccinated is currently accepted as a high-risk cutoff.
- Being unvaccinated or not up to date on COVID-19 vaccinations is also associated with severe disease.
- Obesity, smoking, and lack of physical activity all contribute to more severe COVID-19.
- Other risk factors include preexisting health problems including diabetes mellitus, cancer, organ disease (renal, liver, cardiac, lung), and neurologic problems, including dementia and schizophrenia.
- Pregnancy is also associated with an increased risk for severe COVID-19.
- Worse outcomes have also been noted based on racial, ethnic, and socioeconomic disparities.
- Viral factors may also contribute as rates of hospitalization and death were lower with omicron infection compared to the delta variant.

Antiviral Agents

- Oral antiviral drugs approved for use include *nirmatrelvir-ritonavir* (NMV-r, Paxlovid), which targets SARS-CoV-2 main protease (M^{pro}, $3CL^{pro}$), and *molnupiravir* (Lagevrio), which is a nucleoside analog that becomes incorporated into viral RNA, causing lethal mutations. Prior to the widespread preexisting immunity, NMV-r was shown to result in an 88% decrease in relative risk for hospitalization or death in high-risk adults but no significant difference in low-risk adults (EPIC-HR and EPIC-SR trials). The PANORAMIC trial is currently the largest randomized controlled trial (RCT) in the widespread immunity period and has found no risk reduction for hospitalization or death with molnupiravir, while the results for NMV-r are still pending. Current guidelines recommend NMV-r for outpatients with more than one high-risk factor and within 5 days of symptom onset.
- The ritonavir component of NMV-r inhibits the CYP3A4 pathway to increase NMV levels, but this also results in significant drug-drug interactions. Caution or avoidance is advised in patients taking anticonvulsants, cardiac medications such as amiodarone, pulmonary hypertension (HTN) medications, chemotherapy agents, and immunosuppressants, such as tacrolimus (see National Institutes of Health [NIH] COVID-19 treatment guidelines for full list).
- *Remdesivir* is an adenosine nucleotide analog prodrug that binds to viral RNA-dependent RNA polymerase and terminates RNA transcription. Approved for use in adult and pediatric patients. Outpatients with a risk for severe progression within 7 days of symptom onset to receive infusion for 3 days. Hospitalized patients on low-flow, high-flow nasal cannula (HFNC), or noninvasive ventilation (NIV) should receive treatment for 5 days or discharge. If symptoms are ongoing, an additional 5 days (for a total of 10 days) can be added. Limited data in support of using with severe patients on mechanical ventilator or extracorporeal membrane oxygenation (ECMO). Liver function tests (LFTs) should be monitored, and the drug stopped if alanine aminotransferase (ALT) >10× the upper limit of normal.
- *Anti–SARS-CoV-2 monoclonal antibodies* that target the spike protein were used for the prevention and treatment of omicron variants, but genetic drift has limited further development.
- *Convalescent plasma* has conflicting data, but a recent meta-analysis demonstrates a mortality benefit for immunocompromised patients who are susceptible to refractory infection. However, use is limited by availability.

Management of Severe COVID-19: Hospital Floor/Low-Flow Oxygen

- Management of COVID-19 depends on the current severity of disease and assessment of risk factors for progression to severe disease.
- Patients without hypoxemia but with more than one high-risk factor are treated with antiviral agents (NMV-r for outpatients and remdesivir for inpatients or patients who cannot take NMV-r). Steroid therapy is likely harmful in this group and is not recommended.
- Home medications, including statins, ACE inhibitors, and anticoagulation, can be continued unless there are other indications for stopping.
- Patients who are hypoxemic on low-flow oxygen are treated with remdesivir if presenting within 7 days of symptom onset as well as immunomodulatory therapy with dexamethasone 6 mg/d for 10 days. The RECOVERY trial demonstrated an 18% relative reduction in mortality in these patients treated with dexamethasone.

- If oxygen requirement escalates, consider further adjunctive immunomodulatory treatment with tocilizumab (Actemra, anti–IL-6) or baricitinib (Olumiant, JAK inhibitor).
- For adults with primary COVID-19 admission and no contraindication, we recommend therapeutic anticoagulation with low-molecular-weight heparin (LMWH). D-dimer testing has been proposed as a tool to select patients for treatment, but cutoffs are unclear.
- Routine treatment with empiric antibiotics is not recommended unless there is evidence of bacterial co-infection or diagnostic uncertainty.
- Prone positioning in hypoxemic nonintubated patients has been attempted and demonstrates improved oxygenation and a signal toward decreased rates of intubation, but overall data quality remain poor.

Management of Severe COVID-19: Intensive Care Unit

- Patients who require HFNC or NIV should be treated with remdesivir, dexamethasone 6 mg/d, and either tocilizumab or baricitinib.
- We favor HFNC over NIV, given the risks of lung injury with NIV, but data are limited.
- The timing of intubation remains unclear and has varied over the course of the pandemic. Recent studies suggest a protective benefit to early intubation (first 24 hours) over delayed intubation (>48 hours) after intensive care unit (ICU) admission for patients on HFNC or NIV with clinical worsening. Monitoring of patients for work of breathing and risk for patient self-inflicted lung injury (P-SILI) should also inform the timing of intubation.
- Intubated patients should be treated with dexamethasone 6 mg/d and either tocilizumab or baricitinib. Remdesivir is not indicated unless concern for immunocompromise or persistent viral replication.
- Patients in the ICU have an increased risk of bleeding, and prophylaxis dose anticoagulation is currently recommended.
- We typically advocate for standard acute respiratory distress syndrome (ARDS) ventilator management for patients intubated for COVID-19. This includes low tidal volume ventilation of 4 to 8 mL/kg ideal body weight, target plateau pressure <30 cm H_2O, driving pressure <15, and a conservative fluid strategy. We titrate positive end-expiratory pressure (PEEP) based on a best PEEP trial of oxygenation and compliance, and use prone positioning in patients with a PO_2/FIO_2 <150.
- It has been proposed that there are different presentations of COVID-19 ARDS, with a "type L" characterized by high lung compliance, low ventilation to perfusion ratio suggestive of a possible vasoregulation defect, and low recruitability, and a "type H" phenotype with more inflammatory edema and decreased compliance and high right-to-left shunt. Data demonstrating that targeting these subtypes with different mechanical ventilation strategies impacts outcomes are lacking.
- There is insufficient evidence to support the routine use of ECMO in COVID-19 ARDS. We use venovenous (VV) ECMO in refractory hypoxemia, consistent with our standard ARDS approach. Age >65 and a duration of mechanical ventilation >10 days are associated with poor outcomes.

Long COVID

- The National Academies of Sciences, Engineering, and Medicine have recently defined long COVID as "an infection associated chronic condition that occurs after SARS-CoV-2 infection and is persistent for at 3 months as a continuous, relapsing and remitting or progressive disease state that affects one or more organs."
- It can occur after asymptomatic, mild, or severe SARS-CoV-2 infection.
- Symptoms are diffuse and include fatigue, dyspnea, chest pain, cough, muscle weakness, myalgias, psychological symptoms, and cognitive dysfunction. Symptoms can occur during infection or have a delayed onset weeks or months after infection. There may be significant overlap with post–intensive care syndrome in patients who have recovered from severe COVID-19.
- Studies have also demonstrated a higher risk for autoimmune inflammatory rheumatic diseases in those with COVID-19 compared to controls. Persistent cardiac events, imaging abnormalities, and clotting risk are also present up to a year after infection.

SUGGESTED READING

Baumann Kreuziger L, Sholzberg M, Cushman M. Anticoagulation in hospitalized patients with COVID-19. *Blood.* 2022;140(8):809-814.

COVID-19 Treatment Guidelines Panel. *Coronavirus Disease 2019 (COVID-19) Treatment Guidelines.* National Institutes of Health. https://www.ncbi.nlm.nih.gov/books/NBK570371/pdf/Bookshelf_NBK570371.pdf.

Meyerowitz EA, Scott J, Richterman A, et al. Clinical course and management of COVID-19 in the era of widespread population immunity. *Nat Rev Microbiol.* 2024;22:75-88.

Steiner S, Kratzel A, Barut GT, et al. SARS-CoV-2 biology and host interactions. *Nat Rev Microbiol.* 2024;22:206-225.

Wesley Ely E, Brown LM, Fineberg HV. Long COVID defined. *N Engl J Med.* 2024;391:1-8.

3.12

Pleural Disease

Raghu R. Chivukula

Overview

- Pleural diseases are common in critical care and most often present as *pleural effusion* or *pneumothorax*.
- Understanding the mechanisms underlying pleural fluid (PF) accumulation and air leak syndromes is essential for appropriate management.

Pleural Effusion

Classification

- Pleural effusions are broadly classified according to the underlying mechanism of fluid formation and are distinguished by their PF characteristics.
- Transudates occur due to systemic factors that alter hydrostatic or oncotic pressures, without direct pleural inflammation.
- Exudates result from local pleural inflammation, infection, or malignancy, which increase pleural capillary permeability or impair lymphatic drainage.
- Diagnosis of exudative effusion depends on PF analysis.

Light's Criteria (Standard Method)

- PF/serum protein ratio >0.5
- PF/serum lactate dehydrogenase (LDH) ratio >0.6
- PF LDH >2/3 the upper limit of normal serum LDH

Heffner's Criteria (No Serum Required)

- PF protein >2.9 g/dL
- PF LDH > ~150 U/L
- **Optional:** PF cholesterol >45 mg/dL
- See Table 3.12.1 for additional details.

Transudative effusions

While all transudates reflect an alteration in transpleural pressure gradient, a number of distinct mechanisms may be responsible:

- **Increased hydrostatic pressure**
    - **Representative conditions:** congestive heart failure (most common)
    - **Key features:** bilateral effusions (70%), occasionally unilateral; may appear as "false exudate" after diuresis; albumin gradient >1.2 g/dL supports transudate.
- **Decreased oncotic pressure**
    - **Representative conditions:** nephrotic syndrome, hypoalbuminemia
    - **Key features:** low serum albumin (<2.0 g/dL) and total protein; bilateral, symmetric effusions
- Pressure gradient via diaphragmatic defects
    - **Representative conditions:** hepatic hydrothorax, peritoneal dialysis
    - **Key features:** often right sided
- Abnormal fluid tract or leak
    - **Representative conditions:** urinothorax
    - **Key features:** the only low pH transudate (PF:serum creatinine ratio >1)

Management

- Transudates usually resolve with treatment of the underlying systemic disease.
- Thoracentesis is reserved for diagnostic uncertainty or symptomatic relief.

Exudative effusions

In the intensive care unit (ICU) setting, highest concern is typically for inflammatory or infectious etiologies, most commonly in the setting of known or suspected pneumonia (parapneumonic effusions). The severity of inflammatory/infectious exudates is further stratified by PF and ultrasonographic features:

- Uncomplicated parapneumonic effusion
    - Sterile fluid associated with pneumonia or lung inflammation
    - **PF:** pH >7.2, glucose >60 mg/dL, LDH <1,000 U/L
    - **Ultrasound findings:** typically simple fluid
    - **Management:** antibiotics alone; no drainage required
- Complicated parapneumonic effusion
    - **PF:** pH <7.2 or glucose <60 mg/dL; often loculated or turbid
    - **Ultrasound findings:** may exhibit loculation, septation, or visible debris
    - **Management:** chest-tube drainage in addition to antibiotics
- **Empyema**
    - Pus or positive Gram stain/culture in the pleural space
    - Ultrasound/thoracentesis findings: thick, foul smelling, with debris and loculation
    - Management
        - Broad-spectrum antibiotics
        - Small-bore, "pigtail" (10-14F) chest-tube drainage is often adequate.

TABLE 3.12.1 Transudative Versus Exudative Pleural Effusions

Feature	Transudate	Exudate
Mechanism	Systemic (hydrostatic/oncotic imbalance)	Local inflammation or impaired drainage
PF/serum protein ratio	<0.5	>0.5
PF/serum LDH ratio	<0.6	>0.6
PF LDH	<2/3 ULN	>2/3 ULN
PF appearance	Clear, straw colored	Cloudy, turbid, or purulent
Representative causes	CHF, hepatic hydrothorax, nephrotic syndrome	Pneumonia, malignancy, TB, PE

CHF, congestive heart failure; LDH, lactate dehydrogenase; PE, pulmonary embolism; PF, pleural fluid; TB, tuberculosis; ULN, upper limit of normal.

TABLE 3.12.2 Exudative Effusions

Category	Examples	Notes
Thromboembolic	Pulmonary embolism	Small; resolves with anticoagulation
Malignant	Metastatic carcinoma, mesothelioma	Often recurrent; management may involve pleurodesis or indwelling catheter
Inflammatory/autoimmune	Rheumatoid pleuritis, lupus pleuritis	Distinct biochemical signatures (RA: low glucose, low pH)
Tuberculous	TB pleuritis	Lymphocyte predominant; ADA elevated (>40 U/L)

ADA, adenosine deaminase; RA, rheumatoid arthritis; TB, tuberculosis.

- **Intrapleural fibrinolytics:** tissue plasminogen activator (tPA) (10 mg) + DNase (5 mg) twice daily × 3 days improves drainage and reduces surgical referral.
- Surgical consultation for persistent sepsis or incomplete evacuation

- Less common exudative effusions in the ICU are shown in Table 3.12.2.

Pneumothorax

Classification

- Spontaneous
  - **Primary**—no known lung disease (commonest in tall, thin young men)
  - **Secondary**—underlying lung disease (chronic obstructive pulmonary disease [COPD], Pneumocystis infection)
- **Traumatic:** penetrating/blunt chest trauma or iatrogenic (central line, barotrauma)
- **Tension:** progressive air trapping with mediastinal shift and shock

Diagnosis and Imaging

- Ultrasound
  - **Normal lung:** "seashore sign" on M-mode ultrasound
  - **Pneumothorax:** absence of lung sliding; "Barcode sign" on M-mode ultrasound

TABLE 3.12.3 Pneumothorax Management

Type	Initial Management	Definitive/Recurrent Management
Small, stable PSP	Observation, supplemental O_2	Repeat imaging; outpatient follow-up
Large (>2 cm) or symptomatic PSP	Needle aspiration or small-bore chest tube	Recurrence prevention after second event (pleurodesis vs surgery)
Secondary SP	Small-bore chest tube	Surgical pleurodesis at first event
Tension pneumothorax	*Immediate needle decompression* → chest tube	Treat empirically; do not delay for imaging.

PSP, primary spontaneous pneumothorax; SP, spontaneous pneumothorax.

- **Computed tomography (CT) or upright chest x-ray (CXR):** used when uncertain or for basilar pneumothorax (which may be more challenging to evaluate with ultrasound)

Management

See Table 3.12.3 for additional details.

Persistent Air Leak and Bronchopleural Fistula

- **Definition:** ongoing air leak >5–7 days due to alveolar-pleural or bronchopleural communication
- **Management**
  - Optimize drainage and suction (−20 to −40 cm H_2O)
  - Lower airway pressures on ventilator
  - Endobronchial valves, blood patch, or surgery for persistent leaks

SUGGESTED READINGS

Light RW. *Pleural Diseases*. 6th ed. Wolters Kluwer; 2013.

Rahman NM, Maskell NA, West A, et al. Intrapleural use of tissue plasminogen activator and DNase in pleural infection. *N Engl J Med*. 2011;365(6):518-526.

3.13

Hemoptysis

Raymond C. Parrish and Fayez Kheir

Key Points

- Hemoptysis is the expectoration of blood originating from the lower respiratory tract.
- Historically, hemoptysis has been subdivided as either massive (as >150 mL in a 24-hour period) or submassive based on the volume of blood expectorated per unit time. However, a more clinically relevant definition is based on consequences, including impairment of gas exchange, impact on hemodynamics, and/or airway obstruction, which is useful for clinical decision-making.
- Massive hemoptysis is associated with a high mortality rate approaching 30%, though mortality varies significantly by etiology. Death from hemoptysis is most often due to asphyxia rather than the hemodynamic consequence of hemorrhage.
- The course and tempo of further blood loss in a patient presenting with hemoptysis can be unpredictable; thus, prompt evaluation is key. Life-threatening hemoptysis is best addressed by a multidisciplinary team consisting of specialists in critical care, pulmonology, thoracic surgery, radiology, and anesthesiology.

- Medical management of the causative etiology when possible is preferred. In refractory cases and/or those that present in a life-threatening manner, treatment often consists of one or a combination of bronchoscopic interventions, angiography with embolization, or, rarely, surgical resection.

Etiology

- The vast majority (90%) of hemoptysis originates from neovascularization arising from the bronchial circulation (a high-pressure circuit), with the remainder coming primarily from the pulmonary circulation (a low-pressure circuit).
- Rarely, hemoptysis may originate from aberrant communication between other systemic vessels and the airway tree or pulmonary parenchyma.

Differential Diagnosis

- Infection
  - *Mycobacterial* spp. infection (most commonly *Mycobacterium tuberculosis*)
  - Bacterial pneumonia or bronchitis
  - Fungal infection (including *Aspergillus* spp.)
  - Parasitic infection (most commonly *Paragonimus westermani*)
  - Rarely viral infection (eg, herpes simplex virus pneumonia)
- Malignancy
  - Bronchogenic carcinoma
  - Small cell lung cancer
  - Non–small cell lung cancer
  - Carcinoid tumor
  - Metastases from non-lung primary malignancies
- Airway diseases
  - Bronchiectasis
  - Chronic bronchitis
  - Foreign body aspiration
  - Inhalational injury (such as cocaine use or E-cigarette or Vaping product use-Associated Lung Injury [EVALI])
  - Vascular malformation in or communicating with the airways
- Coagulopathy
  - Acquired due to anticoagulation or antiplatelet medication
  - Acquired due to comorbid conditions (ie, liver disease or renal failure)
  - Primary disorders of coagulation or platelet function
- Elevated pulmonary capillary pressures
  - Pulmonary embolism
  - Pulmonary hypertension
  - Decompensated heart failure
  - Mitral stenosis
- Pulmonary capillaritis (often manifest as diffuse alveolar hemorrhage)
  - Granulomatosis with polyangiitis
  - Anti-glomerular basement membrane (GBM) disease
  - Systemic lupus erythematosus
  - Antiphospholipid antibody syndrome
- Pseudohemoptysis
  - Upper respiratory tract (eg, epistaxis or pharyngeal bleeding)
  - Gastrointestinal tract (hematemesis)
  - *Serratia marcescens* pneumonia (which produces a red pigment)

Initial Evaluation and Stabilization

- Is there evidence of clinical consequence from hemoptysis (ie, tachypnea, wheezing, stridor, tachycardia, hypotension, hypoxemia, or hypercapnia)?
  - If not, can proceed with diagnostic evaluation as below with urgency (inpatient vs outpatient) determined by the duration and tempo of symptoms
  - If so, consider hemoptysis to be potentially life-threatening and proceed with stabilization measures, triage to a higher level of care, and early involvement of a multidisciplinary team, including specialists in critical care, pulmonology, thoracic surgery, radiology, and anesthesiology.
- Establish intravenous access and place the patient on continuous pulse oximetry and cardiac monitoring.
- If laterality of the source of bleeding is known, the patient is able to expectorate effectively, and the patient is mentating appropriately, place the patient in lateral decubitus with the source side down. This attempts to minimize blood pooling in the unaffected lung.
- If the patient is not able to expectorate effectively and/or the patient's mental status is waning to the point that the cough reflex is diminished or absent, proceed with endotracheal intubation.
- Induction of anesthesia should be undertaken cautiously, and agents/timing of administration should be geared toward minimizing further suppression of the cough reflex (or minimizing time to endotracheal tube insertion after the reflex is suppressed). Video laryngoscopy or fiberoptic intubation is strongly recommended to maximize first-pass success.
- Endotracheal intubation is typically best performed with a single-lumen endotracheal tube (at least size 8 mm) rather than a double-lumen endotracheal tube.
  - Double-lumen tubes do offer the potential advantage of being able to isolate the uninvolved lung from the bleeding lung. However, the smaller inner diameter of the bronchial lumens of a double-lumen tube (relative to single-lumen tubes of similar outer diameter) severely limits subsequent bronchoscopic interventions.

Diagnostic Evaluation

- Laboratory
  - All patients should have a full set of labs sent, including complete blood count, prothrombin time, partial thromboplastin time, D-dimer, liver function tests, creatinine, blood urea nitrogen, B-type natriuretic peptide, arterial blood gas, and blood culture. Sputum should be sent for bacterial Gram stain and culture, fungal culture, acid-fast bacilli (AFB) smear and culture, and cytology.
    - If practicing in an area where tuberculosis is endemic and/or patient risk factors are present, strong consideration should be given to further tuberculosis testing and appropriate isolation with airborne pathogen precautions.
  - If vasculitis is suspected, consider sending C-reactive protein (CRP), erythrocyte sedimentation rate (ESR), antinuclear antibody (ANA), anti–double-stranded DNA, antineutrophil cytoplasmic antibody (ANCA), anti-GBM, antiphospholipid testing, and a urinalysis.

  - If cardiac or pulmonary vascular cause is suspected, an electrocardiogram and echocardiogram should additionally be performed.
- Computed tomographic angiography (CTA) (only if patients are clinically stable)
  - Ideally, images should be obtained with contrast bolus in the arterial phase with multiplanar reformation to optimize the chance of distinguishing between bronchial, nonbronchial systemic, or pulmonary circulation as the origin of hemorrhage.
  - CTA of the chest has been shown to have the highest sensitivity for the localization of the source of hemoptysis of all available diagnostic tests, notably superior to that of bronchoscopy.
- Endoscopic
  - Flexible bronchoscopy can be used to directly visualize the source of bleeding (if in the large airways) or localize the source of bleeding to a bronchopulmonary segment and is preferably performed within 48 hours of hemoptysis.
  - Serial lavage with sequential instillation of aliquots of saline is the gold standard assessment for diffuse alveolar hemorrhage. If the return of serial aliquots is progressively bloodier, this confirms a diagnosis of diffuse alveolar hemorrhage.
  - Importantly, bronchoscopy can also facilitate simultaneous therapeutic intervention as detailed further below.
- Endovascular
  - Invasive angiography can be used similarly to CTA to localize the source of bleeding; however, angiography must be performed separately for the bronchial and the pulmonary circulation (if necessary).
  - Importantly, invasive angiography can also facilitate simultaneous therapeutic intervention as detailed further below.

Management

- Medications
  - Correction of coagulopathy is critical if present. However, care should be taken to avoid overly aggressive resuscitation with large volumes of blood products as increased filling pressures in the pulmonary circulation may predispose to further bleeding.
  - Immunosuppression is central to the treatment of vasculitis, with intravenous (IV) corticosteroids being the fastest acting option (eg, IV methylprednisolone 500-1,000 mg daily for up to 5 days).
  - Platelet transfusion if the patient is thrombocytopenic is recommended; however, optimum platelet transfusion target is not well established.
  - Desmopressin (DDAVP) is beneficial for patients with uremic platelet dysfunction (IV or subcutaneously [SQ] DDAVP 0.3-0.4 μg/kg once).
  - If the patient is taking an anticoagulant, prompt reversal has some sparse evidence of benefit and should be considered.
  - Tranexamic acid (TXA) has been shown to be beneficial when administered via nebulization (nebulized TXA 500 mg q8h for up to 5 days); however, there is less clear evidence of benefit from IV administration of TXA as compared to hemorrhage from other sites, such as obstetrical hemorrhage.
- Endoscopic
  - Approach to bronchoscopy
    - Rigid bronchoscopy is recommended for optimum visualization, ability to isolate individual bronchi, and facilitation of the use of the largest range of endoscopic tools. However, rigid bronchoscopy requires specialized training and generally can only be performed in an operating room.
    - Flexible bronchoscopy can be used for therapeutics for hemoptysis and should be considered immediately once the patient is intubated, if the patient cannot be safely moved out of an emergency department or intensive care unit, or if rigid bronchoscopy is not available.
    - Regardless of approach, bronchoscopy uniquely allows for therapeutic aspiration of clotted blood, which may be useful in cases where gas exchange is already impaired prior to the procedure.
  - Topical agents
    - Iced normal saline
    - Epinephrine (use with caution given ventricular arrhythmia risk)
    - TXA
  - Balloon tamponade
    - Via purpose-made endobronchial blocker
    - Alternatively, a Fogarty catheter can be utilized and taped in place along the endotracheal tube; however, these are prone to unintentional migration.
  - Advanced tools
    - Endobronchial covered stents and one-way endobronchial valves have been successfully utilized to "jail off" a source of bleeding and may have particular utility in malignant causes of hemoptysis.
    - Thermal therapies such as electrocautery, argon plasma coagulation, or laser have been shown to stop airway bleeding successfully and durably; however, these technologies necessitate lowering of FIO_2 to minimize the risk of airway fire. Microwave ablation for bleeding tumor is an alternative option and does not require lowering FIO_2. However, such technologies require specialized equipment and training for safe use, which may limit their generalizable utility.
    - Absorbable hemostatic agents (such as oxidized regenerated cellulose) and fibrin or cyanoacrylate glues are also being used to tamponade bleeding and promote clot formation via an endobronchial approach.
- Endovascular
  - Approach
    - Invasive angiography, similar to bronchoscopy, has the benefit of providing an opportunity for diagnosis and treatment in a single procedure.
    - Bronchial artery embolization has a high success rate in achieving immediate and durable hemostasis.
  - Embolization tools
    - Gelfoam
    - Microspheres
    - Coils
  - Stenting
    - In cases where a vessel has been eroded (such as by a tumor) or disrupted (such as following a biopsy or trauma), endovascular stenting with a covered

stent has been reported in bronchial, nonbronchial systemic, and pulmonary circulation with resultant cessation of hemorrhage.

- Surgery
  - Surgical resection for hemoptysis, while often definitive in achieving control of the source of hemorrhage, carries a significant risk of morbidity and mortality (estimated at 6%-35%). There is some evidence to suggest that emergent resection, in particular, carries a higher relative risk of mortality compared to nonemergent resection.
  - Often, patients presenting with hemoptysis have not or cannot be evaluated for their ability to tolerate lung resection with pulmonary function testing, which makes prognostication additionally challenging.
  - Surgical resection should, therefore, be reserved for those patients with hemoptysis refractory to medical, bronchoscopic, and endovascular therapy, or for patients who are otherwise quite healthy for whom surgical resection would provide a definitive and/or curative solution.

SUGGESTED READINGS

Abdulmalak C, Cottenet J, Beltramo G, et al. Haemoptysis in adults: a 5-year study using the French nationwide hospital administrative database. *Eur Respir J*. 2015;46(2):503-511.

Bruzzi JF, Rémy-Jardin M, Delhaye D, Teisseire A, Khalil C, Rémy J. Multi–detector row CT of hemoptysis. *RadioGraphics*. 2006;26(1):3-22.

Collard HR, Schwarz MI. Diffuse alveolar hemorrhage. *Clin Chest Med*. 2004;25(3):583-592.

Cordovilla R, Bollo De Miguel E, Nuñez Ares A, Cosano Povedano FJ, Herráez Ortega I, Jiménez Merchán R. Diagnóstico y tratamiento de la hemoptisis [Diagnosis and treatment of hemoptysis]. *Arch Bronconeumol*. 2016;52(7):368-377.

Fartoukh M, Khoshnood B, Parrot A, et al. Early prediction of in-hospital mortality of patients with hemoptysis: an approach to defining severe hemoptysis. *Respiration*. 2012;83(2):106-114.

Gesthalter Y, Kheir F. Hemoptysis. In: Broaddus VC, Schnapp LM, Stapleton RD, Murray JF, Nadel JA, eds. *Murray and Nadel's Textbook of Respiratory Medicine*. 7th ed. Elsevier; 2022.

Hirshberg B, Biran I, Glazer M, Kramer MR. Hemoptysis: etiology, evaluation, and outcome in a tertiary referral hospital. *Chest*. 1997;112(2):440-444.

Ibrahim WH. Massive haemoptysis: the definition should be revised. *Eur Respir J*. 2008;32(4):1131-1132.

Jean-Baptiste E. Clinical assessment and management of massive hemoptysis. *Crit Care Med*. 2000;28(5):1642-1647.

Khalil A, Soussan M, Mangiapan G, Fartoukh M, Parrot A, Carette MF. Utility of high-resolution chest CT scan in the emergency management of haemoptysis in the intensive care unit: severity, localization and aetiology. *Br J Radiol*. 2007;80(949):21-25.

Knott-Craig CJ, Oostuizen JG, Rossouw G, Joubert JR, Barnard PM. Management and prognosis of massive hemoptysis. Recent experience with 120 patients. *J Thorac Cardiovasc Surg*. 1993;105(3):394-397.

Mal H, Rullon I, Mellot F, et al. Immediate and long-term results of bronchial artery embolization for life-threatening hemoptysis. *Chest*. 1999;115(4):996-1001.

Mondoni M, Carlucci P, Cipolla G, et al. Bronchoscopy to assess patients with hemoptysis: which is the optimal timing? *BMC Pulm Med*. 2019;19(1):36.

Mondoni M, Carlucci P, Job S, et al. Observational, multicentre study on the epidemiology of haemoptysis. *Eur Respir J*. 2018;51(1):1701813.

Ong TH, Eng P. Massive hemoptysis requiring intensive care. *Intensive Care Med*. 2003;29(2):317-320.

Razazi K, Parrot A, Khalil A, et al. Severe haemoptysis in patients with nonsmall cell lung carcinoma. *Eur Respir J*. 2015;45(3):756-764.

Tsoumakidou M, Chrysofakis G, Tsiligianni I, Maltezakis G, Siafakas NM, Tzanakis N. A prospective analysis of 184 hemoptysis cases—diagnostic impact of chest x-ray, computed tomography, bronchoscopy. *Respiration*. 2006;73(6):808-814.

3.14

Upper Airway Diseases and Disorders

Annette A. Wang and Phillip Song

- The upper airway includes multiple anatomic spaces above the trachea, including the nasal cavity, nasopharynx, oral cavity, oropharynx, and larynx.
- Obstruction, swelling, and anatomic distortion of the upper airway can result in difficult mask ventilation and intubation.
- Presentation and physical examination findings can vary, and specialized examinations with flexible endoscopy (nasopharyngoscopy, laryngoscopy, and bronchoscopy) may be necessary for diagnosis and treatment.
- An important consideration in the critical care environment is recognizing potential upper airway complications and planning for adjunct methods of securing the airway.

Key Elements of History and Physical Examination

- The functions of the upper airway are respiration, deglutination, and voice/speech production.
- The head and neck examination should include a thorough examination of the nasal and oral cavity, oropharynx, larynx, voice and speech assessment, and a complete cranial nerve examination.
- The review of symptoms should include voice, swallowing, and breathing complaints.
- Speech changes suggest problems in the oral cavity and oropharynx.
  - Swelling of the base of tongue and pharynx results in a muffled sound or "hot potato" voice quality.
    - Examples include peritonsillar abscess, epiglottitis, Ludwig angina, and neoplasms of the tongue and tonsils.
  - Stertor describes a wet, gurgling sound from the pharynx during breathing and is often related to problems in the oral cavity and oropharynx associated with swallowing and speech symptoms.
    - Tongue and tonsillar swelling from angioedema can also result in stertor.

- The vocal folds provide the sound source for voice production; hoarseness could indicate a laryngeal abnormality.
- Velopharyngeal insufficiency can result in airflow through the nose during speech and is often associated with nasal regurgitation and problems with pharyngeal function.
  - Cerebrovascular accidents and tumors of the pharynx or skull base are potential causes of acquired velopharyngeal insufficiency.
  - Cleft palate is the most common congenital cause of velopharyngeal insufficiency.
- Inspiratory stridor is the result of narrowing or obstruction at the larynx or supraglottis.
- Expiratory stridor usually indicates narrowing below the larynx.
- Trismus can result from spasms of the mastication muscles or limitation in movement in the temporomandibular joint.
  - Typically, an interincisor distance of <3.5 cm is considered trismus.

Risk Factors for Upper Airway Problems

- Head and neck cancers
- Facial and cervical trauma
- Skull base and central nervous system (CNS) tumors
- Radiation treatment
- Smoking, tobacco, and substance abuse
- Surgery for temporomandibular joint, sinuses/septum, tonsils/adenoids, sleep apnea, thyroid, carotid vessels, and anterior cervical spine
- Cardiac, thoracic, and esophageal surgery due to the anatomic path of the recurrent laryngeal nerves

Endoscopic Examination of the Upper Airway

- Nasopharyngoscopy is an important tool to examine the nasal cavity, pharynx, base of tongue, and larynx.
- Elements of nasopharyngoscopy include examination of velopharyngeal movement, assessment of the upper airway spaces (especially the oropharyngeal and supraglottic airway), and vocal fold movement.

Common Problems of the Upper Airway

Oral Cavity

Trauma

- Significant oral trauma includes facial fractures and dental damage, which can result in difficult mask ventilation and airway control.
- Careful assessment of the stability of the fractures, especially for the midface and mandible, and a nasopharyngoscopy to evaluate the upper airway examination are essential for safe management.

Angioedema

- Angioedema is a localized submucosal swelling of fluid into interstitial tissue that most typically involves the mouth, lips, tongue, and throat.
- Self-limiting over 24 to 48 hours; however, may result in airway distress
  - *Mast cell–mediated or histaminergic angioedema* is the result of allergy with release of histamine, resulting in urticaria, pruritus, flushing, edema, and bronchospasm.
  - *Bradykinin-induced angioedema* is commonly seen with angiotensin-converting enzyme (ACE) inhibitors and results in swelling without significant urticaria or bronchospasm.
  - *Hereditary angioedema secondary to C1 inhibitor deficiency* is a rare cause of angioedema, which can lead to upper airway swelling, precipitous airway closures, and asphyxiation.
    - Diagnosis is based on complement testing.

Ludwig Angina

- Ludwig angina is an infection of the floor of mouth, involving the confluent submandibular, sublingual, and submental spaces, that typically arises from an odontogenic or salivary gland infection.
- It is Often a polymicrobial infection that is treated with broad-spectrum antibiotics and careful airway monitoring
- Physical examination findings include thickening and woody induration of the floor of mouth, severe tongue swelling, and edema extending back toward the base of tongue, resulting in upper airway obstruction, drooling, dysphagia, speech changes, and stertor.
- Transoral access is difficult, so nasal intubation or tracheostomy may be necessary.

Oropharynx

- The oropharynx is composed of the base of tongue, pharyngeal walls, tonsils, and soft palate.

Oropharyngeal Dysphagia

- The primary function of the oropharynx is to safely deliver food into the esophagus by contracting the base of tongue, squeezing the pharyngeal muscles, elevating the larynx, and opening the upper esophageal sphincter through the relaxation of the cricopharyngeus muscle.
- Unlike the oral phase of swallowing, which is controlled by the jaw, teeth, and anterior two-thirds of the tongue, the oropharyngeal muscles play a significant role in initiating the involuntary or autonomic swallow.
- The incidence of oropharyngeal dysphagia is very high, especially in older adults, head and neck cancer, neurologic disease, in the critical care setting, and after prolonged intubation.
- Diagnosis is based on videofluoroscopic modified barium swallow or a flexible endoscopic examination of swallowing (FEES) with nasopharyngoscopy.
  - *Penetration* describes food or liquid entering the level of the glottis, below the vocal folds. Patients are at high risk for aspiration when penetration is seen in swallowing studies.
  - *Aspiration* describes food or liquid below the vocal folds into the trachea and upper airway. Patients are at high risk of developing aspiration pneumonia and pulmonary complications.
  - *Silent aspiration* occurs when there is no attempt to cough or expel the aspirated contents. Silent aspiration can occur after prolonged intubation and with advanced pulmonary disease.

- Early recognition and intervention are important, and consultation with speech language pathology and swallowing therapist for a clinical swallowing assessment should be performed early.

Infections of the Oropharynx

- Tonsillitis and peritonsillar abscesses
    - Peritonsillar abscesses can occur as a complication of regular tonsillitis.
        - The abscess is deep to the capsule of the tonsils and between the pharyngeal muscles and can spread into the deeper layers of the neck. Predominant bacteria include group A *Streptococcus*, *Streptococcus anginosus*, *Staphylococcus aureus*, and respiratory anaerobes. Infections are frequently mixed flora. Physical examination shows an asymmetric bulge superior and lateral to the tonsil.
    - Peritonsillar cellulitis or phlegmon is an inflammatory swelling adjacent to the tonsil without a discrete abscess collection.
        - Clinically, it is difficult to distinguish between cellulitis and abscess without attempted needle drainage or imaging. Peritonsillar cellulitis can develop into an abscess requiring drainage.
    - Trismus indicates spread of the abscess and inflammation past the pharyngeal constrictors and into the masseter and pterygoid muscles.
        - Diagnosis can be made with a computed tomography (CT) scan, transoral ultrasound, or an exploratory needle or incisional drainage attempt. Complications include airway swelling as well as spread to adjacent tissue layers and deeper neck planes, including the retropharyngeal space and parapharyngeal space. Treatment is incisional drainage and appropriate antibiotics.
- Parapharyngeal and retropharyngeal space infections
    - Deep neck space infections can cause airway distress and dysphagia.
    - Parapharyngeal space infections can show a bulge on the tonsils and lateral pharyngeal wall with lateral neck swelling.
    - Retropharyngeal space infections can lead to infections into the mediastinum and present with neck rigidity and dysphagia.

Larynx

- The functions of the larynx are to protect the lungs from aspiration, enable the transit of food and liquid into the esophagus, deliver air into the lungs, and produce voice.
- The larynx comprises the epiglottis, hyoid bone, thyroid and cricoid cartilages, arytenoid, cricoarytenoid joint, and true and false vocal folds.
- There are three distinct regions: supraglottis, glottis, and subglottis.
- Innervation of the larynx:
    - The motor supply of the larynx is through the recurrent laryngeal nerve (RLN), which branches from the vagus nerve in the neck. The RLN takes a track under the aortic arch on the left side and the subclavian artery on the right side. The nerve then ascends along the tracheoesophageal groove to enter the larynx between the cricothyroid joints.
    - The long course of the RLN makes it susceptible to injury from the skull base to thoracic conditions from tumors or iatrogenic causes.
        - Rare anatomic variations include a *right non-RLN*, which descends on the right side without looping around the subclavian artery. This variant is associated with the lack of an innominate artery and the passage of the subclavian artery behind the esophagus. A *left non-RLN* is associated with *situs inversus* and *primary ciliary dyskinesia*.
    - The superior laryngeal nerve provides most of the sensation of the larynx and coordinates swallowing and cough.

Laryngeal Fractures

- Laryngeal fractures are rare injuries involving the cartilaginous framework of the larynx—most often the thyroid cartilage, followed by the cricoid and arytenoid cartilages—but have a high mortality rate.
- One common etiology of these injuries is blunt trauma from motor vehicle accidents, though the incidence due to motor vehicle accidents has decreased with the introduction of safety features, such as seatbelts and airbags.
- The first step in management is to establish a secure airway. Early intervention (within 24-48 hours) is associated with improved functional speech, swallowing, and airway patency.

Supraglottic Diseases

- The supraglottis is the region above the vocal folds and includes the epiglottis, aryepiglottic folds, false vocal folds, and laryngeal ventricle. Autoimmune diseases such as polyangiitis, systemic lupus erythematosus, amyloid, sarcoid, and immunoglobulin G4 (IgG4RD)-related disease can involve the supraglottis.
- Epiglottitis and supraglottitis
    - *Haemophilus influenzae* type b (Hib) was the most common bacterium before widespread immunization; *S. aureus* and *streptococci* species are now more common.
    - Symptoms include sore throat, fever, difficulty swallowing, drooling, and stridor. Can progress to rapid airway obstruction from swelling
    - Associated with the "thumb sign" on lateral soft tissue neck x-ray
    - Epiglottic edema can act like a ball valve with intralaryngeal collapse from positive pressure ventilation, making intubation difficult.
- Laryngeal ventricle
    - The laryngeal ventricle is a potential space containing mucus glands and providing lubrication for the true vocal folds.
    - Laryngoceles and sacular cysts
        - Cystic swelling that enlarges within the laryngeal ventricle
            - Swelling can be seen within the false vocal fold as well as widening of the aryepiglottic fold.
        - *Internal laryngoceles* describe a cyst contained within the larynx, *external laryngoceles* spread into the lateral neck, and *combined* has both components.
        - Can enlarge within the larynx, resulting in airway compromise and voice changes
        - Can become infected, forming a laryngopyocele with extension into the deep neck spaces

Glottic Diseases

- The glottis starts at the level of the vocal folds and extends to the lower boundary of the thyroid cartilage and includes the vocal folds, arytenoid cartilage, and interarytenoid region.
- Vocal fold pathology results in voice changes and hoarseness.
  - The vocal folds, especially the posterior region of the medial arytenoid (vocal process) and interarytenoid mucosa, are susceptible to intubation injury and laryngeal stenosis.
  - Vocal fold immobility describes the inability of the vocal folds to move.
    - Unilateral vocal fold paralysis (UVFP) occurs when the mobility of a single vocal fold is impaired by neurologic injury.
      - The clinical features of UVFP are weak, breathy voice quality, early vocal fatigue, reduced cough strength, and aspiration with thin liquids. UVFP is commonly associated with surgery or malignancy, idiopathic, and neurologic disease and impacts quality of life.
      - Overall, surgical iatrogenic injury accounts for ~50% of all UVFP in adults. Of these, thyroid and parathyroid surgeries are responsible for ~1/3 of postsurgical UVFP.
    - Bilateral vocal fold paralysis and immobility result in breathing problems and stridor, while the voice is often normal.
      - Etiologies of bilateral vocal fold paralysis include iatrogenic injury (post-esophageal surgery and thyroidectomy), skull base lesions, and acute neurologic disease (myasthenia gravis and Guillain-Barré syndrome).
    - Glottic stenosis occurs when both vocal folds are unable to separate or abduct, resulting in bilateral vocal fold immobility.
      - Conditions that can result in glottic stenosis include neoplasms, radiation, rheumatologic disorders, bilateral cricoarytenoid joint fixation, posterior glottic stenosis, bilateral vocal fold paralysis, prolonged intubation, and laryngeal trauma.

Subglottic Diseases

- The subglottis is defined by the cricoid cartilage, which is the only area within the respiratory tract that is a complete ring.
- Because the subglottic airway is rigid, it is susceptible to injury from endotracheal tubes (ETTs), especially with overinflated cuffs, which can result in necrosis of the respiratory mucosa and scarring.
- Subglottic stenosis can be associated with trauma, prolonged intubation, tracheostomy, granulomatosis with polyangiitis, infection, and idiopathic subglottic stenosis.

Intubation-Related Injury and Edema

- Laryngeal injury is a frequent complication of intubation, especially with prolonged intubation in critically ill patients.
  - Though there is no consensus, potential risk factors include intubation duration, repeat intubation, ETT size, ETT type, and cuff pressures.
- The proposed mechanism of injury is that the ETT is forced into the posterior glottis by the tongue, which can lead to ulceration and formation of hypertrophic granulation tissue.
- Laryngeal intubation injury may be challenging to diagnose as patients present late in the disease course.
  - Symptoms include dysphonia, pain, dysphagia, and stridor.
  - Signs include laryngeal erythema/edema, ulcerations, granulation tissue, vocal fold immobility, and glottic or subglottic stenosis, among others.
- Diagnosis is clinical and supported by imaging.
  - Speech language therapy assessment of laryngeal function, flexible endoscopic evaluation, videofluoroscopy, and laryngeal videostroboscopy may be helpful.
  - Management strategies include corticosteroid injection, antireflux medication, granulation tissue removal, balloon dilation, vocal fold medialization, and speech and language therapy for voice and swallowing.

Tracheoesophageal Fistula

- Tracheoesophageal fistula (TEF) is a pathologic connection between the trachea and the esophagus.
- Congenital TEFs are rare and often occur with other congenital anomalies involving the heart or genitourinary systems, or as part of CHARGE syndrome or VACTERL association.
- Acquired TEFs can occur with mucosal erosion between the party wall due to prolonged endotracheal intubation, trauma, infections, or malignancy.
- TEFs result in recurrent aspiration pneumonias and require surgical management.

Summary

- Management of upper airway disorders often requires specialty consultation, including speech language pathology, respiratory therapy, and otolaryngology.
- Nasopharyngoscopy and laryngoscopy are the most common assessment tools for the upper airway, and symptoms and changes in the voice, upper airway sounds, and swallowing function should be assessed promptly.
- Difficult laryngeal exposure from narrowing, stenosis, or distortion of laryngeal landmarks can pose serious problems with securing the airway and should be documented early.
- An airway plan including adjuvant methods of oxygenation and ventilation such as high-flow nasal oxygenation, Heliox, bilevel positive airway pressure (BiPAP), supraglottic airway, and surgical airway methods should be discussed once difficult laryngeal exposure is recognized.
- Upper airway disorders have the potential to progress quickly, so early recognition is important.
- Progressive upper airway problems include epiglottitis, angioedema, oropharyngeal and laryngeal hemorrhage, anaphylaxis, laryngeal trauma, inhalation injuries, and iatrogenic injuries secondary to airway manipulation.
- Pulse oximetry is not a reliable indicator of upper airway stenosis and should not be relied upon. Typically, oxygenation will not change until the late stages of airway compromise. Similarly, pulmonary function testing is not a surrogate for the upper airway examination.

SUGGESTED READINGS

American Gastroenterological Association medical position statement on management of oropharyngeal dysphagia. *Gastroenterology*. 1999;116(2): 452-454.

Brodsky MB, Levy MJ, Jedlanek E, et al. Laryngeal injury and upper airway symptoms after oral endotracheal intubation with mechanical ventilation during critical care. *Crit Care Med*. 2018;46(12):2010-2017.

Hartl DM, Crevier-Buchman L, Vaissière J, Brasnu DF. Phonetic effects of paralytic dysphonia. *Ann Otol Rhinol Laryngol*. 2005;114(10):792-798.

Pinho CMR, Jesus LMT, Barney A. Aerodynamic measures of speech in unilateral vocal fold paralysis (UVFP) patients. *Logoped Phoniatr Vocol*. 2012;38(1):19-34.

Shah RK, Roberson DW, Jones DT. Epiglottitis in the Haemophilus influenzae type B vaccine era: changing trends. *Laryngoscope*. 2004; 114(3):557-560.

Skoretz SA, Flowers HL, Martino R. The incidence of dysphagia following endotracheal intubation. *Chest*. 2010;137(3):665-673.

Tovar Padua LJ, Cherry JD. Croup (laryngitis, laryngotracheitis, spasmodic croup, laryngotracheobronchitis, bacterial tracheitis, and laryngotracheobronchopneumonitis) and epiglottitis (supraglottitis). In: Cherry JD, Harrison GJ, Kaplan SL, Steinbach WJ, Hotez PJ, eds. *Feigin and Cherry's Textbook of Pediatric Infectious Diseases*. 8th ed. Vol 1. Elsevier; 2019:175.

3.15

Pulmonary Vasculitic and Autoinflammatory Disorders

Raghu R. Chivukula

General Principles

- A number of autoinflammatory conditions can affect the lung parenchyma and/or vasculature. A subset of such conditions can present acutely or with rapid escalation in severity, leading to intensive care unit (ICU) admission. It is, therefore, important for all intensive care physicians to maintain an index of suspicion for such diagnoses, even though each is individually rare as compared to other forms of respiratory failure, such as pneumonia, pulmonary edema, and acute respiratory distress syndrome (ARDS). Pulmonology and/or rheumatology consultation should be obtained if concern is raised for these entities.
- As lung biopsy is rarely available to establish these diagnoses unequivocally, management frequently depends on a combination of clinical history, computed tomographic (CT) imaging, serologic testing, and bronchoscopy. A unifying feature of several small-vessel disorders of the lung that affect the alveolar circulation is diffuse alveolar hemorrhage (DAH). DAH need not be diffuse with regard to the involved lung but rather implies an alveolar source of bleeding. The diagnosis of DAH is established by bronchoscopy and serial bronchoalveolar lavage (BAL) revealing progressive increase in bloody secretions (and implying an alveolar rather than an airway source of bleeding). DAH may reflect "bland" etiologies (eg, heart failure, anticoagulation) or, conversely, an inflammatory "capillaritis"—distinguishing these requires diagnostic evaluation as outlined for specific disease entities below.

Antineutrophil Cytoplasmic Antibody–Associated Vasculitis

Granulomatosis With Polyangiitis

Clinical Presentation/Imaging

- Chronic sinusitis, nasal septum perforation, otitis media
- Cough, hemoptysis; *cavitating nodules on CT* or nodules on chest x-ray; DAH
- Renal involvement: rapidly progressive (RP) *glomerulonephritis*

Epidemiology

- Peak onset age 40 to 60 years; slight male predominance
- Incidence ~10 to 20 per million/year in North America/ Europe

Diagnostics

- *PR3-ANCA (antineutrophil cytoplasmic antibody)* positive in ~75% of cases
- CT of the chest showing nodules and cavitation
- Biopsy (sinus or lung): necrotizing granulomatous vasculitis

Therapy

- Induction: rituximab + glucocorticoids (Stone et al. 2010)
- Maintenance: azathioprine or rituximab (Yates et al. 2016)

Microscopic Polyangiitis

Clinical Presentation/Imaging

- DAH: dyspnea, new infiltrates on chest x-ray or ground-glass opacities on CT, falling hemoglobin
- Renal: pauci-immune *necrotizing glomerulonephritis* without granulomas

Epidemiology

- Median onset ~50 years; no strong sex bias
- Incidence ~10 per million/year

Diagnostics

- *MPO-ANCA* positive in ~60%
- Bronchoscopy with BAL
- Renal biopsy confirms pauci-immune necrotizing glomerulonephritis.

Therapy

- Induction: cyclophosphamide or rituximab + steroids
- Maintenance: azathioprine, methotrexate, or rituximab

Eosinophilic Granulomatosis With Polyangiitis

Clinical Presentation/Imaging

- Adult-onset asthma, marked peripheral *eosinophilia*
- Pulmonary infiltrates; transient opacities on CT
- Mononeuritis multiplex

Epidemiology

- Mean onset ~40 years; equal sex distribution
- Incidence ~1 to 4 per million/year

Diagnostics

- Complete blood count (CBC): eosinophils >1.5 × 10^9/L
- *MPO-ANCA positive in ~40%, immunoglobulin E (IgE) typically elevated*
- Tissue biopsy (skin or nerve): eosinophil-rich granulomatous vasculitis

Therapy

- Mepolizumab for relapsing/refractory disease
- Cyclophosphamide + steroids for severe manifestations

Anti-Glomerular Basement Membrane Disease (Goodpasture Syndrome)

Clinical Presentation/Imaging

- Hemoptysis and DAH with bilateral infiltrates
- Rapidly progressive *renal failure*

Epidemiology

- Bimodal peaks at 20 to 30 and 60 to 70 years
- Incidence ~1 per million/year

Diagnostics

- Serum *anti-glomerular basement membrane (GBM) antibody* assay (ELISA)
- Renal biopsy: linear IgG/C3 deposition on GBM

Therapy

- Plasma exchange ×14 days + high-dose steroids + cyclophosphamide (Levy et al. 2001)

Immune Complex Vasculitides

System Lupus Erythematosus–Associated Pulmonary Capillaritis

Clinical Presentation/Imaging

- DAH: hemoptysis, anemia, new bilateral infiltrates on chest x-ray or CT
- Typically in patients with other manifestations of *systemic lupus erythematosus (SLE)*

Epidemiology

- Predominantly women (F:M ≈ 9:1); onset 15 to 45 years

Diagnostics

- *High-titer antinuclear antibody (ANA)* and anti–double-strand DNA
- Bronchoscopy with BAL to exclude infection

Therapy

- High-dose steroids ± cyclophosphamide (Zamora et al. 1997)

Immunoglobulin A Vasculitis (Henoch-Schönlein)

Clinical Presentation/Imaging

- Palpable purpura, arthralgias; rare DAH with bilateral infiltrates

Epidemiology

- Peak in children; adult cases more severe

Diagnostics

- Skin or renal biopsy: *IgA deposition*
- Exclude other causes of capillaritis

Therapy

- Supportive care; steroids for severe pulmonary hemorrhage

Medium- and Large-Vessel Vasculitides

Behçet Disease

Clinical Presentation/Imaging

- *Recurrent oral/genital ulcers, uveitis*
- Pulmonary artery aneurysms → massive hemoptysis; computed tomographic angiogram (CTA) shows aneurysms.

Epidemiology

- Young adults 20 to 40 years; more severe in males
- Prevalence 10 to 20 per 100,000 in endemic areas (Turkey and neighboring regions in particular)

Diagnostics

- International Criteria for Behçet's Disease clinical criteria
- CTA for pulmonary vessels

Therapy

- High-dose glucocorticoids + cyclophosphamide
- Tumor necrosis factor-alpha (TNF-α) inhibitors (infliximab) for refractory cases (Seyahi et al. 2015)

Takayasu Arteritis

Clinical Presentation/Imaging

- Constitutional symptoms
- *Pulmonary artery stenosis* causing dyspnea/pulmonary hypertension

Epidemiology

- Women of childbearing age; prevalence ~1 to 2 per million

Diagnostics

- Elevated erythrocyte sedimentation rate/C-reactive protein (ESR/CRP)
- CTA or magnetic resonance angiogram (MRA) demonstrating large-vessel involvement

Therapy

- High-dose steroids
- Methotrexate or azathioprine as steroid-sparing agents

Polyarteritis Nodosa

Clinical Presentation/Imaging

- Systemic symptoms; rare bronchial artery involvement with hemoptysis; CT may show *bronchial artery enlargement.*
- Associated with *hepatitis B virus (HBV) infection*

Epidemiology

- Adults 40 to 60 years; incidence ~2 to 9 per million/year

Diagnostics

- HBV serology
- Biopsy of the affected organ

Therapy

- Steroids + cyclophosphamide; antiviral therapy if HBV associated

Cytokine Storm Syndromes

Hemophagocytic Lymphohistiocytosis

Clinical Presentation/Imaging

- *Fevers*, cytopenias, hyperferritinemia
- *ARDS* and capillary leak; chest imaging shows diffuse bilateral ground-glass opacities.
- *Distributive shock* that can mimic septic shock

Epidemiology

- Primary/genetic in infants; secondary in adults (infection, malignancy)

Diagnostics

- HLH-2004 criteria (fever, splenomegaly, ferritin >500 μg/L, etc)
- Soluble interleukin-2 (IL-2) receptor level
- Bone marrow biopsy: hemophagocytosis
- Epstein-Barr virus (EBV), cytomegalovirus (CMV) serologies, and viral testing

Therapy

- Etoposide + dexamethasone; treat underlying trigger (Henter et al. 2007).
- Management of ARDS with lung-protective ventilation

Macrophage Activation Syndrome

Clinical Presentation/Imaging

- Similar to hemophagocytic lymphohistiocytosis (HLH) in systemic juvenile idiopathic arthritis/adult-onset Still disease (sJIA/AOSD); ARDS with bilateral infiltrates
- Distributive shock that can mimic septic shock

Epidemiology

- Children with sJIA; rare in adults with AOSD

Diagnostics

- Ferritin >684 ng/mL, cytopenias, elevated aspartate aminotransferase (AST)/triglycerides
- Exclude sepsis

Therapy

- High-dose steroids; anakinra for refractory cases (Grom et al. 2016)

Myositis-Related Interstitial Lung Disease

Anti-Aminoacyl tRNA synthetase Syndromes

Clinical Presentation/Imaging

- RP respiratory failure with dyspnea and hypoxemia
- High-resolution CT (HRCT): bilateral ground-glass opacities, consolidation, and traction bronchiectasis
- Systemic features: myalgias, mechanic's hands, Raynaud phenomenon

Epidemiology

- Onset typically in 40s to 50s; slight female predominance
- Incidence ~1 to 2 per 100,000

Diagnostics

- Myositis panel: anti–Jo-1 and other antisynthetase antibodies

- Pulmonary function tests: restrictive pattern with reduced diffusing capacity of the lungs for carbon monoxide (DLCO)
- Lung biopsy if unclear: interstitial pneumonia with inflammatory infiltrates

Therapy

- High-dose corticosteroids for acute interstitial lung disease (ILD) flares
- Immunosuppression: cyclophosphamide or rituximab (per consensus statements)
- Consider lung transplant evaluation

Anti–MDA5 Rapidly Progressive Interstitial Lung Disease

Clinical Presentation/Imaging

- RP respiratory failure with severe hypoxemia; most patients develop ILD within weeks.
- HRCT shows bilateral peripheral ground-glass opacities and perilobular consolidation, often with early traction bronchiectasis.
- "Mechanic's hands," palmar papules or ulcerations, mild rash, or arthritis may coexist (Chen et al. 2023).
- Importantly, there may not be any overt myopathy.

Epidemiology

- Median age ~50 years; slight female predominance
- Originally described in East Asian cohorts, now recognized worldwide
- 6-month survival in RP cases is ≈40% to 45%.

Diagnostics

- Serology: anti-MDA5 antibody by ELISA (often with anti-Ro52 co-positivity)
- Pulmonary workup: pulmonary function tests (PFTs) (restrictive, low DLCO) and HRCT to define pattern
- Histopathology (if needed): surgical biopsy shows diffuse alveolar damage in fulminant cases.
- Muscle evaluation: enzymes and electromyography (EMG)/biopsy may be near normal in amyopathic patients.

Therapy

- High-dose corticosteroids (eg, methylprednisolone pulses) for all patients with RP-ILD
- Combination immunosuppression: calcineurin inhibitor (tacrolimus or cyclosporine) plus cyclophosphamide is associated with improved survival in retrospective series (Gono et al. 2021).
- Rituximab for refractory or steroid-intolerant disease
- Consider lung transplant evaluation.

Drug-Induced Vasculitis

Clinical Presentation/Imaging

- DAH with diffuse infiltrates
- ANCA positivity in the context of drugs like propylthiouracil or hydralazine

Epidemiology

- Rare; associated with specific medications

Diagnostics

- Drug history review; ANCA testing
- Exclude primary vasculitis

Therapy

- Discontinue offending drug; immunosuppression if severe

SUGGESTED READINGS

Chen X, Jiang W, Jin Q, Peng Q, Zhang L, Lin S, Lu X, Liu M, Wang Y, Song A, Feng R, Wang G. Clinical, radiological and pathological features of anti-MDA5 antibody-associated interstitial lung disease. RMD Open. 2023 May;9(2):e003150. doi: 10.1136/rmdopen-2023-003150. PMID: 37258042; PMCID: PMC10255007.

Moreno-Torres V, Martín-Iglesias D, Vivero F, González-Echavarri C, García-Moyano M, Enghelmayer JI, Malfante P, Gaser A, Ruiz-Irastorza G; EPIMAR cohort Investigators. Intravenous cyclophosphamide improves functional outcomes in interstitial lung disease related to idiopathic inflammatory myopathies. Semin Arthritis Rheum. 2023 Apr;59:152164. doi: 10.1016/j.semarthrit.2023.152164. Epub 2023 Jan 11. PMID: 36773521.

Giampietro C, Ridene M, Lequerre T, Costedoat Chalumeau N, Amoura Z, Sellam J, Sibilia J, Bourgeois P, Fautrel B; CRI (Club Rhumatismes et Inflammation). Anakinra in adult-onset Still's disease: long-term treatment in patients resistant to conventional therapy. Arthritis Care Res (Hoboken). 2013 May;65(5):822-6. doi: 10.1002/acr.21901. PMID: 23225779.

Henter JI, Horne A, Aricó M, et al. HLH-2004: diagnostic and therapeutic guidelines for hemophagocytic lymphohistiocytosis. *Pediatr Blood Cancer*. 2007;48(2):124-131.

Liu Y, Jesus AA, Marrero B, et al. Activated STING in a vascular and pulmonary syndrome. *N Engl J Med*. 2014;371(6):507-518.

Stone JH, Merkel PA, Spiera R, et al. Rituximab versus cyclophosphamide for ANCA-associated vasculitis. *N Engl J Med*. 2010;363(3):221-232.

Wechsler ME, Akuthota P, Jayne D, et al. Mepolizumab or placebo for Eosinophilic Granulomatosis with Polyangiitis. *N Engl J Med*. 2017;376(20):1921-1932.

Yates M, Watts RA, Bajema IM, et al. EULAR/ERA-EDTA recommendations for the management of ANCA-associated vasculitis. *Ann Rheum Dis*. 2016;75(9):1583-1594.

Zamora MR, Warner ML, Tuder R, Schwarz MI. Diffuse alveolar hemorrhage and systemic lupus erythematosus. Clinical presentation, histology, survival, and outcome. Medicine (Baltimore). 1997 May;76(3):192-202. doi: 10.1097/00005792-199705000-00005. PMID: 9193454.

3.16

Inhalational Injuries and Tracheobronchitis in the Intensive Care Unit

Raghu R. Chivukula

Overview

- Inhalational injuries are a significant contributor to morbidity and mortality in critically ill patients, particularly those with burns, smoke exposure, or environmental/occupational accidents. They primarily involve injury to the upper and lower airways and can lead to tracheobronchitis, pulmonary edema, and acute respiratory failure.
- Tracheobronchitis in the intensive care unit (ICU) may also result from thermal, chemical, or infectious insults and often complicates mechanical ventilation. Prompt recognition and multidisciplinary management are essential.

Smoke Inhalation

Epidemiology and Pathophysiology

- Common in burn patients; up to 30% of burn victims may have concurrent smoke inhalation injury.
- Injury due to heat, particulate matter, and toxic gases (CO, cyanide, acrolein)
- Damage includes airway edema, bronchorrhea, sloughing of mucosa, and impaired mucociliary clearance.
- May cause upper airway obstruction, chemical pneumonitis, and systemic toxicity (eg, CO/CN poisoning)

Diagnostics

- Clinical signs: hoarseness, singed nasal hairs, soot in oropharynx, stridor, facial burns
- Bronchoscopy is the gold standard for airway visualization.
- Chest imaging: early may be normal; later shows infiltrates or pulmonary edema.
- Labs: COHb (carboxyhemoglobin), lactate (marker of cyanide)

Management

- Transfer to burn center for full evaluation and management
- Early intubation for airway protection in patients with progressive edema
- 100% FiO_2 for CO poisoning until COHb $<5\%$, hyperbaric oxygen can be considered
- Hydroxocobalamin for suspected cyanide toxicity
- Bronchodilators for bronchospasm. Corticosteroids have no proven benefit.
- Pulmonary hygiene: suctioning, chest physiotherapy, nebulized heparin/acetylcysteine in some centers

Thermal Airway Injury

Epidemiology and Pathophysiology

- Usually confined to the upper airway (nasopharynx, oropharynx, larynx); lower tract spared due to efficient heat dissipation
- Mucosal edema and ulceration can rapidly progress to airway obstruction.
- Seen in facial burns, flame exposure, or scalding

Diagnostics

- Immediate evaluation of airway patency
- Laryngoscopy/bronchoscopy to assess supraglottic edema
- Chest imaging often unremarkable initially

Management

- Consider transfer to burn center for full evaluation and management.
- Head-of-bed elevation and humidified oxygen
- Early intubation for high-risk patients; airway edema may preclude later intubation.
- Corticosteroids: controversial; not routinely recommended
- Avoid aggressive fluid resuscitation that may worsen airway edema.

Chemical Inhalation Injury

Epidemiology and Pathophysiology

- Industrial accidents, warfare agents, and accidental exposures
- Water-soluble gases (ammonia, chlorine): damage the upper airways and eyes
- Poorly soluble gases (phosgene): penetrate deeper, cause delayed pulmonary edema
- Mechanisms: mucosal irritation, oxidative stress, capillary leak

Diagnostics

- History of exposure is key.
- Symptoms may be delayed: dyspnea, cough, wheezing, chest tightness.
- Chest x-ray (CXR) may be normal early; can progress to noncardiogenic pulmonary edema.
- Bronchoscopy may reveal inflammation or sloughing.

Management

- Supportive care: oxygen, bronchodilators, airway protection
- Avoid steroids unless severe bronchospasm or acute respiratory distress syndrome (ARDS).
- Nebulized sodium bicarbonate occasionally used in chlorine inhalation (anecdotal benefit)
- Observation for delayed ARDS

Infectious Tracheobronchitis in the Ventilated Intensive Care Unit Patient

Epidemiology and Pathophysiology

- Common in mechanically ventilated patients; may precede or coexist with ventilator-associated pneumonia (VAP)

- Caused by colonization and infection by typical VAP organisms: *Pseudomonas, Klebsiella, Staphylococcus aureus*, etc
- Inflammation without parenchymal infiltrates

Diagnostics

- Clinical: fever, increased secretions, new purulence, elevated white blood cells (WBCs), worsening ventilator parameters
- CXR: no new infiltrate (differentiates from VAP)
- Bronchoscopy with quantitative cultures may be helpful.
- Exclude noninfectious causes (eg, aspiration, obstruction).

Management

- Management per Infectious Diseases Society of America (IDSA) guidelines is identical to VAP with empiric antibiotics targeted to risk profile and prior culture data. De-escalate based on cultures to complete 7-day course.
- Pulmonary hygiene: suctioning, sedation minimization
- Avoid prolonged unnecessary antibiotics to reduce resistance.

Fungal Tracheobronchitis (Eg, *Aspergillus*)

Epidemiology and Pathophysiology

- Occurs in immunocompromised patients (neutropenia, transplant, steroids)
- Airway invasive form of pulmonary aspergillosis
- Subtypes: ulcerative, pseudomembranous, obstructive
- High mortality if untreated

Diagnostics

- Bronchoscopy: visualizes pseudomembranes or ulcerations
- Bronchoalveolar lavage (BAL) with fungal stains and culture, galactomannan
- CT of the chest: may show airway thickening, "halo sign" if parenchymal invasion
- Consider biopsy if diagnosis is unclear.

Management

- Prompt initiation of antifungals with input from Infectious Disease consultants
- Reduce immunosuppression if feasible.
- Airway debridement may be needed.
- Monitor for dissemination.

Postintubation Tracheobronchitis

Epidemiology and Pathophysiology

- Common after prolonged intubation due to mucosal irritation and biofilm formation
- May lead to ulceration, granulation tissue, or later stenosis
- Risk factors: excessive cuff pressure, prolonged ventilation, reflux

Diagnostics

- Bronchoscopy: erythema, ulceration, granulation tissue
- Cough, secretions, occasional hemoptysis postextubation
- Cultures may reveal colonizers or pathogens.

Management

- Pulmonary hygiene and humidification
- Antibiotics only if signs of infection
- Avoidance: proper cuff pressure, early mobilization
- ENT or bronchoscopy follow-up if persistent symptoms

Toxic Epidermal Necrolysis–Associated Tracheobronchitis

Epidemiology and Pathophysiology

- Toxic epidermal necrolysis/Stevens-Johnson syndrome (TEN/SJS) can involve airway epithelium → sloughing, necrosis.
- Life-threatening airway obstruction and infection
- Occurs in 25% to 50% of patients with TEN with mucosal involvement

Diagnostics

- Clinical suspicion in patients with TEN/SJS with respiratory distress
- Bronchoscopy: ulceration, sloughing mucosa
- High risk of pneumonitis or secondary bacterial infection

Management

- Supportive ICU care; early airway protection
- Immunosuppressive therapy for TEN (eg, intravenous immunoglobulin [IVIG], cyclosporine)
- Monitor for secondary infections.
- Aggressive pulmonary toilet and bronchodilation

SUGGESTED READINGS

Koulenti D, Tsigou E, Rello J. Ventilator-associated tracheobronchitis: to treat or not to treat? *Antibiotics (Basel)*. 2020;9(2):51.

Milton-Jones H, Soussi S, Davies R, et al. An international RAND/UCLA expert panel to determine the optimal diagnosis and management of burn inhalation injury. *Crit Care*. 2023;27:459.

Walker PF, Mason AD Jr, Cancio LC, et al. Diagnosis and management of inhalation injury. *Burns*. 2015;41(6):1081-1099.

3.17

Pulmonary Contusion

Joshua S. Ng-Kamstra

Definition

Pulmonary contusion (PC) is a pattern of injury to lung parenchyma resulting from either blunt trauma or a blast wave.

Epidemiology

- PCs are present in about 20% to 30% of patients with thoracic trauma.
- Most PCs occur in the context of rib fractures.
- Among the patients with critical polytrauma, the incidence of PC may be as high as 40%.
- The most common causative mechanism is motor vehicle collision.
- In older or frail individuals, a high-energy mechanism is not required. Low-level falls cause almost 20% of PCs in this population.

Clinical Manifestations

- Symptoms
  - Dyspnea
  - Chest pain from associated chest wall injuries
- Signs
  - Tachypnea
  - Tachycardia
  - Hypoxemia
  - Decreased air entry
  - Coarse breath sounds
  - Hemoptysis
  - Evidence of chest wall injury (eg, bruising, instability)

Pathophysiology

- Local tissue damage occurs immediately at the time of injury, due to the implosion effect (rapid changes in alveolar volume), inertia effects (differential acceleration of tissues), and spallation (injury due to the interaction of a pressure wave with the gas/tissue interface).
- Atelectasis, interstitial edema, alveolar hemorrhage, and the accumulation of protein-rich alveolar fluid worsen over the first 24 to 48 hours, accompanied by neutrophil and fibroblast infiltration.
- Within the area of injury, this leads to decreased compliance and poor gas exchange.
- Increased pulmonary shunt fraction causes hypoxemia.
- An intense activation of the innate immune system causes local and systemic inflammation, mediated by neutrophils, complement, and cytokines, notably interleukin-6.
- Primary alveolar injury heals between days 2 and 7.
- Secondary injury (eg, acute respiratory distress syndrome [ARDS], pneumonia, ventilator-associated lung injury) can markedly prolong the clinical course.

Imaging

- Chest radiograph
  - Contusions appear as haziness or focal consolidations.
  - Clinically significant PCs can often be seen on chest x-ray performed during the initial trauma assessment, though they may take several hours after injury to appear.
  - Radiographic findings can worsen significantly over the first 48 hours as the injury progresses.
- Ultrasound
  - Compared to radiography, ultrasound has a higher sensitivity for diagnosing contusions (92% vs 44%), with similar specificity (89% vs 97%).
  - The clinical significance of radiographically negative but ultrasound-positive contusions is unknown.
- Computed tomography (CT)
  - Gold standard for the detection of PCs
  - For "occult" contusions seen on CT but not on x-ray, clinical outcomes are no worse than having no contusion.
  - In one study, bilateral contusions were shown to have a significant impact on pulmonary complications, in contrast to unilateral contusions.
  - More precisely, the severity of impairment in gas exchange and the risk of progression to ARDS or pneumonia are related to the ratio of contused and total lung volume. A clinically relevant cutoff is 20%.
  - Artificial intelligence models have been developed to automatically calculate this volume.

Differential Diagnosis (Table 3.17.1)

Complications

- Hypoxemic respiratory failure
  - Due to increased shunt fraction
- ARDS
- Pneumonia

Management

- An excellent multimodal regimen of pain control should be instituted to manage pain from associated chest wall injuries. This will allow for deep breathing and coughing. Pain control is discussed in more detail in the next chapter (Section 3.14: Upper Airway Diseases and Disorders).
- Fluid management
  - No evidence exists for strict fluid restriction. Guidelines suggest appropriate resuscitation for hemorrhagic or hypovolemic shock.
  - Avoid excessive fluid administration.
- Pulmonary toilet
  - Ensure adequate pain control to allow for deep breathing and coughing.
  - Incentive spirometry is used to prevent atelectasis, though evidence of clinical effectiveness is limited.
  - Aggressive management of secretions, including frequent suctioning, chest physiotherapy, and early mobilization, may minimize the risk of respiratory failure.
- High-flow oxygen
  - For patients who remain hypoxemic despite the above, a trial of high-flow oxygen may avoid the need for intubation.

TABLE 3.17.1 Timing, radiologic findings, and other features of pulmonary contusions compared to other post-traumatic pulmonary diagnoses

Diagnosis	Time Course Following Injury	Usual Chest X-ray Findings	Usual CT Findings	Distinguishing Features
Pulmonary contusion	Immediate onset, peaks at 1-2 d, improves by 7 d	Diffuse haziness or focal opacity underlying the site of blunt impact	Ground-glass opacities (± subpleural sparing)	
Pneumonia	Onset usually >3 d	Focal opacity	Ground-glass opacities ± dense consolidation	Fever, purulent secretions
ARDS	Onset up to 7 d	Diffuse, patchy opacity	Dependent (more than nondependent) ground-glass opacities with areas of sparing	
Pulmonary embolism	Onset any time following trauma	Normal, may have enlarged pulmonary artery, Hampton hump, Westermark sign	Filling defect in pulmonary artery	Pleuritic chest pain, right heart strain, evidence of deep vein thrombosis, classic ECG findings (rare)
Atelectasis	Onset any time	Linear opacities, segmental or subsegmental collapse	Linear opacities, segmental or subsegmental collapse, displacement of fissures, crowding of vessels	
TRALI	Onset within 6 h of blood product transfusion	Diffuse airspace disease and interstitial edema	Diffuse airspace disease and interstitial edema	Fever
Pulmonary edema	Onset any time	Diffuse increase in interstitial markings, pulmonary vascular redistribution, bronchial cuffing	Ground-glass opacities, septal thickening	Evidence of systemic fluid overload, significant volume loading during resuscitation, history of heart failure, crackles
Aspiration	Onset any time	Dependent airspace opacity	Dependent airspace opacity, debris in airways	Context of altered level of consciousness, impaired swallowing, bowel obstruction or ileus

ARDS, acute respiratory distress syndrome; CT, computed tomography; ECG, electrocardiogram; TRALI, transfusion-related acute lung injury.

- The ROX (Ratio of OXygen) index can be used to risk-stratify patients on standard or high-flow oxygen therapy.
- Noninvasive positive pressure ventilation (NIPPV)
  - If no contraindications exist (eg, active pneumonia, upper gastrointestinal [GI] or airway injury), NIPPV may help reduce shunt fraction resulting from fluid-filled or atelectatic alveoli.
- Ventilation strategy
  - No formal criteria exist to mandate intubation.
  - In the absence of other indications for intubation (eg, concomitant operative injuries, traumatic brain injury, mental status changes), consider the use of the ROX index to predict failure of high-flow oxygen therapy.
  - If mechanical ventilation is required, consider the use of lung-protective strategies early, even in the absence of ARDS.
  - The ARDSnet High PEEP (positive end-expiratory pressure) strategy (or a strategy based on the "Open Lung Concept," characterized by recruitment maneuvers, short expiratory times, and high respiratory rates) has been noted to prevent progression from unilateral PC to ARDS in an animal model, in contrast to the ARDSnet low PEEP strategy.
  - In unilateral contusions, refractory hypoxemia may improve if the patient is positioned with the *uninjured* side down, which may decrease shunt fraction.
  - Extracorporeal membrane oxygenation may be required in refractory cases.
- No evidence exists for prophylactic antibiotics or steroids in this patient population.

Outcomes

- In a study using the National Inpatient Sample, mortality among individuals with unilateral PC was 4.7%, and 9.6% among those with bilateral contusions.
- Mortality and pulmonary complications are related to the proportion of involved lung parenchyma, the burden of bony thoracic trauma, and the overall injury severity.
- A study of survivors of severe chest trauma with PC (>10 months after injury) demonstrated near-normal spirometry.

SUGGESTED READINGS

Bader A, Rahman U, Morris M, et al. Pulmonary contusions in the elderly after blunt trauma: incidence and outcomes. *J Surg Res*. 2018;230:110-116.

Chiumello D, Coppola S, Froio S, Gregoretti C, Consonni D. Noninvasive ventilation in chest trauma: systematic review and meta-analysis. *Intensive Care Med*. 2013;39:1171-1180.

Choi J, Mavrommati K, Li NY, et al. Scalable deep learning algorithm to compute percent pulmonary contusion among patients with rib fractures. *J Trauma Acute Care Surg*. 2022;93:461-466.

Choi J, Tennakoon L, You JG, Kaghazchi A, Forrester JD, Spain DA. Pulmonary contusions in patients with rib fractures: the need to better classify a common injury. *Am J Surg*. 2021;221:211-215.

Cohn SM, Dubose JJ. Pulmonary contusion: an update on recent advances in clinical management. *World J Surg*. 2010;34:1959-1970.
Cornillon A, Balbo J, Coffinet J, et al. The ROX index as a predictor of standard oxygen therapy outcomes in thoracic trauma. *Scand J Trauma Resusc Emerg Med*. 2021;29:81.
de Moya MA, Manolakaki D, Chang Y, et al. Blunt pulmonary contusion: admission computed tomography scan predicts mechanical ventilation. *J Trauma*. 2011;71:1543-1547.
Deunk J, Poels TC, Brink M, et al. The clinical outcome of occult pulmonary contusion on multidetector-row computed tomography in blunt trauma patients. *J Trauma Acute Care Surg*. 2010;68:387.
Finkbeiner R, Krinner S, Langenbach A, Besendörfer M, Schulz-Drost S. Age distribution and concomitant injuries in pulmonary contusion: an analysis based on routine data. *Thorac Cardiovasc Surg*. 2018;66:678-685.
Hosseini M, Ghelichkhani P, Baikpour M, et al. Diagnostic accuracy of ultrasonography and radiography in detection of pulmonary contusion; a systematic review and meta-analysis. *Emergency*. 2015;3:127-136.
Hoth JJ, Wells JD, Jones SE, Yoza BK, McCall CE. Complement mediates a primed inflammatory response after traumatic lung injury. *J Trauma Acute Care Surg*. 2014;76:601-609.
Landeck T, Schwarz H, Hammermüller S, et al. High positive end-expiratory pressure ventilation mitigates the progression from unilateral pulmonary contusion to ARDS: an animal study. *J Trauma Acute Care Surg*. 2024;96:287.
Lee NH, Kim SH, Seo S, et al. Prediction of respiratory complications by quantifying lung contusion volume using chest computed tomography in patients with chest trauma. *Sci Rep*. 2023;13:6387.
Lewis BT, Herr KD, Hamlin SA, et al. Imaging manifestations of chest trauma. *RadioGraphics*. 2021;41:1321-1334.
Požgain Z, Kristek D, Lovrić I, et al. Pulmonary contusions after blunt chest trauma: clinical significance and evaluation of patient management. *Eur J Trauma Emerg Surg*. 2018;44:773-777.
Raghavendran K, Davidson BA, Woytash JA, et al. The evolution of isolated bilateral lung contusion from blunt chest trauma in rats: cellular and cytokine responses. *Shock*. 2005;24:132-138.
Raghavendran K, Notter RH, Davidson BA, Helinski JD, Kunkel SL, Knight PR. Lung contusion: inflammatory mechanisms and interaction with other injuries. *Shock*. 2009;32:122-130.
Sarkar N, Zhang L, Campbell P, et al. Pulmonary contusion: automated deep learning-based quantitative visualization. *Emerg Radiol*. 2023;30:435-441.
Schulz-Drost S, Finkbeiner R, Lefering R, et al. Lung contusion in polytrauma: an analysis of the TraumaRegister DGU. *Thorac Cardiovasc Surg*. 2021;69:735-748.
Simon B, Ebert J, Bokhari F, et al. Management of pulmonary contusion and flail chest: an Eastern Association for the Surgery of Trauma practice management guideline. *J Trauma Acute Care Surg*. 2012;73:S351-S361.
Wang C, Zhang L, Qin T, et al. Extracorporeal membrane oxygenation in trauma patients: a systematic review. *World J Emerg Surg*. 2020;15:51.

3.18

Flail chest and surgical stabilization of rib fractures

Joshua S. Ng-Kamstra

Definition

- Three or more consecutive rib fractures with each rib fractured in more than one place (radiologic flail segment)
- Rib fractures resulting in paradoxical chest wall motion (clinical flail chest)

Epidemiology

- In a US trauma population, diagnosed in about 1% of all patients with an injury severity score (ISS) >9
- In the Netherlands, present in about 4% of patients admitted with rib fractures

Clinical Manifestations

- Signs
  - Segment of chest wall that moves paradoxically relative to the rest of the chest (inward with inspiration, outward with exhalation)
    - Paradoxical motion is not always readily apparent.
  - Visible chest wall deformity
  - Bony crepitus to palpation
  - Splinting with deep respiration
  - Impaired cough
  - Increased work of breathing
  - Hypoxemia
- Symptoms
  - Subjective "clicking" of ribs
  - Severe pain with movement, breathing, or coughing
  - Inability to clear secretions
  - Dyspnea

Anatomic Patterns and Associated Injuries

- Upper (first-third) rib fractures may be associated with vascular injuries, including blunt cerebrovascular injury.
- Middle (fourth-ninth) rib fractures are primarily associated with cardiopulmonary injuries, most commonly pulmonary contusion.
- Lower (9th-12th) injuries are associated with diaphragmatic, hepatic, and splenic injuries.
- Clinical flail can occur in a "central" pattern with paired fractures on either side of the sternum, commonly associated with cardiopulmonary resuscitation (CPR) or steering wheel impacts.
- Fractures of the sternum or cartilage can similarly cause a flail phenomenon in the context of nonsegmental rib fractures in contiguous ribs.

Treatment Modalities

- Analgesia
  - Multimodal (acetaminophen, nonsteroidal antiinflammatory drug [NSAID], gabapentinoids, lidocaine patches, muscle relaxants, opioids)
  - Patient-controlled analgesia in alert patients
  - Epidural analgesia
  - Ketamine

- Intercostal nerve blocks or serratus blocks
- Intercostal cryoablation in operative patients
- Pulmonary toilet
  - Cough training (brace chest with pillow)
  - Oscillatory positive expiratory pressure
  - Frequent suctioning
- Incentive spirometry
- Noninvasive positive pressure ventilation (NIPPV)
  - NIPPV decreases atelectasis and may prevent intubation.
- High-flow oxygen
  - May treat hypoxemia related to underlying pulmonary injury (see Section 3.17: Pulmonary Contusion)
- Mechanical ventilation
  - Indicated for refractory respiratory failure, decreased level of consciousness, or overall traumatic injury burden
- Surgical stabilization

Surgical Stabilization of Rib Fractures

- Indications
  - Flail chest
  - May be indicated for severe nonflail chest wall injury (eg, bicortically displaced ribs, mechanically ventilated patients)
- Outcomes
  - In patients with flail chest, decreases the duration of mechanical ventilation, intensive care unit (ICU) length of stay, ventilator-associated pneumonia rates. No definitive impact on mortality
- Contraindications
  - Shock or ongoing resuscitation
  - Acute myocardial infarction
  - Severe hypoxemia precluding appropriate positioning or single lung ventilation
  - Higher priority injuries requiring emergent management
  - Unstable spine injuries precluding appropriate positioning
  - Traumatic brain injury is not a contraindication as was previously thought.
- Timing
  - As soon as possible, ideally within 72 hours of injury
- Approaches
  - Intrathoracic (placed with video-assisted thoracoscopic surgery)
  - Extrathoracic
    - Muscle-sparing approaches preferred
    - Posterolateral, anterolateral, or subpectoral exposures can be used depending on the location of fractures.
- Adjuncts
  - Cryoablation or intercostal injection of liposomal bupivacaine can provide long-duration pain control following surgical stabilization of rib fractures (SSRF).
- Complications
  - Bleeding
  - Wound infection
  - Hardware infection
  - Hardware failure
  - Winged scapula (long thoracic nerve injury)
  - Pain
  - Nonunion

SUGGESTED READINGS

Dehghan N, de Mestral C, McKee MD, Schemitsch EH, Nathens A. Flail chest injuries: a review of outcomes and treatment practices from the National Trauma Data Bank. *J Trauma Acute Care Surg*. 2014;76:462-468.

Dehghan N, Nauth A, Schemitsch E, et al. Operative vs nonoperative treatment of acute unstable chest wall injuries: a randomized clinical trial. *JAMA Surg*. 2022;157:983-990.

Delaplain PT, Facs SDS, Pieracci FM, et al. Chest wall injury society guideline for ssrf indications, contraindications and timing. https://wjes.biomedcentral.com/articles/10.1186/s13017-024-00559-2.

de Moya M, Nirula R, Biffl W. Rib fixation: who, what, when? *Trauma Surg Acute Care Open*. 2017;2:e000059.

Duggal A, Perez P, Golan E, Tremblay L, Sinuff T. Safety and efficacy of noninvasive ventilation in patients with blunt chest trauma: a systematic review. *Crit Care*. 2013;17:R142.

Fokin AA, Hus N, Wycech J, Rodriguez E, Puente I. Surgical stabilization of rib fractures. *JBJS Essent Surg Tech*. 2020;10:e0032.

Greiffenstein P, Tran MQ, Campeau L. Three common exposures of the chest wall for rib fixation: anatomical considerations. *J Thorac Dis*. 2019;11:S1034-S1043.

Hisamune R, Kobayashi M, Nakasato K, et al. A meta-analysis and trial sequential analysis of randomised controlled trials comparing nonoperative and operative management of chest trauma with multiple rib fractures. *World J Emerg Surg*. 2024;19:11.

Lagazzi E, de Roulet A, Proaño-Zamudio JA, et al. Is severe traumatic brain injury no longer a contraindication for surgical stabilization of rib fractures in patients with multiple rib fractures? A propensity-matched analysis. *J Trauma Acute Care Surg*. 2023;94:823-830.

Marasco SF, Balogh ZJ, Wullschleger ME, et al. Rib fixation in non-ventilator-dependent chest wall injuries: a prospective randomized trial. *J Trauma Acute Care Surg*. 2022;92:1047-1053.

Marasco SF, Davies AR, Cooper J, et al. Prospective randomized controlled trial of operative rib fixation in traumatic flail chest. *J Am Coll Surg*. 2013;216:924-932.

Mukherjee K, Schubl SD, Tominaga G, et al. Non-surgical management and analgesia strategies for older adults with multiple rib fractures: a systematic review, meta-analysis, and practice management guideline from the Eastern Association for the Surgery of Trauma and the Chest Wall Injury Society. *J Trauma Acute Care Surg*. 2023;94:398-410.

Peek J, Beks RB, Hietbrink F, et al. Epidemiology and outcome of rib fractures: a nationwide study in the Netherlands. *Eur J Trauma Emerg Surg*. 2022;48:265-271.

Pieracci FM, Leasia K, Bauman Z, et al. A multicenter, prospective, controlled clinical trial of surgical stabilization of rib fractures in patients with severe, nonflail fracture patterns (Chest Wall Injury Society NONFLAIL). *J Trauma Acute Care Surg*. 2020;88:249-257.

Pieracci FM, Majercik S, Ali-Osman F, et al. Consensus statement: surgical stabilization of rib fractures rib fracture colloquium clinical practice guidelines. *Injury*. 2017;48:307-321.

Prins JTH, Van Lieshout EMM, Ali-Osman F, et al. Outcome after surgical stabilization of rib fractures versus nonoperative treatment in patients with multiple rib fractures and moderate to severe traumatic brain injury (CWIS-TBI). *J Trauma Acute Care Surg*. 2021;90:492.

Stopenski S, Binkley J, Schubl SD, Bauman ZM. Rib fracture management: a review of surgical stabilization, regional analgesia, and intercostal nerve cryoablation. *Surg Pract Sci*. 2022;10:100089.

Sum S-K, Peng Y-C, Yin S-Y, et al. Using an incentive spirometer reduces pulmonary complications in patients with traumatic rib fractures: a randomized controlled trial. *Trials*. 2019;20:797.

Talbot BS, Gange CP, Chaturvedi A, Klionsky N, Hobbs SK, Chaturvedi A. Traumatic Rib injury: patterns, imaging pitfalls, complications, and treatment. *RadioGraphics*. 2017;37:628-651.

3.19

Sleep-Related Breathing Disorders

Raghu R. Chivukula

Introduction

- Sleep-related breathing disorders (SRBDs) are a spectrum of abnormal respiratory patterns that occur during sleep ranging from snoring to hypopnea (reduced ventilation) to apnea (absent ventilation).
- In the United States, ~5% of the general population has obstructive sleep apnea (OSA) syndrome.
- Untreated SRBD results in periods of severe hypercapnia and hypoxemia, leading to neurocognitive and cardiovascular end-organ effects that include systemic hypertension, risk of coronary artery disease, congestive heart failure, and acute ischemic stroke.

Definitions

- Respiratory effort–related arousal (RERA) event: ≥10 seconds event requiring increased respiratory effort to maintain baseline airflow but without significant hypoxemia; arousal from sleep (by electroencephalogram [EEG]) is required.
- Hypopnea event: ≥10 seconds; at least 30% decrease from baseline airflow; at least 4% desaturation
- Apnea event: ≥10 seconds; at least 80% decrease from baseline airflow. Note: Apnea can be obstructive, central, or mixed.
    - Obstructive apnea is due to upper airway collapse with persistent ventilatory efforts.
    - Central apnea is due to a lack of ventilatory efforts (ie, no activation of the diaphragm per electromyography [EMG] measurements).
    - Mixed apnea is a combination of obstructive and central apnea.

Measurements

- Apnea index (AI): total number of apnea events per hour of sleep
- *Apnea-hypopnea index (AHI): total number of apnea and hypopnea events per hour of sleep*, may be subdivided into sleep stages—nonrapid eye movement (NREM) versus rapid eye movement (REM)
- Respiratory disturbance index (RDI): total number of apnea, hypopnea, and RERA events per hour of sleep
- Oxygen desaturation index (ODI): total number of desaturation by >3% to 4% events per hour of sleep
- Fraction of sleep spent below 90% oxygen saturation: total exposure time to hypoxemia
- Mean oxygen saturation: average saturation throughout sleep (inversely related to the risk of cardiovascular disease or glucose intolerance)
- Arousal index: number of arousals per hour of sleep

Epidemiology

- OSA affects men more commonly than women (2-3:1).
- Affects 3% to 5% of adults in the United States, prevalence plateaus in the 60s.
- Risk factors include family history, menopause in females, aging, race, obesity, snoring, smoking, alcohol use, medications, increased neck circumference (>17 inches in men, >16 inches in women), macroglossia, nasal narrowing, low-lying soft palate, retrognathia/micrognathia, enlarged tonsils/adenoids, and mandibular hypoplasia.

Differential Diagnosis

- *Hypoventilation syndromes*
    - Awakeful hypercarbia or elevated serum bicarbonate that is worse during sleep
    - Congenital central alveolar hypoventilation (CCAH): impaired autonomic control of ventilation, failure to respond to hypoxia and hypercapnia triggers, mildly elevated $Paco_2$ during the wakeful period, and markedly elevated $Paco_2$ during NREM sleep
        - Associated with Hirschsprung disease (10%-50%), increased risk of neuroblastoma and ganglioneuroma
    - Obesity-hypoventilation syndrome (OHS): obesity (body mass index [BMI] >30 kg/m^2) and *hypercapnia ($Paco_2$ >45 mm Hg) during the wakeful period* in the absence of other known causes of alveolar hypoventilation (ie, chronic obstructive pulmonary disease [COPD], neuromuscular disease, hypothyroidism, or restrictive lung disease)
        - Often coexist with OSA
        - Associated with symptoms and signs of right heart failure, pulmonary hypertension, polycythemia, and insulin resistance
    - Central sleep apnea syndromes
        - Primary: disturbed sleep with >5 central apnea and hypopnea events per hour and normocarbia during awake time
        - Secondary: high-altitude periodic breathing, medical illness, drug or substance, Cheyne-Stokes breathing (associated with heart failure or stroke)
- OSA syndrome
    - AHI or RDI >15 events per hour in an asymptomatic patient
    - AHI or RDI >5 events per hour in a symptomatic patient (ie, sleepiness, fatigue, inattention, snoring, restless sleep)
    - RERA >5 events per hour with daytime sleepiness (previously known as upper airway resistance syndrome [UARS], now classified as part of OSA syndrome)
    - Diagnosis is established with polysomnography.
        - Severity of OSA is graded based on AHI (mild 5-15; moderate 16-30; or severe >30) and degree of sleep fragmentation, daytime sleepiness, nadir of Sao_2, nocturnal arrhythmias, and concurrent cardiovascular/neurologic disorders.

Key Pathophysiology

- Combination of pressure gradient (between nasal pressure and alveolar pressure) and airway resistance determines airflow.
- Factors: nasal pressure, alveolar pressure, obesity (increased fat deposition), nasal obstruction, micrognathia,

retrognathia, tonsillar/uvular hypertrophy, macroglossia, tissue edema or fibrosis

- Balance between activation of dilator muscles and decreased intraluminal pressure results in upper airway patency.
- Obstruction occurs when airway resistance increases (narrow airway) or in the presence of decreased dilator muscle activation.
- Most common areas of obstruction are behind the palate (retropalatal) or behind the tongue (retrolingual).

Management and Treatment

- *Positive airway pressures (PAPs)*
  - Continuous positive airway pressure (CPAP) provides a single constant positive pressure during the entire respiratory cycle.
  - Bilevel positive airway pressure (BPAP) provides a higher inspiratory positive airway pressure (IPAP) and a lower expiratory positive airway pressure (EPAP) during the respiratory cycle.
  - Autotitrating positive airway pressure (APAP) provides a variable positive airway pressure in response to a change in airflow, a change in circuit pressure, or a vibratory snore (depending on the device-specific algorithms).
  - Adaptive servoventilation provides a variable amount of pressure support superimposed on a low level of CPAP.
    - The pressure support can increase during the hypoventilation period and decrease during the hyperventilation period.
  - Disposable nasal device allows unimpeded inspiration but increased resistance on expiration, generating a positive end-expiratory pressure.
    - Adherence to the device is important (at least 4 hours a night for 70% of nights).
  - Side effects: nasal congestion, dryness, epistaxis, rhinorrhea, sinus discomfort, facial skin irritation, eye irritation, gastric distention, and chest discomfort
  - Oral device
    - Mandibular reposition devices that displace the mandible and tongue forward
    - Tongue-retaining devices that secure the tongue in a soft bulb located anterior to the teeth
    - Oral device has higher preference than the PAP devices but unclear if more effective.
- *Surgery*
  - In patients who have failed PAP and oral devices, or with an obvious upper airway obstructive lesion, uvulopalatopharyngoplasty (UPPP), laser-assisted uvulopalatoplasty, radiofrequency ablation, maxillomandibular advancement (MMA), or tracheostomy
- *Clinical considerations*
  - Patients with OSA have increased likelihood of insulin resistance, systemic hypertension, pulmonary hypertension, ischemic heart disease, nocturnal cardiac arrhythmias, and complications with heart failure and stroke.
  - ~70% of patients undergoing bariatric surgery have OSA.
  - Perioperative airway complications in the setting of OSA are estimated at 17% due to:
    - Difficult tracheal intubation
    - Postoperative atelectasis and splinting leading to shunting
    - Upper airway edema secondary to intubation, resulting in increased airway resistance
    - Medication-related decreased upper airway dilator muscle tone and central respiratory drive
    - Predisposed postoperative arrhythmia, hypertension
  - SRBD is worsened in pregnancy due to estrogen-induced increased nasopharyngeal mucosal edema, resulting in increased upper airway resistance.
    - OSA is associated with fetal growth retardation, fetal death, pregnancy-induced hypertension, pulmonary hypertension, and gestational diabetes.
    - CPAP is safe during pregnancy.

SUGGESTED READINGS

Aurora RN, Chowdhuri S, Ramar K, et al. The treatment of central sleep apnea syndromes in adults: practice parameters with an evidence-based literature review and meta-analyses. *Sleep*. 2012;35(1):17-40.

Benjamin JA, Lewis KE. Sleep-disordered breathing and cardiovascular disease. *Postgrad Med J*. 2008;84(987):15-22.

Berry RB, Budhiraja R, Gottlieb DJ, et al. Rules for scoring respiratory events in sleep: update of the 2007 AASM manual for the scoring of sleep and associated events. Deliberations of the sleep apnea definitions task force of the American Academy of Sleep Medicine. *J Clin Sleep Med*. 2012; 8(5):597-619.

Berry RB, Hill G, Thompson L, McLaurin V. Portable monitoring and autotitration versus polysomnography for the diagnosis and treatment of sleep apnea. *Sleep*. 2008;31(10):1423-1431.

Bose S. Obstructive sleep apnea and perioperative complications. *Chest*. 2008;134(4):890-891.

Bourjeily G, Ankner G, Mohsenin V. Sleep-disordered breathing in pregnancy. *Clin Chest Med*. 2011;32(1):175-189.

Chau EH, Lam D, Wong J, et al. Obesity hypoventilation syndrome: a review of epidemiology, pathophysiology, and perioperative considerations. *Anesthesiology*. 2012;117(1):188-205.

Dempsey JA, Veasey SC, Morgan BJ, O'Donnell CP. Pathophysiology of sleep apnea. *Physiol Rev*. 2010;90(1):47-112.

Gay PC. Sleep and sleep-disordered breathing in the hospitalized patient. *Respir Care*. 2010;55(9):1240-1254.

Jennum P, Riha RL. Epidemiology of sleep apnoea/hypopnoea syndrome and sleep-disordered breathing. *Eur Respir J*. 2009;33(4):907-914.

Kapur VK. Obstructive sleep apnea: diagnosis, epidemiology, and economics. *Respir Care*. 2010;55(9):1155-1167.

Liess BD, Dost JS, Templer JW, Tobias JD. Congenital central alveolar hypoventilation syndrome (Ondine's curse) with survival into adulthood. *Clin Pediatr (Phila)*. 2008;47(9):941-946.

Lurie A. Obstructive sleep apnea in adults: epidemiology, clinical presentation, and treatment options. *Adv Cardiol*. 2011;46:1-42.

Mohsenin V. Sleep-related breathing disorders and risk of stroke. *Stroke*. 2001;32(6):1271-1278.

Portela PC, Fumadó JC, García HQ, Borrego FR. Sleep-disordered breathing and acute stroke. *Cerebrovasc Dis*. 2009;27(suppl 1):104-110.

Richards KC, Anderson WM, Chesson AL Jr, Nagel CL. Sleep-related breathing disorders in patients who are critically ill. *J Cardiovasc Nurs*. 2002;17(1):42-55.

3.20

Pulmonary Imaging

Davit Kocharyan

Anatomy and landmarks

Airway

- The trachea has a length of 10 to 12 cm and consists of 16 to 20 C-shaped cartilaginous rings. At the level of carina (T5), the trachea divides into the right and left main bronchi at an angle of 60 degrees.
    - Pathologies such as left atrial enlargement, subcarinal masses, lymphadenopathy, lobar collapse, or pericardial effusion result in the widening of the carinal angle.
    - In adults, the right main bronchus has a more vertical course, predisposing to a higher incidence of right-sided aspiration.
- The right main bronchus has a more vertical course in adults and averages 2.2 cm in length. It gives rise to the right upper bronchus and bronchus intermedius, which extends peripherally 3 to 4 cm before branching. The bronchus intermedius further bifurcates into right upper and middle lobe bronchi. The right lung contains 10 segmental bronchi.
- The left main bronchus is twice as long as the right main bronchus (5 cm), narrower, and less vertical than the right one. It divides into left upper and left lower bronchi. The left lung contains eight segmental bronchi for the same number of segments.
- Following 6 to 20 divisions, the segmental bronchi branch into cartilage-free bronchioles, which further branch into terminal (or "respiratory") bronchioles.

Lung Parenchyma

- The primary pulmonary lobule consists of alveolar ducts, alveolar sacs, and alveoli, accompanied by their respective blood vessels, nerves, and connective tissue distal to the respiratory bronchioles. This structure is beyond the sensitivity of conventional radiologic resolution.
- The *secondary pulmonary lobule (SPL)* is the primary unit of lung formation from the radiologic perspective. The SPL comprises 30 to 50 primary lobules, has a polyhedral shape, and averages 1 to 2.5 cm in diameter. It is the smallest structural lung unit enclosed in connective tissue that can be visualized on a high-resolution computed tomography (CT) scan.
- The acinus is the gas exchange unit of the lung located distal to the terminal bronchiole. 6 to 12 acini are conjoined together in a single SPL.

Vascular System

- The vascular pedicle is the broad shadow of the main systemic veins and arteries on a frontal chest radiography (CXR). It stretches from the right lateral border of the superior vena cava (SVC), where it crosses the right main bronchus, to the left lateral margin of the left subclavian artery, where it originates from the aortic arch. The normal measurement of the vascular pedicle on an upright posteroanterior CXR is <6 cm.
- Pulmonary arteries (PAs)
    - The main pulmonary artery (MPA) arises in the mediastinum at the level of the pulmonary valve. It extends superiorly and to the left, measuring 4 to 5 cm.
        - Enlargement of the MPA and its descending lobar branches may be indicative of PA hypertension. The typical maximal MPA diameter is 28 mm (measured at its bifurcation).
    - Before leaving the pericardium, the MPA divides into the shorter left and longer right PA at the T5 level.
    - The left PA curves over the left main bronchus before branching into the left upper and interlobar arteries. The right PA travels behind the ascending aorta before bifurcating into ascending and descending (interlobar) trunks in front of the right main bronchus.
    - Bilaterally, the lobar branches give rise to segmental, followed by subsegmental divisions that run along the segmental and subsegmental bronchi, accordingly.
- Each of the lungs is drained by superior and inferior pulmonary veins, which empty into the right atrium.
- Thoracic aorta
    - Four segments comprise the thoracic aorta: the root, ascending, transverse (arch), and descending. The lateral aspect of the aortic arch forms a smooth "knob" above the left hilum.
    - The arch typically has three main branches located anterior to and to the left of the trachea: the brachiocephalic artery, left common carotid artery, and left subclavian artery.

Mediastinum

- Although compartmentalization of the mediastinum carries significant relevance for the diagnostic radiology of mediastinal processes and tumors, no distinct anatomic boundaries separate mediastinal compartments. Hence, pathologic processes can spread unchecked among the compartments.
- The traditional anatomic model has four compartments:
    - Anterior: extends from the sternum to the anterior surface of the pericardium
    - Middle: space between the anterior and posterior pericardium
    - Posterior: bordered by the posterior pericardium and the thoracic spine
    - Superior: space above the aortic arch
- Radiographic anatomy
    - On the posteroanterior CXR, the right mediastinal contour is composed of the right brachiocephalic vein, SVC, and the right atrium.
    - The aortic arch, the pulmonary trunk, and the left ventricle (LV) form the left margin of the mediastinal silhouette.
    - On the lateral radiograph, the right ventricle (RV) and the pulmonary trunk are the most anterior structures, followed by the left atrium, LV, and inferior vena cava (IVC) posteriorly.

Hilum

- The hilum is a concave convergence of the lung and mediastinum that serves as an entry and exit point for the systemic and pulmonary vasculature, bronchi, and lymphatics.
- While major bronchi and blood vessels make up most of the typical hilar opacities on CXR, the majority of what is visualized is PAs because the PAs and bronchi branch out from the hilum together.
  - Although PA enlargement causes hilar expansion, the hila retain their vascular configuration.

Diaphragm

- The diaphragm is the primary respiratory muscle, irrelevant of the body's position. The diaphragmatic innervation originates from C3 to C5 levels via phrenic nerve.
- In 88% of individuals, the right hemidiaphragm is higher than the left by 1.5 to 2 cm.
  - Patients who are obese may exhibit bilaterally high riding diaphragm due to their body habitus, so this should be distinguished from diaphragmatic paresis.

Imaging Modalities

Chest Radiograph

- In the intensive care unit (ICU), CXR is the most widely used modality since it is portable, allows quick acquisition, and provides instant data on a built-in screen. However, recent meta-analyses indicate no relevant effect on mortality or hospitalization length following the elimination of the routine daily CXRs in the ICU.
- The image quality can be significantly compromised due to the anteroposterior (AP) CXR technique commonly employed in the ICU as well as superimposed foreign bodies.

Chest Computed Tomography

- CT is more accurate than CXR in identifying and describing pathologies related to the lungs, pleura, and mediastinum. CT angiography is the first-line modality to assess for pulmonary embolism (PE) in the ICU.
- The inherent limitations of the CT are the need for transportation outside the ICU, risks of intravenous contrast as well as significantly increased radiation

Lung Ultrasound

- The limited sensitivity of CXR and challenges associated with performing CT make lung ultrasound (LUS) an extremely valuable technique for a bedside assessment in the ICU. LUS demonstrated greater diagnostic sensitivity for pulmonary pathologies than CXR in the ICU setting.
- To differentiate between normal versus pathologic conditions, a qualitative LUS relies on the interpretation of artifacts (A- and B-lines) in the context of actual images.
- The BLUE (Bedside Lung Ultrasound in Emergency) protocol combines ultrasound (US) findings to establish different profiles (A, B, C, etc.) for the main pathologic conditions (pneumonia, PE, congestive heart failure [CHF], etc) with an accuracy of >90%.
  - A-profile: predominantly bilateral, anterior A-lines + lung sliding
  - B-profile: anterior lung sliding + lung rockets (≥3 B-lines per scan)
  - C-profile: anterior alveolar consolidation(s)
- Subcutaneous emphysema, calcifications of pleura, large thoracic dressings, pleurodesis, anasarca, and overlying lines and tubes can limit the usability of LUS.

Pulmonary Pathologies

Atelectasis

- Epidemiology
  - The most common reason for lung opacities on CXR in ICU patients is atelectasis.
  - The most affected lobes are the left lower lobe (66%), the right lower lobe (22%), and the right upper lobe (11%).
- Classes of atelectasis
  - The main types of atelectasis and their respective pathophysiologic mechanisms are summarized in Table 3.20.1.
  - There are other patterns of atelectasis based on the anatomic location.
    - Rounded: located juxtapleural and associated with chronic pleural conditions/effusion (mostly seen in posterior lower lobes)
    - Discoid/plate like: located peripherally and can carry clinical significance after general anesthesia because of hypoventilation
    - Diffuse/generalized atelectasis: extensive lung volume loss without distinct indication of linear, segmental, or lobar atelectasis
- CXR findings in atelectasis
  - The radiographic findings of atelectasis can be categorized into direct and indirect signs (Table 3.20.2).
  - Diagnostic utility of air bronchograms
    - In patients with acute lobar collapse, the lack of air bronchogram (branching, linear tubular lucency appearing on the radiograph as the bronchus or bronchiole crosses the airless lung tissue) suggests mucoid impaction (obstruction) as a likely etiology.
    - The presence of an air bronchogram indicates more compression atelectasis since the secretion-filled bronchi in resorptive atelectasis (longstanding obstruction) omit air bronchograms.
    - However, air bronchogram has no diagnostic values in differentiating between atelectasis and pneumonia since it may manifest in either condition.
- CT findings in atelectasis
  - CT features of atelectasis are identical to those on CXR.
  - Volume loss is a frequently identified finding on the CT and is delineated with greater clarity.
  - The rounded atelectasis on CT produces a distinct curving pattern of the adjacent bronchi and pulmonary vessels called the "comet-tail sign."
  - Lobar atelectasis on the CT scan has wedge-shaped contours with the apex oriented toward the origin of the affected bronchus.
  - The contrast-enhanced CT depicts the atelectasis as a rather substantial degree of attenuation of the lung tissue. This helps to differentiate it from a consolidative process like pneumonia, which has a smaller degree of attenuation.

TABLE 3.20.1 Types, Mechanisms, and Etiology of Atelectasis

Type	Mechanism	Etiology
Obstructive or resorption atelectasis (the most common type)	The absorption of air distal to the obstruction of a large or medium-sized airway leads to lobar collapse.	Malpositioned ETT Mucous plugging Strictures/stenosis Aspiration/foreign body Neoplasm Lymphadenopathy
Compressive atelectasis	Intrathoracic and intraabdominal space-occupying processes preventing alveoli aeration	Pleural effusion (most common in ICU) Tension pneumothorax Hemothorax Mass Abdominal distension
Passive/relaxation atelectasis	Equilibration of intrapleural and intraalveolar pressures results in lung volume loss due to the normal elastic recoil.	Simple pneumothorax Diaphragmatic pathologies that decrease the downward force
Cicatrization atelectasis	Retraction of fibrotic lung tissue results in loss of lung volume.	Interstitial fibrosis Radiation therapy Pneumoconioses Bronchiectasis Infections Sarcoidosis
Adhesive atelectasis	Surfactant impairment	ARDS Uremia Pulmonary hemorrhage Radiation pneumonitis Inhalation injury
Gravity dependent	A combination of enhanced perfusion with decreased alveolar volume	Frequently observed in postoperative patients because of shallow breathing

ARDS, acute respiratory distress syndrome; ETT, endotracheal tube; ICU, intensive care unit.

  - CT can determine if a tumor or foreign body is the source of endobronchial obstruction.
- LUS findings in atelectasis
  - The two primary forms of atelectasis that can be identified by LUS are compression atelectasis and resorption atelectasis.
    - In compression (passive) atelectasis, the consolidated lung tissue is visualized inside an anechoic pleural effusion accompanied by the presence of trapped air within the bronchi.
    - A dynamic lung US sign called "lung pulse" (visible heartbeats in the context of absent lung sliding) characterizes resorption (active) atelectasis.

TABLE 3.20.2 Imaging Features of Atelectasis

Direct Signs	Indirect Signs
• Triangular or wedge-shaped opacifications facing the pulmonary hilum with or without an air bronchogram • Crowding of vessels and bronchi • Displacement of interlobar fissures toward the pathology	• Hilar displacement • Narrowing of intercostal spaces on the ipsilateral side • No visualization of an interlobar artery • High-standing hemidiaphragm on the affected side • Mediastinal shift toward the affected hemithorax • Compensatory hyperexpansion of the contralateral lung

  - The presence of "lung pulse" indicates complete atelectasis (sensitivity 93%, specificity 100%) following selective intubation in patients with no baseline respiratory pathologies.
  - Sonographic detection of mediastinal and cardiac shift, along with diaphragmatic displacement, also indicates the diagnosis of atelectasis.
  - Hyperechoic intraparenchymal images visualized within a tissue-like pattern (air bronchograms) are an important diagnostic artifact in differentiating pneumonia versus atelectasis.
  - Dynamic air bronchograms (air within the bronchi moving within the surrounding tissue synchronously with ventilation) rule out atelectasis (sensitivity 64%, specificity 94%) and is highly specific for a ventilator-associated pneumonia (VAP). In the early phase of atelectasis, the air bronchogram is either static or completely absent following air resorption in small airways.

Aspiration

- Pathophysiology and epidemiology
  - Intubation, diminished cough reflex, sedation, and enteric tube feeding all heighten the risk of aspiration in the ICU setting.
  - Even when the endotracheal tube (ETT) cuff is inflated, it is still possible to aspirate around it.
  - The aspiration risk in patients with a tracheostomy tube is twice that of patients with an ETT.

- Radiographic findings
  - Depending on the volume and the character of the aspirate, the clinical picture may present in the form of airway obstruction, chemical pneumonitis, or infectious pneumonia.
  - Dependent regions of the lungs (the posterior segments of the upper lobes, superior and posterior basal segments of the lower lobes) are the most affected areas, hence a central predominance on supine AP CXR.
  - The right lung is more frequently affected than the left because the right mainstem bronchus has a larger diameter and straighter course.
  - The most observed radiographic presentations of aspiration include patchy, poorly defined ground-glass consolidative and nodular opacities that carry a focal or multifocal pattern. It is also common to observe volume loss, bronchiolar impaction, and thickening of the airways. In 10% of cases, the CXR may appear normal depending on the aspirated content.
  - The presence of "tree-in-bud" opacities (centrilobular V- and Y- branching structures) on a CT scan in a dependent distribution is suggestive of aspiration (nonspecific sign).
- Aspiration pneumonitis versus pneumonia
  - In the initial 1 to 2 days of aspiration pneumonitis (Mendelson syndrome), opacities may become more prominent, followed by relatively swift resolution.
  - Aspiration pneumonia should be suspected when opacities persist or increase over several days. Aspiration pneumonia manifests on CT scan as unilateral or bilateral patchy or confluent consolidations with ground-glass opacities involving mostly the dependent lung areas.

Pneumonia

- Epidemiology
  - In the ICU, the diagnosis of pneumonia should be suspected if the CXR demonstrates new or worsening opacities accompanied by purulent sputum, fever, or leukocytosis.
  - Two significant risk factors for pneumonia in the ICU population are aspiration and mechanical ventilation.
  - Mixed anaerobic or aerobic gram-negative bacteria, such as *Pseudomonas aeruginosa*, are the primary cause of pneumonias in ICU.
- Classification schemes
  - Based on the distinct radiomorphologic pattern, there are three forms of inhalational pneumonia: lobar, lobular (bronchopneumonia), and interstitial (Table 3.20.3).
  - Based on the specific clinical setting of acquisition, pneumonia is also categorized into community-acquired (CAP), health care–associated (HCAP), hospital-acquired (HAP), and ventilator-associated pneumonia (VAP) (Table 3.20.4).
    - CAP: pneumonia in patients admitted to the hospital from home or developing during the first 48 hours of admission. CAP subdivides into typical versus atypical pneumonia depending on the clinical picture and causative organism (Table 3.20.4).
    - HCAP: the patient has been hospitalized in the last 90 days, resides in a nursing home, or has received antibiotics, chemotherapy, or wound care within 30 days.
    - HAP: develops ≥48 hours following hospitalization
    - VAP: manifests 48 to 72 hours postintubation

TABLE 3.20.3 Radiomorphologic Patterns of Pneumonia

Histopathology	Pathogenesis	Causative Organism	Imaging Findings
Lobar	The most prevalent pattern in CAP, develops when microorganisms enter the distal airspaces, typically in the subpleural lung	*Streptococcus pneumoniae*, *Klebsiella*, *Legionella*	Peripheral opacity of any size, mostly unifocal and unilateral, progresses to homogeneous consolidation. Air bronchograms are often present, and the infection tends to cross bronchopulmonary segments. Minimal volume loss, positive "bulging fissure" sign (displacement of the adjacent fissure due to lobar expansion), and "spine sign" (the overlying lower lob consolidation causes a paradoxical rise in density of the lower thoracic spine on the lateral CXR), ground-glass opacities near the consolidation can be seen on CT scan.
Bronchopneumonia	Initially, it involves the distal airway followed by extension into the peribronchiolar alveoli, filling them with pus and edema. Bilateral and multifocal processes are more common. The most common type of pneumonia.	*Staphylococcus aureus*, gram-negative organisms, anaerobic bacteria, *Legionella pneumophila*.	The initial radiologic presentation consists of many indistinct, centrilobular nodular opacities measuring 5 to 10 mm. Progressing infection results in the conversion of patchy opacities into multifocal bilateral consolidation, a component of volume loss present, positive "tree-in-bud" sign.
Interstitial	The mainstay of the process is the mononuclear cell infiltration around the bronchial and bronchiolar walls and further extension into the alveolar interstitium.	Viral organisms and *Mycoplasma pneumoniae*	Reticulonodular and nodular opacities on CT represent bronchial wall thickening and bronchiolitis, positive "tree-in-bud" sign, interlobular septal thickening, and ground-glass opacities with patchy distribution, atelectasis.

CAP, community-acquired pneumonia; CT, computed tomography; CXR, chest radiography.

TABLE 3.20.4 Imaging Findings in CAP/HAP/VAP

Clinical Setting	Causative Organism	Imaging Findings
Typical CAP	*Streptococcus, Staphylococcus, Haemophilus, Klebsiella, Pseudomonas, Legionella, Moraxella*	New patchy or nodular opacities, lobar, sublobar, or multifocal consolidations, lobar or bronchopneumonia pattern
Atypical CAP	*Mycoplasma, Chlamydia*, viruses, *Coxiella*	Multifocal or diffuse reticulonodular opacities on CXR, patchy ground glass, or interstitial pattern on CT scan
HAP	*Staphylococcus aureus*, MRSA, gram-negative bacilli	Nonspecific findings, unilateral or bilateral consolidations
VAP	*S. aureus*, MRSA, *Enterobacter, Pseudomonas aeruginosa, Escherichia coli*	Bronchopneumonia, consisting of multifocal bilateral areas of consolidation, opacities in nondependent lung areas on CT scan

CAP, community-acquired pneumonia; CT, computed tomography; CXR, chest radiography; HAP, hospital-acquired pneumonia; MRSA, methicillin-resistant *Staphylococcus aureus*; VAP, ventilator-associated pneumonia.

- Based on the causative agent, pneumonia can be bacterial, viral, or fungal.
  - Bacterial: as noted in the previous section and Tables 3.20.3 and 3.20.4
  - Viral: interstitial pneumonia is the classic radiographic pattern related to viral infection.
  - Fungal: *Aspergillus* infection can manifest as either angioinvasive disease or aspergilloma (fungal ball), the former often in the setting of immunocompromise, and the latter often with underlying structural lung disease such as bronchiectasis. Aspergilloma manifests as a round opacity within a cavity or cyst. A "halo sign" (ground-glass opacity surrounding the lesion) on CT scan is suggestive of angioinvasive aspergillosis. *Pneumocystis jirovecii* pneumonia (PJP) typically presents with bilateral perihilar or diffuse symmetric opacities that might be finely granular, reticular, or ground glass in nature. Cystic lesions (pneumatocele) may develop in up to 50% of cases, predisposing patients to pneumothorax (PTX).

Hematogenous Pneumonia

- Epidemiology
  - Most commonly affects intravenous (IV) drug users or those with infected central catheters via seeding of septic emboli
- CXR and CT findings
  - Both the CT and CXR reveal peripherally distributed multiple, poorly defined nodules and wedge-shaped consolidations in the middle and lower lung zones.
  - The nodules tend to cavitate and have a basilar predominance, reflecting the apicobasal gradient of the pulmonary blood flow.
  - A CT scan may often demonstrate nodule-associated pulmonary vasculature known as the "feeding vessel sign."
- LUS findings
  - On LUS, pneumonia can be characterized by B′-profile (B-profile + abolished lung sliding), A/B profile (half A at one lung and half B-profile at another) and C-profile.
  - A dynamic linear/arborescent air bronchogram is indicative of VAP/CAP and has a positive predictive value of 86%.
  - Small subpleural, echo-poor consolidation with irregular margins on LUS is called the "Shred sign" and has a sensitivity of 86% in detecting pneumonia.
  - Uniform texture of consolidation on LUS that resembles abdominal parenchyma is known as a "tissue-like pattern" (sensitivity/specificity >95% in detecting pneumonia).

Acute Respiratory Distress Syndrome

- Definition and classification
  - Defined as diffuse, acute onset (within 1 week) inflammatory lung injury presenting with significant hypoxia and bilateral radiographic opacities of noncardiogenic origin
  - Direct (ie, pneumonia, aspiration) versus secondary (ie, sepsis, trauma, pancreatitis)
    - When acute respiratory distress syndrome (ARDS) is secondary to pulmonary injury, there is a predominance of nondependent, asymmetric, patchy, ground-glass and dense consolidative opacities on the CT scan (atypical CT pattern).
    - Conversely, extrapulmonary causes of ARDS typically present as symmetric, widespread ground-glass opacities with AP density gradient (most dense posteriorly).
- Time course of radiographic findings
  - There is a delay in radiologic abnormalities relative to the clinical manifestation by >12 hours (up to 24 hours) following the inciting injury. This can distinguish ARDS from cardiogenic/hypervolemic edema, where radiographic changes (large pleural effusions, an enlarged heart, a widened vascular pedicle, an upper lobe vascular redistribution) usually coincide with clinical symptoms.
  - The pathophysiology of ARDS ascends through three overlapping and progressive stages, which are reflected in radiologic findings (Table 3.20.5).
- LUS findings in ARDS
  - Nonhomogeneous B-line distribution with spared lung regions (A/B profile), irregular pleural margins, and decreased lung sliding (B′-profile), or subpleural consolidations (C-profile)

Hydrostatic Pulmonary Edema

- The mechanism of hydrostatic pulmonary edema (HPE) is an elevated pulmonary venous pressure due to left-sided heart failure (most common cause), renal failure, liver failure, or fluid overload.

TABLE 3.20.5 ARDS Stages and Imaging Findings

Phase	Pathophysiology	CXR Findings	CT Findings
Exudative Days 1-7	Extravasation of circulating fluid into the interstitium and alveolar space results in collapse in the most dependent parts of the lungs, right-to-left shunt.	It may be normal in the first 24 h, elevated hemidiaphragm, decreased lung volumes, pulmonary edema (early phase). Bilateral diffuse, patchy opacities, over time opacities become confluent, "white lung" in extreme cases, air bronchograms (intermediate phase).	Heterogeneous lung involvement, ground-glass opacities with superimposed thickened interstitial/interlobular septa ("crazy paving," nonspecific) CT scan cannot reliably identify the early exudative phase.
Proliferative Days 8-14	Fibroblast migration, a proliferation of type II pneumocytes, increased collagen secretion, and hyaline membrane formation	Coarse reticular opacities, inhomogeneous pattern, bullous hyperinflation	Patchy opacities progress to consolidation, primarily affecting the lower lobes, ground-glass, and reticular opacities; progression of focal opacities points to superimposed pneumonia.
Fibrotic >2 wk	Continued collagen deposition, destruction of alveolar spaces, and fibrosis	Interstitial appearance: indistinct vascular margins, thickening of peribronchial and perivascular connective tissue	Replacement of ground-glass and consolidative opacities with coarse reticular opacities, pleural thickening, cysts of varying sizes, traction bronchiectasis, honeycombing, and architectural distortion

ARDS, acute respiratory distress syndrome; CT, computed tomography; CXR, chest radiography.

- Grades of HPE and associated CXR findings (recognizing that these exist on a continuum and coexist frequently)
  - Grade 1: pulmonary venous hypertension (pulmonary capillary wedge pressure [PCWP] ~12-18). On CXR, the characteristic pattern of early HPE is cephalization of the pulmonary veins, widened vascular pedicle (>6 cm), and cardiomegaly (cardiothoracic ratio >50%). Widening of the vascular pedicle (usually toward the right side) by 1 cm correlates with estimated expansion of intravascular volume by 2 L.
  - Grade 2: interstitial pulmonary edema (PCWP ~18-25). On CXR, peribronchial cuffing, fissural thickening, and vascular indistinctness. With a rise of pulmonary capillary pressure, interlobular septal thickening (Kerley A/B lines) and small pleural effusions can develop.
  - Grade 3: alveolar pulmonary edema (PCWP >25). Ground-glass opacities emerge, followed by the development of consolidative opacities. Airspace HPE can exhibit a central, nongravitational distribution, preserving the peripheral lung (bat wing or butterfly edema, <10% of cases). Although the findings are usually bilateral and symmetric, conditions such as emphysema or acute mitral regurgitation can result in an uneven distribution of pulmonary edema.
- CT correlates of HPE
  - CT scan has higher accuracy in identifying early manifestations of HPE, such as ground-glass opacities, airway, and interlobular septal thickening.
  - Ground-glass opacities have a gravity-dependent and peripheral appearance on the CT scan.
  - CT scan is more sensitive than CXR in detecting small pleural effusions and is more accurate in defining the extent and location of consolidation.
- LUS in pulmonary edema
  - LUS can help to differentiate pulmonary edema from other potential causes of respiratory distress, such as pneumonia, ARDS, or chronic interstitial lung disease.
  - A diffuse B-profile along with a regular thin pleura, normal sliding, and potential bilateral pleural effusion points to cardiogenic pulmonary edema (HPE).

Pleural Effusion

- The two main types of pleural effusion are transudates and exudates.
  - Elevated hydrostatic pressure in the capillary bed and reduced oncotic pressure are the main mechanisms causing transudates (CHF, hypoalbuminemia, end-stage renal disease [ESRD]).
  - A secondary increase in microvascular permeability due to infections, inflammation, or neoplasms results in exudates (pneumonia, pleural tumors).
- Upright CXR findings in pleural effusion
  - The characteristic features of pleural effusion on the semi- or full upright radiograph are lack of diaphragmatic delineation, blunting of the costophrenic angles, and increased basilar opacities.
  - The upright lateral projection is more sensitive in detecting small pleural effusions and can identify as little as 50 to 75 mL of pleural fluid in the posterior costophrenic angle. On the frontal CXR, >200 mL of fluid are required to blunt the lateral costophrenic angle, 200 mL is necessary to observe a "meniscus sign," and hemidiaphragm obliteration is thought to require at least 500 mL.
  - In subpulmonic pleural effusion, the lateral costophrenic angle may retain its sharpness until a significant volume of fluid has accumulated and subsequently spills into it. The opacity of a subpulmonic effusion can also mimic the contour of the diaphragm, leaving an impression of an "elevated diaphragm."
- Supine CXR findings in pleural effusion
  - On supine CXR, effusions can be identified with an accuracy of 67% to 95%, but supine CXR tends to underestimate pleural fluid volume.

- Larger effusions on a supine CXR are identified by haziness or veil-like opacification due to layering pleural fluid and preserved vascular shadows. Pleural effusion may appear in the shape of an apical cap or cause thickening of the minor fissure.

- CT findings in pleural effusion
  - CT scan has higher sensitivity and specificity in detecting small pleural effusions. Contrast-enhanced CT scans have better visualization for pleural effusions and can help differentiate them from adjacent parenchymal abnormalities.
  - The classic pattern of free-flowing pleural effusion on the CT is a sickle-shaped opacity in the most dependent part of the thoracic cavity, the posterior costophrenic sulci.
- Imaging findings in complicated pleural effusions
  - A uniform opacity with a convex border is a characteristic feature of loculated pleural effusion, which is usually exudative. Loculated fluid has fixed morphology and does not obey the rules of gravity, regardless of the patient's position. On CT scans, loculated effusions appear in a lenticular shape with smooth margins, scalloped borders, and uniform attenuation.
  - On CXR, empyema has smooth margins that are convex to the lung in contrast to transudative pleural effusion that is concave to the lung. On CT, empyema features sharply defined margins, bowing of vessels and bronchi away from the lesion, whereas the lung abscess has a less discrete boundary with lung tissue. While empyemas have an elliptic shape, smooth inner surface, and obtuse angle with pleura, abscesses are rounder, with relatively thick walls and acute angle with pleura. The hallmark of empyema on contrast-enhanced CT is the "split pleura" sign—enhanced, separated, and thickened layers of visceral and parietal pleura encircling a tense, bulging, lenticular fluid collection.
- LUS for pleural effusion
  - LUS is a reliable tool for diagnosing, quantifying, and assessing the characteristics of pleural effusions and has higher sensitivity and specificity for identifying and quantifying pleural effusion than bedside CXR.
  - Whether free flowing or loculated, most pleural effusions have hypoechoic/anechoic pattern with a distinct echogenic line that differentiates the visceral pleura from the lung parenchyma.
  - Internal fibrin strands or septation characterize the echotexture of exudative effusion, whereas a transudate is typically homogeneously anechoic.
  - The volume of pleural effusion can be estimated by measuring the maximal distance between the pleural layers at the end of expiration (Balik): V (mL)=20 × Sep (mm).

Pneumothorax

- CXR findings in PTX
  - The findings of PTX on CXR are contingent upon the imaging position since air will travel to the nondependent parts of the chest: in an upright position, the gas will accumulate in apicolateral portions of the chest.
  - The primary criterion in an upright position is the identification of the separated visceral pleura as a fine, curvilinear reflection, with increased radiolucency between the chest wall and the separated visceral pleural line.
  - In a supine CXR, air predominantly accumulates along the anterior mediastinal structures and subpulmonic regions. The supine CXR significantly underestimates the actual size of PTX and is far less sensitive compared to erect CXR. Indirect signs of PTX on a supine CXR include increased radiolucency of the ipsilateral lung, the deep sulcus sign (a deep, radiolucent lateral costophrenic sulcus), and sharp delineation of cardiomediastinal and diaphragmatic borders.
  - Tension PTX has additional radiographic features: contralateral mediastinal shift and ipsilateral lung collapse, inversion of the ipsilateral diaphragm, ipsilateral flattening of the cardiac boundaries, hyperlucent hemithorax and enhanced thoracic volume, and/or widened ipsilateral intercostal space.
- LUS in PTX requires a two-step approach to establish the diagnosis.
  - The initial step is to detect A′-profile (very sensitive but not specific): A-profile + abolished lung sliding
  - The detection of the lung point is the second essential step following the detection of A′-profile. The lung point is a pathognomonic sign for PTX, and in the M mode, it indicates the transition from the seashore to stratosphere sign.
  - If implemented correctly, the LUS can have very high sensitivity (>95%) and specificity (>91%) in diagnosing PTX (both are superior to bedside CXR).

Pulmonary Embolism

- CXR in PE
  - CXR is false negative in 40% of cases and, therefore, plays no role in the diagnosis of PE.
  - Nonspecific, indirect signs on CXR include atelectasis, pleural effusion, peripheral oligemia (Westermark sign), elevated hemidiaphragm, Hampton hump (a wedge-shaped subpleural infarction), and prominent central PAs (Fleischner sign).
- CT pulmonary angiography (CTPA) in PE
  - Given its high accuracy (sensitivity 83% and specificity 96%), CTPA is the modality of choice in patients with clinically suspected acute PE.
  - The direct diagnostic criteria of PE on CT scans include complete arterial occlusion resulting in lack of opacification of the entire lumen (vessel cutoff sign), enlarged vascular diameter of the same order of arteries due to the clot burden, clearly defined central arterial filling defect encompassed by contrast media (railway track sign), and partial eccentric filling defect in peripheral arteries where the embolus forms an acute angle with the arterial wall.
  - Acute right heart overload results from a substantial increase in PA pressure owing to an obstruction of >30% of pulmonary circulation.
  - The prognostically significant signs indicating increased pressures on the right side of the heart include RV-to-LV ratio >1, flattening or bulging of interventricular septum toward the left, and dilatation of PA and coronary sinus.

Supporting Devices

- *ETT*
  - The ETT tip should be positioned 4 ± 2 cm above the carina when the patient's head is in a neutral position.
  - Neck flexion leads to caudal displacement of the ETT, measuring up to 2 cm, whereas neck extension may result in superior migration by the same distance.
  - In the case of mainstem intubation (10% of urgently performed ICU intubations), the CXR will show hyperinflation of the ipsilateral lung with a contralateral shift of the mediastinum.
    - The CXR may also demonstrate signs of atelectasis, consolidation, and opacification in combination with volume loss on the contralateral side.
  - Right mainstem intubation occurs more frequently due to the more vertical orientation of the right mainstem bronchus.
  - The tip of a tracheostomy tube should be projected approximately at the T3 level, and the tube diameter should be approximately two-thirds that of the trachea.
- Catheters and tubes
  - The SVC is formed by the convergence of the right and left brachiocephalic veins at the level of the first intercostal space, right to the midline.
  - The optimal position of a central venous catheter (CVC) tip is just above the junction of the SVC and the right atrium (cavo-atrial junction), central to the venous valves.
    - On CXR, it correlates to a level of ~4 cm below the carina.
  - In up to one-third of cases, CVCs are malpositioned at the time of insertion.
  - Common aberrant locations include the internal jugular vein, the right atrium/RV, the contralateral subclavian vein, the ipsilateral artery, the IVC, and extrathoracic sites.
    - Inadequately low placement within the right atrium may lead to cardiac dysrhythmia and mechanical irritation of the tricuspid valve.
    - If the catheter is not positioned exactly at the right mediastinal border but is instead observed to extend toward the aortic arch, an intraarterial placement should be suspected.
    - The posterior orientation of the catheter tip indicates its placement into the azygos vein.
    - If the catheter tip is positioned against the lateral wall of the SVC, the excessive focal pressure on the venous wall may result in perforation (rare).
  - For optimal placement, a PA catheter should be positioned in the proximal right/left PA or proximal interlobar PA.
    - On CXR, the tip typically sits in the right PA, 1 cm to the right of the spine.
    - When the catheter tip is placed centrally in the proximal pulmonary trunk, catheter pulsation may cause irritation to the pulmonary valve.
    - Pulmonary infarction may occur distal to the tip of the catheter if it is advanced too far since the diameter of the catheter gets closer to that of the PA it sits in.
    - The PA catheter should be retracted if it extends beyond the pulmonary hilum on the CXR.
  - The proper position of the chest tube on CXR depends on whether it is meant to evacuate air or fluid.
    - Since air accumulates anteriorly and superiorly, the optimal orientation of the chest tube is toward the apex in the context of PTX.
    - Most fluid collections are gravity dependent; therefore, pleural fluid evacuation requires inferiorly directed chest tube placement, positioned just above the diaphragm.
  - The proximal side hole on the chest tube marked by an interruption of the radiopaque identification line should be positioned medial to the inner margin of the ribs on CXR.
  - The major complications of chest tube misplacement (10%) include insertion into the lung parenchyma, mediastinum, or transdiaphragmatic insertion into the liver or spleen.
  - The intraparenchymal chest tube insertion may lead to pulmonary contusion, which manifests as a new opacity around the insertion site on CXR.

SUGGESTED READINGS

Bentz MR, Primack SL. Intensive care unit imaging. *Clin Chest Med*. 2015;36(2):219-234, viii.

Breitkopf R, Treml B, Rajsic S. Lung sonography in critical care medicine. *Diagnostics (Basel)*. 2022;12(6):1405.

Brogi E, Gargani L, Bignami E, et al. Thoracic ultrasound for pleural effusion in the intensive care unit: a narrative review from diagnosis to treatment. *Crit Care*. 2017;21:325.

Collins J, Stern EJ. *Chest Radiology: The Essentials*. 3rd ed. Wolters Kluwer Health; 2015.

Dickman E, Terentiev V, Likourezos A, Derman A, Haines L. Extension of the thoracic spine sign. *J Ultrasound Med*. 2015;34(9):1555-1561.

Digumarthy SR. *Problem Solving in Chest Imaging E-Book*. 1st ed. Elsevier; 2019.

Garg M, Prabhakar N, Kiruthika P, et al. Imaging of pneumonia: an overview. *Curr Radiol Rep*. 2017;5(4):16.

Gulati A, Balasubramanya R. Lung imaging. In: *StatPearls* [Internet]. StatPearls Publishing; 2023. Accessed June 19, 2024. https://www.ncbi.nlm.nih.gov/books/NBK558976/

Hill JR, Horner PE, Primack SL. ICU imaging. *Clin Chest Med*. 2008;29(1):59-76, vi.

Kvetan V, Oropello JM, Pastores SM, eds. *Critical Care*. 1st ed. McGraw-Hill Education LLC; 2016.

Lichtenstein DA. BLUE-protocol and FALLS-protocol: two applications of lung ultrasound in the critically ill. *Chest*. 2015;147(6):1659-1670.

Lichtenstein DA, Mezière GA. Relevance of lung ultrasound in the diagnosis of acute respiratory failure. *Chest*. 2008;134(1):117-125.

Parker MS, Rosado-de-Christenson ML, Abbott GF. *Chest Imaging Case Atlas*. 2nd ed. Thieme; 2012.

Mojoli F, Bouhemad B, Mongodi S, Lichtenstein D. Lung ultrasound for critically ill patients. *Am J Respir Crit Care Med*. 2019;199(6):701-714.

Rocca E, Zanza C, Longhitano Y, et al. Lung ultrasound in critical care and emergency medicine: clinical review. *Adv Respir Med*. 2023;91(3):203-223.

Rubinowitz AN, Siegel MD, Tocino I. Thoracic imaging in the ICU. *Crit Care Clin*. 2007;23(3):539-573.

Schaefer-Prokop C. *Critical Care Radiology*. Thieme; 2011.

Shepard JAO, McLoud TC, eds. *Thoracic Imaging*. 3rd ed. Elsevier; 2019.

Stefanidis K, Dimopoulos S, Nanas S. Basic principles and current applications of lung ultrasonography in the intensive care unit. *Respirology*. 2011;16(2):249-256.

Villasana-Gomez G, Toussie D, Kaufman B, et al. Chest intensive care unit imaging: pearls and pitfalls. *Clin Chest Med*. 2024;45(2):213-235.

Walker C. *Muller's Imaging of the Chest E-Book: Expert Radiology Series*. 2nd ed. Elsevier; 2018.

Wormanns D. *Diagnostic Imaging of the Chest*. Thieme; 2020.

3.21

Pharmacologic Therapies for Pulmonary Disorders

Natasha Lopez

Beta Agonist

- Short-acting inhaled beta-2 agonist
  - Albuterol, levalbuterol
    - First-line therapy for asthma and chronic obstructive pulmonary disease (COPD) exacerbations
    - Albuterol is the most frequently used, loses beta-2 selectivity at higher doses. Can use multiple inhalations during the first hour, can also deliver as continuous nebulization
    - Levalbuterol is a highly selective beta-2 agonist, potentially less tachycardia, but clinical trials demonstrated minimal difference compared to albuterol.
    - Meter-dose inhaler (MDI) or nebulization dosage forms. MDI with a spacer and nebulization have comparable improvements in lung function and hospitalization risk. Can be administered in ventilated patients, with MDIs requiring twice the standard dose
    - Nebulization preferred in patients who are breathless, unable to take deep breaths, or altered mental status
    - Side effects often dose related, including tachycardia, tremors, hypokalemia, and type B lactic acidosis (rare)
- Short-acting inhaled nonselective beta agonist
  - Epinephrine (ie, racemic epinephrine)
    - Stimulates alpha, beta-1, and beta-2 receptors, resulting in bronchodilation
    - Available as racemic epinephrine 2.25% nebulization solution or MDI
    - Not for routine management and treatment of asthma or COPD due to side-effect profile (tachycardia, hypertension); consider in acute anaphylaxis with edema
- Long-acting inhaled beta-2 agonist
  - Olodaterol, salmeterol
    - Used in the chronic treatment of asthma and in COPD if combined with an inhaled corticosteroid. No role in acute exacerbations
- Parenteral beta agonist
  - Epinephrine, terbutaline
    - Terbutaline acts specifically on beta-2 receptors versus epinephrine stimulates alpha, beta-1, and beta-2 receptors, resulting in a higher side-effect profile.
    - Epinephrine can be administered intravenously (IV), intramuscularly (IM), or subcutaneously (SC); terbutaline is administered SC.
    - Not recommended due to the risk of adverse effects (arrhythmias, tachycardia, increased blood pressure) and no benefit compared to inhaled beta-2 agonist. Consider in anaphylactic-induced asthma exacerbation

Anticholinergic

- Short-acting inhaled
  - Ipratropium bromide
    - Use combination with beta-2 agonist in severe asthma exacerbations and as first-line therapy in COPD exacerbations
    - MDI or nebulizer, in acute exacerbation can be given every 20 minutes for 3 doses; combination of albuterol with ipratropium commercially available
    - Side effects: dry mouth, anisocoria can occur when nebulized
- Long-acting inhaled
  - Aclidinium, umeclidinium, tiotropium
    - No role in the acute exacerbation setting

Corticosteroids

- Systemic glucocorticoids
  - Dexamethasone, methylprednisolone, prednisone, prednisolone
    - Recommended for moderate-to-severe asthma and COPD exacerbations
    - Initially administer IV, can be converted to oral (PO) when patient can reliably take and absorb oral medications. IV and PO are bioequivalent.
    - Dosage, duration, and tapering are variable based on indication and case-specific factors.
    - Side effects: hyperglycemia, fluid retention, hypertension, neuropsychiatric (insomnia, psychosis), gastritis/gastrointestinal bleeding, myopathy, leukocytosis
- Inhaled glucocorticoids
  - Betamethasone, budesonide, fluticasone
    - High-dose inhaled is not an alternative for oral in acute exacerbation due to variable inhaled absorption. Adding inhaled to systemic has no additive benefit in the acute setting.

Magnesium

- Bronchodilator effect due to the inhibition of calcium influx into airway smooth muscle cells
- Administered as a single dose 2 g IV over 20 minutes
- Adjunct to first-line therapy and/or refractory asthma cases; evidence suggests decreased hospitalization in acute asthma exacerbation. Caution in patients with renal impairment, bradycardia, and myasthenia gravis

Methylxanthines

- Aminophylline, theophylline
  - Nonselective phosphodiesterase inhibitors induced bronchodilation and increased diaphragmatic contraction.
  - Administer IV bolus followed by continuous infusion (aminophylline, theophylline) or PO (theophylline). Drug level monitoring needed due to narrow therapeutic index.

- Only consider in refractory asthma due to the risk of adverse effects (atrial/ventricular arrhythmias, seizures, nausea/vomiting), no role in acute COPD exacerbation

Phosphodiesterase Type 4 Inhibitor Therapy

- Roflumilast
  - No role in the acute setting. Approved for the reduction of exacerbations of patients with COPD

Anesthetic Agents

- Inhaled halothane, isoflurane, sevoflurane
  - Promotes bronchodilation, decreases airway responsiveness, and attenuates bronchospasm. Evidence for use is limited to case reports for refractory status asthmaticus.
  - Requires specialized equipment and monitoring on standard mechanical ventilators with a full-time anesthesiologist available at bedside
- Ketamine
  - Bronchodilation is promoted through inhibition of endogenous catecholamine reuptake, resulting in decreased lower airway resistance and increased lung compliance in asthmatics.
  - Evidence for use is limited to case reports for refractory status asthmaticus. Spontaneous ventilation is generally preserved.
  - Side effects: tachycardia, hypertension, hypersalivation, nystagmus, emergence phenomena (visual/auditory hallucination, delirium, dysphoria)

Leukotriene Inhibitors

- Montelukast, zafirlukast
  - No role in acute exacerbation unless triggered by overproduction of leukotrienes (eg, nonsteroidal antiinflammatory drug [NSAID]-induced exacerbation). Can continue chronic therapy during an exacerbation
  - IV formulation not available in the United States, oral dosage can be crushed for feeding tube administration.

Oxygen

- COPD exacerbations
  - Administer to keep a Pao_2 of 60 to 70 mm Hg to target or Spo_2 of 88% to 92%.
  - Oxygenation above this may not offer much benefit and may worsen hypercarbia.
- Pneumothorax
  - Placing patients on 100% O_2 decreases nitrogen concentrations and can increase the resorption rate of the pneumothorax.

Inhaled Helium-Oxygen Mixture

- Low density of helium generates less airway resistance, resulting in decreased work of breathing, leading to improved ventilation.
- Evidence does not support routine usage; no benefit compared to standard therapies (oxygen, noninvasive ventilation) in asthma or COPD exacerbations.

Pulmonary Arterial Hypertension

Prostacyclin and Prostacyclin Receptor Agonist

- Epoprostenol (IV, inhaled), iloprost (inhaled), selexipag (PO), treprostinil (PO, IV, inhaled, SC)
  - Induces vasodilation (systemic and pulmonary for IV, SC, PO formulations), inhibits proliferation and platelet aggregation
  - Continuous infusion epoprostenol has been shown to improved pulmonary hemodynamics, 6-minute walk distance (6MWD), and survival in severe pulmonary arterial hypertension (PAH).
  - Epoprostenol IV or inhaled can be considered for acute lowering of pulmonary vascular resistance (PVR). Inhaled administration allows selective pulmonary vasodilation without systemic hypotension.
  - Iloprost and treprostinil inhaled require specific delivery systems; in the intensive care unit (ICU), therapy can be transitioned to inhaled epoprostenol or nitric oxide.
  - Side effects: hypotension (IV, SC, PO formulations), infection (IV, SC formulation), headache, nausea, diarrhea, jaw pain. Side effects often limit dose titration.

Nitric Oxide-Cyclic Guanosine Monophosphate Enhancers

- Cyclic guanosine monophosphate (cGMP) phosphodiesterase 5 (PDE5) inhibitors
  - Sildenafil (IV, PO), tadalafil (PO)
    - Prevents degradation of cGMP, resulting in vasodilation and inhibiting proliferation
    - Long-term therapy for World Health Organization (WHO) group I; improves pulmonary hemodynamics, exercise capacity, symptoms, and time to clinical worsening. Sildenafil's shorter half-life allows faster dose titration in the acute setting.
    - Side effects: hypotension (avoid nitrates and riociguat), rebound PAH with abrupt discontinuation
- Soluble guanylate cyclase (sGC) stimulant
  - Riociguat (PO)
    - Stimulates sGC both with and independent of nitric oxide, resulting in vasodilation
    - Therapy for WHO groups I and IV (chronic thromboembolic pulmonary hypertension); can be continued in the ICU, but the long half-life and hypotension limit the use for acute management.
    - Side effects: hypotension (avoid nitrates and with PDE5 inhibitors), bleeding, teratogenic
- Nitric oxide (inhaled)
  - Selective pulmonary vasodilator resulting in reduced PVR without systemic hypotension
  - Consider for acute lowering of PVR in the ICU
  - Side effects: methemoglobinemia, rebound PAH with abrupt discontinuation

Endothelin Receptor Antagonist

- Ambrisentan (PO), bosentan (PO), macitentan (PO)
  - Blocks endothelin-induced pulmonary vasoconstriction and proliferation

- Therapy for WHO group I; endothelin receptor antagonist (ERA) therapy should be continued in the ICU, but limited utility for initiating acute management.
- Improves symptoms, exercise tolerance, pulmonary hemodynamics, WHO functional class, time to clinical worsening
- Side effects: teratogenic, hepatotoxicity with bosentan, peripheral edema

Calcium Channel Blockers

- Amlodipine (PO), diltiazem (IV, PO), nifedipine (PO)
  - Initiate in WHO group I with a positive vasoreactivity test
  - Side effects: hypotension, bradycardia with diltiazem, peripheral edema.

Transforming Growth Factor-Beta Pathway Modulation

- Sotatercept (SC)
  - Additive therapy in WHO group I for long-term improvement of PVR, 6MWD, and time to clinical worsening
  - No role in the acute setting or continuation in the ICU based on the drug onset ~7 days, half-life ~24 days, and clinical outcomes observed at 24 weeks

SUGGESTED READINGS

Agustí A, Celli BR, Criner GJ, et al. Global initiative for chronic obstructive lung disease 2023 report: GOLD executive summary. *Am J Respir Crit Care Med*. 2023;207(7):819-837.

Barnett CF, O'Brien C, De Marco T. Critical care management of the patient with pulmonary hypertension. *Eur Heart J Acute Cardiovasc Care*. 2022;11(1):77-83.

Barst RJ, Rich S, Bourge RC, Langleben D, Uretsky BF, Blackburn SD. A comparison of continuous intravenous epoprostenol (prostacyclin) with conventional therapy for primary pulmonary hypertension. *N Engl J Med*. 1996;334(5):296-301.

Ding Z, Li X, Lu Y, et al. A randomized, controlled multicentric study of inhaled budesonide and intravenous methylprednisolone in the treatment on acute exacerbation of chronic obstructive pulmonary disease. *Respir Med*. 2016;121:39-47.

Epperson J, Athar ZM, Arshad M, Chen EY. Ketamine as an adjunct therapy in acute severe asthma: an in-depth review of efficacy and clinical implications. *Cureus*. 2024;16(6):e62483.

Garner O, Ramey JS, Hanania NA. Management of life-threatening asthma. *Chest*. 2022;162(4):747-756.

Global Initiative for Asthma. *Global Strategy for Asthma Management and Prevention, 2024*. Global Initiative for Asthma; Updated May 2024.

Humbert M, Kovacs G, Hoeper MM, et al. 2022 ESC/ERS guidelines for the diagnosis and treatment of pulmonary hypertension. *Eur Respir J*. 2023; 61(1):2200879.

Jin Q, Chen D, Zhang X, et al. Medical management of pulmonary arterial hypertension: current approaches and investigational drugs. *Pharmaceutics*. 2023;15(6):1579.

Kew KM, Kirtchuk L, Michell CI, Griffiths B; The Cochrane Collaboration. Intravenous magnesium sulfate for treating adults with acute asthma in the emergency department. *Cochrane Database Syst Rev*. 2014;2014: CD010909.

Khan KS, Jawaid S, Memon UA, et al. Management of chronic obstructive pulmonary disease (COPD) exacerbations in hospitalized patients from admission to discharge: a comprehensive review of therapeutic interventions. *Cureus*. 2023;15(8):e43694.

Kiser TH, Allen RR, Valuck RJ, Moss M, Vandivier RW. Outcomes associated with corticosteroid dosage in critically ill patients with acute exacerbations of chronic obstructive pulmonary disease. *Am J Respir Crit Care Med*. 2014;189(9):1052-1064.

Leuppi JD, Schuetz P, Bingisser R, et al. Short-term vs conventional glucocorticoid therapy in acute exacerbations of chronic obstructive pulmonary disease: the REDUCE randomized clinical trial. *JAMA*. 2013; 309(21):2223.

Ni H, Aye SZ, Naing C; Cochrane Airways Group. Magnesium sulfate for acute exacerbations of chronic obstructive pulmonary disease. *Cochrane Database Syst Rev*. 2022;5(5):CD013506.

Papadopoulou E, Bin Safar S, Khalil A, et al. Inhaled *versus* systemic corticosteroids for acute exacerbations of COPD: a systematic review and meta-analysis. *Eur Respir Rev*. 2024;33(171):230151.

Tobias JD. Inhalational anesthesia: basic pharmacology, end organ effects, and applications in the treatment of status asthmaticus. *J Intensive Care Med*. 2009;24(6):361-371.

Van Geffen WH, Douma WR, Slebos DJ, Kerstjens HA; Cochrane Airways Group. Bronchodilators delivered by nebuliser versus pMDI with spacer or DPI for exacerbations of COPD. *Cochrane Database Syst Rev*. 2016;2016(8):CD011826.

Walters JA, Tan DJ, White CJ, Wood-Baker R; Cochrane Airways Group. Different durations of corticosteroid therapy for exacerbations of chronic obstructive pulmonary disease. *Cochrane Database Syst Rev*. 2018; 3(3):CD006897.

3.22

Thoracic Surgery Postoperative Management and Perioperative Complications

Philicia Moonsamy

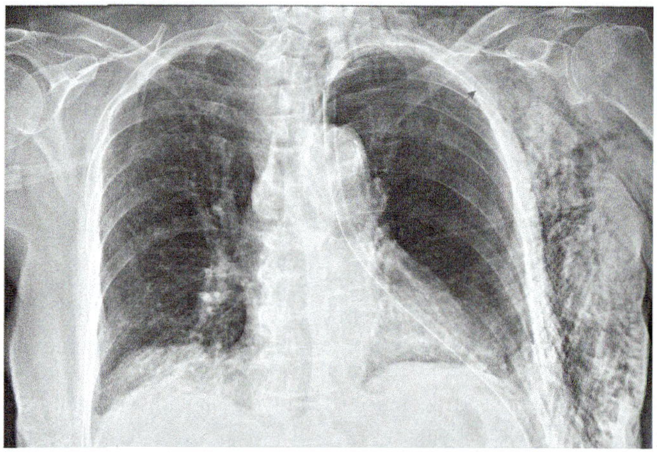

FIGURE 3.22.1 **Patient with pneumothorax (*arrows*) and subcutaneous emphysema after left upper lobectomy.**

Overview

- Increasing adoption of minimally invasive techniques in thoracic surgery has significantly reduced the incidence of postoperative complications compared to traditional open thoracotomy.
- Since 2019, robotic assisted thoracic surgery (RATS) has become the most common approach to anatomic lung resection nationally. Here, we outline the most common postoperative complications in modern-day thoracic surgery patients.

Air Leak

- Prolonged air leak, defined as a leak lasting >5 days, is the most common complication after pulmonary resection.
- Air leaks after thoracic surgery usually arise from the lung parenchyma (alveolar-pleural fistula) and generally do not lead to respiratory failure.
- Reducing the time on positive pressure ventilation to minimize peak airway pressures decreases the incidence of air leak; therefore, it is important for thoracic surgery patients to be extubated in the operating room.
- Preventive measures include creation of a pleural tent after upper lobectomy, buttressing the bronchial stump with a muscle flap, suture closure of identified leaks in the operating room, and the use of sealants such as polyethylene glycol.
- Given the communication between the colonized lung and the pleural space, patients with prolonged air leaks are at risk for developing an empyema.

Diagnosis

- The presence and size of the air leak is easily assessed in the chest drainage system by identifying bubbling into the water seal chamber during expiration.
- The presence of an air leak precludes removal of the chest tube, which would result in the development of a pneumothorax.
- Patients with increasing subcutaneous emphysema on examination or on chest x-ray should be carefully examined for an air leak (Figure 3.22.1).

Treatment

- Nearly all parenchymal air leaks will resolve with chest tube drainage and time.
- The presence of an air leak does not necessitate applying suction to the chest tube—the amount of suction applied should be the lowest amount that keeps the lung expanded and prevents the accumulation of subcutaneous emphysema. As with all fistula management, suction should be minimized and chest tubes should be kept to water seal as long as a large pneumothorax does not develop.
- Clinicians may hasten resolution of air leaks by introducing sclerosing agents into the pleural space for pleurodesis. This can be done via the patient's chest tube or in the operating room.
    - Commonly used agents: talc, doxycycline, bleomycin, or autologous blood
- An air leak that develops suddenly or one that increases to become present throughout the respiratory cycle indicates the development of a bronchopleural fistula (BPF), with air leaking from the bronchial stump after lobectomy or pneumonectomy. This can lead to imminent respiratory compromise; therefore, management is very different than with parenchymal air leaks and requires operative management with repair and autologous tissue coverage.
    - BPF management is discussed further in section "Postpneumonectomy Complications."

Postpneumonectomy Perioperative Complications

- Pneumonectomy carries a significantly higher risk of perioperative morbidity and mortality compared to other pulmonary resections.
- Management of the postpneumonectomy space is surgeon specific, with some opting not to place a chest tube. When a chest tube is placed, it may be clamped or placed to a chest drainage system on water seal. The chest tube can be unclamped to evaluate for bleeding or to equalize the intrathoracic pressure if there is excessive mediastinal shift causing hemodynamic compromise. Suction should never be applied to the chest tube as this can cause shifting of the mediastinum and cardiac herniation, leading to hemodynamic collapse.
- The pneumonectomy space gradually fills with fluid in the weeks after surgery. Over time, further expected anatomic changes include hyperinflation of the remaining

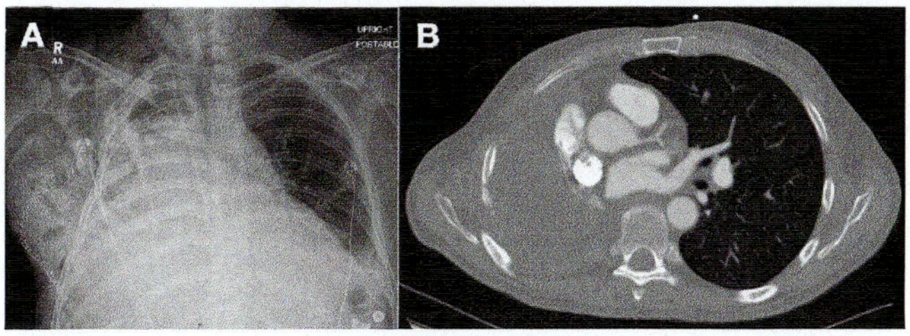

FIGURE 3.22.2 Expected radiographic changes in the postpneumonectomy period. (A) Fluid filling the pneumonectomy space in the immediate postoperative period. **(B)** The postpneumonectomy space fills completely with fluid in the weeks after surgery.

lung, elevation of the hemidiaphragm, and gradual shift of the mediastinum toward the pneumonectomy space (Figure 3.22.2).

Postpneumonectomy Pulmonary Edema

- Development of pulmonary edema in the remaining lung is a potentially devastating complication that can quickly lead to acute respiratory distress syndrome (ARDS) with a high associated mortality (>50%).
- Patients who undergo right pneumonectomy are at higher risk.
- Although previous dogma stressed positive fluid balance as the main driver, the exact cause is unknown. Most modern literature cite multifactorial causes including barotrauma or high delivered oxygen concentration during single-lung ventilation in the operating room, perioperative fluid overload, and reperfusion injury to the remaining lung.
- Early treatment and diagnosis are imperative. Characteristic chest x-ray findings include extensive airspace opacities similar to those seen in ARDS with Kerley lines, peribronchial cuffing, and haziness of vessel outlines.
- One prospective study found that intraoperative administration of 250 mg of methylprednisolone just before pulmonary artery ligation decreased the incidence of postpneumonectomy pulmonary edema.
- Treatment is supportive starting with supplemental oxygen and diuresis to prevent fluid overload. Mechanical ventilation is often required and should be delivered with lung-protective ventilation strategies using low-tidal volumes of 6 mL/kg of predicted body weight and ensuring plateau pressures are <30 cm H_2O. Nitrous oxide has been shown to improve oxygenation, especially in cases of pulmonary hypertension. Finally, extracorporeal membrane oxygenation (ECMO) may be required in refractory cases.

Bronchopleural Fistula

- BPF can develop early in the first postoperative week or late in the following weeks to months due to bronchial stump dehiscence. Both situations are surgical emergencies.
- Risk factors include longer residual bronchial stump, residual tumor at the stump, previous radiation, age >60, and prolonged ventilation.
- Since the bronchial stump after right pneumonectomy is longer and more exposed than on the left, this complication is more frequent after right pneumonectomy. The left bronchial stump usually retracts under the arch of the aorta and is protected.
- The timing of the development of a BPF determines management. Early BPF occurs within 2 weeks of surgery and is not associated with empyema. Patients who develop an early BPF should be taken back to the operating room for repair and autologous tissue coverage. Late BPF occurs >2 weeks after surgery and is associated with the development of an empyema because the pneumonectomy space has filled with fluid by this time.
- Patients with a late BPF present with a new air-fluid level in the pneumonectomy cavity and associated clinical symptoms of empyema and sepsis, such as fever, leukocytosis, and hemodynamic instability. This is a critical care emergency and should be tackled as follows:
    - Position the patient such that the pneumonectomy side is dependent in order to protect the remaining lung from soilage via the airway.
    - Place a chest tube expeditiously to drain the empyema in the pneumonectomy space and protect the contralateral lung. Send the fluid for Gram stain and culture.
    - Initiate broad-spectrum antibiotics.
    - The patient should be urgently taken back to the operating room for bronchoscopy and exploration of the pneumonectomy space with washout and debridement of all infected tissues. The bronchial stump should not be repaired in an infected field, and the chest should be left open with an Eloesser flap for further debridement.
    - Once the patient has stabilized and source control has been achieved, the patient can return to the operating room for repair of the bronchial stump and buttress with autologous tissue.

Hemorrhage

- Hypotension after surgery should always raise suspicion for bleeding.
- Chest tube output of >1 L in an hour or 200 mL/h for 4 hours are indications to return to the operating room for exploration.
- Always obtain a chest x-ray to assess for retained hemothorax in patients with low chest tube output where bleeding is suspected, since low output can be falsely reassuring.

Pneumonia

- Thoracic surgery patients are at particularly high risk for developing pneumonia and mucous plugging after surgery.
- Pain with respiration leading to poor pulmonary toilet and a change in chest wall mechanics, especially after thoracotomy, are the main drivers of this problem.
- Atelectasis causes a ventilation/perfusion mismatch and can result in hypoxemia and respiratory decline.

Treatment

- Early ambulation, encouraging the patient to cough, and effective pain control are the mainstays of both prevention and treatment of mucous plugging and pneumonia in thoracic surgery patients.

- Chest physiotherapy and inhaled mucolytics are useful adjuncts to improve pulmonary toilet.
- Prior to the initiation of antibiotics, blood and sputum cultures should be sent. If the patient is unable to cough to produce sputum, a bronchoalveolar lavage (BAL) can be obtained with bronchoscopy. Surgeons may have sent a preoperative BAL before lung resection, which can guide choice of antibiotics. Antibiotic coverage should initially be broad but ultimately tailored to the cultures.

Atrial Fibrillation

- Atrial fibrillation is the most common arrhythmia following lung resection, with an incidence of 33% after lobectomy.
- Risk factors include age over 70, male sex, prior arrhythmia, larger amount of lung resected (highest risk after pneumonectomy), and blood transfusion. Thoracic surgeons often prescribe prophylactic beta-blocker postoperatively for patients with these risk factors.

Diagnosis and Workup

- In addition to a 12-lead electrocardiogram (ECG), labs including complete blood count (CBC) and basic metabolic panel (BMP) should be obtained.
- A chest x-ray should also be obtained to rule out worsening pneumothorax as a precipitating factor for new-onset atrial fibrillation.

Treatment

- Initial management includes repleting electrolytes, focusing on achieving serum magnesium >2 mg/dL and serum potassium >4 mmol/L.
- Further treatment is guided by the patient's hemodynamics:
  - Hemodynamically unstable patients must be transferred to the intensive care unit (ICU) and electrically cardioverted.
  - Hemodynamically stable patients should be chemically converted with rate control drugs. The first-line agent is a beta-1 selective blocker, most commonly metoprolol. Calcium channel blockers such as diltiazem can also be used as a second agent or as a primary agent in patients who have a contraindication to beta-blockers, such as severe chronic obstructive pulmonary disease (COPD). Amiodarone can be used safely in thoracic surgery patients but should be avoided in pneumonectomy patients or patients with severe underlying lung disease due to the risk of pulmonary toxicity. Finally, digoxin may be used in recalcitrant cases.

Recurrent Laryngeal Nerve Injury

- Injury to the recurrent laryngeal nerve (RLN) can occur during dissection under the aortic arch during left upper lobectomy or during dissection around the trachea while harvesting lymph node station 4R in the right chest.
- Patients with RLN paresis or paralysis are at increased risk for aspiration, which can be a devastating complication in thoracic surgery patients who already have some degree of respiratory compromise after surgery.

Diagnosis

- RLN injury should be suspected in patients who have a weak cough and develop a hoarse or weak voice after surgery.
- The diagnosis is made by direct visualization of the vocal cords with fiberoptic laryngoscopy, which reveals lack of movement of the affected vocal cord during coughing or phonation.

Treatment

- Paralysis is usually temporary due to thermal injury with a structurally intact nerve. Therefore, initial treatment is directed at reestablishing normal glottic anatomy by injecting collagen to medialize the affected vocal cord.
- Patients should be treated early in their course to prevent further complications such as aspiration and mucous plugging from poor pulmonary toilet.

Chyle Leak

- Lymph node dissection is a step in all lung resection techniques. Therefore, these patients are at increased risk for postoperative chyle leak. The leak usually arises from the dissected lymph node bed and not from the thoracic duct itself.

Diagnosis

- High nonbloody chest tube output after thoracic surgery should raise clinical suspicious for chyle leak.
- The diagnosis can usually be made clinically by the identification of milky chest tube output after the patient has started eating fat-containing food. However, about 30% of chylothoraces present without the classic milky appearance.
- If the patient is unable to eat or if the chest tube output remains high despite diuresis, the fluid can be tested for triglycerides, lymphocytes, and chylomicrons. Triglyceride level >110 mg/dL, lymphocyte count >90%, or any detection of chylomicrons in the fluid is diagnostic of chyle.

Treatment

- The treatment strategy is guided by the volume of the chyle leak (Figure 3.22.3).
  - Low output chylothorax is defined as <10 mL/kg/d, high output is >12 mL/kg/d or >1.1 L/d.
- Low output chylothorax is treated with dietary modifications and pharmacologic therapy alone for up to 2 weeks (octreotide: 100 µg subcutaneously [SC] every 6-8 hours or 50-200 µg intravenously [IV] every 8 hours and midodrine: 2.5-10 mg orally [po] every 8 hours).
  - Patients should kept nil per os (NPO) with immediate initiation of total parenteral nutrition (TPN) until the chest tube output decreases, at which time patients can be transitioned to a low-fat diet of < 20 g/d.
- Failure of nonoperative management or high output chylothorax should be treated with thoracic duct ligation via the right chest or lymphangiogram with thoracic duct embolization (TDE).
- Pleurodesis by introducing a sclerosing agent such as talc into the pleural space can be considered in refractory cases or when other interventions are contraindicated.

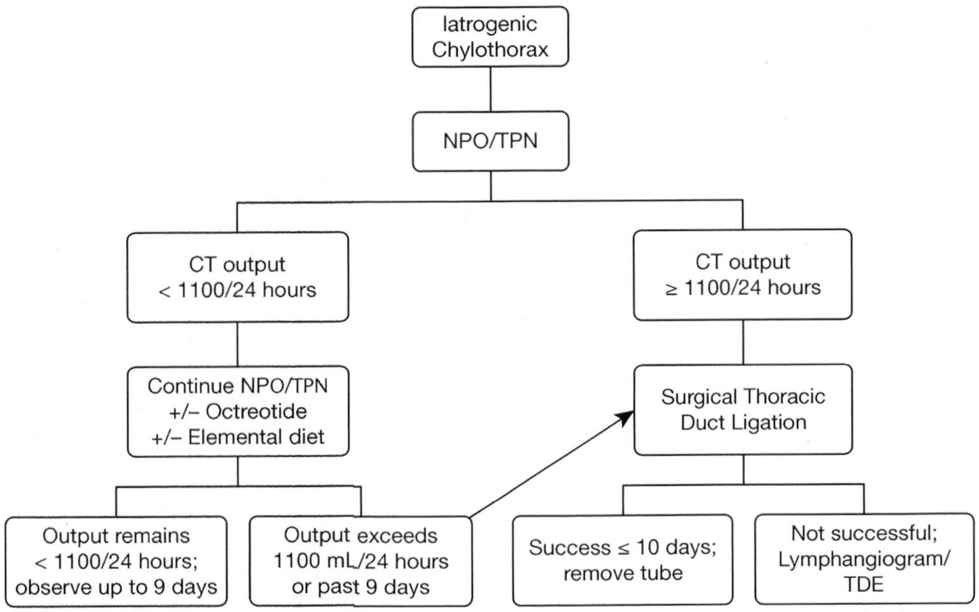

FIGURE 3.22.3 Treatment algorithm for iatrogenic chylothorax. CT, computed tomography; NPO, nil per os; TDE, thoracic duct embolization; TPN, total parenteral nutrition.

SUGGESTED READINGS

Groth SS, Burt BM, Sugarbaker DJ. Management of complications after pneumonectomy. *Thorac Surg Clin*. 2015;25(3):335-348.

Iyer A, Yadav S. Postoperative care and complications after thoracic surgery. In: Firstenberg MS, ed. *Principles and Practice of Cardiothoracic Surgery*. IntechOpen; 2013:57.

Little AG, Merrill WH, eds. *Complications in Cardiothoracic Surgery: Avoidance and Treatment*. John Wiley & Sons; 2011.

LoCicero J III, Feins RH, Colson YL, et al. *Shield's General Thoracic Surgery*. 8th ed. Lippincott Williams & Wilkins; 2019.

Mathisen DJ, Morse C. *Master Techniques in Surgery: Thoracic Surgery: Transplantation, Tracheal Resections, Mediastinal Tumors, Extended Thoracic Resections*. Lippincott Williams & Wilkins; 2014.

Mathisen DJ, Morse C. *Thoracic Surgery: Lung Resections, Bronchoplasty*. Lippincott Williams & Wilkins; 2014.

Seitlinger J, Fiore A, Grande AM, et al. Major complications of thoracic surgery. In: Aseni P, Grande AM, Leppäniemi A, Chiara O, eds. *The High-Risk Surgical Patient*. Cham: Springer International Publishing; 2023:527-536.

Shapiro M, Swanson SJ, Wright CD, et al. Predictors of major morbidity and mortality after pneumonectomy utilizing the Society for Thoracic Surgeons General Thoracic Surgery Database. *Ann Thorac Surg*. 2010;90(3):927-935.

Ziarnik E, Grogan EL. Postlobectomy early complications. *Thorac Surg Clin*. 2015;25(3):355-364.

3.23

Veno-Venous Extracorporeal Membrane Oxygenation

John Fountain, Eduardo M.H. Padrao, and Jonah Rubin

Venovenous extracorporeal membrane oxygen (V-V ECMO) is a form of advanced life support for patients with hypoxemic and/or hypercapnic respiratory failure in whom conventional interventions have failed. V-V ECMO provides respiratory support by pumping venous blood through a membrane/artificial lung (also called an oxygenator) and returning it to the venous circulation. The membrane lung both oxygenates and clears carbon dioxide (CO_2) from venous blood. An alternate form of extracorporeal life support (ECLS), termed *extracorporeal CO_2 removal* ($ECCO_2R$), prioritizes CO_2 removal over oxygenation using lower flows but is otherwise mechanically similar. In contrast to venoarterial (VA) ECMO, which is not discussed in this chapter, V-V ECMO provides no hemodynamic support (with the exception of configurations in which the return cannula sits in the pulmonary artery, discussed later).

A multidisciplinary team is essential for the successful implementation of an ECMO program, consisting of physicians, respiratory therapists, perfusionists, nurses, and often palliative and spiritual care.

Indications

- Severe respiratory failure as a bridge to recovery or transplant
    - ECMO does not treat the underlying respiratory pathology.
    - In some cases, ECMO may be used as a bridge to decision regarding transplant candidacy.

- No universally accepted criteria for identifying which patients, and at what stage of illness, would benefit from ECMO
- ECMO centers each develop their own processes to make such candidacy determinations.
- As a guide, the following indications, published by the Extracorporeal Life Support Organization (ELSO), may be considered:
  - Hypoxemic respiratory failure (Pao_2/Fio_2 <80 mm Hg), after optimal medical management, including, in the absence of contraindications, a trial of prone positioning
  - Hypercapnic respiratory failure (pH <7.25), despite optimal conventional mechanical ventilation (respiratory rate 35 bpm and plateau pressure [P_{plat}] ≤30 cm H_2O)
  - Ventilatory support as a bridge to lung transplantation or primary graft dysfunction following lung transplant

Contraindications

- Given the complex candidacy criteria and multidisciplinary nature of V-V ECMO, decisions regarding candidacy should be made by multiple collaborating clinicians.
- *Absolute contraindications*
  - Since ECMO is a bridge and not a therapy, its absolute contraindications are any conditions for which recovery or transplant are not possible.
    - As the possibility of recovery is often difficult to predict, ECMO is increasingly seen as having no absolute contraindications, since each factor must be evaluated independently in the context of the individual patient.
  - Factors that are associated with poor outcomes are generally considered relative contraindications.
- *Relative contraindications* (including, but not limited to, the following)
  - Advanced age
  - Invasive mechanical ventilation >7 days
  - Systemic or central nervous system bleeding
  - Immunosuppression
  - Metastatic cancer or other condition with a prognosis of <1 year

Extracorporeal Membrane Oxygen Circuit

The V-V ECMO circuit comprises:

- Drainage and reinfusion cannulae
- Pump
- Membrane lung (or "oxygenator")
- Blender
- Heat exchanger
- Flow and pressure sensors

Configurations

There are multiple possible cannulation configurations, dictated by anatomic considerations, patient stability, flow requirements, and anticipated duration of ECMO support.

- Drainage (also called inflow or venous) cannulae are often placed in a femoral vein.
- Return (also called outflow or arterial—even in V-V ECMO) cannulae may be placed in an internal jugular (IJ), subclavian, or femoral vein.
- In patients who are cannulated in an emergent situation, femoral-femoral venous cannulation may be the most practical.
- Newer dual-lumen single cannulae perform both drainage and reinfusion through a single cannula with two internal channels, placed in the IJ vein.
  - The IJV size limits the maximal diameter of such cannulae, which, in turn, limits maximal achievable flow.
  - In patients who can be effectively supported with such cannulae, awake ECMO and physical rehabilitation may be more readily achieved.
    - This is particularly important for transplant candidates, for whom physical rehabilitation on ECMO has been associated with better outcomes.
  - The ProTek Duo is a particular dual-lumen single cannula that is placed in the IJ and terminates in the pulmonary artery.
    - By bypassing the right ventricle, this configuration provides mechanical circulatory support for the right ventricle—violating the aforementioned principle that V-V ECMO provides no hemodynamic support.
    - V-V ECMO via a ProTek Duo is often called V-P ECMO since the return cannula terminates in the pulmonary artery.
  - Such cannulae are more stable given their deep placement, which may allow for safer ambulation when able and indicated.
- In cases where V-V ECMO support is inadequate to meet the patient's respiratory demands, or the patient needs additional hemodynamic support, additional limbs can be added.
  - Examples include:
    - VV-V ECMO (two venous drainage cannulae, one venous reinfusion cannula)
    - V-AV ECMO (one venous drainage cannula with one venous reinfusion cannula and one arterial reinfusion cannula)

Cannulation

- Centers vary in policies regarding who cannulates patients to ECMO, and with what degree of training.
- Intensivists, cardiac anesthesiologists, cardiac or thoracic surgeons, advanced practice providers, and others perform cannulations in various institutions.
- During cannulation, a one-time bolus of heparin is generally administered to prevent clotting in the circuit.
- Initiation of V-V ECMO can lead to transient hypotension due to a vasodilatory response, which clinicians should anticipate.
  - Some administer a one-time dose of steroids (such as hydrocortisone 100 mg) to offset this effect.

Management

Settings

The following parameters are set on the ECMO circuit:

- Pump
  - Flow rate: usually set by rotations per minute (RPM) to achieve a given flow, measured in liters per minute (LPM)
- Membrane lung
  - Fraction of delivered o_2 (Fdo_2)
  - Sweep gas flow rate (measured in LPM)
- Temperature

Initiation

- Initial ECMO settings vary based upon the patient's clinical status. In general, the following settings are appropriate for initiation:
  - Flow rate at least 3 LPM (typical range 3-7 LPM)
    - Vo_2 can be estimated to target a more precise flow rate; the Do_2/Vo_2 ratio must be >2:1, which is the point at which oxygen consumption is dependent upon oxygen delivery (supply dependence).
  - Fdo_2 1.0
  - Sweep gas between 1 and 10 LPM
    - In patients with severe respiratory acidosis, $Paco_2$ should be gradually reduced due to an increased risk of intracerebral hemorrhage with rapid reduction.
  - An arterial blood gas should be obtained shortly after initiating ECMO to facilitate further titration.

Daily Monitoring

- Cannulae
  - Fibrin/clots
  - Kinking
  - Surgical site/positioning/sutures
- Pump—RPM, LPM
- Membrane lung
  - dP, defined as the difference between the pre- and postmembrane pressures
    - This must be cross-referenced with LPM, as increases in flow will lead to an increase in pressure.
  - Pre- and postmembrane oxygen saturation or blood gas checks

For patients on ECMO, multiple laboratories should be checked routinely and with clinical changes, including

- Complete blood count (CBC)
- Routine chemistries
- Arterial blood gas
- Coagulation studies
- Markers of hemolysis, including lactate dehydrogenase (LDH), bilirubin, and/or plasma-free hemoglobin

Circuit Dysfunction/Troubleshooting

Preparedness for circuit dysfunction ranges from monitoring to necessitating emergent circuit exchange. Generally, a second circuit should be primed and ready at the bedside at all times in case of circuit emergencies.

- *Chatter (or chugging)* is a visible shaking of the cannulae, caused by intermittent reductions in flow rates through the drainage line due to temporary occlusion of one or more ports on the drainage cannula or kinking of the drainage line.
  - May be caused by
    - Intravascular volume depletion
    - Drainage flow rates too high for the cannulated vessel
  - Management includes volume resuscitation if intravascular volume depletion is suspected and further fluid is tolerated, or reduction in drainage flow rate if able. Otherwise, adjustment of the cannula positioning or placement of an additional venous drainage cannula may be considered.
  - Cutouts (temporary no-flow) result if the flow through the drainage limb abruptly ceases, and represent collapse of the cannulated vessel
- *Cannula migration*
  - Over time and with movement, the ECMO cannulae may migrate from their original position, which may lead to impaired venous drainage or recirculation (see later).
  - Daily x-rays can help identify early cannula migration.
- *Recirculation* is a phenomenon in which oxygenated blood returning via the reinfusion cannula is drained by the drainage cannula before it reaches the systemic circulation, leading to inefficiency.
  - Some amount of recirculation is unavoidable, but clinically significant amounts will lead to hypoxemia.
  - May be caused by a close proximity of drainage and reinfusion cannulae, high intrathoracic pressure, and high-flow rates. Cannulae can be kept 10 cm apart to help limit this.
  - Monitored by checking the premembrane lung oxygen saturation (termed $SpreO_2$), which should be much lower than the postmembrane lung oxygen saturation, and can be compared to a venous blood gas
- *Circuit air*
  - Air may be entrained due to the loss of cannula integrity (eg, cracking), malposition, or cavitation (high negative pressure that draws gas out of solution), or introduced via another procedure (such as placing a central line). The management of air entrainment depends on its location.
  - Premembrane gas may be aspirated from the cannula at the nearest access site.
  - The membrane lung acts as a trap, and in most cases, air should not pass beyond the membrane lung if the source is premembrane (except in cases where a large amount of gas is entrained).
    - Gas within the membrane lung may be aspirated if it is a small amount. Large amounts may necessitate membrane lung exchange.
    - This may result in immediate membrane lung failure requiring an emergency circuit exchange.
  - Postmembrane air introduction is at the highest risk of systemic air embolization.
    - To remove air, both limbs should be clamped and the air aspirated from the nearest access site.
      - While the limbs are clamped, patients are likely to need increased hemodynamic and respiratory support.
- *Membrane lung malfunction*
  - Should be suspected when postmembrane blood gas indicates inadequate oxygenation despite Fdo_2 1.0, there is evidence of membrane thrombus (rising dP), or hemolysis
  - In cases where membrane lung malfunction is suspected, it should be replaced before it becomes an emergency.
- *Pump malfunction*
  - In the rare instance that the pump itself fails, both limbs should be clamped while the pump is evaluated.
    - A hand crank may be used while the pump is evaluated to provide flow after unclamping.
  - As earlier, a backup circuit should be ready at bedside at all times to facilitate rapid exchange.
- *Accidental decannulation*
  - Clamp both limbs immediately, hold pressure at insertion sites, and assess need for emergency recannulation.

Liberation

- *Bridge to transplant*
  - Continued need for V-V ECMO determined in the operating room (OR) posttransplant
  - For patients who remain on ECMO after a lung transplant, they would now be classified as a "bridge to recovery."
- *Bridge to recovery*
  - Timing
    - Readiness for liberation should be assessed regularly.
    - Clues that a patient may be ready for liberation include improvements in respiratory mechanics, oxygen saturations, and imaging.
  - Protocol
    - In contrast to V-A ECMO, V-V ECMO support may be weaned without changes in flow rate.
    - Institutional protocols vary in how ECMO is weaned. Some will wean Fdo_2 and sweep in a stepwise manner as ventilator settings (respiratory rate, tidal volume, Fio_2) are increased. Some are purely clinician driven.
    - All liberation protocols culminate in a "capping trial" in which the sweep gas is turned off completely, essentially turning "off" the membrane lung.
      - An arterial blood gas should be checked to assess gas exchange shortly after capping.
    - If ventilation and oxygenation are adequate with acceptable ventilator settings for a sustained period of time, patients should proceed to decannulation.

Non-Extracorporeal Membrane Oxygen Management

Mechanical Ventilation

- Minimal data guide appropriate ventilator management for patients on V-V ECMO.
- The following parameters were used in the EOLIA trial, but are not necessarily the recommended approach:
  - P_{plat} <25
  - Driving pressure <15
    - Tidal volume will be determined by lung compliance in a pressure control mode, or may be set at a low volume in a volume control mode.
  - Respiratory rate (RR) <10
  - Positive end-expiratory pressure (PEEP) >10
  - Fio_2 0.30 to 0.50
- In patients cannulated to V-V ECMO as a bridge to transplant, extubation may be pursued to facilitate early mobilization and participation with physical therapy, given the potential wait for an available organ.
- Some are studying early extubation and awake ECMO for patients on a bridge to recovery.

Renal Replacement Therapy

- Indications and timing for renal replacement therapy (RRT) are the same as for non-ECMO patients.
- Both continuous and intermittent hemodialysis can be considered, and indications are similar to non-ECMO patients. Peritoneal dialysis can also be used, usually in patients already on that modality.
- The RRT system can be set up as:
  - System with an independent RRT machine (requires an additional catheter only for dialysis)
  - In-line hemofilter (the filter is placed within the ECMO system but with no RRT machine)
  - In-system prepump RRT machine
  - In-system postpump RRT machine
  - In-system with the RRT access line postpump and return line prepump

Other Management Considerations

- The ECMO circuit alters the pharmacology of many medications, including sedatives. Proper dosing should be confirmed with a pharmacist.
- ECMO itself may cause immunosuppression, and the temperature regulator may mask a fever. This should be considered when assessing for infection.
- Traditionally, patients on ECMO are anticoagulated to avoid circuit clotting. With newer modern equipment that may be less prone to clotting, ongoing studies are evaluating the optimal amount, if any, of systemic anticoagulation for patients on ECMO. Institutional protocols will vary.
- Transportation outside the intensive care unit (ICU) is inherently risky and should be carefully considered and planned.

Complications

- *Infection*
  - Patients on ECMO have a higher risk of infection compared to other critically ill patients. Signs and symptoms of infection may be difficult to assess, given circuit temperature regulation and multiple potential etiologies of leukocytosis.
- *Bleeding*
  - Most common complication in the setting of anticoagulation, thrombocytopenia, and platelet dysfunction in patients on ECMO
  - Initial management involves reduction in anticoagulation, transfusion of platelets, and transfusion of antifibrinolytics (if fibrinolysis is a concern). Stopping anticoagulation is only recommended when initial measures fail.
    - In cases where anticoagulation is held, flow rates can be increased to reduce circuit clot formation.
  - Common sites of bleeding
    - Cannulation sites are the most common source of bleeding, and this can be a sign of loose cannulae, which are at higher risk of dislodgement.
      - Direct pressure should be applied, and additional sutures may be necessary.
      - If bleeding persists, the site may need to be surgically explored.
    - Surgical site bleeding in patients who underwent surgery is the second most common source of bleeding.
      - The site should be evaluated and pressure held if accessible.
      - Surgical exploration may be necessary.
    - Gastrointestinal bleeding should be treated with local measures (endoscopy or angiography) whenever possible.
    - Patients on ECMO are also at substantially higher risk of intracerebral hemorrhage. A thorough neurologic examination should be performed at regular intervals.
- *Thrombocytopenia*
  - Patients on ECMO have multiple etiologies for thrombocytopenia, including disseminated intravascular

coagulation (DIC), heparin-induced thrombocytopenia (HIT), consumption, sequestration, sepsis, critical illness, and medication induced.
  - Centers vary in protocols regarding platelet transfusion thresholds.
- *Hemolysis*
  - Usually a consequence of high pressure in the systems due to clot and/or fibrin deposition or turbulent flow
    - Different circuits and pumps are optimized for specific flows, which may affect the likelihood of hemolysis.
    - The circuit may need to be replaced when clot or fibrin is suspected to be causing hemolysis.
    - Non-ECMO causes of hemolysis should be investigated depending on patients' comorbidities and clinical manifestations.
- *Systemic thrombosis*
  - Venous thromboembolism
    - Common in patients on ECMO. Risk factors include infection, duration of ECLS, and the absence of anticoagulation.
      - Deep venous thrombosis (DVT) is often identified in the inferior vena cava, related to the cannulae.
    - If DVT or pulmonary embolism is diagnosed, anticoagulation is the mainstay of treatment.
- *Vascular complications*
  - Acute limb ischemia, more commonly seen in V-A ECMO, though can also be seen in V-V ECMO
    - Potential mechanisms in V-V ECMO include embolization, high-dose vasopressors, peripheral artery disease, or venous gangrene due to obstruction of the femoral vein by the venous cannula.
      - In the appropriate patient, HIT should be considered.
    - Management includes anticoagulation and treating reversible causes or aggravating factors when possible (high-dose pressors, acidosis, hypotension, etc).
  - Other complications include arteriovenous fistulas.
- *Cerebrovascular accident*
  - Often difficult to diagnose due to sedation and difficulty in obtaining imaging
  - As earlier, intracranial hemorrhage is the most common cause of stroke in patients on ECMO. It is usually extensive and may be fatal. This can necessitate discontinuation of ECMO and neurosurgical consultation.
  - Ischemic stroke is less common but also occurs. Etiology can be cardioembolic, atheroembolic, or an air embolism.
    - There are no formal guidelines for stroke management in patients on ECMO.
      - Thrombolysis is contraindicated.

Evidence Surrounding the Use of Venovenous Extracorporeal Membrane Oxygen and Extracorporeal CO_2 Removal

Venovenous Extracorporeal Membrane Oxygen

- CESAR (2009)
  - Methods: prospective, multicenter (the United Kingdom), randomized controlled trial, nonblinded
  - Population: adult patients with reversible severe respiratory failure on mechanical ventilation (Murray score ≥3 or pH <7.2 despite optimized ventilation)
  - Intervention: transfer to ECMO-capable center with consideration for ECMO.
  - Control: standard of care
  - Results: significant difference in death or severe disability at 6 months (37% in intervention arm vs 53% in control group, $P = .03$)
  - Limitations
    - Data for three patients were missing, and depending on the outcomes of these patients, the results may have been neutral.
    - Intervention is transfer to an ECMO center as opposed to being cannulated to ECMO (only 76% of patients underwent ECMO).
    - Lack of standard-of-care protocol (less patients in control group had lung-protective ventilation)
- EOLIA (2018)
  - Methods: prospective, multicenter (64 centers in France), randomized controlled trial, nonblinded
  - Population: adult patients with acute respiratory distress syndrome (ARDS), on optimized mechanical ventilation for <7 days, with P/F <50 for >3 hours; P/F <80 for >6 hours; or pH <7.25 with $Paco_2$ >60 for >6 hours. A total of 249 patients were included.
  - Intervention: VV ECMO
  - Control: standard of care (appropriate lung-protective ventilation and as-needed neuromuscular blockade, PEEP titration, inhaled nitric oxide [iNO], recruitment maneuvers, and prone positioning)
  - Results: no difference in mortality at day 60 (35% in intervention arm vs 46% in control group, $P = .09$). Lower relative risk of treatment failure (0.62, 95% confidence interval [CI] = 0.47-0.82; $P < .001$)
  - Limitations
    - Underpowered (sample was calculated with inflated predicted mortality)
    - Trial stopped early due to futility.
    - High crossover rate in the control group (increasing type I error)
    - Lack of blinding
    - Slow recruitment

Extracorporeal CO_2 Removal

- REST (2021)
  - Methods: prospective, multicenter (51 centers in the United Kingdom), randomized controlled trial, nonblinded
  - Population: adult patients with acute hypoxemic respiratory failure (<48 hours) on mechanical ventilation, with P/F <150. A total of 412 patients were included.
  - Intervention: $ECCO_2R$
  - Control: standard of care (appropriate lung-protective ventilation and PEEP titration by PEEP table)
  - Results: no difference in mortality at day 90 (41.5% in intervention arm vs 39.5% in control group, $P = .68$)
  - Limitations
    - Low rate of prone positioning
    - Lack of blinding
    - Stopped early due to futility
    - Sites with little experience using $ECCO_2R$

SUGGESTED READINGS

Cavayas YA, Munshi L, Del Sorbo L, Fan E. The early change in $Paco_2$ after extracorporeal membrane oxygenation initiation is associated with neurological complications. *Am J Respir Crit Care Med.* 2020;201(12):1525-1535.

Combes A, Hajage D, Capellier G, et al. Extracorporeal membrane oxygenation for severe acute respiratory distress syndrome. *N Engl J Med.* 2018;378(21):1965-1975.

McNamee JJ, Gillies MA, Barrett NA, et al. Effect of lower tidal volume ventilation facilitated by extracorporeal carbon dioxide removal vs standard care ventilation on 90-day mortality in patients with acute hypoxemic respiratory failure: the REST randomized clinical trial [published correction appears in *JAMA.* 2022;327(1):86]. *JAMA.* 2021;326(11):1013-1023.

Peek GJ, Mugford M, Tiruvoipati R, et al. Efficacy and economic assessment of conventional ventilatory support versus extracorporeal membrane oxygenation for severe adult respiratory failure (CESAR): A multicentre randomised controlled trial. Lancet. 2009; 374(9698), 1351–1363

Tipograf Y, Salna M, Minko E, et al. Outcomes of extracorporeal membrane oxygenation as a bridge to lung transplantation. *Ann Thorac Surg.* 2019;107(5):1456-1463.

Tonna JE, Abrams D, Brodie D, et al. Management of adult patients supported with venovenous extracorporeal membrane oxygenation (VV ECMO): guideline from the Extracorporeal Life Support Organization (ELSO). *ASAIO J.* 2021;67(6):601-610.

SECTION 4

Gastrointestinal and Hepatobiliary

Section Editor: Casey M. Luckhurst

4.1

Abdominal Compartment Syndrome

Mary M. Leech and Katherine H. Albutt

Definition

Abdominal perfusion pressure = mean arterial pressure − intra-abdominal pressure (APP = MAP − IAP).

- Normal IAP is 0 to 5 mm Hg.
- Intra-abdominal hypertension refers to acute or chronic IAP elevation, typically >12 mm Hg, without evidence of end-organ dysfunction (although there may be subclinical changes present).
- Abdominal compartment syndrome (ACS) refers to the clinical presentation of sustained severely increased IAP >20 mm Hg resulting in end-organ dysfunction.

Common Causes to Remember

- Massive resuscitation and transfusions leading to bowel wall edema
- Intraperitoneal and/or retroperitoneal hemorrhage
- Bowel distention due to obstruction or ileus
- Bowel reperfusion injury from ischemia of any cause
- Ascites or similar space-occupying intra-abdominal process, mass, or fluid
- Inflammatory processes resulting in bowel wall edema and widespread capillary leak, for example, sepsis or acute pancreatitis
- Loss of domain/abdominal closure under tension

Types of Abdominal Compartment Syndrome

- Primary: primary etiology lies within the abdomen (eg, excessive bowel wall edema or distention).
- Secondary: from external causes (eg, circumferential burn eschar)
- Tertiary: recurrent ACS after initial treatment of primary or secondary ACS
- Acute: for example, acute bowel wall edema from massive resuscitation
- Chronic: for example, late stages of cirrhosis with massive ascites

Epidemiology

- Incidence of intra-abdominal hypertension in intensive care units (ICUs) can be up to 50%.
- Incidence of *true* compartment syndrome in ICU patients is 1% to 14%.
- Measuring and detecting IAP requires a high index of provider suspicion.

Key Pathophysiology

- Upward displacement of the diaphragm results in decreased thoracic volumes and pulmonary compliance, which lead to an increase in peak airway pressures, ventilation and perfusion mismatch, hypoxia, hypercapnia, and acidosis. This can devolve into concomitant acute respiratory distress syndrome.
- Compression of the inferior vena cava (IVC) results in decreased cardiac venous return and increased peripheral vascular resistance. As a result, blood pressure, cardiac output, cardiac index, and right atrial and pulmonary artery occlusion pressures decrease. Peripherally, this backup of blood from IVC compression causes end-organ venous congestion and ischemia.

- Direct compression of the kidneys and obstruction of venous outflow result in a decrease in the glomerular filtration rate and urine output.
- Compression of the mesenteric vasculature leads to a decrease in splanchnic perfusion, mesenteric venous hypertension, intestinal edema, and visceral edema.
- Elevated central venous pressure interferes with cerebral venous outflow and results in increased intracranial pressure.

Clinical Manifestations

- Distended, tense abdomen
- Hypoxia, hypercapnia, and high peak inspiratory pressures with decreased compliance in the mechanically ventilated patients
- Shortness of breath in extubated patients
- Elevated central venous and pulmonary capillary wedge pressures
- Oliguria and eventually anuria with worsening acute kidney injury
- Decreased cardiac output, hypotension, acidosis, increasing vasopressor requirements
- Decreased intestinal, renal, hepatic blood flow
- Signs of increased intracranial pressure

Diagnosis/Measurement of Intra-abdominal Pressure

- Bladder pressure is an indirect measure of intraperitoneal pressure.
- A total of 50 mL of sterile saline is instilled into the bladder via a Foley catheter with the drainage tube clamped, while the aspiration port is attached to a pressure transducer (zeroed at the level of the pubic symphysis, Figure 4.1.1). The patient must be paralyzed and flat for this measurement to be valid.

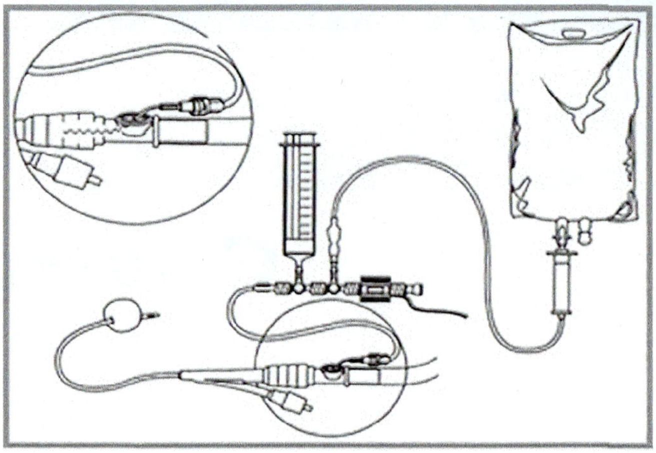

FIGURE 4.1.1 **Repeat frequently (every 4-6 hours).** Monitor the trend.

Management and Treatment

- Reversing the underlying cause is also critical.
- Maximal medical management includes nasogastric tube decompression, muscle paralysis, diuresis, and rectal tube placement. Paracentesis and/or intra-abdominal drainage can be considered prior to decompression. Escharotomy should be done for constrictive burn eschars.
- Surgical decompression via laparotomy is typically definitive! Indications to proceed to the surgery (rather than rely on nonoperative management alone) include hemodynamic instability, prolonged anuria, inability to ventilate despite increasing pressures, concern for bowel ischemia, and inability to rapidly reverse the underlying cause (eg, in patients with severe burns). The abdomen is left open (usually with a negative pressure Vac dressing) until the etiology of the ACS improves. There are some notable risks associated with this delayed closure, including ventral hernias, fluid and electrolyte derangements, odds of renal failure, and development of enterocutaneous fistula.

SUGGESTED READINGS

Joynt GM, Wai JK. Intra-abdominal hypertension and abdominal compartment syndrome—making progress? *Anaesth Intensive Care*. 2012;40(1):11-13.

Khan S, Verma AK, Ahmad SM, et al. Analyzing intra-abdominal pressures and outcomes in patients undergoing emergency laparotomy. *J Emerg Trauma Shock*. 2010;3(4):318-325.

Kirkpatrick AW, Roberts DJ, De Waele J, et al. Intra-abdominal hypertension and the abdominal compartment syndrome: updated consensus definitions and clinical practice guidelines from the World Society of the Abdominal Compartment Syndrome. *Intensive Care Med*. 2013;39(7):1190-1206.

Raeburn CD, Moore EE, Biffl WL, et al. The abdominal compartment syndrome is a morbid complication of postinjury damage control surgery. *Am J Surg*. 2001;182(6):542-546.

4.2

Acute Pancreatitis

Robert D. Sinyard and Katherine H. Albutt

- Acute pancreatitis (AP) is an inflammatory disease of the pancreas.
- It can be divided into three severity categories:
  - Mild AP: characterized by the absence of organ failure and severe systemic complications
  - Moderately severe AP: characterized by local complications, with or without organ failure that lasts <48 hours
  - Severe acute pancreatitis (SAP): characterized by failure of one or more organ systems that lasts for >48 hours
- It can be divided into two broad classifications.
  - Interstitial edematous pancreatitis: characterized by inflammation of the pancreas and/or surrounding tissues without evidence of tissue necrosis
  - Necrotizing pancreatitis: characterized by inflammation associated with pancreatic parenchymal or peripancreatic necrosis

Common Causes to Remember (Table 4.2.1)

Epidemiology

- Increasing incidence, ranging from 5 to 35 cases per 100,000 population

TABLE 4.2.1 Common and Rare Causes of Acute Pancreatitis

Common Causes *(70%-80%)*	**Rare Causes** *(Investigate if common ones excluded)*
• Alcohol (~35%): most common cause in men, usually recurrent acute flares	• Metabolic: hypercalcemia (>12-14 mg/dL), hypertriglyceridemia (>1,000 mg/dL)
• *Gallstones* (~45%): most common cause in women, usually small stones (<5 mm)	• Medications: antiretrovirals, thiazides, furosemide, sulfa drugs, tetracycline, metronidazole, valproic acid, 6-MP (consider those on chemotherapy)
• Post-endoscopic retrograde cholangiopancreatography (ERCP)	• Infections: mumps, hepatitis B, HIV/AIDS, coxsackie, mycoplasma, salmonella, legionella
• Idiopathic (10%-20%) → minimal risk of recurrence	• Perforated peptic ulcer • Postsurgical, posttraumatic
• Microlithiasis, stone debris, or sludge	• Obstructive: pancreas divisum, ampullary/pancreatic tumors
• Sphincter of Oddi dysfunction	• Other: ischemic, autoimmune, hereditary

- Moderately severe or severe pancreatitis accounts for 15% to 25% of all cases.
- Mortality in AP is under 5%, with a lower mortality in patients with interstitial pancreatitis as compared with those with necrotizing pancreatitis.
- Only 3% to 7% of patients with cholelithiasis and 10% of alcoholics develop AP.

Key Pathophysiology

- Unregulated protease activation within pancreatic acinar cells
- Protective mechanisms (enzyme compartmentalization, specific trypsin inhibitors such as serine protease inhibitor Kazal type 1 [SPINK1], low intracellular Ca^{2+}) are overwhelmed.
- Trypsinogen converted to trypsin, leading to activation of pancreatic proteases (phospholipase A2, chymotrypsin, elastase), complement, kallikrein-kinin, pro-inflammatory interleukins (TNFα, IL-1, IL-6, IL-8), coagulation, and fibrinolysis
- Autodigestion of the gland (with or without systemic inflammatory response syndrome [SIRS])
- Mechanisms of trypsin activation depend on etiology, which is largely debated.
  - Mechanical causes: gallstones, tumors, endoscopic retrograde cholangiopancreatography (ERCP), trauma, pancreas divisum
    - Obstruction of the ampulla by gallstone, edema following stone passage, tumor (pancreatic or ampullary), or high resistance given accessory pancreatic duct (of Santorini) in pancreas divisum ultimately lead to increased intrapancreatic duct pressures and/or reflux of bile into the pancreatic duct during transient ampulla obstruction.
  - Systemic causes: EtOH, drugs, hypertriglyceridemia, hypercalcemia, infections, and toxins, with exact mechanism of pancreatic enzymatic autoactivation unclear

Diagnosis

- AP is diagnosed by the presence of at least two of the three following criteria:
  - Acute abdominal pain consistent with the disease
  - Biochemical evidence of AP (serum lipase >3× upper limit of normal)
  - Characteristic findings on abdominal imaging (computed tomography [CT] or magnetic resonance imaging [MRI])
- Clinical
  - Epigastric pain, sometimes radiating to the back or shoulder, accompanied by nausea and/or vomiting, is the most common clinical presentation.
  - Signs of shock in fulminant attacks
  - Tenderness with abdominal palpation +/− guarding
  - Jaundice if there is concurrent biliary obstruction
  - Palpable abdominal mass if a pancreatic collection or pseudocyst is present
  - Ecchymosis of the periumbilical (Cullen sign), flank area (Grey-Turner sign), or inguinal ecchymoses (Fox sign) is rare and nonspecific (suggesting retroperitoneal hemorrhage).

- Laboratory
  - Serum lipase >3 times the upper limit of normal is sensitive and specific for the diagnosis of AP if clinical signs are also present.
  - Serum amylase levels are no longer recommended, given limitations in sensitivity and negative predictive value.
  - ALT >3 times the upper limit of normal may be specific for gallstone pancreatitis.
- Imaging findings
  - Imaging is not necessary to make the diagnosis if the clinical picture and serum tests are consistent with AP.
  - Gold standard imaging modality: abdominal CT with intravenous (IV) contrast
    - Most useful at presentation to identify potential alternative diagnoses
    - Useful later in the course of disease to identify acute peripancreatic collections or acute necrotic collections
  - Abdominal ultrasound
    - Most sensitive modality for identifying cholelithiasis; can also identify common bile duct dilatation
    - Gallstones confirm the etiology of gallstone pancreatitis in the absence of a more apparent cause.
    - If seen, the pancreas may appear edematous with significant nonorganized surrounding fluid.
  - Endoscopic ultrasound is the most accurate modality for choledocholithiasis but is invasive and rarely necessary.
  - Magnetic resonance cholangiopancreatography may also identify anatomical abnormalities (pancreas divisum, malignancy/cystic ductal obstruction) as well as the presence or absence of gallstones.

Severity Scoring

- *No system is superior, and severity scoring should not replace clinical judgment and dynamic assessment.*
- C-reactive protein ≥150 mg/L at 48 hours distinguishes mild versus severe attack.
- Apache II: useful index to classify the severity of the disease, but cumbersome to use
- Ranson criteria: require 48 hours of clinical information to calculate (Table 4.2.2)
- CT severity index: estimates the degree of necrosis and predicts higher morbidity and mortality. IV contrast is necessary (Table 4.2.3).

TABLE 4.2.2 Ranson Criteria

At Presentation, At 48 h	Prognosis	
Age >55 y; Hematocrit (HTC) drop >10%	*Number of criteria*	*Mortality (%)*
WBC >16,000/dL; BUN rise >5 mg/dL	0-2	<5
Glucose >200 mg/dL; Base deficit >4 mEq/L	3-4	15-20
ALT >250 U/dL; Ca <8 mEq/L	5-6	40
LDH >350 IU; Pao_2 <60 mm Hg	≥7	>99
Estimated fluid sequestration >6 L		

ALT, alanine transaminase; BUN, blood urea nitrogen; LDH, lactate dehydrogenase; WBC, white blood cell.

- Bedside index of severity in acute pancreatitis (BISAP)
  - BUN ≥25 mg/dL
  - Impaired mental status
  - SIRS
  - Age >60 years
  - Pleural effusion
  - Similar predictive ability for mortality as Apache II
- Harmless acute pancreatitis score (HAPS)
  - Rebound tenderness/guarding
  - Creatinine ≥2 mg/dL
  - Hematocrit >43% in men and >39.6% in women
  - Can be calculated within 30 minutes of admission
  - 98% predictive ability of patients with a benign course if all three parameters are negative

Differential Diagnosis

- Other causes of epigastric/right upper quadrant abdominal pain: acute cholecystitis, perforated viscus, peptic ulcer, mesenteric ischemia, small bowel obstruction, ruptured abdominal aortic aneurysm (AAA), acute myocardial infarction (MI), pneumonia

Management and Treatment

- Fluid resuscitation
  - Patients with SAP need intensive care unit (ICU)-level monitoring for management of end-organ dysfunction
  - Fluid resuscitation is critical and should be goal directed and targeted to end-organ perfusion parameters (ie, mean arterial pressure [MAP], urinary output, serial ultrasound). The goal is to restore intravascular volume for end-organ perfusion and to avoid secondary pancreatic injury due to hypoperfusion.
    - Underresuscitation may lead to renal dysfunction and systemic hypoperfusion.
    - Overresuscitation may lead to acute respiratory distress syndrome (ARDS) and abdominal compartment syndrome.
    - Lactated Ringer has been shown to be superior to normal saline by reducing inflammatory mediator production.
- Pain control
  - IV opiates are standard.
  - Morphine has not been shown to cause or exacerbate AP attacks despite concerns for sphincter of Oddi dysfunction.
- Nutritional support
  - *Early enteral feeding has been shown to be safe and is the standard of care.*
  - Patients not expected to resume oral feedings for 5 to 7 days (eg, severe attacks) should receive nutritional support.
  - *Enteral feeding is the preferred mode of nutritional support,* as it prevents atrophy of the intestinal mucosa and bacterial translocation, thus leading to improved mortality, lower incidence of organ failure, systemic infection, need for surgery, and potentially a reduction in length of stay.
  - Oral or nasogastric feeding can be tried first, with jejunal feeding reserved for patients who cannot tolerate these approaches.

TABLE 4.2.3 Balthazar (CT) Severity Index

CT Grade	Inflammatory Process	Points	Necrosis (%)	Points	Prognosis	
A	Normal pancreas	0	None	0	*Score*	*Mortality (%)*
B	Enlarged pancreas, contour Irregularity, homogeneous attenuation	1	<30	2	0-3	3
C	Peripancreatic haziness	2	30-50	4	4-6	6
D	Single peripancreatic fluid collection	3	>50	6	7-10	17
E	≥2 peripancreatic fluid collections or gas in the pancreas/retroperitoneum	4				

CT, computed tomography.

- Total parenteral nutrition (TPN) is reserved only for those patients unable to tolerate enteral feeding.
  - Avoid TPN administration as an adjunct to enteral feedings as it has been associated with a higher mortality, increased infectious complications, and longer ICU and hospital length of stay.
- Antibiotic prophylaxis
  - Consensus guidelines recommend against the use of prophylactic antibiotics in patients with AP, even those with presumed sterile necrosis.
  - No mortality benefit or decrease in infectious complications
- ERCP
  - This is not indicated in mild and non-gallstone pancreatitis.
  - *Early (within 48 hours) ERCP is only indicated in patients with pancreatitis with concomitant cholangitis secondary to persistent choledocholithiasis.*
  - In patients without obstructive jaundice, early ERCP does not show a clear benefit and should be avoided as it can worsen pancreatitis.
- Interventional management
  - *The only clear indication for intervention is infected pancreatic or peripancreatic necrosis.*
  - Whenever infected necrosis is suspected, a CT scan with IV contrast is the best first test.
  - Infection can be proven by the presence of gas in pancreatic necrosis on CT scan or by fine-needle aspiration (FNA) with Gram stain and culture of the necrosis.
  - In a severely ill patient with suspected infected necrosis, intervention should be performed even in the absence of definite proof of infection.
  - When infection is proven or suspected, the first intervention should be antibiotic administration (a carbapenem is standard) and followed by interventional management.
  - Other indications for intervention include ongoing gastric, intestinal or biliary obstruction, persistent pain, and failure to thrive.
  - *Interventions should be delayed until at least 4 to 6 weeks* after the onset of pancreatitis whenever possible (allows for the development of a rind around a pancreatic pseudocyst or walled-off necrosis [WON]).
  - Currently, there are three well-established approaches for the management of pancreatic necrosis—surgical, percutaneous, and endoscopic. Once the decision is made for intervention, the choice of modality is individualized and based on multiple factors, including the location and extent of necrosis, communication with pancreatic duct, presence of pancreatic duct stricture or biliary obstruction, hemodynamic status, and overall fitness of the patient.
  - The progression from less invasive drainage procedures to more invasive surgical debridement is termed the *step-up approach and* has been proven to reduce the incidence of multiorgan failure.
  - Surgical techniques include video-assisted retroperitoneal debridement (VARD), sinus tract endoscopy (STE), surgical transgastric necrosectomy, and open transperitoneal necrosectomy.
  - Omission or delay of cholecystectomy in gallstone pancreatitis is associated with increased risk of recurrent attacks. The standard of care is cholecystectomy during index admission. In very severe disease, the timing of cholecystectomy should be determined by patient and disease-specific factors.

Outcomes

- Mortality: 2% to 3% overall, may be up to 30% in SAP with infected necrosis
- Complications
  - Systemic
    - Acute lung injury (ALI)/ARDS, multiorgan failure, coagulopathy/disseminated intravascular coagulation (DIC), acute renal failure (usually prerenal, confers worse prognosis)
    - Severe hypocalcemia
  - Pancreatic fluid collections (Table 4.2.4)
    - Acute peripancreatic fluid collection (<4 weeks from symptom onset) consists of homogeneous simple peripancreatic fluid without a well-defined wall.
    - Acute necrotic collections (4 weeks from symptom onset) may be intrapancreatic or in the peripancreatic tissue and are more heterogeneous without a well-defined wall.
    - With time (>4 weeks), these collections develop a rind and become pseudocysts (homogeneous collections with a discrete wall) or WON (heterogeneous solid and liquid collection with a discrete wall) at which point intervention can be considered (Table 4.2.5).
    - Pancreatic fistulas (17%-76% of severe cases)
      - High volume and amylase content coming from the pancreatic drains are indicative of pancreatic fistula formation.
      - Treatment is conservative.

TABLE 4.2.4 Classification of Pancreatic Fluid Collections

	Collection Type	Timing After Onset of Symptoms	Imaging Appearance
Interstitial edematous pancreatitis	Acute peripancreatic fluid collection (APFC)	0-4 wk	Homogeneous Fluid filled Nonencapsulated Extrapancreatic
	Pancreatic pseudocyst	>4 wk	Homogeneous Fluid filled Encapsulated ("mature") Extrapancreatic
Acute necrotizing pancreatitis	Acute necrotic collection (ANC)	0-4 wk	Heterogeneous Fluid and solid components Nonencapsulated Extrapancreatic or intrapancreatic
	Walled-off necrosis (WON)	>4 wk	Heterogeneous Fluid and solid components Encapsulated Extrapancreatic or intrapancreatic

      - Endoscopic transpapillary stenting may be as safe and decrease the time to fistula closure by decompressing the pancreatic duct.
- Other
    - Type 3c diabetes—acquired blood glucose dysregulation secondary to loss of pancreatic parenchyma
    - Pleural effusion/pancreatic ascites (consider evaluation for pancreatic duct disruption)
    - Exocrine pancreatic insufficiency—requires per oral enzyme replacement therapy (PERT)
    - Splenic/mesenteric/portal vein thrombosis with gastric varices (requires immediate initiation of therapeutic anticoagulation with transition to longer term therapy for at least 3-6 months pending suspected etiology and symptom resolution)
    - Disconnected pancreatic duct syndrome—typically requires endoscopic or surgical intervention

TABLE 4.2.5 Indications for Intervention

APFC/ANC	Sterile WON—Asymptomatic	Sterile WON—Symptomatic	Infected WON
Clinical deterioration with concern for infection after attempt at antibiotics alone	None	Gastric/intestinal/biliary obstruction Persistent pain and/or failure to thrive	Documented or suspected infection of WON

WON, walled-off necrosis.

SUGGESTED READINGS

Aboulian A, Chan T, Yaghoubian A, et al. Early cholecystectomy safely decreases hospital stay in patients with mild gallstone pancreatitis: a randomized prospective study. *Ann Surg*. 2010;251:615-619.

Al-Omran M, Albalawi ZH, Tashkandi MF, et al. Enteral versus parenteral nutrition for acute pancreatitis. *Cochrane Database Syst Rev*. 2010;1:CD002837.

Bakker OJ, van Baal MC, van Santvoort HC, et al. Endoscopic transpapillary stenting or conservative treatment for pancreatic fistulas in necrotizing pancreatitis: multicenter series and literature review. *Ann Surg*. 2011;253:961-967.

Banks PA, Freeman ML. Practice guidelines in acute pancreatitis. *Am J Gastroenterol*. 2006;101:2379-2400.

Bernhardt A, Kortgen A, Niesel H, et al. Using epidural anesthesia in patients with acute pancreatitis—prospective study of 121 patients. *Anaesthesiol Reanim*. 2002;27:16-22.

Besselink MG, van Santvoort HC, Buskens E, et al. Probiotic prophylaxis in predicted severe acute pancreatitis: a randomised, double-blind, placebo-controlled trial. *Lancet*. 2008;371:651-659.

Bradley EL 3rd. A clinically based classification system for acute pancreatitis: summary of the International Symposium on Acute Pancreatitis, Atlanta, GA, September 11 through 13, 1992. *Arch Surg*. 1993;128:586-590.

Cannon JW, Callery MP, Vollmer CM Jr. Diagnosis and management of pancreatic pseudocysts: what is the evidence? *J Am Coll Surg*. 2009;209:385-393.

Casaer MP, Mesotten D, Hermans G, et al. Early versus late parenteral nutrition in critically ill adults. *N Engl J Med*. 2011;365:506-517.

Eatock FC, Chong P, Menezes N, et al. A randomized study of early nasogastric versus nasojejunal feeding in severe acute pancreatitis. *Am J Gastroenterol*. 2005;100:432-439.

Everhart JE, Ruhl CE. Burden of digestive diseases in the United States part III: liver, biliary tract, and pancreas. *Gastroenterology*. 2009;136:1134-1144.

Fagenholz PJ, Castillo CF, Harris NS, et al. Increasing United States hospital admissions for acute pancreatitis, 1988–2003. *Ann Epidemiol*. 2007;17:491-497.

Fagenholz PJ, Fernandez-del Castillo C, Harris NS, et al. National study of United States emergency department visits for acute pancreatitis, 1993–2003. *BMC Emerg Med*. 2007;7:1.

Forsmark CE, Baillie J. AGA institute technical review on acute pancreatitis. *Gastroenterology*. 2007;132:2022-2044.

Frey CF, Zhou H, Harvey DJ, et al. The incidence and case-fatality rates of acute biliary, alcoholic, and idiopathic pancreatitis in California, 1994–2001. *Pancreas*. 2006;33:336-344.

Frossard JL, Steer ML, Pastor CM. Acute pancreatitis. *Lancet*. 2008;371:143-152.

Gardner TB, Vege SS, Pearson RK, et al. Fluid resuscitation in acute pancreatitis. *Clin Gastroenterol Hepatol*. 2008;6:1070-1076.

Hernandez V, Pascual I, Almela P, et al. Recurrence of acute gallstone pancreatitis and relationship with cholecystectomy or endoscopic sphincterotomy. *Am J Gastroenterol*. 2004;99:2417-2423.

Jacobson BC, Vander Vliet MB, Hughes MD, et al. A prospective, randomized trial of clear liquids versus low-fat solid diet as the initial meal in mild acute pancreatitis. *Clin Gastroenterol Hepatol*. 2007;5:946-951; quiz 886.

Jensen EH, Borja-Cacho D, Al-Refaie WB, Vickers SM. *Exocrine Pancreas*. Elsevier Saunders; 2007.

Kutsogiannis J, Alberda C, Gramlich L, et al. Early use of supplemental parenteral nutrition in critically ill patients: results of an international multicenter observational study. *Crit Care Med*. 2011;39:2691-2699.

McClave SA, Dryden GW. Issues of nutritional support for the patient with acute pancreatitis. *Semin Gastrointest Dis*. 2002;13:154-160.

Meng WB, Li X, Li YM, et al. Three initial diets for management of mild acute pancreatitis: a meta-analysis. *World J Gastroenterol*. 2011;17:4235-4241.

Mofidi R, Suttie SA, Patil PV, et al. The value of procalcitonin at predicting the severity of acute pancreatitis and development of infected pancreatic necrosis: systematic review. *Surgery*. 2009;146:72-81.

Moraes JM, Felga GE, Chebli LA, et al. A full solid diet as the initial meal in mild acute pancreatitis is safe and result in a shorter length of hospitalization: results from a prospective, randomized, controlled, double-blind clinical trial. *J Clin Gastroenterol*. 2010;44:517-522.

Munsell MA, Buscaglia JM. Acute pancreatitis. *J Hosp Med*. 2010;5:241-250.

Petrov MS, van Santvoort HC, Besselink MG, et al. Early endoscopic retrograde cholangiopancreatography versus conservative management in acute biliary pancreatitis without cholangitis: a meta-analysis of randomized trials. *Ann Surg*. 2008;247:250-257.

Quan H, Wang X, Guo C. A meta-analysis of enteral nutrition and total parenteral nutrition in patients with acute pancreatitis. *Gastroenterol Res Pract*. 2011;2011:698248.

Sathiaraj E, Murthy S, Mansard MJ, et al. Clinical trial: oral feeding with a soft diet compared with clear liquid diet as initial meal in mild acute pancreatitis. *Aliment Pharmacol Ther*. 2008;28:777-781.

van Santvoort HC, Besselink MG, Bakker OJ, et al. A step-up approach or open necrosectomy for necrotizing pancreatitis. *N Engl J Med*. 2010;362:1491-1502.

van Santvoort HC, Besselink MG, de Vries AC, et al. Early endoscopic retrograde cholangiopancreatography in predicted severe acute biliary pancreatitis: a prospective multicenter study. *Ann Surg*. 2009;250:68-75.

Vege S, Yadav D, Chari S. *Pancreatitis*. Blackwell Publishing; 2007.

Vege SS, Gardner TB, Chari ST, et al. Low mortality and high morbidity in severe acute pancreatitis without organ failure: a case for revising the Atlanta classification to include "moderately severe acute pancreatitis." *Am J Gastroenterol*. 2009;104:710-715.

Villatoro E, Mulla M, Larvin M. Antibiotic therapy for prophylaxis against infection of pancreatic necrosis in acute pancreatitis. *Cochrane Database Syst Rev*. 2010;5:CD002941.

Wilson CT, de Moya MA. Cholecystectomy for acute gallstone pancreatitis: early vs delayed approach. *Scand J Surg*. 2010;99:81-85.

Wu BU, Conwell DL. Update in acute pancreatitis. *Curr Gastroenterol Rep*. 2010;12:83-90.

Wu BU, Hwang JQ, Gardner TH, et al. Lactated Ringer's solution reduces systemic inflammation compared with saline in patients with acute pancreatitis. *Clin Gastroenterol Hepatol*. 2011;9:710-717.e711.

Yadav D, Lowenfels AB. Trends in the epidemiology of the first attack of acute pancreatitis: a systematic review. *Pancreas*. 2006;33:323-330.

4.3

Hepatic Dysfunction and Hyperbilirubinemia

Christine Zachek and Jay Luther

Definitions

- Acute liver failure (ALF): severe acute liver injury with hepatic encephalopathy and coagulopathy (elevated international normalized ratio [INR] ≥1.5) without preexisting liver disease. Duration of symptoms is typically <26 weeks.
- Acute on chronic liver failure (ACLF): acute decompensation in patients with preexisting liver disease. No consensus definition, but various professional societies include extrahepatic organ failure (eg, renal dysfunction, hepatic encephalopathy, coagulopathy, circulatory and respiratory failure) to grade ACLF and access mortality risk.
- Secondary hepatic dysfunction: acquired liver injury without underlying liver disease. No clear definition but can result from the hypoxia/ischemia (shock), cholestatic dysfunction, drug-induced liver injury (DILI), and inflammation.
- Cholestasis: impaired bile conjugation or secretion due to altered hepatocellular transport or impaired excretion due to extrahepatic bile duct obstruction. Total bilirubin >2 mg/dL is commonly used as a practical cutoff.
- Jaundice: yellow discoloration of the sclera, skin, and mucus membranes (usually seen when total bilirubin >2 mg/dL)
- Indirect hyperbilirubinemia: elevated unconjugated bilirubin due to increased production (hemolysis), reduced hepatic uptake, or impaired conjugation
- Direct hyperbilirubinemia: elevated conjugated bilirubin due to biliary obstruction, intrahepatic cholestasis, or defective excretion

Epidemiology

- Secondary hepatic dysfunction in intensive care unit (ICU) patients is common, frequently multifactorial, and can have important prognostic implications.
  - 11% to 36% of ICU patients develop cholestasis, with an overall mortality ranging between 27% and 48%.
- **Risk factors** for developing liver dysfunction in the ICU include shock, major surgery, sepsis (particularly gram-negative infections), and the use of total parenteral nutrition (TPN).

Common Etiologies of Hepatic Dysfunction

Extrahepatic Biliary Duct Obstruction

- Choledocholithiasis
- Primary sclerosing cholangitis
- Traumatic or iatrogenic injury to the common bile duct (CBD)
- Acute pancreatitis
- Malignancy

Increased Bilirubin Production

- Massive transfusion
- Resorption of blood collections
- Acute hemolysis (eg, disseminated intravascular coagulation [DIC] or immune-mediated hemolysis)

Impaired Bilirubin Excretion

- DILI
- Viral hepatitis
- Alcohol-associated hepatitis
- Liver trauma/biloma
- Sepsis/ischemic hepatitis ("shock liver")
- TPN

Hyperbilirubinemia

History

- Drug or toxin exposure, alcohol consumption
- Recent trauma
- Past surgical history, especially abdominal surgeries
- Potential hepatitis exposures (ie, recent travel, intravenous drug use)

Physical Examination

Classic findings like Murphy or Courvoisier sign are unlikely to be appreciated in patients who are sedated or have undergone recent surgery.

Initial Laboratory Studies

- Serum bilirubin (total and direct), aspartate aminotransferase/alanine aminotransferase (AST/ALT), alkaline phosphatase (AP), prothrombin time/INR, albumin

Unconjugated (Indirect) Hyperbilirubinemia

- Tests of hemolysis (haptoglobin, lactate dehydrogenase [LDH], reticulocyte count) and consider imaging for concealed hematomas (such as retroperitoneal bleeds)
- Underlying conditions like congestive heart failure (CHF), Gilbert syndrome, and certain medications can also cause an isolated indirect hyperbilirubinemia.

Cholestatic or Obstructive Pattern

- AP disproportionally elevated; near-normal AST/ALT
- +/− conjugated (direct) hyperbilirubinemia
  - Imaging: abdominal ultrasound for evidence of cholecystitis, choledocholithiasis, or ductal dilatation
  - Computed tomography/endoscopic retrograde cholangiopancreatography/magnetic resonance cholangiopancreatography (CT/ERCP/MRCP) as indicated

Hepatocellular Injury Pattern

- ALT/AST disproportionally elevated
  - Viral hepatitis serologies (including hepatitis A immunoglobulin M [IgM] antibody, hepatitis B surface antigen and core antibody, and hepatitis C RNA)
  - Toxicology screen (acetaminophen levels)
  - Consider abdominal ultrasound with vascular studies to evaluate for Budd-Chiari syndrome.
  - Hepatology consult for unusual causes including Wilson disease, autoimmune hepatitis, and rare causes of viral hepatitis

Differential Diagnosis

Hypoxic Liver Injury

- Epidemiology
  - Occurs in 12% to 22% of ICU patients with shock
  - Also known as "shock liver" or "ischemic hepatitis," although shock is NOT essential as cases have been described resulting from CHF, acute circulatory failure, and/or acute respiratory failure
- Diagnosis
  - Appropriate clinical setting with cardiac, respiratory, or circulatory failure
  - An acute increase in AST/ALT levels (>5 to >20 times the upper limit of normal)
  - Exclusion of other causes of hepatocellular damage
  - Histologic pattern of centrilobar necrosis on liver biopsy (rarely required)
- Key pathophysiology
  - The common feature is reduced oxygen delivery to hepatocytes—hypoperfusion, increased metabolic demand, systemic hypoxia, impaired oxygen extraction—induce a mismatch of oxygen supply and demand that leads to cell death.
  - Most cases are multifactorial, but acute heart failure and cardiogenic shock are the most common underlying conditions, present in up to 70% of cases.
  - AST/ALT levels rapidly increase after the initial insult, peaking at ~24 hours, and normalizing in 10 to 15 days.
- Management and treatment
  - Management of hypoxic hepatitis is supportive—aim to provide adequate hemodynamic support and reverse the underlying insult.
    - Co-occurring respiratory failure and renal failure are common, necessitating mechanical ventilation in 70% to 80% of patients and renal replacement therapy (RRT) in 41%.
  - Advanced dialysis device systems have been used experimentally in patients with hypoxic liver injury, but more research is needed to guide practice.
- Outcomes
  - Hypoxic liver injury carries a 28-day mortality of 40% to 60% and 1-year mortality of 75%.
  - Poor prognostic indicators include elevated INR, prolonged hepatic dysfunction, septic shock, underlying liver disease, and multisystem organ failure.

Sepsis/Multiple Organ Failure

- Epidemiology
  - Septic shock is the most common cause of cholestasis in ICU patients.
  - The most common source is intraabdominal infections, but hyperbilirubinemia has been documented with meningitis, endocarditis, pneumonia, and urinary tract infections.
- Key pathophysiology
  - Hepatic dysfunction from sepsis is multifactorial and can be divided into two phases:
    1. Hypoperfusion: reduced blood flow, increased tissue oxygen demand, and inability of hepatocytes to effectively extract oxygen
    2. Hepatocellular dysfunction and cholestasis:
       - Increased intestinal permeability → increased hepatic concentrations of endotoxins and inflammatory cytokines → disruption of bile transport mechanisms and cellular architecture → impaired bile flow and cholestasis
       - Increased bilirubin load from hemolysis, trauma, hematomas
       - Hepatic microthrombi can impair cellular function and bile flow.
- Management and treatment
  - There is no specific diagnostic test, given the multifactorial nature of sepsis-induced liver dysfunction. Typical laboratory values include a conjugated hyperbilirubinemia and modestly elevated AP (2-3 times normal).

- Treatment is primarily aimed at the underlying cause of sepsis, with aggressive resuscitation, early and appropriate antibiotics, and adequate source control.

Total Parenteral Nutrition

- Epidemiology
  - The reported incidence of parenteral nutrition–related liver dysfunction is highly variable in the literature ranging from 15% to 40%, with one recent study among critically ill patients reporting ~30% on TPN experienced hepatic dysfunction.
  - Risk factors: daily calorie intake >25 kcal/kg, early initiation of parental nutrition, and sepsis
- Key Pathophysiology
  - The most common form of TPN-induced injury is hepatic steatosis and, occasionally, cholestasis. Liver dysfunction can range from mildly elevated aminotransferase levels to steatosis and fibrosis.
  - Liver histology shows periportal fat that may progress to panlobular steatosis in more severe cases.
  - The mechanisms leading to TPN-induced liver dysfunction are incompletely understood; however, possible contributing factors may include:
    - High insulin-to-glucagon ratio that increases lipolysis and accumulation of fatty acids in hepatocytes
    - Bowel rest leading to intestinal bacterial overgrowth, hepatic steatosis, and cholestasis
    - Fatty acid metabolites of lipid emulsions can cause inflammation and oxidative stress.
  - TPN-induced hepatic dysfunction is typically self-limited and resolves after stopping TPN.
- Management and Treatment
  - TPN-induced liver dysfunction is generally self-limited. There is no specific treatment beyond discontinuing TPN.
    - Use enteral nutrition whenever possible.
    - Avoid early (within 1 week) initiation of TPN, even if that means "underfeeding" the patient. There is strong evidence that late initiation of TPN is associated with better outcomes.
    - Avoid excessive calories and avoid dextrose as the sole carbohydrate.

Summary

- Secondary hepatic dysfunction is common in critically ill patients, and new-onset hepatic dysfunction in the ICU is associated with an increased risk of mortality.
- Treatment is largely supportive; however, it is important to exclude treatable causes early.

SUGGESTED READINGS

Caser MP, Mesotten D, Hermans G, et al. Early versus late parenteral nutrition in critically ill adults. *N Engl J Med*. 2011;365:506-517.

Horvatits T, Drolz A, Trauner M, Fuhrmann V. Liver injury and failure in critical illness. *Hepatology*. 2019;70(6):2204-2215.

Lescot T, Karvellas C, Beaussier M, Magder S. Acquired liver injury in the intensive care unit. *Anesthesiology*. 2012;117(4):898-904.

Mitra A, Ahn J. Liver disease in patients on total parenteral nutrition. *Clin Liver Dis*. 2017;21(4):687-695.

Perez Ruiz de Garibay A, Kortgen A, Leonhardt J, Zipprich A, Bauer M. Critical care hepatology: definitions, incidence, prognosis and role of liver failure in critically ill patients. *Crit Care*. 2022;26(1):289.

Strnad P, Tacke F, Koch A, Trautwein C. Liver—guardian, modifier and target of sepsis. *Nat Rev Gastroenterol Hepatol*. 2017;14(1):55-66.

Van Eldere A, Pirani T. Liver intensive care for the general intensivist. *Anaesthesia*. 2023;78(7):884-901.

4.4

Hepatic Encephalopathy

Christine Zachek and Jay Luther

Definition

- Hepatic encephalopathy (HE) is a neuropsychiatric disorder defined as brain dysfunction caused by liver insufficiency and/or portosystemic shunting.
- Dysfunction ranges from subtle, subclinical findings to coma. HE can include personality changes, impaired cognitive function, motor abnormalities, and altered consciousness.
- *See* Table 4.4.1 *for additional details.*

Classification

- Type A: HE associated with acute liver failure (ALF)
- Type B: HE associated with portosystemic bypass without liver disease
- Type C: HE associated with chronic liver disease
- Newer classification schemes incorporate symptom severity, time course, and precipitating factors in addition to the abovementioned underlying disease process.

TABLE 4.4.1 West Haven Criteria for Grading Hepatic Encephalopathy

Grade	Features
0	No encephalopathy, testing without evidence of mental change
1	Lack of awareness, euphoria or anxiety, shortened attention span, impairment of addition or subtraction, altered sleep
2	Disorientation to time, obvious personality change, inappropriate behavior, lethargy or apathy
3	Somnolence to stupor, responsive to stimuli, confusion, gross disorientation, bizarre behavior
4	Coma

Adapted from Vilstrup H, Amodio P, Bajaj J, et al. Hepatic encephalopathy in chronic liver disease: 2014 practice guideline by the American Association for the Study of Liver Diseases and the European Association for the Study of the Liver. *Hepatology*. 2014;60(2):715-735.

Main Precipitating Factors of Hepatic Encephalopathy

- Increased nitrogen load
  - Gastrointestinal (GI) bleeding
  - Excessive dietary protein intake
  - Constipation
  - Renal failure
- Metabolic disorders
  - Hyponatremia (astrocyte swelling)
  - Hypokalemia (increase in renal NH_3)
  - Metabolic alkalosis (increased NH_3 diffusion across the blood-brain barrier [BBB])
  - Hypoxemia
  - Hypovolemia (diuretics, diarrhea)
  - Hypoglycemia
- Medications
  - Narcotics
  - Benzodiazepines
  - Sedatives
  - Diuretics
- Miscellaneous
  - Bacterial infection
  - Surgery
  - Superimposed acute liver dysfunction (viral, drug induced, alcoholic hepatitis, hepatocellular carcinoma, vascular occlusion)
  - Progressively worsening liver disease
  - Transjugular intrahepatic portosystemic shunt (TIPS)

Epidemiology

- The incidence and prevalence of type C HE depend on the sensitivity of the diagnostic criteria. Prevalence estimates for minimal or covert HE in patients with cirrhosis range from 20% to 80%.
- Overt HE will occur in 30% to 40% of patients with cirrhosis at some point in their clinical course; 10% to 14% have overt HE at the time of cirrhosis diagnosis.
- Patients undergoing a TIPS procedure have a significantly higher risk of developing HE, with the 1-year incidence being between 10% and 50% depending on patient selection.

Key Pathophysiology

- The pathophysiology of HE is complex and incompletely understood but likely reflects a combination of accumulation of neurotoxins and increased permeability of the BBB. Several predominant theories are listed below.
- Ammonia
  - Ammonia is primarily produced as the result of protein digestion in the gut, where it enters the portal circulation and is converted to urea in the liver via the urea cycle.
  - In the presence of liver dysfunction, ammonia accumulates and enters the systemic circulation.
  - Elevated levels of NH_3 cross into the BBB and accumulate in astrocytes.
  - Astrocytes normally take up glutamate, a major neurotransmitter, and convert it into glutamine (a reaction that requires NH_3).
  - In the presence of excess NH_3, excessive amounts of glutamine accumulate in the astrocytes, leading to cell swelling.
  - Astrocyte swelling and cerebral edema impair neuronal communication, leading to neurologic dysfunction.
  - It is important to note that there is poor correlation between blood NH_3 levels and the severity of HE, particularly in chronic liver disease.
- Systemic inflammation (resulting from hepatitis, gut bacterial translocation, other infections, and hyperammonemia) can trigger oxidative stress, which can increase the BBB permeability.
- Metals serve as cofactors for enzymatic reactions. Manganese accumulation in the basal ganglia has been implicated in the psychomotor impairment associated with HE. Zinc supplementation (in patients with deficiency) has improved neurocognitive function in patients with HE.
- Alterations in neurotransmitters, such as increased *GABA (γ-aminobutyric acid)* tone and glutamate-induced *N*-methyl-D-aspartate (NMDA) stimulation, have also been implicated as a mechanism for HE. Patients with HE may have increased levels of neurosteroids that activate GABA receptors, causing neuroinhibition.

Differential Diagnosis

- HE is a predominantly clinical diagnosis.
- Neurologic changes can vary from subtle mental function changes (sleep disturbance, inattention, memory difficulty) to confusion, lethargy, and coma.
- Neurologic signs may include asterixis, hyperreflexia, and clonus.
- Serum ammonia measurements are not part of the diagnostic criteria and are not specific for HE.
- Arterial ammonia levels can also help risk-stratify patients with ALF and assess responses to treatment interventions.

Differential Diagnosis in Patients With Cirrhosis

- *See* Table 4.4.2.

Management and Treatment

Acute therapy involves ensuring airway protection, identification of precipitating causes, and lowering ammonia levels.

- Identification and treatment of precipitating causes
  - Bacterial infections: initiate empiric antibiotics while awaiting diagnostic workup, covering organisms commonly isolated in spontaneous bacterial peritonitis (SBP), including *Escherichia coli*, *Klebsiella pneumonia*, and *Streptococcus pneumoniae*.
  - Metabolic disturbances: identify and correct factors such as dehydration, metabolic alkalosis, hyponatremia, and hypokalemia.
  - GI bleeding: stool examination for occult blood and nasogastric tube placement may be necessary to rule out small quantities of GI bleeding.
- Treatment principles for type C HE (associated with chronic liver disease)
  - Decrease intestinal ammonia production
    - Nonabsorbable disaccharides
      - Lactulose is first line for the treatment of HE. Administration of lactulose increases intestinal

TABLE 4.4.2 Cirrhosis: Etiology and Diagnostic Method

Etiology	Diagnostic Method
Neurologic lesions • Hemorrhage (subdural, subarachnoid, intracerebral) • Infarction • Mass lesions (abscesses, brain tumors) • Meningitis • Encephalitis • Epilepsy, postictal state • Psychiatric disorders	CT scan, MRI, arteriography Lumbar puncture HSV, arbovirus serologies EEG

Toxic encephalopathy
• Alcohol
  • Acute intoxication
  • Withdrawal syndrome
  • Wernicke syndrome
	Blood/urine toxicologic screens

Metabolic encephalopathy
• Hypoxia, hypercapnia
• Hypoglycemia, ketoacidosis
• Acute renal insufficiency
• Hyponatremia
  • Endocrine dysfunction (thyroid, adrenal)
  • Vitamin B_{12} deficiency
	Clinical context, relevant lab tests

CT, computed tomography; EEG, electroencephalogram; HSV, herpes simplex virus; MRI, magnetic resonance imaging.

transit, acidifies bowel contents, and traps NH_3 by converting it into the poorly absorbed ammonium (NH_4^+) ion.
  - Guidelines recommend starting dosing at 25 mL every 1 to 2 hours, titrated to two to three semisoft bowel movements a day.
- Antibiotics
  - Rifaximin decreases intestinal NH_3 production by their bactericidal effects on enteric bacteria.
  - Evidence most supports the use of rifaximin in addition to lactulose to prevent recurrence of HE. The literature suggests that the combination of lactulose and rifaximin improves HE, reduces hospital stays, and decreases sepsis-related mortality, but more quality data are needed.
  - The dose of rifaximin is 550 mg 2 times daily (bid).
- Dietary protein and amino acids
  - It is no longer recommended to decrease dietary protein content in type C HE, as this further worsens the patient's typically poor baseline nutritional status.
  - There have been a number of trials of branched-chain amino acid (BCAA) supplementation to improve HE symptoms, but more evidence is needed.

○ Other treatments
- Patients who develop intractable HE in the presence of large portosystemic shunts (such as after a TIPS procedure) may be considered for partial occlusion or embolization of these shunts. The benefit of the procedure must be weighed against the potential risk of worsening variceal bleeding. Of note, prophylactic rifaximin prior to TIPS decreases the risk of overt HE postprocedure.
- Liver transplantation: patients with end-stage liver disease and recurrent or persistent HE should be evaluated for transplant candidacy.

● Treatment principles for type A HE (associated with ALF)

○ Assess for cerebral edema and increased intracranial pressure (ICP)
- Serum ammonia in patients with ALF <75 μM rarely develops intracranial hypertension (ICH), whereas arterial ammonia levels of >100 μM on admission represent an independent risk factor for the development of high-grade HE, and a level of >200 μM predicts ICH.
- Noncontrast head computed tomography (CT) can demonstrate features of cerebral edema.
- Elevated the head of bed to 30 degrees
- Sedation to treat ventilator dyssynchrony
- Hypertonic saline or mannitol therapy
- Consider placement of an ICP monitor in severe, high-grade cases (carries risk of hemorrhage and infection)
- Avoidance of fever

○ Continuous renal replacement therapy (CRRT) may be indicated to manage the metabolic disturbances, elevated ammonia, and hypervolemia associated with ALF.

○ Evaluation for liver transplantation

Outcomes

- Even while receiving preventive therapy, the risk of recurrent HE episodes is high—42% risk of recurrence within 1 year and 46% risk within 6 months for those with recurrent overt HE.
- The first episode of HE in a patient with cirrhosis marks a turning point in the evolution of their disease with 1- to 3-year survivals of 42% and 23%, respectively. Posttransplant survival rates at 1 and 3 years are 80% and 70%, respectively.

SUGGESTED READINGS

Bureau C, Thabut D, Jezequel C, et al. The use of rifaximin in the prevention of overt hepatic encephalopathy after transjugular intrahepatic portosystemic shunt: a randomized controlled trial. *Ann Intern Med.* 2021;174(5):633-640.

European Association for the Study of the Liver. EASL Clinical Practice Guidelines on the management of hepatic encephalopathy. *J Hepatol.* 2022;77(3):807-824.

Rose CF, Amodio P, Bajaj JS, et al. Hepatic encephalopathy: novel insights into classification, pathophysiology and therapy. *J Hepatol.* 2020;73(6): 1526-1547.

Vilstrup H, Amodio P, Bajaj J, et al. Hepatic encephalopathy in chronic liver disease: 2014 Practice Guideline by the American Association for the Study of Liver Diseases and the European Association for the Study of the Liver. *Hepatology.* 2014;60(2):715-35.

Wijdicks EF. Hepatic encephalopathy. *N Engl J Med.* 2016;375(17): 1660-1670.

4.5

Hepatorenal Syndrome

Scott Moses and Danielle L. Saly

Hepatorenal Syndrome

- Acute, severe form of kidney dysfunction mediated by cirrhosis
- Diagnosis of exclusion when alternative etiologies of acute kidney injury (AKI) are ruled out, such as prerenal causes and acute tubular necrosis.

Epidemiology

Uncommon cause of AKI in the cirrhosis population, ~12% of total AKI diagnoses in the cirrhotic population in most series

Key Pathophysiology

- Cirrhosis → portal hypertension → splanchnic vasodilation → endogenous vasodilator production (nitric oxide) → severe arterial underfilling → stimulation of vasoconstrictor systems (catecholamine release, renin-angiotensin-aldosterone, antidiuretic hormone) → maladaptive renal vasoconstriction → decreased glomerular filtration rate (GFR) → hepatorenal syndrome (HRS)
- Previously two types of HRS described: type 1 HRS and type 2 HRS
- Type 1 defined by acute, rapid decline in GFR; type 2 defined by slow, gradual decline in GFR
- Terminology now changing depending on the severity and chronicity of renal dysfunction
- Previous type 1 HRS now classified as HRS-AKI
- Previous type 2 HRS now encompasses less severe, subacute, and chronic cirrhosis–related decrements in GFR. Proposed terminology for this includes HRS-nonacute kidney injury (HRS-nAKI), HRS-acute kidney disease (HRS-AKD; used for kidney dysfunction lasting 7-90 days), or HRS-chronic kidney disease (HRS-CKD; for kidney dysfunction >90 days).

Hepatorenal Syndrome-Acute Kidney Injury Diagnostic Criteria

- Must meet all criteria
- Diagnosis of cirrhosis with ascites present
- A rise in serum creatinine (Cr) by ≥0.3 mg/dL (≥26.5 μmol/L) within 48 hours, or an increase in serum Cr to ≥1.5 times baseline in the prior 7 days; this definition is in line with the Kidney Disease: Improving Global Outcomes (KDIGO) Cr criteria for AKI.
- Urine volume is not used as most patients with cirrhosis will be oliguric at baseline.
- Lack of evidence for an alternative cause of AKI
- No response to volume expansion with albumin (1 g/kg of 25% albumin up to 100 g/24 hours) and cessation of diuretics for 48 hours

Differential Diagnosis

- HRS-AKI is a diagnosis of exclusion.
  - Essential to rule out other causes of AKI which include:
    - Prerenal AKI
    - Acute tubular necrosis
    - Nephrotoxic drug exposure
    - Glomerulonephritis
    - Parenchymal renal disease and structural abnormalities

When to Suspect Hepatorenal Syndrome-Acute Kidney Injury

- Abrupt decline in GFR in a patient with cirrhosis and ascites
- No hypertension
- Normal urine sediment
- Minimal or no proteinuria
- Low urine sodium levels (<20 mmol/L)

Common Precipitants

- Infection, commonly spontaneous bacterial peritonitis
- Large-volume paracentesis without adequate albumin resuscitation and subsequent fluid shifts
- Excessive diuresis
- Alcoholic hepatitis
- Gastrointestinal (GI) bleeding
- Significant diarrhea, often in the context of increased lactulose use

Management

- Evaluate for infection and initiate treatment if present.
- Avoid volume depletion by holding diuretics, monitoring GI losses (especially in patients on high-dose lactulose with diarrhea), and transfusing red blood cells for active bleeding.
- The only definitive treatment is liver transplantation.
- Medical therapy is used as a bridge to transplant.
- The cornerstone of medical management is vasoconstrictor therapy to increase splanchnic vascular tone.
- Terlipressin is the agent of choice; it is a prodrug of vasopressin.
- Terlipressin is contraindicated with worsening respiratory symptoms, hypoxia, prior severe vascular disease, or any active signs of ischemia (myocardial, peripheral vascular, or mesenteric). Not typically used for patients with Cr >5 mg/dL.
- If terlipressin is not available or contraindicated, norepinephrine can be used in the intensive care unit (ICU).
- Midodrine can also be used in combination with octreotide in patients not eligible for transfer to the ICU.
- Vasoconstrictor therapy is used in combination with volume expansion with 25% albumin in patients who do not have signs of hypervolemia.

Duration of Treatment

- Vasoconstrictor therapy and albumin usually continued for 14 days; albumin should only be used if no signs of intravascular volume overload.
- Therapy is usually stopped if:
  - 14 days of therapy completed
  - No change in serum Cr in 3 days
  - Improvement in serum Cr to within 0.3 mg/dL of baseline

- Patient initiated on renal replacement therapy
- Patient undergoes liver transplantation
- Serious adverse events during treatment

Outcomes

- Terlipressin does not affect transplant-free survival.
- Even with medical treatment, survival of HRS-AKI is measured in days to weeks in all series.
- Without a transplant, prognosis is poor.
- 90-day mortality of 50%
- If initiated on renal replacement therapy, mortality is 85% at 6 months without transplant.

SUGGESTED READINGS

Allegretti AS, Patidar KR, Ma AT, Cullaro G. From past to present to future: terlipressin and hepatorenal syndrome-acute kidney injury. *Hepatology*. 2025;81(6):1878-1897.

Angeli P, Garcia-Tsao G, Nadim MK, Parikh CR. News in pathophysiology, definition and classification of hepatorenal syndrome: a step beyond the International Club of Ascites (ICA) consensus document. *J Hepatol*. 2019;71(4):811-822.

Angeli P, Gines P, Wong F, et al; International Club of Ascites. Diagnosis and management of acute kidney injury in patients with cirrhosis: revised consensus recommendations of the International Club of Ascites. *Gut*. 2015;64(4):531-537.

Biggins SW, Angeli P, Garcia-Tsao G, et al. Diagnosis, evaluation, and management of ascites, spontaneous bacterial peritonitis and hepatorenal syndrome: 2021 practice guidance by the American Association for the Study of Liver Diseases. *Hepatology*. 2021;74(2):1014-1048.

European Association for the Study of the Liver. EASL clinical practice guidelines for the management of patients with decompensated cirrhosis [*J Hepatol*. 2018;69(5):1207]. *J Hepatol*. 2018;69(2):406-460.

Ginès P, Schrier RW. Renal failure in cirrhosis [*N Engl J Med*. 2011;364(4):389]. *N Engl J Med*. 2009;361(13):1279-1290.

Martín-Llahí M, Pépin MN, Guevara M, et al; TAHRS Investigators. Terlipressin and albumin vs albumin in patients with cirrhosis and hepatorenal syndrome: a randomized study. *Gastroenterology*. 2008;134(5):1352-1359.

Nadim MK, Kellum JA, Forni L, et al. Acute kidney injury in patients with cirrhosis: Acute Disease Quality Initiative (ADQI) and International Club of Ascites (ICA) joint multidisciplinary consensus meeting. *J HEPATOL*. 2024;81(1):163-183.

Sort P, Navasa M, Arroyo V, et al. Effect of intravenous albumin on renal impairment and mortality in patients with cirrhosis and spontaneous bacterial peritonitis. *N Engl J Med*. 1999;341(6):403-409.

4.6

Bowel Ischemia and Perforation

Casey M. Luckhurst

Definition

Gastrointestinal perforation refers to the complete penetration of the wall of the stomach, small intestine, or large intestine, allowing intestinal contents to flow into the peritoneal cavity.

Key Pathophysiology

- Peptic ulcer perforation occurs when the injurious effects of acid and pepsin overwhelm the mucosal barrier and acid suppression therapy has not been instituted or is inadequate to control the local acid environment.
- In mechanical obstruction (obstructing tumor, volvulus, bowel herniation) without vascular compromise, ingested fluid and food, digestive secretions, and gas accumulate above the level of the obstruction, leading to proximal bowel overdistention, ischemia, and perforation.
- Intestinal ischemia (associated with hernia, obstruction, volvulus, intussusception, vascular compromise) can progress to infarction, gangrene, and perforation rapidly, with a time course depending on the etiology and severity.
- Traumatic (blunt or penetrating) or iatrogenic perforations can also occur (surgical or endoscopic).

Common Causes to Remember

- Severe peptic ulcer disease
- Malignancy
- Appendicitis
- Diverticulitis
- Volvulus (small bowel or colonic)
- Severe inflammatory bowel disease
- Toxic megacolon
- Bowel obstruction
- Mesenteric ischemia (arterial or venous)
- Trauma
- Iatrogenic
- Symptoms and signs
    - Hollow viscus perforation may present with localized or systemic signs and symptoms.
    - Contained perforations may present with typical signs of infection (fever, leukocytosis), as well as focal tenderness to palpation in the anatomic region.
    - Free perforations will result in peritonitis, which can lead to systemic signs of infection, including tachycardia, hypotension, and end-organ malperfusion (acute kidney injury, lactic acidosis, altered mental status).

Diagnosis

- Clinical examination—signs/symptoms of infection coupled with abdominal examination with focal or diffuse tenderness, rebound tenderness, guarding
- Laboratory evaluation: nonspecific but may include leukocytosis, metabolic acidosis
- Plain films: free air in the subdiaphragmatic space can be identified (Figure 4.6.1).
- Cross-sectional imaging: abdominal CT may provide information about the location of the perforation (localized bowel wall thickening, mesenteric and soft tissue stranding adjacent to the perforation) (Figure 4.6.2).

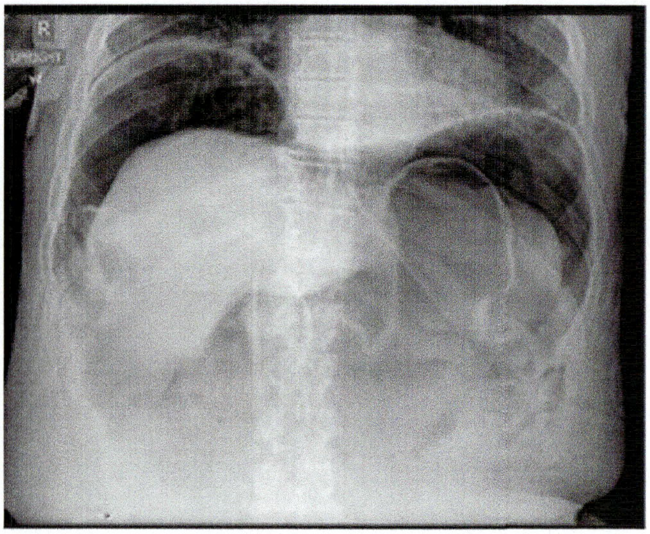

FIGURE 4.6.1 Free air under the diaphragm after iatrogenic duodenal perforation.

- Many times, the exact location may be difficult to diagnose on CT, but secondary signs (free air, free fluid, hyper-enhancing peritoneum, rim-enhancing fluid collections) are sufficient for diagnosis.
- Use of intravenous (IV) contrast, if not contraindicated, improves sensitivity in diagnosis and visualization of the anatomy. It is necessary for a diagnosis of mesenteric ischemia (typically CT angiography for arterial ischemia as compared with normal CT with IV contrast).
- Oral contrast can be helpful in identifying the location of a hollow viscus perforation, particularly the foregut (esophagus, stomach, duodenum, and proximal jejunum).

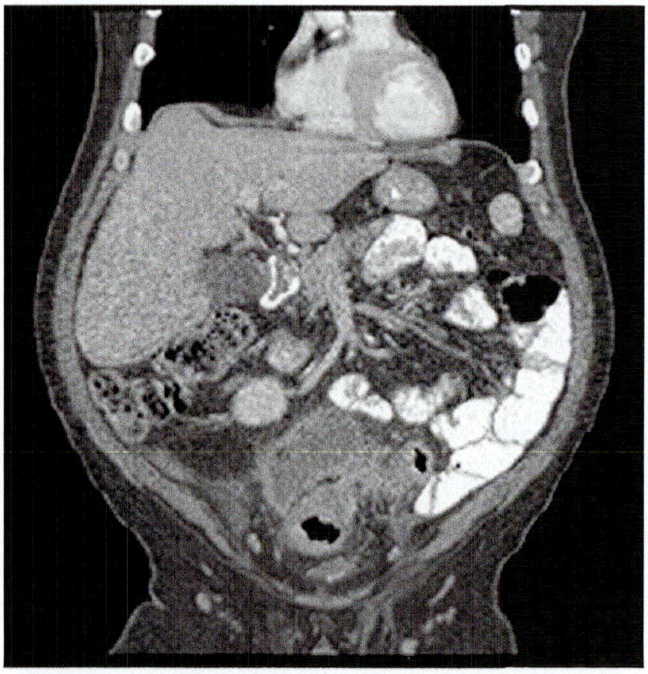

FIGURE 4.6.2 Localized sigmoid wall thickening, adjacent soft tissue stranding, and abscess in the lower abdomen with acute diverticulitis.

- Rectal contrast can be used if concerns for colonic perforation, although this is uncomfortable for the patient, more difficult to administer, and not routinely done as it rarely changes clinical management.

Management and Treatment

- Initial management with resuscitation
  - Medical management includes
    - Restoring intravascular volume
    - Initiation of vasopressors if needed for organ perfusion
    - Administration of broad-spectrum antibiotics for enteric coverage
    - Prompt surgical consultation
- Perforated ulcer disease may be managed operatively or nonoperatively depending on the location of the perforation, whether or not it is contained, and the clinical presentation of the patient (stable vs unstable).
- The management of ischemia or perforation secondary to malignancy is complex, and prompt surgical consultation is warranted as well as involvement of the patient's oncologist, if previously diagnosed. This is an opportunity to utilize multidisciplinary care and shared decision-making.
- Appendicitis is typically managed surgically, although it may be managed nonoperatively depending on the surgical anatomy, initial presentation of the patient, and patient preference.
  - In uncomplicated appendicitis, some data suggest that nonoperative management with antibiotics alone is feasible, although the failure and recurrence rates range from 30% to 50%.
  - Perforated appendicitis with abscess formation is typically managed with percutaneous drain placement, IV antibiotics, and discussion of interval appendectomy once the acute illness has resolved.
- On the contrary, diverticulitis is typically managed with IV antibiotics, and surgery is avoided unless there are clinical signs of decompensation.
- Bowel obstructions are typically managed nonoperatively in the absence of concern for ischemia. If there is failure to resolve or concern for the development of ischemia, surgery is warranted.
- The management of a volvulus depends on the anatomic location, with small bowel and cecal volvulus typically requiring surgical intervention, whereas a sigmoid colonic volvulus can be managed endoscopically in the absence of evidence of perforation or ischemia.
- Surgical evaluation is warranted in cases of toxic megacolon, fulminant colitis, and concern for failure of medical management of inflammatory bowel disease.
- Mesenteric ischemia may present as arterial or venous ischemia. Both disease processes require multidisciplinary management with general surgery, vascular surgery, and, sometimes, interventional radiology. Expeditious initiation of anticoagulation is warranted in the absence of contraindications. Surgical intervention may be warranted to restore arterial inflow or to address bowel ischemia.
  - Extensive venous thrombosis leading to venous ischemia is a complex disease to manage, and multidisciplinary involvement with the aforementioned consultations and hematology is warranted.

- Traumatic hollow viscus injury is almost exclusively managed operatively, with outcomes strongly dependent on prompt diagnosis and treatment.
- Similar to other processes mentioned previously, iatrogenic perforation, commonly in the setting of endoscopy, is managed based on the clinical presentation of the patient, with some cases treated medically and others requiring prompt surgical intervention.
- Broad-spectrum antibiotics, bowel rest, and percutaneous drainage of extraluminal collections may be used for the clinically well patient with localized peritoneal irritation.
- In disseminated peritonitis, surgical exploration with cavity washout is usually warranted. Perforations may be patched (gastroduodenal), primarily repaired (intestinal), excised (gastric, intestinal), or proximally diverted (diverticulitis).

Acknowledgments

We gratefully acknowledge the contributions of previous edition author, George Kasotakis, as portions of those chapters have been retained in this revision.

SUGGESTED READINGS

Beckham H, Whitlow CB. The medical and nonoperative treatment of diverticulitis. *Clin Colon Rectal Surg*. 2009;22(3):155-160.

Castellví J, Pi F, Sueiras A, et al. Colonoscopic perforation: useful parameters for early diagnosis and conservative treatment. *Int J Colorectal Dis*. 2011;26(9):1183-1190.

Horn AE, Ufberg JW. Appendicitis, diverticulitis and colitis. *Emerg Med Clin North Am*. 2011;29(2):347-368.

Rafferty J, Shellito P, Hyman NH, et al. Practice parameters for sigmoid diverticulitis. *Dis Colon Rectum*. 2006;49(7):939-944.

Spirt MJ. Complicated intra-abdominal infections: a focus on appendicitis and diverticulitis. *Postgrad Med*. 2012;122(1):39.

4.7

Acute Mesenteric Ischemia

Srihari K. Lella and Jahan Mohebali

Definition

- Acute mesenteric ischemia (AMI) is caused by a sudden decrease in perfusion to the small and/or large bowel, resulting in a mismatch of metabolic supply and demand, with an ultimate risk of bowel necrosis.

Epidemiology

- AMI is rare: Its incidence increases with age and is reported to be around 1.09/100,000 person-years.
- AMI is most common after the sixth decade of life, especially in patients with peripheral or coronary atherosclerosis.
- AMI affects women 3 times as frequently as men.

Key Pathophysiology

- The mesenteric blood supply is derived from three major arteries:
  - The celiac artery
  - The superior mesenteric artery (SMA = most commonly implicated vessel)
  - The inferior mesenteric artery (IMA)
- The mesenteric arterial cascade involves an extensive collateral circulation connecting the major mesenteric vessels to each other as well as to the systemic circulation.
- The probability of intestinal ischemia depends upon the adequacy of systemic and collateral perfusion, the number and caliber of affected vessels, and the duration of the insult.
- Typically, only one-fifth of the mesenteric capillaries are open at any given time, through which normal oxygen consumption can be maintained.
- As a result, mesenteric vasculature can compensate for up to a 75% acute reduction in perfusion for as long as 12 hours through increased oxygen extraction at the tissue level and increased collateral circulation.
- Despite the extensive collateral mesenteric circulation, prolonged bowel hypoperfusion results in vasoconstriction, thus ultimately reducing collateral flow.
- Prolonged ischemia results in disruption of the intestinal mucosal barrier, primarily from reactive oxygen species and polymorphonuclear neutrophils, which can further result in the systemic release of intracellular breakdown products and an increase in anaerobic metabolism.
- AMI affects mucosal surfaces first due to the higher mucosal metabolic demand, and this clinically presents with malabsorption and heme-positive diarrhea.
- Ischemic damage is due to both hypoxic and reperfusion injury, often with vasoconstriction persisting after restoration of blood flow.

Etiology and Risk Factors

- The etiology of AMI may be categorized as
  - Mesenteric arterial embolism
  - Mesenteric arterial thrombosis
  - Nonocclusive mesenteric ischemia
  - Mesenteric venous thrombosis
- Mesenteric arterial embolism
  - 40% to 50% of cases of AMI are from an embolism, which historically was thought to be the most common cause.
  - Primary source of embolization is cardiac.
  - Occlusion usually at a branch of the SMA distal to the middle colic artery and the first few jejunal branches, resulting in relative sparing of the proximal jejunum and distal large bowel
  - Risk factors
    - Cardiac arrhythmia (eg, atrial fibrillation)
    - Myocardial infarction/ventricular aneurysm
    - Low ejection fraction (congestive heart failure, cardiomyopathy)

        - Recent cardiac or aortic catheterization
        - Recent cardiac valve replacement
        - Endocarditis
        - Atrial septal defect (resulting in paradoxical embolus)
        - Aortic aneurysm or mural thrombi
- Mesenteric arterial thrombosis
    - Recent studies demonstrate this to be the most common cause of AMI, accounting for >50% of cases.
    - Most common cause is acute thrombosis of a chronic atherosclerotic lesion.
    - Occlusion usually occurs at the origin of the mesenteric vessel (SMA or celiac).
    - Less common causes include arterial dissection, arterial aneurysm, vasculitis, and iatrogenic injury (ie, intraoperative).
    - Risk factors
        - Known atherosclerosis/vascular disease
        - Abdominal trauma
        - Infection
        - In-stent restenosis of previously treated lesion or hyperplasia of prior bypass graft
- Nonocclusive mesenteric ischemia
    - 20% of cases, but it has the highest mortality rate.
    - Difficult to diagnose and treat due to association with multisystem organ failure
    - Occurs most commonly due to a global reduction in cardiac output
    - Underlying etiology is due to vasospasm, which may persist even after the inciting event is corrected.
    - Risk factors
        - Hypovolemia
        - Sepsis
        - Aortic insufficiency
        - Status post cardiac surgery
        - Digoxin use (may result in splanchnic vasoconstriction)
        - Cocaine abuse
        - Vasoactive medications (epinephrine, norepinephrine, vasopressin)
- Mesenteric venous thrombosis
    - 5% to 10% of cases
    - Usually associated with the existence of a hypercoagulable state
    - Risk factors
        - Malignancy
        - Inherited coagulopathy and other forms of thrombophilia (ie, factor V Leiden, factor C, or factor S deficiency)
        - Oral contraceptive use
        - Portal hypertension
        - Nephrotic syndrome
        - History of prior deep venous thrombosis or pulmonary embolus

Diagnosis

- History and physical examination

❑ ***History and physical examination alone are notoriously nonsensitive and nonspecific for AMI.***

    - Embolic AMI: sudden onset of severe periumbilical pain, typically out of proportion to physical examination findings
    - Arterial thrombosis, however, can occur more insidiously, with 95% of patients reporting a 24-hour history of vague abdominal pain.
    - Nonocclusive mesenteric ischemia can have more atypical presentation as these patients tend to be critically ill and may have concurrent multiorgan failure.
    - Symptoms may also be accompanied by anorexia, vomiting, and melena.
    - Patients with transmural bowel necrosis can present with peritonitis, tachycardia, hypotension, fevers, and other signs/symptoms of sepsis.
    - AMI may be mistaken for another pathology, resulting in delay in diagnosis and treatment, which increases morbidity and mortality.
    - If AMI is suspected, prompt workup and imaging should be obtained to confirm the diagnosis and proceed with treatment.
- Laboratories
    - No single serologic value is diagnostic or prognostic, but a common presentation includes:
        - Leukocytosis with left shift
        - Hemoconcentration
        - Anion gap metabolic acidosis (lactic acidosis)
        - High amylase, aspartate aminotransferase, and lactate dehydrogenase
        - Elevated urinary and plasma intestinal fatty acid–binding protein
            - Lab abnormalities may not be present in some patients and, when abnormal, tend to be nonspecific.
- Imaging studies
    - Plain abdominal radiographs
        - Neither sensitive nor specific for mesenteric ischemia; normal in up to 25% of patients with ischemic bowel
        - Significant findings include "thumbprinting" suggestive of intestinal wall edema, pneumatosis intestinalis suggestive of bowel wall necrosis, or pneumoperitoneum suggestive of bowel perforation.
    - Doppler-flow ultrasonography
        - Useful in identifying proximal SMA and celiac lesions
        - Role may be limited in acute settings due to the inability to assess lesions distal to the proximal vessel (eg, distal SMA emboli) and to determine bowel malperfusion.
        - Often technically limited due to interference from air-filled bowel
        - Requires trained technologist
    - Computed tomographic angiography (CTA)
        - Can evaluate for both acute and chronic mesenteric ischemia with high sensitivity and specificity (>90%)
        - Allows for visualization of bowel wall thickening, pneumatosis intestinalis, and portal venous gas
        - Higher accuracy for thromboembolic etiologies versus nonocclusive ischemia
        - Can also be used to rule out other causes of acute abdomen
    - Mesenteric angiography
        - Previous gold standard imaging modality to diagnose AMI

        - Early angiography (within 12 hours of event) associated with improved survival
        - Allows simultaneous intervention to restore blood flow
    - Magnetic resonance angiography (MRA)
        - Can evaluate for stenosis as well as nonatherosclerotic pathologies (eg, fibromuscular dysplasia)
        - Avoids ionizing radiation, but makes study lengthy and may not be feasible in the emergent evaluation of patients
- Intraoperative diagnosis
    - Exploratory laparotomy is the gold standard and is required for suspicion of any bowel infarction.

Treatment and Management

- Goal of treatment is restoration of mesenteric perfusion and resection of necrotic bowel.
    - Aggressive hemodynamic monitoring and support (isotonic fluids and/or vasopressors)
    - Broad-spectrum intravenous (IV) antibiotics (coverage for enteric flora with concerns for bowel perforation or bacterial translocation)
    - Immediate therapeutic IV anticoagulation
    - Correction of electrolyte and acid-base abnormalities
    - Mesenteric arteriography
        - Hypotension or hypovolemia may lead to false-positive studies.
        - Therapeutic options include intra-arterial vasodilators (papaverine), thrombolytic agents, angioplasty, stenting, and thromboembolectomy.
    - Consider surgery for emergent situations when there is suspicion of intestinal infarction or perforation.
- Mesenteric arterial embolism
    - Surgical embolectomy versus local thrombolytic therapy
        - Surgical embolectomy
            - SMA is exposed at the base of the transverse mesocolon, and the patient is systemically heparinized if not already done so.
            - Arteriotomy is made over the SMA, and a balloon-tipped embolectomy (Fogarty) catheter is passed proximally and distally.
            - If Fogarty cannot be passed distally, thrombotic material may be "milked" out by pressing the mesentery on either side.
            - Tissue plasminogen activator (TPA) can be infused through arteriotomy distally, if the thrombus is incompletely removed.
            - Extraction of the thrombus proximally should result in torrential inflow of blood.
            - Arteriotomy can be closed primarily or patched as needed and flow reestablished.
            - Examination for infarcted bowel is performed 20 to 30 minutes following revascularization.
            - The abdomen may be left open with a temporary abdominal closure device to allow for a second-look laparotomy within 24 to 48 hours to assess the evolution of bowel ischemia.
        - Local thrombolytic therapy
            - Although previously described, thrombolysis alone can be risky due to the time required to achieve result; its primary use is as adjunctive therapy to eliminate residual thrombus burden.
            - Thrombolysis is contraindicated if the patient has an open abdomen, recent surgery, or if further surgery is required.
            - TPA can exacerbate bleeding from the intestinal mucosa.
            - Surgical intervention is mandatory if no resolution within several hours or with worsening clinical status.
    - Long-term anticoagulation to prevent future embolic events
- Mesenteric arterial thrombosis
    - Therapy requires treatment of both the acute thrombus and the underlying atherosclerotic lesion that resulted in the acute thrombosis.
    - Similar to embolic pathology, there should be a low threshold to explore the abdomen to examine the bowel.
    - Endovascular revascularization is now more prevalent than open revascularization for mesenteric thrombosis.
    - As lesions are typically in the proximal SMA or celiac artery, they are often treated with angioplasty and stenting, which can be performed antegrade or retrograde.
    - In rare instances, a bypass from the aorta or the left or right common iliac artery to the distal SMA may be required.
        - Antegrade bypass off the aorta provides for straighter graft orientation but requires, at least, partial clamping of the supraceliac aorta, which can result in significant hemodynamic changes.
        - Retrograde bypass off the iliac artery avoids aortic cross-clamping but can be prone to kinking with lower patency rates.
    - Long-term antiplatelet agents may reduce the risk of recurrence.
- Mesenteric venous thrombosis
    - Initial management with heparin anticoagulation and workup for a hypercoagulable state
    - Additional supportive management with antibiotic therapy, nasogastric tube decompression, fluid resuscitation, analgesics, and total parenteral nutrition may be required.
    - Close observation with serial abdominal examinations is warranted; prompt laparotomy is necessary for any suspicion of infarcted bowel.
    - Small reports of successful venous thrombolysis; insufficient data to recommend thrombolysis over standard therapy
    - Prevention of recurrence with long-term anticoagulation
- Nonocclusive mesenteric ischemia
    - Primary therapy is reversal of the underlying condition: optimize cardiac output, decrease vasopressors and other offending agents, and provide supportive care.
    - Successful use of local intra-arterial angiographic papaverine infusion has been reported, but evidence is conflicting, with the risk of worsening hypotension in already hemodynamically labile patients.
    - IV glucagon has been described to increase cardiac output and transmural flow to the small and large intestine while decreasing gastrointestinal (GI) motility and secretory function, but evidence is limited.
    - Long-term management with standard-dose aspirin

Outcomes

- Reported mortality approximates 60% to 70%.
  - Range is from 20% with early diagnosis and management to >70% following bowel infarction.
  - Diagnosis prior to infarction is the single strongest predictor of survival.
  - Other predictors of mortality are advanced age, poor functional status, and prior cardiac surgery.
- Reported 30-day postoperative morbidity approximates 60%.
  - Pulmonary and infectious complications are the most common.

Acknowledgments

We gratefully acknowledge the contributions of previous edition author(s), Lauren Steffel and Haytham M.A. Kaafarani, as portions of those chapters have been retained in this revision.

SUGGESTED READINGS

Boley SJ, Brandt LJ, Sammartano RJ. History of mesenteric ischemia: the evolution of a diagnosis and management. *Surg Clin North Am*. 1997;77(2):275-288.

Cho JS, Carr JA, Jacobsen G, et al. Long-term outcome after mesenteric artery reconstruction: a 37-year experience. *J Vasc Surg*. 2002;35(3):453-460.

Demirpolat G, Oran I, Tamsel S, et al. Acute mesenteric ischemia: endovascular therapy. *Abdom Imaging*. 2007;32(3):299-303.

Evennett NJ, Petrov MS, Mittal A, et al. Systematic review and pooled estimates for the diagnostic accuracy of serological markers for intestinal ischemia. *World J Surg*. 2009;33(7):1374-1383.

Gupta PK, Natarajan B, Gupta H, et al. Morbidity and mortality after bowel resection for acute mesenteric ischemia. *Surgery*. 2011;150(4):779-787.

Huerta C, Rivero E, Montoro MA, et al. Risk factors for intestinal ischaemia among patients registered in a UK primary care database: a nested case-control study. *Aliment Pharmacol Ther*. 2011;33(8):969-978.

Klein HM, Lensing R, Klosterhalfen B, et al. Diagnostic imaging of mesenteric infarction. *Radiology*. 1995;197:79-82.

Kumar, S, Sarr MG, Kamath PS. Mesenteric venous thrombosis. *N Engl J Med*. 2001;345(23):1683-1688.

McKinsey JF, Gewertz BL. Acute mesenteric ischemia. *Surg Clin North Am*. 1997;77:307-318.

Ofer A, Abadi S, Nitecki S, et al. Multidetector CT angiography in the evaluation of acute mesenteric ischemia. *Eur Radiol*. 2009;19(1):24-30.

Oldenburg WA, Lau LL, Rodenberg TJ, et al. Acute mesenteric ischemia: a clinical review. *Arch Intern Med*. 2004;164:1054-1062.

Park WM, Gloviczki P, Cherry KJ Jr, et al. Contemporary management of acute mesenteric ischemia: factors associated with survival. *J Vasc Surg*. 2002;35(3):445-452.

Schoots IG, Levi MM, Reekers JA, et al. Thrombolytic therapy for acute superior mesenteric artery occlusion. *J Vasc Interv Radiol*. 2005;16(3):317-329.

Vicente DC, Kazmers A. Acute mesenteric ischemia. *Curr Opin Cardiol*. 1999;14(5):453-458.

Wyers MC, Powell RJ, Nolan BW, et al. Retrograde mesenteric stenting during laparotomy for acute occlusive mesenteric ischemia. *J Vasc Surg*. 2007;45(2):269.

Zettervall SL, Lo RC, Soden PA, et al. Trends in treatment and mortality for mesenteric ischemia in the United States from 2000 to 2012. *Ann Vasc Surg*. 2017;42;111-119.

4.8

Gastrointestinal Bleeding

Cara Hannigan

- Gastrointestinal (GI) bleeding is a common medical emergency.
- Upper GI bleeding (UGIB) accounts for ~70% of cases.
  - Estimated to occur in 80 to 150 out of 100,000 people each year
- Jejunoileal bleeding accounts for <5% of cases.
- Lower GI bleeding (LGIB) accounts for ~25% of cases.
  - Estimated to occur in 20.5 to 27 cases per 100,000 people each year
- Incidence increases with age and is higher in men than in women.

Clinical Presentation

- **Melena**: black, tarry stools resulting from digestion of blood in the stomach
- **Hematemesis**: vomiting of blood, which can range from bright red (indicating active bleeding) to coffee-ground appearance (indicating partially digested blood)
- **Hematochezia**: passage of fresh, bright red blood through the rectum, which can occur if bleeding is brisk
- **Symptoms**: can include abdominal pain, changes in bowel habits, and signs of anemia (eg, fatigue, weakness, pallor)
- **Asymptomatic iron deficiency anemia**: GI bleed is a common cause of unexplained anemia (Table 4.8.1).

Diagnosis

- Diagnosis facilitated by nasogastric lavage
  - Bloody aspirate indicates UGIB.
  - Can assess rate of ongoing bleeding
  - 20% of those with nonbloody aspirate are bleeding from upper GI source.

TABLE 4.8.1 Causes of GI Bleeding

Upper GI Bleeding (Proximal to the Ligament of Treitz)	Lower GI Bleeding (Distal to Ligament of Treitz)
Peptic ulcer disease	Diverticular disease
Esophageal varices	Angiodysplasia
Gastritis	Colorectal polyps and malignancies
Malignancies	Inflammatory bowel disease
Mallory-Weiss tear	Ischemic colitis
Arteriovenous malformations	Anorectal conditions
Dieulafoy lesion	Infectious colitis

GI, gastrointestinal.

- Diagnosis facilitated by rectal examination
  - Presence of fresh blood
  - Guaiac-positive stool
  - Can identify hemorrhoidal bleeds, anal masses, or fissures
- Urgent endoscopy (esophagogastroduodenoscopy [EGD] or colonoscopy) within 24 hours essential for localization and intervention
  - Push enteroscopy or double-balloon enteroscopy for suspected small bowel source
  - Capsule endoscopy for stable unlocalized bleeds
- Imaging studies may be considered when there is no obvious source.
  - Computed tomographic (CT) angiography can detect bleeding 0.3 to 0.5 mL/min.
  - Tagged red blood cell (RBC) scan 0.1 to 0.35 mL/min
    - Low-spatial resolution with accuracy 40% to 60%
  - Angiography can detect bleeding 0.5 to 1.0 mL/min.
    - Provoked angiography can increase the likelihood of localization.
    - Can be combined with therapeutic treatment

Complications of Gastrointestinal Bleeding

- Rebleeding
- Hypovolemic shock
- Death
- Iron deficiency anemia
- Coagulopathy

Upper Gastrointestinal Bleeding

Causes

- **Peptic ulcer disease (PUD)**
  - Most common cause of UGIB
  - Occur in the stomach or the duodenum (most likely)
  - Risk factors include *Helicobacter pylori* infection, nonsteroidal antiinflammatory drugs (NSAIDs) use, steroid use, and smoking.
- **Esophageal varices**
  - Seen in patients with cirrhosis and portal hypertension
  - These enlarged veins in the esophagus are prone to rupture, causing severe bleeding.
  - Higher risk of rebleeding and need for transfusion
- **Gastritis**
  - Inflammation and irritation of the stomach lining
  - Occurs secondary to acid injury combined with ischemia
  - Risk factors include alcohol use, NSAIDs, stress, and *H. pylori* infection, burns, head injury, ventilator dependence >48 hours.
  - Prophylactic treatment for at-risk patients: proton pump inhibitor (PPI) or H_2 blocker
  - Low risk of significant bleeding
- **Malignancies**
  - Friable lesions in the stomach or esophagus, particularly if the tumor erodes into blood vessels
- **Mallory-Weiss tears**
  - Tears in the mucosa and submucosa at the gastroesophageal junction, typically caused by severe retching or vomiting
  - Common in alcoholics
  - Over 90% self-limited
- **Arteriovenous malformations (AVMs)**
  - Abnormal connections between arteries and veins in the GI tract can lead to bleeding.
- **Dieulafoy lesion**
  - Tortuous large artery in the stomach submucosa that can erode and cause sudden, severe bleeding

Diagnosis

- **Endoscopy**: EGD can visualize the entire esophagus, stomach, and duodenum to identify the bleeding source and potentially perform therapeutic interventions.
  - If bleeding recurrence after initial endoscopic treatment, then repeat endoscopy is recommended.
- **Laboratory tests**
  - Complete blood count (CBC) to assess for anemia.
    - Hematocrit is unreliable as a diagnostic measure in the acute setting.
  - Coagulation studies to assess for coagulopathy
  - Elevated blood urea nitrogen (BUN) level can occur due to digestion of hemoglobin.
- **Imaging**: in cases where endoscopy is inconclusive or unavailable, imaging studies like angiography or tagged RBC scan may be considered.

Management

- **Resuscitation**: initial management focuses on stabilizing the patient's hemodynamic status with intravenous fluids and blood products as needed.
- **Endoscopic therapy**: allows direct visualization of the bleeding source and enables therapeutic interventions such as:
    - Injection of epinephrine
    - Thermal coagulation
    - Application of hemostatic clips.
    - Banding of varices
    - Sclerotherapy of varices
  - Successful in 75% of cases (Table 4.8.2)
- **Pharmacologic therapy**
  - Includes PPIs to suppress gastric acid production
  - Triple or quadruple therapy for *H. pylori*
  - Antibiotics (ceftriaxone) 5 to 7 days for variceal bleeding
  - Octreotide 5 days for variceal bleeding (splanchnic vasoconstriction)
- **Angiography and embolization:** for cases of ongoing bleeding with a localized target vessel
  - Embolization with coils or fibrin glue
  - Transjugular intrahepatic portosystemic shunt (TIPS) for variceal bleed

TABLE 4.8.2 Forest Classification of Endoscopic Findings and Rebleeding Risks

Stage	Characteristics	Rebleeding (%)
Ia	Spurting bleed	60-100
Ib	Oozing bleed	50
IIa	Nonbleeding visible vessel	40-50
IIb	Adherent clot	20-30
IIc	Flat spot in ulcer crater	7-10
III	Clean base ulcer	3-5

- **Surgical intervention**: resection of tissue or vessel ligation indicated for:
  - Persistent or severe bleeding not amenable to endoscopic or percutaneous management
  - Failure of endoscopic, pharmacologic, or percutaneous management
  - Massive bleeding causing hemodynamic instability
  - Bleeding in the setting of a resectable malignancy

Jejunoileal Bleeding

Causes

- **Angiodysplasia**
  - Abnormal, fragile blood vessels in the mucosa
- **Malignancies**
  - **Gastrointestinal stromal tumors (GISTs)**: can occur in the stomach or small intestine and may cause bleeding due to their propensity to ulcerate or erode blood vessels
- **Inflammatory conditions**
  - **Crohn disease**: chronic inflammation in the small intestine can lead to ulceration and subsequent bleeding.
- **Ischemic enteritis**: reduced blood flow to the small intestine can cause tissue damage.
- **Meckel diverticulum**: a congenital outpouching of the small intestine that may contain ectopic gastric or pancreatic tissue, prone to ulceration
- **Small bowel varices**: rare but can occur in the setting of portal hypertension

Diagnosis

- **Challenges in diagnosis**: jejunoileal bleeding poses diagnostic challenges since it is beyond the reach of standard upper and lower scopes and requires specialized endoscopic techniques.
  - **Capsule endoscopy**: a pill-sized camera that captures images as it travels through the GI tract
  - **Double-balloon enteroscopy**: utilizes two balloons, one at the tip of the enteroscope and one on the over tube, to anchor and advance the scope through the small intestine
  - **Push enteroscopy**: endoscopic examination using a longer scope to reach the proximal jejunum, allowing direct visualization and potential intervention
- **Radiologic studies**: may include CT angiography or mesenteric angiography to detect active bleeding and potentially guide therapeutic interventions

Management

- **Endoscopic interventions**: techniques such as injection of epinephrine, thermal coagulation, or clipping may be used for hemostasis.
- **Pharmacologic management**: based on the etiology of the bleed, therapies such as immunosuppressants or antiinflammatory agents may be employed to control inflammation and reduce the risk of recurrent bleeding.
- **Surgical intervention**: reserved for cases of severe or refractory bleeding, or when a definitive surgical approach is necessary, such as resection of a tumor

Lower Gastrointestinal Bleeding

Causes

- **Diverticular disease**
  - Most common cause of LGIB
  - Diverticula are small pouches that can form in the colon wall.
  - Bleeding occurs when these pouches become inflamed and/or rupture.
  - Most common in the left colon
  - 75% of bleeds stop spontaneously.
  - 10% rebleed in 1 year, 50% rebleed in 10 years
- **Angiodysplasia**
  - Abnormal, fragile blood vessels in the colon mucosa can bleed spontaneously.
  - More likely in people aged >50 due to acquired degenerative lesions secondary to progressive dilation of normal vessels in the submucosa.
- **Colorectal polyps and malignancies**
  - Benign growths (polyps) or malignant tumors (cancer) in the colon or rectum can cause bleeding, particularly with larger lesions.
  - Typically presents as a slow chronic bleed
- **Inflammatory bowel disease (IBD)**
  - Ulcerative colitis and Crohn disease can cause inflammation and ulceration in the intestinal lining.
- **Ischemic colitis**
  - Reduced blood flow to the colon due to arterial blockage or low blood pressure can cause ischemic injury and subsequent bleeding.
- **Anorectal conditions**
  - Conditions such as hemorrhoids, anal fissures, perianal abscesses, and masses can cause bleeding during bowel movements.
- **Infectious colitis**
  - Bacterial, viral, or parasitic infections of the colon can lead to inflammation.
  - *Escherichia coli, Clostridium difficile, Yersinia enterocolitica, Campylobacter, Shigella*

Diagnosis

- **Colonoscopy**: can visualize the entire colon and rectum to identify the bleeding source and potentially perform therapeutic interventions
- **Flexible sigmoidoscopy**: limited to examining the distal colon and rectum
- **Rectal examination and anoscopy**: limited examination but can quickly diagnose without the need for sedation
- **Stool studies**: occult blood testing to detect microscopic bleeding
- **Laboratory tests**
  - CBC to assess for anemia.
    - Hematocrit is unreliable as a diagnostic measure in the acute setting.
  - Coagulation studies to assess for coagulopathy
- **Imaging**: in cases where colonoscopy is inconclusive or unavailable, imaging studies like angiography or tagged RBC scan may be considered.

Management

- **Resuscitation**: similar to UGIB, initial management focuses on stabilizing the patient with intravenous fluids and blood products as needed.

- **Endoscopic therapy**: colonoscopy and sigmoidoscopy are utilized for hemostasis and diagnosis.
  - Injection of epinephrine
  - Thermal coagulation
  - Application of hemostatic clips
  - Banding of hemorrhoids
  - Sclerotherapy of hemorrhoids
  - Cold or hot snare polypectomy
  - Endoscopic submucosal resection
- **Pharmacologic therapies**: treatments may include
  - Antibiotics for infectious colitis
  - Antiinflammatory agents for IBD
  - Biologic therapies for IBD
- **Angiography and embolization:** for cases of ongoing bleeding with a localized target vessel
  - Embolization with coils or fibrin glue
- **Surgical intervention**: resection of tissue or vessel ligation indicated for:
  - Persistent or severe bleeding not amenable to endoscopic or percutaneous management
  - Failure of endoscopic, pharmacologic, or percutaneous management
  - Massive bleeding causing hemodynamic instability
  - Bleeding in the setting of a resectable malignancy

Outcomes

- Most GI bleeding stops spontaneously.
- 15% have ongoing major bleeding requiring emergent resuscitation.
- Mortality is >5%.
  - Single leading cause for morbidity and mortality is multiorgan failure from inadequate resuscitation.
- Risk factors for adverse outcomes
  - Age >60 years
  - Comorbid disease
  - Renal failure
  - Liver disease
  - Cardiac disease
  - Respiratory insufficiency
  - Magnitude of hemorrhage
  - Systolic blood pressure <100 mm Hg on presentation
  - Transfusion requirement

Conclusions

- GI bleeding requires prompt diagnosis and intervention.
- Advances in medical, endoscopic, percutaneous, and surgical therapies continue to refine management strategies, emphasizing the importance of multidisciplinary care.

SUGGESTED READINGS

Adegboyega T, Rivadeneira D. Lower GI bleeding: an update on incidences and causes. *Clin Colon Rectal Surg*. 2020;33(1):28-34.

Chalasani N, Kahi C, Francois F, et al. Improved patient survival after acute variceal bleeding: a multicenter, cohort study. *Am J Gastroenterol*. 2003;98:653-659.

Chung IK, Kim EJ, Lee MS, et al. Endoscopic factors predisposing to rebleeding following endoscopic hemostasis in bleeding peptic ulcers. *Endoscopy*. 2001;33:969-975.

Costable NJ, Greenwald DA. Upper gastrointestinal bleeding. *Clin Geriatr Med*. 2021;37(1):155-172.

Guglielmi A, Ruzzenente A, Sandri M, et al. Risk assessment and prediction of rebleeding in bleeding gastroduodenal ulcer. *Endoscopy*. 2002;34:778-786.

Gunjan D, Sharma V, Rana SS, Bhasin DK. Small bowel bleeding: a comprehensive review. *Gastroenterol Rep (Oxf)*. 2014;2(4):262-275.

Jung K, Moon W. Role of endoscopy in acute gastrointestinal bleeding in real clinical practice: an evidence-based review. *World J Gastrointest Endosc*. 2019;11(2):68-83.

Kamboj AK, Hoversten P, Leggett CL. Upper gastrointestinal bleeding: etiologies and management. *Mayo Clin Proc*. 2019;94(4):697-703.

Khuroo MS, Farahat KL, Kagevi IE. Treatment with proton pump inhibitors in acute non-variceal upper gastrointestinal bleeding: a meta-analysis. *J Gastroenterol Hepatol*. 2005;20:11-25.

Mohammed Ilyas MI, Szilagy EJ. Management of diverticular bleeding: evaluation, stabilization, intervention, and recurrence of bleeding and indications for resection after control of bleeding. *Clin Colon Rectal Surg*. 2018;31(4):243-250.

Riha HM, Wilkinson R, Twilla J, et al. Octreotide added to a proton pump inhibitor versus a proton pump inhibitor alone in nonvariceal upper-gastrointestinal bleeds. *Ann Pharmacother*. 2019;53(8):794-800.

Sudan R, Brandt C, Cox ML, Bendersky V, Ignacio R. ACS/ASE Medical Student Core Curriculum Gastrointestinal Hemorrhage.

4.9

Malabsorption in the Critically Ill Patient

Kiran Dyamenahalli and John O. Hwabejire

Overview

- *Definition:* malabsorption is defined as defective digestion and/or absorption of nutrients. It can be global (affecting all substrates) or partial (limited to specific nutrients).
- *Significance in critical illness:* malabsorption is a common and often underdiagnosed issue in critically ill patients, contributing to malnutrition, delayed recovery, and increased morbidity and mortality. Factors unique to critical illness, such as systemic inflammation, gut ischemia, altered motility, and specific interventions (medications, surgery), can precipitate or exacerbate malabsorption.
- *Clinical manifestations*
  - *Gastrointestinal symptoms:* diarrhea (often the most prominent symptom, though not always indicative of malabsorption alone), steatorrhea, abdominal distension, pain, flatulence, nausea, vomiting, and intolerance to enteral feeding. Undigested food particles in stool may be observed.
  - *Systemic signs and symptoms:* weight loss (can be masked by fluid resuscitation), muscle wasting, edema/anasarca (due to protein-calorie malnutrition), specific nutrient

deficiency signs (eg, anemia from iron/B_{12}/folate deficiency, coagulopathy from vitamin K deficiency, bone pain/fractures from calcium/vitamin D deficiency, neurologic symptoms from thiamine/B_{12} deficiency)

Etiology and Differential Diagnosis

Malabsorption in the critically ill patients is often multifactorial and can result from:

- *Luminal factors (impaired digestion)*
  - Exocrine pancreatic insufficiency (eg, severe pancreatitis, pancreatic surgery, sepsis-induced dysfunction)
  - Chronic cholestasis or biliary obstruction (impaired fat digestion)
  - Small intestinal bacterial overgrowth (SIBO) (deconjugation of bile salts, mucosal damage)
  - Gastric acid suppression (eg, proton pump inhibitors), potentially contributing to SIBO and impaired B_{12}/iron absorption
- *Mucosal factors (impaired absorption)*
  - Intestinal ischemia (global or segmental, due to low-flow states, vasopressors, or vascular events)
  - Gut edema (secondary to systemic inflammation, fluid overload, hypoalbuminemia), impairing villous function
  - Inflammatory conditions (eg, severe sepsis-induced enteropathy, inflammatory bowel disease [IBD] flare, radiation enteritis)
  - Infections (eg, *Clostridioides difficile*, cytomegalovirus [CMV], parasitic infections like *Giardia*, tropical sprue, Whipple disease, AIDS-related enteropathies)
  - Celiac disease (though less likely to present acutely in critical illness unless previously undiagnosed or triggered)
  - Specific enzyme deficiencies (eg, lactase deficiency, sometimes acquired)
- *Structural/anatomic factors*
  - Short-bowel syndrome (SBS) (due to extensive resection from trauma, ischemia, Crohn, etc)
  - Fistulas (bypassing absorptive surface)
  - Strictures or partial obstructions (can lead to SIBO)
  - Postsurgical anatomy (eg, gastric bypass, gastrectomy, intestinal resections)
- *Motility disorders*
  - Ileus (postoperative, sepsis related, medication induced—opioids, anticholinergics). While primarily affecting transit, severe ileus can impair mixing and absorption and contribute significantly to feeding intolerance.
  - Gastroparesis
- *Medication effects*
  - Antibiotics (altering gut microbiome, *C. difficile* infection)
  - Opioids (reduce motility, contribute to ileus and constipation, potentially affecting transit)
  - Laxatives (overuse)
  - Chemotherapy
  - Certain antivirals or antifungals

Diagnostic Approach

The diagnostic workup should be guided by the clinical presentation and suspected underlying etiology, considering the limitations and feasibility of tests in the critically ill setting.

- *Clinical assessment:* detailed history (including prior surgeries, chronic illnesses, medications), physical examination (abdominal distension, bowel sounds, signs of nutrient deficiencies)
- *Stool tests*
  - *Macroscopic examination:* volume, consistency, presence of undigested food
  - *Microscopic examination:* fecal leukocytes (inflammation), ova and parasites (infectious etiology), Sudan stain for fecal fat (qualitative assessment of steatorrhea)
  - *Quantitative fecal fat:* 72-hour stool collection for fat quantification remains the gold standard for steatorrhea (>7 g/24 hours on a 100-g fat diet) but is often impractical in the intensive care unit (ICU).
  - *Stool elastase-1:* noninvasive marker for pancreatic exocrine insufficiency (PEI); low levels suggest significant dysfunction.
  - *Stool pH:* low pH (<5.5) suggests carbohydrate malabsorption.
  - *Stool cultures/polymerase chain reaction (PCR):* to rule out bacterial or viral enteritis, including *C. difficile*
- *Blood tests*
  - *Complete blood count:* anemia (type can suggest specific deficiencies—microcytic for iron, macrocytic for B_{12}/folate). Eosinophilia may suggest a parasitic infection.
  - *Electrolytes and renal function:* assess hydration and electrolyte imbalances (hypokalemia, hypomagnesemia common with diarrhea)
  - *Liver function tests:* elevated bilirubin/alkaline phosphatase in cholestasis
  - *Nutrient levels:* serum albumin/prealbumin (markers of protein status, though affected by inflammation), iron studies, ferritin, vitamin B_{12}, folate, 25-hydroxyvitamin D, fat-soluble vitamins (A, E, K), calcium, magnesium, zinc. Prothrombin time/international normalized ratio (INR) may be elevated in vitamin K deficiency.
  - *Inflammatory markers:* C-reactive reaction (CRP), procalcitonin
  - *Specific antibodies:* tissue transglutaminase (tTG) or immunoglobulin A (IgA) antiendomysial (EMA) antibodies for celiac disease (less reliable in acute illness)
- *Imaging*
  - *Abdominal radiographs:* can show dilated loops in ileus or obstruction, air-fluid levels
  - *Computed tomography (CT) or magnetic resonance imaging (MRI) of the abdomen/pelvis:* useful for identifying structural abnormalities (strictures, fistulas, masses), IBD activity, pancreatic pathology, or signs of ischemia (bowel wall thickening, pneumatosis)
  - *Small bowel follow-through or enteroclysis:* can delineate mucosal detail, strictures, fistulas, or motility issues, but requires patient cooperation and is less common in the intubated ICU patient
- *Endoscopy/colonoscopy with biopsy*
  - *Upper endoscopy with small bowel biopsy:* gold standard for diagnosing mucosal diseases like celiac disease, tropical sprue, or infectious enteritis. Can also obtain aspirates for SIBO diagnosis
  - *Colonoscopy with biopsy:* for evaluating IBD or infectious colitis

- *Breath tests*
  - *Hydrogen/methane breath tests (eg, lactulose or glucose):* used to diagnose SIBO, though can be affected by gut motility and recent antibiotic use. Less reliable in critically ill patients with dysmotility
  - *C-D-xylose breath test:* alternative for SIBO diagnosis, less affected by transit time

Management and Treatment

Management in the critically ill patients focuses on addressing the underlying cause, supporting nutritional status, and managing symptoms and complications.

- *Treat the underlying etiology:* this is paramount (eg, managing sepsis, improving gut perfusion, treating infections, addressing surgical issues).
- *Nutritional support*
  - *Early enteral nutrition (EN):* preferred route if the gut is accessible and functional. Start cautiously and advance slowly, monitoring for intolerance (high residuals, vomiting, abdominal distension, increased stool output).
  - *Formula selection:* consider polymeric formulas initially. Semi-elemental or elemental formulas (predigested nutrients, lower fat) may be better tolerated in severe malabsorption (eg, SBS, severe pancreatic insufficiency, gut ischemia). High-protein formulas are essential in critical illness.
  - *Feeding route:* postpyloric feeding (nasojejunal or gastrostomy/jejunostomy tube) may improve tolerance in patients with gastroparesis or high aspiration risk.
  - *Pancreatic enzyme replacement therapy (PERT):* indicated for documented or highly suspected PEI, especially with steatorrhea. Administer with meals/feeds.
  - *Parenteral nutrition (PN):* indicated when EN is not feasible, insufficient to meet nutritional needs, or contraindicated for an extended period (eg, prolonged ileus, high-output fistula, severe malabsorption refractory to EN). PN carries risks (infection, liver complications, gut atrophy) and should be used judiciously.
- *Symptom management*
  - *Diarrhea*
    - Rule out infectious causes before using antimotility agents.
    - Address underlying cause (eg, treating SIBO with antibiotics).
    - Consider fiber supplements (soluble fiber) to bulk stool.
    - Antimotility agents (loperamide, diphenoxylate/atropine) can be used cautiously after infection has been ruled out but may worsen ileus.
    - Octreotide may be used in severe, refractory secretory diarrhea (eg, high-output fistulas, certain tumors) but can worsen gut ischemia.
  - *SIBO:* treat with broad-spectrum antibiotics targeting enteric aerobes and anaerobes (eg, rifaximin, metronidazole, ciprofloxacin, doxycycline). Cycles may be needed.
- *Correction of nutrient deficiencies*
  - Aggressive repletion of fluid and electrolytes
  - Supplementation of vitamins (especially fat-soluble A, D, E, K, and water-soluble B_{12}, folate, thiamine) and minerals (iron, calcium, magnesium, zinc). Parenteral repletion may be necessary in severe malabsorption.
- *Management of complications:* address issues like dehydration, electrolyte imbalances, catheter-related infections (with PN), and metabolic bone disease.

Specific Considerations in Critically Ill Subpopulations

Malabsorption in the Critically Ill Surgical Patient

- Common due to postoperative ileus, gut manipulation, resections leading to short bowel, anastomotic leaks, or preexisting conditions like IBD or malignancy
- Bariatric surgery patients are at high risk for specific nutrient deficiencies and altered anatomy affecting absorption and tolerance.

Ileus

- A common cause of feeding intolerance and a potential contributor to malabsorption in critical illness
- Characterized by impaired gut motility without mechanical obstruction
- Causes include surgery (postoperative ileus), inflammation (sepsis, pancreatitis, peritonitis), medications (opioids), electrolyte abnormalities (hypokalemia, hypomagnesemia), and critical illness itself.
- Management focuses on addressing the underlying cause, limiting opioids, judicious use of prokinetic agents (eg, metoclopramide, erythromycin—use with caution due to side effects and limited evidence in critical illness), and delaying EN until some bowel function returns, or using postpyloric feeds.

Short-Bowel Syndrome

- Defined by insufficient remaining small intestine length and function, leading to malabsorption, diarrhea, and nutritional deficiencies
- Common causes in the critical illness context: extensive bowel resection for ischemia, trauma, complicated IBD, or volvulus
- *Management in ICU:* aggressive fluid and electrolyte repletion, PN initiation early to meet needs, cautious introduction of EN to promote adaptation, gastric acid suppression, management of diarrhea (loperamide, potentially octreotide in severe cases), prevention/treatment of SIBO, and vigilant monitoring/repletion of macro- and micronutrients
- *Complications:* liver disease (PN-associated), SIBO, nephrolithiasis (oxalate), gastric hypersecretion, catheter-related issues

Small Intestine Bacterial Overgrowth

- Excessive bacterial proliferation in the small intestine, often due to stasis (ileus, strictures, dysmotility), impaired host defenses, or altered anatomy (blind loops, diverticula)
- Contributes to malabsorption (bile salt deconjugation, mucosal damage), diarrhea, and potentially D-lactic acidosis

- Diagnosis in ICU can be challenging (breath tests affected by motility, jejunal aspirate invasive). Often suspected based on clinical picture (diarrhea, bloating, feeding intolerance) in patients with risk factors
- Management: treat underlying cause if possible, cyclic antibiotics (eg, rifaximin, metronidazole), nutritional support

Pancreatic Exocrine Insufficiency

- Impaired secretion of pancreatic enzymes needed for digestion, commonly seen after severe pancreatitis, pancreatic surgery, or in severe critical illness
- Leads to malabsorption of fats, proteins, and carbohydrates, particularly fats (steatorrhea)
- Diagnosis: fecal elastase-1 is a practical test in stable patients but often diagnosed presumptively in ICU based on history (pancreatitis) and symptoms (steatorrhea, feeding intolerance).
- Management: PERT administered with enteral feeds is the mainstay. Use of semi-elemental formulas may help. Ensure adequate nutritional intake.

Malabsorption in the Critically Ill Bariatric Patient

- Patients postbariatric surgery (especially Roux-en-Y gastric bypass [RYGB] and biliopancreatic diversion [BPD]) have altered anatomy predisposing to malabsorption and specific nutrient deficiencies (protein, iron, B_{12}, folate, calcium, vitamin D, fat-soluble vitamins, trace elements like copper, zinc, thiamine).
- Critical illness exacerbates these risks due to increased metabolic demand, decreased intake, and potential for complications (anastomotic issues, ulcers, strictures, SIBO).
- Management requires high index of suspicion for deficiencies, aggressive screening and repletion (often requiring parenteral vitamins/minerals), careful consideration of feeding route and formula, and management of potential surgical complications. Thiamine repletion is crucial, especially with vomiting or before glucose administration.

Outcomes

- Malabsorption in the critically ill patients is associated with worse outcomes, including prolonged ICU stay, increased complications (infections, wound healing issues), and higher mortality.
- Early identification, diagnosis, and aggressive nutritional and specific therapeutic interventions are crucial to mitigate the negative impact of malabsorption in this vulnerable population. Prognosis depends heavily on the underlying critical illness and the specific cause and severity of malabsorption.

SUGGESTED READINGS

Alhazzani W, Moller MH, Arabi YM, et al. Guidelines for the provision and assessment of nutrition support therapy in the adult critically ill patient: Society of Critical Care Medicine (SCCM) and American Society for Parenteral and Enteral Nutrition (A.S.P.E.N.). *Crit Care Med*. 2016:44(2):390-438.

Biasco G, Basili V, Caletti E, et al. Gastrointestinal dysfunction in the critically ill patient. *World J Crit Care Med*. 2021;10(5):213-224.

Boullata JI, Platt V. Intestinal dysfunction and malabsorption in the critically ill. In Cresci G, ed. *Nutrition Support for the Critically Ill Patient*. American Society for Parenteral and Enteral Nutrition; 2015: 155-170.

Chapple LA, Chapman MJ, Summers MJ, et al. Gastrointestinal dysfunction in critical illness: association with enteral feeding intolerance and ventilator-free days. *Nutrients*. 2021;13(10):3638.

Davies AR, Morrison SS, Bailey MJ, et al. A multicenter, randomized controlled trial comparing early nasojejunal with nasogastric feeding in critically ill patients. *Crit Care Med*. 2012;40(10):2840-2846.

Kelly CP, LaMont JT. Clostridioides difficile Infection—more difficult than ever. *N Engl J Med*. 2008;359(18):1932-1940.

Khalid I, Doshi P, DiGiovine B. Factors associated with, and prediction of, feeding intolerance in adult critically ill patients. *JPEN J Parenter Enteral Nutr*. 2010;34(1):15-21.

Kumpf VJ. Nutrition support therapy in adult patients with short bowel syndrome. *Nutr Clin Pract*. 2018;33(6):724-737.

McClave SA, Taylor BE, Martindale Z, et al. Guidelines for the provision and assessment of nutrition support therapy in the adult critically ill patient: Society of Critical Care Medicine (SCCM) and American Society for Parenteral and Enteral Nutrition (A.S.P.E.N.). *JPEN J Parenter Enteral Nutr*. 2016;40(2):159-211.

Miller KR, McClave SA. The gut in critical illness: role in organ failure. *Curr Opin Crit Care*. 2015;21(2):145-151.

Pimentel M, Saad RJ, Long MD, et al. ACG clinical guideline: small intestinal bacterial overgrowth. *Am J Gastroenterol*. 2020;115(2):165-178.

Reintam Blaser A, Malbrain MLNG, Starkopf J, et al. Gastrointestinal dysfunction in the critically ill: a systematic review of definitions and clinical incidence. *Intensive Care Med*. 2016;42(11):1684-1694.

Remer T, O'Leary K, Rust B. Management of pancreatic exocrine insufficiency. *Clin Gastroenterol Hepatol*. 2020;18(6):1257-1264.

Singer P, Blaser AR, Berger MM, et al. ESPEN guideline on clinical nutrition in the intensive care unit. *Clin Nutr*. 2019;38(2):48-73.

Ukleja A. Malabsorption in the critically ill patient. *Crit Care Clin*. 2015; 31(3):477-488.

Volkert D, Chourdakis M, Faxen-Irving G, et al. ESPEN guidelines on nutrition in dementia and Parkinson's disease. *Clin Nutr*. 2015;34(6): 1052-1073.

White RH, Wood AJ, Quigley EMM. Nutritional consequences of bariatric surgery. *Gastroenterol Clin North Am*. 2017;46(3):553-567.

4.10

Ileus and Acute Colonic Pseudoobstruction (Ogilvie Syndrome)

Kiran Dyamenahalli and John O. Hwabejire

- Intestinal motility disorders can lead to various clinical manifestations, broadly attributed to ileus or intestinal pseudo-obstruction.
- *Ileus* generally refers to a functional impairment of intestinal transit, most commonly encountered as *postoperative ileus* (POI) after surgical procedures, presenting as abdominal distension and intolerance of oral intake.
- *Intestinal pseudo-obstruction* describes a clinical syndrome of mechanical bowel obstruction symptoms but without an anatomic occluding lesion, resulting from severe impairment of intestinal propulsion. It can be acute (like Ogilvie syndrome) or chronic.

Definitions

- *Ileus (functional ileus):* a temporary, nonmechanical impairment of intestinal transit due to neural or muscular dysfunction. Bowel contents fail to move forward despite the absence of a physical blockage.
- *POI:* expected, transient bowel dysmotility following surgery, particularly abdominal procedures
  - Typically involves initial delay in gastric and colonic emptying (hours) followed by recovery of small bowel function (within 24-48 hours), and later recovery of gastric and colonic function (within 48-72 hours)
  - Considered a normal physiologic response in its initial phase
- *Prolonged or paralytic ileus:* pathologic continuation of POI beyond the expected recovery period (often defined as the inability to tolerate oral intake or the absence of bowel function beyond 3-6 days postabdominal surgery)
  - Often suggests an underlying complication (eg, intra-abdominal sepsis, anastomotic leak, electrolyte imbalance, prolonged opioid use)
  - May sometimes be referred to as secondary POI when caused by a specific complication
- *Intestinal pseudo-obstruction:* a syndrome characterized by signs and symptoms of mechanical bowel obstruction despite the absence of an occluding lesion detected by radiologic or surgical exploration
  - Caused by disorders of intestinal smooth muscle (myopathy) or the nerves controlling it (neuropathy)
  - *Acute colonic pseudo-obstruction (ACPO)/Ogilvie syndrome:* acquired, acute massive dilation of the colon, typically the right colon and cecum, in the absence of mechanical obstruction
    - Most often seen in hospitalized, older, or debilitated patients with multiple comorbidities
    - Associated with recent surgery (especially nonabdominal), trauma, infections, cardiac events, respiratory failure, metabolic derangements, and certain medications
  - *Chronic intestinal pseudo-obstruction (CIPO):* a rare, chronic disorder characterized by recurrent episodes resembling mechanical obstruction due to severe, persistent dysmotility affecting segments of or the entire gastrointestinal (GI) tract
    - Can be primary (idiopathic, often congenital or genetic) or secondary (due to systemic diseases such as scleroderma, amyloidosis, muscular dystrophy, paraneoplastic syndromes, endocrine disorders, or chronic use of certain medications)

Epidemiology

- *PO):* extremely common after abdominal and retroperitoneal surgery
  - Incidence varies widely (3%-35%) depending on the surgical type and definition used.
  - Higher incidence after colorectal surgery (up to 25% of hemicolectomies for prolonged ileus)
- *Impact of prolonged ileus:* a major source of postoperative morbidity
  - Increases hospital length of stay (LOS) by ~5 days on average
  - Associated with increased health care costs
  - Increases readmission rates significantly (up to 10-fold)
- *ACPO (Ogilvie syndrome):* less common than POI
  - Incidence varies depending on the patient population: ~0.1% of all surgery patients, higher in specific groups like critically ill burn patients (0.3%), patients who are with trauma (0.05%).
  - Patients are typically older (mean age >60 years) and have significant underlying medical issues; ~60% are institutionalized or chronically ill.

Key Pathophysiology

- At its core, ileus and pseudo-obstruction involve a disruption of the complex interplay between the enteric nervous system (ENS), central nervous system (CNS), smooth muscle cells, immune cells, and humoral factors that regulate gut motility.
- *Pathophysiology of POI*
  - A complex, multifactorial process initiated by surgical stress and manipulation
  - Involves both neural reflexes and local inflammatory responses
  - *Early phase (neural reflexes)*
    - Rapid onset (minutes to hours post-op)
    - Direct stimulation of afferent nerves in the mesentery and peritoneum during manipulation activates spinal reflex arcs.
    - Increased sympathetic output and decreased parasympathetic tone inhibit intestinal smooth muscle contraction and secretion
    - Involves pathways mediated by corticotropin-releasing factor (CRF) in the hypothalamus and adrenergic signaling

        - Nonadrenergic, noncholinergic (NANC) inhibitory neurotransmitters, such as nitric oxide (NO), vasoactive intestinal peptide (VIP), and neuropeptide Y (NPY), are released from ENS neurons, further suppressing motility.
    - *Late phase (inflammatory response)*
        - Develops hours after surgery and is responsible for sustained dysmotility and prolonged ileus
        - Intestinal manipulation triggers a local inflammatory cascade in the muscularis externa.
        - Release of damage-associated molecular patterns (DAMPs) from the injured tissues activates innate immune cells such as mast cells and macrophages residing in the muscularis.
        - These cells release pro-inflammatory cytokines (eg, tumor necrosis factor alpha [TNF-α], interleukin-6 [IL-6], IL-1β), chemokines, and mediators like prostaglandins (via cyclooxygenase-2 [COX-2]) and NO (via inducible nitric oxide synthase [iNOS]).
        - Recruitment of circulating leukocytes (neutrophils, monocytes) to the gut wall further amplifies inflammation.
        - Inflammatory mediators directly impair smooth muscle contractility and disrupt neuromuscular transmission within the ENS.
        - Increased vascular permeability contributes to bowel wall edema, which can also impair motility.
    - *Systemic factors contributing to POI*
        - *Opioids:* potent inhibitors of gut motility. Activate mu-opioid receptors throughout the GI tract, suppressing acetylcholine release from cholinergic neurons and increasing NANC inhibitory tone. This is a major preventable cause of prolonged ileus.
        - *Anesthetics:* while volatile anesthetics transiently inhibit motility, their effect is usually short-lived and less significant contributor to prolonged POI compared to opioids.
        - *Electrolyte imbalances:* hypokalemia, hypomagnesemia, and hyponatremia can impair smooth muscle function.
        - *Sepsis or systemic inflammatory response:* inflammation outside the manipulated gut can also suppress motility.
        - *Perioperative fluid management:* excessive fluid administration can lead to bowel wall edema, potentially delaying recovery of function.
- *Pathophysiology of ACPO (Ogilvie syndrome)*
    - Primarily related to an acquired imbalance in autonomic regulation of colonic motility
    - Often triggered by an underlying medical condition that disrupts autonomic input to the colon
    - Proposed mechanisms include:
        - Increased sympathetic tone or decreased parasympathetic tone, leading to inhibition of propulsive contractions
        - Specific conditions (eg, trauma, sepsis, cardiac ischemia, respiratory failure) or medications (eg, opioids, anticholinergics, calcium channel blockers) disrupt autonomic pathways.
        - Impaired release or action of NANC neurotransmitters like NO may contribute to failure of haustral relaxation.
    - Unlike POI, it often involves isolated or predominant colonic dilation, sparing the small bowel (though functional small bowel changes can occur).
- *Pathophysiology of CIPO*
    - Involves irreversible damage or dysfunction of the ENS (neuropathy) or intestinal smooth muscle (myopathy)
    - Can be primary (eg, related to genetic mutations affecting enteric neurons or smooth muscle) or secondary to systemic diseases
    - Results in widespread or localized failure of coordinated peristalsis

Clinical Presentation and Diagnosis

- *Symptoms (common to ileus and pseudo-obstruction)*
    - Abdominal distension (most prominent symptom)
    - Diffuse or poorly localized abdominal pain (usually noncolicky in simple ileus or Ogilvie, may be colicky if partial obstruction is considered, or in CIPO exacerbations)
    - Nausea and vomiting (often bilious)
    - Inability to tolerate oral intake
    - Obstipation (inability to pass stool or flatus) is common; some patients may pass small amounts of liquid stool.
- *Physical examination*
    - Generalized abdominal distension is characteristic.
    - Tympany on percussion
    - Bowel sounds are typically absent or hypoactive in significant ileus or Ogilvie; they can be variable in CIPO depending on the underlying pattern of dysmotility. Unlike mechanical obstruction, hyperactive or high-pitched bowel sounds are usually absent.
    - Tenderness is usually mild and diffuse in uncomplicated ileus or Ogilvie; localized tenderness, guarding, or rebound suggests a complication (eg, perforation, ischemia) or an alternative diagnosis (eg, abscess).
- *Imaging studies:* essential for differentiating functional obstruction from mechanical obstruction and assessing severity
    - *Plain abdominal radiographs (supine and upright views)*
        - Show dilated bowel loops with air-fluid levels
        - In general ileus/POI: dilated loops in both small and large bowels may be present, often with air distributed throughout the colon.
        - In small bowel obstruction (SBO): dilated loops primarily in the small bowel with numerous air-fluid levels, often a transition point may be suggested, and the colon is typically decompressed or contains minimal gas distally.
        - In Ogilvie syndrome: characterized by marked dilation of the colon, predominantly the cecum and right colon, often extending variably to the transverse or descending colon. The haustral pattern is typically preserved (distinguishing it from toxic megacolon, which loses haustrations). Absence of a mechanical cutoff sign. Small bowel may be normal or mildly dilated due to functional backup.
        - Upright views are crucial for visualizing air-fluid levels and free air (suggesting perforation).
    - *Computed tomography (CT) scan (with oral and/or intravenous [IV] contrast)*

    - The imaging modality of choice to confirm the diagnosis and rule out mechanical obstruction or other intra-abdominal pathology
    - Provides detailed visualization of bowel loops, wall thickness, mesentery, and surrounding structures
    - Reliably differentiates mechanical obstruction (showing a distinct transition point) from functional ileus or pseudo-obstruction (showing diffuse dilation without a transition point)
    - Identifies underlying causes or complications such as intra-abdominal abscess, hematoma, pancreatitis, tumor, adhesions, or ischemic changes
  - *Water-soluble contrast studies (eg, Gastrografin enema or oral follow-through)*
    - Can be helpful in select cases to confirm the absence of a mechanical obstruction, particularly in suspected partial SBO or distal colonic obstruction not clearly visualized on CT
    - Contrast should flow freely past the point of suspected obstruction in ileus or pseudo-obstruction.
    - *Caution:* barium contrast should generally be avoided if obstruction or perforation is suspected due to the risk of inspissation proximal to an obstruction or severe mediastinitis/peritonitis if leakage occurs.

Differential Diagnosis

- It is paramount to distinguish ileus and pseudo-obstruction from mechanical bowel obstruction or other conditions causing abdominal distension and altered bowel function, as management differs significantly.
- *Key differential diagnoses*
  - *Mechanical SBO:* adhesions (most common cause), hernia (external or internal), stricture (Crohn, radiation), tumor, gallstone ileus, bezoar. Typically presents with colicky pain, vomiting, abdominal distension, and often hyperactive bowel sounds initially, followed by hypoactive sounds. Imaging shows dilated small bowel with a transition point and a decompressed colon.
  - *Mechanical large bowel obstruction (LBO):* colorectal cancer (most common), diverticular stricture, volvulus (sigmoid, cecal), fecal impaction, extrinsic compression. Presents with abdominal distension, pain, absolute constipation. Imaging shows dilated colon proximal to the obstruction; small bowel dilation occurs later if the ileocecal valve is competent.
  - *Toxic megacolon:* severe colonic dilation with signs of systemic toxicity, usually a complication of inflammatory bowel disease (IBD) or *Clostridioides difficile* infection. Differs from Ogilvie by the presence of systemic toxicity, frequent diarrhea (initially), and loss of haustrations on imaging
  - *Ischemic colitis:* can cause abdominal pain, distension, and bloody diarrhea. Imaging may show thickened bowel wall. Severe ischemia can progress to necrosis and perforation.
  - *Intra-abdominal sepsis:* abscess (eg, appendiceal, diverticular, surgical), peritonitis, pancreatitis. Often associated with fever, localized or generalized abdominal pain, and signs of systemic inflammation, which can also induce a secondary ileus
  - *Retroperitoneal processes:* hematoma, infection, tumors irritating adjacent bowel
  - *Severe electrolyte imbalances:* hypokalemia, hypomagnesemia
  - *Severe systemic illness:* sepsis, pneumonia, myocardial infarction, renal failure (common precipitants of Ogilvie syndrome)
  - *Medications:* opioids, anticholinergics, calcium channel blockers, phenothiazines, vinca alkaloids
  - *Spinal cord injury or disease:* can affect autonomic innervation of the bowel

Management and Treatment

- Management strategies differ for POI, prolonged ileus/pseudo-obstruction, and CIPO.
- *General/supportive measures (applicable to ileus and pseudo-obstruction)*
  - *Identify and correct underlying causes:* crucial step. Address electrolyte abnormalities, discontinue causative medications (especially opioids, anticholinergics), and treat sepsis or other medical conditions.
  - *Bowel rest (NPO):* withhold oral intake to prevent further distension, nausea, and vomiting.
  - *IV fluid resuscitation and electrolyte correction:* maintain hydration and correct electrolyte imbalances that can impair gut motility.
  - *Nasogastric (NG) decompression:* indicated for significant nausea, vomiting, or abdominal distension to reduce patient discomfort and prevent aspiration. *Routine* postoperative NG decompression without specific indications is not recommended as it has not been shown to shorten ileus duration and may increase pulmonary complications.
  - *Ambulation:* early and regular ambulation is encouraged for general postoperative recovery (pulmonary toilet, deep venous thrombosis [DVT] prophylaxis, preventing deconditioning), although its direct impact on shortening *prolonged* ileus duration is not strongly evidenced.
- *Management and prevention of POI*
  - *Focus on prevention (Enhanced Recovery After Surgery—ERAS principles)*
    - *Minimally invasive surgery:* laparoscopic and robotic approaches cause less tissue trauma and inflammation compared to open surgery, leading to faster return of bowel function.
    - *Opioid-sparing analgesia*
      - *Epidural analgesia:* thoracic epidural analgesia (eg, bupivacaine ± low-dose opioid) effectively reduces POI duration, likely by blocking sympathetic afferents and limiting systemic opioid exposure. Optimal placement is midthoracic (T6-T9) and continued for 2 to 3 days postoperatively.
      - *Multimodal analgesia:* utilizing combinations of nonopioid pain medications (nonsteroidal antiinflammatory drugs [NSAIDs]/ketorolac, acetaminophen, gabapentin, ketamine) reduces total opioid requirement and thus limits opioid-induced gut dysmotility.
      - *Local/regional anesthesia:* local infiltration at the incision site, transversus abdominis plane (TAP)

blocks, or wound catheters can provide significant pain control, reducing systemic opioid needs.
- *Peripherally acting mu-opioid receptor antagonists (PAMORAs)*
  - Block the constipating effects of opioids in the gut wall without crossing the blood-brain barrier (preserving central analgesia)
  - Alvimopan is approved for accelerating the recovery of bowel function after bowel resection surgery. Administered orally before surgery and continued postoperatively. Studies show reduced time to bowel function recovery and shorter LOS. Contraindicated in patients who have received therapeutic opioids for >7 consecutive days prior to the dose.
  - Methylnaltrexone is a different PAMORA primarily used for opioid-induced constipation in palliative care, less evidence for POI.
- *Goal-directed fluid management:* avoiding fluid overload minimizes bowel wall edema.
- *Early enteral feeding:* initiating small, clear liquids or light diet as soon as the patient is able can stimulate gut motility and is generally safe and beneficial postoperatively, decreasing infectious complications and LOS compared to prolonged NPO status. Contraindicated with persistent nausea/vomiting or signs of obstruction

- *Treatment of established prolonged POI*
  - Rule out and manage underlying complications (abscess, leak).
  - Continue supportive care (NPO, IV fluids, NG if needed, ambulation).
  - Discontinue or minimize opioids.
  - PAMORAs (eg, alvimopan) are primarily preventive, less evidence for treating established prolonged ileus.
  - Conventional prokinetics (metoclopramide, erythromycin): generally ineffective for established POI and not routinely recommended
  - Laxatives/stimulants (eg, bisacodyl suppository): some evidence for modest benefit in preventing or reducing duration, but less proven for treating established prolonged ileus
  - Chewing gum: stimulates cephalic-vagal reflex and motility. Studies are conflicting, but it is a safe, inexpensive option sometimes used as an adjunct.

- *Management of ACPO (Ogilvie syndrome)*
  - *Conservative management*
    - Identify and remove inciting factors (medications, underlying illness).
    - NPO, IV fluids, electrolyte correction
    - Serial abdominal examinations and plain radiographs (or CT) every 12 to 24 hours to monitor cecal diameter
    - Rectal tube placement may help decompress the sigmoid or rectum if distended.
    - *Threshold for active decompression:* intervention is generally indicated if the cecal diameter is >9 to 10 cm or if the patient shows signs of worsening distension, significant pain, or early ischemia, especially after 24 to 48 hours of conservative management. A cecal diameter >12 cm carries a high risk of perforation and mandates prompt decompression.
  - *Pharmacologic decompression*
    - *Neostigmine:* an acetylcholinesterase inhibitor that increases parasympathetic tone and stimulates colonic motility
      - Highly effective first-line treatment for Ogilvie syndrome without mechanical obstruction
      - Response rate 60% to 90% within 30 minutes
      - Typical dose: 2.0 mg IV (some protocols suggest starting with 1.0 mg to assess tolerance)
      - Requires continuous cardiac monitoring due to the risk of bradycardia and hypotension. Atropine should be readily available to counteract these side effects.
      - Other potential side effects: salivation, lacrimation, nausea, vomiting, abdominal cramping
      - Contraindications: mechanical bowel obstruction, bradycardia (<40 bpm), hypotension, active bronchospasm, renal insufficiency, recent myocardial infarction, or elevated creatinine
      - Recurrence occurs in up to 40% of patients and may require repeat neostigmine or endoscopic decompression.
    - Other agents (metoclopramide, erythromycin, PAMORAs) are generally *ineffective* for Ogilvie syndrome.
  - *Endoscopic decompression*
    - Indicated for patients who fail to respond to neostigmine or have contraindications to it
    - Colonoscopic decompression can successfully decompress the colon in many cases.
    - Associated with a risk of perforation (1%-5%, higher in unprepared bowel or presence of ischemia)
    - Placement of a decompressive colonic tube or stent via colonoscopy may not only reduce recurrence but also carry risks.
  - *Surgical management*
    - Reserved for patients with complications (perforation, ischemia) or failure of both medical and endoscopic decompression
    - Options include tube cecostomy (less favored due to morbidity/recurrence but an option in critically ill) or colectomy.
    - Subtotal colectomy with ileostomy is often necessary, especially in cases of perforation or recurrent dilation, to definitively remove the dilated segment and prevent recurrence.

Outcomes and Complications

- *POI:* primarily associated with increased hospital stay, higher costs, and delayed recovery. Prolonged POI can contribute to malnutrition, pulmonary complications (due to reduced mobility and aspiration risk), and patient discomfort.
- *ACPO (Ogilvie syndrome)*
  - Mortality is significantly influenced by the patient's underlying comorbidities and the development of complications.
  - Mortality rates range from 15% in uncomplicated cases treated early to over 30% with complications.
  - The primary feared complication is colonic ischemia and *perforation*, which dramatically increases mortality (reported mortality up to 40%-50% with perforation).

- Risk of perforation correlates strongly with the degree and duration of colonic dilation.
  - Risk is low if cecal diameter is <12 cm.
  - Risk rises significantly once cecal diameter exceeds 12 cm and with prolonged dilation (>48-72 hours).
- Earlier decompression (pharmacologic or endoscopic), ideally within 48 to 72 hours of significant dilation or when the threshold diameter is reached, is associated with better outcomes and reduced risk of perforation compared to delayed intervention.
- Recurrence after successful decompression (medical or endoscopic) is common (up to 40%) and requires repeat treatment.

- *CIPO:* associated with significant morbidity, including malnutrition (often requiring parenteral nutrition), recurrent hospitalizations, chronic pain, and reduced quality of life. Prognosis varies depending on the underlying cause and severity.

SUGGESTED READINGS

Bharucha AE, Knowles CH, Camilleri M, et al. Bowel obstruction. *Gastroenterology*. 2015;149(5):1107-1116.e2.

Choi MK, Otegbeye O, Bechtold ML. Nutrition and functional gastrointestinal disorders: a 2023 update. *World J Gastroenterol*. 2023;29(4):605-621.

De Giorgio R, Tack J. Chronic intestinal pseudo-obstruction. *Orphanet J Rare Dis*. 2008;3:33.

Gustafsson UO, Scott MJ, Schwenk W, et al. Guidelines for perioperative care in elective colonic surgery: Enhanced Recovery After Surgery (ERAS®) society recommendations: 2018. *World J Surg*. 2019;43(3):659-695.

Hoshino N, Uemura K, Kiyama T, et al. Daikenchuto for reducing postoperative ileus in patients undergoing elective abdominal surgery. *Cochrane Database Syst Rev*. 2018;4(4):CD012271.

Jain A, Patel P. Postoperative ileus. In: *StatPearls* [Internet]. StatPearls Publishing; 2025.

Kamalpour M, Lee H. Acute colonic pseudo-obstruction (Ogilvie syndrome): a review. *Clin Colon Rectal Surg*. 2020;33(4):242-248.

Livingston EH. Diagnosis and management of small bowel obstruction. *JAMA*. 2019;322(9):865-866.

Luckey A, Livingston E, Tache Y. Postoperative ileus: the clinical problem and methods of investigation. *Ann Surg*. 2003;237(1):9-17.

Markides G, Kudchadkar S, Suhocki P, et al. Management of acute colonic pseudo-obstruction: a systematic review and meta-analysis. *Am J Surg*. 2015;210(5):887-896.e1.

Neal MD, Hall DE, Sun Y, et al. Development and validation of a postoperative ileus risk score to facilitate enhanced recovery. *JAMA Surg*. 2017;152(4):371-378.

Parrish CR. Ileus. In: Feldman M, Friedman LS, Brandt LJ, eds. *Sleisenger and Fordtran's Gastrointestinal and Liver Disease*. 11th ed. Elsevier; 2021; 2039.

Quah GS, Eslick GD, Cox MR. The efficacy of neostigmine in the treatment of acute colonic pseudo-obstruction: a systematic review and meta-analysis of randomized controlled trials. *Colorectal Dis*. 2018;20(6): 487-495.

Rawlins L, Dobbs B, King T, et al. The economic impact of prolonged postoperative ileus after major abdominal surgery. *Surg Endosc*. 2021; 35(1):147-154.

Rodriguez-Lago I, Jiménez-Moya A, Sáez-González E, et al. Clinical management of chronic intestinal pseudo-obstruction: a narrative review. *World J Gastroenterol*. 2021;27(23):3354-3366.

Stakenborg N, De Coen K, Tack J, et al. Opioid-induced constipation and postoperative ileus: from pathophysiology to contemporary management. *J Neurogastroenterol Motil*. 2020;26(4):415-430.

Vanek VW, Al-Salti M. Acute pseudo-obstruction of the colon (Ogilvie's syndrome): analysis of 400 cases. *Dis Colon Rectum*. 1986;29(3):203-210.

Weledji EP, Ngowe MN. Intestinal obstruction. *Medicine (Baltimore)*. 2018;97(36):e12001.

Young-Fadok TM. Postoperative ileus. *Clin Colon Rectal Surg*. 2008;21(1): 34-39.

4.11

Clostridium difficile and Toxic Megacolon

Thomas Peponis

Clostridium difficile Infection

- *Clostridioides difficile* (previously called *Clostridium difficile*) is an anaerobic, Gram-positive bacillus.
- Many people are asymptomatic carriers, and colonization does not necessarily mean infection.
- It is most commonly transmitted via the fecal-oral route.
- Antibiotic therapy can alter the bacterial composition of colonic microbiota.

This can lead to the overgrowth of *C. difficile* and subsequent release of toxins (enterotoxin and cytotoxin) that cause mucosal inflammation and damage.

- Risk factors
  - Most important
    - Previous exposure to antibiotics (frequently clindamycin, fluoroquinolones, penicillins, and cephalosporins)
    - Advanced age: There is a higher rate among patients older than 65.
    - Hospitalization or residence in a long-term care facility
    - Contact with the health care environment
  - Other
    - Severe underlying disease
    - Inflammatory bowel disease (particularly ulcerative colitis)
    - Immunosuppression
    - Use of acid-suppressing medications, and specifically proton pump inhibitors, has been implicated.

Epidemiology

- *C. difficile* is the most common cause of nosocomial infectious diarrhea. It also accounts for 15% to 30% of cases of antibiotic-associated diarrhea.
- Colonization with *C. difficile* is common and occurs in 4% to 15% of otherwise healthy adults, up to 21% of hospitalized adults, and up to 30% of residents in long-term care facilities.

- Between 2001 and 2012, there was a 43% increase in the incidence of *C. difficile* infection. However, between 2011 and 2017, studies have shown a 24% decrease, likely secondary to health care–driven initiatives focusing on infection control.
- 3% to 5% of patients with *C. difficile* infection will develop fulminant colitis.

Key Pathophysiology

- Transmission of *C. difficile* occurs from person to person via the fecal-oral route.
- About 20% of all hospitalized adults are carriers of *C. difficile (colonized but asymptomatic).*
- *C. difficile* is an anaerobic, Gram-positive, spore-forming, toxin-producing bacillus. It can exist in both spore and vegetative forms.
- When outside the colon, it survives in spore form, which is resistant to heat, acid, and antibiotics.
- The spores can be converted to the fully functional, vegetative, toxin-producing form when inside the colon.
- *C. difficile* becomes pathogenic when it starts releasing exotoxins.
- Its two exotoxins that mediate colitis and diarrhea are toxin A (enterotoxin) and toxin B (cytotoxin); both toxins adhere to receptors on the colonocyte brush border and cause necrosis and shedding of these cells into the lumen.
- Toxin B is essential for the virulence of *C. difficile* and is ~10 times more potent than toxin A in mediating colonic mucosal damage.
- The inflammation may ultimately result in toxic megacolon and septic shock.
- Many recent *C. difficile* outbreaks involved a hypervirulent strain, NAP1/BI/027; this strain has hypersporulation capacity and produces an additional "binary" toxin.

Diagnosis

- Clinical findings
  - Most common symptom is diarrhea.
  - *C. difficile* infection can be categorized as mild, severe, or fulminant.
  - Severe *C. difficile* infection if white blood cell (WBC) >15,000 cells/mm^3, or serum creatinine >1.5 mg/dL
  - Fulminant infection when meeting criteria for severe *C. difficile* infection plus hypotension, or septic shock, or ileus, or megacolon on imaging
- Laboratory tests
- Stool testing is the most accurate way to diagnose C. difficile infection.
- Only patients with symptoms suggestive of active *C. difficile* infection should be tested (three or more unformed stools in 24 hours).
- Testing patients with formed stools is rarely indicated.
    - No single test is highly sensitive and specific at the same time to definitively differentiate between colonization (asymptomatic carrier) and *C. difficile* infection.
    - Two-step testing is usually recommended.
    - Stool culture is very sensitive; however, it cannot differentiate between active infection and asymptomatic colonization. In addition, it is time-consuming, therefore not commonly used.
    - Enzyme immunoassays that detect toxins A and B, which are produced by the organism, usually result quickly and have high specificity but are lacking in sensitivity.
    - Testing for glutamate dehydrogenase (GDH), an enzyme produced by both toxigenic and nontoxigenic strains, is very sensitive and can be used as a screening tool. If positive, it needs to be followed by a test with high specificity, such as enzyme immunoassays for toxins. Nucleic acid amplification testing (NAAT) detects chromosomal toxic genes and is also quite sensitive, but not as specific, hence frequently combined with one of the aforementioned tests as part of the two-step testing to confirm the infection.
    - A reasonable algorithm followed by many centers includes screening with either NAAT or GDH testing and confirming *C. difficile* infection with a toxin enzyme immunoassay.
    - In patients with ileus, consideration should be given to rectal swabs for polymerase chain reaction (PCR) testing if clinical suspicion is high.
- Imaging findings
  - A computed tomography (CT) scan of the abdomen/pelvis is not essential in diagnosing *C. difficile* colitis and should not be used for that purpose.
  - Severe/complicated *C. difficile* infection will most commonly appear as pancolitis with pancolonic wall thickening on CT scan.
- Endoscopic findings
  - Routine endoscopic evaluation to diagnose or determine the extent of colitis is not recommended.
  - Pseudomembranes are pathognomonic of *C. difficile* colitis but are only found in about 50% of patients.
  - Colonoscopic evaluation carries the risk of perforation and should be used judiciously.
  - It can help differentiate among various colitides, including cytomegalovirus (CMV), *C. difficile*, inflammatory bowel disease, ischemic colitis, and graft-versus-host disease.

Management and Treatment

- General principles
  - Stop the inciting antimicrobial agents as soon as possible.
  - Implement infection control policies.
  - Avoid the use of antidiarrheal agents.
- Medical
  - First episode
  - Mild-to-moderate *C. difficile* infection
    - Vancomycin 125 mg orally every 6 hours for 10 days
    - Or fidaxomicin 200 mg twice a day for 10 days
  - Severe *C. difficile* infection (initial episode)
    - Same as above, plus bezlotoxumab 10 mg/kg infusion can be considered as an adjunct treatment for high-risk patients. Bezlotoxumab is an antitoxin B monoclonal antibody.
  - Fulminant *C. difficile* infection
    - Vancomycin 500 mg orally every 6 hours and metronidazole 500 mg intravenously every 8 hours

- In patients with ileus, consider adding vancomycin per rectum (500 mg of vancomycin in 100 mL saline per rectum every 6 hours).
- Second episode
- Mild-to-moderate *C. difficile* infection
    - If vancomycin had been used for the initial episode, then fidaxomicin 200 mg twice a day for 10 days or prolonged vancomycin with taper and pulse.
    - If fidaxomicin had been used for the initial episode, then use prolonged vancomycin with taper and pulse.
- Severe-complicated or fulminant *C. difficile* infection (second episode)
- Vancomycin 500 mg orally every 6 hours and metronidazole 500 mg intravenously every 8 hours
- Third or subsequent episode
- 10-day course of vancomycin followed by fecal microbiota transplantation, if available
- If fecal microbiota transplantation is not available, then prolonged vancomycin with taper and pulse or fidaxomicin, or rifaximin.
    - Fecal microbiota transplantation
    - With fecal microbiota transplantation, microorganisms from healthy donor stool are infused into the intestine of the patient to restore their colonic microbiota.
    - This can be delivered either via colonoscopy, nasogastric tube, or enema.
    - Delivery by colonoscopy is the preferred approach.
    - Success rates vary from 60% to 90% in most studies.

- Surgical treatment principles
    - Fulminant *C. difficile* infection: patients with *C. difficile* infection who develop signs of systemic toxicity need admission to the intensive care unit (ICU).
        - A surgical consult is warranted in all cases of severe-complicated or fulminant disease.
        - If patients with systemic disease do not improve with medical therapy or the colon perforates, prompt surgery can be lifesaving.
        - The current standard of care is a subtotal colectomy, during which almost the entire colon, except for the rectum and distal sigmoid, is removed, and an end ileostomy is created.
        - Surgery in this setting is associated with high morbidity and mortality rates.
        - A surgical alternative to a subtotal colectomy would be a diverting loop ileostomy with antegrade colonic antibiotic (usually vancomycin) lavage.
        - A recent meta-analysis comparing the two surgical options found no differences in terms of postoperative mortality and morbidity but higher stoma reversal rates in the diverting ileostomy group.

Outcomes

- *C. difficile* infection recurs in about 13% of patients with community-associated infection. Recurrence rates are higher, ~21%, in patients with health care–associated infections.
- Mortality is also higher in patients with health care–associated infections, with the risk of death within 30 days being ~9%.
- Mortality is significantly higher among patients with fulminant *C. difficile* colitis, and in some studies, the rate is higher than 50%.
- Although end ileostomies after a subtotal colectomy are reversible, many patients will end up with a permanent ileostomy for various reasons.

SUGGESTED READINGS

Brandt LJ, Reddy SS. Fecal microbiota transplantation for recurrent Clostridium difficile infection. *J Clin Gastroenterol*. 2011;45(suppl):S159-S67.

Butala P, Divino CM. Surgical aspects of fulminant Clostridium difficile colitis. *Am J Surg*. 2010;200(1):131-135.

Efron PA, Mazuski JE. Clostridium difficile colitis. *Surg Clin North Am*. 2009;89(2):483-500.

Gough E, Shaikh H, Manges AR. Systematic review of intestinal microbiota transplantation (fecal bacteriotherapy) for recurrent Clostridium difficile infection. *Clin Infect Dis*. 2011;53(10):994-1002.

Guh AY, Mu Y, Winston LG, et al. Trends in US burden of Clostridioides difficile infections and outcomes. *N Engl J Med*. 2020;382(14):1320-1330.

Jaber MR, Olafsson S, Fung WL, Reeves ME. Clinical review of the management of fulminant Clostridium difficile infection. *Am J Gastroenterol*. 2008;103(12):3195-3203.

Kelly CR, Fischer M, Allegretti JR, et al. ACG Clinical Guidelines: Prevention, diagnosis, and treatment of Clostridioides difficile infections. *Am J Gastroenterol*. 2021;116(6):1124-1147.

Kelly CP, LaMont JT. Clostridium difficile—more difficult than ever. *Engl J Med*. 2008;359(18):1932-1940.

Kirkpatrick ID, Greenberg HM. Evaluating the CT diagnosis of Clostridium difficile colitis: should CT guide therapy? *AJR Am J Roentgenol*. 2001;176(3):635-639.

Lessa FC, Mu Y, Bamberg WM, et al. Burden of Clostridium difficile infection in the United States. *N Engl J Med*. 2015;372:825-834.

Loo VG, Bourgault AM, Poirier L, et al. Host and pathogen factors for Clostridium difficile infection and colonization. *N Engl J Med*. 2011;365(18):1693-1703.

Neal MD, Alverdy JC, Hall DE, Simmons RL, Zuckerbraun BS. Diverting loop ileostomy and colonic lavage: an alternative to total abdominal colectomy for the treatment of severe, complicated Clostridium difficile associated disease. *Ann Surg*. 2011;254(3):423-427.

Poylin V, Hawkins AT, Bhama AR, et al. The American Society of Colon and Rectal Surgeons Clinical Practice Guidelines for the management of Clostridioides difficile infection. *Dis Colon Rectum*. 2021;64(6):650-668.

Sailhamer EA, Carson K, Chang Y, et al. Fulminant Clostridium difficile colitis: patterns of care and predictors of mortality. *Arch Surg*. 2009;144(5):433-439.

Wilcox MH, Gerding DN, Poxton IR, et al; MODIFY I and MODIFY II Investigators. Bezlotoxumab for prevention of recurrent Clostridium difficile infection. *N Engl J Med*. 2017;376(4):305-317.

4.12

Gastrointestinal and Intra-Abdominal Infections

Lydia Maurer and George Velmahos

Initial Evaluation and Resuscitation

- In a patient with suspected intra-abdominal infection, promptly evaluate the patient's ABCs (airway, breathing, circulation) and obtain large-bore peripheral intravenous (IV) access.
- Consider initiating transfer to a monitored or intensive care setting.
- Perform a thorough cardiopulmonary and abdominal examination, including a hernia examination and rectal examination (as appropriate).
- In accordance with surviving sepsis guidelines, initiate fluid resuscitation with crystalloid at 30 mL/kg within 3 hours, targeting a mean arterial pressure >65 mm Hg.
- Send initial laboratory tests, including complete blood count, basic metabolic panel, liver function tests (LFTs), lactate, lipase, coagulation factors, type and screen, blood cultures, and arterial or venous blood gas.
- Initiate broad-spectrum antibiotic therapy covering common intra-abdominal pathogens, in alignment with local antibiograms and hospital antibiotic stewardship guidelines to cover Gram positives (including methicillin-resistant *Staphylococcus aureus* [MRSA]), Gram negatives (including *Pseudomonas*), and anaerobes.
- Common initial regimens include vancomycin + cefepime + flagyl and vancomycin + piperacillin-tazobactam.

Workup of Suspected Intra-Abdominal Infection

- Concurrent with initial laboratory investigations, resuscitation, and transferring the patient to the appropriate level of care if necessary, order imaging in concordance with the patient's history, physical examination, and labs.
- An upright chest and abdominal radiograph may show free air, bearing in mind that the sensitivity of abdominal x-ray for free air is ~70%. It can also show a bowel gas pattern to suggest ileus, bowel obstruction, or volvulus.
- For suspected right upper quadrant (RUQ) pathology (acute cholecystitis, choledocholithiasis, cholangitis), an RUQ ultrasound (US) at the bedside may prove useful.
- A computed tomography (CT) scan of the abdomen and pelvis with IV contrast can expose a wide range of intra-abdominal pathology. The absence of IV contrast reduces accuracy significantly but may be justified in preexisting renal impairment. If preexisting renal function was normal, IV contrast does not exacerbate infection-related renal dysfunction. Oral contrast is not necessary in most cases, unless an upper gastrointestinal (GI) perforation is suspected. It may cause delays and risk aspiration.

Esophagus, Stomach, and Duodenum

- Esophageal perforation
  - Common etiologies include recent endoscopy or esophageal surgery, excess alcohol consumption with vomiting (Boerhaave syndrome), known malignancy, and foreign body impaction in the setting of prior esophageal narrowing (stricture, achalasia, etc.), among others.
  - Workup includes fluoroscopic swallow study or CT esophagogram. Water-soluble contrast over barium may cause severe pneumonitis and should be used with caution.
  - Treatment depends somewhat on the location of perforation, but generally includes a combination of broad-spectrum antibiotics (including antifungal coverage), primary repair or esophageal stent placement, and neck or chest drainage.
- Perforated peptic ulcer disease (PUD)
  - Primary risk factors are nonsteroidal antiinflammatory drug (NSAID) use, smoking, and *Helicobacter pylori* infection.
  - Workup generally includes computed tomography (CT) of the abdomen/pelvis with IV and oral contrast (if possible), and patients should be tested for *H. pylori* to guide post-op treatment. Absence of oral contrast extravasation does not preclude a perforation, if extraluminal gas is identified or a high index of clinical suspicion exists.
  - Management includes broad-spectrum antibiotics, including antifungals, nasogastric tube placement, proton pump inhibitors, and a surgery consult for possible open or laparoscopic repair.
  - Gastroduodenal perforations may be managed nonoperatively if the patient is physiologically stable and there is no significant oral contrast extravasation.

Liver and Gallbladder

- Acute cholecystitis
  - Gallbladder inflammation results from occlusion of the cystic duct with gallstones or sludge (calculous cholecystitis), impaired gallbladder emptying in the absence of stones (acalculous cholecystitis), or impaired vascular supply (also acalculous cholecystitis).
  - Workup includes RUQ US, which may identify gallbladder wall thickening, pericholecystic fluid, gallstones, and a sonographic Murphy sign (RUQ tenderness upon pressing the US probe over the gallbladder). The absence of gallstones does not mean the absence of acute cholecystitis in the right clinical scenario, as stones may be in the acalculous form of the inflammatory process or simply not detected by the US.
  - Acalculous cholecystitis can be more definitively diagnosed with a hepatobiliary iminodiacetic acid (HIDA) scan demonstrating gallbladder ejection fraction <35%; however, while more sensitive than US for acalculous cholecystitis, the sensitivity of HIDA is ≤70%.
  - A CT scan improves the diagnostic accuracy of RUQ US by demonstrating similar findings. In uncertain cases, US and CT should be considered complementary tests.

- Cholecystitis is initially an inflammatory process, which can progress to transmural ischemia and necrosis, undergo superinfection by enteric Gram negatives and anaerobes, and, in severe cases, cause emphysematous cholecystitis and perforation.
- In the patient who is septic with suspected or confirmed cholecystitis, antibiotics targeting Gram negatives and anaerobes should be initiated, and surgery should be consulted to discuss interventions such as cholecystectomy versus percutaneous cholecystostomy tube placement.
- Internal stenting, either transmural or transcystic, is advanced choice for patients who have temporary or permanent contraindications for surgery.

- Cholangitis
  - Bacterial infection of the biliary tree that can be quite severe and rapidly progress to septic shock if not treated expeditiously
  - Common risk factors include previous biliary tract interventions (eg, recent endoscopic retrograde cholangiopancreatography [ERCP]), gallstones (causing choledocholithiasis), history of primary sclerosing cholangitis, and biliary obstruction from stricture, malignancy, or parasites.
  - Classic diagnostic features include the Charcot triad (jaundice, RUQ pain, fever) or Reynold pentad (jaundice, RUQ pain, fever, hypotension, altered mental status).
  - Highest sensitivity and specificity for diagnosis with Tokyo guidelines—at least two out of three Charcot criteria + leukocytosis + abnormal LFTs + imaging w/biliary dilation
  - RUQ US can demonstrate biliary dilation and stones. CT is more sensitive for dilated ducts and pericholecystic inflammation, but not for stones. Magnetic resonance cholangiopancreatography (MRCP) is the most sensitive for stones in the common bile duct, but not always feasible or available.
  - Prompt management should include IV antibiotics covering Gram negatives and anaerobes (particularly with biliary penetration, including piperacillin-tazobactam, fluoroquinolones, carbapenems), consult to GI for ERCP, and consult to surgery for cholecystectomy prior to discharge.
- Liver abscess
  - Common risk factors are infections or other abnormalities in the biliary tract, trauma, hepatic artery angioembolization, and previous intraoperative damage to the right hepatic artery.
  - Diagnosed by CT of the abdomen/pelvis with IV contrast showing an abscess
  - Common organisms are enteric Gram negatives and anaerobes, including *Entamoeba histolytica* (cause of "amoebic abscess"); echinococcal cysts can occur in patients traveling from Southeast Asia, predominantly.
  - Stool test for *Entamoeba* can be performed, along with serology for *Echinococcus* if suggested by clinical history.
  - Initiate empiric IV antibiotics covering Gram negatives and anaerobes (including metronidazole to cover *E. histolytica*), albendazole if echinococcal cyst; consult to surgery and/or interventional radiologist (IR) for percutaneous drainage.

Pancreas and Spleen

- Infected pancreatic necrosis
  - The spectrum of acute pancreatitis ranges from an easily managed inflammation to the most severe, life-threatening form. Necrotizing pancreatitis (NP) is not necessarily infected but can easily become so, especially after iatrogenic manipulation or secondary superinfection.
  - Patients who develop NP should be cared for at tertiary care centers by multidisciplinary teams accustomed to managing patients with NP.
  - NP should be suspected with worsening of the clinical picture, septic shock, or gas in peripancreatic collections on imaging tests.
  - Workup includes CT of the abdomen/pelvis with IV contrast, and initial management may include endoscopic transgastric necrosectomy and/or IR drain placement (as determined by a multidisciplinary team in accordance with the "step-up" approach), along with broad-spectrum IV antibiotic management.
  - Additional complications that can arise in patients with infected pancreatic necrosis include: bowel perforation, vascular pseudoaneurysm formation and bleeding, and fistula formation.
- Splenic abscess
  - Most common causes include hematogenous spread from sepsis, infective endocarditis, or contiguous spread from a local infectious nidus such as infected pancreatic necrosis or diverticulitis.
  - Diagnosed by CT of the abdomen/pelvis showing a rim-enhancing unilocular or multilocular collection
  - Initial management includes IV antibiotics covering Gram positives, Gram negatives, and anaerobes.
  - For the patient in septic shock with rapid clinical decline, definitive treatment is a splenectomy.
  - For hemodynamically stable patients, percutaneous aspiration or drain placement may be effective options for drainage of abscesses that are radiographically accessible.

Small Intestine

- Small intestinal diverticulitis
  - Occurs when sac-like areas of mucosa herniate through the wall of the small intestine and become inflamed, resulting in pain, bleeding, or perforation
  - A Meckel diverticulum is the most common form of small bowel diverticular disease. It is a remnant of the omphalomesenteric duct with gastric, pancreatic, and intestinal mucosa.
  - At times, small bowel diverticulitis (including inflammation of a Meckel diverticulum) can be visualized on a CT scan, although often the diagnosis is established intraoperatively and unexpectedly.
  - In cases of local inflammation of non-Meckel small bowel diverticulitis, treatment with antibiotics, serial examinations, and bowel rest is also a reasonable strategy—with close monitoring for perforation.

Colon and Rectum

- Appendicitis
  - Diagnosed by US (more common in pediatrics) or CT of the abdomen/pelvis. US demonstrates a dilated, noncompressible, blind-ending loop in the right lower quadrant.

CT is more sensitive and specific and can show evidence of perforation or alternative diagnoses.
  - Patients should be started on IV antibiotics for Gram negatives and anaerobes, and general surgery should be consulted to discuss surgery with the patient.
  - Large, randomized studies suggest noninferior outcomes with antibiotics versus surgery, except in the presence of an appendicolith in which a higher proportion of patients required operative management in the first 24 hours. One in three patients treated with antibiotics had their appendix removed within 90 days.
- Diverticulitis
  - Uncomplicated diverticulitis occurs with inflammation and often focal perforation of a colonic diverticulum (sac-like outpouching), generally in the sigmoid colon.
  - Patients generally present with left lower quadrant or suprapubic pain.
  - Diagnosed by CT scan showing inflammation of the sigmoid colon in the presence of diverticuli, with or without foci of air visible around the sigmoid
  - Complicated diverticulitis describes a spectrum of disease from inflammation of the colon plus an area of unorganized fluid (phlegmon) and air outside the sigmoid colon (Hinchey Ia) to diffuse feculent peritonitis (Hinchey IV).
  - For patients with uncomplicated diverticulitis without systemic signs of infection, outcomes are similar between treatment with and without antibiotics.
  - Patients with signs of systemic infection (fever, other abnormal inflammatory parameters or vital signs) and those with complicated disease should be started on IV antibiotics covering Gram negatives and anaerobes.
  - Surgery should be consulted and follow the patient, and patients who worsen despite antibiotics, along with those with diffuse peritonitis, should generally be considered for an urgent sigmoid colectomy.
- Infectious colitis
  - Patients with clinical suspicion for colitis, including profuse diarrhea and abdominal pain, should be worked up for an infectious etiology, of which the causes can be bacterial, viral, or parasitic. Other noninfectious etiologies, including inflammatory and ischemic, should also be considered as clinically appropriate.
  - Clinical history should include a comprehensive exposure history, including travel, sick contacts, food exposures, ingestion of contaminated water, and exposure to daycare centers.
  - With severe abdominal pain plus profuse diarrhea, an abdominal CT should be obtained to look for signs of perforation, ischemia, or other etiologies.
  - Workup includes stool ova and parasites, *Clostridium difficile*, and studies for any other specific infections for which the patient has risk factors (eg, *Cryptosporidium, Salmonella, Shigella, Campylobacter, Giardia*, cytomegalovirus [CMV], tuberculosis [TB]), including sexually transmitted infections.
  - Treatment should include bowel rest, resuscitation, serial abdominal examinations, and medication to treat the appropriate etiology. Surgery should be consulted with worsening abdominal examination, evidence of peritonitis, or hemodynamic instability.
- Perirectal and perianal abscesses
  - If clinical suspicion for perirectal/perianal abscess by history, or in the patient with undifferentiated septic shock, perform a thorough perianal and rectal examination looking for areas of erythema, induration, and fluctuance.
  - If a patient is symptomatic and a perianal abscess is not identified on physical examination, obtain a CT of the abdomen/pelvis with IV contrast.
  - Management of perirectal and perianal abscesses is surgical drainage at the bedside or in the operating room (OR). Patients with surrounding cellulitis or immunosuppressed status may also be treated with antibiotics targeting Gram negatives and anaerobes.
  - One out of three patients who have a perianal abscess drained will subsequently develop a fistula-in-ano and, therefore, should be given anticipatory guidance and referred to a colorectal surgeon for follow-up.

SUGGESTED READINGS

Dellinger RP, Carlet JM, Masur H, et al. Surviving Sepsis Campaign guidelines for management of severe sepsis and septic shock. *Crit Care Med*. 2004; 32(3):858-873.

Ferraioli G, Brunetti E, Gulizia R, Mariani G, Marone P, Filice C. Management of splenic abscess: report on 16 cases from a single center. *Int J Infect Dis*. 2009;13(4):524-530.

Hall J, Hardiman K, Lee S, et al. The American Society of Colon and Rectal Surgeons clinical practice guidelines for the treatment of left-sided colonic diverticulitis. *Dis Colon Rectum*. 2020;63(6):728-747.

Lardière-Deguelte S, Ragot E, Amroun K, et al. Hepatic abscess: diagnosis and management. *J Visc Surg*. 2015;152(4):231-243.

Mantas D, Kykalos S, Patsouras D, Kouraklis G. Small intestine diverticula: is there anything new? *World J Gastrointest Surg*. 2011;3(4):49-53.

Mariat G, Mahul P, Prévôt N, et al. Contribution of ultrasonography and cholescintigraphy to the diagnosis of acute acalculous cholecystitis in intensive care unit patients. *Intensive Care Med*. 2000;26(11):1658-1663.

Maurer LR, Fagenholz PJ. Contemporary surgical management of pancreatic necrosis. *JAMA Surg*. 2023;158(1):81-88.

Miura F, Takada T, Kawarada Y, et al. Flowcharts for the diagnosis and treatment of acute cholangitis and cholecystitis: Tokyo Guidelines. *J Hepatobiliary Pancreat Surg*. 2007;14(1):27-34.

Sahnan K, Askari A, Adegbola SO, et al. Persistent fistula after anorectal abscess drainage: local experience of 11 years. *Dis Colon Rectum*. 2019; 62(3):327-332.

Shaish H, Ream J, Huang C, et al. Diagnostic accuracy of unenhanced computed tomography for evaluation of acute abdominal pain in the emergency department. *JAMA Surg*. 2023;158(7):e231112.

Shane AL, Mody RK, Crump JA, et al. 2017 Infectious Diseases Society of America clinical practice guidelines for the diagnosis and management of infectious diarrhea. *Clin Infect Dis*. 2017;65(12):e45-e80.

Søreide K, Thorsen K, Harrison EM, et al. Perforated peptic ulcer. *Lancet*. 2015;386(10000):1288.

The Coda Collaborative. A randomized trial comparing antibiotics with appendectomy for appendicitis. *N Engl J Med*. 2020;383(20):1907-1919.

Thorsen K, Glomsaker TB, von Meer A, Søreide K, Søreide JA. Trends in diagnosis and surgical management of patients with perforated peptic ulcer. *J Gastrointest Surg*. 2011;15(8):1329-1335.

Williams LMS, Walker GR, Loewenherz JW, Gidel LT. Association of contrast and acute kidney injury in the critically ill: a propensity-matched study. *Chest*. 2020;157(4):866-876.

Younes Z, Johnson DA. The spectrum of spontaneous and iatrogenic esophageal injury: perforations, Mallory-Weiss tears, and hematomas. *J Clin Gastroenterol*. 1999;29(4):306-317.

4.13

Inflammatory Bowel Disease

Grace C. Lee

- Inflammatory conditions of the gastrointestinal (GI) tract; may have extraintestinal manifestations
- The cause is unknown; genetic, immunologic, and environmental factors have been implicated.
- Surgery is reserved for the treatment of complications or severe, medically refractory disease.
- *Crohn disease (CD)*
  - Can involve any part of the GI tract
  - Most commonly involves the terminal ileum, small bowel, colon, and anus
  - Chronic, relapsing, and often granulomatous inflammatory disease
  - Usually noncontinuous regional enteritis "skip lesions" that are transmural
  - Often associated with enteric and perianal fistulas and strictures
- *Ulcerative colitis (UC)*
  - Involves large bowel only
  - Usually continuous from the rectum and extends proximally
  - Limited only to the mucosa of the rectum and colon
  - Surgery can be curative—removing the colon and rectum cures the disease.

Epidemiology

- Incidence of inflammatory bowel disease (IBD) has been rising around the world—increased from 3.7 million people in 1990 to 6.8 million in 2017.
- Highest rates of IBD are in North America.
- Bimodal incidence peaks between 15 to 30 and 50 to 70 years of age.
- Family history is present in 10% to 30% of patients with IBD, more common in CD.

Key Pathophysiology

- Environmental factors felt to trigger an overactive or deregulated immune response to bacteria in the intestinal lumen in those with a genetic predisposition
- Idiopathic disease, thought to be autoimmune in nature, with complex interactions between genetics, environment exposures, immunologic factors, and microbiome
- CD: various genes implicated, including *NOD2*, *IL-23*, and autophagy-related 16-like 1 (*ATG16L1*), which play a role in innate immunity and regulation of the epithelial barrier.
- UC: triggered by an environmental factor, including alterations in the intestinal microbiome. Defect in the regulatory mechanism of mucosal immunity results in autoreactivity against colonic epithelial cells, limiting disease to the mucosa only.

Diagnosis

- Crohn's Disease
  - Differential diagnosis: UC, diverticulitis, acute infectious ileitis or colitis, acute appendicitis, colorectal cancer, lymphoma, tuberculosis, irritable bowel syndrome
  - Characterized as inflammatory, fibrostenotic, or penetrating/fistulizing phenotype
  - Clinical presentation
    - Typically presents with abdominal pain (86%), diarrhea (78%), and hematochezia (49%)
    - Fatigue, fever, weight loss, and growth failure in younger patients may also be present.
    - Perianal abscesses and fistulas may precede bowel symptoms. Approximately one-third of patients with CD have perianal fistulizing disease.
    - 30% will have extraintestinal symptoms, such as arthropathy, dermatologic (pyoderma gangrenosum and erythema nodosum), and uveitis.
  - Evaluation
    - Disease is not limited to any portion of the GI tract. Distal ileum and colon are most commonly involved, followed by small bowel alone.
    - Colonoscopy with entrance into the terminal ileum is standard. Inflammation of the terminal ileum may confirm the diagnosis and help differentiate from UC. Up to 35% will have skip lesions, with a cobblestone appearance.
    - Upper endoscopy can be used to evaluate for CD in the proximal GI tract.
    - Endoscopic scoring systems (such as the Crohn's Disease Endoscopic Index of Severity [CDEIS] and the Simple Endoscopic Score for Crohn's Disease [SES-CD]) are useful for quantifying the distribution and severity of Crohn inflammation.
    - Biopsies show chronic inflammation, often transmural, and aggregation of macrophages forming noncaseating granulomas. Granulomas are the most specific finding, but not always identified, and are not required for diagnosis. Must still rule out infectious causes.
    - Capsule endoscopy can be used to identify occult small bowel CD; however, should not be used if there is concern for small bowel strictures.
    - Laboratory values
      - Markers of inflammation, such as serum erythrocyte sedimentation rate (ESR), serum C-reactive protein (CRP), and fecal calprotectin, are often elevated.
  - Imaging
    - Computed tomography/magnetic resonance (CT/MR) enterography: commonly used; MR enterography avoids radiation.
    - Caution with levels of radiation exposure in younger patients. Chronicity of disease leads to frequent imaging.
    - Upper GI series with small bowel follow-through can identify strictures in the small bowel.
- Ulcerative Colitis
  - Differential diagnosis: CD, diverticulitis, colorectal cancer, infectious colitis, pseudomembranous colitis, ischemic colitis, radiation-induced colitis, irritable bowel syndrome

- Clinical presentation
  - Common symptoms include diarrhea, abdominal cramping, rectal bleeding, urgency, tenesmus, and nocturnal bowel movements.
  - >30% have extraintestinal manifestations; often associated with primary sclerosing cholangitis.
  - Evaluation
    - Typical endoscopic findings coupled with history can help establish a diagnosis. Biopsy can be confirmatory.
    - Colonoscopy demonstrates continuous mucosal involvement from the rectum up through the colon. Friable, edematous mucosa is typical. Findings of chronic inflammation and crypt abscesses on biopsy are common.
    - The terminal ileum is usually not inflamed, helping to distinguish UC from CD; however, ~10% of patients with UC have "backwash ileitis" from inflammation in the ascending colon.
    - Document extent of disease: Montreal classification is (1) proctitis, (2) left-sided colitis, or (3) extensive colitis (extension proximal to splenic flexure).
    - Endoscopic scoring systems (such as the Mayo Score and the Ulcerative Colitis Endoscopic Index of Severity [UCEIS]) are useful for quantifying the distribution and severity of UC inflammation.
    - Laboratory values
      - Like in CD, markers of inflammation such as serum ESR, serum CRP, and fecal calprotectin are often elevated. Fecal calprotectin can be used to assess response to therapy and relapse.
    - Imaging
      - Imaging is not always necessary, but CT scans can be helpful in evaluating for toxic megacolon and ruling out colon perforations.
      - CT and MR enterography can also be helpful in distinguishing UC from CD.
- ***Differentiating UC and CD***
  - Clinical manifestations for both UC and CD overlap.
  - 10% of patients with IBD have the indeterminate type.
  - Both can have extraintestinal manifestations and may develop characteristic skin lesions (erythema nodosum, pyoderma gangrenosum).
  - UC is limited to the colon and rectum, while CD can involve any portion of the GI tract. UC does not involve the small bowel; therefore, terminal ileal inflammation on colonoscopy is often indicative of CD.
  - UC involves the rectum, while CD can spare the rectum.
  - Perianal disease is associated with CD, with "elephant ear" anal skin tags, perianal abscesses, and perianal fistulas.
  - Histologically, CD is transmural and often forms granulomas. CD also tends to form enteric and perianal fistulas, due to the transmural nature of the disease.

Management and Treatment

- The goals of therapy are to control symptoms and improve the quality of life by healing the mucosa and preventing disease progression, complications, or colorectal cancer.
- Therapies are directed toward *inducing* remission when a patient is first diagnosed and then *maintaining* remission.
- CD can be treated, not cured. UC can be cured with surgery (total proctocolectomy) if medical therapy fails.

Crohn's Disease

- **Medical management**
  - Nonsteroidal antiinflammatory drugs (NSAIDs) may worsen disease activity and should be avoided when possible.
  - Smoking increases the risks of disease recurrence; smoking cessation should be encouraged.
  - Mild-to-moderate CD
    - Can often be treated with oral medications as an outpatient
    - Sulfasalazine can be used to treat mild-to-moderate colonic CD.
    - Budesonide 9 mg daily can be used for inducing remission in patients with ileocecal CD, without systemic steroid side effects.
    - Antibiotics are not recommended as primary therapy for CD.
  - Moderate-to-severe CD
    - Oral steroids (prednisone) are effective for inducing remission and can be used short term.
    - Thiopurines (azathioprine and 6-mercaptopurine) can be used to maintain remission and avoid long-term steroid use, with a 60% to 70% response rate. They are not effective to induce remission.
    - Methotrexate can be used in patients with steroid-dependent CD, for maintaining remission.
    - Anti-tumor necrosis factor (TNF) agents (infliximab, adalimumab, certolizumab) are effective for inducing and maintaining remission in patients refractory to thiopurines, methotrexate, and steroids. Response rate is ~80%.
    - Combination therapy of infliximab with immunomodulators (thiopurines) is effective.
    - Newer biologics such as vedolizumab (anti-integrin) and ustekinumab (anti-interleukin) may be used in patients with CD who have failed treatment with other therapies.
    - Infliximab is often used as first-line therapy for patients with perianal and enteric fistulizing CD.
  - Severe and fulminant CD
    - Intravenous (IV) steroids and infliximab are often used to treat patients with severe disease, often in the inpatient setting.
- **Surgical management**
  - Perianal disease: perianal abscesses should be drained at the bedside or in the operating room. Perianal fistulas are often managed with seton placement. Fistulotomies and formal fistula repairs can be complicated by nonhealing wounds in patients with CD and anal inflammation.
  - Intra-abdominal abscesses (most commonly abscess near ileal disease): antibiotics and percutaneous drainage, followed by induction of remission with steroids and infliximab. Surgery with resection of involved intestinal segments for failed medical management
  - Terminal ileal disease causing small bowel obstruction: most common cause of surgery in patients with CD.

Conservative therapy with resuscitation, nasogastric decompression, and IV steroids is often successful. Ileocolic resection is indicated for patients who fail medical therapy. The Kono-S ileocolic anastomosis with mesenteric exclusion has been suggested to decrease rates of Crohn recurrence. In patients who are severely malnourished, active smokers, or on long-term high-dose steroids, ileostomies are sometimes considered.
- Small bowel strictures: endoscopic dilation can be considered for short-segment fibrotic small bowel strictures. Success rates are 90%; however, recurrence is high (40%-70%), and one-third of patients go on to require small bowel resection or strictureplasty.
- Severe acute/fulminant colitis or toxic megacolon: *Clostridioides difficile* and cytomegalovirus (CMV) colitis should be excluded. Total abdominal colectomy with end ileostomy is indicated if medical therapy fails or if there is evidence of colonic perforation.
- ~30% to 55% of patients with CD require bowel resection.
- Surgical considerations: minimize bowel resection length to avoid short bowel syndrome, utilize strictureplasty when possible.

Ulcerative Colitis

- **Medical management**
  - Mildly to moderately active UC/proctitis
    - 5-aminosalicylic acid (5-ASA) enemas are used to induce and maintain remission. Can be combined with oral 5-ASA
    - Budesonide 9 mg daily can be added to induce remission in patients who do not respond to 5-ASA.
    - Patients with UC who do not respond to 5-ASA can also be treated with oral systemic corticosteroids to induce remission. Oral steroids should not be used to maintain remission.
  - Moderately to severely active UC
    - Budesonide or oral systemic corticosteroids can be used to induce remission. Steroids should not be used to maintain remission.
    - Anti-TNF agents (infliximab or adalimumab) can be used to induce and maintain remission. Can combine with azathioprine
    - In patients who fail anti-TNF therapy, vedolizumab or tofacitinib can be used to induce and maintain remission.
  - Acute severe UC
    - Often hospitalized, consider surgical consult
    - Test for *C. difficile* infection (stool test) and CMV infection (endoscopic biopsies)
    - No evidence for routine use of antibiotics
    - IV corticosteroids (methylprednisolone 60 mg/d or hydrocortisone 100 mg 3-4× per day) to induce remission
    - If fails to respond to IV steroids by 3 to 5 days, then add rescue therapy with infliximab or cyclosporine.
- **Surgical management**
  - UC can be surgically cured with total proctocolectomy, which removes all areas of disease.
  - Indications: medically refractory disease, colonic perforation, toxic megacolon, fulminant colitis, severe hemorrhage, invisible dysplasia, endoscopically unresectable dysplasia, and carcinoma
  - There is a 20% colectomy rate reported with first-time severe colitis requiring hospitalization. An additional 6% required subsequent colectomy during the following 3 months.
  - Urgent or emergent surgery often entails total abdominal colectomy with end ileostomy. There is a risk of rectal stump dehiscence, which can be mitigated with the placement of a rectal tube, creation of mucus fistula, or implanting the rectal stump in the subcutaneous tissues.
  - Younger patients with good anal sphincter function and no suspicion of CD are candidates for restoration of intestinal continuity with an ileoanal J pouch, in which the terminal ileum is used to create a neo-rectum reservoir.
  - Patients who are not candidates for J pouches can undergo total proctocolectomy with end ileostomy, or total abdominal colectomy with end ileostomy followed by completion proctectomy.

Colorectal Cancer Screening in Ulcerative Colitis and Crohn Colitis

- Colorectal cancer risks: incidence 2% to 5% by 10 years, 20% by 20 years; 1% to 2% per year if disease is present over 10 years
- Colorectal cancer risk is higher for patients with longer duration of disease, primary sclerosing cholangitis, and family history of colorectal cancer.
- Surveillance colonoscopy starting 8 years after the diagnosis of UC or Crohn colitis, then every 1 to 3 years. Multiple colon biopsies required at regular intervals. Chromoendoscopy can be used to improve the detection of dysplastic areas.
- Indications for surgery: colorectal cancer, dysplasia that is not endoscopically resectable, and "invisible" dysplasia on random biopsies
- Surgery usually entails total colectomy or total proctocolectomy. Segmental colectomy is not recommended because 14% to 40% of patients with Crohn colitis who undergo segmental colorectal cancer resection develop metachronous colorectal cancer.

Specific Critical Care Considerations in Patients With Inflammatory Bowel Disease

- Both UC and CD have elevated risks of thromboembolic events. Deep venous thrombosis (DVT) prophylaxis should be administered while hospitalized, and extended DVT prophylaxis considered for postoperative patients.
- Concomitant *C. difficile* and CMV infections must be ruled out in patients admitted with IBD flares. *C. difficile* is associated with higher rates of mortality in patients with UC.
- Check hemoglobin levels, consider IV iron infusions; patients with IBD are often anemic.
- Patients with IBD are often severely malnourished—and are at risk for refeeding syndrome with resumption of enteral nutrition.

- Patients who have been steroid dependent are at risk for adrenal insufficiency, which can manifest with vague symptoms (nausea, abdominal pain, lethargy) as well as hypotension.
- High-dose steroids can mask colonic perforations. Low threshold to reimage if suspicion for colonic perforation in patient not improving with medical therapy, even in the absence of peritonitis on examination.

SUGGESTED READINGS

Abraham C, Cho JH. Inflammatory bowel disease. *N Engl J Med*. 2009;361:2066-2078.

Devlin SM, Panaccione R. Evolving inflammatory bowel disease treatment paradigms: top-down versus step-up. *Gastroenterol Clin North Am*. 2009;38:577-594.

Holubar SD, Lightner AL, Poylin V, et al. The American Society of Colon and Rectal Surgeons clinical practice guidelines for the surgical management of ulcerative colitis. *Dis Colon Rectum*. 2021;64:783-804.

Kappelman MD, Horvath-Puho E, Sandler RS, et al. Thromboembolic risk among Danish children and adults with inflammatory bowel diseases: a population-based nationwide study. *Gut*. 2011;60(7):937.

Le Berre C, Honap S, Peyrin-Biroulet L. Ulcerative colitis. *Lancet*. 2023;402:571-584.

Lichtenstein GR, Loftus EV, Isaacs KL, Regueiro MD, Gerson LB, Sands BE. ACG clinical guideline: management of Crohn's disease in adults. *Am J Gastroenterol*. 2018;113:481-517.

Lightner AL, Vogel JD, Carmichael JC, et al. The American Society of Colon and Rectal Surgeons clinical practice guidelines for the surgical management of Crohn's disease. *Dis Colon Rectum*. 2020;63:1028-1052.

Loftus EV, Sandborn WJ. Epidemiology of inflammatory bowel disease. *Gastroenterol Clin North Am*. 2002;31:1-20.

Luglio G, Rispo A, Imperatore N, et al. Surgical prevention of anastomotic recurrence by excluding mesentery in Crohn's disease: the SuPREMe-CD study—a randomized clinical trial. *Ann Surg*. 2020;272:210-217.

Peyrin-Biroulet L, Deltenre P, de Suray N, Branche J, Sandborn WJ, Colombel JF. Efficacy and safety of tumor necrosis factor antagonists in Crohn's disease: meta-analysis of placebo-controlled trials. *Clin Gastroenterol Hepatol*. 2008;6(6):644-653.

Rubin DT, Ananthakrishnan AN, Siegel CA, Sauer BG, Long MD. ACG clinical guideline: ulcerative colitis in adults. *Am J Gastroenterol*. 2019;114:384-413.

Rutgeerts P, Sandborn WJ, Feagan BG, et al. Infliximab for induction and maintenance therapy for ulcerative colitis. *N Engl J Med*. 2005;353:2462-2476.

Torres J, Mehandru S, Colombel JF, Peyrin-Biroulet L. Crohn's disease. *Lancet*. 2017;389:1741-1755.

Velayos FS, Loftus EV Jr, Jess T, et al. Predictive and protective factors associated with colorectal cancer in ulcerative colitis: a case-control study. *Gastroenterology*. 2006;130(7):1941-1949.

Xavier RJ, Podolsky DK. Unravelling the pathogenesis of inflammatory bowel disease. *Nature*. 2007;448(7152):427-434.

4.14

Vascular Diseases of the Small Bowel

Srihari K. Lella and Jahan Mohebali

Credit to previous edition chapter by Robert Crawford, MD that has been updated.

Mesenteric Venous Thrombosis

- Primary mesenteric venous thrombosis (MVT) is spontaneous, idiopathic thrombosis of the mesenteric veins without association with another disease or etiologic factor.
- 90% of MVTs are due to a secondary etiology.
- MVT is a rare and potentially lethal type of mesenteric ischemia.
- Often leads to intestinal infarction due to a delay in diagnosis
- Most often affects the superior mesenteric vein, rarely the inferior mesenteric vein (see Table 4.14.1)

Epidemiology

- Accounts for 10% to 15% of all cases of mesenteric ischemia
- Slightly more common in males than in females
- Accounts for 0.006% of hospital admissions
- Venous thrombosis is found in 0.001% of patients undergoing exploration due to vague abdominal symptoms.

TABLE 4.14.1 Risk Factors for Acute Mesenteric Venous Thrombosis

Intra-abdominal infection	Blunt or penetrating abdominal trauma
Hepatic cirrhosis	Abdominal surgery (eg, postsplenectomy)
Smoking history	Malignancy
Oral contraceptive pill usage	Factor V Leiden
Protein C/S deficiency	Intra-abdominal inflammatory states (eg, pancreatitis)
Congestive heart failure	Increased abdominal pressure/ abdominal compartment syndrome

Key Pathophysiology

- Listed as primary/idiopathic (due to thrombotic disorders) or secondary (caused by another disease process)
- Initial thrombosis of the mesenteric venous system, due to the abovementioned risk factors, usually occurs in the superior mesenteric vein
- Venous congestion leads to an influx of third-space fluid into the bowel wall.
- Bowel edema coupled with decreased outflow secondary to thrombosis prevents arterial inflow, leading to ischemia and necrosis.
- Majority of morbidity and mortality associated with the amount of bowel necrosis

Differential Diagnosis

- Signs and symptoms: 4 weeks is classified as acute MVT, while >4 weeks is classified as chronic MVT.
  - Abdominal pain, nausea, and vomiting

- Distended abdomen
- Leukocytosis
- Metabolic acidosis
- Guaiac-positive stool
- Palpable abdominal mass
- Peritoneal signs

- Pain evolves over 5 to 7 days due to prolonged ileus.
- Any intra-abdominal process that can cause vague to severe abdominal pain
  - Pancreatitis
  - Gastric/duodenal ulcer
  - Inflammatory bowel disease
  - Biliary pathology
  - Arterial mesenteric ischemia, embolic or thrombotic
  - Malignancy
  - Infection (enteritis, colitis)
  - Spontaneous intestinal perforation
  - Diverticulitis
  - Mesenteric adenitis
  - Pelvic inflammatory disease

Management and Treatment

- Potentially preventable by identifying patients at risk (ie, hypercoagulable states)
- High index of suspicion with initial presentation to prevent morbidity and mortality of intestinal necrosis
- Immediate anticoagulation with systemic heparin
- Nil per os (NPO)
- Gastric decompression via nasogastric tube
- Resuscitative fluids
- Antibiotics for bacterial translocation and/or sepsis
- Surgery may be necessary to confirm the diagnosis and can be therapeutic in the setting of bowel infarction.
- Thrombectomy and local lytic therapy can be used at specialized centers in more severe cases.

Outcomes

- Mortality rate 20% to 50% (range due to the degree of bowel injury)
- High recurrence rate within 30 days postoperatively if the underlying causative agent remains present

Arteriovenous Malformation

- Abnormal connection between a vein and an artery in which blood does not flow through a capillary bed but rather directly from artery to vein
- Usually a congenital anomaly due to arrested development during various stages of embryogenesis
- Associated with aortic stenosis
- "Dieulafoy lesion": an arteriovenous malformation (AVM), usually in the upper stomach, that is prone to bleeding
- Risk factors: believed to be genetic, specific transmission patterns remain unknown

Epidemiology

- ~1.4/100,000 per year are detected in the United States.
- Only 12% of people with AVM will exhibit symptoms, which vary in severity.
- Equal rate in males and females; no racial predilection identified

Pathophysiology

- Due to the lack of a capillary network, blood flows directly from high to low pressure.
- Excessive strain is conveyed to the venous wall that can lead to rupture.
  - As high pressure enters the vein with a smaller wall thickness, the risk of rupture increases.
- Symptoms are associated with the location of the AVM within the body and would present with anemia of any severity and associated physiologic disturbances.

Differential Diagnosis

- Can occur anywhere in the body, including the intestines
- Once bleeding or hemorrhage ensues, the identification of an AVM can be made.
- Includes any cause of upper or lower gastrointestinal bleeding
  - Varices
  - Bleeding gastric or duodenal ulcer
  - Mallory-Weiss tear
  - Gastritis
  - Diverticulosis/diverticulitis
  - Hemorrhoids
  - Polyps
  - Malignancy
  - Infectious enteritis or colitis
  - Inflammatory bowel disease
  - Anal fissure

Management and Treatment

- AVM identified as a result of intestinal bleeding or hemorrhage
  - Aggressive intravenous resuscitation with fluids and/or blood products
  - Identification of the location of malformation
    - Endoscopic ultrasound
    - Endoscopic therapy: clipping, sclerotherapy, cautery, epinephrine injection
    - Angiography may be of use if endoscopic treatment is unsuccessful.
    - Surgery (resection of the affected portion) reserved for AVM refractory to less invasive means.

Embolic and Thrombotic Mesenteric Arterial Disease

This entity results in mesenteric ischemia caused by intracardiac thrombosis, cardiac valve vegetations, hypercoagulable state, or atherosclerotic disease. (See section "Mesenteric Ischemia".)

Acknowledgments

We gratefully acknowledge the contributions of previous edition author(s), Robert Crawford, as portions of those chapters have been retained in this revision.

SUGGESTED READINGS

Akhras J, Patel P, Tobi M. Dieulafoy's lesion-like bleeding: an underrecognized cause of upper gastrointestinal hemorrhage in patients with advanced liver disease. *Dig Dis Sci*. 2007;52(3):722-726.

Batur P, Stewart WJ, Isaacson JH. Increased prevalence of aortic stenosis in patients with arteriovenous malformations of the gastrointestinal tract in Heyde syndrome. *Arch Intern Med*. 2003;163(15):1821-1824.

Bradbury MS, Kavanagh PV, Bechtold RE, et al. Mesenteric venous thrombosis: diagnosis and noninvasive imaging. *Radiographics*. 2002;22(3): 527-541.

Fallah MA, Prakash C, Edmundowicz S. Acute gastrointestinal bleeding. *Med Clin North Am*. 2000;84(5):1183-1208.

Kumar S, Sarr MG, Kamath PS. Mesenteric venous thrombosis. *N Engl J Med*. 2001;345(23):1683-688.

Lee Y, Walmsley R, Leong R, Sung J. Dieulafoy's lesion. *Gastrointest Endosc*. 2003;58(2):236-243.

Schoots IG, Koffeman GI, Legemate DA, et al. Systematic review of survival after acute mesenteric ischaemia according to disease aetiology. *Br J Surg*. 2004;91(1):17-27.

Stabile BE, Stamos MJ. Surgical management of gastrointestinal bleeding. *Gastroenterol Clin North Am*. 2000;29(1):189-222.

4.15

Obesity

Eran Brauner

Definition

Obesity is defined as a body mass index (BMI) ≥30 kg/m^2.

Epidemiology

- Obesity is an exploding epidemic in the Western world and the United States.
- In 2022, all US states and territories had an obesity prevalence >20%.
  - 22 states had an obesity prevalence between 30% and 35%.
  - 19 states had an obesity prevalence between 35% and 40%.
- Many adults with obesity have other serious chronic diseases.
  - 58% have high blood.
  - 23% have diabetes.
- In 2019, obesity was related to nearly $173 billion in medical expenditures.
- Obesity affects some groups more than others, including non-Hispanic Black adults and adults with less education.

Key Pathophysiology

- Cardiovascular
  - Typical physiologic effects of obesity include:
    - Increased blood volume, stroke volume, and cardiac output
    - Increased left ventricular (LV) and left atrial (LA) filling pressures
    - LV hypertrophy and LA enlargement; and increased risk for LV dysfunction. Ventricular dilatation and diastolic dysfunction (obesity cardiomyopathy)
  - This can manifest as left or right heart failure with signs of pulmonary edema, fatigue, or generalized edema.
  - Hyperinsulinemic states decrease natriuretic peptide levels, increase renal sympathetic activity; increased renal-angiotensin-aldosterone system leads to hypertensive state.
  - Atrial fibrillation is a frequent complication of obesity, either as a result of LA enlargement and increased feeling pressure or autonomic dysregulation.
  - Pulmonary hypertension secondary to elevated LA pressure, hypoxia from obstructive sleep apnea (OSA), and hypoventilation syndrome or chronic thromboembolism
  - Ischemic heart disease due to cardiac hypertrophy, chronically augmented preload, higher wall tension, and, therefore, inadequate blood supply to meet myocardial oxygen demands
  - In addition, hypertension, hypercholesterolemia, and, typically, an unhealthy diet produce coronary atherosclerosis.
- Respiratory
  - Increase oxygen consumption up to 60% and carbon dioxide production and increase work of breathing
    - Resulting in compensatory increase in neural respiratory drive, and when this fails, obesity hyperventilation syndrome (OHS) ensues, resulting in hypercapnia and hypoxemia
    - Increased airway resistance from parapharyngeal adipose tissue renders the upper airway susceptible to collapse, as seen in OSA.
    - Increased baseline pleural pressure from abdominal and chest wall adiposity results in reduced expiratory reserve volume and functional residual capacity.
    - As a result, these patients are susceptible to collapse of peripheral-dependent airways, atelectasis, and tidal ventilation below the lower inflection point of the inspiratory pressure-volume curve, with a corresponding decrease in lung compliance.
    - Because dependent perfusion is increased in some patients with obesity, concomitant basilar atelectasis may cause $\dot{V}/\dot{Q}$ mismatch and resultant hypoxemia.
    - Elevated risk of acute respiratory distress syndrome (ARDS), possibly related to the baseline $\dot{V}/\dot{Q}$ mismatch, atelectrauma, or pro-inflammatory response from adipose tissue
    - Severe obesity may also substantially increase the metabolic demand of breathing.
    - Obesity is a risk factor for difficult intubation and difficult mask ventilation.
- Coagulation
  - Obesity is associated with increased risk of venous thromboembolism (VTE). This may be due to:
    - Increase circulating procoagulant factors, pro-inflammatory and hypofibrinogenic state, low antithrombin III levels, and decreased fibrinolytic activity
    - Slow venous return related to immobility and increased intra-abdominal pressure
    - Inadequate dosing of prophylactic anticoagulants may play an additional role.

- Nutrition
  - Despite sufficient caloric intake, many patients who are obese remain malnourished, with a high rate of micronutrient deficiencies.
  - Obesity may occur with increased normal or low muscle mass.
  - Although low muscle mass and sarcopenia occur mainly with aging, it can be substantial and not immediately obvious in the critically ill patient with higher BMI.
  - Patients who are obese with critical illness, like those who are not obese, are at risk for loss of muscle mass.
- Endocrine
  - Endocrine abnormalities are frequently associated with obesity, even if it is not clear whether there is causality or association.
  - Insulin resistance and type 2 diabetes mellitus are common.
  - Hypothyroidism should be suspected.
  - Hormones such as insulin, corticosterone, and aldosterone are found in increased quantities.
- Renal
  - Obesity is a risk factor for chronic kidney disease (CKD). The mechanism for this includes subclinical CKD, intra-abdominal hypertension, and alteration in baseline and evoked circulating inflammatory mediators and adipokines.
  - Increased renal perfusion and glomerular hyperfiltration augment intraglomerular pressure and sodium reabsorption, leading to glomerulomegaly and focal sclerosis.
  - High BMI is an independent risk factor for acute kidney injury (AKI).
- Immune system and infection
  - Adipose tissue produces several hormones (adipokines) and inflammatory mediators, resulting in chronic inflammation.
  - Obesity may be a risk factor for bloodstream infections, pneumonia, and soft tissue infections in hospitalized and critically ill patients.
    - Potential contributing factors include altered cellular immunity, increased use of central venous catheter, prolonged urinary catheter, and inadequate antibiotic dosing.

Management and Treatment

- General
  - The obvious goal is to reduce weight by decreasing caloric intake and increasing energy expenditure.
  - Changes in diet and lifestyle are not realistic during acute diseases.
  - Surgical management by means of gastric restrictive operations or other alternatives has been effective but is not a choice for critically ill patients.
- Respiratory
  - Intubation
    - Due to an elevated Mallampati score, limited mouth opening, and reduce cervical mobility, one should expect difficult intubation.
    - Often, mask ventilation requires two providers for the task.
    - To limit desaturation, preoxygenation must be optimized and allow at least 5 minutes of noninvasive ventilation (NIV) in a sitting position.
    - Preoxygenating with high-flow nasal cannula (HFNC) combined with NIV may be more effective at reducing oxygen desaturation compared to NIV alone in this population.
    - Reverse Trendelenburg position at 30 degree or 25 degree head-up positioning both for preoxygenation and for postintubation recruitment maneuver
  - Mechanical ventilation
    - Protective ventilation should be applied as in patients who are not obese.
    - During mechanical ventilation, the tidal volume delivered should be estimated based on ideal body weight (IBW) (6 mL/kg).
    - Calculations according to actual body weight (ActBW) may result in inappropriately aggressive alveolar inflation and barotraumas.
    - Methods to improve ventilation in the patient who are obese include reverse Trendelenburg position and higher levels of positive end-expiratory pressure (PEEP) up to 10 or even 15 cm H_2O.
    - Respiratory rate (RR) to achieve CO_2 of 35 to 45 mm Hg or pH >7.25
    - Recruitment maneuvers (40-50 cm H_2O) followed by PEEP 10 cm H_2O during anesthesia and paralysis
  - Patient who is obese with ARDS
    - Volume normalized to the ARDSnet protocol predicted body weight based on height and sex.
    - Plateau pressure <30 cm H_2O remains the standard (higher level of plateau pressure not necessarily reflect elevated transpulmonary pressure).
    - When available, esophageal manometry of transpulmonary pressure may help determine the contribution of the chest wall to total respiratory compliance.
    - Prone position (if PO_2/FIO_2 <150 mm Hg) is safe, efficient, and may benefit the patient who is obese, more than those who are not obese.
    - Reverse Trendelenburg can help avoid complications of increased abdominal pressure.
    - Extracorporeal membrane oxygenation (ECMO) can also be safely used in patients who are obese with ARDS and is associated with similar or improved outcomes compared with those who are not obese.
  - Extubation
    - Extubating to continuous positive airway pressure (CPAP) or other forms of noninvasive positive pressure ventilation (NIPPV), especially in patients with comorbidities and or OSA/HS (hypopnea syndrome) and hypercarbia during spontaneous breathing trials
- Cardiovascular
  - Accurate hemodynamic monitoring is a key.
  - Oscillometric pressure measurements are less accurate, and invasive blood pressure (BP) monitoring should be used for hemodynamically unstable patients.
  - Noninvasive cardiac output measurements are also inaccurate in patients who are obese.
  - Transthoracic echocardiography will often have poor acoustic windows. Transesophageal echocardiography may be warranted.

- The treatment considerations here are no different than for patient who is not obese with hypertension/hypotension and cardiomyopathy. With few considerations:
  - Fluid resuscitation in the obese should account for both the increased blood volume and the risk of fluid overload and heart failure.
  - Using adjusted body weight (AdjBW = IBW + 0.4 (ActBW-IBW)) to guide initial resuscitation may result in better outcome.
    - Vasoactive drugs should be titrated to their clinical effect rather than using weight-based dosing.
- A high index of suspicion should exist for the possibility of myocardial ischemia, and when possible, the coronary system should be evaluated before high-risk procedures.

- Coagulation
  - Thromboprophylaxis is an integral part of the treatment strategy.
    - Standard fixed prophylactic doses of unfractionated and low-molecular-weight heparin (LMWH) typically do not offer acceptable levels of antithrombotic activity.
    - Because of the increased volume of distribution and possible poor absorption by the large subcutaneous tissue, the standard doses are not sufficient.
    - The optimal dosage and dosage intervals are unknown; some practice uses anti-Xa levels of 0.3 to 0.5 U/mL as a surrogate.
    - Some suggested LMWH of 40 to 60 mg 2 times daily (bid) or 60 mg once a day (qd) or 0.5 mg/kg qd or bid.
  - Sequential compression devices offer theoretical benefit, but the compliance with correct application is low.
  - Early ambulation remains important.
  - There should be increased vigilance and a lowered threshold for VTE monitoring and diagnosis.
    - Venous duplex ultrasonography is used for monitoring of extremity thrombosis, but the images can be suboptimal, compromising its sensitivity.
    - Similar challenges exist with computed tomography (CT) for the diagnosis of suspected pulmonary embolism.
- Nutrition
  - A common problem is to restrict nutrition on the belief that the patient who is obese is overfed.
  - Per American Society for Parenteral and Enteral Nutrition (ASPEN) guidelines:
    - Caloric intake of 11 to 14 kcal/kg of actual ActBW/d for BMI 30 to 50 kg/m^2 and 22 to 25 kcal/kg of IBW/d if BMI >50 kg/m^2
    - Protein target of 2 to 2.5g/kg of IBW/d
    - Adjustment of nutrition according to serum markers such as glucose, urea, and triglyceride is the same as for patients who are not obese (see ASPEN guidelines).
  - Calorimetry and nitrogen balance calculations are useful.
- Drug absorption
  - The enteral absorption is typically normal, but the parenteral may vary widely because of changes in volume of distribution and organ dysfunctions that impair metabolism and clearance, especially in the critically ill patient.
  - Lipophilic agents are distributed over larger volumes, and dosing should be adjusted for drugs such as aminoglycosides, quinolones, benzodiazepines, and calcium channel blockers.
  - Because the net effect of the different interactions may be unpredictable, a one-size-fits-all approach is not justified, and all drugs should be closely monitored.
  - AdjBW is likely to be more relevant than IBW or ActBW for both hydrophilic and lipophilic drugs calculations.
- Renal
  - Using ActBW to apply the oliguria criteria may lead to false-positive diagnosis of AKI.
  - For estimated glomerular filtration rate (GFR), the CKD epidemiology collaboration equation is currently the best validated tool for patients who are obese.
  - Cystatin C (CC) has been proposed as an alternative biomarker for estimating GFR as it is less influenced by muscle mass than creatinine.
  - In morbidly obese individuals, serum CC may be elevated due to adipose tissue production and low-grade inflammation, independent of actual kidney function, leading to overestimation of kidney dysfunction.
    - When available, combined creatinine-cystatin C equations (eg, CKD-EPI creatinine + cystatin C) may provide a more accurate GFR estimate in this population.
- Immunity and infection
  - Same as for patients who are not obese; frequent assessment and prompt removal of all indwelling catheter, Tight glucose monitoring, avoiding hypothermia and appropriate antibiotic dosing
- Other factors to consider
  - Ultrasound guidance for intravenous (IV) insertion should be the standard of care for both peripheral and central.
    - Femoral axis has been shown to increase the risk of infection should be used when no other available sites.
  - Incorrect blood BP cuff size may affect accuracy.
  - Increased radiation dose for CT and x-rays may mitigate the noise and radiation scattered caused by subcutaneous adipose tissue.
  - Standard of care is recommended for pressure ulcer prevention, including regular positioning and frequent checks for early pressure injury.
- Glucagon-like peptide-1 receptor (GLP-1) receptor agonists (RAs) in the critically ill patient
  - The increasing prevalence of obesity and type 2 diabetes has led to a surge in the use of long-acting . Examples: liraglutide, semaglutide, dulaglutide, exenatide
  - Mechanism of action: enhance glucose-dependent insulin secretion, suppress glucagon release, slow gastric emptying, promote satiety and lead to weight loss, and enhance glucose control
  - Implications in critically ill patients
    - Hypoglycemia: may occur when used in combination with insulin
    - Delayed gastric emptying: can complicate enteral feeding and postoperative ileus. May affect the interpretation of gastric residual volumes. Can impair absorption of oral medications and increase the risk of aspiration
    - Renal considerations: exenatide is contraindicated in end-stage renal disease (ESRD) or severe renal impairment. Vomiting and dehydration may exacerbate renal dysfunction.

- Pharmacokinetics: long-acting GLP-1 RAs, such as semaglutide, have prolonged half-lives (~7 days), and its effect may persist throughout the patient's intensive care unit (ICU) stay.

Outcomes

- Trauma: most studies report worse outcomes in patients who are obese compared to their nonobese counterparts.
  - Obesity is an independent factor for mortality in blunt traumatic patients.
  - It seems that obesity is associated with a specific pattern of injuries, according to which patients who are obese tend to suffer more chest and extremity injuries but fewer head injuries.
- Emergency and elective surgery: there is an increased incidence of complications related to obesity, particularly wound infections, pneumonia, and bacteremia.

SUGGESTED READINGS

Anderson MR, Shashaty MGS. Impact of obesity in critical illness. *Chest*. 2021;160(6):2135-2145.

Ayalon I, Bodilly L, Kaplan J. The impact of obesity on critical illnesses. *Shock*. 2021;56(5):691-700.

Brown CVR, Neville AL, Rhee P, Salim A, Velmahos GC, Demetriades D. The impact of obesity on the outcomes of 1,153 critically injured blunt trauma patients. *J Trauma*. 2005;59:1048-1051.

Brown CVR, Velmahos GC. The consequences of obesity on trauma, emergency surgery, and surgical critical care. *World J Emerg Surg*. 2006;1:27-32.

Centers for Disease Control and Prevention. Obesity and overweight: resources. http://www.cdc.gov/obesity/resources/index.html

McClave SA, Taylor BE, Martindale RG, et al; Society of Critical Care Medicine; American Society for Parenteral and Enteral Nutrition. Guidelines for the provision and assessment of nutrition support therapy in the adult critically ill patient: Society of Critical Care Medicine (SCCM) and American Society for Parenteral and Enteral Nutrition (A.S.P.E.N.). *JPEN J Parenter Enteral Nutr*. 2016;40(2):159-211.

Schetz M, De Jong A, Deane AM, et al. Obesity in the critically ill: a narrative review. *Intensive Care Med*. 2019;45(6):757-769.

4.16

Gastrointestinal Diagnostic Modalities

Robert D. Sinyard and Casey M. Luckhurst

Conditions

- Critically ill patients often require diagnostic studies for gastrointestinal (GI) disorders that may be the primary driver of their illness or sequelae of other illnesses. Common reasons to pursue diagnostic imaging include:
  - Concern for intra-abdominal infection
  - Concern for GI bleeding
  - Assessment of bowel absorption and/or motility for the purposes of medical administration or nutritional support
  - Concern for noninfectious acute intraperitoneal process (eg, pancreatitis, ureteral injury)

Bedside Diagnostics

- Drain studies
  - Surgical patients may have preoperative or postoperative drains in place that can provide insight into intra-abdominal processes.
    - Following pancreatic/splenic surgery: consider drain amylase for evaluation of pancreatic anastomotic or tail leak.
    - Following urologic, colorectal, or renal trauma: consider sending a drain creatinine (Cr) and comparing it to serum Cr.
    - Following foregut or thoracic surgery: consider sending fluid for triglycerides or chylomicron levels concerning for a chyle leak.
  - Pressure and temperature monitoring
    - Some Foley catheters can be placed, which enable temperature monitoring or intra-abdominal pressure monitoring.
    - Patients undergoing cooling or warming for different clinical illnesses may benefit from this type of more invasive temperature monitoring.
    - Patients with concerns for abdominal compartment syndrome (ACS) may undergo regular bladder pressure transduction (pressures of ≥20 mm Hg are associated with organ failure), though diagnosis of ACS and decision for therapy require an understanding of the entire clinical picture.
  - Peritoneal sampling
    - Patients with abdominal ascites without existing drains in place may benefit from bedside paracentesis for diagnostic or therapeutic purposes.
  - Biopsy
    - Though uncommon, occasional bedside or image-guided biopsy may offer diagnostic benefit that affects the care of critically ill patients, particularly as it relates to major medication decisions or goals of care discussions (eg, organ rejection, malignant bowel obstruction).

Assessments of Bowel Absorption and Motility

- Motility studies
  - GI motility is often affected by critical illness, and diagnostic options in the setting of critical illness may alter clinical decision-making.
  - Motility can be assessed using formal studies such as capsule or radioactive compound study time as well as gastric emptying studies, though these are uncommon in an intensive care unit (ICU) setting.

- More commonly, diagnostics such as Gastrografin administration with follow-up KUB (kidneys, ureters, bladder) or measurement of gastric residuals may help assess for motility or resolving GI obstruction.
  - Gastrografin challenge involves administration of nondilute Gastrografin via a nasogastric (NG) tube, followed by clamping of the NG tube for ~1 hour. An abdominal x-ray (XR) 4 to 6 hours later that demonstrates contrast passage through the small bowel into the colon helps demonstrate appropriate motility and/or resolution of a small bowel obstruction. Notably, only patients who are awake and able to be seated upright or standing should undergo this trial, given the risk for aspiration when the NG is clamped. Aspiration of Gastrografin can cause severe chemical pneumonitis.
- Absorption measurement
  - Assessing enteral absorption can help with decisions regarding the route of medication administration and nutritional support.
  - Administration of acetaminophen followed by blood-level measurements of acetaminophen at 30 to 60 minutes can provide rough estimates for adequate versus inadequate enteral absorption.

Endoscopic Diagnostics

- Upper and lower endoscopy, both of which can be performed in the operating room, endoscopy suite, or at bedside in the ICU, can have both diagnostic and therapeutic benefits for critically ill patients.
  - Upper endoscopy
    - For patients with significant GI bleeding originating from the foregut, upper endoscopy is typically first-line diagnostic modality.
      - Upper endoscopy is able to identify gastritis, malignancy, peptic ulcer disease, Dieulafoy lesions, antral vascular ectasia, and hemobilia.
    - Upper endoscopy with adjuncts such as endoscopic retrograde cholangiopancreatography and endoscopic ultrasound (U/S) may be helpful for evaluation of biliary or pancreatic pathology, with additional benefits of concomitant therapeutic intervention.
  - Lower endoscopy
    - For patients with lower GI bleeding, rigid or flexible proctoscopy as well as colonoscopy are first-line therapies, though often limited by inadequate bowel preparation, particularly in critically ill patients. Lower endoscopy may also diagnose infectious (cytomegalovirus [CMV] colitis, pseudomembranous colitis) or inflammatory conditions (Crohn, ulcerative colitis).
    - Common etiologies for lower GI bleeding in critically ill patients include ischemic colitis, diverticulosis, malignancy, hemorrhoids, and inflammatory bowel disease.
    - Beyond potential therapeutic maneuvers, endoscopic evaluation of the lower GI tract may also provide additional diagnostic benefit with localization and endoscopic tattooing of problematic lesions that may require surgical intervention.

Imaging Modalities (Computed Tomography, Magnetic Resonance, X-Ray, Nuclear, Ultrasound)

- Most GI pathologies in critically ill patients utilize imaging modalities as part of the diagnostic workup. An overview of the varying modalities with potential indications is briefly described below.
  - Computed tomography (CT)
    - Abdominal and pelvic CT images with intravenous (IV) contrast provide excellent insight into evolving intra-abdominal processes as they provide insight into tissue perfusion, edema/inflammation, intra-abdominal fluid collections, luminal dilation, and extraluminal gas.
    - CT angiography (arteriography or venography) is particularly helpful for the diagnosis of intra-abdominal pathology arising from vascular sources (mesenteric ischemia due to peripheral arterial disease or mesenteric thrombosis) as well as for intra-abdominal hemorrhage. Angiography is also particularly helpful for surgical planning if endovascular techniques are to be utilized.
    - If concerns exist for intraluminal processes, including obstruction, perforation, or fistula, the addition of enteral contrast may also be helpful.
    - Notably, noncontrasted CT images of the abdomen are rarely useful, and an effort should be made to provide IV contrast whenever possible. Consider prehydration for patients with a glomerular filtration rate (GFR) <30 or pretreatment for those with listed allergies.
    - The genitourinary system may be studied with add-ons to the standard CT with IV contrast. First, delayed images may be obtained (typically 8-10 minutes after IV contrast administration). This time interval allows for contrast filtration by the kidneys, and subsequent images help identify pathology of the renal collecting system as well as the ureters. Separately, contrast provided via a Foley catheter followed by clamping of the catheter helps distend the bladder and may enable identification of bladder pathology, especially traumatic injuries.
  - Magnetic resonance imaging (MRI)
    - Though more difficult to obtain on critically ill patients due to the length of scan time, MRI may be particularly useful for the diagnosis of GI pathology involving the pancreaticobiliary system (specifically magnetic resonance cholangiopancreatography), given high sensitivity for intraductal stone disease as well as pancreatic ductal integrity.
  - XR
    - Given their ability to be performed at bedside, XRs or "plain film" images have utility in rapid diagnosis of pneumoperitoneum, GI tube dislodgment, and ileus versus obstruction. Additionally, bedside XRs provide crucial information regarding tube placement (endotracheal tubes, enteric tubes, thoracostomy tubes, etc).

- Fluoroscopic examinations such as upper GI series may also be useful for evaluating foregut integrity and motility (eg, esophageal dysmotility, duodenal perforation).
- U/S
  - U/S of the abdomen can provide diagnostic insight into GI pathology and, importantly, can be repeated as needed if clinical conditions change.
  - A right upper quadrant U/S often provides insight into hepatobiliary pathology such as gallbladder disease (calculous or acalculous cholecystitis), biliary obstruction (cholangitis), and hepatic vascular abnormalities (portal/hepatic vein thrombosis, hepatic arterial insufficiency, pseudoaneurysm).
  - A bedside (point-of-care) U/S of the abdomen may be useful for patients with suspected abdominal trauma to evaluate for free fluid in the setting of possible intra-abdominal hemorrhage. Nontrauma patients, particularly postoperative patients, may also benefit from a FAST (Focused Assessment with Sonography in Trauma) examination to evaluate for intra-abdominal hemorrhage. Point-of-care U/S also allows for sampling of intra-abdominal fluid in the setting of ascites and evaluation for spontaneous peritonitis.
  - Finally, duplex capabilities allow for ultrasonographic assessment of mesenteric vasculature for the evaluation of acute or chronic arterial disease of the bowel as well as splenic, hepatic, and renal vasculature.
- Nuclear studies
  - In some instances, nuclear studies may be helpful for diagnostic purposes, such as a hepatobiliary iminodiacetic acid (HIDA) scan, for the evaluation of acalculous cholecystitis or biliary dyskinesia.
  - Tagged red blood cell scans may also be useful for critically ill patients with GI bleeds that have been unable to be localized via additional diagnostic methods.

Gastrointestinal Laboratory Analyses

- Coagulation studies (prothrombin time/international normalized ratio [PT/INR], partial thromboplastin time [PTT], bleeding time) may provide diagnostic insight when considering hepatic synthetic function as well as potential etiologies for postoperative or intraluminal GI bleeding.
- Nutritional laboratory assessment (albumin, prealbumin, transferrin, retinal binding protein), though limited by the acute inflammatory response of critical illness, may provide diagnostic benefit for critically ill patients when making decisions regarding the need for enteral/parenteral support or resuscitation and diuresis management.
- Stool assessments (*Clostridioides difficile* toxin assays, fecal ova and parasite testing, or fecal fat/elastase) may provide diagnostic benefit for infectious or malabsorptive conditions.
- Serologies (*Helicobacter pylori*, inflammatory bowel disease panels, or tissue transglutaminase immunoglobulin A [IgA]) are rarely used in critical care scenarios.
- Liver function tests (LFTs) are helpful evaluative tools for evaluating both prior and ongoing hepatocyte damage. Rising direct bilirubin levels may indicate biliary obstruction, whereas indirect hyperbilirubinemia may indicate hemolysis, hematoma resorption, hepatic congestion, or impaired conjugation.
- Tumor markers such as carcinoembryonic antigen (CEA) (colorectal) and CA 19-9 (pancreatic) may be helpful for initial diagnosis of a malignancy or monitoring for recurrence.

SUGGESTED READINGS

American College of Radiology. *ACR Appropriateness Criteria®: imaging of acute abdominal pain in the ICU setting*. https://www.acr.org/Clinical-Resources/ACR-Appropriateness-Criteria

Banks PA, Freeman ML; Practice Parameters Committee of the American College of Gastroenterology. Practice guidelines in acute pancreatitis. *Am J Gastroenterol*. 2006;101(10):2379-2400.

Droege ME, Rhoades AG, Droege CA, et al. Clinical experience, characteristics, and performance of an acetaminophen absorption test in critically ill patients. *Am J Ther*. 2023;30(2):e95-e102.

Howarth, Douglas. (2006). The Role of Nuclear Medicine in the Detection of Acute Gastrointestinal Bleeding. Seminars in nuclear medicine. 36. 133-46. 10.1053/j.semnuclmed.2005.11.001.

Kirkpatrick AW, Roberts DJ, De Waele J, et al. Intra-abdominal hypertension and the abdominal compartment syndrome: updated consensus definitions and clinical practice guidelines from the World Society of the Abdominal Compartment Syndrome. *Intensive Care Med*. 2013;39(7):1190-1206.

Kwo PY, Cohen SM, Lim JK. ACG clinical guideline: evaluation of abnormal liver chemistries. *Am J Gastroenterol*. 2017;112(1):18-35.

Laine L, Barkun AN, Saltzman JR, Martel M, Leontiadis GI. ACG clinical guideline: upper gastrointestinal and ulcer bleeding. *Am J Gastroenterol*. 2021;116(5):899-917.

Levine, M.S. (2006). Radiological Imaging of the Upper Gastrointestinal Tract. In: Faigel, D.O., Kochman, M.L. (eds) Endoscopic Oncology. Humana Press. https://doi.org/10.1007/978-1-59745-172-7_7

Mariani G, Boni G, Barreca M, Bellini M, Fattori B, AlSharif A, et al. Radionuclide gastroesophageal motor studies. J Nucl Med. 2004 Jun;45(6):1004-28.

Strate LL, Gralnek IM. ACG clinical guideline: management of patients with acute lower gastrointestinal bleeding. *Am J Gastroenterol*. 2016;111(5):755-764.

Tilsed JV, Casamassima A, Kurihara H, Mariani D, Martinez I, Pereira J, Ponchietti L, Shamiyeh A, Al-Ayoubi F, Barco LA, Ceolin M, D'Almeida AJ, Hilario S, Olavarria AL, Ozmen MM, Pinheiro LF, Poeze M, Triantos G, Fuentes FT, Sierra SU, Soreide K, Yanar H. ESTES guidelines: acute mesenteric ischaemia. Eur J Trauma Emerg Surg. 2016 Apr;42(2):253-70.

4.17

Pharmacologic Therapies for Gastrointestinal Disorders

Gianna Lauren Casal and Matthew Bartek

The organization of this section reflects commonly encountered gastrointestinal (GI) manifestations in the intensive care unit (ICU). The chapter is organized in tables based on disease process and options for pharmacologic management.

Nausea/Vomiting

- A multimodal strategy, combining agents acting on different neurochemical pathways, can provide superior symptom control and potentially reduce individual drug side effects.
- Aggressive fluid and electrolyte replacement are fundamental supportive measures.
- *See Table 4.17.1 for more detailed management.*

Dysmotility

- Highly prevalent in critically ill patients (up to 60%), particularly when on mechanical ventilation
- Can lead to complications like feeding intolerance, regurgitation, aspiration, pneumonia, fluid sequestration, delayed nutrient delivery, and bacterial translocation
- Contributing factors include sepsis and other inflammatory states, electrolytes, imbalances, and medication-induced dysmotility.
- Combination therapy can be synergistic.
- Dysmotility is common in critically ill patients and may manifest as feeding intolerance, ileus, or pseudo-obstruction.
- Pharmacologic therapy is directed at stimulating gut motility while addressing underlying contributing factors, such as electrolyte disturbances, hyperglycemia, and the use of opioids or sedatives.
- *See Table 4.17.2 for more detailed management.*

TABLE 4.17.1 Nausea/Vomiting

Drug Class	Mechanism of Action	Side Effects	Considerations
	Treatment		
5HT3 antagonists Ondansetron Olanzapine Metoclopramide	Antiserotonergic peripherally via vagus nerve and centrally via chemoreceptor trigger zone (CTZ)	• Headache • Constipation • QTc prolongation	
Dopamine antagonists Chlorpromazine Droperidol Haloperidol Prochlorperazine Olanzapine Metoclopramide	Antidopaminergic via CTZ	• Extrapyramidal symptoms • QTc prolongation • CNS depression	
Antihistamines Diphenhydramine Meclizine	Inhibit histamine and muscarinic receptors involved in emesis	• CNS depression	• Anticholinergic effects
Benzodiazepines Diazepam Lorazepam Midazolam	GABA-mediated reduction of serotonin and dopamine on CTZ	• CNS and respiratory depression • Hypotension	• Risk of delirium
Corticosteroid Dexamethasone	Inhibition of prostaglandin synthesis, reduced endogenous opioid release, decreased serotonin	• Hyperglycemia	
NK1 receptor antagonists Aprepitant Fosaprepitant	Inhibits substance P and neurokinin 1 receptors	• Fatigue • Diarrhea	• Augments antiemetic effect of corticosteroids and 5HT3 antagonists
Anticholinergics Scopolamine	Block acetylcholine from muscarinic receptors involved in central vomiting center and vestibular system	• Delirium • Urinary retention • Blurry vision • Diaphoresis • Constipation • Xerostomia	

CNS, central nervous system.

TABLE 4.17.2 Dysmotility

Drug	Mechanism of Action	Side Effects	Dosing
Metoclopramide	Dopamine antagonism in GIT, sensitizes GIT to acetylcholine	• Extrapyramidal symptoms • QTc prolongation	IV/PO: 5-10 mg bid-qid; 5 mg if CrCl < 40 mL/min
Erythromycin	Motilin receptor agonist	• QTc prolongation	IV: 3 mg/kg q8h PO: 250 mg erythromycin *base* q8h

bid, 2 times daily; CrCl, creatinine clearance; GIT, gastrointestinal tract; IV, intravenous; PO, oral; q, every; qid, 4 times daily.

Gastritis, Peptic Ulcer Disease, Stress Ulceration

- Management is focused on the prevention of stress ulceration in the ICU.
- Identify if patients have an indication for stress ulcer prophylaxis.
  - Risk factors for the development of ulcers include mechanical ventilation >48 hours and coagulopathy (defined by thrombocytopenia, elevated international normalized ratio [INR], or elevated partial thromboplastin time [PTT]).
  - Other well-documented risk factors include traumatic brain injury/spinal cord injury, high-dose steroids, shock states, and chronic liver failure.
- Critically ill patients receiving enteral nutrition, including tube feeds (and on mechanical ventilation), have shown no difference in incidence of GI bleed when comparing patients receiving stress ulcer prophylaxis to patients receiving placebo/no prophylaxis, but did find a higher incidence of pneumonia in patients receiving stress ulcer prophylaxis.
- For stress ulcer prophylaxis: use the lowest dose for the shortest duration of time; inappropriate continuation leading to long-term side effects and outcomes has been well documented.
- *See Table 4.17.3 for more detailed management.*

Constipation

- Common complication in the ICU, affecting up to 85% of patients.
- Multifactorial arising from shock, the use of sedatives and opioids, and electrolyte and dietary changes
- *See Table 4.17.4 for more detailed management.*

Diarrhea

- Ensure workup of etiology as antidiarrheal can worsen certain processes, especially infectious.
- *See Table 4.17.5 for more detailed management.*

Upper Gastrointestinal Bleed

- Upper GI bleeding is managed with prompt resuscitation, early endoscopic evaluation, and adjunctive pharmacologic therapy.
  - In patients with suspected variceal bleeding, vasoactive agents (eg, octreotide) and prophylactic antibiotics are started empirically.
- Management of coagulopathy or reversal of anticoagulation may be necessary at the time of suspected upper GI bleed.
- Pharmacologic therapy should be combined with endoscopic and resuscitative measures, as no drug alone is definitive therapy.
- *See Table 4.17.6 for more detailed management.*

TABLE 4.17.3 Gastritis, Peptic Ulcer Disease, Stress Ulceration

Drug Class	Mechanism of Action	Side Effects	Considerations
Histamine 2 receptor antagonists Famotidine Ranitidine	Reversibly binds H_2 receptors on gastric parietal cells inhibiting production and secretion of gastric acid	• Agitation • Thrombocytopenia	• May reduce absorption of drugs requiring acidic environment (ART, transplant medications, levothyroxine) • Use lowest dose for shortest duration
Proton pump inhibitors Esomeprazole Lansoprazole Omeprazole Pantoprazole	Irreversibly bind H^+/K^+-ATPase pump, which inhibits gastric acid secretion	• *Clostridium difficile* • Electrolyte malabsorption • Osteoporosis • Pneumonia • Dementia • Kidney disease	
Antacids Aluminum hydroxide Calcium carbonate Magnesium oxide	Neutralize gastric acid	• Poor taste • Hypermagnesemia	• Caution in renal impairment • May reduce absorption of drugs requiring acidic environment (ART, transplant medications, levothyroxine)
Protectant Sucralfate	Complexes with positively charged proteins to form viscous adhesive that forms a protective layer against peptic acid, bile salts, and pepsin	• Generally well tolerated	

ART, antiretroviral therapy.

TABLE 4.17.4 Constipation

Drug	Mechanism of Action	Side Effects
Bulking agents Fiber Methylcellulose	Retain water in stool for optimizing volume and consistency	• Flatulence • Abdominal distension
Osmotics Polyethylene glycol Lactulose Magnesium	Luminal water binding	• Bloating
Lubricant Mineral oil	Decreases water absorption and lubricates intestine to facilitate passage	• Abdominal cramping • Oily leakage
Stimulant Bisacodyl Senna	Stimulate peristalsis and motility via intestinal mucosa	• Abdominal cramping
Softener Docusate	Incorporates water and fat at stool interface to soften	
Opioid-induced constipation		
Opioid antagonist Methylnaltrexone Naloxegol	Peripheral mu antagonist inhibits opioids binding in GIT and reducing motility.	• Risk of GI perforation with methylnaltrexone if known obstruction

GI, gastrointestinal.

TABLE 4.17.5 Diarrhea

Drug Class	Mechanism of Action	Side Effects
Cations Aluminum Bismuth	• Reduce fluid secretion into bowel • Antiinflammatory via inhibition of prostaglandin synthesis • Antimicrobial	• Dark stool
Opioids Loperamide Diphenoxylate Tincture of opium	• Inhibition of mu opioid receptor in GIT, resulting in peristalsis and increased gastric time	• QTc prolongation with loperamide
Somatostatin analogs Octreotide	• Inhibits gastric motility, pancreatic secretions, and intestinal absorption • Generally administered subcutaneously	• Can cause hyperglycemia and cholelithiasis
Anticholinergics Atropine Hyoscyamine	• Blocks acetylcholine from binding parasympathetic sites in smooth muscle	• See anticholinergic side effects above
Bile acid sequestrants	• Forms insoluble complex with bile acids for fecal excretion • Inhibit intestinal bile salt enterohepatic reuptake	• Malabsorption of fat-soluble vitamins/folate • Hypertriglyceridemia

GIT, gastrointestinal transit.

TABLE 4.17.6 Upper Gastrointestinal Bleed

Drug Class	Mechanism of Action	Considerations
Treatment of esophageal varices		
Somatostatin analogs Octreotide	• Vasoconstriction of splanchnic blood flow and reduced portal pressures	• Use primarily in esophageal varices as 50 μg bolus followed by continuous infusion 50 μg/h
Secondary prophylaxis of esophageal varices		
Beta-blockers Nadolol Propranolol	• Reduce portal pressure	• Esophageal varices
Treatment of upper GI bleed		
Proton pump inhibitors	See Gastritis	
Alternatives for upper GI bleed with refractory hemorrhagic shock		
Antifibrinolytics Aminocaproic acid Tranexamic acid (TXA)	• Inhibits proteolytic activity of plasmin and reversibly displaces plasminogen from fibrin leading to inhibition of fibrinolysis	• TXA in renal impairment can lead to seizures

GI, gastrointestinal.

SUGGESTED READINGS

Bugaev N, Bhattacharya B, Chiu WC, et al. Promotility agents for the treatment of ileus in adult surgical patients: a practice management guideline from the Eastern Association for the Surgery of Trauma. *J Trauma Acute Care Surg*. 2019;87(4):922-934.

Chang L, Chey WD, Imdad A, et al. American Gastroenterological Association-American College of Gastroenterology clinical practice guideline: pharmacological management of chronic idiopathic constipation. *Gastroenterology*. 2023;164(7):1086-1106.

Heckroth M, Luckett RT, Moser C, Parajuli D, Abell TL. Nausea and vomiting in 2021: a comprehensive update. *J Clin Gastroenterol*. 2021;55(4):279-299.

Huang HB, Jiang W, Wang CY, Qin HY, Du B. Stress ulcer prophylaxis in intensive care unit patients receiving enteral nutrition: a systematic review and meta-analysis. *Crit Care*. 2018;22(1):20.

Kaplan DE, Ripoll C, Thiele M, et al. AASLD practice guidance on risk stratification and management of portal hypertension and varices in cirrhosis. *Hepatology*. 2024;79(5):1180-1211.

Palmowski L, von Busch A, Unterberg M, et al. Timely cessation of proton pump inhibitors in critically ill patients impacts morbidity and mortality: a propensity score-matched cohort study. *Crit Care Med*. 2024;52(2):190-199.

Semrad CE. Approach to the patient with diarrhea and malabsorption. *Goldman's Cecil Medicine*. 2012;895-913.

4.18

Gastrointestinal and Abdominal Postoperative Management and Perioperative Complications

Matthew Elson and Jonathan Parks

Postoperative Management

- Traditionally, patients routinely kept NPO and on intravenous fluids until return of bowel function, on bedrest, and with tubes/drains in place for long periods
- Enhanced Recovery After Surgery (ERAS) protocols are now the standard of care in numerous subspecialties—reduce hospital length of stay and complications by 30% to 50%.
  - Allow patients to have carbohydrate-based drinks up to 2 hours prior to an operation instead of prolonged preoperative fasting
  - Focus on minimally invasive laparoscopic and robotic-assisted techniques, when able
  - Minimization of intraoperative and postoperative intravenous fluids
  - Avoidance and/or early removal of tubes/drains
  - Early postoperative mobilization
  - Ability to start oral (PO) intake on postoperative day zero, regardless of bowel function

Perioperative Complications

- Postoperative ileus/early postoperative bowel obstruction
  - Present with abdominal distention, nausea/vomiting, abdominal discomfort, and lack of bowel function
  - Risk factors include prolonged operative time, extensive bowel manipulation, bowel resection/anastomosis, narcotic use, and electrolyte abnormalities.
  - Ileus that occurs after initial return of bowel function may signal an intra-abdominal infection or anastomotic leak.
  - Diagnosis confirmed with plain abdominal radiograph or computed tomography (CT) scan.
  - Ileus often self-resolves within 2 to 4 days; sometimes requires decompression with a nasogastric tube.
  - Complete, high-grade mechanical obstruction requires reoperative intervention.
- Anastomotic leak
  - Risk factors include ischemia, technical error, tension, distal obstruction, infection, the emergent nature of the operation, malnutrition, and immunosuppression.
  - Can present with fever, abdominal pain, leukocytosis, or ileus and progress toward sepsis, shock, and peritonitis
  - Abdominal CT with PO contrast is most commonly used for diagnosis in hemodynamically stable patients.
  - Small, contained leaks in stable patients can be managed with bowel rest, antibiotics, and radiologically guided drain placement.
  - Unstable patients require operative intervention.
- Stoma complications
  - If not properly sited, can be bothersome to patients when it sits within a skin fold or along the pant line
  - Dehydration and electrolyte abnormalities can result from high ostomy output.
  - Skin irritation/dermatitis if ostomy appliance not fitted properly
  - Stoma retraction if bowel is under tension when brought up to the abdominal wall
  - Stoma necrosis from compromised blood supply during ostomy creation—mild ischemia may only result in mucosal sloughing/duskiness, but requires reoperation if necrosis goes down past the level of the fascia
  - Stomal prolapse often worrisome to patients but does not require intervention if bowel is reducible.
  - Parastomal hernias can result in bowel obstruction, incarceration, and strangulation.
- Surgical site infection
  - Classified as superficial (skin, subcutaneous tissue), deep (fascia, muscle), and organ space infections
  - *Staph aureus* is the most common pathogen.
  - Incidence related to the level of surgical wound contamination and the presence of risk factors such as obesity, diabetes, and smoking
  - Increases the risk of other complications, such as hernia formation and fascial dehiscence
  - Superficial infections can often be treated simply by opening the incision, but deeper infections may require antibiotics and operative debridement.
  - Prophylactic antibiotic dosing prior to skin incision is frequently used for prevention.
- Seroma/hematoma
  - Seromas are sterile collections of clear, serous fluid; often result when dead space within the operative field not properly reapproximated, such as during flap creation; small collections can be observed, but larger collections and ones that become infected require drainage.
  - Hematomas are more prone to infection; often result from inadequate hemostasis or the use of antiplatelet/anticoagulant medications postoperatively; can often be observed but may require intervention if expanding, causing hemodynamic instability, if infected, or causing necrosis of the overlying skin.
- Wound dehiscence
  - Separation of the *fascial* layers of an incision
  - Can be related to technical errors in closure, fascial ischemia/necrosis, wound infection, malnutrition, immunosuppression, and abdominal distention
  - Can present as a sudden rush of salmon-colored fluid from the incision, often with a ripping sensation; evisceration of abdominal contents makes the diagnosis obvious
  - A small dehiscence can be managed conservatively, but larger ones require operative intervention, ensuring any infection is adequately treated; bowel evisceration is a surgical emergency.

- Enterocutaneous fistula (ECF)
  - One of the most dreaded complications for both surgeons and patients
  - Represent an abnormal connection between the gastrointestinal mucosa and the skin
  - Often results after a missed bowel injury, anastomotic leak, or technical error when closing an incision
  - Risk factors include the presence of a foreign body, radiation, infection, inflammatory bowel disease, neoplasia, distal obstruction, and steroid use.
  - The key points of initial management include control of sepsis, dehydration, and electrolyte abnormalities, along with wound care for skin protection and effluent measurement.
  - Low-output fistulas (<500 mL/d) can often be managed expectantly and frequently close with time.
  - High-output fistulas can require prolonged bowel rest (NPO), nutrition supplementation with total parental nutrition (TPN), administration of somatostatin analogues such as octreotide to reduce secretions, and even delayed operative repair (>6 months).

SUGGESTED READINGS

Dawes AJ, Gahagan JV. Stoma complications. *Clin Colon Rectal Surg*. 2023;37(6):387-397.

Ljungqvist O, Scott M, Fearon KC. Enhanced recovery after surgery: a review. *JAMA Surg*. 2017;152(3):292-298.

Scarborough JE, Mantyh CR, Sun Z, Migaly J. Combined mechanical and oral antibiotic bowel preparation reduces incisional surgical site infection and anastomotic leak rates after elective colorectal resection. *Ann Surg*. 2015;262(2):331-337.

Seidelman JL, Mantyh CR, Anderson DJ. Surgical site infection prevention: a review. *JAMA*. 2023;329(3):244-252.

Townsend JCM, Beauchamp RD, Evers BM, Mattox KL. Surgical complications. In: Townsend CM Jr, Beauchamp RD, Evers BM, Mattox KL, eds. *Sabiston Textbook of Surgery*. 20th ed. Elsevier; 2016.

SECTION 5

Renal

Section Editor: Edward A. Bittner

5.1

Acute Kidney Injury

John Bryant and Christina Anne Jelly

Definition

- Increase in serum creatinine (Cr) ≥0.3 mg/dL within 48 hours
- Increase in serum Cr ≥1.5 × baseline, which is known or presumed to have occurred within the prior 7 days
- Urine output (UOP) <0.5 mL/kg/h for 6 hours (Table 5.1.1)
- Several definitions have been proposed by national and international societies to define acute kidney injury (AKI). It is important to understand the differences and potential pitfalls of commonly used definitions.
    - RIFLE (Risk, Injury, Failure, Loss of kidney function, and End-stage kidney disease): one of the early definitions (2004) that grades severity based on UOP and serum Cr. Studies have shown that patients in all of the RIFLE classifications have higher mortality than intensive care unit (ICU) patients without AKI.
    - AKIN (Acute Kidney Injury Network): published in 2007. Unlike RIFLE criteria, AKIN does not require a baseline serum Cr to be used. However, stage III in AKIN staging can be variable based on local renal replacement therapy (RRT) practices. RIFLE and AKIN criteria have been shown to be diagnostically similar in ICU patients.
    - KDIGO (Kidney Disease Improving Global Outcomes): in an effort to consolidate guidelines, KDIGO, a global organization, proposed criteria in 2012, which encompass RIFLE and AKIN. KDIGO gives a specific timeline and simplifies the identification of patients with stage III AKI.
- UOP may better predict mortality in the ICU than serum Cr in AKI. The definition of AKI does not delineate the multiple etiologies that may cause AKI.

TABLE 5.1.1 Acute Dialysis Quality Initiative (ADQI) Criteria (Also Referred to as RIFLE Criteria)

Risk	Increase in serum creatinine ≥1.5 × baseline or decrease in GFR ≥25%	UOP <0.5 mL/kg/h × 6 h
Injury	Increase in serum creatinine ≥2.0 × baseline or decrease in GFR ≥50%	UOP <0.5 mL/kg/h × 12 h
Failure	Increase in serum creatinine ≥3.0 × baseline or decrease in GFR ≥75% OR absolute serum creatinine 4.0 mg/dL with an acute rise of at least 0.5 mg/dL	UOP <0.3 mL/kg/h × 24 h OR anuria × 12 h
Loss[a]	Complete loss of renal function >4 wk	Requiring RRT >4 wk
ESRD[a]	End-stage renal disease (>3 mo)	Requiring RRT >3 mo

ESRD, end-stage renal disease; GFR, glomerular filtration rate; RRT, renal replacement therapy; UOP, urine output.
[a]Loss and ESRD are excluded from certain studies as clinical outcomes rather than diagnostic criteria.

Epidemiology

- Affects 5% to 25% of patients in the ICU
- Median age 67
- Sepsis is the most common contributing condition, followed by major surgery, cardiogenic shock, hypovolemia, and medications.
- Causes can be divided into prerenal (due to renal hypoperfusion), intrinsic (disease of the renal parenchyma), or postrenal (collecting system obstruction)

Key Pathophysiology

- Renal blood flow (RBF)—at baseline ~1.1 L/min or ~20% of cardiac output
- Autoregulation maintains RBF (and therefore glomerular filtration rate [GFR]) remarkably stable at systolic body pressure (SBP) ranging from 90 to 200 mm Hg
- Myogenic = ↑ perfusion pressure causes ↑ stretch of smooth muscle in afferent arterioles, which causes smooth muscle contraction (calcium mediated), which results in ↑ resistance and ↓ RBF.
- Tubuloglomerular feedback = ↑ RBF causes ↑ delivery of sodium to the macula densa, which leads to the release of local vasoconstrictors (likely adenosine), which results in ↑ resistance and ↓ RBF.
- Sympathetic nervous system (SNS) = SNS activation (hemorrhage, surgery, etc) causes release of norepinephrine,

which causes renal vasoconstriction and mesangial cell contraction, which ↓ RBF > ↓ GFR.

- Renin-angiotensin = renin secretion is controlled by (1) intrarenal baroreceptors, (2) macula densa, (3) renal sympathetic nerves, and (4) beta-1 activation on granular cells. (Recall renin degrades angiotensinogen to angiotensin I, which is then converted to angiotensin II in the lung.)
  - Angiotensin II causes (1) vasoconstriction, (2) mesangial cell contraction, (3) aldosterone secretion, (4) increased thirst, (5) Na^+ reabsorption in the proximal tubule, and (6) antidiuretic hormone (ADH) secretion.

Differential Diagnosis

Prerenal	Intrinsic Renal			Postrenal
	Glomerular	TI	Vascular	
Hypovolemia (GI loss, Insensible loss, bleeding, diuretics, renal salt wasting)	Anti-GBM	ATN	Vasculitides	Nephrolithiasis
CHF	ANCA+ (MPAN, Churg-Strauss, granulomatosis with polyangiitis)	AIN	TTP/HUS	Obstructing clot
Cirrhosis	Immune complex/decreased complement (PSGN, SLE, MPGN, Cryo, shunt nephritis)	Drugs	Malignant HTN	Malignancy
Nephrotic Syndrome	Immune complex/normal complement (IgA nephropathy, HSP)	Crystalluria	Preeclampsia	Foley dysfunction
Sepsis		Contrast	Scleroderma	BPH
NSAIDs/COX-2 inhibitors		Multiple myeloma	Atheroembolic	Retroperitoneal fibrosis
ACEI/ARB		Sarcoid	Antiphospholipid antibody syndrome (APLS)	Postsurgical
Hypercalcemia (causing blunted ADH response and hypovolemia)		Rhabdomyolysis	Bilateral renal artery/vein thrombosis	Medications
Renal artery stenosis		Infection		
		TINU (tubulointerstitial nephritis and uveitis)		
		IgG4		

ACEI, angiotensin-converting enzyme inhibitor; AIN, acute interstitial nephritis; ANCA, antineutrophil cytoplasmic antibody; ARB, angiotensin receptor blocker; ATN, acute tubular necrosis; BPH, benign prostatic hyperplasia; CHF, congestive heart failure; COX-2, cyclooxygenase-2; GBM, glioblastoma multiforme; GI, gastrointestinal; HTN, hypertension; HUS, hemolytic uremic syndrome; IgG4, immunoglobulin G4; MPAN, mitochondrial membrane protein-associated neurodegeneration; MPGN, membranoproliferative glomerulonephritis; NSAIDs, nonsteroidal antiinflammatory drugs; PSGN, poststreptococcal glomerulonephritis; SLE, systemic lupus erythematosus; TTP, thrombotic thrombocytopenic purpura.

Diagnosis

History

- Exposure: hypotension, medications, intravenous (IV) contrast, transfusions
- Illness/injury: surgery, infection, illness, rash

Labs

- Blood urine nitrogen (BUN)/Cr
  - BUN rising out of proportion to Cr → prerenal, upper gastrointestinal bleeding (UGIB), sepsis, corticosteroids, tube feeds
  - Cr rising out of proportion to BUN → rhabdomyolysis
- Fractional excretion of sodium (FENa)
  - <1% = prerenal, contrast-induced nephropathy (CIN), pigment nephropathy
  - >2% = ATN
- FEBUN (more useful than FENa if concurrent diuretic use or chronic kidney disease [CKD])
  - <35% = prerenal
- Urine dipstick
  - 3+ protein = consider nephrotic syndrome
  - +Blood, 0 red blood cells (RBCs) = consider myoglobinuria
- Urine sediment
  - Muddy brown casts (epithelial cells) → ATN
  - RBC casts/dysmorphic RBC → glomerulonephritis (GN)
  - White blood cell (WBC) casts → AIN (or pyelonephritis)

Uniform standards for defining and classifying AKI have been developed by a multidisciplinary collaborative network and are summarized in Table 5.1.2.

Special Cases

- Creatine kinase (CK) → rhabdomyolysis (polytrauma, crush injury)
- Uric acid → tumor lysis (lymphoma, leukemia, metastatic cancer, eg, melanoma)
- Urine eosinophils >1% may suggest AIN (sensitivity 40%, specificity 72%, positive predictive value [PPV] 38%).
- Peripheral smear → if schistocytes, consider TTP

TABLE 5.1.2 Acute Kidney Injury Network (AKIN) Criteria

Stage 1	Increase in serum creatinine ≥0.3 mg/dL or increase ≥1.5-2-fold from baseline	UOP <0.5 mL/kg/h for >6 h
Stage 2	Increase in serum creatinine >2-2.99-fold from baseline	UOP <0.5 mL/kg/h for >12 h
Stage 3	Increase in serum creatinine to ≥3-fold from baseline or serum creatinine ≥4.0 mg/dL with an acute rise of at least 0.5 mg/dL or initiation of RRT	UOP <0.3 mL/kg/h for >24 h OR anuria for 12 h

Either serum creatinine or UOP criteria are sufficient to establish the diagnosis.
RRT, renal replacement therapy; UOP, urine output.

- Serum protein electrophoresis (SPEP) + serum free light chain (FLC) → evaluate for multiple myeloma (urine protein electrophoresis [UPEP] only adds minimal value in detection of amyloidosis)
- ANA, ANCA, anti-GBM, antistreptolysin O (ASLO), cryocrit, C3/C4 → glomerular disease
- Ultrasound → evaluate for hydronephrosis and/or chronicity of renal disease
- Electrolytes → monitor for need for RRT

Management and Treatment

- Optimize volume status
- Support hemodynamics
- Avoid nephrotoxins (contrast, NSAIDs, ACEI/ARB, calcineurin inhibitors, aminoglycosides, fleets enema)
- Renally dose all medications: antibiotics, opioids, heparin
- If serum Cr rises >1.5 mg/dL in 24 hours, assume estimated GFR (GFR) <15.
- RRT
  - One of the most critical decisions when managing AKI is the decision to initiate RRT. The most common criterion for RRT is severe oliguria or anuria, which is not responsive to diuretic therapy. Timing of RRT may be variable depending on institutional practice patterns.
  - Other indications for RRT include acidosis (pH <7.15), electrolyte abnormalities, toxin ingestion, volume overload, and uremia ("AEIOU").
  - Timing of initiation RRT (early vs late) is still being studied and is controversial. Two landmark randomized controlled trials of note (AKIKI and ELAIN) compared early versus late initiation of RRT. AKIKI showed no difference in mortality, while ELAIN did show early RRT reduced mortality in the first 90 days. It is important to note there were several differences studies, including sample size (larger in AKIKI), design (AKIKI multicenter vs single center in ELAIN), and definitions of early dialysis.

Treatment in Special Cases

- GN: methylprednisolone 0.5 to 1 g IV × 3 days ± cyclophosphamide or mycophenolate mofetil ± plasmapheresis
- Scleroderma renal crisis: titrate captopril to maximum tolerated dose
- TTP: plasma exchange (consult with blood bank)
- Rhabdomyolysis: IV fluid (±mannitol, ±bicarbonate = limited evidence)
- AIN: stop offending medications, consider steroids.
- Drug crystals: stop drug, alkalinize urine, fomepizole for ethylene glycol.
- Obstruction: alpha-antagonist, 5-alpha-reductase inhibitor, percutaneous nephrostomy

SUGGESTED READINGS

Gaudry S, Hajage D, Schortgen F, et al. Initiation strategies for renal-replacement therapy in the intensive care unit. *N Engl J Med*. 2016;375:122-133.

Mandelbaum T, Scott DJ, Lee J, et al. Outcome of critically ill patients with acute kidney injury using the AKIN criteria. *Crit Care Med*. 2011;39(12):2659-2664.

Perazella MA, Bomback AS. Urinary eosinophils in AIN: farewell to an old biomarker? *Clin J Am Soc Nephrol*. 2013;8(11):1841-1843.

Petejova N, Martinek A. Acute kidney injury due to rhabdomyolysis and renal replacement therapy: a critical review. *Crit Care*. 2014;18(3):224.

Pickkers P, Darmon M, Hoste E, et al. Acute kidney injury in the critically ill: an updated review on pathophysiology and management. *Intensive Care Med*. 2021;47(8):835-850.

Zarbock A, Kellum JA, Schmidt C et al. Effect of early vs delayed initiation of renal replacement therapy on mortality in critically ill patients with acute kidney injury: the ELAIN randomized clinical trial. *JAMA*. 2016;315(20):2190-2199.

5.2

Infections of the Urinary Tract

Levi Zehr and Daniel W. Johnson

Definitions

- Uncomplicated urinary tract infection (UTI)
  - Localized to urethra/bladder: urethritis, acute simple cystitis
  - Features: dysuria, urinary urgency, urinary frequency, suprapubic pain
- Complicated UTI
  - Infection beyond bladder: prostatitis, upper urinary tract, pyelonephritis, perinephric abscess
  - Features: fever, chills, rigors, significant fatigue or malaise, flank pain, costovertebral angle tenderness on examination, pelvic/perineal pain in men (prostatitis)
- Catheter-associated urinary tract infection (CAUTI)
  - IDSA criteria: urethral/suprapubic/condom catheter used in past the 48 hours AND UTI signs or symptoms AND bacteriuria (≥1,000 CFU/mL) AND no other source of infection
- Intensive care unit (ICU)-acquired UTI
  - Symptoms and positive urine cultures (≤2 species) at ≥48 hours of ICU admission

Epidemiology

- Overall: *Escherichia coli* (75%-95%), *Proteus mirabilis*, *Klebsiella pneumoniae*, *Staphylococcus saprophyticus*, rarely *Staphylococcus aureus*
- ICU setting
  - *E. coli* 24%, *P. aeruginosa* 10%, *Klebsiella* spp. 10%, *Enterococcus* spp. 10%, *P. mirabilis* 4%, *Staphylococcus* spp. 4%
  - Incidence 10% to 25%. Bacteriuria incidence 3% to 8% per catheter day, 25% develop CAUTI
  - <1% of CAUTIs progress to bacteremia.
  - *Candida* spp. removed from UTI definition, treatment advised if multisite cultures

Key Pathophysiology

- Ascending urethral bacterial colonization and migration, pili and flagella, biofilm and immune system evasion, damage to epithelium and tissues with toxins and proteases
- CAUTI uropathogens
  - 2/3 ascend urethral-catheter space (~80% for Gram-positive cocci [GPC], ~55% for Gram-negative cocci [GNR]) versus 1/3 ascend catheter lumen. Biofilm formation can limit immune and antibiotic clearance.

Management and Treatment

- Urinalysis (UA): pyuria (white blood cell [WBC] >10/mm^3) very sensitive unless neutropenic, positive nitrites 100% specific, WBC casts suggest renal involvement.
- Urine culture (often with >100,000 CFU/mL)
- Ultrasound (US) if urinary obstruction suspected
- Computed tomography (CT) of the abdomen/pelvis wo/w intravenous (IV) contrast if suspected nephrolithiasis and/or obstruction
- Uncomplicated UTI
  - Nitrofurantoin, trimethoprim-sulfamethoxazole (TMP-SMX), fosfomycin
- Complicated UTI
  - Inadequate response after 48 to 72 hours of antibiotics: investigate for infectious complications and abnormal anatomy.
  - Agent/duration adjusted for presenting illness severity, comorbidities, local resistance patterns. Narrow based on
  - Oral, inpatient: fluoroquinolone
  - IV, inpatient
    - Standard spectrum: third-generation cephalosporin, fluoroquinolone
    - Broad spectrum: fourth-generation cephalosporin, extended-spectrum penicillin, carbapenem
    - Critically ill: antipseudomonal carbapenem plus vancomycin
- CAUTI
  - Replace catheter followed by urine culture, pyuria is nondiagnostic.
  - 7 to 14 days for symptomatic and/or complicated, longer if fever persists >72 hours
  - Prevent by limiting catheter days

SUGGESTED READINGS

American College of Radiology. *ACR Appropriateness Criteria®: acute pyelonephritis*. Accessed June 25, 2024. https://acsearch.acr.org/docs/69489/Narrative/

Gupta K, Hooton TM, Naber KG, et al; Infectious Diseases Society of America; European Society for Microbiology and Infectious Diseases. International clinical practice guidelines for the treatment of acute uncomplicated cystitis and pyelonephritis in women: a 2010 update by the Infectious Diseases Society of America and the European Society for Microbiology and Infectious Diseases. *Clin Infect Dis*. 2011;52(5):e103-e120.

Hooton TM, Bradley SF, Cardenas DD, et al. Diagnosis, prevention, and treatment of catheter-associated urinary tract infection in adults: 2009 International Clinical Practice Guidelines from the Infectious Diseases Society of America. *Clin Infect Dis*. 2010;50(5):625-663.

Patel PK, Advani SD, Kofman AD, et al. Strategies to prevent catheter-associated urinary tract infections in acute-care hospitals: 2022 update. *Infect Control Hosp Epidemiol*. 2023;44(8):1209-1231.

Weiner LM, Webb AK, Limbago B, et al. Antimicrobial-resistant pathogens associated with healthcare-associated infections: summary of data reported to the National Healthcare Safety Network at the Centers for Disease Control and Prevention, 2011-2014. *Infect Control Hosp Epidemiol*. 2016;37(11):1288-1301.

5.3

Acid-Base Physiology and Disorders

Lukas H. Matern

Diagnosis of Primary Acid-Base Disorders

- The diagnosis of acid-base disorders can often be simplified to three steps:
  1. Identify the primary acid-base disturbance.
  2. Check for compensation.
  3. Assess for secondary acid-base disorders.
- Arterial blood pH is tightly regulated between 7.35 and 7.45 in healthy, nonpregnant adults.
- Abnormalities of arterial blood pH are defined as follows:
  - pH <7.35 indicates acidemia, representing the accumulation of acids (including carbon dioxide) and/or the loss of bicarbonate.
  - pH >7.45 indicates alkalemia, representing a loss of normal acids (including carbon dioxide) and/or abnormal retention of bicarbonate.
- If acidemia (pH <7.35) is present:
  - An arterial carbon dioxide tension ($Paco_2$) >40 mm Hg indicates a primary respiratory acidosis.
    - The acuity or chronicity of respiratory acid-base disorders may be determined by assessing the degree of metabolic compensation via renal bicarbonate handling (see next section).
  - A serum bicarbonate concentration ($[HCO_3^-]$) <24 mEq/L indicates a primary metabolic acidosis.
- If alkalemia (pH >7.45) is present:
  - $Paco_2$ <40 mm Hg indicates a primary respiratory alkalosis.
  - $[HCO_3^-]$ >24 mEq/L indicates a primary metabolic alkalosis.

Formulae for Compensatory Changes

- Respiratory acidosis (assuming intact renal function)
  - If acute:
    - pH change: Δ $Paco_2$ + 10 mm Hg $\rightarrow$ Δ pH − 0.08
    - Metabolic compensation: Δ $Paco_2$ + 10 mm Hg $\rightarrow$ Δ $[HCO_3^-]$ + 1 mEq/L
  - If chronic:
    - pH change: Δ $Paco_2$ + 10 mm Hg $\rightarrow$ Δ pH − 0.03
    - Metabolic compensation: Δ $Paco_2$ + 10 mm Hg $\rightarrow$ Δ $[HCO_3^-]$ + 4 mEq/L
- Respiratory alkalosis (assuming intact renal function)
  - If acute:
    - pH change: Δ $Paco_2$ − 10 mm Hg $\rightarrow$ Δ pH + 0.08
    - Metabolic compensation: Δ $Paco_2$ − 10 mm Hg $\rightarrow$ Δ $[HCO_3^-]$ − 2 mEq/L
  - If chronic:
    - pH change: Δ $Paco_2$ − 10 mm Hg $\rightarrow$ Δ pH + 0.03
    - Metabolic compensation: Δ $Paco_2$ − 10 mm Hg $\rightarrow$ Δ $[HCO_3^-]$ − 5 mEq/L
- Metabolic acidosis (assuming spontaneous ventilation)
  - pH change: Δ $[HCO_3^-]]$ − 6 mEq/L $\rightarrow$ Δ pH − 0.10
  - Respiratory compensation: Δ $Paco_2$ = 1.5 • Δ $[HCO_3^-]$ + 8 ± 2
    - This key relationship is called the Winters formula.
    - Respiratory compensation is limited by physical fitness and central nervous system function.
- Metabolic alkalosis (assuming spontaneous ventilation)
  - pH change: Δ $[HCO_3^-]$ + 6 mEq/L $\rightarrow$ Δ pH + 0.10
  - Respiratory compensation: Δ $[HCO_3^-]$ + 1 mEq/L $\rightarrow$ $Paco_2$ + 0.7 mm Hg
    - Compensatory hypoventilation may be limited beyond $Paco_2$ >55 mm Hg.

Diagnosing Secondary Acid-Base Disorders

- Any significant mismatch between the degree of pH disturbance and compensatory changes should prompt evaluation for secondary acid-base disorders.
  - For example, inadequate respiratory compensation for a metabolic acidosis (ie, $Paco_2$ elevated relative to the expected value) suggests a secondary respiratory acidosis (eg, due to altered mental status or respiratory muscle fatigue).
- Different forms of metabolic acidosis can be characterized based on the anion gap (AG), which may also uncover secondary acid-base disorders.
  - AG = $[Na^+]$ − $[HCO_3^-]$ − $[Cl^-]$
  - A normal AG is around 12 mEq/L, whereas an elevated AG is often defined as >16 mEq/L.
  - If the AG is elevated—even in the presence of alkalemia—an AG metabolic acidosis must be present, indicating the accumulation of abnormal acids (eg, lactate, ketones) in the blood.
  - The AG must be corrected upward by 2.5 mEq/L for every 1 g/dL decrease in measured serum albumin below 4 g/dL.
- If AG ≤16 in the setting of a metabolic acidosis, the patient is said to have a non-AG (or normal AG) metabolic acidosis.
  - A non-AG metabolic acidosis is generally due to abnormal wasting or depletion of serum bicarbonate.
- If the patient has an AG metabolic acidosis, correct the measured serum bicarbonate for the AG to detect additional "buried" metabolic disorders.
  - Corrected $[HCO_3^-]$ = (AG − 12) + measured $[HCO_3^-]$
    - If the corrected $[HCO_3^-]$ >26 mEq/L, a concurrent metabolic alkalosis is present.
    - If the corrected $[HCO_3^-]$ <22 mEq/L, a concurrent non-AG metabolic acidosis is present.
    - If the corrected $[HCO_3^-]$ =22 to 26 mEq/L, an isolated AG metabolic acidosis is likely.
  - Other formulae, such as the gap-gap or Δ/Δ quotient, function interchangeably with the equation for corrected bicarbonate.

Determining the Causes of Acid-Base Disorders

- Goal in respiratory acidosis: determine why the patient is hypoventilating.
  - Common causes: altered mental status (eg, sedation, encephalopathy, neurologic injury), obstructive lung disease, mechanical airway obstruction, and restrictive lung disease (eg, interstitial lung disease, splinting, phrenic nerve injury)
  - A respiratory acidosis may also be exacerbated in hypermetabolic states (eg, fever), in which the production of CO_2 is augmented.
- Goal in respiratory alkalosis: determine why the patient is hyperventilating.
  - Common causes: anxiety, pain, sepsis, liver disease, pregnancy, iatrogenic hyperventilation, pulmonary embolism, and salicylate toxicity
- Goal in AG metabolic acidosis: determine which abnormal acids are accumulating.
  - Consider the MUDPILES mnemonic: methanol ingestion, uremia, diabetic ketoacidosis, propylene glycol administration or paraldehyde toxicity, isoniazid use, lactic acidosis, ethylene glycol ingestion, and salicylate toxicity.
    - Also consider metformin bioaccumulation and rhabdomyolysis, which are associated with lactic acidosis.
    - Ethanol toxicity may cause both lactic acidosis and ketoacidosis.
    - States of starvation may be associated with ketoacidosis, which can be exacerbated by certain drugs (eg, sodium-glucose cotransporter 2 [SGLT-2] inhibitors).
  - Consider checking lactate, serum ketones (eg, beta-hydroxybutyrate), urine toxicology, renal function tests, and salicylate levels.
  - Calculation of the osmolal gap may be helpful in detecting abnormal osmolytes, which may suggest certain toxic ingestions.
    - Osmolal gap = measured serum osmolality − $(2 \cdot [Na^+] + \text{glucose}/18 + \text{BUN}/2.8)$ (where BUN is blood urea nitrogen)
    - If the osmolal gap is >10 mOsm/kg, assess for toxic alcohols (eg, ethanol, methanol, or ethylene glycol).
- Goal in non-AG metabolic acidosis: determine how the patient is losing bicarbonate and/or retaining chloride.
  - Common causes: hyperalimentation, adrenal insufficiency, renal tubular acidosis (RTA), diarrhea, acetazolamide use, spironolactone use, and excess saline administration
  - Calculate the urine anion gap (UAG) to further pinpoint causes of bicarbonate loss.
  - $UAG = [Na^+]_{urine} + [K^+]_{urine} - [Cl^-]_{urine}$
    - UAG <0 mEq/L indicates extrarenal and especially intestinal causes (eg, diarrhea or enterocutaneous fistulae).
    - UAG >0 mEq/L indicates renal causes (especially RTA type 1 or 4).
- Goal in metabolic alkalosis: determine why the patient is retaining bicarbonate and/or losing chloride.
  - Assess volume status, blood pressure, and urine chloride concentration ($[Cl^-]_{urine}$).
  - Elevated blood pressure and hypervolemia may be more suggestive of saline-unresponsive processes (eg, hyperaldosteronism), which often manifest with evidence of volume retention.
    - Conversely, hypovolemia may occur in saline-responsive etiologies or iatrogenic "contraction" alkalosis (especially from overdiuresis).
  - $[Cl^-]_{urine}$ <20 mEq/L suggests a saline-responsive etiology, which may sometimes be accompanied by relative hypochloremia.
    - The differential may include hyperemesis, excess nasogastric tube suctioning, diuretic use, and posthypercapnia syndrome.
  - $[Cl^-]_{urine}$ >20 mEq/L suggests a saline-unresponsive etiology.
    - The differential may include states of excess mineralocorticoid (Conn syndrome, Cushing disease, exogenous steroid use), licorice ingestion, Liddle syndrome, Bartter or Gitelman syndromes, milk-alkali syndrome, and laxative abuse.

Treatment Approaches

- Treatment goal in respiratory acidosis: support ventilation to remove accumulated $Paco_2$.
  - Provide ventilatory assistance with an increased minute ventilation.
    - If mechanical ventilation is inadequate or ineffective, consider a trial of extracorporeal CO_2 removal.
  - Treat pain interfering with effective ventilation (eg, consider placement of an epidural or regional anesthetic for rib fractures).
  - Treat restrictive lung disease as able (eg, drain large pleural effusions).
  - Provide diuresis for pulmonary edema.
  - Of note, a buffer such as tromethamine (THAM) may aid in temporizing a severe respiratory acidosis.
    - Bicarbonate administration is not recommended, as it may increase $Paco_2$ via carbonic anhydrase-mediated interconversion of HCO_3^- with CO_2.
- Treatment goal in respiratory alkalosis: remove reversible stimuli causing hyperventilation.
  - Treat pain and anxiety (eg, administer benzodiazepines for a panic episode).
  - Correct any associated hypoxemia.
  - Avoid iatrogenic overventilation.
- Treatment goals in metabolic acidosis: stop the production or accumulation of abnormal acids and/or restore serum bicarbonate.
  - If the AG is elevated, identify and correct the underlying acid-generating process.
    - Supportive renal replacement therapy may be needed for profound acidemia, severe toxidromes, or symptomatic uremia.
    - Sodium bicarbonate administration is not recommended in most patients with an AG metabolic acidosis (see later).
  - If the AG is normal, consider repleting bicarbonate while addressing causes of bicarbonate loss.
- Treatment goals in metabolic alkalosis: restore correct volume imbalances, administer saline, and/or prevent further bicarbonate retention.

- If $[Cl^-]_{urine}$ <20 mEq/L (saline-responsive), give saline while repleting K^+ as needed.
- If $[Cl^-]_{urine}$ >20 mEq/L (saline-unresponsive), consider a trial of spironolactone to counteract possible mineralocorticoid excess.
  - If a contraction alkalosis appears likely, consider a diuretic holiday or the addition of acetazolamide.
- Important notes on sodium bicarbonate administration in acidosis:
  - Sodium bicarbonate may transiently elevate serum pH, but it is associated with physiologic adverse effects including:
    - Rebound alkalemia after correction of the underlying acidosis
    - Reduced cardiac contractility due to intracellular acidosis and hypocalcemia
    - Impaired oxygen delivery due to a leftward shift of the oxyhemoglobin dissociation curve
    - Hypernatremia or volume overload, depending on the concentration and volume of bicarbonate infused
  - Unless the patient has a non-AG metabolic acidosis, it is prudent to reserve bicarbonate boluses for patients with critical acidemia and refractoriness to catecholamine vasopressors.
    - The BICAR-ICU trial concluded that bicarbonate infusions may reduce mortality and avert the need for renal replacement therapy in a small subgroup of patients with severe metabolic acidosis and renal impairment.
  - If bicarbonate repletion is indicated, the arterial base deficit may be used to guide administration using the estimated bicarbonate space.
    - The bicarbonate space is defined as the percentage of total body water (in liters, equal to total body weight in kilograms) into which a bolus of sodium bicarbonate will distribute, usually 20% to 40%.
    - Thus: bicarbonate dose required = base deficit • total body water • bicarbonate space
    - Incremental dosing of bicarbonate guided by repeated blood gas analysis is a prudent approach.

Strong Ion Difference/Stewart Model

- Stewart derived three independent variables to explain acid-base physiology based on blood plasma:
  - Strong ion difference (SID)
    - Strong ions are derived from compounds that fully dissociate at physiologic pH.
    - The SID is the difference between the sum of the concentrations of all dissociated cations and all dissociated anions and is roughly equal to 40 mEq/L.
    - $SID = [Na^+] + [K^+] + [Ca^{2+}] + [Mg^{2+}] - [Cl^-] - [Xa^-]$
    - SID can be approximated as $[Na^+] + [K^+] - [Cl^-]$, where $[Xa^-]$ represents other unmeasured strong anions.
  - Weak acids $[A_{tot}^-]$
    - Strong acids [HB] completely dissociate at physiologic pH into $[H^+]$ and $[B^-]$.
    - Weak acids [HA] only partially dissociate into $[H^+]$ and $[A^-]$.
    - The sum of the concentrations of these weak acids is represented as $[A_{tot}^-]$.
    - These compounds represent the buffer activity of the system, including proteins (primarily albumin), sulfates, and phosphates.
  - $Paco_2$
    - Links the metabolic and respiratory processes where dissolved plasma CO_2 is regulated by ventilation
- In this model, $[H^+]$ and pH are dependent variables derived from the abovementioned independent variables (primarily SID).
- Deficit or excess of water in plasma will concentrate or dilute the strong cations and anions equally and, therefore, increase or reduce the SID.

❑ ***This model may more effectively account for acidosis (excess of unmeasured anions such as lactate or ketones) that would otherwise be obscured by the alkalinizing effect of hypoalbuminemia (deficit of weak acid) commonly seen in intensive care unit (ICU) patients but is not commonly used, nor has it been shown to affect clinical outcomes.***

  - This model also does not account for the hemoglobin concentration since its only example is the plasma.
- Clinical application
  - Metabolic alkalosis
    - Low $[A_{tot}^-]$
  - Decreased albumin: from critical illness, cirrhosis, or nephrotic syndrome
    - High SID
  - Increased $[Na^+]$
    - Decreased water in plasma or concentration alkalosis
    - Excess mineralocorticoid (Conn, Cushing, steroids, licorice, Liddle, Bartter, Gitelman)
    - Milk-alkali syndrome
    - Refeeding syndrome/total parenteral nutrition (TPN)
  - Decreased $[Cl^-]$
    - Vomiting
    - Diuretics
    - Nasogastric loss tube (NGT) losses
  - Metabolic acidosis
    - Low SID
  - Increased $[Cl^-]$ from NaCl infusion (hyperchloremic acidosis)
  - Decreased $[Na^+]$ from increased water in plasma or dilutional acidosis
  - High $[A_{tot}^-]$
  - Increased organic acids (lactate, ketones, formate, salicylate), sulfates, albumin, or phosphates
    - Check the strong ion gap (SIG)
  - $SIG = SID_{app} - SID_{eff} = [Xa^-]$
  - SID_{app} = Apparent SID = $[Na^+] + [K^+] + [Ca^{2+}] + [Mg^{2+}] - [Cl^-]$
  - SID_{eff} = Effective SID = $[protein] + [PO_3^4] + [HCO_3^-]$
    - SIG >0
      - ❑ Increase in unaccounted anions (lactate, ketones, formate, methanol, salicylates)
    - SIG = 0
      - ❑ Increased $[Cl^-]$ secondary to NaCl infusion, RTA
  - Respiratory alkalosis and acidosis: given $Paco_2$ is an independent variable.

SUGGESTED READINGS

Achanti A, Szerlip HM. Acid-base disorders in the critically ill patient. *Clin J Am Soc Nephrol*. 2023;18(1):102-112.

Al-Jaghbeer M, Kellum JA. Acid-base disturbances in intensive care patients: etiology, pathophysiology and treatment. *Nephrol Dial Transplant*. 2015;30(7):1104-1111.

Jaber S, Paugam C, Futier E, et al. Sodium bicarbonate therapy for patients with severe metabolic acidaemia in the intensive care unit (BICAR-ICU): a multicentre, open-label, randomised controlled, phase 3 trial. *Lancet*. 2018;392(10163):2440.

5.4

Renal Replacement Therapy

Luke Tseng and Edward A. Bittner

Overview

- Encompasses a variety of techniques used to substitute renal function in the setting of acute kidney injury (AKI), most commonly acute tubular necrosis (ATN), or chronic kidney disease (CKD)
- Most important functions are solute clearance and volume removal.
- AKI requiring renal replacement therapy (RRT) may be associated with mortality >50%.

Convection Versus Diffusion

- RRT modalities may use either one or both mechanisms.
- Both convection and diffusion involve blood passing through a filter that contains a semipermeable membrane.
- The fluid that leaves the filter is termed *ultrafiltrate* or *effluent*.
- Convection
  - The primary mechanism for hemofiltration-based modalities
  - Transmembrane pressure drives bulk water movement across the membrane from a high-pressure blood compartment to a low-pressure ultrafiltrate compartment.
  - Bulk water movement drags solutes along with it to clear solute from the blood, thus termed "solvent drag."
  - Effectively clears the blood of small molecules (eg, urea, electrolytes), "middle molecules" (eg, cytokines), and volume
  - Due to clearance of proinflammatory cytokines, there is a theoretical benefit in sepsis; notably, the literature has not shown any benefit for initiating RRT for the sole purpose of accelerating resolution of sepsis.
  - The lost blood volume from bulk water movement will need to be replaced with replacement fluid to maintain fluid balance.
- Diffusion
  - The primary mechanism for hemodialysis-based modalities
  - In the filter, dialysate fluid runs countercurrent to blood flow.
  - Solute is cleared as it diffuses along its concentration gradient from the blood compartment to the dialysate/ultrafiltrate compartment.
  - Results in solute clearance with minimal change in blood volume

Modalities

- Intermittent hemodialysis (IHD)
  - Typically used in the outpatient setting for patients with CKD or for inpatients who are hemodynamically stable
  - Requires a specialized dialysis nurse
  - Uses diffusion to clear solute; ultrafiltration can be used to remove volume
  - Administered in short sessions, 3 to 6 hours per session, 3 to 4 times per week.
  - Higher blood flow rates, 350 to 400 mL/min
  - Allows for quick, efficient clearance of solutes and toxins
  - Clearance is related to blood flow rate.
  - Less effective for volume removal, since volume reaccumulates between sessions
  - Quick and efficient solute clearance can lead to significant fluid shifts, hemodynamic instability, and disequilibrium syndrome from cerebral edema.
- Continuous renal replacement therapy (CRRT)
  - Used in the intensive care unit (ICU) to provide RRT for patients who are hemodynamically unstable
  - Can be operated by a trained bedside nurse
  - Lower blood flow rates, 100 to 250 mL/min
  - Clearance is related to effluent flow rate—the sum of ultrafiltrate fluid driven by convection and the dialysate flow rate (if being used).
  - Three main types, none of which has been shown to be superior—continuous venovenous hemofiltration (CVVH), continuous venovenous hemodialysis (CVVHD), and continuous venovenous hemodiafiltration (CVVHDF)
  - CVVH
    - Relies on convection to clear solute (via solvent drag) and volume
    - Relatively high amount of convection is required to clear solute, so replacement fluid is administered to replace volume losses.
      - Replacement fluid approximates physiologic electrolyte balance.
      - Different formulations may differ in specific electrolyte levels, such as potassium and phosphate (eg, PrismaSol has 4K, 2K, or 0K options; Phoxillum contains phosphate).
      - Replacement fluid can be administered prefilter or postfilter.

- Prefilter: dilutes blood entering filter, which reduces the risk of filter clotting but may make clearance less efficient
- Postfilter: allows for more efficient solute clearance but increases the risk of filter clotting due to hemoconcentration as blood passes through the filter
  - Net negative fluid balance can be achieved by administering less replacement fluid than the effluent flow rate (ie, fluid that is lost during ultrafiltration); thus, the net ultrafiltration rate determines fluid balance.
- CVVHD
  - Relies on diffusion to clear solute; there is a countercurrent flow of dialysate fluid
  - Does not require replacement fluid
- CVVHDF
  - Combines CVVH and CVVHD
  - Uses both dialysate fluid and replacement fluid
- Slow continuous ultrafiltration (SCUF)
  - A special form of CRRT that uses convection at low blood and effluent flow rates to enable gentle volume removal
  - No replacement fluid is used; volume is removed, but solute is not efficiently cleared.
  - Used when volume overload is the only issue
- Prolonged intermittent renal replacement therapy (PIRRT)
  - These are hybrid forms of RRT that may be used for critically ill patients in centers without access to CRRT.
  - Typically involves dialysis being performed for 6 to 12 hours per session, 4 to 7 times a week
  - Examples include slow low-efficiency daily dialysis (SLEDD) and sustained low-efficiency dialysis (SLED).
  - Accelerated venovenous hemofiltration (AVVH)
    - A hybrid modality that is used at Massachusetts General Hospital (MGH) to transition from CRRT to IHD
    - Sessions run for 8 to 10 hours at night.
    - Allows for more patient mobility during the day and a more gradual transition from CRRT to IHD as hemodynamic stability is achieved and maintained

Intermittent Hemodialysis Versus Continuous Renal Replacement Therapy

- CRRT is thought to be more hemodynamically tolerable in critically ill patients with hemodynamic instability and is recommended as first line for this population by KDIGO (Kidney Disease: Improving Global Outcomes).
- In patients who are hemodynamically stable or only requiring low-dose vasopressors, existing data suggest that there is no difference in mortality or renal recovery between IHD and CRRT.
- Of note, these data are of variable quality due to relatively small sample sizes in trials, inconsistent definitions of hypotension and hemodynamic instability, and frequent exclusion of patients with shock or high vasopressor requirements.
- In facilities with limited access to CRRT, it may also be reasonable to trial hybrid therapies, such as SLED.
- There is no strong data to suggest superiority of any single modality of CRRT—choice between CVVH versus CVVHD versus CVVHDF will likely depend on provider preference, institutional culture, and other patient-specific factors.
- CRRT is preferred to IHD in the setting of elevated intracranial pressure (see section "Indications").

Indications

- Classic urgent indications:
  - Refractory metabolic acidosis
    - Of note, lactic acid is poorly cleared by CRRT; therefore, treating the underlying cause of lactic acidosis remains paramount.
  - Refractory electrolyte abnormalities, for example, hyperkalemia with electrocardiogram (ECG) changes
  - Toxic ingestion, for example, lithium, toxic alcohols, metformin, salicylates
    - IHD is preferred for this indication due to more efficient clearance.
  - Volume overload, specifically severe pulmonary edema
    - CRRT is preferred; if IHD is used, volume can reaccumulate between sessions.
  - Uremic complications, for example, pericarditis, bleeding, encephalopathy
    - More commonly seen in CKD than in AKI
- CRRT-specific indications:
  - CRRT is preferred for patients with intracranial hypertension; IHD can rapidly correct uremia, leading to a rapid decrease in serum osmolarity and worsening cerebral edema.
  - Intracranial bleeding or severe transient brain attack (TBI) with other indications for dialysis
  - Acute liver failure: CRRT can assist with the gentle clearance of ammonia.
  - Severe hyponatremia or hypernatremia: CRRT can provide more gradual serum sodium correction.
  - Severe tumor lysis syndrome: CRRT is more effective than IHD at clearing phosphate.

Timing for Initiation

- If the patient meets any of the classic urgent indications earlier, RRT should be initiated.
- The controversy around timing pertains to patients who have severe AKI but do not yet meet any urgent indication.
  - Many randomized controlled trials (RCTs) have been conducted to answer this question: in patients with severe AKI, should RRT be initiated early (prior to the onset of strict indications or complications), or deferred until a hard indication is present?
  - ELAIN trial (2016)—a single-center trial that found mortality benefit with early initiation of RRT in surgical ICU patients with stage 2 AKI
  - AKIKI trial (2016), IDEAL-ICU trial (2018), STARRT-AKI trial (2020)—large, multicenter trials that found no difference in mortality between early and standard (delayed) initiation of RRT in patients with severe AKI; a significant percentage of patients in the delayed cohorts did not even require RRT.
  - AKIKI-2 trial (2021)—compared delayed initiation to more delayed initiation (oliguria >72 hours or blood urea nitrogen [BUN] >140 mg/dL) and found that more delayed initiation increased mortality

- Currently, the evidence suggests that delayed initiation of RRT in patients with severe AKI and no urgent indication for dialysis is safe (so long as the delay is not excessively prolonged) and may spare unnecessary RRT.

Dosing

- For IHD, dose is determined by the rate of urea clearance; dose can be increased by increasing clearance per session and the number of sessions per week.
- For CRRT, dose is expressed as the effluent flow rate.
  - RCTs have been conducted to determine the optimal dose.
  - ATN trial (2008)—included both IHD and CRRT patients; found that intensive therapy (higher dose) did not have any improvement in mortality or renal recovery compared to less intensive dosing
  - RENAL trial (2009)—focused on CVVHD patients; between intensive (40 mL/kg/h) versus less intensive (25 mL/kg/h) dosage, there was no difference in mortality or renal recovery.
  - In summary, there is likely no benefit to higher effluent flow rates; higher effluent flow rates are also associated with higher rates of hypophosphatemia, hypokalemia, and, possibly, prolonged ventilator weaning.
  - KDIGO recommends an effluent flow rate of 20 to 25 mL/kg/h.
  - In practice, the prescription should be written higher, for an effluent rate of 25 to 30 mL/kg/h, to account for daily treatment interruptions, such as filter clotting or circuit disconnection for patient transport, imaging studies, and procedures.

Vascular Access

- Most common vascular access for newly initiated CRRT is a temporary, nontunneled, large-bore, two-lumen dialysis catheter.
  - Placed in a central vein
  - In order of preference: right internal jugular (IJ) vein > common femoral vein > left IJ vein > subclavian vein
    - Right IJ vein—straight path to the cavoatrial junction; 16 cm catheter
    - Common femoral vein—also relatively straight path; no increased risk of infection unless the patient is obese; 24 cm catheter
    - Left IJ vein—flow may be suboptimal due to less straight path to the cavoatrial junction; 20 cm catheter.
    - Subclavian vein—generally avoided due to the risk of venous stenosis, which may compromise future arteriovenous (AV) fistula creation if long-term dialysis is needed
  - Typically has a red "arterial" port and a blue "venous" port
    - Arterial port
      - Named as such due to the historical use of arterial access to drive blood flow to the machine
      - Nowadays refers to the proximal port, which siphons blood from the patient to the machine, driven by a pump in the machine
    - Venous port
      - Refers to the distal port through which blood is returned from the machine to the patient
    - With this configuration, unfiltered blood is drawn proximally, then filtered by the machine, and returned to the patient distally; if the ports are "flipped" (ie, blood is siphoned distally and returned to the patient proximally), there would be recirculation, which reduces efficiency.
- If the RRT course is anticipated to be >1 to 3 weeks, tunneled dialysis catheter placement should be considered to decrease the risk of infection and improve patient comfort.
- AV fistulas can be used for IHD, but not for CRRT.
  - In CRRT, the continuous nature of therapy leads to the risk of needle dislodgement and exsanguination; low-flow rates may also lead to thrombosis of fistula.

Anticoagulation

- For CRRT, there is a risk for filter clotting due to relatively low blood flow rates.
- Regional citrate anticoagulation
  - Recommended as first line by KDIGO
  - Infusion of citrate prefilter chelates calcium and prevents filter clotting.
  - Citrate-calcium complex may be lost in ultrafiltrate, so postfilter infusion of calcium is required to prevent hypocalcemia.
  - Circuit and serum ionized calcium should be monitored closely.
  - With normal liver function, citrate is metabolized to bicarbonate, so metabolic alkalosis is a potential side effect.
  - Caution in liver failure—citrate metabolism may be impaired, leading instead to anion gap metabolic acidosis.
- Heparin
  - In patients with low bleeding risk, systemic infusion of unfractionated heparin is an option.
  - Contraindicated in heparin-induced thrombocytopenia (HIT)
- No anticoagulation
  - For patients with high bleeding risk
  - Requires high vigilance due to the risk of filter clotting and frequent interruptions in treatment
  - Risk of filter clotting can be reduced by infusing replacement fluid prefilter for CVVH, using higher blood flow rates, or opting for CVVHD over CVVH to minimize filtration fraction (ratio of ultrafiltration to blood flow).

Complications

- Vascular access: pneumothorax, hematoma, line infection, venous thrombosis, central vein stenosis, air embolism, catheter dysfunction
- Filter clotting
  - Most common complication in CRRT
  - Commonly due to catheter dysfunction leading to inadequate flow
  - If not able to restore flow promptly, may lead to loss of blood extracorporeally in the circuit
- Hypotension: common with initiation of therapy and may be exacerbated by targeting net negative ultrafiltration
- Hypothermia: importantly, this may mask fever in patients at risk for sepsis.
- Electrolyte derangements: particularly hypophosphatemia, which may lead to prolonged ventilator weaning; may require switching to phosphate-containing replacement fluid

- Incorrect medication dosing: may lead to over- or underdosing of important medications such as antimicrobials; may be complicated by unanticipated circuit downtime (eg, due to filter clotting), leading to unpredictable drug levels; consult with pharmacist
- Potential micronutrient losses

Discontinuation

- Once hemodynamic stability has been established, CRRT can be weaned to IHD for patients who remain dialysis dependent.
  - At MGH, it is common practice to wean gradually from CRRT to AVVH to IHD.
- Renal recovery is suggested by spontaneous daily urine output >500 mL to 1 L per day and spontaneous reduction in BUN and creatinine.

SUGGESTED READINGS

Allegretti AS, Endres P, Parris T, et al. Accelerated venovenous hemofiltration as a transitional renal replacement therapy in the intensive care unit. *Am J Nephrol*. 2020;51(4):318-326.

Barbar SD, Clere-Jehl R, Bourredjem A, et al; IDEAL-ICU Trial Investigators and the CRICS TRIGGERSEP Network. Timing of renal-replacement therapy in patients with acute kidney injury and sepsis. *N Engl J Med*. 2018;379(15):1431-1442.

Bellomo R, Cass A, Cole L, et al; RENAL Replacement Therapy Study Investigators. Intensity of continuous renal-replacement therapy in critically ill patients. *N Engl J Med*. 2009;361(17):1627-1638.

Côté JM, Koyner JL, Murray PT. Renal replacement therapy for acute kidney injury in the intensive care unit. In: Hall JB, Schmidt GA, Wood LDH, eds. *Principles of Critical Care*. 5th ed. McGraw-Hill Education; 2024:1064-1075.

Gaudry S, Hajage D, Martin-Lefevre L, et al; AKIKI-2 Investigators. Delayed versus more-delayed strategy for renal replacement therapy initiation in critically ill patients with severe acute kidney injury: a multicenter randomized trial. *JAMA Intern Med*. 2021;181(2):153-162.

Gaudry S, Hajage D, Schortgen F, et al. Initiation strategies for renal-replacement therapy in the intensive care unit. *N Engl J Med*. 2016;375(2):122-133.

Gaudry S, Palevsky PM, Dreyfuss D. Extracorporeal kidney-replacement therapy for acute kidney injury. *N Engl J Med*. 2022;386(10):964-975.

Hoste EAJ, Vanommeslaeghe F. Basic Principles of Renal Replacement Therapy. In: Vincent JL, Abraham E, Kochanek PM, Moore FA, eds. *Textbook of Critical Care*. 8th ed.: Elsevier; 2023:233-239.e3.

Kidney Disease: Improving Global Outcomes (KDIGO) Acute Kidney Injury Work Group. KDIGO clinical practice guideline for acute kidney injury. *Kidney Int Suppl*. 2012;2(1):1-138.

Ostermann M, Bellomo R, Burdmann EA, et al. Controversies in acute kidney injury: conclusions from a Kidney Disease: Improving Global Outcomes (KDIGO) Conference. *Kidney Int*. 2020;98(2):294-309.

Palevsky PM, Zhang JH, O'Connor TZ, et al; VA/NIH Acute Renal Failure Trial Network. intensity of renal replacement therapy in critically ill patients with acute kidney injury. *N Engl J Med*. 2008;359(7):7-20.

Schefold JC, von Haehling S, Pschowski R, et al. The effect of continuous versus intermittent renal replacement therapy on the outcome of critically ill patients with acute renal failure (CONVINT): a prospective randomized controlled trial. *Crit Care*. 2014;18(1):R11.

Tandukar S, Palevsky PM. Continuous renal replacement therapy: who, when, why, and how. *Chest*. 2019;155(3):626-638.

Teixeira JP, Davenport A, Kashani K, et al. Continuous kidney replacement therapies: core curriculum 2025. *Am J Kidney Dis*. 2025;85(6):767-786.

Tolwani A. Continuous renal-replacement therapy for acute kidney injury. *N Engl J Med*. 2012;367(26):2505-2514.

Zarbock A, Kellum JA, Schmidt C, et al. Effect of early vs delayed initiation of renal replacement therapy on mortality in critically ill patients with acute kidney injury: the ELAIN randomized clinical trial. *JAMA*. 2016;315(20):2190-2199.

5.5

Renal Imaging and Other Diagnostic Modalities

Emily Anne Smith Bergbower and Elizabeth Cox Williams

This chapter reviews the most common renal imaging platforms and provides guidance to intensivists in studies regarding mechanisms, function, usefulness, and cost (Table 5.5.1).

The X-Ray or "Plain Film"

- Plain films of the abdomen are readily available and easily obtained. Often, the imaging can be done with a portable machine at bedside in the intensive care unit (ICU) or emergency department (ED). It is a pertinent first imaging test to be conducted as part of an initial workup for relevant chief complaints.
- The densities of the kidney and surrounding soft tissue structures are similar, limiting anatomic assessment. Depending on position and body habitus, the evaluator of the plain film may be able to estimate kidney length and shape.
- Calcifications along the renal tract are usually well visualized with plain film, but this modality may be limited for small renal stones (<5 mm).

TABLE 5.5.1 Imaging Has Been Split Into Five General Categories for Consideration

	X-Ray	Ultrasound	CT	MRI	Nuclear
Ease	+++	+++	++	+	+
Cost	+	+	++	+++	+++
Speed	+++	+++	++	±	+
Anatomic depth	±	++	++	+++	+
Complex patient factors	±	–	+	++	++

The x-ray category includes plain film radiography, excretory urography, and traditional renal angiography. For this grading scale, +++ pertains to high, ++ to intermediate, and + or ± to low or minimal. A specific note should be made regarding the category of complex patient factors. This includes considerations such as radiation exposure, contrast administration, patient anxiety and discomfort, travel from bedside to scanner, and length of imaging time.

CT, computed tomography; MRI, magnetic resonance imaging.

- Gas bubbles can be seen in the region of the renal parenchyma and collecting system on plain film in patients with conditions such as emphysematous pyelonephritis. If gas is noted on plain film, further imaging by computed tomography (CT) should be obtained.
- This imaging modality provides no information on renal function.
- Patients undergoing x-ray are exposed to low levels of radiation.

Enhancing X-Ray #1: Excretory Urography or the "Intravenous Pyelogram"

- While reliant on x-ray imaging, performing excretory urography is more complex than taking a single plain film. For this technique, patients are administered intravenous (IV) water-soluble iodinated contrast dye, and x-rays are taken sequentially at specific timed intervals. As the kidney filters the contrast dye, it passes into the urine and enhances various structures, leading to optimal assessment with sequential imaging.
- Excretory urography provides a greater depth of anatomic assessment than the plain film alone. With the addition of contrast, the course of the ureters can be visualized, as well as anatomic variants in kidney shape/structure.
- Excretory urography can be useful for diagnosing renal papillary necrosis, upper urinary tract tumors, and ureteric obstruction. In the case of obstruction, a delay in contrast excretion can delineate the site.
- Retrograde pyelography is a similar concept to excretory urography. Instead of IV contrast, a catheter is placed in the ureter and contrast is administered retrograde into the collecting system.
- IV contrast dye is not totally benign and can precipitate allergic reactions. A careful history and premedication, if necessary, can decrease this risk.
- Excretory urography with serial imaging by plain film is rarely performed due to the advent of CT imaging.

Enhancing X-Ray #2: Renal Angiography

- This modality is reliant on sequential, timed x-ray images after the administration of contrast into the renal artery.
- Although largely phased out by the advent of CT angiography, renal angiography was once a key technique for evaluating the renal vasculature. Occlusion, stenosis, aneurysms, and arteriovenous (AV) malformations can all be diagnosed using renal angiography.
- While the serial imaging portion is straightforward, this test requires femoral arterial access, which carries risks of arterial injury, hemorrhage, infection, and damage to surrounding structures.

Ultrasound

- For this imaging modality, high-frequency sound waves are generated by an ultrasound (US) machine and emitted by a transducer. These waves are then reflected back to the transducer at varying speeds and intensity (essentially, acoustic impedance), allowing for the production of an image.
- The degree of echogenicity creates varying levels of brightness in the US image, permitting accurate interpretation and clinical diagnosis.
- Anatomic assessment of the kidneys by US provides more accurate information than x-ray evaluation. Kidney size and shape can be easily and reliably ascertained, as well as visualization of the renal parenchyma and the renal pelvis.
- US is a useful imaging modality for the detection of hydronephrosis, renal stones or calcifications, tumors, cysts, and congenital anomalies.
- US is noninvasive, does not require radiation or contrast, and produces images in real time. As a standalone technique, it does not assess renal function.
- Imaging can be done at the bedside and requires only a portable machine.
- Accuracy and image quality are operator dependent.

Enhancing Ultrasound #1: Doppler

- The addition of Doppler to US testing provides key information about blood flow in the renal arteries and veins as well as in the kidney itself.
- There are three forms of Doppler to consider: color, power, and spectral. Color Doppler provides data on the directionality and magnitude of flow. Power Doppler increases the US machine's sensitivity to slow flow at the expense of directional information but can provide insight into perfusion and the microvasculature. Finally, spectral Doppler reveals directionality, speed, and relative flow during systole and diastole. This method allows for the velocity of flow over time to be displayed as a waveform.
- Overall, Doppler is particularly useful in the assessment of suspected or known renovascular anomalies, such as stenosis, aneurysm, or AV fistula. It can also provide key information on renal blood flow in patients with dissections or trauma and evaluate for thrombosis.
- Doppler is a critical imaging modality for the immediate postoperative period following renal transplant to assess directionality and velocity of flow.
- Doppler technology is integrated into US machine.

Enhancing Ultrasound #2: Microbubble Contrast

- Microbubbles are small phospholipid shells that contain inert gas, such as perfluorocarbon, sulfur hexafluoride, or nitrogen gas.
- Microbubble contrast is injected IV, and the kidney is imaged by US once the microbubbles have reached the renal vasculature. The bubbles are compressible and oscillate when exposed to the US beam, producing a nonlinear response that affects backscatter and enhances vascular contrast.
- This imaging modality can be extremely useful for better characterizing renal masses.
- This form of contrast is quite safe. The gas contained in the circulating shells is exhaled and does not require filtration or secretion.

Computed Tomography

- CT imaging relies upon x-ray imaging taken at varying angles and computer processing to produce cross-sectional images.

- The x-rays that pass through the body vary in intensity due to tissue density.
- This imaging modality is rapid but requires transport to a dedicated scanner.
- While CT imaging can be performed with and without water-soluble iodinated IV contrast, the "dry" CT (without) is limited in its evaluation. The dry CT allows for strong delineation of conditions such as renal stones or hydronephrosis, but the addition of contrast provides strong characterization of renal anatomic structure and function.
- This type of imaging modality lends itself to multiphase imaging protocols, in which images are acquired at fixed points in time after contrast administration.

Enhancing the Computed Tomography: Urography and Angiography

- CT urography (CTU) is the modern alternative to excretory urography/IV pyelography. In this protocol, multiphase imaging of the kidney is obtained once contrast has entered the collecting system. Protocols vary by hospital.
- CT angiography (CTA) is the modern alternative to renal angiography. Here, the IV contrast administered serves to best assess the renal artery, which permits for close assessment of bleeding, stenosis, or any vascular anomalies. This study is easy and fast to perform and usually only requires a single acquisition.

Magnetic Resonance Imaging

- Magnetic resonance imaging (MRI) modality relies on the alignment of the body's hydrogen protons in response to the MRI machine's powerful magnet. The addition of radio waves to the magnetic field directed at the patient will cause these protons to resonate and enter a higher energy state. When the source of radiofrequency pulses is turned off and the protons return to a relaxed state, signals will be emitted by the protons and detected by coils in the MRI machine. Signals can be converted by computer processing into images.
- MRI protocols vary to highlight different pathologies and change the contrast of the image. This is referred to as a "sequence."
- Magnet strength (generally 1.5-3 T) directly correlates to the quality of spatial resolution of the resulting image.
- MRI can be enhanced with gadolinium-based contrast media. In the presence of chronic kidney disease, *nephrogenic systemic fibrosis* is a rare and feared complication of gadolinium-based contrast agents. Newer MRI contrast preparations carry a much lower risk of causing this condition.
- MRI is an expensive imaging modality that requires longer acquisition times, requiring the patient to lie still in a confined space for an extended period of time. Motion can easily degrade MRI.
- All patients must be screened for MRI safety according to established protocols. Some patients may be unable to undergo MRI due to metallic implants that are not compatible with the strong magnetic field.

Enhancing the Magnetic Resonance Imaging: Urography and Angiogram

- MR urography (MRU) is a similar concept to the previously discussed excretory urography and CTU. There are two types for intensivists to consider. The first is the static fluid-sensitive form, which is T2 weighted. This method serves to image a fluid-filled urinary system in which the urine itself intrinsically acts as the contrast medium. The second type is T1 weighted and shows the urinary system after gadolinium contrast has been administered.
- MRU is more frequently performed in pediatric patients in whom radiation exposure from CT is avoided.
- MR angiogram (MRA) is similar in concept to the previously discussed types of angiography. Here, the MRI protocol is adjusted to accentuate the arteries. It can be performed with and without contrast.

Nuclear Medicine or "Renal Scintigraphy"

- In nuclear medicine, renal imaging can allow for assessment of renal function, anatomy, structure, and perfusion.
- This modality is dependent on the injection of a labeled radiotracer that is specific for what is being evaluated. The three primary radiotracers are technetium-99m (Tc-99m) MAG3, Tc-99m diethylene triamine pentaacetic acid (DTPA), and Tc-99m dimercaptosuccinic acid (DMSA).
- Imaging will be either dynamic or static. In dynamic imaging, a series of images will be collected at timed intervals, and images will reflect the passage of the radiotracer through the vasculature. Overall, the primary goal will be to assess perfusion to the kidneys and the excretion of tracer through the collecting system. Tc-99m MAG3 and Tc-99m DTPA are the two radiotracers used in dynamic imaging. Of special note, Tc-99m DTPA allows for concurrent glomerular filtration rate (GFR) measurement.
- In static imaging, images will be acquired at a specific delayed time point to assess anatomy, specifically of the renal cortex. Radiotracer Tc-99m DMSA is used for this modality, and it is retained in renal tubular cells. This method is particularly useful for the evaluation of renal scarring.
- While renal scintigraphy is a very useful form of imaging that provides functional information and quantitative data, it requires trained operators and specific equipment, including the radiotracers. Additionally, testing can take up to an hour.

Positron Emission Tomography

- As an aside, this chapter will touch briefly on the positron emission tomography (PET) scan, which is generally not useful for an evaluation of the renal system.
- PET relies on an F-fluorodeoxyglucose (FDG) tracer, which is renally excreted. Often, there is too much of a signal, and this can obscure renal tumors.
- Research is ongoing related to its usefulness, and the presented line of thought may be changing under certain conditions.

SUGGESTED READINGS

Bertolotto M, Bucci S, Valentino M, Curro F, Sachs C, Cova MA. Contrast-enhanced ultrasound for characterizing renal masses. *Eur J Radiol*. 2018; 105:41-48.

Brisbane W, Bailey MR, Sorensen MD. An overview of kidney stone imaging techniques. *Nat Rev Urol*. 2016;13(11):654-662.

Francis ST, Selby NM, Taal MW. Magnetic resonance imaging to evaluate kidney structure, function, and pathology: moving toward clinical application. *Am J Kidney Dis*. 2023;82(4):491-504.

Furlow B. Computed tomography of renal masses in adults. *Radiol Technol*. 2016;87(3):305CT-325CT.

Hartman R, Kawashima A, Takahashi N, et al. Applications of dual-energy CT in urologic imaging: an update. *Radiol Clin North Am*. 2012;50(2): 191-205.

Innes GD, Wishart I, Lau T, Islam A, Gourlay K, Scheuermeyer FX. Can plain film radiography improve the emergency department detection of clinically important urinary stones? *Am J Emerg Med*. 2021;50: 449-454.

Keramida G, James JM, Prescott MC, Peters AM. Pitfalls and limitations of radionuclide renal imaging in adults. *Semin Nucl Med*. 2015;45(5): 428-439.

Klibanov AL. Microbubble contrast agents: targeted ultrasound imaging and ultrasound-assisted drug-delivery applications. *Invest Radiol*. 2006; 41(3):354-362.

Lerman LO, Rodriguez-Porcel M, Romero JC. The development of x-ray imaging to study renal function. *Kidney Int*. 1999;55(2):400-416.

Lindenberg L, Mena E, Choyke PL, Bouchelouche K. PET imaging in renal cancer. *Curr Opin Oncol*. 2019;31(3):216-221.

Liu PS, Platt JF. CT angiography of the renal circulation. *Radiol Clin North Am*. 2010;48(2):347-365, viii-vix.

O'Connor OJ, Maher MM. CT urography. *AJR Am J Roentgenol*. 2010; 195(5):W320-W324.

Platt JF. Doppler ultrasound of the kidney. *Semin Ultrasound CT MR*. 1997;18(1):22-32.

Soares GM, Murphy TP, Singha MS, Parada A, Jaff M. Renal artery duplex ultrasonography as a screening and surveillance tool to detect renal artery stenosis: a comparison with current reference standard imaging. *J Ultrasound Med*. 2006;25(3):293-298.

5.6

Pharmacologic Therapies for Renal Disorders

Danielle Leahy and John Klick

Diuretics

- Loop diuretics: inhibit Na-K-2Cl channel in the medullary thick ascending limb to decrease Na and Cl reabsorption
  - Side effects: hypovolemia, hypotension, ↓Na/↑Na, ↓K, ↓Mg, ↓Ca, ↑glucose, ↑urate, ototoxicity, azotemia, metabolic alkalosis
  - Dose equivalents: furosemide oral (PO):furosemide intravenous (IV):torsemide:bumetanide (40:20:20:1)
  - Higher doses may be needed in renal dysfunction to achieve the therapeutic effect.
    - Furosemide (Lasix)
      - Duration of action: PO 6 hours, IV 2 hours
      - Initial dose 10 to 40 mg PO/IV qd (once a day) (PO:IV dose 2:1)
      - IV bolus maximum 160 to 200 mg, maximum daily 400 to 600 mg
      - Infusion 40 mg IV load followed by 5 to 40 mg/h
    - Torsemide (Demadex)
      - Duration of action: 12 to 16 hours
      - Initial dose 10 to 20 mg PO/IV qd to 2 times daily (bid)
      - IV bolus maximum 100 to 200 mg, maximum daily 200 mg
      - Infusion 20 mg IV load followed by 5 to 20 mg/h
    - Bumetanide (Bumex)
      - Duration of action: 6 to 8 hours
      - Initial dose 0.5 mg PO/IV qd up to 1 mg bid
      - IV bolus maximum 4 to 8 mg, maximum daily 10 mg
      - Infusion 1 mg IV load followed by 0.5 to 2 mg/h
    - Ethacrynic acid (Edecrin)—non-sulfa, less ototoxicity
      - Duration of action: PO 6 hours, IV 2 hours
      - Initial dose 50 mg PO qd to bid, 25 to 100 mg IV
      - IV bolus maximum 100 mg, maximum daily 400 mg
      - Not used as an infusion
- Thiazide diuretics: inhibit Na-Cl channel in the distal tubule
  - Side effects: ↓Na, ↓K, ↓Mg, ↑Ca, ↑urate, ↑glucose
    - Hydrochlorothiazide (Hydrodiuril)
      - Duration of action: 6 to 12 hours
      - Initial dose: 12.5 to 25 mg PO qd to bid
      - Maximum daily 200 mg
      - Give 30 minutes before loop diuretic; no IV form
    - Metolazone (Zaroxolyn)
      - Duration of action: 12 to 24 hours
      - Initial dose: 1.25 to 10 mg PO qd or 5 mg bid
      - Maximum daily 20 mg
      - No IV form
    - Chlorothiazide (Diuril)
      - Duration of action: 2 hours
      - Initial dose: 125 to 500 mg IV qd to q8h
      - IV bolus maximum 1,000 mg, maximum daily 2,000 mg
      - Not used as an infusion
- Aldosterone antagonist: blocks aldosterone binding to mineralocorticoid receptor leading to decreased sodium reabsorption and potassium excretion in the distal tubule and collecting duct
  - Side effects: hyperkalemia, gynecomastia
    - Spironolactone (Aldactone)
      - Duration of action: 48 to 72 hours
      - Initial dose: 12.5 to 25 mg PO qd to bid
      - Maximum daily 200 mg
      - No IV form
- Carbonic anhydrase inhibitor: prevents bicarbonate reabsorption in the proximal convoluted tubule, thereby increasing sodium excretion
  - Side effects: hyperglycemia, hypokalemia, hepatic encephalopathy
    - Acetazolamide (Diamox)
      - Duration of action: 4 to 5 hours
      - Initial dose: 125 to 500 mg IV qd to q6h

- IV bolus maximum 500 mg, maximum daily 2,000 mg
- Not used as an infusion
- Helpful in the treatment of the contraction alkalosis seen with the use of other diuretics

- Osmotic diuretics: cause free water loss by increased osmotic gradient in the renal tubules
  - Side effects: hyponatremia followed by hypernatremia, headache, nausea/vomiting
    - Mannitol
      - Duration of action: 3 to 6 hours
      - Initial dose: test dose 0.2 g/kg or typically 20 to 100 g
      - Urgent intracranial pressure (ICP) reduction: 1 to 2 g/kg of 20% solution
      - Maximum daily 100 g
      - Most commonly used as an infusion
- Antidiuretic hormone (ADH) antagonists: inhibit ADH action of inserting water channels into the collecting tubule by interfering with intracellular messaging (effectively causing nephrogenic diabetes insipidus)
  - Side effects: bone/teeth abnormalities in children, sunlight sensitivity
    - Demeclocycline (Declomycin)
      - Common dose: 600 to 1,200 mg/d PO divided doses
      - Off-label use for syndrome of inappropriate antidiuretic hormone secretion (SIADH)
      - Not available IV
- Vasopressin receptor antagonists: block the binding of arginine vasopressin (AVP), also known as antidiuretic hormone (ADH), to V1A, V1B, and V2 receptors
  - Side effects: thirst, polyuria, hypernatremia, dry mouth, CYP 3A4 interactions → liver injury
    - Tolvaptan (Samsca): selective V2 antagonist, suppresses insertion of aquaporin channels in the collecting duct, causing increased free water excretion
      - Common dose: 15 to 90 mg PO
      - Approved for short-term use in resistant hypervolemic and euvolemic hyponatremia and rapidly progressive autosomal dominant polycystic kidney disease (ADPKD)
      - Not available IV

Buffers

Commonly used to treat acidosis of varying causes, although evidence of their effectiveness is limited; treating the underlying cause is always preferred.

- Sodium bicarbonate
  - Dissociates into Na^+ and HCO_2^-, which can bind free H^+ to raise pH
  - Bicarbonate administration generates CO_2 (which can rapidly diffuse into cells); if ventilation is fixed, may actually exacerbate intracellular acidosis
  - Bicarbonate unlikely to improve hemodynamics or response to pressors
  - Supplementation used as treatment in renal tubular acidosis
  - Side effects: hypernatremia, hyperosmolality, may stimulate lactate production
- *Tris* (hydroxymethyl)-aminomethane (THAM)
  - Reduces arterial $[H^+]$ without producing CO_2
  - Protonated THAM is renally excreted.
  - May improve acidosis in patients with acute respiratory distress syndrome/acute lung injury (ARDS/ALI) with permissive hypercapnia
  - Adverse effects: hypoglycemia, hyperkalemia, extravasation-related necrosis

Dopamine

Endogenous catecholamine (precursor to norepinephrine and epinephrine)

Regulator of renal blood flow and salt and water reabsorption via renal proximal tubule through action on dopamine D1 and D2 receptors

Exogenous infusion activates a variety of receptors in dose-dependent manner:

- Low dose (1-3 μg/kg/min): D1 receptor activation → increased natriuresis, diuresis, and renal blood flow (via renal vasodilation)
- Intermediate dose (3-10 μg/kg/min): activates beta-1 and beta-2 (plus D1) → increases renal blood flow by increasing cardiac output
- High dose (>10 μg/kg/min): activates alpha receptors (plus beta-1, beta-2, and D1) → increased systemic vascular resistance (SVR), pulmonary vascular resistance (PVR), decreased renal blood flow
- Side effects: arrhythmia, tissue necrosis with extravasation, increased myocardial oxygen demand
- Nephroprotective effects in acute kidney injury (AKI) (via increased renal blood flow) remain a controversial topic.

Selective D1 Dopamine Receptor Agonists

- Binds to D1 receptors in blood vessels → activates adenylyl cyclase → increases intracellular cyclic adenosine monophosphate (cAMP) → smooth muscle relaxation
- Decreases vascular resistance in systemic and renal arteries, promoting increased renal blood flow, diuresis, and natriuresis
- May have beneficial effects on renal function for patients at risk for AKI

Fenoldopam (Corlopam)

- Does not cross blood-brain barrier, therefore no central D1 activation
- Short-term (<48 hours) IV infusion to treat in-hospital hypertensive emergency
- Side effects: dizziness, cardiac dysrhythmias, hypokalemia, headache
- Onset of action: 5 minutes
- Initial dose: 0.01 to 0.3 μg/kg/min (increase every 15 minutes by 0.05-0.1 until target blood pressure is achieved)
- Max dose: 1.6 μg/kg/min infusion

SUGGESTED READINGS

Addison JD, Peterson EJ, Meyenburg L. Intravenous or oral acetazolamide for treatment of diuretic-induced alkalosis in patients with heart failure. *Ann Pharmacother*. 2023;57(11):1241-1247.

Coppola S, Caccioppola A, Froio S, Chiumello D. Sodium bicarbonate in different critically ill conditions: from physiology to clinical practice. *Anesthesiology*. 2021;134(5):774-783.

Gehlbach BK, Schmidt GA. Bench-to-bedside review: treating acid-base abnormalities in the intensive care unit—the role of buffers. *Crit Care*. 2004;8(4):259-265.

Gheorghiade M, Gattis WA, O'Connor CM, et al. Effects of Tolvaptan, a vasopressin antagonist, in patients hospitalized with worsening heart failure: a randomized controlled trial. *JAMA*. 2004;291:1963-1971.

Heidenreich PA, Bozkurt B, Aguilar D, et al. 2022 AHA/ACC/HFSA guideline for the management of heart failure: a report of the American College of Cardiology/American Heart Association Joint Committee on Clinical Practice Guidelines. *Circulation*. 2022;145(18):e895-e1032.

Kallet RH, Jasmer RM, Luce JM, Lin LH, Marks JD. The treatment of acidosis in acute lung injury with tris-hydroxymethylaminomethane (THAM). *Am J Respir Crit Care Med*. 2000;161:1149-1153.

Noce A, Marrone G, Rovella V, et al. Fenoldopam mesylate: a narrative review of its use in acute kidney injury. *Curr Pharm Biotechnol*. 2019; 20(5):366-375.

Verbalis JG, Adler S, Schrier RW, et al. Efficacy and safety of oral Tolvaptan therapy in patients with the syndrome of inappropriate antidiuretic hormone secretion. *Eur J Endo*. 2011;164:725-732.

Sarafidis PA., Georgianos PI, Lasaridis AN. Diuretics in clinical practice. Part I: mechanisms of action, pharmacological effects and clinical indications of diuretic compounds. *Expert Opin Drug Saf*. 2010;9(2): 243-257.

5.7

Pharmacologic Implications of Altered Renal Clearance

Takashi Sakano and Jeffrey W. Cannon

Key Points

- Kidneys are important for the elimination of toxins and are composed of functional units called nephrons.
- Many medications are subject to renal clearance, and dose modifications may be necessary when renal clearance is altered.
- *Renal clearance* is defined as the theoretical plasma volume from which a substance is eliminated by the kidneys per unit time (mL/min).
- $C_X = U_X * V/P_X$, where C_X: clearance of *X*; U_X: urine concentration of *X*; *V*: urine flow rate; and P_X: plasma concentration of *X*.
- Renal clearance is composed of glomerular filtration, tubular secretion, and tubular reabsorption.
- Blood that flows through the nephron is filtered at the level of the glomerulus, and substances can undergo secretion and reabsorption in the renal tubules.
- Renal dysfunction can impair glomerular filtration, tubular secretion, and/or tubular reabsorption.
- Glomerular filtration
  - Determinants of glomerular filtration include glomerular blood flow, hydrostatic and oncotic pressure, integrity of the Bowman capsule, and molecular size and weight of the filtered substance.
  - Substances must be in their unbound form to undergo glomerular filtration.
- Tubular secretion
  - Utilizes active transporters: organic anion transporter (OAT), organic cation transporter (OCT), and adenosine triphosphate (ATP)-binding cassette (ABC) transporters
  - Active secretion of a drug may be reduced by a second substance that inhibits or competes for the same transporter, or by a reduction in transporter function and/or expression as occurs in kidney dysfunction.
- Tubular reabsorption
  - Tubular reabsorption occurs by active transport and passive reabsorption.
  - Active reabsorption occurs by OAT, OCT, and sodium-dependent transporters.
  - Determinants of passive reabsorption include lipid solubility, ionization state, and molecular size and weight.
  - Ionization states of drugs may be modified by altering the urine pH.
  - Similar to tubular secretion, reabsorption may be reduced by a second substance that inhibits or competes for the same transporter, or by a reduction in transporter function and/or expression as occurs in kidney dysfunction.
  - Glomerular filtration rate (GFR) is used as a measure of kidney function and is commonly estimated by creatinine and cystatin-C–based formulas.
- Key pathophysiology
  - Change affecting glomerular filtration, tubular secretion, and/or tubular reabsorption can alter renal clearance.
  - With altered renal clearance, care must be taken to determine if clearance is increased or decreased.
  - Decreased renal clearance can be from chronic kidney disease or acute kidney injury.
  - Injury to nephrons can result in reduced function of the kidney to clear drugs from blood.
  - Increased renal clearance can occur in young patients and in patients with hypermetabolic pathologies (burns, sepsis, etc).
  - Sepsis and large burns can cause endothelial leakage and/or increased cardiac output, thereby increasing flow and filtration through nephrons and decreasing reabsorption.
- Management and treatment
  - With changes in renal clearance, renally eliminated drugs need to be prescribed and titrated accordingly.
  - The simplest solution for medication selection in altered renal clearance is to choose a medication that is not renally cleared.
  - When this is not feasible, the medication must be adjusted for changes in renal clearance.
  - Medication adjustments for renal clearance are often accomplished by changing the dosing frequency and/or the dosage strength.
  - Examples of renally eliminated classes of drugs include antimicrobial agents, analgesics, anticoagulants, and neuromuscular blockers, among others.

SUGGESTED READINGS

Buxton IO. Pharmacokinetics: the dynamics of drug absorption, distribution, metabolism, and elimination. In: Brunton LL, Knollmann BC, eds. *Goodman & Gilman's: The Pharmacological Basis of Therapeutics*. 14th ed. McGraw-Hill Education; 2023:29-73.

Jang SM, Infante S, Abdi Pour A. Drug dosing considerations in critically ill patients receiving continuous renal replacement therapy. *Pharmacy (Basel)*. 2020;8(1):18.

Kohan DE, Rosenberg ME. Drug dosing considerations in patients with acute kidney injury and chronic kidney disease. In: Taal MW, Chertow GM, Marsden PA, Skorecki K, Yu ASL, Brenner BM, eds. *Brenner and Rector's The Kidney*. 11th ed. Elsevier; 2020:1989-2014.

Lea-Henry TN, Carland JE, Stocker SL, et al. Clinical pharmacokinetics in kidney disease: fundamental principles. *Clin J Am Soc Nephrol*. 2018; 13(7):1085-1095.

5.8

Genitourinary Emergencies

Luke Tseng and Edward A. Bittner

Overview

- Can be grouped based on etiology
  - Obstructive—acute urinary retention, obstructive uropathy
  - Infectious—obstructive pyelonephritis, Fournier gangrene
  - Ischemic—testicular torsion, ischemic priapism, paraphimosis
  - Traumatic—kidney, ureter, bladder, urethra, genitalia
- All urologic emergencies should be managed expeditiously with early urologic consultation.

Obstructive Etiology

- Acute urinary retention
  - Mechanism: usually due to underlying benign prostatic hyperplasia (BPH) with an acute inciting event, such as medications (eg, opioids, antihistamines, anticholinergics), neuraxial anesthesia, or recent trauma (eg, recent Foley catheter placement)
  - Presentation: inability to void, suprapubic pressure; may be asymptomatic
  - Diagnosis: bladder scanner reading >400 mL
    - Caution—bladder scanner may erroneously read intraabdominal fluid (eg, ascites) as urine volume.
  - Management: bladder decompression with urethral catheterization
    - 16F Foley catheter is typically first line.
    - If BPH is suspected, place 18F or 20F catheter (increased rigidity is better able to bypass the prostate) or coudé catheter (curved tip).
    - If urethral stricture is suspected, place a smaller catheter, for example, 12F or 14F.
    - If gross hematuria or passage of blood clots, place a 22F or 24F three-way catheter for continuous bladder irrigation to prevent occlusion by blood clots.
    - If initial attempts are unsuccessful, limit further attempts and consult urology—may require flexible cystoscopy, placement of catheter over guidewire, or suprapubic catheter.
    - Alpha-antagonist (eg, tamsulosin) should be started 24 to 72 hours prior to removing catheter and attempting voiding trial.
- Obstructive uropathy
  - Only considered an emergency if there is complete occlusion of urinary flow (eg, bilateral obstructing ureteral stones or ureteral stone in a patient with solitary kidney), or superinfection of urine leading to urosepsis (see section "Infectious Etiology")
  - Mechanism: precipitation of minerals, most commonly calcium oxalate or calcium phosphate (less commonly ammonium magnesium phosphate, uric acid, or cystine); some risk factors include dehydration, diabetes, metabolic syndrome, primary hyperparathyroidism, and recurrent urinary tract infection.
  - Presentation: colicky flank pain, hematuria, nausea, vomiting; oliguria if obstructive; fever +/− hypotension if superinfected stone
  - Diagnosis: computed tomography (CT) of the abdomen/pelvis without intravenous (IV) contrast may demonstrate stones with associated hydronephrosis or hydroureter.
  - Management: emergent ureteral stent placement to allow for urinary diversion; once stabilized, can return for definitive treatment with laser lithotripsy

Infectious Etiology

- Obstructive pyelonephritis
  - Mechanism: ureteral stone obstructs urinary flow, leading to ascending urinary infection that can involve the renal pelvis and parenchyma.
  - Presentation: flank pain, fever, leukocytosis; hypotension with elevated lactate may be concerning for urosepsis evolving to septic shock.
  - Diagnosis: urinalysis with bacteriuria, +white blood cells (WBCs), +leukocyte esterase, +/− nitrites; CT of the abdomen/pelvis without IV contrast demonstrating obstructive stone; gas in the collecting system or parenchyma may be concerning for emphysematous pyelonephritis; imaging may also demonstrate perinephric abscess.
  - Management: broad-spectrum antibiotics + emergent decompression with either percutaneous nephrostomy or ureteral stenting
    - Studies have not shown superiority of one decompression technique over the other.

- For patients who are septic, there may be a preference for percutaneous nephrostomy, since it does not require general anesthesia.
- Once the infection has resolved and the patient has improved clinically, the patient can return for definitive stone management (ie, laser lithotripsy); early lithotripsy should be avoided due to the risk of causing urothelial trauma, which may worsen bacterial translocation.
- If CT imaging was concerning for emphysematous pyelonephritis, which is a necrotizing infection, it is reasonable to initially treat with percutaneous nephrostomy and broad-spectrum antibiotics; if the patient does not improve clinically, low threshold to proceed with partial or total nephrectomy.

- Fournier gangrene
  - Mechanism: necrotizing bacterial infection that involves the genitalia and perineum and spreads along deep fascial planes; risk factors include obesity, diabetes, and immunosuppression; infection can progress quickly.
  - Presentation: perineal pain, erythema, possibly visible purple/black necrosis and palpable crepitus; constitutional symptoms, fever, hypotension
  - Diagnosis: CT imaging demonstrating subcutaneous air; importantly, if the patient is unstable and examination is concerning for Fournier gangrene, operative management should proceed without imaging.
  - Management: broad-spectrum antibiotics and emergent surgical debridement of all necrotic tissue
    - Wound should be left open for drainage (perhaps with wound vac), and patient may return to the operating room (OR) in 24 to 48 hours for repeat examination and possibly additional debridement.
    - Once source control has been obtained and infection has been treated, patient may need extensive reconstructive surgery.

Ischemic Etiology

- Testicular torsion
  - Mechanism: testicle rotates within tunica vaginalis, leading to compression of arterial blood supply and testicular ischemia.
    - Often associated with "bell clapper" deformity—high attachment of the tunica vaginalis to the spermatic cord, leaving the testis free to rotate
    - Rotation of the testis may also be more likely with the presence of a mass, such as lymphoma.
  - Presentation: intense testicular pain; testicle may be palpated higher in scrotum; loss of cremasteric reflex (upward movement of testis when the ipsilateral inner thigh is palpated)
  - Diagnosis: testicular Doppler ultrasound demonstrating lack of blood flow
    - Of note, if there is a high enough clinical suspicion based on examination, operative intervention should not be delayed for imaging.
    - Rate of testicular salvage is 95% if detorsed within 6 hours; by 12 hours, the testicle is unlikely to be salvageable.
  - Management: emergent surgical detorsion
    - Manual detorsion at the bedside can be attempted while awaiting operative management; affected testis should be rotated away from midline (as if opening a book); even if successful, should still proceed to the OR for definitive management.
    - Surgical management involves exposing and untwisting the testicle.
    - The testicle is then examined—if deemed viable, proceed with orchiopexy; if necrotic, proceed with orchiectomy.
    - Orchiopexy should also be performed on the contralateral, unaffected testis to reduce the risk of torsion in the future.
- Ischemic priapism
  - Mechanism: unwanted erection lasting >4 hours; prolonged tumescence of corpora cavernosa leads to compromise of venous outflow and ischemia; can be conceptualized as compartment syndrome of the penis
    - Primary risk factor is sickle cell disease; other risk factors include trazodone and intracavernosal injections; phosphodiesterase type 5 (PDE-5) inhibitors (eg, sildenafil) are unlikely to cause ischemic priapism.
    - In contrast, nonischemic priapism is not an emergency; this is a high-flow state, which does not typically present as pain; may be due to trauma or congenital atrioventricular (AV) fistulas.
  - Presentation: rigid, painful erection; can progress to gangrene
  - Diagnosis: cavernosal blood gas demonstrating hypoxemia, hypercapnia, and acidemia
  - Management: emergent decompression via intracavernosal aspiration of blood (5 mL)
    - Followed by intracavernosal injection of phenylephrine; can be repeated every 5 minutes until detumescence is achieved
    - If phenylephrine injections are unsuccessful, may proceed with operative shunt creation (eg, between corpora cavernosa and glans) to facilitate decompression
- Paraphimosis
  - Mechanism: in uncircumcised males, the foreskin may be retracted for a prolonged time, leading to a tourniquet-like effect, causing edema to develop and an inability to reduce the foreskin; can progress to ischemia and necrosis.
    - Oftentimes an iatrogenic complication—the foreskin is retracted for urethral catheter placement and may not be reduced completely afterward.
  - Presentation: painful, edematous, retracted foreskin; skin discoloration would suggest ischemia.
  - Diagnosis: history and physical examination are sufficient.
  - Management: attempt manual reduction of foreskin.
    - Apply ice and steady pressure on the glans and foreskin to reduce edema; then, while continuing to apply pressure on the glans, reduce the foreskin.
    - If manual reduction is unsuccessful, will need operative reduction; can be forceps assisted, or may require dorsal slit procedure to relieve constriction, followed by delayed circumcision

Traumatic Etiology

- General principles
  - If hemodynamically unstable, proceed promptly with damage control surgery.

- If hemodynamically stable, nonoperative management is preferred; for hemodynamically stable but bleeding patients, angioembolization may be an option.

- Kidney
  - Mechanism: rapid deceleration injury, blunt injury, penetrating injury (gunshot or stab)
  - Presentation: flank ecchymosis, hematuria, +/− hemodynamic instability
  - Diagnosis: CT of the abdomen/pelvis with IV contrast
    - American Association for the Surgery of Trauma (AAST) grades
      - Grade I: subcapsular hematoma or parenchymal contusion
      - Grade II: perirenal hematoma, laceration <1 cm
      - Grade III: laceration >1 cm, active bleeding
      - Grade IV: laceration into collecting system with active urinary extravasation, ureteropelvic junction (UPJ) disruption, active bleeding beyond Gerota fascia
      - Grade V: shattered or devascularized kidney
    - Grades I to III are considered low grade; grades IV to V are high grade.
  - Management
    - If hemodynamically unstable, proceed with damage control surgery.
    - If hemodynamically stable, trial nonoperative management.
      - High-grade injuries (AAST IV or V) with continued slow bleeding may be candidates for angiography with embolization.
      - Should be closely monitored for 48 to 72 hours
      - Patients with high-grade injuries may develop refractory renovascular hypertension, which may be an indication for delayed nephrectomy.
- Ureter
  - Mechanism: ureteral injury is relatively rare; most commonly due to ballistic injury or sudden deceleration
  - Presentation: hematuria
  - Diagnosis: CT of the abdomen/pelvis with delayed phase (to evaluate urine flow)
  - Management
    - If discovered during damage control surgery, best to divert urine with nephrostomy or ureterostomy; can proceed with delayed repair once stable
    - For minor ureteral contusion or incomplete transection, place ureteral stent.
    - For complete transection, will need surgical repair/reconstruction
- Bladder
  - Mechanism: pelvic fracture, typically blunt trauma
  - Presentation: hematuria, suprapubic tenderness, difficulty voiding
  - Diagnosis: CT cystography
    - Extraperitoneal injury: urinary extravasation into extraperitoneal space
    - Intraperitoneal injury: typically involves dome of the bladder, with urinary extravasation into the peritoneum
  - Management
    - Extraperitoneal injury: nonoperative management with urethral catheter
    - Intraperitoneal injury: requires surgical repair due to the risk for peritonitis
- Urethra
  - Mechanism: blunt trauma
    - Anterior urethral injury—anterior to urogenital diaphragm; usually due to straddle injury
    - Posterior urethral injury—posterior to urogenital diaphragm; usually due to pelvic fracture
  - Presentation: blood at urethral meatus, scrotal/perineal hematoma
  - Diagnosis: retrograde urethrogram
    - For a patient with pelvic fracture and blood at the urethral meatus, do not attempt urethral catheter placement due to high risk for occult urethral injury and placing catheter in a false tract; perform retrograde urethrogram first.
    - Retrograde urethrogram showing contrast extravasation confirms urethral injury.
    - For women—retrograde urethrogram cannot be easily performed; if there is high index of suspicion, proceed with flexible cystourethroscopy.
  - Management: bladder decompression followed by surgical repair
    - For complete urethral injury or posterior urethral injury, place suprapubic catheter.
    - For partial or anterior urethral injury, a single attempt at urethral catheterization is reasonable; low threshold for urologic assistance.
    - Surgical repair may be delayed if the patient is unstable.
- Genitalia
  - Penile fracture
    - Mechanism: laceration of the tunica albuginea during sexual intercourse, leading to popping sensation and rapid detumescence
    - Presentation: discolored, swollen penis; penile hematoma may present as "eggplant deformity."
    - Diagnosis: history and physical examination are usually sufficient; if diagnosis remains unclear, can pursue ultrasound or magnetic resonance imaging (MRI) to demonstrate disruption of tunica albuginea.
    - Management: prompt surgical exploration and repair may prevent erectile dysfunction.
      - Involves exposure of corpora cavernosa, evacuation of hematoma, and repair of tunica albuginea
      - If concurrent urethral injury, that should be repaired as well with urethral catheter left in place.
  - Scrotal trauma
    - Mechanism: blunt or penetrating injury
    - Presentation: pain, ecchymosis, swelling
    - Diagnosis: proceed to OR if testicular rupture is suspected; otherwise can acquire testicular Doppler ultrasound to evaluate the extent of injury and viability of testis
    - Management
      - Minor injury can be managed conservatively.
      - If expanding hematoma, concern for testicular rupture or ischemia, or penetrating mechanism, then proceed with urgent surgical exploration, debridement, and testicular salvage versus orchiectomy depending on viability.

SUGGESTED READINGS

American College of Surgeons. *Best Practices Guidelines: Management of Genitourinary Injuries*. American College of Surgeons; 2025.

Coccolini F, Moore EE, Kluger Y, et al. Kidney and uro-trauma: WSES-AAST guidelines. *World J Emerg Surg*. 2019;14:54.

Ludvigson AE, Beaule LT. Urologic emergencies. *Surg Clin North Am*. 2016;96(3):407-424.

Manjunath AS, Hofer MD. Urologic emergencies. *Med Clin North Am*. 2018;102(2):373-385.

Scheidt MJ, Nikolaidis P, Dogra V, et al. ACR Appropriateness Criteria® radiologic management of urinary tract obstruction. *J Am Coll Radiol*. 2020;17(5 suppl):S281-S292.

SECTION 6

Hematology/Oncology

Section Editors: Raghu R. Chivukula and Casey M. Luckhurst

6.1

Anemia

Richard A. Newcomb

Disease of low hemoglobin concentration or low red blood cell (RBC) count characterized by:

- Decreased production/hypoproliferation
- Ineffective erythropoiesis
- Decreased red cell survival

Common Causes to Remember (Table 6.1.1)

Epidemiology

- RBC lifespan ~120 days
- Etiology of anemia in intensive care unit (ICU) patients is often multifactorial.
- Incidence in ICU patients between 29% and 37%
- 44% of ICU patients in the United States will receive one blood transfusion during their ICU stay.

TABLE 6.1.1 Common Causes of Anemia
1. Blood loss
• Gastrointestinal bleed
• Coagulation disorder
• Surgical procedures
• Phlebotomy
• Extracorporeal circuit disruption (extracorporeal membrane oxygenation [ECMO], continuous venovenous hemofiltration [CVVH])
2. Bone marrow depression
3. Nutritional disorder
4. Red blood cell destruction

Key Pathophysiology

- Hemodilution
- Blood loss
  - Phlebotomy
  - Hemorrhage
  - Disruption of extracorporeal circuit
- Reduced RBC survival and production
- Iron metabolism
- B_{12}/folate metabolism
- Decreased erythropoietin concentration
- Abnormal red cell maturation

Anemia in the Critically Ill

Critical illness → blood loss and/or decreased production → immune activation → decreased iron → decreased erythropoiesis

Differential Diagnosis

- Iron deficiency anemia
  - Most common cause of anemia
  - Patients with iron deficiency anemia have longer ICU stays.
- Hemolytic anemia (RBC destruction)
  - RBC problem: intracellular
    - Intrinsic: hemoglobinopathy (sickle cell disease), enzyme deficiency (G6PD deficiency)
    - Extrinsic: infection (malaria, *Babesia*, *Clostridium perfringens*)
  - RBC problem: membrane
    - Intrinsic: cirrhosis/Zieve syndrome, paroxysmal nocturnal hemoglobinuria
    - Extrinsic: autoimmune hemolytic anemia (warm/cold)
  - Blood vessel problem: microangiopathic hemolytic anemia
    - Disseminated intravascular coagulopathy
    - Thrombotic microangiopathy (transplant associated, medication)
    - Hemolytic uremia syndrome (*Escherichia coli* associated, atypical)
- Blood loss

Management and Treatment

See Section 17: Transfusion Therapy.

- Blood transfusions
- Erythropoietin therapy

SUGGESTED READINGS

Henry ML, Garner WL, Fabri PJ. Iatrogenic anemia. *Am J Surg*. 1986;151:362.

Shander A. Anemia in the critically ill. *Crit Care Clin*. 2004;20:159-178.

Vincent JL, Baron JF, Reinhart K, et al. Anemia and blood transfusion in critically ill patients. *JAMA*. 2002;288:1499-1507.

von Ahsen N, Muller C, Serke S, Frei U, Eckardt KU. Important role of nondiagnostic blood loss and blunted erythropoietic response in the anemia of medical intensive care patients. *Crit Care Med*. 1999;27:2630-2639.

Walsh TS, Saleh E. Anemia during critical illness. *BJA*. 2006;97:278-291.

6.2

Thrombocytopenia

Debbie Jiang

Severity

- Mild: 100 to 149 × 10⁹/L
- Moderate: 50 to 99 × 10⁹/L
- Severe: <50 × 10⁹/L
  - Risk of spontaneous bleeding increases when <10 × 10⁹/L.

Causes of Hospital-Acquired Thrombocytopenia by Mechanism (Table 6.2.1)

Epidemiology

- Up to 50% of patients in the intensive care unit (ICU) develop thrombocytopenia.

TABLE 6.2.1 Hospital-Acquired Thrombocytopenia by Mechanism

Mechanism	Examples
1. *Dilution*	• Fluid resuscitation • Gestational thrombocytopenia
2. *Splenic sequestration*	
3. *Increased consumption*	• Significant blood loss • Massive blunt trauma • Postoperative • DIC • Thrombotic microangiopathy (TTP, complement-mediated HUS) • Extracorporeal circuit
4. *Decreased production*	• Toxin (alcohol) • Infection (viral [eg, HIV, HCV], sepsis from any source) • Iatrogenic (radiation, chemotherapy, linezolid, valproic acid) • Marrow disease (MDS, leukemia, infiltration) • Liver disease • Nutrient deficiency (vitamin B_{12}, folate, copper)
5. *Accelerated destruction*	• Immune thrombocytopenia (ITP) • Drug-induced ITP (antibiotics, quinine) • Heparin-induced thrombocytopenia (HIT) • Vaccine-induced immune thrombotic thrombocytopenia (VITT) • Posttransfusion purpura

DIC, disseminated intravascular coagulation; HCV, hepatitis C virus; HUS, hemolytic uremic syndrome; MDS, myelodysplastic syndrome; TTP, thrombotic thrombocytopenic purpura.

- Hospital-acquired thrombocytopenia is associated with increased length of stay, morbidity, and mortality.
- Most common causes
  - ~50% sepsis, myelosuppression, or disseminated intravascular coagulation (DIC)
  - ~15 to 20% drug related: can be iatrogenic marrow suppression or drug-induced immune thrombocytopenia (ITP)
  - ~15% liver disease/splenomegaly

Key Pathophysiology

- Platelet lifespan: 7 to 10 days
- Dilutional—transfusion of crystalloid, packed cells, and/or fresh frozen plasma (FFP) without replacing platelets
- Splenic sequestration—normal spleen holds 1/3 of body's platelets. Up to ~90% can be sequestered in massive splenomegaly.
- Consumption—platelets used up in thrombus formation. Schistocytes on blood smear indicate microvascular platelet thrombus formation, resulting in microangiopathic hemolytic anemia (MAHA), as seen in thrombotic microangiopathies (TMAs) and DIC.
- Underproduction—due to bone marrow disease (expect disturbance of other cell lines) or liver disease (impaired thrombopoietin production)
- Destruction—accelerated antibody clearance. Takes ~5 to 10 days for thrombocytopenia to manifest due to the time for antibody formation
- Thrombosis + thrombocytopenia has a limited differential and is usually due to an urgent condition: heparin-induced thrombocytopenia (HIT), vaccine-induced immune thrombotic thrombocytopenia (VITT), DIC, antiphospholipid syndrome, TMA.

Evaluation

- History: ask about bleeding, new medications and supplements, infectious symptoms.
- Examination: look for bleeding (ecchymoses, petechiae, mucosal bleeding), hepatosplenomegaly, lymphadenopathy, signs of thrombosis.
- Labs
  - Complete blood count (CBC) and differential—other cytopenias or cytoses?
  - Smear—rule out pseudothrombocytopenia, schistocytes
  - DIC panel

Differential Diagnosis

The differential diagnosis of thrombocytopenia is broad, but the most likely etiology can be ascertained through careful evaluation of the clinical context, physical examination, and laboratory findings (Figure 6.2.1).

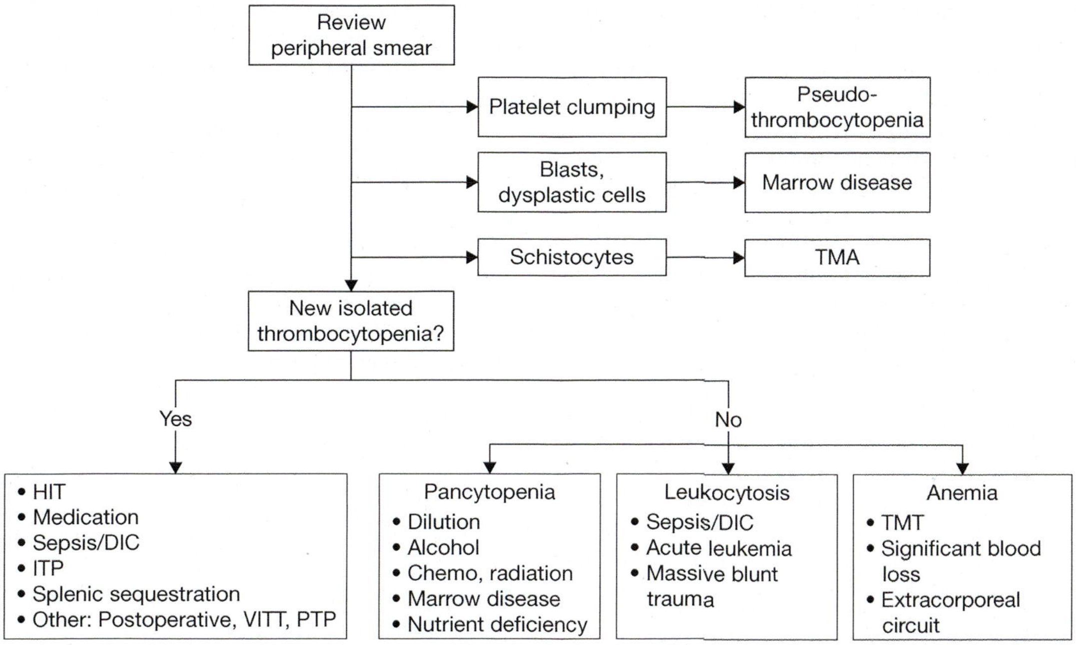

FIGURE 6.2.1 Diagnostic approach to determining the underlying etiology of thrombocytopenia. DIC, disseminated intravascular coagulation; HIT, heparin-induced thrombocytopenia; ITP, immune thrombocytopenia; PTP, posttransfusion purpura; TMA, thrombotic microangiopathy; TMT, transcranial magnetic stimulation; VITT, vaccine-induced immune thrombotic thrombocytopenia.

- Sepsis and DIC
  - Sepsis alone can cause inflammatory myelosuppression, leading to thrombocytopenia.
  - DIC (often triggered by sepsis) leads to consumptive thrombocytopenia through abnormally hyperactive coagulation.
- Medications
  - Drug-induced ITP (DITP) occurs after ~1 week of exposure to offending agent and returns to normal levels after ~1 week of discontinuing the drug.
  - Common offenders
    - Anticonvulsants (carbamazepine, phenytoin)
    - Cinchona alkaloids (quinine, quinidine)
    - H_2 antagonists (cimetidine)
    - Antibiotics (beta-lactams, vancomycin, rifampin, sulfonamides)
    - Platelet inhibitors (abciximab, eptifibatide): rapid onset, ~3 days
    - Antirheumatics (gold salts)
    - Immune checkpoint inhibitors (pembrolizumab, nivolumab)
    - Analgesics (naproxen, diclofenac, acetaminophen)
  - Rarely, medications directly suppress bone marrow: linezolid, valproic acid, daptomycin.
- HIT
  - Antibodies to platelet factor 4 (PF4) complexed with heparin
    - Classically presents after 5 to 10 days of heparin exposure
    - Or within 1 day if recent heparin exposure (within 100 days)
  - Highly prothrombotic. Can be venous (deep venous thrombosis [DVT], pulmonary embolism [PE]) or arterial (limb artery, stroke, myocardial infarction [MI])
  - Occurs in 0.2 to 5% of heparin-treated adults
  - Risk factors
    - Unfractionated heparin > low-molecular-weight heparin >> fondaparinux
    - Female
    - Age (>40 years)
    - Surgical > medical patient
  - Calculate 4T score to estimate pretest probability.
  - HIT antibody testing
    - ELISA looks for PF4-heparin antibodies. Sensitive but not specific. Optical density (OD) strongly predictive. HIT is rarely diagnosed in those with OD <1.0.
    - Serotonin release assay (SRA): functional assay. Sensitive and specific; used for confirmation
- ITP
  - Autoimmune disorder characterized by isolated thrombocytopenia and bleeding (petechiae, mucocutaneous bleeding)
  - Primary or secondary from underlying disease (eg, autoimmune disorder, lymphoma)
  - Unlike sepsis, HIT, primary TMAs, patient often looks well.
- Posttransfusion purpura (PTP)
  - Extremely rare, but life-threatening
  - Immune-mediated, severe thrombocytopenia triggered by recent (within ~5-12 days) blood transfusion

Thrombotic Microangiopathies

- Thrombotic thrombocytopenic purpura (TTP)
  - Severe deficiency of ADAMTS13, the protease that cleaves large von Willebrand factor (vWF) multimers
  - Large vWF multimers → widespread platelet-rich thrombus deposition in microvasculature → MAHA (schistocytes) + thrombocytopenia
  - Suspect if see schistocytes + thrombocytopenia ± neurologic symptoms (confusion, stroke)

- Classic "pentad" (thrombocytopenia, MAHA, fever, altered mental status, and renal insufficiency) is rarely seen.
- Complement-mediated TMA (previously atypical hemolytic uremic syndrome [HUS])
  - Hallmark = renal failure
  - Uncontrolled complement activation → microvascular platelet thrombus deposition, especially in kidney
  - Does not respond to plasma exchange
- Shiga toxin–mediated HUS
  - Preceded by a gastrointestinal illness from Shiga-producing *Escherichia coli*, *Shigella*
  - Often after exposure to undercooked meat, contaminated vegetables

Management and Treatment

- General principles for platelet transfusion
  - Platelet $<10 \times 10^9$/L (increased risk of spontaneous bleeding)
  - Platelet $<50 \times 10^9$/L if bleeding or high risk of bleeding (surgery, needs anticoagulation)
- Sepsis and DIC
  - Treat underlying
  - Supportive blood product transfusion (cryoprecipitate for fibrinogen 100-150)
- Medications
  - Remove offending agent. Platelet count should recover within ~1 week.
  - Add medication to allergy list if drug-induced ITP is confirmed by platelet recovery after withdrawal of agent and/or drug-dependent platelet antibody testing.
- HIT: remove all heparin exposure (including heparin, catheters, and flushes).
  - Start nonheparin agent (argatroban, bivalirudin, direct oral anticoagulant [DOAC]).
  - Evaluate for thrombosis.
  - Avoid platelet transfusion (theoretical risk of triggering a thrombotic event).
  - Add heparin to allergy list; lifelong avoidance.
- ITP
  - Corticosteroids are mainstay of first-line treatment.
  - Intravenous immune globulin (IVIg) can be used for critical thrombocytopenia requiring rapid recovery.
- TTP
  - Therapeutic plasma exchange for immune-mediated TTP: removes anti-ADAMTS13 antibody and repletes ADAMTS13
  - Give FFP to replenish ADAMTS13 until plasma exchange can be initiated.
  - Avoid platelet transfusion unless clinically relevant bleeding or procedure with significant bleeding risk is required.
  - Immunosuppression: glucocorticoids + rituximab reduces rate of relapse.
  - Caplacizumab, an anti-VWF antibody, may be used in severe cases.
- Complement-mediated HUS: anticomplement therapy (eculizumab, ravulizumab)
- Shiga toxin HUS: supportive. If hypovolemic, fluids reduce the risk of requiring renal replacement therapy. Avoid nonsteroidal antiinflammatory drugs (NSAIDs).

SUGGESTED READINGS

Arnold DM, Patriquin CJ, Nazy I. Thrombotic microangiopathies: a general approach to diagnosis and management. *CMAJ*. 2017;189(4):E153-E159.

Bakchoul T, Marini I. Drug-associated thrombocytopenia. *Hematology*. 2018;2018(1):576-583.

Greinacher A. Heparin-induced thrombocytopenia. *N Engl J Med*. 2015; 373(3):252-261.

Greinacher A, Selleng S. How I evaluate and treat thrombocytopenia in the intensive care unit patient. *Blood*. 2016;128(26):3032-3042.

6.3 Thrombocytosis

Debbie Jiang

- Thrombocytosis = platelet count >450,000

Common Causes to Remember (Table 6.3.1)

Epidemiology

- ~85% reactive/secondary and 10% to 15% primary

Key Pathophysiology

- Reactive: secondary condition extrinsically stimulates platelet production, primarily mediated by inflammatory cytokines (eg, interleukin-6 [IL-6]).
- Primary/autonomous: increase in thrombopoiesis from inherited mutation (familial) or acquired mutation resulting in clonal expansion (classically involving *JAK2*, *MPL*, or *CALR*)

TABLE 6.3.1 Common Causes of Thrombocytosis

Reactive/Secondary	Autonomous/Primary

• Infection
• Inflammation: vasculitis, inflammatory bowel disease, connective tissue disease, pancreatitis
• Asplenia
• Cancer
• Iron deficiency
• Drugs (ATRA, epinephrine, vincristine, thrombopoietin receptor agonists)
• Recovery ("rebound") after surgery, severe bleeding, or chemotherapy
• Severe trauma, burns
	• Familial thrombocytosis
	• Acquired, clonal
	  • Myeloproliferative neoplasm (MPN): Essential thrombocythemia, polycythemia vera, primary myelofibrosis
	  • Chronic myeloid leukemia
	  • Myelodysplastic syndrome/MPN overlap

Differential Diagnosis

- Reactive/secondary thrombocytosis
  - Suspect if clinically apparent systemic disease
  - Elevated acute-phase reactants (erythrocyte sedimentation rate [ESR], C-reactive protein [CRP])
  - Transient, self-limited
- Myeloproliferative
  - More likely to have complications (bleeding, thrombosis).
  - Splenomegaly is more common.
  - "Giant" platelets are more often seen on a peripheral blood smear.
  - Abnormalities may occur in other cell lines (leukocytosis, erythrocytosis, or anemia).
  - Persistent

Management and Treatment

- Reactive/secondary
  - Identify and treat the underlying disease process.
- Myeloproliferative
  - Treat primary hematologic process (eg, cytoreduction with hydroxyurea for high-risk myeloproliferative neoplasm [MPN], tyrosine kinase inhibitor such as imatinib for chronic myeloid leukemia [CML]).
  - Aspirin 81 mg daily for thrombosis prevention.
  - Significantly elevated platelet count (>1,000 × 10^9/L) may result in acquired von Willebrand disease (vWD).

SUGGESTED READINGS

Kaushansky K. Hereditary and reactive thrombocytosis. In: Kaushansky K, Prchal JT, Burns LJ, Lichtman MA, Levi M, Linch DC, eds. *Williams Hematology*. 10th ed. McGraw-Hill; 2021;535-536.

Shafer AI. Thrombocytosis. *N Engl J Med*. 2004;350:2122-2129.

6.4

Neutropenia

Richard A. Newcomb

Definition

- Disease of a decreased number of neutrophils characterized by
  - Absolute neutrophil count (ANC) <1,500/mm^3
  - Classified as mild (1,000-1,500), moderate (500-1,000), or severe (<500)
  - Risk of infection increases as ANC decreases.
  - Common features include fevers and infections.
- Severe neutropenia and increased risk of severe infections occur when the ANC <500/mm^3.

Common Causes to Remember (Table 6.4.1)

TABLE 6.4.1 Common Causes of Neutropenia

Decreased Production	Increased Destruction (Extrinsic Factors)
• Intrinsic disorders of proliferation and maturation • Bone marrow problems	• Autoimmune neutropenia • Chemotherapy agents
• Hereditary disorders (Duffy-null–associated neutrophil count, familial neutropenia, congenital neutropenia) • Hematologic malignancies • Toxins (radiation, alcohol, arsenic) • Nutritional deficiencies (B_{12}, folate, copper)	• Hypersplenism • Drugs (phenytoin, flecainide, indomethacin, propylthiouracil, clozapine, antibiotics including penicillin, cephalosporins, trimethoprim-sulfamethoxazole, vancomycin, ganciclovir, and iron chelators) • Infections (viral, bacterial, fungal)

Epidemiology

- Females > males
- Older > young
- African Americans > Whites

Key Pathophysiology

- Neutrophils are an imperative component of the host defense system.
- Oral mucosal ulceration and gingivitis are common problems, as bacteria overwhelm the oral pharynx in those who are neutropenic.
- Neutropenia secondary to chemotherapy drugs tends to result in the most severe infections.
  - Infections can be severe, necessitating intensive care unit (ICU) admission.
    - Usually secondary to "neutropenic fever"
  - Oral pharynx and gastrointestinal tract can be severely affected.
- Patients with chronic neutropenia tend to have functional monocytes and intact immune function.
  - Infections tend to be less severe as compared to those with neutropenia caused by chemotherapy.
- It is important to note that normal, systemic signs of infection may be blunted in the setting of neutropenia, but they will present with fever, possibly as their only marker of inflammation and infection.
  - Caution with medicines that blunt fevers, including acetaminophen, nonsteroidal antiinflammatory drugs, and corticosteroids.

Differential Diagnosis

- Any patient who is neutropenic must be thoroughly worked up, as they often simply present with a fever.
  - Fever of unknown origin

- Drug induced
- Infection: bacterial, viral, fungal
- Complete blood cell (CBC) with differential and evaluation of a peripheral blood smear
- Shock and respiratory failure are the leading causes for neutropenic admissions to the ICU.

Management and Treatment

- If a specific drug is the assumed offending agent, remove it immediately.
- In the setting of neutropenia and fever, a comprehensive infectious workup includes blood cultures and antimicrobial coverage.
  - For all patients, Gram-negative rods, including *Pseudomonas* coverage
  - For patients with shock or concern for line infection, pneumonia, or severe mucositis, add Gram-positive cocci coverage (staph and strep).
  - For patients with persistent fever after 72 hours or prolonged neutropenia (>2-4 weeks) prior to fever, consider antifungal coverage.
  - For all patients, review prior culture data and history of antimicrobial-resistant pathogens to inform antibiotic selection.
- Hematopoietic growth factors
  - Granulocyte colony–stimulating factor—increases neutrophil count and function
    - Avoid use in patients with active myeloid malignancy (eg, acute myeloid leukemia, myelodysplastic neoplasm) without consulting hematology/oncology.
- Isolation rooms: positive pressure room

SUGGESTED READINGS

Bhatt V, Saleem A. Review: drug induced neutropenia—pathophysiology, clinical features, and management. *Ann Clin Lab Sci*. 2004;34(2):131-137.

Boxer LA. How to approach neutropenia. *Hematology Am Soc Hematol Educ Program*. 2012;2012:174-182.

Valent P. Low blood counts: immune mediated, idiopathic, or myelodysplasia. *Hematology Am Soc Hematol Educ Program*. 2012;2012:485-491.

Zimmer AJ, Freifeld AG. Optimal management of neutropenic fever in patients with cancer. *J Oncol Pract*. 2019;15(1):19-24.

6.5

Hemoglobinopathies

Miriam A. Osei and Sharl Azar

- Inherited group of genetic disorders due to quantitative or qualitative defects in globin chain synthesis of hemoglobin (Hb) and include
  - Sickle cell disease (SCD)
  - Thalassemias

Epidemiology

- Hereditary hemoglobinopathies are clustered in areas where malaria is endemic. The mutation has been preserved in the genome as it can confer some protection against malaria.
- 8 million individuals living with SCD worldwide; 500,000 births annually; 75% of births in Sub-Saharan Africa (Table 6.5.1)
- 1 out of every 365 African American births in the United States with SCD; 1 out of every 16,300 Hispanic American births

TABLE 6.5.1 Ethnic Groups Commonly Affected by Hereditary Hemoglobinopathies

Hemoglobinopathies	Ethnic Groups
Sickle cell disease	Africans, Greeks, Southern Italians, Turks, Arabs, Indians
Alpha-thalassemia	Chinese, Taiwanese, South-East Asian, Cypriot, Greek, Turkish, Sardinian
Beta-thalassemia	All ethnic groups, except Northern Europeans

- 8% of African American births with sickle cell trait
- 1.3 million individuals living with thalassemia worldwide; 5% to 7% of the world population are carriers of some form of thalassemia trait.
- 1.35/100,000 persons with thalassemia in the United States
- 10% to 15% of people from the Mediterranean and Southeast Asia have beta-thalassemia.

Key Pathophysiology

- Hb is made of globin polypeptide chains arranged in a tetramer.
  - The tetramer is typically divided into two alpha chains and two beta chains.
- Each Hb polypeptide chain interacts with one heme moiety and an iron atom in the ferrous state.
  - Each heme-ferrous complex can bind one oxygen molecule.
  - Therefore, each Hb tetramer can bind four oxygen molecules.
- Mutations in the amino acid sequences of the alpha or beta chains can cause disease and clinical symptoms.
  - Known areas of mutations that cause clinical symptoms include (1) a key histidine in the F helix; (2) connections between the alpha1 and beta1 subunits; and (3) connections between the alpha1 and beta2 subunits.
- Types of Hb
  - During the first trimester, the fetus has primarily embryonic Hbs: Gower 1, Gower 2, and Portland 1.
  - By 34 to 36 weeks of gestation, fetal hemoglobin (Hb F) comprises 90% to 95%, with the rest represented by adult hemoglobin (Hb A).
  - At term, Hb F comprises 53% to 95%, with Hb A comprising around 20% to 30% of total Hb.
  - Persistently elevated Hb F is seen in hemoglobinopathies, but can also be seen in the following infants:
    - Small for gestational age

        - Chronic hypoxia
        - Trisomy 13
    - Hb F levels stay elevated during the neonatal period and decrease to <3% by 6 months of life.
    - At birth, the infant starts producing hemoglobin A2 (Hb A2) and reaches adult levels by 6 months.
    - Because of the predominance of alpha chain Hbs in infancy, typically alpha chain hemoglobinopathies present in the neonatal period, whereas beta chain abnormalities present after 3 months of age.
- Common pathway for hereditary hemoglobinopathies
    - Point mutations in the amino acids associated with the alpha or beta chains will produce clinical syndromes if they alter solubility and/or oxygen-binding affinity.
    - This leads to an inadequate supply of Hb, which leads to the destruction of red cells and associated precursors. Depending on the number and location of mutations, clinical severity can range from in utero death (eg, hydrops fetalis) to asymptomatic carriers with mild anemia.
- Specific hereditary hemoglobinopathies
    - *SCD:* caused by a mutation in the beta chain that changes the sixth amino acid from glutamic acid to valine (Hb S)
        - Pathophysiology: when deoxygenated, Hb S polymerizes, forming long, rigid rods inside red blood cells (RBCs), which leads to the characteristic "sickle" shape of the RBC. Sickled RBCs are less flexible, more adherent to blood vessel endothelium, and occlude capillary vessels, leading to tissue ischemia, microinfarction of organs, and pain. Furthermore, hemolysis occurs as the body attempts to digest the polymers, leading to significantly reduced lifespan of sickled RBCs (~10-20 compared to the usual 120 days) and causing chronic hemolytic anemia. The changes to red cell structure, distensibility, rheology, and interactions with inflammatory cells and the surrounding vasculature all collectively account for the complex manifestations of SCD.
    - *Thalassemia:* caused by mutations in alpha or beta chain subunits that decrease the quantity of the affected subunit
        - Pathophysiology: a reduced supply of the affected subunit causes decreased production and accumulation of the other subunits. Heterozygous individuals typically only manifest with mild anemia.
        - Homozygous individuals typically have more severe anemia, since the red cell precursors are destroyed in the bone marrow, with the few red cells that survive ultimately destroyed by the spleen. This leads to a profound hemolytic anemia. The body adapts by hypertrophy of the bone marrow, causing characteristic bone abnormalities in patients, such as "chipmunk" facies.
    - *Unstable Hbs:* rare, inherited mutations that decrease solubility of Hb and typically precipitate to form inclusion bodies in red cells called Heinz bodies. The spleen removes these Heinz bodies, leaving defective RBCs (bite cells or degmacytes), which are subsequently destroyed by the body at a rapid rate. As a result, even patients who are heterozygous are symptomatic.
- Acquired Hb abnormalities
    - Patients with acquired Hb abnormalities typically have normal genetics related to the structure of Hb and thus produce normal Hb molecules, but those proteins are then impacted by toxins.

Differential Diagnosis

- The differential diagnosis for anemia is large; however, consider testing for hemoglobinopathies in patients with the following:
    - History of hydrops fetalis during pregnancy
    - Unexplained anemia and splenomegaly
    - Neonatal or infantile anemia with Hb F
    - Neonatal or infantile anemia with low Hb A
    - Unexplained microcytosis
    - Clinical features suggestive of sickle cell
    - Unexplained hemolysis
    - Unexplained irregularly contracted cells
    - Unexplained cyanosis with normal oxygen saturations

Diagnosis

- Hereditary
    - Cellulose acetate electrophoresis is a quick and inexpensive initial test but does not screen for certain variants.
    - Agar gel electrophoresis is a good follow-up study that is able to identify other variants not screened by cellulose acetate electrophoresis.
    - High-pressure liquid chromatography (HPLC): some variants cannot be detected by either electrophoresis technique and will require HPLC. Also suitable for beta-thalassemia carrier detection because it can quantify Hb A2 and Hb F.
    - Further genetic testing, including alpha and beta globin gene sequencing, is available to determine the specific genetic variant and especially for definitive diagnosis of the thalassemias.
- Acquired
    - Tests for carboxyhemoglobin, methemoglobin, and sulfhemoglobin are readily available and should be sent in the right clinical scenario.

Presentation, Management, and Treatment

    - SCD: most patients are anemic with reactive bone marrow and a pronounced reticulocytosis. In critical care settings, patients could present with any or all of the following:
    - *Acute vaso-occlusive pain episodes (VOEs):* sudden onset of severe pain that can vary in location of the body, severity, and duration, with identifiable (weather changes, dehydration, stress) or no identifiable (majority of the time) trigger
        - The international gold standard for the assessment of pain is the patient report as there is no definitive objective measure of sickle cell pain or its severity.
        - It is important to ensure that the pain is not masking other potentially life-threatening complications of SCD (see later).
        - Treatment is supportive and should be initiated rapidly with multimodal pain control, including

intravenous (IV) opioids, hydration with IV, and oral (PO) fluids, but being careful not to overhydrate, and individualized for each patient and reassessed frequently,
    - The American Society of Hematology recommends a door-to-first-dose of pain medication time of no >60 minutes
  - *Acute chest syndrome (ACS):* life-threatening complication that presents with new radiodensity on chest imaging and fever or respiratory symptoms (hypoxemia, cough, etc)
    - Most likely, it is caused by a combination of many underlying pathogenic processes, including pneumonia, pulmonary infarction, fat embolism, bone marrow infarction, and/or myocardial infarction.
    - Incentive spirometry at the beginning of hospitalizations should be used to reduce the risk of developing ACS.
    - Commonly occurs a few days into hospitalization for an acute VOE and can evolve rapidly; thus, close monitoring for the development of ACS during hospitalizations is important.
    - Treatment includes admission to a monitored setting and may require admission to the intensive care unit. It requires adequate pain control, judicious hydration to avoid pulmonary edema, oxygen therapy that may escalate to include mechanical ventilation, empiric antibiotics for community-acquired pneumonia with atypical bacteria coverage, and transfusions, particularly exchange transfusions to decrease the Hb S percent.
  - *Splenic sequestration crisis:* potentially life-threatening complication that presents with an acute drop in Hb level (~2 g/dL drop), abdominal pain, and splenomegaly
    - Typically, patients with sickle cell auto-infarct their spleen in childhood.
    - However, the spleen can persist, and an acute sickle cell crisis could occlude venous outflow from the spleen, causing severe anemia.
    - Patients with Hb SC or Hb S/B+ thalassemia subtypes are more likely to retain their spleen into adulthood.
    - These patients typically require transfusions and an emergent splenectomy.
    - Reticulocytosis is often preserved in splenic sequestration, allowing it to be better differentiated from an aplastic crisis.
  - *Aplastic crisis:* patients present with an acute anemia and a decreased reticulocytosis.
    - Aplastic crisis is from bone marrow suppression, most commonly by infection with parvovirus B19A.
    - Management includes close monitoring and transfusions as needed.
    - Most cases resolve with supportive care.
  - *Infections:* patients are susceptible to encapsulated organisms because of the loss of their spleen.
    - The classic infection, but not most common infection, is osteomyelitis from *Salmonella* species.
    - Treatment is with antibiotics, and vaccination against encapsulated organisms is essential to reducing the frequency of these infections.
    - Independent of splenic physiology, patients with SCD can have irregular immunoglobulin G (IgG) and IgM antibody responses, along with defects in the alternative complement pathway.
  - *Anemia:* patients with sickle cell are typically chronically anemic and can tolerate very low Hbs with episodes of acute worsening due to other complications.
    - Transfusion thresholds should be determined by the clinical scenario and not on preset numbers, given the risk of complications with transfusions themselves.
    - Generally, consider a transfusion if there is a >2 g/dL drop from patient's baseline Hb or if there are significant symptoms of worsening anemia such as dyspnea or tachycardia.
  - *Hyperhemolytic crisis:* presents with sudden exacerbation of hemolysis with worsening anemia despite ongoing reticulocytosis
    - Underlying mechanism not fully understood, although complement activation implicated and commonly seen in cases of delayed hemolytic transfusion reaction following transfusions
    - Management includes transfusion with compatible blood, complement inhibitors, and immunosuppressive therapies.
  - *Stroke:* patients with SCD are at increased risk of strokes, with about a quarter having had a stroke by age 45.
    - Management of acute stroke includes transfusion, particularly prompt exchange transfusion.
    - Chronically, individuals who have had a stroke are treated with serial simple or exchange transfusions to prevent a second stroke.
  - *Other end-organ ischemia:* patients could present with retinal detachments, retinal vessel occlusions, acute renal infarction/failure, aseptic necrosis of bones and joints, priapism, pulmonary hypertension, venous thromboembolisms, and chronic leg ulcers.
    - In the chronic care setting, patients are treated with the critical disease-modifying therapy, hydroxyurea, and other therapies that decrease VOEs (L-glutamine) and increase Hb (voxelotor).
    - Transformative therapy includes bone marrow transplantation and recently approved gene therapy.
- Beta-thalassemias
  - Beta-thalassemia has a wide spectrum of disease, with most individuals with mild to no symptoms. Definitions include:
    - Beta-thalassemia major (transfusion dependent thalassemia, TDT): requires intensive transfusion therapy to survive
    - Beta-thalassemia intermedia (non-transfusion dependent thalassemia, NTDT): patients can survive without transfusions but may require them at least intermittently throughout their lives.
    - Beta-thalassemia minor/trait: asymptomatic
  - Patients can present with hepatosplenomegaly, gallstones, chronic leg ulcers, anemia, and high-output cardiomyopathy.
  - Patients with severe disease are usually malnourished from increased caloric requirements, increased susceptibility to infections, and will require chronic transfusions to improve oxygen delivery and suppress erythropoiesis.
  - Target hemoglobin is 9.5 - 10.5 g/dL.
  - Most severe cases will develop iron overload and have shortened lifespan, warranting iron chelation.

- Iron should not be supplemented in these patients because of ineffective erythropoiesis, especially since they can easily be misdiagnosed with iron deficiency anemia.
- Splenectomy should be considered in patients who require a high volume of transfusions.
- Treatment includes luspatercept, bone marrow transplantation, and gene therapy.

- Alpha-thalassemias: similarly, a wide spectrum of disease with definitions including:
  - Alpha-thalassemia-2 trait: one locus deleted, asymptomatic
  - Alpha-thalassemia-1 trait: two loci deleted, asymptomatic
  - Thalassemia-intermedia (Hb H disease): caused by a three-locus deletion. Symptomatic anemia; usually will not need transfusions until later in adulthood
  - Hydrops fetalis: caused by all four loci deleted (Hb Bart), leading to in utero death
  - Treatment is similar to beta-thalassemia in symptomatic individuals.
- Methemoglobinemia
  - Caused by toxins that oxidize iron to the ferric state, which has a very high affinity for oxygen and prevents oxygen delivery
  - Heme in the ferric state is bluish, and as a result, patients typically present bluish, similar to cyanosis.
  - As a result, patients present with hypoxic symptoms, blue, but with normal oxygen saturation. Blood can appear muddy.
  - Cerebral ischemia occurs at levels >15%, and death >60%.
  - Treatment is with 1 mg/kg IV of methylene blue (give blue to blue), although caution is required in individuals with G6PD deficiency.
    - Mild cases can be treated with PO methylene blue or ascorbic acid (300-600 mg/d).
- Unstable Hbs: these patients might require a splenectomy to correct anemia.
  - Many of these patients will present with severe anemia, splenomegaly, chronic leg ulcers, and early biliary disease.

SUGGESTED READINGS

DeBaun MR, Jordan LC, King AA, et al. American Society of Hematology 2020 guidelines for sickle cell disease: prevention, diagnosis, and treatment of cerebrovascular disease in children and adults. *Blood Adv*. 2020;4(8):1554-1588.

Kavanagh PL, Fasipe TA, Wun T. Sickle cell disease: a review. *JAMA*. 2022;328(1):57-68.

Langer AL. Beta-thalassemia. In: Adam MP, Feldman J, Mirzaa GM, et al, eds. *GeneReviews®* [Internet]. University of Washington; 1993-2024. https://www.ncbi.nlm.nih.gov/books/NBK1426/

Madu AJ, Ugwu AO, Efobi C. Hyperhaemolytic syndrome in sickle cell disease: clearing the cobwebs. *Med Princ Pract*. 2021;30(3):236-243.

Musallam KM, Taher AT, Cappellini MD, et al. Alpha-thalassemia: a practical overview. *Blood Rev*. 2024;64:101165.

Yee ME, Bakshi N, Graciaa SH, et al. Incidence of invasive haemophilus influenzae infections in children with sickle cell disease. *Pediatr Blood Cancer*. 2019;66(6):e27642.

6.6

Hematopoietic Cell Transplantation

Richard A. Newcomb

Definition

- Infusion of hematopoietic stem and progenitor cells to the patient (recipient) intravenously (IV)
  - Allogeneic transplant: from a donor
    - Goals
      - Consolidation therapy for high-risk hematologic malignancies and provision of "graft-versus-malignancy" effect
      - Restoration of normal hematopoiesis and immune function in patients with bone marrow failure, hemoglobinopathies, or immunodeficiencies
    - Donors
      - Related (siblings, parents, children)
      - Unrelated (volunteers through registries)
      - Umbilical cord (donor banks)
    - Donor human leukocyte antigen (HLA) match
      - HLA match is an important consideration.
      - Preference is typically for a full match at A, B, C, DRB1, and DQB1.
      - With the advent of posttransplant cyclophosphamide, HLA-mismatched transplants are feasible, safe, and effective and have expanded access to transplant for patients of non-European ancestry.
    - Stem cell sources and considerations
      - Peripheral blood: faster engraftment, preferred for patients with cancer, more graft-versus-host disease (GVHD)
      - Bone marrow: slower engraftment, higher risk of graft failure, less chronic GVHD
      - Umbilical cord: slower engraftment, historically more infectious complications, available across ancestral groups
    - Conditioning intensity
      - Myeloablative
      - Reduced intensity
    - Improvements in the treatment of hematologic malignancy, transplant procedures, and supportive care have significantly reduced nonrelapse mortality.
      - Reduced infection rates, liver and kidney dysfunction, GVHD, recurrence of malignant conditions, and overall transplant-related mortality

- Autologous transplant: from the patient
  - Use the patients' own stem cells from their bone marrow or peripheral blood to restore hematopoiesis after high-dose chemotherapy
    - Need to ensure the "graft" (transplanted cells) does not contain tumor cells
      - "Purging" = in vivo treatment with chemotherapy
- The goal is to reestablish marrow function in a patient after receipt of high-dose chemotherapy.

Diseases Treated With Bone Marrow Transplant/Stem Cell Transplant

- Acute leukemia (acute lymphoblastic leukemia [ALL], acute myeloid leukemia [AML])
- Chronic leukemia (chronic lymphocytic leukemia [CLL], chronic myeloid leukemia [CML])
- Hodgkin disease
- Non-Hodgkin lymphoma
- Multiple myeloma
- Myelodysplastic syndromes
- Aplastic anemia
- Hemoglobinopathies (thalassemia and sickle cell disease)
- Immunodeficiency disorders (severe combined immunodeficiency [SCID], Wiskott-Aldrich syndrome, Chediak-Higashi syndrome)

Complications

- Infections
  - Bacterial
  - Invasive fungal
    - Patients should receive prophylaxis with fluconazole for the first 100 days.
    - Secondary to delayed engraftment (more commonly seen with cord blood donor)
    - Seen in patients afflicted with acute and chronic GVHD that are being treated with steroids
  - Cytomegalovirus (CMV) reactivation: can detect CMV in the blood of the transplant recipient, but there is NO evidence of disease.
    - Seen at 15 to 100 days posttransplant
    - Patient or donor was seropositive for CMV pretransplant.
    - Risk is found in patients with compromised cellular immunity.
      - Those with acute GVHD or those who received a T-cell–depleted transplant
    - Prevention: letermovir in CMV-seropositive recipients
    - Treatment: IV ganciclovir or foscarnet
  - CMV disease: hepatitis, gastroenteritis or colitis, pneumonitis (mortality up to 50%)
  - *Pneumocystis jirovecii* pneumonia (PJP)
    - Prophylaxis with bactrim, dapsone, or atovaquone
- Veno-occlusive disease/sinusoidal occlusion syndrome
  - Onset within 3 weeks of conditioning (typically myeloablative)
  - Weight gain, ascites, tender hepatomegaly, and elevated bilirubin
  - Right upper quadrant ultrasound with Doppler shows reversal of vascular flow.
  - Secondary to injury to the sinusoidal endothelial cells in the liver
    - Characterized by the loss of sinusoidal wall integrity with consequent sinusoidal congestive obstruction
  - The liver appears marbled and bluish red in color; the cut surface appears congested (dilated sinusoids filled with red blood cells [RBCs]).
  - Hepatorenal failure ensues.
  - Supportive therapy (renal replacement therapy) and defibrotide can be tried in patients with multisystem organ failure.
- Pulmonary complications
  - Idiopathic pneumonia syndrome
    - Onset after 3 weeks posttransplant
    - Dry cough, dyspnea, hypoxemia, and nodular radiographic infiltrates (>90% of patients will have diffuse infiltrates on chest x-ray [CXR])
    - Diagnose with bronchioalveolar lavage (BAL) and biopsies, which will demonstrate alveolar damage, pneumonia, and interstitial lymphocytic inflammation
    - Treatment is mainly supportive, and prevention and treatment of infections
      - Corticosteroids
      - Etanercept
    - Incidence ~10% with an unfortunately high mortality rate
  - Diffuse alveolar hemorrhage
    - Onset in the first 30 days posttransplant
    - Cough, dyspnea, fever, hypoxemia, infiltrates on CXR involving the middle and lower lung zones
    - Hemoptysis is rare.
    - Diagnosis is confirmed with >20% hemosiderin-laden macrophages on BAL in the absence of infection.
    - Treatment is supportive (mechanical ventilation) and corticosteroids.
    - Incidence ~5% with an unfortunately high mortality rate
  - Periengraftment respiratory distress syndrome
    - Onset within 5 days
    - Skin rash, pulmonary infiltrates (noninfectious), hypoxemia, fever, capillary leak, and diarrhea
    - Treatment with corticosteroids usually leads to rapid clinical improvement.
- Graft-versus-host disease (GVHD)
  - Arises when donor T cells respond to genetically defined proteins on host cells, namely, HLAs
  - Can develop even with HLA identity between the donor and the recipient
  - Acute (day 0-100)
    - Skin
      - Grade depends on the area involved.
      - Maculopapular rash
    - Gastrointestinal (GI) tract
      - Grade depends on the volume of diarrhea.
      - Based on clinical criteria
      - Nausea, anorexia, abdominal pain, diarrhea
      - Confirm with biopsies; however, cannot be excluded as there can be patches of normal tissue
    - Liver
      - Grade depends on bilirubin level.
    - Treat with high-dose corticosteroids.

- Steroid refractory: ruxolitinib; preference remains for clinical trial if available.
- Infection is the leading cause of death.
- Chronic (day 100-on)
  - Can affect almost any part of the body
  - Skin, nails, mouth, eyes, muscles, joints, GI tract, liver, lungs, kidneys, heart, bone marrow
  - Pathophysiology is multifactorial, with dysregulated T-cell activation (TH2) and often the development of fibrosis.
  - Treatment paradigms have changed recently.
    - First-line systemic therapy: corticosteroids
    - Steroid-refractory disease: three recent Food and Drug Administration (FDA) approvals:
      - Ruxolitinib
      - Belumosudil
      - Ibrutinib
  - Response to treatment is unpredictable.
  - Course is determined by the severity and extent of the associated immunodeficiency.
    - ~50% have limited disease and good prognosis.
    - In patients with extensive disease, up to 60% will respond to treatment and can eventually discontinue immunosuppressive therapy.
    - Unfortunately, the remaining patients tend to succumb to opportunistic infections or require long-term immunosuppressive therapy.

SUGGESTED READINGS

Ho VT, Linden E, Revta C, Richardson PG. Hepatic veno-occlusive disease after hematopoietic stem cell transplantation: review and update on the use of defibrotide. *Semin Thromb Hemost*. 2007;33(4):373-388.

Jamy O, Zeiser R, Chen YB. Novel developments in the prophylaxis and treatment of acute GVHD. *Blood*. 2023;142(12):1037-1046.

Jenkins P, Johnston LJ, Pickham D, Chang B, Rizk N, Tierney DK. Intensive care utilization for hematopoietic cell transplant recipients. *Biol Blood Marrow Transplant*. 2015;21(11):2023-2027.

Rubia-Brandt L. Sinusoidal obstruction syndrome. *Clin Liver Dis*. 2010;14(4):651-668.

Vande Vusse LK, Madtes DK. Early onset noninfectious pulmonary syndromes after hematopoietic cell transplantation. *Clin Chest Med*. 2017;38(2):233-248.

Zeiser R, Blazar BR. Acute graft-versus-host disease—biologic process, prevention, and therapy. *N Engl J Med*. 2017;377(22):2167-2179.

Zeiser R, Blazar BR. Pathophysiology of chronic graft-versus-host disease and therapeutic targets. *N Engl J Med*. 2017;377(26):2565-2579.

6.7

Tumor Lysis Syndrome

Brandon J. Aubrey and Andrew M. Brunner

Tumor lysis syndrome (TLS) is a potentially life-threatening oncologic emergency that occurs when a large number of cancer cells die rapidly, releasing intracellular contents into the bloodstream to cause a range of metabolic disturbances, including hyperuricemia, hyperphosphatemia, hypocalcemia, hyperkalemia, and acute kidney injury.

Key Points

- TLS-related metabolic derangements can quickly lead to renal failure, cardiac arrhythmias, and seizures and may become life-threatening if not promptly treated.
- Recognizing risk factors for TLS allows implementation of close laboratory monitoring, prophylactic treatment, and early interventions to prevent complications.
- Timing: onset is typically within 12 to 72 hours of initiating cytotoxic therapy, peaks at around 2 to 3 days after starting therapy, and resolves within 5 to 7 days with appropriate supportive care.
- Aggressive hydration, effective urate-lowering therapy, and careful management of electrolyte disturbances (including hemodialysis when required) have significantly improved patient outcomes.
- TLS can be an early, life-threatening complication of potentially curative cancer therapy that may require critical care support when severe.

Pathophysiology

- TLS is driven by the release of intracellular contents (uric acid, potassium, phosphate, nucleic acids) caused by the death of cells within rapidly proliferating tumors.
- TLS may be due to (1) spontaneous cell death within a large, proliferative tumor, and/or (2) exposure of cancer cells to cytotoxic therapy that induces widespread cell death.
- Hyperuricemia: uric acid is poorly soluble and precipitates more readily at an acidic pH. High blood levels of uric acid lead to precipitation of urate crystals within renal tubules, causing tubule obstruction and inflammation that then leads to acute kidney injury.
- Hyperphosphatemia: elevated phosphate levels drive the precipitation of calcium-phosphate crystals, leading to secondary hypocalcemia. Precipitation of calcium-phosphate crystals within the kidney, and other soft tissues, causes end-organ damage.
- Release of nucleic acids, tissue factor, cytokines, and other intracellular factors into circulation can activate the coagulation system and precipitate (or worsen) disseminated intravascular coagulation (DIC). TLS and DIC are distinct entities but often occur together and have overlapping pathophysiology.

Risk Factors

- TLS risk relates to:
  - Tumor properties (disease type, rapid cell proliferation, and tumor bulk)
  - Drug effects (treatment with drugs that induce cell death and necrosis)
- Disease types associated with increased TLS risk: acute myeloid leukemia, acute lymphoblastic leukemia, lymphoblastic lymphoma, Burkitt lymphoma/leukemia, diffuse large B-cell lymphoma, and chronic lymphocytic leukemia (when treated with the BCL2 inhibitor venetoclax). TLS can occasionally be associated with solid organ cancers, including small cell lung cancer, germ cell tumors, high-grade neuroendocrine tumors, or other tumor types displaying highly aggressive features and large tumor bulk.
- Tumor bulk and high proliferative rate are inferred by a markedly elevated lactate dehydrogenase (LDH), uric acid, and/or white cell count and may be directly demonstrated on imaging studies.
- Hyperuricemia: pretreatment uric acid levels are highly predictive for TLS risk after initiating cytotoxic therapy. Uric acid levels are generally proportional to tumor burden, tumor proliferation, and baseline levels of spontaneous TLS. Pretreatment uric acid level >7.5 mg/dL predicts for moderate-to-high risk of developing TLS.
- TLS can be precipitated by any cytotoxic medication: chemotherapy, steroids, BCL2-targeting drugs (venetoclax), and a growing number of novel targeted therapies.

Diagnostic Criteria

- Cairo-Bishop diagnostic criteria
  - Laboratory TLS (≥2 of the following criteria):
    - Uric acid ≥8.0 mg/dL or ≥25% increase from baseline
    - Potassium ≥6.0 mEq/L or ≥25% increase from baseline
    - Phosphate ≥4.5 mg/dL or ≥25% increase from baseline
    - Calcium ≤7.0 mg/dL or ≥25% decrease from baseline
  - Clinical TLS: laboratory criteria listed here plus one clinical criterion that can include acute kidney injury (creatinine [Cr] ≥1.5 × upper limit of normal), cardiac arrhythmia, sudden death or seizure.

Prophylaxis for Tumor Lysis Syndrome

- Uric acid–lowering therapy
  - Allopurinol inhibits xanthine oxidase, preventing the formation of new uric acid from purines. It takes 1 to 3 days for the therapeutic effect and does not allow for the removal of existing uric acid.
  - Rasburicase is an enzyme that rapidly converts uric acid into allantoin, a highly soluble and easily excreted substance (onset of urate-lowering effect is <4 hours).
- Allopurinol is used in routine clinical practice when there is a clinical concern for TLS.
- Rasburicase indications: there are no universally accepted clinical or laboratory findings to guide the use of rasburicase. Generally, rasburicase will be considered in the setting of high-grade malignancy with laboratory evidence of TLS and uric acid level ≥8.0 mg/dL.
- Rasburicase carries a risk of oxidative hemolysis that may be catastrophic in patients with glucose-6-phosphate dehydrogenase (G6PD) deficiency.
- Prephase treatment: initial period of treatment with lower intensity cytotoxic therapy to reduce the extent of cell death upon initiation of full-dose intensive chemotherapy
- Leukapheresis: procedure to remove white cells through extracorporeal, automated cell separation to rapidly lower the white cell count in patients with leukemia and clinical concern for leukostasis. There is currently no high-level evidence to support the routine use of leukapheresis in the setting of hyperleukocytosis to reduce the risk of TLS. However, this may be considered according to local practice guidelines.

Management of Established Tumor Lysis Syndrome

- Close clinical and laboratory monitoring with frequent measurement of serum electrolytes, renal function, cardiac monitoring, and careful assessment of patient clinical fluid status
- Aggressive hydration with normal saline to maintain excretion of uric acid and phosphate aiming for urine output >100 mL/h with the use of loop diuretics to maintain diuresis and augment potassium excretion as necessary. Lactated Ringer solution is generally avoided because it contains calcium and may exacerbate calcium-phosphate deposition.
- Hyperphosphatemia: treat with phosphate binders (sevelamer or calcium acetate), and patients may require dialysis when hyperphosphatemia is severe.
- Hypocalcemia: reflects compensation for hyperphosphatemia and should not be treated unless severe or symptomatic (calcium replacement can exacerbate calcium-phosphate precipitation, tissue deposition, and renal damage)
- Hyperuricemia: ongoing treatment with allopurinol and rasburicase, as indicated. Alkalinization is not routinely recommended to reduce urate crystal deposition and should only be used for the treatment of metabolic acidosis.
- Hyperkalemia: aggressive monitoring and management of potassium levels according to standard guidelines. Interventions may include, but are not limited to, hydration and loop diuretics, insulin and dextrose, potassium-binding resins, and dialysis when severe and refractory to medical treatment.
- Indications for dialysis:
  - Severe and/or refractory hyperkalemia
  - Severe and/or refractory hyperphosphatemia. Considered when the calcium-phosphate product is >70 mg^2/dL^2
  - Severe, symptomatic hypocalcemia (tetany, seizures, or cardiac instability) failing medical management
  - Volume overload—may be due to the combination of worsening kidney injury and excessive fluid administration
  - Other general indications for renal replacement therapy: anuria/oliguria, uremia, and metabolic acidosis

Outcomes

- Prior to the improved understanding of TLS pathophysiology and the implementation of effective supportive care, including the use of urate-lowering agents, mortality in TLS was reported to approach 80% in some patient populations. In current practice, with aggressive monitoring and early intervention, outcomes are much improved, and mortality rates are significantly lower.

SUGGESTED READINGS

Cairo MS, Coiffier B, Reiter A, Younes A, Panel TLSE. Recommendations for the evaluation of risk and prophylaxis of tumour lysis syndrome (TLS) in adults and children with malignant diseases: an expert TLS panel consensus. *Br J Haematol*. 2010;149(4):578-586.

Howard SC, Jones DP, Pui CH. The tumor lysis syndrome. *N Engl J Med*. 2011;364(19):1844-1854.

6.8

Solid Tumors

Devan Cote

Definition

- Critically ill patients with solid tumors (ie, nonhematologic malignancies) represent a complicated subgroup of intensive care unit (ICU) patients requiring extensive coordination among specialized teams, including oncology, surgery, interventional radiology, and palliative care.
- According to the American Cancer Society, the top six contributors to cancer-related mortality in the United States are solid tumors, shown in Table 6.8.1.
- About 1 in 20 patients diagnosed with a solid tumor will require ICU admission within 2 years of diagnosis.
- Reasons for ICU admission may include cancer progression, elective or emergent surgery, treatment complications, and exacerbations of comorbid illnesses.
- In a large European ICU cohort, 13% of patients had solid tumors, of which 25% were metastatic. Among patients with solid tumors, 70% of admissions were surgical, 63% required mechanical ventilation, 42% had sepsis, and 40% required vasopressors.

Prognosis

- Owing to advances in cancer care and ICU care, the mortality of critically ill patients with solid tumors approaches that of the cancer-free ICU population, depending primarily on the severity of organ failure rather than oncologic stage.
    - According to 2016 SCCM triage guidelines, the decision to admit patients with cancer to the ICU should be made on the same criteria as all critically ill patients, with careful consideration of their long-term prognosis.
    - In a systematic review, mechanical ventilation requirement had the highest association with mortality.
    - Mortality tends to be highest for emergency medical admissions and lowest for elective surgical admissions.
- ICU admission should not be restricted based on the presence of metastatic disease alone.
    - Among a cohort of patients with metastatic solid tumors with unplanned ICU admissions, as many as 37% were home at 90-day follow-up.
- In general, patients with solid tumors have more favorable ICU outcomes than patients with hematologic malignancies.

TABLE 6.8.1 Deadliest Cancers, American Cancer Society 2024

Tumor	Projected US Deaths 2024 (%)
Lung and bronchus	125,070 (20.4)
Colon and rectum	53,010 (8.7)
Pancreas	51,750 (8.5)
Breast	42,780 (7.0)
Prostate	35,250 (5.8)
Liver and intrahepatic bile duct	29,840 (4.9)

Respiratory Failure

- Acute respiratory failure and sepsis are the most common indications for unplanned ICU admission among patients with solid tumors.
- Respiratory failure carries a high mortality in this population, especially when mechanical ventilation is required.
- The differential diagnosis of respiratory failure in patients with solid tumors includes pneumonia, drug-induced pulmonary toxicity, radiation pneumonitis, pulmonary embolism, and cardiogenic causes.
- Pneumonia
    - Pneumonia is the most common cause of respiratory failure in patients with solid tumors.
    - Bacterial pneumonias are most common. Severe viral and fungal pneumonias may also occur, especially in the immunocompromised.
    - The increased susceptibility of patients with cancer to pneumonia is multifactorial, encompassing anatomic factors (eg, obstructive lung cancer), poor airway protection (eg, dysphagia, opioid requirements), disease- and treatment-related immunosuppression, and malnutrition.
    - Patients with cancer undergoing chemotherapy are at risk for nosocomial infections, severe presentations of community-acquired infections (eg, influenza, SARS-CoV-2), and opportunistic infections (eg, pneumocystis, aspergillus, herpes viruses).
        - Risk factors for pneumocystis jirovecii pneumonia (PJP) include lymphopenia <400/μL, chronic corticosteroids, autoimmunity, advanced age, and

exposure to anticancer agents including everolimus, temozolomide, anthracyclines, gemcitabine, cyclophosphamide, and 5-fluorouracil.

- For patients on corticosteroids amounting to ≥20 mg prednisone equivalents daily for >1 month anticipated duration, empiric PJP prophylaxis with trimethoprim-sulfamethoxazole (TMP-SMX) should be considered.
- Invasive aspergillosis may arise in patients with solid tumors with underlying lung conditions, on corticosteroids, and with prior chest radiotherapy.

- In formulating empiric antimicrobial regimens, attention should be given to exposure to community-acquired and nosocomial organisms, immunocompromised status, prior culture data, and local resistance patterns.
- Initial workup may include chest imaging, blood and respiratory cultures, respiratory virus polymerase chain reaction (PCR) (including SARS-CoV-2 and influenza), fungal biomarkers (galactomannan [bronchoalveolar lavage or BAL fluid or serum] for aspergillus; and beta-D-glucan [serum] for PJP and others), urinary antigen testing (*Legionella* and *Pneumococcus*), and methicillin-resistant *Staphylococcus aureus* (MRSA) nasal PCR screening.
- In cases of diagnostic uncertainty, a targeted or random BAL is indicated. BAL studies may include Gram stain and culture, cell count with differential, PJP (conventional staining methods or PCR), cytomegalovirus (CMV) PCR, fungal wet prep, fungal culture, galactomannan (*Aspergillus*), mycobacterial culture, *Legionella* culture, and cytology (eg, tumor cells, viral inclusion bodies).

- Drug-induced pulmonary toxicity
  - Drug-induced interstitial lung disease (ILD) is the most common pulmonary adverse effect of cancer drugs.
  - Drug-induced pulmonary toxicity presents a diagnostic challenge as it is a diagnosis of exclusion.
  - High-resolution computed tomography is recommended to evaluate for treatment-related ILD due to its high sensitivity.
  - Radiographic patterns are highly variable and include nonspecific ground-glass opacities or consolidations, hypersensitivity pneumonitis, bilateral coalescent opacities as seen in acute respiratory distress syndrome (ARDS), usual interstitial pneumonia, nonspecific interstitial pneumonia, organizing pneumonia, and eosinophilic pneumonia.
  - The diagnosis may also be supported by BAL differential cell counts, the presence of elevated inflammatory markers, and the presence of peripheral eosinophilia.
  - A list of anticancer drugs implicated in pulmonary toxicity is shown in Table 6.8.2.
  - When drug-induced lung disease is suspected, clinical tools such as PNEUMOTOX (https://www.pneumotox.com/) can aid in the identification of the most likely culprit medication.
  - In addition to cessation of the suspected trigger agent, corticosteroids are a mainstay of treatment, especially in the critically ill. In cases of severe hypoxemia, pulse-dose steroids can be considered after infectious causes have been ruled out (eg, methylprednisolone 500 mg daily for 3 days). Prednisone (eg, 1 mg/kg daily) is generally continued until clinical improvement or determination of steroid refractoriness. In the steroid refractory, additional immunosuppressants (eg, intravenous [IV] immunoglobulin, infliximab) may be considered under the direction of subspecialty consultants. In the steroid responsive, a steroid taper over several weeks can be initiated after resolution of critical illness while observing for signs of relapse.

TABLE 6.8.2 Anticancer Drugs With Pulmonary Toxicity

Drug Class	Examples
Cytotoxic chemotherapy	Paclitaxel, gemcitabine, bleomycin, cyclophosphamide, methotrexate, carmustine, irinotecan
VEGF inhibitor	Bevacizumab
Tyrosine kinase inhibitor	Gefitinib, erlotinib, afatinib
mTOR inhibitor	Everolimus, sirolimus, temsirolimus
Immune checkpoint inhibitor	Pembrolizumab, nivolumab, ipilimumab, atezolizumab, durvalumab
MAB-drug conjugate	Trastuzumab-emtansine, trastuzumab-deruxtecan

MAB, monoclonal antibody; mTOR, mammalian target of rapamycin; VEGF, vascular endothelial growth factor.

- Radiation pneumonitis
  - Radiation pneumonitis may present within 6 months of completion of radiation therapy (eg, stereotactic body radiation therapy for lung cancer or adjuvant radiation therapy for breast cancer).
  - Unilateral pneumonitis is the most typical presentation, although the inflammation may generalize diffusely in more severe cases.
  - Management involves corticosteroids and supportive care.
  - Patients with a remote history of lung radiation may exhibit recall pneumonitis in response to systemic therapy, in which inflammation is triggered in the previous radiation bed. It is generally corticosteroid responsive.
- Supportive care
  - Supportive care for the patient with cancer in respiratory failure includes oxygen supplementation, assisted airway clearance, high-flow nasal cannula (HFNC) in early respiratory failure in effort to prevent intubation, transient use of noninvasive positive pressure ventilation (NIPPV) for rapidly reversible etiologies (eg, cardiogenic pulmonary edema), and invasive mechanical ventilation.
  - While HFNC and NIPPV may prevent intubation, they do not offer airway protection and are not inherently lung- protective. In patients with ARDS, late intubation can lead to worse outcomes.
  - The decision to intubate should be based on the patient's goals of care, severity of illness, and clinical trajectory.
  - In patients with cancer with respiratory failure, it is important to support patients and families in their decisions by establishing goals of care early in the course of critical illness, including a duration of time-limited maximal ICU supportive care, and whether tracheostomy is indicated and would be acceptable to the patient.

- In these discussions, severity of organ failure, functional status prior to admission, surgical candidacy, oncologic stage, and suitability for further oncologic treatment are important prognostic factors. Therefore, organized multidisciplinary communication from critical care, oncology, surgery, palliative care, and other consulting teams is essential.

Sepsis and Neutropenia

- As in the general ICU population, outcomes of sepsis in patients with solid tumors have improved over the past few decades.
- Although more common among patients with hematologic malignancies, febrile neutropenia remains a serious adverse effect of cytotoxic chemotherapy in patients with solid tumors.
- Febrile neutropenia is defined by a temperature >38 °C and absolute neutrophil count <500/μL. As signs of inflammation are attenuated in neutropenia, fever may be the only symptom of serious underlying infection.
- In a large single-center retrospective study of 9,018 patients with solid tumors who initiated chemotherapy in 2010 to 2016, 9.4% experienced febrile neutropenia during their initial chemotherapy course and 3.7% required ICU admission (Aagaard et al., 2020). The most common tumors in the febrile neutropenia group were ovarian (15.5%), breast (14.7%), non–small cell lung (14.7%), and gastric (11.4%).
- According to IDSA guidelines, initiation of hematopoietic growth factors (eg, granulocyte/macrophage colony–stimulating factor) for febrile neutropenia is not generally recommended (see Section 6.4: Neutropenia).

Chemotherapy and Radiotherapy in the Intensive Care Unit

- In the acute setting, radiation therapy may be indicated for severe tumor-related complications, including tumor hemorrhage, spinal cord compression, brain metastases, vascular compression, and airway obstruction.
- Occasionally, critically ill patients with solid tumor require chemotherapy in the ICU, especially when cancer progression is the suspected driver of critical illness.
- Solid tumor emergencies requiring chemotherapy administration in the ICU include airway obstruction and malignant pericardial and pleural effusions.
- Patients receiving chemotherapy in the ICU are more likely to have advanced disease and to be receiving initiation chemotherapy.
- The intent of chemotherapy may be for cure or palliation.
- Among 83 patients with solid tumor receiving chemotherapy in the ICU at Memorial Sloan Kettering, 27% had thoracic tumors, 24% genitourinary, 18% breast, 8.4% head and neck, 7.2% melanoma, and 7.2% sarcoma.

Special Considerations

- Palliative care
  - Patients with cancer in the ICU present complex pain and symptom management needs, including nausea, anorexia, constipation, and fatigue. Palliative care teams specialize in addressing these challenges in addition to aiding patients and families with advanced care planning and coping with illness.
  - In a randomized trial, patients with metastatic non–small cell lung cancer assigned to early palliative care were found to have improved survival despite having less aggressive care at the end of life.
  - Symptomatic management of recurrent malignant ascites and pleural effusions can be achieved with long-term drainage systems (eg, PleurX).
- Hematologic
  - All patients with cancer are at increased risk for venous thromboembolism (VTE). In the ICU, chemical VTE prophylaxis should be a priority, and pulmonary embolism should remain a top differential consideration for changes in clinical status.
  - Patients with cancer undergoing treatment are susceptible to cytopenias and coagulopathy requiring targeted transfusions and hematopoietic growth factors when indicated. In the bleeding patient, modalities to achieve hemostasis include endoscopic interventions, angioembolization, surgery, and radiotherapy.
- Cardiac
  - Exposure to anthracycline drugs (eg, breast cancer, sarcomas) increases the risk of cardiomyopathy.
  - Pericardial effusion is a complication of malignancy progression (eg, breast, lung, melanoma) and exposure to immune checkpoint inhibitors (eg, pembrolizumab, nivolumab, atezolizumab), potentially causing hemodynamic instability.
- Airway management
  - In the patient with head and neck cancer, airway intervention may be complicated by trismus, oropharyngeal bleeding, copious secretions, airway edema, and distortion of normal anatomy secondary to tumor burden, radiation changes, and flap reconstruction. In these patients with difficult airways, fiberoptic intubation and emergent tracheostomy may be required (see Section 30.1: Emergent Airway Management).
  - Hemoptysis is a complication of primary lung cancer and metastases often involving the airways and bronchial circulation. Management of the patient with significant hemoptysis includes endotracheal intubation, fiberoptic examination to identify the source lesion, fiberoptic intervention by subspecialty teams (eg, interventional pulmonology), and, in severe cases, bronchial artery embolization by interventional radiology. In severe cases, lung isolation may be necessary to minimize the spread of blood to unaffected airways. This can be achieved with deliberate mainstem intubation, double-lumen endotracheal tubes, and bronchial blockers (see Section 3.14: Upper Airway Diseases and Disorders).
- Access complications
  - Many patients with cancer undergoing chemotherapy have intermediate- and long-term central venous access devices (eg, peripherally inserted central catheters and tunneled lines) that are associated with thrombosis and infection.
- Malnutrition
  - In patients at risk for refeeding syndrome, thiamine should be supplemented while monitoring phosphate, magnesium, and calcium.
  - Malnourished patients are at increased risk of healing complications, including wound dehiscence and gastrointestinal anastomotic leaks.

- Tumor lysis syndrome
  - While tumor lysis syndrome (see Section 6.7: Leukemia, Lymphoma, and Tumor Lysis Syndrome) is more common in hematologic malignancies, it is a known complication in patients with solid tumors, especially in patients with advanced disease initiating chemotherapy.
  - The most common tumors in one systematic review included hepatocellular carcinoma, lung cancer, and melanoma.
- Paraneoplastic syndromes
  - Paraneoplastic syndromes should be considered in the investigation of unexplained neurologic, endocrine, or rheumatologic signs and symptoms.
- Drug complications
  - As the catalog of anticancer drugs grows, recognizing adverse effects becomes increasingly challenging, where the input of oncologists and pharmacists is indispensable.
  - In patients with exposure to bleomycin (eg, testicular cancer, germ cell tumors, squamous cell carcinoma), minimizing FIO_2 may reduce bleomycin-induced pulmonary toxicity.
- Endocrine
  - Adrenal insufficiency may occur due to central nervous system (CNS) disease, chronic steroid use, or adrenal metastases.
  - Cerebral salt wasting may be caused by brain tumors or as a complication of craniotomy.
  - Diabetes insipidus and panhypopituitarism may complicate pituitary surgery.
  - Tyrosine kinase inhibitors are associated with thyroid dysfunction.
- Infectious disease
  - Patients with cancer are at risk for health care–acquired organisms.
  - Patients with cancer undergoing cytotoxic chemotherapy may be significantly immunosuppressed. Opportunistic infections should be considered.

SUGGESTED READINGS

Aagaard T, Reekie J, Jorgensen M, et al. Mortality and admission to intensive care units after febrile neutropenia in patients with cancer. *Cancer Med.* 2020;9(9):3033-3042.

Camus P. *PNEUMOTOX*. The Drug-Induced Respiratory Disease Website. https://www.pneumotox.com/

Dai HP, Ma F, Ren YH, Chen SS, Li YQ. Expert consensus on the diagnosis and treatment of anticancer drug-induced interstitial lung disease. *Curr Med Sci.* 2023;43(1):1-12.

Dandachi D, Wilson Dib R, Fernandez-Cruz A, et al. Invasive pulmonary aspergillosis in patients with solid tumours: risk factors and predictors of clinical outcomes. *Ann Med.* 2018;50(8):713-720.

Davidson KR, Ha DM, Schwarz MI, Chan ED. Bronchoalveolar lavage as a diagnostic procedure: a review of known cellular and molecular findings in various lung diseases. *J Thorac Dis.* 2020;12(9):4991-5019.

Ferreyro BL, Munshi L. Acute respiratory failure in the oncologic patient: new era, new issues. *Annual Update in Intensive Care and Emergency Medicine 2019.* 2018;31-45.

Freifeld AG, Bow EJ, Sepkowitz KA, et al. Clinical practice guideline for the use of antimicrobial agents in neutropenic patients with cancer: 2010 update by the Infectious Diseases Society of America. *Clin Infect Dis.* 2011;52(4):e56-e93.

Gonzalez F, Starka R, Ducros L, et al. Critically ill metastatic cancer patients returning home after unplanned ICU stay: an observational, multicentre retrospective study. *Ann Intensive Care.* 2023;13(1):73.

Kalil AC, Metersky ML, Klompas M, et al. Management of adults with hospital-acquired and ventilator-associated pneumonia: 2016 clinical practice guidelines by the Infectious Diseases Society of America and the American Thoracic Society. *Clin Infect Dis.* 2016;63(5):e61-e111.

Leoni D, Encina B, Rello J. Managing the oncologic patient with suspected pneumonia in the intensive care unit. *Expert Rev Anti Infect Ther.* 2016;14(10):943-960.

Metlay JP, Waterer GW, Long AC, et al. Diagnosis and treatment of adults with community-acquired pneumonia. An official clinical practice guideline of the American Thoracic Society and Infectious Diseases Society of America. *Am J Respir Crit Care Med.* 2019;200(7):e45-e67.

Nates JL, Nunnally M, Kleinpell R, et al. ICU admission, discharge, and triage guidelines: a framework to enhance clinical operations, development of institutional policies, and further research. *Crit Care Med.* 2016; 44(8):1553-1602.

Park SY, Lim SY, Um SW, et al. Outcome and predictors of mortality in patients requiring invasive mechanical ventilation due to acute respiratory failure while undergoing ambulatory chemotherapy for solid cancers. *Support Care Cancer.* 2013;21(6):1647-1653.

Pene F, Percheron S, Lemiale V, et al. Temporal changes in management and outcome of septic shock in patients with malignancies in the intensive care unit. *Crit Care Med.* 2008;36(3):690-696.

Puxty K, McLoone P, Quasim T, Kinsella J, Morrison D. Survival in solid cancer patients following intensive care unit admission. *Intensive Care Med.* 2014;40(10):1409-1428.

Puxty K, McLoone P, Quasim T, Sloan B, Kinsella J, Morrison DS. Risk of critical illness among patients with solid cancers: a population-based observational study. *JAMA Oncol.* 2015;1(8):1078-1085.

Rabello LS, Silva JR, Azevedo LC, et al. Clinical outcomes and microbiological characteristics of severe pneumonia in cancer patients: a prospective cohort study. *PLoS One.* 2015;10(3):e0120544.

Shaz D, Pastores SM, Dayal L, et al. Analysis of intent and reason for oncologic therapy administration in cancer patients admitted to the intensive care unit. *J Intensive Care Med.* 2022;37(10):1305-1311.

Shaz DJ, Pastores SM, Goldman DA, et al. Characteristics and outcomes of patients with solid tumors receiving chemotherapy in the intensive care unit. *Support Care Cancer.* 2020;28(8):3855-3865.

Siegel RL, Giaquinto AN, Jemal A. Cancer statistics, 2024. *CA Cancer J Clin.* 2024;74(1):12-49.

Singer ED, Faiz SA, Qdaisat A, et al. Hemoptysis in cancer patients. *Cancers (Basel).* 2023;15(19):4765.

Sklar MC, Mohammed A, Orchanian-Cheff A, et al. The impact of high-flow nasal oxygen in the immunocompromised critically ill: a systematic review and meta-analysis. *Respir Care.* 2018;63(12):1555-1566.

Taccone FS, Artigas AA, Sprung CL, Moreno R, Sakr Y, Vincent JL. Characteristics and outcomes of cancer patients in European ICUs. *Crit Care.* 2009;13(1):R15.

Temel JS, Greer JA, Muzikansky A, et al. Early palliative care for patients with metastatic non-small-cell lung cancer. *N Engl J Med.* 2010;363(8): 733-742.

Worth LJ, Dooley MJ, Seymour JF, et al. An analysis of the utilisation of chemoprophylaxis against *Pneumocystis jirovecii* pneumonia in patients with malignancy receiving corticosteroid therapy at a cancer hospital. *Br J Cancer.* 2005;92(5):867-872.

6.9

Critical Care Management of Severe Immune-Related Adverse Events

Chia-Yun Wu, Maysa Vilbert, and Kerry Reynolds

Overview

- In the dynamic landscape of cancer treatment, we are currently witnessing a transformative era because of advancements in immunotherapy. By leveraging the body's own immune defenses, particularly through immune checkpoint inhibitors (ICIs), we are achieving significant reductions in tumor burden and, in select cases and cancer types, achieving enduring remissions. This progress is underscored by the Food and Drug Administration (FDA)'s approval of over 120 indications for the 15 approved ICIs, with numerous additional agents and combinations advancing through clinical development (Table 6.9.1).
- These therapeutic gains are often tempered by immune-related adverse events (irAEs), reflecting autoinflammatory sequelae of immune activation. From our clinical experience, these toxicities can manifest across nearly every organ system, ranging from mild dermatologic symptoms like rash or pruritus, to severe and potentially life-threatening complications affecting the skin, gastrointestinal (GI) tract, lungs, heart, nervous system, or endocrine glands, to name several. This complexity is further amplified by the unpredictable nature of irAEs. In addition, multiple organs can be affected simultaneously, often manifesting in unusual ways (atypical patterns) that can make diagnosis and treatment challenging.
- The increasing use of immunotherapy in cancer treatment comes with an increase in side effects, known as immune-related adverse events (irAEs). There is a critical need for all health care providers to be equipped to identify and manage these unique clinical presentations. The severity of irAEs is graded from mild to moderate using the Common Terminology Criteria for Adverse Events (CTCAE). In general, grade 3 irAEs require hospitalization, while grade 4 irAEs are life-threatening and require intensive care. Some examples of irAEs are explained herein.

TABLE 6.9.1 FDA-Approved Immune Checkpoint Inhibitors

Mechanism	Drug Name
CTLA-4 blockade	Ipilimumab, tremelimumab
PD-1 blockade	Nivolumab, pembrolizumab, cemiplimab, dostarlimab, retifanlimab, toripalimab, penpulimab
PD-L1 blockade	Atezolizumab, durvalumab, avelumab, cosibelimab
LAG-3 blockade	Relatlimab

CTLA-4, cytotoxic T-lymphocyte antigen 4; FDA, Food and Drug Administration; LAG-3, lymphocyte-activation gene 3; PD-1, programmed death 1; PD-L1, programmed death-ligand 1.

Immune Checkpoint Inhibitor Colitis

- Definitions
  - Grading diarrhea (CTCAE 5.0)
    - Grade 1: increase in <4 stools per day over baseline
    - Grade 2: increase in four to six stools per day over baseline, limiting activities of daily life
    - Grade 3: increase in seven or more stools per day over baseline, limiting self-care
    - Grade 4: life-threatening consequences
    - Grade 5: death
  - Colitis is characterized by inflammation of the colon, most frequently presents with diarrhea. Additional presenting symptoms may include anemia (prevalence of 16.7%), rectal bleeding (6.2%), and abdominal pain (5.2%). Atypical presentations, particularly rectal bleeding, warrant endoscopic evaluation to exclude malignancy or other etiologies.
  - In cases with upper GI involvement, nausea can occur in 12% to 25% of patients.
  - Intestinal perforation can occur in ~1% of cases.
- Epidemiology
  - Combination cytotoxic T-lymphocyte antigen 4/programmed death 1 (CTLA-4/PD-1) therapy has the highest risk of colitis at 16% (11% being grade ≥3), followed by CTLA-4 inhibitors at 8% (5% being grade 3) and PD-1/PD-L1 (programmed death-ligand 1) inhibitors at 1%.
  - Median time to onset is 5 to 10 weeks, although early-onset diarrhea can be seen with combination therapy (ICI-chemo, ICI-tyrosine kinase inhibitor, ICI-ICI).
  - Risk factors include nonsteroidal antiinflammatory drugs (NSAIDs), gut microbiome enriched with bacteria of the phylum Firmicutes, and a history of inflammatory bowel disease.
- Key pathophysiology
  - Tissue-resident $CD8^+$ T cells are present in the healthy colon. Activation of these cells leads to subsequent recruitment of additional CD8 and CD4 T-cell populations from the blood.
  - Colitis is associated with the differentiation of CD8 tissue-resident memory cells to cytotoxic effector cells and the enrichment of CTLA-4^+ T-regulatory cells.
  - These T cells express high levels of CXCR6 and CXCR3 chemokine receptor genes.
  - T-cell interferon (IFN)-γ expression and IFN-γ–inducible genes are strongly increased in ICI colitis.
- Differential diagnosis
  - Immune-mediated gastroenterocolitis, intestinal infection, inflammatory bowel disease, thyroid dysfunction, and celiac disease
  - Workup (imaging and clinical assessment)
    - Review concomitant medications (proton pump inhibitors [PPIs], NSAIDs, laxatives, antibiotics, probiotics).
    - Blood (complete blood count [CBC], comprehensive metabolic panel [CMP], and thyroid-stimulating hormone [TSH]) and stool tests (culture, *Clostridioides difficile*, ova and parasite, cytomegalovirus [CMV], other viral etiologies). Tissue-transglutaminase anti-bodies (Abs) with total immunoglobulin A (IgA) level to rule out new-onset celiac disease
    - Fecal calprotectin: informs disease activity. Elevation is associated with mucosal damage and normalization

with healing. However, it may be elevated due to cancer-related luminal inflammation.
  - Computed tomography (CT) scan of the abdomen and pelvis: fluid-filled colonic distension, bowel wall thickening, and mesenteric vessel engorgement are common features. CT can be negative. Colitis more frequently involves the descending colon.
  - Endoscopic/colonoscopy/flexible sigmoidoscopy: severity assessment; the presence of ulceration may suggest a steroid-refractory course and require an early second immunosuppressant.
- **Management and treatment**
  - For patients with grade ≥2 diarrhea diagnosed with immune-related colitis, hold ICI treatment and begin oral (po) prednisone at 0.5 to 1 mg/kg/d until symptoms improve. Once improvement is seen to grade 1, start tapering the dose by 10 mg per week. For grade ≥3, start prednisone or methylprednisolone at 1 to 2 mg/kg/d and consider hospitalization.
  - If there is no improvement after >48 to 72 hours, the condition is termed *steroid refractory*, and a second-line immunosuppressant is necessary.
  - Second-line therapies for refractory (persistent symptoms after 3 days) and resistant cases (improvement followed by symptoms flare), are needed in 30-45% of patients, and include:
    - Infliximab (preferred)
    - Vedolizumab
  - Third-line immunosuppressants (needed in about 10% of patients)
    - Infliximab or vedolizumab if they were not used as second-line treatments
    - Interleukin-12 (IL-12) and IL-23 blocking Ab ustekinumab
    - JAK inhibitor tofacitinib (life-threatening situation)
    - Fecal microbiota transplantation (investigational and in clinical trial at MD Anderson)
  - Prior to immunosuppressants, patients should be tested for tuberculosis, hepatitis B, and HIV.
- **Outcomes**
  - Symptoms are expected to improve in days.
  - Colitis can reoccur in about one-third of patients rechallenged with ICI.
  - GI toxicities have been associated with improved survival and cancer-related outcomes.

Immune Checkpoint Inhibitor Myocarditis, Myositis, and Myasthenia

- Definitions
  - Typical symptoms for myocarditis: chest pain, shortness of breath, fatigue, palpitations, syncope
  - Severe cases can present with heart block, heart failure, cardiogenic shock, or sudden death.
  - Evaluate for concomitant myositis and myasthenia gravis (overlap syndrome).
    - Typical symptoms: myalgias, muscle weakness, bulbar involvement (ptosis, diplopia, dysphagia), and/or respiratory muscle weakness
  - Diagnosis: either pathohistologic or clinical diagnosis based on 2022 International Cardio-Oncology Society (IC-OS) consensus in Table 6.9.2

TABLE 6.9.2 ICI Myocarditi: Pathohistologic and Clinical Diagnosis

Pathohistologic diagnosis	**Endomyocardial biopsy (EMB)** shows inflammatory infiltrate with myocardial necrosis.
Clinical diagnosis	**Troponin elevation** with 1 major criterion or 2 minor criteria
	Major criteria: cardiac magnetic resonance (CMR) diagnostic for acute myocarditis based on modified Lake Louise criteria
	Minor criteria: clinical symptoms, arrhythmia, left ventricular systolic dysfunction, other irAEs, or suggestive CMR

ICI, immune checkpoint inhibitor; irAEs, immune-related adverse events.

  - The median onset time: 5 to 6 weeks, but can range from 2 to 54 weeks
- Epidemiology
  - Overall incidence: 1% to 1.7%. Combination ICI therapy (such as nivolumab plus relatlimab) may carry a higher risk of ICI myocarditis compared with single ICI therapy.
  - A pharmacovigilance study showed concurrent noncardiac irAEs occurred in 42%, most commonly myositis (25%) and myasthenia gravis (11%).
- Key pathophysiology
  - Characterized by a patchy, heterogeneous lymphohistiocytic infiltrate in the myocardium, which includes $CD4^+$ T cell, $CD8^+$ T cell, mononuclear phagocytes, and dendritic cells
  - In preclinical models, CTLA-4 signaling and IFN-γ/JAK2/STAT1 signaling also play a critical role.
- Differential diagnosis
  - Acute coronary syndrome, pulmonary embolism, viral myocarditis, and malignant pericarditis
  - Workup
    - Troponin, creatine phosphokinase (CPK) (to rule out concurrent myositis), TSH/T4 (rule out hypothyroidism), and NT-proBNP
    - Electrocardiogram (ECG), chest x-ray (CXR)
    - Echocardiogram: in half of ICI myocarditis cases, left ventricular ejection fraction is preserved.
    - Consider cardiac CT or coronary angiography to help with differential diagnosis if coronary artery disease (CAD) is suspected.
    - Cardiac magnetic resonance (CMR) with and without contrast: noninvasive, but less sensitive for myocarditis than endomyocardial biopsy (EMB)
    - EMB is the gold standard, should be considered when the diagnosis is uncertain (ie, cardiac magnetic resonance imaging [MRI] is negative) or when patients do not respond to initial therapy.
    - For patients concerning for overlap syndrome: pulmonary function assessment with negative inspiratory force (NIF) and vital capacity, autoantibody testing for myositis and myasthenia gravis Abs (acetylcholine receptor (AChR) blocking, modulating, and binding Abs; antistriated muscle Abs) and MuSK Ab, and electromyography
- Management and treatment
  - Cardiology consult and neurology consult (if overlap syndrome)

- Start pulsed-dose corticosteroids (intravenous [IV] methylprednisolone 1 g/d for 3-5 days).
  - ATRIUM trial ongoing: a phase 3 randomized, placebo-controlled trial, to assess the efficacy of adding abatacept (10 mg/kg) compared to placebo + steroids in patients with ICI myocarditis
  - Improvement (in both symptoms and troponin levels) is expected in the first 24 to 48 hours after initiation of steroids.
  - If improved, taper to prednisone 1.5 mg/kg, then by 10 mg weekly.
  - If there is no improvement within 24 to 48 hours, the condition is considered steroid refractory, and additional immunosuppression should be added.
- Second-line immunosuppression
  - Abatacept outside clinical trials: 500 mg every 2 weeks for five doses (dosing per American Society of Clinical Oncology [ASCO] guidelines)
  - Mycophenolate 500 mg to 1,000 mg twice daily (bid)
  - Ruxolitinib up to 15 mg bid (dosing per a case report published by Nguyen LS, et al, and a case series published by Salem JE, et al)
  - Antithymocyte globulin (ATG)
  - Alemtuzumab 30 mg IV single dose
- Frequently monitor troponin levels during hospitalization until clinical and biochemical improvement.

- Outcomes
  - High troponin levels (eg, ≥1.5 ng/mL): elevated troponin levels are associated with an increased risk of major adverse cardiac events (MACEs) and poorer survival.
  - MACEs: approximately half of patients experience MACE, including hemodynamically significant complete heart block, cardiogenic shock, cardiac arrest, and cardiovascular death.
  - High mortality rate: mortality rate ranges from 25% to 50%, often due to refractory arrhythmia or cardiogenic shock. In patients with concurrent overlap syndrome, the mortality rate may be as high as 35% to 60%.
  - Permanent discontinuation of ICI therapy. The appropriateness of rechallenging remains unknown and, given the severity of myocarditis, is not recommended

Neurologic Immune-Related Adverse Events

- Definitions
  - Neurologic irAEs include a vast spectrum of diseases:
  - irMeningitis, irEncephalitis, irDemyelinating disease, irVasculitis, irNeuropathy, irNeuromuscular junction disorders, and irMyopathy
  - They usually occur within the first 3 months after starting ICI, with a median time to onset of 4 weeks (1-68 weeks).
    - irMeningitis is more frequently associated with anti–CTLA-4 and combination ICI. Patients may present with headache, photophobia, neck stiffness, nausea and vomiting, and low-grade fever. Mental status is often normal.
    - irEncephalitis may present with confusion, altered mental status and behavior, agitation, speech abnormalities, seizures, weakness, and gait instability. Anti–PD-(L)1 monotherapy, whether used either alone or in combination, carries a higher risk of encephalitis compared to anti–CTLA-4 therapy.
    - IrNeuromuscular conditions such as myasthenia gravis are characterized by marked fatigable or fluctuating muscle weakness, including ptosis, double vision, dysphagia, dysarthria, facial muscle weakness, head drop or neck weakness, and dyspnea due to diaphragmatic weakness. The overlapping syndrome of myasthenia gravis, myositis, and myocarditis is discussed earlier.
    - irNeuropathy—peripheral neuropathies that have a variety of presentations, including cranial neuropathies (especially of the facial and abducens nerves), painful small-fiber neuropathy, and sensorimotor syndrome, such as Guillain-Barré syndrome. The latter is more common with anti–CTLA-4 and combination therapies. Besides the classical symptoms of ascending and progressive muscle weakness, sensory loss, areflexia, dysregulation of autonomic nerves may also occur.
    - irDemyelinating disease includes multiple sclerosis, transverse myelitis, acute disseminated encephalomyelitis, optic neuritis, and neuromyelitis optica.

- Epidemiology
  - The overall incidence is 4% in patients treated with CTLA-4 inhibitors, 6% with PD-1/PD-L1 blockage, and 12% with the combination of PD1 plus CTLA-4 inhibitors.
  - Grade ≥3 occurs in <1% of patients, but they can be fatal or cause permanent neurologic impairment.

- Key pathophysiology
  - In irEncephalitis, patients may develop neural-specific autoantibodies, such as anti–Ma-2 and anti-Hu, which are also observed in paraneoplastic syndromes.
  - irMyasthenia gravis, positive Abs against AChR are reported in about 60% of patients with generalized weakness and more frequently in those with prior myasthenia gravis.

- Differential diagnosis
  - The initial workup is focused on ruling out central nervous system progressive disease or leptomeningeal metastasis, infectious disease, seizure activity, hypophysitis (in the case of headache), paraneoplastic neurologic syndromes, and metabolic alterations causing neurologic symptoms.
  - General diagnostic workup includes brain and/or spine MRI with and without contrast, lumbar puncture (LP) with cerebrospinal fluid (CSF) analysis studies including opening pressure, cell count/differential; protein, glucose; oligoclonal bands and IgG index; cytology (rule out leptomeningeal disease) and/or flow cytometry depending on malignancy; Gram stain/culture; herpes simplex virus (HSV) polymerase chain reaction (PCR), varicella-zoster virus (VZV) PCR, other infectious studies (viral, etc) as indicated along with CBCs and metabolic panel, thyroid panel, adrenocorticotropic hormone (ACTH), and cortisol.
  - Additional specific workup recommendations for patients suspected of:
    - irEncephalitis: autoimmune encephalopathy and paraneoplastic panels of blood and CSF and electroencephalogram (EEG).
    - irMyasthenia gravis: Ab testing for myasthenia gravis (AChR or modulating Ab or MuSK Ab)—the

absence of Abs does not rule out the syndrome and evaluation for concurrent myositis (CK) and myocarditis (troponin). Inflammatory markers (erythrocyte sedimentation rate [ESR] and C-reactive protein [CRP]). Nerve conduction studies and electromyography (EMG). Pulmonary function testing with NIF and forced vital capacity (FVC). Stop medications that can worsen myasthenia, such as beta-blockers, IV magnesium, fluoroquinolones, aminoglycosides, and macrolide antibiotics.
    - irNeuropathy: Guillain-Barré syndrome: MRI of the spine to rule out a compressive lesion; imaging may show nerve root enhancement and thickening. LP may reveal lymphocytic pleocytosis and elevated protein, EMG/nerve conduction studies, and ganglioside Ab panel of blood and CSF.
    - Non–Guillain-Barré suspected peripheral neuropathy: consider all above plus blood work with B_{12}, serum protein electrophoresis (SPEP), hemoglobin A_{1c}, B_6, ESR, CRP, and folic acid.
- Management and treatment
  - Consulting a neurologist for all patients with serious neurologic irAEs. General recommendations:
    - In case of severe symptoms (grade 3-4), patients should be treated with IV methylprednisolone 2 to 4 mg/kg/d and inpatient or intensive care unit (ICU) admission.
  - Specific recommendations
    - Patients with encephalitis should receive IV acyclovir until PCR results are obtained and negative. Then, consider pulsed-dose methylprednisolone 1 g IV daily for 3 to 5 days and IV immunoglobulin (IVIG) (2 g/kg in divided doses over the course of 5 days). Those who do not respond to pulsed-dose corticosteroids should receive rituximab (375/m^2 weekly infusion for 4 weeks).
    - Consider empiric antiviral (IV acyclovir) and antibacterial therapy until CSF results are negative for suspected aseptic meningitis.
    - Patients diagnosed with Guillain-Barré syndrome should start IVIG (0.4 g/kg/d for 5 days for a total of 2 g/kg) or plasmapheresis. Pulse steroid (methylprednisolone 1 g daily for 5 days) may also be added to IVIG or plasmapheresis. Permanently discontinue ICI therapy. Important to continue frequent neurologic and pulmonary function assessments.
    - Painful peripheral neuropathy should be managed with gabapentin, pregabalin, or duloxetine.
    - For patients diagnosed with myasthenia gravis: pyridostigmine 30 mg po 3 times a day, progressively increasing to 120 mg po 4 times a day. Wean pyridostigmine and steroids based on symptom improvement and in collaboration with the neurologist.
    - For patients with grade 3 or 4 myasthenia gravis, consider admission to the ICU for respiratory monitoring. Consider IVIG 2 g/kg over 5 days (0.4 g/kg/d) or plasmapheresis for 5 days. If refractory, consider adding rituximab.
- Outcomes
  - Neurologic irAEs and myocarditis have higher mortality rates than other irAEs.

Immune Checkpoint Inhibitor-Erosive Mucocutaneous Disease, Stevens-Johnson Syndrome/Toxic Epidermal Necrolysis–Like Subtype

- Definitions
  - Characteristics
    - Acute onset, quickly evolving (over maximum of 2 weeks) toward painful skin erosive plaques with positive Nikolsky sign
    - May be associated with mucosal involvement (nasal-oral and urogenital areas)
    - Ocular mucosa is often spared.
  - In diseases causing full-thickness epidermal necrosis, there is a distinct entity of a generalized bullous eruption mimicking Stevens-Johnson syndrome/toxic epidermal necrolysis (SJS/TEN) in patients receiving ICIs: Progressive immunotherapy-related mucocutaneous eruption (PIRME)
    - Compared to classic SJS/TEN, PIRME has delayed onset, mild initial morphologic presentation, benign clinical course, and favorable treatment response.
    - Often associated with recently initiated concomitant medications, suggesting a two-hit mechanism (ICI reduces immune tolerance and induces sensitivity to subsequent drug exposures)
    - Besides full-thickness epidermal necrosis, a distinct interface dermatitis is frequently seen.
- Epidemiology
  - Rare complication, occurs in $<1\%$ of patients receiving ICI treatment
  - Median onset time: 25 to 28 days
- Key pathophysiology
  - Histopathologic evaluation reveals full-thickness epidermal necrosis and subsequent epidermal detachment, in the absence of immunoglobulin deposition.
- Differential diagnosis
  - Other severe cutaneous adverse reactions (SCARs) to drugs, such as drug reaction with eosinophilia and systemic symptoms (DRESS)
    - In DRESS, systemic involvement and lymphadenopathy are frequently present; no sheet-like detachment; infrequent or mild mucosal involvement
  - Erythema multiforme (EM) with mucosal involvement
    - In EM, there are typical target lesions; extremity predominance; no flaccid bulla or sheet-like skin detachment
  - Toxic shock syndrome: may have positive blood culture and fever; nonspecific histopathology
  - Paraneoplastic pemphigus: can be associated with underlying tumor; chronic course; Abs against desmoglein 3 and plakins
- Management and treatment
  - Monitor for serious complications such as volume depletion/electrolyte disturbance, hypothermia, infection, and high output cardiac failure.
  - Prednisone/IV methylprednisolone 1 to 2 mg/kg/d (usually need a higher dose) (1.5 mg/kg minimum)
  - Second-line immunosuppression may be considered in severe or steroid-unresponsive cases (new blistering lesions or new detached/detachable skin): IVIG 1 g/kg/d

for 3 to 4 days, etanercept/tumor necrosis factor (TNF) inhibitor or cyclosporine can be considered. Special considerations as follows:
  - For patients without severe sepsis or renal insufficiency, prefer etanercept/TNF inhibitor or pulse steroid + IVIG
  - For patients with severe sepsis, prefer steroid-sparing agents.
  - For patients with renal insufficiency, avoid cyclosporine.
- The potential benefits of immunosuppression overweigh the risk of infection, except for patients with severe infection.

- Outcomes
  - Mortality rates: ranging from benign course with favorable treatment response for PIRME to 10% for SJS and 50% for TEN
  - SCORTEN score, calculated on day 1 and day 3 of admission, is a severity of illness score validated for SJS and TEN.
    - It includes seven independent risk factors for death with equal weighting: age ≥40 years, malignancy, tachycardia ≥120/min, body surface area (BSA) ≥10%, serum urea >10 mmol/L (>28 mg/dL), serum glucose >14 mmol/L (>252 mg/dL) and bicarbonate <20 mmol/L.
    - Hospital mortality rate according to SCORTEN score: score 0 to 1: 3%; score 2: 12%; score 3: 35%; score 4: 58%; score ≥5: 90%

Adrenal Crisis Secondary to Immune Checkpoint Inhibitor

- Definitions
  - Adrenal crisis can occur in patients with primary adrenal insufficiency (AI) (ICI-adrenalitis) or secondary/central AI (ICI-hypophysitis).
  - Symptoms
    - Predominant manifestation: hypotension
    - Nonspecific symptoms: nausea, vomiting, abdominal pain, weakness, headache, and confusion
  - Diagnosis of AI
    - Morning (6-8 AM) cortisol <3 μg/dL
    - ACTH level. In secondary AI, ACTH levels are low, whereas in primary AI, ACTH levels are high.
    - If ACTH normal or non-diagnostic, perform cosyntropin (ACTH) stimulation test. Cortisol level <15 μg/dL measured at baseline, 30 and 60 minutes after cosyntropin administration is consistent with primary AI.
    - Cosyntropin (ACTH) stimulation test, indicated by a cortisol level 30 to 60 minutes after cosyntropin administration of <15 μg/dL
  - Median time to ICI-hypophysitis onset: occurs later after PD-1/PD-L1 inhibitors (25.8 weeks), compared to CTLA-4 inhibitors (9.3 weeks) or combination CTLA-4/PD-1 (12.5 weeks)
- Epidemiology
  - ICI-hypophysitis: more commonly seen with CTLA-4 inhibitors or combination therapy (4%-13.6%) than with PD-1/PD-L1 inhibitors therapy (0.5%-1%)
  - ICI-adrenalitis: rare, <1%
- Key pathophysiology
  - ICI-hypophysitis induced by CTLA-4 inhibitors: possible direct targeting of CTLA-4 expressing on anterior pituitary cells and development of antipituitary Abs → trigger Ab-dependent cell-mediated cytotoxicity (ADCC) and the classic complement pathway
  - Mechanisms behind ICI-induced hypophysitis by PD-1/PD-L1 inhibitors and ICI-adrenalitis remain unknown.
- Differential diagnosis
  - In secondary AI, ACTH levels are low, whereas in primary AI, ACTH levels are high.
  - Primary AI: autoimmune adrenalitis (such as polyglandular autoimmune syndrome), infectious adrenalitis (such as tuberculosis, fungal, and HIV infection), adrenal metastasis, adrenal hemorrhage, and medication (such as ketoconazole, fluconazole, and mitotane)
  - Central AI: pituitary tumor/metastasis, pituitary surgery/radiation, pituitary destroyed by infection (tuberculosis or histoplasmosis), medication (chronic high-dose glucocorticoid)
- Management and treatment
  - Monitor hemodynamics, electrolytes, and fluid status.
  - Stress dose steroids in adrenal crisis: hydrocortisone 100 mg, followed by 50 mg q6 to 8h
  - Taper to physiologic maintenance over 5 to 7 days when clinical status improves: hydrocortisone 15 to 20 mg (divided doses; 2/3 AM, 1/3 early PM) or prednisone 5 mg qd.
  - Sick dose with any future minor illness: 2 to 3 times of steroid maintenance dose for 3 days
  - Fludrocortisone (0.05-0.1 mg/d) in addition to hydrocortisone/prednisone is necessary in ICI-adrenalitis.
  - Initiate adrenal replacement prior to other hormone (such as thyroid hormone) replacement to avoid adrenal crisis.
  - Rare to have any evidence of diabetes insipidus but if present, normal saline ≥2 L or monitored free water replacement; repeat fluid bolus as needed
- Outcomes
  - Likely require lifelong physiologic hormone replacement
  - ICI therapy can be resumed once patient is stabilized on replacement hormones.

Immune Checkpoint Inhibitor Hypothyroidism

- Definitions
  - Myxedema coma can occur in patients with primary hypothyroidism (ICI-thyroiditis) and central hypothyroidism (ICI-hypophysitis).
  - Clinical presentation of decompensated hypothyroidism
    - Altered mental status, hypothermia, hypotension, bradycardia, hypoventilation, hyponatremia, hypoglycemia
    - Puffy hands and face, swollen lips, and an enlarged tongue secondary to nonpitting edema
  - Diagnosis
    - T4: usually very low
    - TSH: high (in primary hypothyroidism) or low to normal (in central hypothyroidism)
  - Possible precipitants: infection, myocardial infarction, surgery, and sedative drugs (esp. opioids) in a poorly controlled hypothyroid patient
- Epidemiology
  - Hypothyroidism more commonly associated with anti–PD-1 drugs or ICI combination: 15% in ICI combination, 8% in PD-1/PD-L1 blockade, while 3% in anti–CTLA-4 blockade

- Grade ≥3 hypothyroidism is rare, occurring in roughly 0% to 2% of patients.
- Myxedema coma is case reportable, likely due to earlier awareness and early diagnosis of hypothyroidism.

- Key pathophysiology
  - Remains unknown. Thyroid irAEs may involve cellular immune (T-cell infiltration and activation), humoral immune (B cell and autoantibodies), genetic susceptibility (upregulating HLA-DR), and cytokine (increased IFN-γ and IL-2; decreased IL-10).
- Differential diagnosis
  - Adrenal crisis, heart failure, sepsis, hepatic encephalopathy
  - Workup:
    - TSH, free T4, cortisol
    - Na, glucose, arterial blood gas (ABG), ECG
    - To rule out other etiology: CXR, blood culture, CBC, liver function tests (LFTs)
- Management and treatment
  - Life-threatening emergency requiring admission and endocrinology consultation
  - Draw cortisol and empirically treat AI: hydrocortisone 100 mg q8h until exclusion of AI. Give steroids BEFORE thyroid hormone replacement to avoid precipitating possible adrenal crisis (according to American Thyroid Association guidelines).
  - Thyroid hormone replacement (according to American Thyroid Association guidelines)
    - Levothyroxine (T4): loading dose 200 to 400 μg IV followed by 50-100 μg IV qd until able to take T4 po; daily replacement dose: 1.6 μg/kg/d po, reduced to 75% if IV administered
    - Liothyronine (T3): loading dose 5 to 20 μg followed by 2.5 to 10 μg q8h (in myxedema)
    - Monitor FT4 and T3 q1-2 days, avoiding very high T3 levels.
  - Supportive measures, such as mechanical ventilation, fluids and vasopressor drugs for hypotension, IV dextrose, and monitoring for arrhythmia
- Outcomes
  - Life-threatening form of hypothyroidism with a mortality rate ranging from 25% to 60%
  - Clinical and biochemical improvement typically occur within a week after adequate treatment.
  - ICI therapy can be resumed once patient is stabilized on replacement hormones and symptoms resolve to baseline.

SUGGESTED READINGS

Abdel-Rahman O, Elhalawani H, Fouad M. Risk of gastrointestinal complications in cancer patients treated with immune checkpoint inhibitors: a meta-analysis. *Immunotherapy*. 2015;7:1213-1227.

Abu-Sbeih H, Ali FS, Wang Y. Clinical review on the utility of fecal microbiota transplantation in immunocompromised patients. *Curr Gastroenterol Rep*. 2019;21:8.

Abu-Sbeih H, Tang T, Ali FS, et al. The impact of immune checkpoint inhibitor-related adverse events and their immunosuppressive treatment on patients' outcomes. *J Immunother Precis Oncol*. 2018;1:7-18.

Arnaud-Coffin P, Maillet D, Gan HK, et al. A systematic review of adverse events in randomized trials assessing immune checkpoint inhibitors. *Int J Cancer*. 2019;145:639-648.

Balaji A, Hsu M, Lin CT, et al. Steroid-refractory PD-(L)1 pneumonitis: incidence, clinical features, treatment, and outcomes. *J Immunother Cancer*. 2021;9:e001731.

Beattie J, Rizvi H, Fuentes P, et al. Success and failure of additional immune modulators in steroid-refractory/resistant pneumonitis related to immune checkpoint blockade. *J Immunother Cancer*. 2021;9:e001884.

Benatar M, McDermott MP, Sanders DB, et al. Efficacy of prednisone for the treatment of ocular myasthenia (epitome): a randomized, controlled trial. *Muscle Nerve*. 2016;53:363-369.

Blum SM, Zlotoff DA, Smith NP, et al. Immune responses in checkpoint myocarditis across heart, blood, and tumor. *bioRxiv [Preprint]*. 2023: 2023.09.15.557794.

Brahmer JR, Abu-Sbeih H, Ascierto PA, et al. Society for Immunotherapy of Cancer (SITC) clinical practice guideline on immune checkpoint inhibitor-related adverse events. *J Immunother Cancer*. 2021;9(6):e002435.

Burton LB, Eskian M, Guidon AC, Reynolds KL. A review of neurotoxicities associated with immunotherapy and a framework for evaluation. *Neurooncol Adv*. 2021;3(suppl 5):v108-v120.

Chang HC, Wang TJ, Lin MH, et al. A review of the systemic treatment of Stevens-Johnson syndrome and toxic epidermal necrolysis. *Biomedicines*. 2022;10(9):2105.

Chaput N, Lepage P, Coutzac C, et al. Baseline gut microbiota predicts clinical response and colitis in metastatic melanoma patients treated with ipilimumab. *Ann Oncol*. 2017;28:1368-1379.

Chen ST, Semenov YR, Alloo A, et al. Defining D-irAEs: consensus-based disease definitions for the diagnosis of dermatologic adverse events from immune checkpoint inhibitor therapy. *J Immunother Cancer*. 2024; 12(4):e007675.

Coutzac C, Adam J, Soularue E, et al. Colon immune-related adverse events: anti-CTLA-4 and anti-PD-1 blockade induce distinct immunopathological entities. *J Crohns Colitis*. 2017;11:1238-1246.

Cuzzubbo S, Javeri F, Tissier M, et al. Neurological adverse events associated with immune checkpoint inhibitors: review of the literature. *Eur J Cancer*. 2017;73:1-8.

Delaunay M, Prevot G, Collot S, et al. Management of pulmonary toxicity associated with immune checkpoint inhibitors. *Eur Respir Rev*. 2019; 28(154):190012.

Dubey D, David WS, Amato AA, et al. Varied phenotypes and management of immune checkpoint inhibitor-associated neuropathies. *Neurology*. 2019;93:e1093-e1103.

Dubey D, David W, Reynolds K, et al. Immune checkpoint inhibitor related neurologic adverse events: clinical spectrum, management and outcomes (S21.003). *Neurology*. 2019;92:S21.003.

Dubin K, Callahan MK, Ren B, et al. Intestinal microbiome analyses identify melanoma patients at risk for checkpoint-blockade-induced colitis. *Nat Commun*. 2016;7:10391.

Esfahani K, Hudson M, Batist G. Tofacitinib for refractory immune-related colitis from PD-1 therapy. *N Engl J Med*. 2020;382:2374-2375.

Faje A, Reynolds K, Zubiri L, et al. Hypophysitis secondary to nivolumab and pembrolizumab is a clinical entity distinct from ipilimumab-associated hypophysitis. *Eur J Endocrinol*. 2019;181(3):211-219.

Galant-Swafford J, Troesch A, Tran L, et al. Landscape of immune related pneumonitis in cancer patients with asthma being treated with immune checkpoint blockade. *Oncology*. 2020;98:123-130.

Gardin T, Longbrake EE. Inducing or "Unmasking" autoimmunity? The role of immune checkpoint therapy in propagating neurologic immune-related adverse events. *Neurology*. 2021;96(16):733-734.

Guégan S, Bastuji-Garin S, Poszepczynska-Guigné E, et al. Performance of the SCORTEN during the first five days of hospitalization to predict the prognosis of epidermal necrolysis. *J Invest Dermatol*. 2006;126(2):272-276.

Gupta A, De Felice KM, Loftus EV, et al. Systematic review: colitis associated with anti-CTLA-4 therapy. *Aliment Pharmacol Ther*. 2015;42:406-417.

Haanen J, Obeid M, Spain L, et al. Management of toxicities from immunotherapy: ESMO Clinical Practice Guideline for diagnosis, treatment and follow-up. *Ann Oncol*. 2022;33(12):1217-1238.

Hughes RA, Mehndiratta MM, Rajabally YA. Corticosteroids for chronic inflammatory demyelinating polyradiculoneuropathy. *Cochrane Database Syst Rev*. 2017;11:CD002062.

Hughes RAC, Swan AV, Raphaël J-C, et al. Immunotherapy for Guillain-Barré syndrome: a systematic review. *Brain*. 2007;130:2245-2257.

Johnson DB, Manouchehri A, Haugh AM, et al. Neurologic toxicity associated with immune checkpoint inhibitors: a pharmacovigilance study. *J Immunother Cancer*. 2019;7:134.

Jonklaas J, Bianco AC, Bauer AJ, et al. Guidelines for the treatment of hypothyroidism: prepared by the American Thyroid Association task force on thyroid hormone replacement. *Thyroid*. 2014;24(12):1670-1751.

Kuo AM, Markova A. High grade dermatologic adverse events associated with immune checkpoint blockade for cancer. *Front Med (Lausanne)*. 2022;9:898790.

Lenti MV, Ribaldone DG, Borrelli de Andreis F, et al. A 1-year follow-up study on checkpoint inhibitor-induced colitis: results from a European consortium. *ESMO Open*. 2024;9(7):103632.

Luoma AM, Suo S, Williams HL, et al. Molecular pathways of colon inflammation induced by cancer immunotherapy. *Cell*. 2020;182(3): 655-671.e22.

Lyon AR, López-Fernández T, Couch LS, et al. 2022 ESC Guidelines on cardio-oncology developed in collaboration with the European Hematology Association (EHA), the European Society for Therapeutic Radiology and Oncology (ESTRO) and the International Cardio-Oncology Society (IC-OS). *Eur Heart J*. 2022;43(41):4229-4361.

Mahmood SS, Fradley MG, Cohen JV, et al. Myocarditis in patients treated with immune checkpoint inhibitors. *J Am Coll Cardiol*. 2018; 71(16):1755-1764.

Manson G, Maria ATJ, Poizeau F, et al. Worsening and newly diagnosed paraneoplastic syndromes following anti-PD-1 or anti-PD-L1 immunotherapies, a descriptive study. *J Immunother Cancer*. 2019;7:337.

Marini A, Bernardini A, Gigli GL, et al. Neurologic adverse events of immune checkpoint inhibitors: a systematic review. *Neurology*. 2021; 96(16):754-766.

Martins F, Sofiya L, Sykiotis GP, et al. Adverse effects of immune checkpoint inhibitors: epidemiology, management and surveillance. *Nat Rev Clin Oncol*. 2019;16:563-580.

Molina GE, Yu Z, Foreman RK, et al. Generalized bullous mucocutaneous eruption mimicking Stevens-Johnson syndrome in the setting of immune checkpoint inhibition: a multicenter case series. *J Am Acad Dermatol*. 2020;83(5):1475-1477.

Moslehi JJ, Salem JE, Sosman JA, et al. Increased reporting of fatal immune checkpoint inhibitor-associated myocarditis. *Lancet*. 2018; 391(10124):933.

Naidoo J, Wang X, Woo KM, et al. Pneumonitis in patients treated with anti-programmed death-1/programmed death ligand 1 therapy. *J Clin Oncol*. 2017;35:709-717.

Nguyen LS, Bretagne M, Arrondeau J, et al. Reversal of immune-checkpoint inhibitor fulminant myocarditis using personalized-dose-adjusted abatacept and ruxolitinib: proof of concept. *J Immunother Cancer*. 2022; 10(4):e004699.

Nishino M, Giobbie-Hurder A, Hatabu H, et al. Incidence of programmed cell death 1 inhibitor-related pneumonitis in patients with advanced cancer: a systematic review and meta-analysis. *JAMA Oncol*. 2016;2:1607-1616.

Nosadini M, Mohammad SS, Ramanathan S, et al. Immune therapy in autoimmune encephalitis: a systematic review. *Expert Rev Neurother*. 2015;15:1391-1419.

O'Leary CL, Pierce N, Patel SP, Naidoo J. Immune-related toxicity in NSCLC: current state-of-the-art and emerging clinical challenges. *J Thorac Oncol*. 2024;19(3):395-408.

Petri CR, Patell R, Batalini F, et al. Severe pulmonary toxicity from immune checkpoint inhibitor treated successfully with intravenous immunoglobulin: case report and review of the literature. *Respir Med Case Rep*. 2019;27:100834.

Qin Q, Patel VG, Wang B, et al. Type, timing, and patient characteristics associated with immune-related adverse event development in patients with advanced solid tumors treated with immune checkpoint inhibitors. *J Clin Oncol*. 2020;38:e15160.

Reynolds KL, Guidon AC. Diagnosis and management of immune checkpoint inhibitor-associated neurologic toxicity: illustrative case and review of the literature. *Oncologist*. 2019;24:435-443.

Reynolds KL, Zlotoff DA, Mooradian M, et al. Abatacept for immune checkpoint inhibitor associated myocarditis (ATRIUM): phase 3, investigator-initiated, randomized, placebo-controlled study to evaluate the efficacy and safety of abatacept compared to placebo in hospitalized patients with immune checkpoint inhibitor associated myocarditis. *JCO*. 2023;41:TPS2680.

Safa H, Johnson DH, Trinh VA, et al. Immune checkpoint inhibitor-related myasthenia gravis: single center experience and systematic review of the literature. *J Immunother Cancer*. 2019;7(1):319.

Salem JE, Bretagne M, Abbar B, et al. Abatacept/ruxolitinib and screening for concomitant respiratory muscle failure to mitigate fatality of immune-checkpoint inhibitor myocarditis. *Cancer Discov*. 2023;13(5):1100-1115.

Satoh TK, Neulinger MM, Stadler PC, et al. Immune checkpoint inhibitor-induced epidermal necrolysis: a narrative review evaluating demographics, clinical features, and culprit medications. *J Dermatol*. 2024;51(1):3-11.

Schneider BJ, Naidoo J, Santomasso BD, et al. Management of immune-related adverse events in patients treated with immune checkpoint inhibitor therapy: ASCO guideline update [published correction appears in *J Clin Oncol*. 2022;40(3):315]. *J Clin Oncol*. 2021;39(36):4073-4126.

Schneider-Gold C, Gajdos P, Toyka KV, et al. Corticosteroids for myasthenia gravis. *Cochrane Database Syst Rev*. 2005;150.

Spain L, Walls G, Julve M, et al. Neurotoxicity from immune-checkpoint inhibition in the treatment of melanoma: a single centre experience and review of the literature. *Ann Oncol*. 2017;28:377-385.

Stroud CR, Hegde A, Cherry C, Naqash AR, et al. Tocilizumab for the management of immune mediated adverse events secondary to PD-1 blockade. *J Oncol Pharm Pract*. 2019;25:e21712.

Suresh K, Naidoo J, Zhong Q, et al. The alveolar immune cell landscape is dysregulated in checkpoint inhibitor pneumonitis. *J Clin Invest*. 2019; 129:4305-4315.

Suresh K, Voong KR, Shankar B, et al. Pneumonitis in non-small cell lung cancer patients receiving immune checkpoint immunotherapy: incidence and risk factors. *J Thorac Oncol*. 2018;13:1930-1939.

Tang SQ, Tang LL, Mao YP, et al. The pattern of time to onset and resolution of immune-related adverse events caused by immune checkpoint inhibitors in cancer: a pooled analysis of 23 clinical trials and 8,436 patients. *Cancer Res Treat*. 2021;53:339-354.

Tawbi HA, Schadendorf D, Lipson EJ, et al. Relatlimab and nivolumab versus nivolumab in untreated advanced melanoma. *N Engl J Med*. 2022;386(1):24-34.

Thomas AS, Ma W, Wang Y. Ustekinumab for refractory colitis associated with immune checkpoint inhibitors. *N Engl J Med*. 2021;384:581-583.

Thomas MF, Slowikowski K, Manakongtreecheep K, et al. Single-cell transcriptomic analyses reveal distinct immune cell contributions to epithelial barrier dysfunction in checkpoint inhibitor colitis. *Nat Med*. 2024;30(5):1349-1362.

Toyozawa R, Haratake N, Toyokawa G, et al. Atezolizumab-induced aseptic meningitis in patients with NSCLC. *JTO Clin Res Rep*. 2020;1:100012.

Wang Y, Abu-Sbeih H, Mao E, et al. Endoscopic and histologic features of immune checkpoint inhibitor-related colitis. *Inflamm Bowel Dis*. 2018; 24:1695-1705.

Wang DY, Salem JE, Cohen JV, et al. Fatal toxic effects associated with immune checkpoint inhibitors: a systematic review and meta-analysis. *JAMA Oncol*. 2018;4:1721-1728.

Wang DY, Ye F, Zhao S, et al. Incidence of immune checkpoint inhibitor-related colitis in solid tumor patients: a systematic review and meta-analysis. *Oncoimmunology*. 2017;6:e1344805.

Wang Y, Wiesnoski DH, Helmink BA, et al. Fecal microbiota transplantation for refractory immune checkpoint inhibitor-associated colitis. *Nat Med*. 2018;24:1804-1808.

Wang Y, Zhou S, Yang F, et al. Treatment-related adverse events of PD-1 and PD-L1 inhibitors in clinical trials: a systematic review and meta-analysis. *JAMA Oncol*. 2019;5:1008-1019.

Wei SC, Meijers WC, Axelrod ML, et al. A genetic mouse model recapitulates immune checkpoint inhibitor-associated myocarditis and supports a mechanism-based therapeutic intervention. *Cancer Discov*. 2021; 11(3):614-625.

Zhan L, Feng HF, Liu HQ, et al. Immune checkpoint inhibitors-related thyroid dysfunction: epidemiology, clinical presentation, possible pathogenesis, and management. *Front Endocrinol (Lausanne)*. 2021;12:649863.

Zou F, Wang X, Glitza Oliva IC, et al. Fecal calprotectin concentration to assess endoscopic and histologic remission in patients with cancer with immune-mediated diarrhea and colitis. *J Immunother Cancer*. 2021; 9:e002058.

6.10

Coagulopathy

Andrea Ansari and Jarone Lee

Definition

- Disorder of one or more of the factors involved in the coagulation cascade that causes dysfunction in clotting

Common Causes to Remember (Table 6.10.1)

Epidemiology

- Prolonged prothrombin time (PT) and partial thromboplastin time (PTT) are seen in 14% to 28% of intensive care unit (ICU) patients.
- Thrombocytopenia (<150,000/μL) occurs in 35% to 44% of medical ICU patients.
- An estimated 1% to 3% of patients on warfarin develop a major bleed per year.

Key Pathophysiology

- During normal physiologic processes, primary hemostasis occurs when the endothelium is damaged, inflammatory cytokines are released, and platelets bind to the endothelium and each other to form a primary platelet plug.
- Secondary hemostasis involves the activation of the coagulation cascade extrinsically by tissue factor (thromboplastin) released at the site of endothelial injury and intrinsically by platelets and collagen activating factor XII.
- Both pathways lead to a common pathway, with the formation of thrombin and a fibrin clot.

TABLE 6.10.1 Common Causes of Coagulopathy

Inherited	Acquired
• Hemophilia A (factor VIII deficiency) • Hemophilia B (Christmas disease, factor IX deficiency) • Hemophilia C (factor XI deficiency, Rosenthal syndrome) • von Willebrand disease	• Vitamin K antagonists • Specific factor inhibitors • Autoantibodies to specific factors • Heparin • Trauma • Sepsis • Liver disease • Uremia • Acquired von Willebrand disease

- Hemophilia A occurs from a deficiency of factor VIII (FVIII), which, in the majority of cases, is an X-linked recessive disorder.
- Hemophilia B occurs from a deficiency of factor IX; it is also an X-linked recessive disorder.
- von Willebrand factor (vWF) enhances the binding of platelets to the endothelium, and to each other; however, it is also bound to FVIII.
  - A deficiency in vWF can, therefore, lead to increased degradation of free circulating FVIII, as well as poor adherence of platelets.
- Warfarin is a vitamin K antagonist (VKA), and it inhibits the production of factors II, VII, IX, and X.
- Direct oral anticoagulants (DOACs) are inhibitors of specific coagulation factors.
  - Dabigatran is a direct thrombin (factor IIa) inhibitor (DTI).
  - Factor Xa inhibitors include rivaroxaban, apixaban, edoxaban, and betrixaban.
- Parenteral DTIs include argatroban and bivalirudin.
- Heparin and low-molecular-weight heparin (LMWH) bind to antithrombin and increase its binding to thrombin and factor Xa, leading to inactivation of the two enzymes.
- Pregnancy, autoimmune diseases, and malignancy can lead to autoantibodies against specific factors.
  - These are very rare; autoantibodies to FVIII are the most common.
- Protein C degrades factor V and FVIII in the coagulation cascade, inhibits tissue factor, and reduces the release of inflammatory mediators.
- During sepsis and septic shock, inflammatory cytokines cause activation of the coagulation cascade, which, in turn, activates the intrinsic pathway and further consumption of coagulation factors.
- Trauma initially causes vascular injury and initiation of the coagulation cascade. This is often followed by a diffuse inflammatory response, acidemia, and hypothermia, leading to a mixed coagulopathy.
  - Iatrogenic hemodilution can contribute to the coagulopathy in trauma.
- It was long believed that the inability to synthesize clotting factors caused the coagulopathy of liver disease; however, recent evidence suggests that patients with cirrhosis are in a paradoxical prothrombotic state with an elevated rate of thrombin generation.
  - The endotoxemia of severe liver disease is postulated to increase tissue factor and vWF release.
  - It appears that cirrhosis may increase the risk of both thrombosis and bleeding.
- PT measures the extrinsic and common pathways, thereby assessing the activity of tissue factor and factors VII, X, V, II (prothrombin), and I (fibrinogen).
- PTT measures the intrinsic pathway but is less sensitive than the PT for the common pathway.
  - Factors XII, XI, IX, and VIII are part of the extrinsic pathway.

Differential Diagnosis

- These are often overlapping disease processes, but the following chart can help differentiate the different causes of a coagulopathy:

PT Prolonged	PTT Prolonged	Both Prolonged	Neither Prolonged
Factor VII deficiency	Factor VIII, IX, XI deficiency	Factor X, V, II deficiency	Thrombocytopenia
Mild vitamin K deficiency	Unfractionated heparin	Severe vitamin K deficiency	Uremia
Mild liver disease	Inhibiting antibodies	VKAs	Antiplatelet therapy and platelet dysfunction
Low VKA	Antiphospholipid antibody	Liver failure	
	von Willebrand disease	Massive bleeding	
	DOACs	DTIs	

  - Thrombocytopenia—typically presents with mucosal or cutaneous bleeding (gingival or epistaxis), rather than the intramuscular, intra-articular, or deep soft tissue bleeding seen with factors related to coagulopathies
  - Disseminated intravascular coagulation (DIC)—activation of coagulation leading to intravascular fibrin, followed by small- and medium-vessel thrombosis that leads to organ dysfunction
    - Bleeding is actually a late finding in DIC after platelets and coagulation factors have been consumed.

Management and Treatment

- Hemophilia A or B
  - Patients who are bleeding or at risk of bleeding need to have the missing factor replaced.
  - The percent of factor replacement necessary depends on the site of injury and the degree of bleeding.
  - Patients with hemophilia A on emicizumab should still be given factor replacement.
  - For critically ill patients with trauma or any patient with severe bleeding, 100% factor activity is the target level.
    - 1 U/kg of factor VIII increases the factor activity by 2%, 50 U/kg of factor is needed to achieve 100%.
    - 1 U/kg of factor IX increases factor activity by 1%; 100 U/kg of factor is needed to achieve 100%.
    - Head injury is the most common cause of death among patients with hemophilia, and even those with head injury without intracranial injury on computed tomography scan should be increased to a 50% activity level.
    - Recommendation for patients undergoing major surgery: raise activity levels to a goal of 100% but a minimum of 60% and maintain at 30% to 50% for 10 to 14 days after.
    - Factor VIII has a half-life of 8 to 12 hours; so, maintenance dosing will give half the initial dose every 12 hours.
      - The half-life of factor IX is longer at 18 hours.
      - Ideally, repeat dosing should be based on factor levels posttreatment.
    - Because of the multiple transfusions, 20% to 30% of patients can develop inhibitors to factor VIII or IX.
      - These patients should be treated in close consultation with a hematologist.
- Platelet transfusion
  - Thrombocytopenia and platelet transfusion are addressed in another chapter, but they are an integral part of the coagulation cascade.
  - Platelet transfusions are indicated when platelet counts are <10,000/μL, <50,000/μL with active bleeding and for surgical procedures, or <100,000 with central nervous system bleeding and before neurosurgery or ocular surgery.
- VKA reversal guidelines
  - 4-factor prothrombin complex concentrate (4F-PCC)
  - Fixed dose of 1,000 U for patients with actively bleeding
  - International normalized ratio (INR) and weight-based dosing for intracranial hemorrhage
    - 25 U/kg for INR 2≤4
    - 35 U/kg for INR 4 to 6
    - 50 U/kg for INR >6
  - Alternative is fresh frozen plasma (FFP) 10 to 30 mL/kg if PCC is contraindicated or unavailable.
- DOAC reversal guidelines
  - Factor Xa inhibitors
    - Andexanet alpha approved for rivaroxaban and apixaban
    - PCC 25 to 50 U/kg alternative agent
  - Direct thrombin inhibitors
    - Idarucizumab or 4F-PCC 25 to 50 U/kg for reversal of dabigatran
    - Recombinant FVIIa (rFVIIa) 70 to 90 μg/kg for reversal of argatroban, bivalirudin, or fondaparinux
- Trauma
  - Tranexamic acid (TXA) blocks the conversion of plasminogen to plasmin, which is involved in fibrinolysis and breaking up clots.
  - Plasmin is also an inflammatory mediator.
  - The PATCH trial demonstrated a significant improvement in mortality at 24 hours (9.7% vs 14.1%) and 28 days (17.3% vs 21.8%), but not at 6 months, when TXA was given versus placebo within 3 hours of injury to patients with major trauma and a COAST score >3.
    - The dose was 1 g over 10 minutes at the scene of the trauma or en route to the hospital, followed by 1 g over 8 hours.
    - There was no difference in the primary outcome of survival with a favorable functional outcome.
    - No other secondary outcomes were found to have significant differences, including the occurrence of venous thromboembolism (VTE) and transfusion.
  - The CONTROL trial showed no benefit to rFVIIa when given within 12 hours to patients with bleeding trauma.
- Coagulopathy in the critically ill
  - Most importantly, identify and treat the underlying cause.

- FFP contains all coagulation factors, but its use should be limited to patients with active bleeding or a high risk of bleeding.
- PCC does not provide all coagulation factors, so it should be prioritized for use in cases where the large volumes of plasma cannot be tolerated or for reversal of previously discussed anticoagulants.
- DDAVP (desmopressin) induces the release of vWF and can thereby increase platelet binding, as well as the concentration of FVIII.
    - For these reasons, it is considered the first-line treatment of von Willebrand disease.
- rFVIIa has never been shown to improve clinically relevant outcomes but has been associated with an increase in thrombotic complications, especially arterial thrombosis.
    - There are rare circumstances where FVIIa can be considered a rescue therapy.

Outcomes

- Intracranial hemorrhage is the most severe hemorrhagic complication in people with hemophilia, with a lifetime risk of 3% to 13% and a mortality of 30% despite advances in factor replacement therapy.
- Thrombocytopenia is an independent predictor of ICU mortality, with a relative risk (RR) of 1.9 to 4.2 in various studies.

SUGGESTED READINGS

Aldhaeefi M, Badreldin HA, Alsuwayyid F, et al. Practical guide for anticoagulant and antiplatelet reversal in clinical practice. *Pharmacy (Basel)*. 2023;11(1):34.

Drews RE. Critical issues in hematology: anemia, thrombocytopenia, coagulopathy, and blood product transfusions in critically ill patients. *Clin Chest Med*. 2003;24(4):607-622.

Eikelboom JW, Weitz JI. New anticoagulants. *Circulation*. 2010;121(13):1523-1532.

Ferro D, Angelico F, Caldwell SH, Violi F. Bleeding and thrombosis in cirrhotic patients: what really matters? *Dig Liver Dis*. 2012;44(4):275-279.

Fowler H, Lacey R, Keaney J, Kay-Jones C, Martlew V, Thachil J. Emergency and out of hours care of patients with inherited bleeding disorders. *Haemophilia*. 2012;18(3):e126-e131.

Franchini M, Frattini F, Crestani S, Bonfanti C. Haemophilia B: current pharmacotherapy and future directions. *Expert Opin Pharmacother*. 2012;13(14):2053-2063.

Hart DP, Matino D, Astermark J, et al. International consensus recommendations on the management of people with haemophilia B. *Ther Adv Hematol*. 2022;13:20406207221085202.

Hess JR, Brohi K, Dutton RP, et al. The coagulopathy of trauma: a review of mechanisms. *J Trauma: Injury Infect Crit Care*. 2008;65(4):748-754.

Holbrook A, Schulman S, Witt DM, et al. Evidence-based management of anticoagulant therapy: antithrombotic therapy and prevention of thrombosis, 9th ed: American College of Chest Physicians Evidence-Based Clinical Practice Guidelines. *Chest*. 2012;141(2 suppl):e152S-e184S.

Hoots WK. Emergency management in hemophilia. In: Lee CA, Berntorp EE, Hoots WK, eds. *Textbook of Hemophilia*. 2nd ed. Wiley-Blackwell; 2010:394.

Kumar A, Mhaskar R, Grossman BJ, et al; AABB Platelet Transfusion Guidelines Panel. Platelet transfusion: a systematic review of the clinical evidence. *Transfusion*. 2015;55(5):1116-1127; quiz 1115.

Levi M, Opal SM. Coagulation abnormalities in critically ill patients. *Crit Care*. 2006;10(4):222.

Levi M, Schultz M. Coagulopathy and platelet disorders in critically ill patients. *Minerva Anestesiol*. 2010;76(10):851-859.

Maegele M. The European perspective on the management of acute major hemorrhage and coagulopathy after trauma: summary of the 2019 updated European guideline. *J Clin Med*. 2021;10(2):362.

Maegele M. Update on the pathophysiology and management of acute trauma hemorrhage and trauma-induced coagulopathy based upon viscoelastic testing. *Clin Exp Emerg Med*. 2024;11(3):259-267.

Marx JA, Hockberger RS, Walls RM, et al, eds. *Rosen's Emergency Medicine: Concepts and Clinical Practice*. Mosby/Elsevier; 2010.

Papageorgiou C, Jourdi G, Adjambri E, et al. Disseminated intravascular coagulation: an update on pathogenesis, diagnosis, and therapeutic strategies. *Clin Appl Thromb Hemost*. 2018;24(9_suppl):8S-28S.

PATCH-Trauma Investigators and the ANZICS Clinical Trials Group; Gruen RL, Mitra B, Bernard SA, et al. Prehospital tranexamic acid for severe trauma. *N Engl J Med*. 2023;389(2):127-136.

Peyvandi F, Klamroth R, Carcao M, et al. Management of bleeding disorders in adults. *Haemophilia*. 2012;18:24-36.

Pollack CV Jr. New oral anticoagulants in the ED setting: a review. *Am J Emerg Med*. 2012;30(9):2046-2054.

Pollack CV Jr, Reilly PA, Eikelboom J, et al. Idarucizumab for dabigatran reversal. *N Engl J Med*. 2015;373(6):511-520.

Retter A, Hunt BJ. Consumptive coagulopathy in the ICU. *Hematology Am Soc Hematol Educ Program*. 2023;2023(1):754-760.

Roberts I, Shakur H, Afolabi A, et al. The importance of early treatment with tranexamic acid in bleeding trauma patients: an exploratory analysis of the CRASH-2 randomised controlled trial. *Lancet*. 2011;377(9771):1096-1101, 1101.e1-e2.

Roy AM, Konda M, Goel A, Sasapu A. Epidemiology and factors affecting mortality of hospitalized patients with disseminated intravascular coagulation in the United States. *Blood*. 2019;134(supplement_1):2404.

Saba HI, Tran DQ. Challenges and successes in the treatment of hemophilia: the story of a patient with severe hemophilia A and high-titer inhibitors. *J Blood Med*. 2011;3:17-23.

Sborov DW, Rodgers GM. Acquired hemophilia A: a current review of autoantibody disease. *Clin Adv Hematol Oncol*. 2012;10(1):19-27.

Shakur H, Roberts I, Bautista R, et al. Effects of tranexamic acid on death, vascular occlusive events, and blood transfusion in trauma patients with significant haemorrhage (CRASH-2): a randomised, placebo-controlled trial. *Lancet*. 2010;376(9734):23-32.

Zanon E, Pasca S, Demartis F, et al. Intracranial haemorrhage in haemophilia patients is still an open issue: the final results of the Italian EMO.REC registry. *J Clin Med*. 2022;11(7):1969.

6.11

Hematology Diagnostic Modalities

Raghu R. Chivukula

General Principles

Hematologic abnormalities are common in critical illness and frequently require specialized testing to establish a diagnosis and management plan. In this chapter, we review the common assays that all intensivists should be familiar with. Complex hematologic disorders should prompt hematology consultation.

Anemia and Hemolysis

Peripheral Blood Smear

- Indication: identify schistocytes, spherocytes
- Principle: microscopic morphology of stained blood smear
- Interpretation: abnormal shapes indicate hemolysis or malignancy. Schistocytes suggest microangiopathic hemolytic anemia. Spherocytes suggest immune-mediated hemolysis.

Reticulocyte Count

- Indication: differentiate hemolysis versus marrow failure
- Principle: supravital stain or flow cytometry quantifies immature red blood cells (RBCs).
- Interpretation: elevated suggests hemolysis; low suggests inadequate production.

Lactate Dehydrogenase and Haptoglobin

- Indication: detect hemolysis biochemically
- Principle: lactate dehydrogenase (LDH) is an abundant RBC protein that is liberated when RBCs are lysed; haptoglobin binds free hemoglobin (Hb).
- Interpretation: high LDH, low haptoglobin confirms hemolysis.

Indirect Bilirubin

- Indication: assess unconjugated bilirubin in hemolysis
- Principle: hemolysis generates bilirubin that is subsequently conjugated by the liver. Rapid production of bilirubin (such as in hemolysis), therefore, preferentially elevates the unconjugated fraction.
- Interpretation: elevated indirect bilirubin indicates RBC breakdown.

Direct Antiglobulin Test ("Direct Coombs'")

- Indication: evaluate immune-mediated hemolysis
- Principle: detection of immunoglobulin G (IgG) or complement on RBC surface via agglutination
- Interpretation: positive indicates autoimmune hemolysis.

Cell-Free Hemoglobin

- Indication: monitor hemolysis in extracorporeal membrane oxygenation (ECMO) or massive transfusion
- Principle: spectrophotometric and immunoassay measurements
- Interpretation: elevated free Hb with low haptoglobin indicates hemolysis.

Coagulation and Fibrinolysis

Prothrombin Time/International Normalized Ratio

- Indication: monitor warfarin and evaluate the extrinsic pathway
- Principle: tissue factor initiates clot; time measured optically.
- Interpretation: prolonged prothrombin time/international normalized ratio (PT/INR) indicates factor deficiency or anticoagulation.

Activated Partial Thromboplastin Time

- Indication: monitor heparin and assess the intrinsic pathway
- Principle: activator plus phospholipid initiates clot; time measured
- Interpretation: prolongation suggests heparin effect or factor deficiency.

Fibrinogen Level

- Indication: assess disseminated intravascular coagulation (DIC) and bleeding risks
- Principle: Clauss assay measures clotting time inversely proportional to fibrinogen.
- Interpretation: low levels indicate consumption or dilution, suggestive of DIC.

D-dimer

- Indication: rule out thrombosis (eg, venous thromboembolism/pulmonary embolism [VTE/PE]) and support DIC diagnosis
- Principle: immunoassay for fibrin degradation products
- Interpretation: elevated in thrombosis, but nonspecific (acute phase reactant). Low D-dimer argues against significant ongoing thrombosis.

Thrombin Time

- Indication: suspect fibrinogen dysfunction
- Principle: thrombin added to plasma; measures fibrin formation time
- Interpretation: prolonged thrombin time (TT) indicates dysfibrinogenemia or inhibitors.

Anti-Xa Assay

- Indication: monitor heparinoid levels in situations where prothrombin time (PTT) is unreliable
- Principle: chromogenic substrate measures residual factor Xa activity.
- Interpretation: results typically correlate with anticoagulant activity, but fundamentally reflect drug level rather than physiologic effect per se.

Point-of-Care and Viscoelastic Testing

Activated Clotting Time

- Indication: rapid assessment of heparin activity (typically in catheterization lab, operating room)
- Principle: whole blood is activated and the time to clot formation is directly assessed within a cartridge.
- Interpretation: therapeutic time is typically 250 to 300 seconds (from baseline of 100-120 seconds).

Thromboelastography/Rotational Thromboelastography

- Indication: guide blood product transfusion in bleeding patients
- Principle: measures clot kinetics and strength in whole blood
- Interpretation: parameters (R, α, MA, LY30) direct specific therapy. R time reflects clot initiation (depends most on clotting factors). α-Angle reflects the speed of clot strengthening (depends most on fibrinogen). MA reflects peak clot strength (depends most on platelet activity). LY30 reflects clot breakdown (depends on fibrinolysis).

Platelet Function Assay100

- Indication: evaluate platelet function and antiplatelet therapy
- Principle: measures time to occlusion or aggregation in response to agonists
- Interpretation: prolonged times indicate dysfunction or drug effect.

Thrombosis and Hypercoagulability

Heparin-Induced Thrombocytopenia Antibody ELISA (Heparin-PF4)

- Indication: suspect heparin-induced thrombocytopenia (HIT) based on "4T score"
- Principle: detects PF4-heparin complex antibodies via ELISA
- Interpretation: positive requires functional assay confirmation.

Serotonin Release Assay

- Indication: confirm HIT after positive ELISA
- Principle: measures serotonin release from activated donor platelets
- Interpretation: positive confirms HIT diagnosis.

ADAMTS13 Activity Assay

- Indication: diagnose thrombotic thrombocytopenic purpura (TTP) versus other microangiopathies
- Principle: fluorescent substrate assay for von Willebrand factor (vWF) cleavage; inhibitor detection
- Interpretation: activity <10% supports TTP.

Antiphospholipid Panel

- Indication: evaluate unexplained thrombosis or pregnancy loss
- Principle: functional assays and ELISAs for antiphospholipid antibodies ("lupus anticoagulant")
- Interpretation: persistent positivity confirms antiphospholipid syndrome (APS) (use with caution in critically ill as may be nonspecific).

SUGGESTED READINGS

Cuker A. Clinical and laboratory diagnosis of heparin-induced thrombocytopenia: an integrated approach. *Semin Thromb Hemost*. 2014;40(1):106-114.

Lassila R. Platelet function tests in bleeding disorders. *Semin Thromb Hemost*. 2016;42(3):185-190.

Samuel S, Allison TA, Sharaf S, et al. Antifactor Xa levels vs. activated partial thromboplastin time for monitoring unfractionated heparin. A pilot study. *J Clin Pharm Ther*. 2016;41(5):499-502.

Shih AW, McFarlane A, Verhovsek M. Haptoglobin testing in hemolysis: measurement and interpretation. *Am J Hematol*. 2014;89(4):443-447.

6.12

Disseminated Intravascular Coagulopathy

Andrea Ansari and Jarone Lee

Definition

The systemic activation of coagulation resulting in a disturbance in the balance between procoagulants and inhibitors, thrombus formation, and lysis, causing an acquired coagulopathy.

Common Causes to Remember (Table 6.12.1)

Epidemiology

- Occurs in ~1% of hospital admissions, but the occurrence varies significantly
- Occurs in 10% to 30% of intensive care unit (ICU) patients

TABLE 6.12.1 Common Causes of Disseminated Intravascular Coagulopathy

• Sepsis or severe infection • Trauma • Malignancy (especially myeloproliferative and lymphoproliferative) • Toxicologic	• Placental abruption/amniotic fluid embolism • Organ destruction (pancreatitis, hepatic failure) • Immunologic reactions • Vascular abnormalities

- Occurs in 10% to 30% of patients following out-of-hospital cardiac arrest
- Occurs in 30% to 40% of patients with head trauma
- Occurs in 10% of patients with solid tumors
- Occurs in ~30% to 60% of patients with severe sepsis

Key Pathophysiology

- Disseminated intravascular coagulopathy (DIC) always occurs secondary to an underlying disorder.
- An underlying disease process activates pro-inflammatory cytokines, which further stimulate monocytes and endothelial cells to express tissue factor and more cytokines.
- Tissue factor initiates the extrinsic pathway by activating factor VII.
- The intrinsic pathway can be activated by cell-free DNA but is thought to be less involved in DIC.
- Impairment of all major anticoagulant pathways (antithrombin III, protein C, and tissue factor pathway inhibitor) leads to uncontrolled coagulation.
- The combination of increased tissue factor and impaired anticoagulation leads to intravascular fibrin formation.
- Additionally, the fibrinolytic system is initially depressed by elevated levels of plasminogen activator inhibitor-1, and fibrin cannot be broken down and removed.
- Widespread microvascular deposition of fibrin leads to thrombosis with further consumption of platelets and coagulation factors, and eventually organ dysfunction from worsening thrombosis.
- Progressive thrombocytopenia and consumptive coagulopathy increase the risk of bleeding in these patients.
- Red blood cells (RBCs) can be sheared by fibrin and thrombi in blood vessels, leading to hemolytic anemia.
- During fibrinolysis, plasmin cleaves cross-linked fibrin several times, resulting in the formation of fibrin degradation products and D-dimers.
- There are five scoring systems for the diagnosis of DIC: International Society on Thrombosis and Haemostasis (ISTH), Korean Society on Thrombosis and Hemostasis (KSTH), Japanese Association for Acute Medicine (JAAM), Revised JAAM (R-JAAM), and Japanese Ministry of Health and Welfare (JMHW).
  - One comparative study of the scoring systems found KSTH had the highest sensitivity and R-JAAM had the highest specificity.

Differential Diagnosis

- Thrombotic thrombocytopenic purpura (TTP)—typically results from an impairment of ADAMTS-13, which normally cleaves Von Willebrand factor (vWF), but when it is not present, it leads to ultra-large vWF and the activation of platelets and thrombosis.
  - Prothrombin time/partial thromboplastin time (PT/PTT) should not be elevated in patients with TTP.
- Hemolytic uremic syndrome—similar to TTP and in the same spectrum but usually occurs in children
- Heparin-induced thrombocytopenia (HIT)—when receiving heparin, some patients develop antibodies to platelet antigens, which can directly activate platelets, causing thrombosis and decreasing platelet count.
  - Many patients in the hospital are on heparin or low-molecular-weight heparin (LMWH) for thromboembolic prophylaxis, and many of these same patients have disease processes that can increase the risk of DIC.
  - HIT antibodies and serotonin release assays can be helpful in differentiating HIT from DIC.
- Severe liver disease—it can be difficult to differentiate from DIC; however, factor VIII, fibrinogen, fibrin split products, including D-dimer, and platelets are more likely to be normal.
  - DIC is an acute consumptive process, so these laboratory values will change more acutely.
  - Trending values over time can be helpful in the diagnosis, especially since platelets should not drop precipitously in liver disease.

Management and Treatment

- First and foremost, treat the underlying disorder.
- There is minimal high-quality research, so most of this is expert opinion.
- Once the underlying disorder is adequately treated, DIC may still worsen.
- Platelet transfusion
  - If the patient is actively bleeding or at high risk of bleeding (recent surgery or due to undergo an invasive procedure) with platelets <50,000/μL, platelet transfusion is recommended.
  - Nonbleeding patients should not be transfused unless platelets are <10 to 20,000/μL (based on chemotherapy trials, not DIC).
- Fresh frozen plasma (FFP)
  - If a patient with DIC is actively bleeding or has a high risk of bleeding with an elevated PT/PTT (>1.5 times normal) or fibrinogen <1.5 g/dL, FFP is recommended.
  - It should not be given routinely for patients with elevated PT/PTT.
  - Initial suggested transfusion dose is 15 mL/kg.
- Prothrombin complex concentrate (PCC)
  - Can be given for the same indications as FFP; however, it does not contain fibrinogen or all the clotting factors.
  - FFP is preferable to PCC unless the patient cannot tolerate the larger volume of FFP.
- Fibrinogen concentrate or cryoprecipitate
  - Recommended for actively bleeding patients with persistent severe hypofibrinogenemia (<1.5 g/dL)
- Recombinant factor VIIa
  - Guidelines caution its use in severe, life-threatening bleeding.
- Unfractionated heparin and LMWH
  - Recommended for thromboembolic prophylaxis in nonbleeding patients with DIC
  - Do not stop prophylaxis in patients who are showing signs of developing DIC with abnormal coagulation parameters.
  - Consider therapeutic doses of heparin/LMWH in nonbleeding patients where thrombosis predominates (severe purpura fulminans).
  - Only recommended in patients with inherited or acquired antithrombin deficiency
- Antithrombin concentrate
  - Has demonstrated improvements in coagulation parameters in multiple studies
  - A large, multicenter randomized controlled trial of antithrombin in severe sepsis showed no improvement in mortality; however, subgroup analysis in the group that did not receive heparin and developed DIC showed

improved mortality (25.4% vs 40%) with antithrombin, and it also increased the risk of major bleeding.

- Activated protein C (APC)
  - Protein C degrades factor V and factor VIII in the coagulation cascade, inhibits tissue factor, and reduces the release of inflammatory mediators.
  - APC was shown to improve mortality versus placebo (24.7% vs 30.8%) in the treatment of patients with severe sepsis and organ dysfunction.
  - Subgroup analysis later showed the highest benefit in patients with DIC.
  - The ADDRESS study showed no improvement in mortality in patients with sepsis with lower disease severity (APACHE-II <25), and the RESOLVE study showed no decrease in mortality in pediatric patients with sepsis.
  - The PROWESS-SHOCK study group showed no significant benefit of APC in patients with septic shock.
  - APC was taken off the market on October 2011 after the PROWESS-SHOCK study was completed.
- Recombinant human thrombomodulin
  - Binds to thrombin, inactivating thrombin's role in coagulation and also activating protein C
  - Has been shown to increase resolution of DIC compared to heparin in one study and reduce organ failure compared to placebo in another, but has never significantly decreased mortality
- Recombinant tissue factor pathway inhibitor
  - No significant benefit seen in patients with severe sepsis
- Antifibrinolytic agents
  - The coagulopathy of acute promyelocytic leukemia (AML-M3) responds well to all-*trans*-retinoic acid, and tranexamic acid has been shown to improve mortality from bleeding when given within the first 3 hours of trauma.

Outcomes

- Major bleeding (intracranial, intrathoracic, intra-abdominal, or requiring packed RBC transfusion) occurs in 5% to 12% of patients.
- In patients with sepsis, the presence of DIC nearly doubles the mortality.
- Acute DIC in severe sepsis, trauma, and burns is associated with a high mortality rate varying from ~40% to 80%.

SUGGESTED READINGS

Abraham E, Laterre P-F, Garg R, et al. Drotrecogin alfa (activated) for adults with severe sepsis and a low risk of death. *N Engl J Med*. 2005;353(13):1332-1341.

Adelborg K, Larsen JB, Hvas AM. Disseminated intravascular coagulation: epidemiology, biomarkers, and management. *Br J Haematol*. 2021; 192(5):803-818.

Bernard GR, Vincent J-L, Laterre P-F, et al. Efficacy and safety of recombinant human activated protein C for severe sepsis. *N Engl J Med*. 2001; 344(10):699-709.

Di Nisio M, Baudo F, Cosmi B, et al. Diagnosis and treatment of disseminated intravascular coagulation: guidelines of the Italian Society for Haemostasis and Thrombosis (SISET). *Thromb Res*. 2012;129(5):e177-e184.

Kienast J, Juers M, Wiedermann CJ, et al. Treatment effects of high-dose antithrombin without concomitant heparin in patients with severe sepsis with or without disseminated intravascular coagulation. *J Thromb Haemost*. 2006;4(1):90-97.

Levi M. Disseminated intravascular coagulation. *Crit Care Med*. 2007; 35(9):2191-2195.

Levi M, Schultz M. Coagulopathy and platelet disorders in critically ill patients. *Minerva Anestesiol*. 2010;76(10):851-859.

Levi M, Toh CH, Thachil J, Watson HG; British Committee for Standards in Haematology. Guidelines for the diagnosis and management of disseminated intravascular coagulation. *Br J Haematol*. 2009;145(1):24-33.

Matsuda T. Clinical aspects of DIC—disseminated intravascular coagulation. *Pol J Pharmacol*. 1996;48(1):73-75.

Nadel S, Goldstein B, Williams MD, et al. Drotrecogin alfa (activated) in children with severe sepsis: a multicentre phase III randomised controlled trial. *Lancet*. 2007;369(9564):836-843.

Popescu NI, Lupu C, Lupu F. Disseminated intravascular coagulation and its immune mechanisms. *Blood*. 2022;139(13):1973-1986.

Ranieri VM, Thompson BT, Barie PS, et al. Drotrecogin alfa (activated) in adults with septic shock. *N Engl J Med*. 2012;366(22):2055-2064.

Wada H, Thachil J, Di Nisio M, et al. Guidance for diagnosis and treatment of DIC from harmonization of the recommendations from three guidelines. *J Thromb Haemost*. 2013;4(11):761-767.

Warren BL, Eid A, Singer P, et al. Caring for the critically ill patient: high-dose antithrombin III in severe sepsis: a randomized controlled trial. *JAMA*. 2001;286(15):1869-1878.

Zafar A, Naeem F, Khalid MZ, Awan S, Riaz MM, Mahmood SBZ. Comparison of five different disseminated intravascular coagulation criteria in predicting mortality in patients with sepsis. *PLoS One*. 2024;19(3):e0295050.

6.13

Hypercoagulable States

Amory de Roulet and David B. Sykes

Key Points

- Virchow triad of risk factors: hypercoagulable state, stasis of flow, endothelial damage
- Most critically ill patients have risk factors for hypercoagulable disorders.
- Recent major surgery and trauma are additional risk factors for venous thromboembolism (VTE).
- Severe COVID (inpatient hospitalization) is associated with thrombosis.

Overview

- Venous clots are common in the critically ill.
- Arterial clots are less common in the critically ill and should prompt a workup for underlying hematologic disorders.
- Routine testing for inherited thrombophilia testing for inpatients is generally not helpful.
  - It rarely alters the immediate management of patients.
  - Diagnostic tests can be confounded by critical illness.

Tests Confounded by Critical Illness

- Lupus anticoagulant
- Protein C
- Protein S
- Antithrombin

Tests That Are Reliable in the Setting of Critical Illness

- Antiplatelet PF4 antibody (heparin-induced thrombocytopenia [HIT])
- JAK2V617F mutation testing (especially for arterial thrombosis)
- Flow cytometry for paroxysmal nocturnal hemoglobinuria (PNH) (especially for intra-abdominal or cerebral sinus thrombosis)
- Anticardiolipin antibodies (antiphospholipid antibody syndrome [APLAS])
- Anti-beta2-glycoprotein 1 antibodies (APLAS)
- Factor V Leiden (do not send routinely on inpatients)
- Prothrombin gene mutation (do not send routinely on inpatients)

Other Testing

- D-Dimer
  - Degradation product of cross-linked fibrin.
  - A high D-dimer can be indicative of augmented fibrinolysis (by plasmin).
  - A useful test in the outpatient and emergency department setting
  - Rarely useful in critically ill inpatients as many conditions elevate the D-dimer
- Antithrombin (AT3)
  - Serine protease inhibitor synthesized in the liver
  - Natural anticoagulant that regulates coagulation by inhibiting thrombin and activated clotting factors
  - AT3 is often low in the critically ill inpatient.
    - Liver dysfunction leads to decreased synthesis (eg, cirrhosis).
    - AT3 is consumed in many settings (eg, disseminated intravascular coagulation [DIC], sepsis, trauma, malignancy, extracorporeal membrane oxygenation [ECMO]).

Pathophysiology

- Common risk factors [** denotes the largest independent risk factors]
  - Recent surgery**
  - Trauma**
  - Tobacco smoking
  - High estrogen state: oral contraceptive pill (OCP), pregnancy
  - Malignancy
  - Advanced liver disease can be a risk factor for both bleeding and clotting.
  - Elevated body mass index (BMI)
- Acquired
  - HIT (both arterial and venous thrombosis)
    - Platelet count decreases 5 to 10 days after heparin initiation.
  - DIC
  - PNH
  - Myeloproliferative neoplasm (MPN)
  - APLAS
  - COVID-19 infection is associated with "thrombo-inflammation," including endothelial damage, high D-dimer, high von Willebrand factor (vWF) Ag activity, and high factor VIII activity.

Diagnostic Considerations

- A personal history of VTE is a strong risk factor for future VTE.
- Family VTE history of first-degree relatives should be obtained.
- Labs: baseline prothrombin time/international normalized ratio (PT/INR), activated partial thromboplastin time (aPTT), fibrinogen, D-dimer
- ** In the critically ill inpatient, the D-dimer can be elevated for myriad reasons. Therefore, it can be quite a helpful test if it is LOW, but not necessarily helpful if it is HIGH**.

Treatment

- Venous and arterial clots are treated with anticoagulation.
- Arterial clots are platelet rich and benefit from an antiplatelet agent (eg, aspirin [ASA], Plavix).
- Anticoagulation
  - Choice of anticoagulant depends on the clinical context:
    - Intravenous (IV): heparin | $t_{1/2}$ = 60 to 90 minutes
    - IV: argatroban | $t_{1/2}$ = 45 minutes
    - IV: bivalirudin | $t_{1/2}$ = 25 minutes
    - Subcutaneous (SQ): low-molecular-weight heparin (LMWH) | $t_{1/2}$ = 3 to 7 hours
    - SQ: fondaparinux | $t_{1/2}$ = 17 to 21 hours
    - Oral (PO): apixaban | $t_{1/2}$ = 9 to 14 hours
    - PO: rivaroxaban | $t_{1/2}$ = 5 to 9 hours
    - PO: dabigatran | $t_{1/2}$ = 12 to 17 hours
- *Special consideration*: When initiating warfarin, the patient should already be therapeutically anticoagulated with another agent (eg, heparin) and the two agents continued together until the PT/INR is within therapeutic range.
- Anticoagulation contraindications
  - Absolute: active bleeding, major trauma
  - Relative: immediately perioperative or periprocedural (if high risk for bleeding), recent bleeding, intracranial or spinal tumors, stable aortic dissection, aortic aneurysm with severe hypertension
  - Long-term risk calculator: HAS-BLED
- Duration of anticoagulation
  - VTE (deep venous thrombosis/pulmonary embolism [DVT/PE])
    - Provoked thrombosis: 3 to 6 months
    - Unprovoked: consider long term
  - Arterial thrombosis: long-term management is beyond the scope of this chapter.

SUGGESTED READINGS

Anderson JA, Weitz JI. Hypercoagulable states. *Crit Care Clin*. 2011;27(4):933-952.

Gorog DA, Storey RF, Gurbel PA, et al. Current and novel biomarkers of thrombotic risk in COVID-19: a consensus statement from the International COVID-19 thrombosis biomarkers colloquium. *Nat Rev Cardiol*. 2022;19(7):475-495.

May JE, Moll S. Unexplained arterial thrombosis: approach to diagnosis and treatment. *Hematology Am Soc Hematol Educ Program*. 2021;2021(1):76-84.

6.14

Coagulation Management Strategies

Amory de Roulet and David B. Sykes

Background

- Coagulopathies are acquired bleeding disorders characterized by abnormal hemostasis.
- Multiple etiologies: anticoagulation therapy, disseminated intravascular coagulation (DIC), sepsis, liver dysfunction, massive bleeding

Key Points

- It is important to consider, diagnose, and rapidly intervene.
- Basic labs: prothrombin time/international normalized ratio (PT/INR), activated partial thromboplastin time (aPTT), fibrinogen, D-dimer
- Low fibrinogen (hypofibrinogenemia) is strongly associated with mortality.
- Thromboelastography (TEG)

Acute Bleeding/Trauma-Induced Coagulopathy

- Trauma-induced coagulopathy (TIC) results from the dilution and consumption of clotting factors as well as the effect of high levels of citrate from blood product transfusion.
- The usefulness of common labs (PT/INR, PTT, and fibrinogen) is questionable during active bleeding due to the delay between test and result times.
- Defining TIC with a single laboratory measurement is imprecise.
- Point-of-care testing with bedside viscoelastic tests (TEG, rotational thromboelastometry [ROTEM]) can provide real-time information (~10 minutes).
    - Measurements include: speed of thrombin generation (reaction time), speed of clot formation (alpha angle), maximum clot strength (maximum amplitude), magnitude of fibrinolysis (LY30), platelet function, presence of heparin, and presence of thrombin inhibitors
    - Goal-directed coagulation management algorithms may have increased efficiency and show reduced mortality when compared to fixed massive transfusion protocols.
- Hypofibrinogenemia
    - Fibrinogen is the earliest depleted factor in coagulopathy, and hypofibrinogenemia (<150 mg/dL) is associated with mortality in patients with acute bleeding.
    - Fibrinogen can be repleted with cryoprecipitate, prothrombin complex concentrate (PCC), and fresh frozen plasma (FFP).
    - Fibrinolysis activation following severe injury is common.
        - Tranexamic acid (TXA) inhibits hyperfibrinolysis and decreases blood transfusion needs and mortality.

Sepsis-Induced Coagulopathy and Disseminated Intravascular Coagulation

- An acquired syndrome characterized by the intravascular activation of coagulation arising from sepsis, trauma, or malignancy. Patients can be both coagulopathic and hypercoagulable (ie, bleeding and clotting).
- Diagnostic criteria: multiple scoring systems based on a combination of clinical and laboratory data: elevated Sequential Organ Failure Assessment (SOFA) score, hypofibrinogenemia, elevated PT/INR, elevated D-dimer, and thrombocytopenia
    - Standard coagulation tests (PT/INR, PTT) are often normal until late in the disease process. Viscoelastic testing (TEG and ROTEM) is considered more sensitive and specific for coagulopathies in sepsis.
- There are no established therapies or guidelines for the management of sepsis-induced coagulopathy (SIC)/DIC.
- Treatment options include repletion of fibrinogen to >150 mg/dL combined with anticoagulation. Other unproven options include antithrombin, activated protein C (PC), FFP, and recombinant thrombomodulin, though these are all controversial.

Coagulopathy in Cirrhosis

- Advanced liver dysfunction can lead to several problems:
    - Decreased synthesis of procoagulant factors (prolonging the PT/INR and aPTT)
    - Decreased synthesis of natural anticoagulant factors (AT3, PC, protein S [PS])
    - Decreased synthesis of fibrinogen + increased fibrinolysis
    - Increased levels of von Willebrand factor
    - Portal hypertension → esophageal varices → bleeding
    - Decreased synthesis of thrombopoietin → thrombocytopenia
    - Portal hypertension → splenomegaly → platelet sequestration → thrombocytopenia
- Laboratory testing has significant limitations:
    - Increased INR and aPTT do not reflect the decreased levels of AT3, PC, and PS.
    - Viscoelastic tests have not yet been validated in patients with cirrhosis.
    - Recommended reading includes the 2019 American Gastroenterological Association (AGA) Clinical Practice Update.

Anticoagulant Reversal

- Warfarin (vitamin K antagonist [VKA])
    - Elevated INR without bleeding
        - Hold warfarin.
        - Consider low-dose oral vitamin K (eg, 50-100 μg).

- Minor bleeding
  - Oral vitamin K (eg, 10 mg, takes ~24 hours for full reversal)
  - Intravenous vitamin K (eg, 1 mg, slightly faster than oral)
- Major bleeding
  - Intravenous vitamin K
  - PCC
  - FFP (higher volume than PCC, requires >6 units of FFP to replace ~50% of factors)

- Direct oral anticoagulant (DOAC)
  - Risk of serious bleeding is slightly lower with DOACs than with warfarin.
  - Specific reversal agents
    - Apixaban and rivaroxaban: andexanet alfa
      - Recombinant factor Xa (FXa) decoy
      - Expensive, short half-life
    - Dabigatran: idarucizumab
      - Monoclonal antibody with high affinity for dabigatran
      - Short half-life = 45 minutes
  - Nonspecific reversal agents
    - PCCs
      - 4-factor PCC (KCENTRA) contains FII, FIX, FX, and FVII as well as small amounts of PC and PS
      - Unproven efficacy.

SUGGESTED READINGS

CRASH-3 Trial Collaborators. Effects of tranexamic acid on death, disability, vascular occlusive events and other morbidities in patients with acute traumatic brain injury (CRASH-3): a randomised, placebo-controlled trial. *Lancet*. 2019;394:1713-1723.

Geeraedts LM Jr, Demiral H, Schaap NP, Kamphuisen PW, Pompe JC, Frolke JP. 'Blind' transfusion of blood products in exsanguinating trauma patients. *Resuscitation*. 2007;73:382-388.

Hill R, Han TS, Lubomirova I, Math N, Bentley P, Sharma P. Prothrombin complex concentrates are superior to fresh frozen plasma for emergency reversal of vitamin K antagonists: a meta-analysis in 2606 subjects. *Drugs*. 2019;79:1557-1565.

Inata Y. Should we treat sepsis-induced DIC with anticoagulants? *J. Intensive Care*. 2020;8:18.

Kustos SA, Fasinu PS. Direct-acting oral anticoagulants and their reversal agents—an update. *Medicines (Basel)*. 2019;6:103.

O'Leary JG, Greenberg CS, Patton HM, Caldwell SH. AGA Clinical Practice Update: coagulation in cirrhosis. *Gastroenterology*. 2019;157(1):34-43.e1.

Roberts I, Shakur H, Afolabi A, et al. Effects of a high-dose 24-h infusion of tranexamic acid on death and thromboembolic events in patients with acute gastrointestinal bleeding (HALT-IT): an international randomised, double-blind, placebo-controlled trial. *Lancet*. 2020;395:1927-1936.

Rourke C, Curry N, Khan S, et al. Fibrinogen levels during trauma hemorrhage, response to replacement therapy, and association with patient outcomes. *J Thromb Haemost*. 2012;10:1342-1351.

6.15

Complications of Immunosuppressive Drugs

Davit Kocharyan

In the United States, over 29,000 transplants are performed annually, with the kidney being the most commonly transplanted organ, followed by the liver, heart, and lung. Effective immunosuppressive agents are the primary contributors to the substantial improvement in survival rates in solid organ transplantation (SOT). Nonetheless, long-term survival following SOT is affected by factors such as chronic rejection, cardiovascular diseases, and complications of chronic immunosuppression (IS), discussed herein. In parallel, while not the primary focus of this chapter, many of the same drugs are employed routinely in the management of autoimmune and rheumatologic conditions and, therefore, share similar toxicity profiles in those contexts.

Alloimmunity

The alloimmune response requires recognition of "non-self" tissue followed by activation and clonal expansion of alloreactive lymphocytes.

- Allorecognition occurs via multiple mechanisms.
  - In the direct pathway, the T cells of the recipient directly recognize intact allogeneic human leukocyte antigens (HLAs) presented on the donor cell. Without IS, this recognition leads to acute cellular rejection due to a large number of recipient T cells triggered by graft antigens.
  - In the indirect pathway, donor HLA-derived peptides are presented to T cells by the recipient's antigen-presenting cells (APCs). The indirect pathway is responsible for chronic or late acute rejection.
- Activation and proliferation of T cells through a three-signal model initiates the cascade of events leading to allorecognition and graft rejection. This mechanism provides a framework for understanding the specific targets of immunosuppressive medications.
  - Signal 1—Alloantigen recognition: APCs engage T-cell receptors, initiating T-cell activation through three signaling pathways: calcium calcineurin, NF-κB, and RAS-MAPK.
  - Signal 2—Lymphocyte activation and co-stimulation: interactions between costimulatory molecules and their ligands enhance interleukin-2 (IL-2) production and subsequent T-cell proliferation.
  - Signal 3—Clonal expansion: IL-2 binds to the CD25 receptor on activated T cells and promotes their proliferation and differentiation into effector cells, contributing to graft rejection.
- In addition to T cells, activated B cells produce alloantibodies targeting donor HLA antigens and contributing to graft rejection.

Principles and Stages of Solid Organ Transplantation Immunosuppression

- Protocols for clinical IS vary based on the organ.
  - In liver transplant, adequate IS can be sustained on low-dose calcineurin inhibitor (CNI) monotherapy.
  - Conversely, patients undergoing isolated kidney transplant could require a triple-drug regimen.
  - Irrespective of the organ system, the three phases of transplant IS are induction, maintenance, and anti-rejection therapy.
- The induction phase usually spans from just before organ implantation to 30 to 60 days posttransplant.
  - More aggressive immunomodulating therapy is required during this stage since the alloreactivity is at its peak.
  - Steroid-based regimens make up the majority of induction treatments, but depleting antibodies, such as antithymocyte globulin (ATG), may be used in highly sensitized patients.
- The maintenance phase starts following the induction phase and continues for the rest of the lifecycle of the patient or the allograft.
  - The primary objectives in this phase are to reduce exposure to immunosuppressive agents while ensuring an adequate graft function, mainly through the use of CNIs.
  - The goal of chronic IS is to preserve the allograft function by balancing between the dampened immune response and the potential side effects of immunosuppressive agents.
  - To optimize dose, boost the synergistic effect, and reduce the side effects, the current regimens of IS often include three agents targeting various parts of the immune system.
  - IS is gradually tapered to sustain adequate therapeutic levels.
- The treatment of the rejection episodes can vary and depend on the specific pathway associated with organ rejection.
  - In liver transplantation, graft rejection is predominantly T-cell mediated, while antibody-mediated rejection is of greater concern in renal transplantation.
  - Mild-to-moderate T-cell rejection can often be managed through dose adjustment of maintenance IS agents or a pulsed dose of corticosteroids.
  - Antibody-mediated rejection episodes may require a more aggressive approach, such as anti-CD20 antibody therapy combined with plasmapheresis.

Classification and Mechanisms of Action

The classification of immunosuppressive agents is based on different approaches: induction versus maintenance, biologic versus pharmacologic, mechanistic, and site of action (Figure 6.15.1). Table 6.15.1 summarizes common immunosuppressive drugs and mechanisms of action.

Immunosuppression Complications—General Principles

- The chronic administration of immunosuppressive agents results in two groups of adverse events: drug-related side effects and IS-related complications. IS-related complications are divided into two categories: infections and malignancies.
- Infections
  - Both opportunistic and conventional infections are the primary cause of graft failure, death, and morbidity in the first year following SOT. The risk of infections depends on the "net state of IS," which is a combination of individual predisposing factors and an immunosuppressive regimen.
  - The extent of net IS delineates the three overlapping phases of posttransplant infection risk:
    - Early perioperative phase (1 month) when IS is not yet entirely effective. Since IS is not at its peak in the first month, the infections arising during this period are primarily related to:
      - Technical complications of surgery: bleeding, strictures, anastomotic leaks, graft injury
      - Hospital-acquired infections: aspiration pneumonia, *Clostridium difficile* colitis, catheter-related bloodstream infections (CRBSIs), and wound infections
      - Recipient-originated infection: *Aspergillus*, *Pseudomonas*, methicillin-resistant *Staphylococcus aureus* (MRSA), vancomycin-resistant *Enterococcus* (VRE)

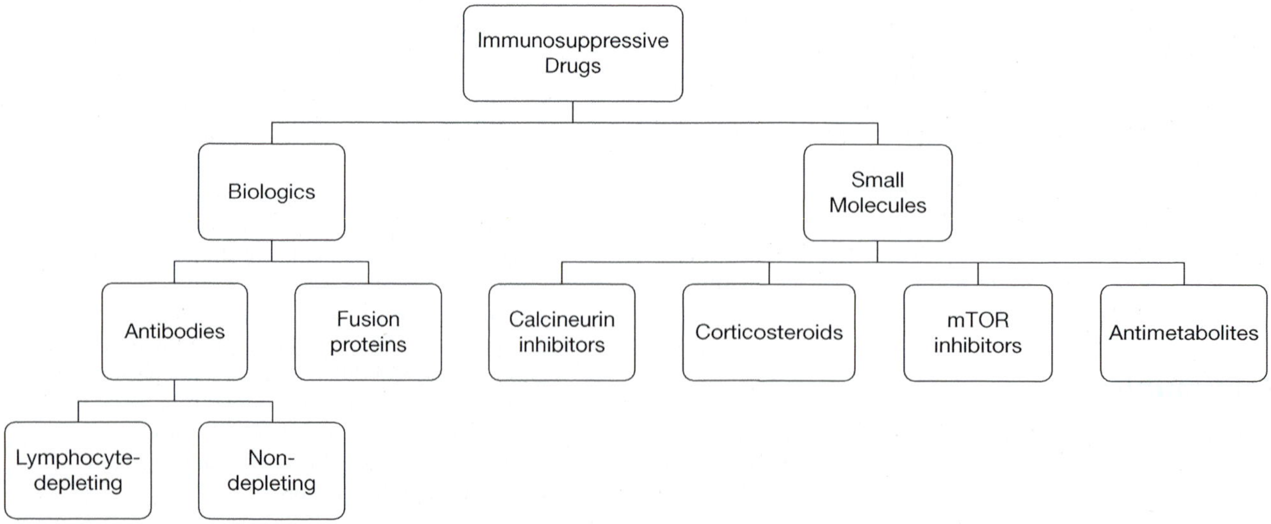

FIGURE 6.15.1 Pharmaceutical classification of major immunosuppressive drug families.

TABLE 6.15.1 Mechanisms of Common IS Agents

Medication Group	Examples	Mechanism of Action
Corticosteroids	Prednisone Prednisolone Methylprednisolone	Pleiotropic effects: ↓ Transcription of cytokine genes in APCs → ↓ IL-2, IL-6, TNF-α; ↑ regulation of antiinflammatory protein lipocortin and IL-10, T-lymphocyte apoptosis
Calcineurin inhibitors (CNIs)	Tacrolimus Cyclosporine	Inhibition of Ca/calmodulin-activated phosphatase → ↓NFAT → ↓ IL-2/INF-γ → ↓ T-cell activation, ↓ Signal 2
Antimetabolites	Azathioprine Mycophenolic acid	Block de novo purine synthesis → ↓ DNA/RNA synthesis → ↓Clonal expansion of T/B cells
mTOR inhibitors	Sirolimus Everolimus	Binds to FK506BP12 in the cytoplasm → ↓mTOR kinase → ↓IL-2–driven T-cell proliferation, ↓ Signal 3
Antibodies—depleting (polyclonal)	Antithymocyte globulin (ATG)	Depletion and receptor modulation of $CD4^+$ T cells, ↓ Signals 1,2,3
Antibodies—depleting (monoclonal)	Rituximab Alemtuzumab Muromonab (OKT3): withdrawn from the market	↓ $CD20^+$ B cells ↓ $CD52^+$ T/B cells ↓ $CD3^+$ T cells, ↓ Signal 1
Antibodies—nondepleting (chimeric, monoclonal)	Basiliximab Daclizumab	Block IL-2 receptors → ↓ T-cell proliferation, ↓ Signal 3
Fusion protein, costimulatory blocker	Abatacept Belatacept	↓ CD28-CD80/B7 costimulatory signal → ↓ T-cell activation ↓ Signal 2 (co-stimulation)

APCs, antigen-presenting cells; IFN, interferon; IL, interleukin; IS, immunosuppression; mTOR, mammalian target of rapamycin; TNF, tumor necrosis factor.

    - Donor-originated infections: herpes simplex virus (HSV), human immunodeficiency virus (HIV), parasites, non-albicans *Candida* species
  - The intermediate phase (1-6 months posttransplant) is when IS reaches its peak. The intermediate phase carries the highest risk of opportunistic infections and reactivation of latent pathogens since IS is at its peak:
    - Without prophylaxis: cytomegalovirus (CMV), Epstein-Barr virus (EBV), varicella-zoster virus (VZV), hepatitis B virus (HBV), hepatitis C virus (HCV), *Mycobacterium* tuberculosis
    - Opportunistic infections: *Aspergillus*, *Candida*, pneumocystis pneumonia (PCP), *Toxoplasma*, *Legionella*, *Listeria*, *Nocardia*, *Histoplasma*, *Coccidioides*, *Cryptococcus*
    - With PCP and antiviral prophylaxis: BK polyomavirus, nephropathy, HCV, adenovirus, influenza, *Cryptococcus*
  - The late phase (>6 months posttransplant) reflects the taper of IS, making the risk of infection comparable to that of the general population, with community-acquired pathogens being most common.
    - *Aspergillus*, *Mucor* species, HSV encephalitis, JC polyomavirus infection
    - However, the PACIFIC trial did not demonstrate a significant correlation between the long-term immunosuppressive therapy (excluding chemotherapy) and higher or lower intensive care unit (ICU)/3-month mortality rates among patients admitted for septic shock.
    - Another study showed that in critically ill renal transplant recipients admitted to the ICU, reducing IS may lower rates of infectious complications without substantially increasing the risk of sensitization, rejection, or graft failure.

- Malignancies
  - Posttransplant malignancies represent the third leading cause of mortality (varies between 10% and 20%) among immunocompromised SOT recipients, following cardiovascular disease and infections.
  - Compared to the general population, SOT recipients have a 2- to 3-fold higher likelihood of developing malignancies that escalates over time due to the direct pro-oncogenic effects of prolonged IS, ineffective immunosurveillance of tumor cells, and a rise in pro-oncogenic viral-driven cancers.
  - Posttransplant malignancies may be categorized into three groups according to their origin and pathogenesis: de novo cancers, donor-related cancers, and recurrent cancers.
    - The most common de novo malignancies are non-melanoma skin cancer, posttransplant lymphoproliferative disorder (PTLD), and anogenital cancers.
    - Renal cell carcinoma and malignant melanoma are mostly donor related.
    - The commonly recurring malignancies are hepatocellular cancer (HCC) and cholangiocarcinoma.
  - The specifics of the immunosuppressive regimen affect the risk of malignancy.
    - T-cell–depleting agents, such as ATGs and belatacept, is linked to an elevated risk of EBV-driven posttransplant PTLD. ~50% of PTLD cases respond to reduction or withdrawal of IS, making prompt and aggressive IS reduction the initial therapeutic intervention upon diagnosis.
    - Corticosteroids exert a direct pro-oncogenic effect on lymphoid cells while concurrently compromising immunosurveillance. Prolonged exposure to glucocorticoids for ≥1 month is linked to a 1.5-fold increase in the risk of basal cell cancer and a >2-fold increase in the risk of squamous cell cancer.

- Azathioprine impairs postreplicative DNA-mismatch repair, thereby amplifying ultraviolet (UV)-induced DNA damage and increasing the risk of nonmelanoma skin cancers.
- CNIs promote carcinogenesis by impairing DNA repair and apoptosis, upregulating tumor growth factor (TGF)-beta (enhancing invasiveness and metastasis) and vascular endothelial growth factor (VEGF) (stimulating angiogenesis), while suppressing IL-2 production by helper T cells.

Drug-Specific Adverse Effects

Corticosteroids

Since the inception of transplantation, corticosteroids have been a cornerstone of IS, acting through genomic and nongenomic mechanisms. The ability to target various sites of the immune system also makes pulse steroids a highly effective tool in the treatment of acute allograft rejection episodes. However, the long-term administration of steroids carries numerous well-known side effects, summarized in Table 6.15.2.

Calcineurin Inhibitors

- CNIs play a crucial role in immunosuppressive therapy, especially for long-term maintenance across nearly all transplant protocols. Tacrolimus, a more potent agent than cyclosporine (CsA), is the preferred CNI in modern regimens.
- Metabolism and pharmacokinetics
  - Cyclosporine and tacrolimus undergo extensive metabolism through the hepatic cytochrome CYP3A4, leading to critical implications for drug-drug interactions (Table 6.15.3).
  - CNIs are commonly administered twice daily, with therapeutic monitoring based on trough levels measured prior to the next scheduled dose. Therapeutic trough levels vary based on time since transplantation, previous rejection episodes, the type of transplanted organ, and concurrent immunosuppressive therapy. The therapeutic trough levels for tacrolimus are generally maintained between 3 and 12 ng/mL, with toxicity risk increasing at concentrations exceeding 20 to 25 ng/mL.
- CNIs are associated with well-known long-term adverse effects, including neurotoxicity, renal dysfunction, metabolic syndrome, vasculopathy, and malignancy, discussed later.
- Neurotoxicity
  - Epidemiology: 7% to 32% of cases and is typically more common and severe with tacrolimus than with cyclosporine

TABLE 6.15.3 Common Drug Interactions of IS Agents

Group/ Immunosuppressive Agent	Common Drug Interactions
CNIs (cyclosporine, tacrolimus)	↑ Levels with: macrolides (azithromycin, erythromycin, clarithromycin), antifungals (azoles in particular), dihydropyridine calcium channel blockers, metoclopramide, grapefruit, HAART ↓ Levels with: phenytoin, carbamazepine isoniazid, rifampicin, sevelamer, efavirenz, tocilizumab
mTOR inhibitors (sirolimus, everolimus)	↑ Levels with: similar to CNIs, fusidic acid, ↑Toxicity with CNIs
Antimetabolite (mycophenolate mofetil [MMF])	↑ Levels with: acyclovir, valganciclovir ↓ Levels with: PPI, quinolone antibiotics ↓ Absorption when used with cyclosporine
Antimetabolite (azathioprine/AZA)	↑ Levels with: allopurinol (xanthine oxidase degrades metabolites of AZA), febuxostat ↓ Anticoagulant effect of warfarin
Corticosteroids	Low-grade interactions
Co-stimulator blocker	No clinically relevant drug interactions
Antibodies (basiliximab, ATG)	No relevant drug interactions; ↑ risk of infection with live vaccinations

ATG, antithymocyte globulin; AZA, azathioprine; CNIs, calcineurin inhibitors; HAART, highly active antiretroviral therapy; IS, immunosuppression; mTOR, mammalian target of rapamycin; PPI, proton pump inhibitor.

TABLE 6.15.2 Adverse Effects of Glucocorticoids

Organ System	Side Effects	Mechanisms of Common Side Effects
Cardiovascular	Electrolyte disarrays, fluid retention, hypertension, increased levels of total cholesterol, triglycerides, and decreased HDL	Salt and water retention, regulation of vascular smooth muscle receptors HTN
GI	Gastritis, PUD, GI bleeding, pancreatitis	Prostaglandin synthesis, acid secretion
Endocrine	DM, Cushing syndrome, obesity, dyslipidemia, adrenal insufficiency, hirsutism	Insulin production/gluconeogenesis/peripheral glucose consumption DM Activity acetyl-CoA carboxylase HDL
Musculoskeletal/skin	Osteoporosis, avascular bone necrosis, myopathy, bruising, impaired wound healing	Osteoblast differentiation/osteoclast formation, Ca absorption in GI tract/Ca excretion Osteoporosis
Ophthalmic	Cataracts, glaucoma, exophthalmos	Morphological and functional changes in the trabecular meshwork
Psychiatric	Psychosis, depression, insomnia, mood swings	Regulation of the serotonin system, Regulation of the dopamine system
Infectious	Increased susceptibility to infections, especially fungal	Cell-mediated immunity

DM, diabetes mellitus; GI, gastrointestinal; HDL, high-density lipoprotein; HTN, hypertension; PUD, peptic ulcer disease.

- Signs/symptoms: headaches, migraines, and fine tremors (mild, dose dependent); cognitive impairment and brain atrophy (more severe, chronic); posterior reversible encephalopathy syndrome (PRES) is at the spectrum of the most severe CNI-induced neurotoxicity.
  - The clinical manifestation of PRES has a broad spectrum of symptoms, ranging from headache and seizures to altered mental status and visual loss.
  - Neuroimaging in PRES provides a distinctive pattern of white matter vasogenic edema predominantly affecting the posterior occipital and parietal lobes (Figure 6.15.2).
- Management
  - Reduction or elimination of CNI
  - Monitoring and supplementing serum magnesium is recommended in CNI-related PRES (CNIs can cause hypomagnesemia, which reduces seizure threshold and increases vasospasm risk).

- Nephrotoxicity
  - Epidemiology: ~20% of patients develop chronic kidney dysfunction by 5 years. Although the prevalence of nephrotoxicity is significantly higher at supratherapeutic calcineurin levels, it may manifest at therapeutic drug levels as well.
  - Mechanism: CNI-induced kidney injury results from endothelial damage and arteriolar vasoconstriction, leading to renal hypoperfusion and chronic ischemia. An imbalance between vasodilators (PGE2 and NO) and vasoconstrictors (thromboxane and endothelin) leads to vasospasm of afferent arterioles.
  - Management
    - Reducing the CNI dose or temporarily discontinuing treatment can often reverse acute toxicity.
    - Chronic nephrotoxicity is characterized by a sustained increase in serum creatinine lasting ≥3 months and typically progresses without intervention.
    - Management of CNI nephrotoxicity involves lower plasma CNI levels combined with a mammalian target of rapamycin (mTOR) inhibitor or mycophenolate mofetil (MMF).
- Metabolic syndrome
  - CNIs are linked to hyperlipidemia, new-onset diabetes mellitus (NODM), hypertension, and cardiovascular disease.
  - Management
    - Reduced CNI dose, with or without the addition of MMF or an mTOR inhibitor, can be utilized for the management of NODM.
    - Steroid-free regimens have been correlated with a lower risk of NODM.
    - The first-line treatment of CNI-induced hypertension is amlodipine with diuretics and angiotensin-converting enzyme (ACE) inhibitors, considered second-line options if dual therapy is required.

mTOR Inhibitors

- Rapamycin (sirolimus) is a macrolide antibiotic derived from *Streptomyces hygroscopicus*. Everolimus, a sirolimus derivative, exhibits enhanced bioavailability and shorter half-life (22 vs 60 hours).
- The primary rationale for using mTOR inhibitors is to mitigate the nephrotoxic and neurotoxic effects associated with CNIs. However, they are not free of specific long-term adverse effects.
  - In comparison to CNIs, mTOR inhibitors demonstrate a higher incidence of myelosuppression, manifested by anemia, leukopenia, and thrombocytopenia.

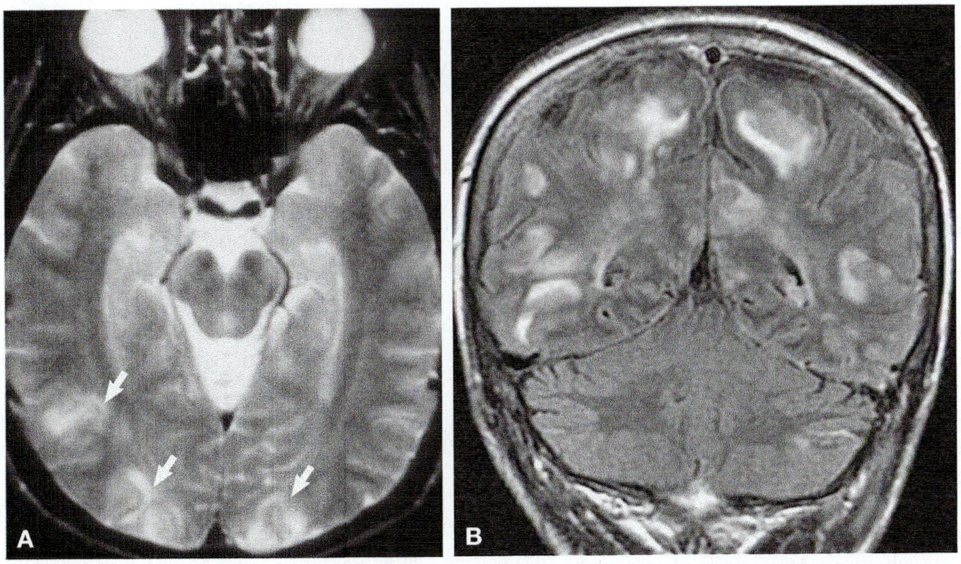

Figure 6.15.2. Posterior Reversible Encephalopathy Syndrome (PRES). A 43-year-old transplant patient who was being treated with cyclosporine presented with visual disturbances and confusion. Axial (A) and coronal (B) T2WIs reveal patchy areas of cortically based signal abnormality within the parietooccipital lobes (arrows), corresponding to the posterior vascular distribution. These findings are in keeping with dysfunction of vascular permeability, the result of a combination of endothelial toxicity and elevated blood pressure. Both clinical symptoms and imaging findings resolved after the cyclosporine doses were reduced. (From Klein J, Vinson EN, Brant WE, Helms CA. *Brant and Helms' Fundamentals of Diagnostic Radiology*. 4th ed. Wolters Kluwer; 2019. Figure 7.16.)

- Proteinuria
- Rates of hyperlipidemia are significantly higher compared to CNIs.
- Increased risk of wound complications
- Oral ulcers, occurring in up to 40% of treated patients

- Management
  - Dose reduction or withdrawal of mTOR inhibitor and initiation of granulocyte colony-stimulating factor are indicated in severe cases of neutropenia.
  - Topical corticosteroid with a dental paste directly to oral ulcers

Antimetabolites

- Signs/symptoms
  - Gastrointestinal (GI) side effects such as nausea, vomiting, diarrhea, abdominal cramps, and anorexia are most common.
  - Myelosuppression, typically manifesting as leukopenia and (less frequently) anemia
- Epidemiology: common, requiring dose reduction or discontinuation of MMF in up to 50% of patients
- Mechanism: mitotic inhibition of rapidly proliferating tissues
- Management
  - Dose splitting (eg, instead of 1,000 mg 2 times daily [bid], 500 mg 3 times daily [qid]), dose reduction, or discontinuation
  - The enteric-coated mycophenolate sodium enables delayed release of mycophenolic acid, the active form of MMF, potentially mitigating GI side effects.
  - In cases of severe neutropenia, granulocyte colony-stimulating factor can be administered.

Biologic Agents

- ATG
  - Short-term adverse effects of ATG treatment include flulike symptoms known as cytokine release syndrome. In extreme cases, it is characterized by fever, tachycardia, dyspnea, chest discomfort, and pulmonary edema. The syndrome is more common after the initial dose and subsides after repeated administration.
  - Premedication with acetaminophen, antihistamines, and corticosteroids generally alleviates the symptoms.
  - Serum sickness, characterized by urticarial rash and arthralgias, may develop in some patients, especially those with prior exposure to ATG.
  - Adverse effects also include leukopenia and potentially increased risk of infections (CMV, *Pneumocystis jirovecii* [PCJ]).
- Anti-CD52 monoclonal antibodies
  - Serve as depleting agents in the induction therapy of SOT, as well as in the management of autoimmune conditions
  - Some studies demonstrated an increased incidence of malignancy and infections in recipients treated with alemtuzumab.
  - Alemtuzumab has also been associated with severe recurrent hepatitis C in liver transplant recipients.
- IL-2 receptor inhibitors
  - Basiliximab and daclizumab are well-tolerated agents that do not induce infusion-related reactions or long-term adverse effects such as nephrotoxicity.
  - IL-2 receptor inhibitors are not associated with elevated risks of infection or malignancy.

6.16

Complications of Chemotherapy

Davit Kocharyan

Background

Chemotherapy employs cytotoxic agents to inhibit tumor growth by targeting rapidly proliferating cells, disrupting DNA, RNA, or protein synthesis, or by impairing the function of existing macromolecules. However, chemotherapy's lack of selectivity also affects normal cells, leading to toxic side effects.

- Epidemiology
  - ~5% to 10% of patients with cancer experience life-threatening complications requiring intensive care unit (ICU) admission, and patients with malignancies comprise ~15% to 20% of ICU admissions.
  - Recent data indicate a significant increase in ICU survival rates for critically ill patients with cancer, reaching ~50% to 60% versus 20% to 30% in the past. Although ICU patients with cancer still expire at a higher rate compared to noncancer patients, their survival rates are now approaching those of similarly sick noncancer patients.
- The toxicity profiles of chemotherapeutic agents vary by class. Classes of chemotherapy vary:
  - By use setting
    - Neoadjuvant: administered before the primary therapeutic intervention
    - Adjuvant: administered in addition to primary therapy to suppress or eradicate residual occult cancer cells
  - By the goal of treatment
    - Curative: aims (with other modalities) to fully eradicate cancer cells from the body
    - Palliative: aims to improve quality of life by relieving symptoms, particularly in metastatic disease
  - By cell-level effect
    - Cell cycle–specific agents (act only at specific phases of the cell cycle)
    - Cell cycle–nonspecific agents (include the resting phase)

- By mechanism
  - Alkylating agents, antimetabolites, antitumor antibiotics, mitotic inhibitors, topoisomerase inhibitors, biologics, hormonal agents, and miscellaneous agents

Table 6.16.1 summarizes the toxicities and mechanisms of action of common chemotherapeutic agents.

Myelosuppression

- Definition: myelosuppression, defined as anemia, neutropenia, and thrombocytopenia, is the most common dose-limiting toxicity of cytotoxic chemotherapy, caused by bone marrow suppression.
- Epidemiology
  - Between 10% and 50% of patients with solid tumors and over 80% of those with hematologic malignancies experience febrile neutropenia during chemotherapy.
  - Patients with solid tumors receiving chemotherapy typically experience neutropenia lasting <7 days, whereas in those with hematologic malignancies, it may last ≥2 weeks.
- Mechanism
  - Direct bone marrow toxicity of cytotoxic chemotherapy
  - Facilitates translocation and expansion of gastrointestinal (GI) flora into the bloodstream, leading to neutropenic fever
- Presentation: most commonly with fever in the setting of neutropenia
  - Febrile neutropenia is characterized by a single oral temperature >38.3 °C or a sustained temperature >38.0 °C for ≥1 hour in a patient with absolute neutrophil count (ANC) <500 cells/mL or an anticipated decline to <500 cells/mL within 48 hours.
- Evaluation
  - Blood cultures are mandatory.
  - Additional cultures as available or indicated by clinical presentation
- Management
  - Empiric antibiotics per local susceptibility patterns: typically fourth generation cephalosporins or equivalent broad-spectrum agents with *Pseudomonas* coverage. Vancomycin is added if indwelling catheters are present and typically for septic shock.

TABLE 6.16.1 Toxicities/Side Effects of Common Chemotherapeutic Agents

Drug Name (Chemotherapy Group/Subgroup)	Mechanism of Action	Common Toxicities/Side Effects
Cyclophosphamide, ifosfamide (alkylating agent/nitrogen mustard)	Production of reactive alkyl group ($R\text{-}CH_2^+$) Binds to nucleophilic sites on proteins and nucleic acids DNA replication and transcription	Myelosuppression, neutropenia, anemia, thrombocytopenia, hemorrhagic cystitis (use mesna to mitigate), NV, infertility
Carboplatin, cisplatin (alkylating agents/platinum analogs)	Formation of intrastrand and interstrand DNA cross-links with the platinum molecule, resulting in strand breakage during replication	Hemorrhage, thrombocytopenia, nephrotoxicity/neurotoxicity, diarrhea, alopecia, NV
Methotrexate, pemetrexed (antimetabolites/folate antagonist)	Inhibition of dihydrofolate reductase Disruption of nucleotide synthesis in a cell cycle–dependent manner	Myelosuppression, mucositis, hepatotoxicity, nephrotoxicity, skin reactions Toxicity mitigation: hydration and urinary alkalinization, leucovorin rescue
Cytarabine (antimetabolites/cytosine arabinoside)	A nucleotide analog that, upon activation to its triphosphate form, inhibits DNA polymerase, incorporates into DNA and RNA, and disrupts cell cycle progression at the G1-S transition.	Myelosuppression; immunosuppression; CNS, cardiac, and pulmonary toxicity
Cladribine (antimetabolites/purine analog)	Phosphorylated by deoxycytidine kinase and incorporated into DNA, leading to strand breaks	Fatigue, headache; skin rash; nausea; bone marrow suppression; infection; fever
5-Fluorouracil (antimetabolites/pyrimidine analog)	The active metabolite, F-dUMP, forms a stable covalent complex with thymidylate synthase in the presence of reduced folate, thereby inhibiting DNA synthesis and repair.	GI issues, leukopenia, thrombocytopenia, hemorrhage, NV
Gemcitabine (antimetabolites/cytidine analogs)	Cell cycle–dependent and S-phase–specific cytotoxicity, likely because of inhibition of DNA polymerase	Myelosuppression, NV, liver enzyme elevations, and interstitial pneumonitis
Paclitaxel (antimitotic agents/taxanes)	Prevents tubulin depolymerization in the mitotic spindle, leading to apoptosis in proliferating cells, M-phase specific	Myelosuppression, predominantly neutropenia, peripheral neuropathy, hypersensitivity
Vinblastine, vincristine (antimitotic agents/vinca alkaloids)	Inhibition of tubulin polymerization, hence mitosis, G2-phase specific	Myelosuppression, especially leukopenia, peripheral neuropathy (both motor and sensory), SIADH, and angina pectoris (rare)
Irinotecan, topotecan (topoisomerase inhibitors)	A topoisomerase I inhibition results in the disruption of both transcription and replication	Myelosuppression, thrombocytopenia, diarrhea

(continued)

TABLE 6.16.1 Toxicities/Side Effects of Common Chemotherapeutic Agents (*continued*)

Drug Name (Chemotherapy Group/Subgroup)	Mechanism of Action	Common Toxicities/Side Effects
Doxorubicin, daunorubicin (topoisomerase inhibitors; anthracycline antitumor antibiotics)	Pleiotropic effects such as oxidative stress, topoisomerase II inhibition, and mitochondrial dysfunction	Myelosuppression, alopecia, NV, diarrhea, stomatitis, skin rash, hyperpigmentation Cardiotoxicity is common with doxorubicin: it can be mitigated by dexrazoxane or by longer infusions.
Etoposide (topoisomerase inhibitor)	Topoisomerase II inhibitor, partially cell cycle dependent	Myelosuppression, NV, stomatitis, diarrhea, hepatic toxicity
Bleomycin (antitumor antibiotic)	Causes direct breakage in DNA strands in both healthy and cancerous cells	Pulmonary toxicity, reversible and irreversible pulmonary fibrosis, hyperpigmentation, fever, chills, rash, exfoliation, anorexia, NV, myelosuppression
L-Asparaginase	An enzyme naturally sourced from *Escherichia coli* or *Erwinia carotovora* that hydrolyzes asparagine, an amino acid critical for the growth of rapidly dividing cells	Hypersensitivity reactions, including anaphylaxis, coagulopathy, abdominal cramps, anorexia, elevated LFTs
Rituximab (biologic)	A monoclonal antibody targeting the CD20-positive B cells	Infusion-related symptoms, fever, chills, malaise
Trastuzumab (biologic)	A monoclonal antibody targeting the Her2/neu growth factor receptor, frequently overexpressed in invasive breast carcinomas	Uncommon acute cardiotoxicity, not recommended to use with doxorubicin, acute fever, chills, NV
Imatinib	Bcr-Abl tyrosine kinase inhibitor with additional activity against PDGF, c-Kit, and SCF receptors	Edema, ascites, chest pain, fatigue, cutaneous rash, elevated LDH, GI symptoms (nausea, diarrhea), muscle cramps, and increased serum creatinine and hepatic enzyme levels
Tamoxifen (hormone/selective estrogen receptor modulator)	Nonsteroidal antiestrogen, cytostatic effects on estrogen-dependent and estrogen-independent cancer cells	Well-tolerated, constitutional symptoms such as hot flashes, sweating, mood changes, weight gain or loss, menstrual changes, including significant vaginal bleeding, venous thromboembolism
Hydroxyurea (miscellaneous)	Ribonucleotide reductase inhibitor that impedes the conversion of ribonucleotides to deoxyribonucleotides required for DNA synthesis; exhibits cell cycle–dependent activity	Myelosuppression, dermatologic reactions, hyperuricemia
Tretinoin, *all-trans retinoic acid* (miscellaneous)	Promotes differentiation and apoptosis of malignant promyelocytes in acute promyelocytic leukemia	Teratogenic, retinoic acid syndrome (ever, chest pain, dyspnea, hypoxia, pulmonary infiltrates, pleural or pericardial effusions), exfoliation, xerostomia

CNS, central nervous system; GI, gastrointestinal; LDH, lactate dehydrogenase; LFTs, liver function tests; NV, nausea and vomiting; SIADH, syndrome of inappropriate antidiuretic hormone secretion.

- In patients with acute leukemia, high-dose corticosteroid therapy, or following allogeneic hematopoietic stem cell transplantation, empiric antifungal therapy is typically considered on day 4 of a persistent fever in conjunction with infectious disease consultants.
- Antibiotic therapy is typically continued until the patient becomes afebrile and achieves myeloid recovery, defined by ANC ≥ 500/μL.
- Transfusion and bone marrow stimulatory agents:
  - Prophylactic administration of granulocyte colony-stimulating factor reduces both the nadir and the duration of neutropenia in relatively high-risk patients.
  - Recent guidelines recommend blood transfusion for hemoglobin (Hgb) levels ≤7 g/dL.
  - Platelet transfusion threshold of 10,000/μL in afebrile patients and 20,000/μL in the presence of fever or active bleeding/procedural bleeding risk.

Cardiotoxicity

- Classification
  - Primary (type I, irreversible) cardiomyopathy resulting from cumulative dose–dependent direct cardiomyocyte injury
  - Secondary (type II, reversible) cardiomyopathy resulting from alterations in perfusion, neural input, or hormonal milieu
  - Myocarditis (type III), characterized by inflammatory cell infiltration into the myocardium
- Anthracyclines
  - Epidemiology: <5% of treated patients
  - Presentation
    - Type 1 cardiotoxicity, characterized by electrocardiogram (ECG) changes (20%-30%), arrhythmias (up to 3%), reduced ejection fraction, and symptomatic heart failure

- Acute anthracycline-induced cardiotoxicity pathologically resembles toxic myocarditis, characterized by cardiomyocyte injury, inflammatory infiltrates, and interstitial edema.
  - Management
    - Beta-blockers and angiotensin-converting enzyme (ACE) inhibitors do not prevent a decline in ejection fraction.
    - Dexrazoxane is indicated for patients receiving cumulative doxorubicin doses exceeding 300 mg/m^2; however, it is not effective in managing anthracycline-induced acute heart failure.
- 5-Fluorouracil (5-FU)
  - Epidemiology: 20% to 30% of treated patients; bolus delivery is associated with lower risk compared to continuous infusion.
  - Presentation
    - Type 2 toxicity: induction of widespread and profound coronary microvascular vasoconstriction
    - Patients receiving 5-FU infusion may develop chest discomfort, acute hypotension, or dyspnea, with ECG findings indicative of myocardial ischemia.
  - Management
    - immediate discontinuation of infusion and management of acute coronary syndrome with appropriate monitoring
- Trastuzumab
  - Epidemiology
    - 15% to 20% of patients experienced trastuzumab-associated cardiotoxicity.
    - <5% heart failure rate as monotherapy but up to 25% when combined with another agent
  - Presentation: predominantly left-sided heart failure (non–dose dependent)
  - Management
    - Left ventricular ejection fraction (LVEF) should be evaluated prior to therapy initiation and monitored periodically throughout treatment.
    - Trastuzumab should be withheld for a minimum of 4 weeks if LVEF decreases by >10% from baseline.
- Cyclophosphamide
  - Epidemiology: 7% to 28% of patients receiving high-dose cyclophosphamide, most commonly during the conditioning phase of stem cell transplantation (dose dependent)
  - Presentation: predominantly myocarditic/pericarditic
    - Endothelial dysfunction and coronary vasospasm, resulting in left ventricular impairment that may progress to pericarditis or hemorrhagic myocarditis
    - Can lead to pericardial effusion, including cases of acute, life-threatening tamponade

Pulmonary Toxicity

- Chemotherapy-induced pulmonary toxicity primarily arises from direct injury to pneumocytes or the alveolar-capillary endothelium, immune-mediated mechanisms, and capillary leak.
- Common radiologic patterns of drug-induced toxicity include:
  - Interstitial infiltrates (bleomycin, methotrexate, taxanes, platinums, rituximab, gemcitabine)
  - Diffuse alveolar damage (bleomycin, busulfan, mitomycin, cyclophosphamide)
  - Nonspecific interstitial pneumonia (methotrexate, bleomycin)
  - Eosinophilic pneumonia (methotrexate, bleomycin)
  - Cryptogenic organizing pneumonia (bleomycin, cyclophosphamide, methotrexate)
  - Pulmonary hemorrhage (high-dose cyclophosphamide, mitomycin, bevacizumab)
  - Hypersensitivity pneumonitis (methotrexate)
  - Pulmonary hypertension and edema (gemcitabine)
  - Late-onset fibrotic lung disease (bleomycin)
- General management
  - Discontinuing the causative agent
  - Pulmonology consultation
  - Lung-protective mechanical ventilation for hypoxemia meeting acute respiratory distress syndrome (ARDS) criteria
  - Avoiding high FIO_2, especially in cases of bleomycin and mitomycin C toxicity
  - Systemic steroids at 0.5 to 1.0 mg/kg/d depending on severity
  - Diuretics can be considered in noncardiogenic pulmonary edema.
- All-*trans* retinoic acid (ATRA), though not a cytotoxic chemotherapeutic agent, may induce differentiation syndrome.
  - Characterized by rapid maturation of blasts into neutrophils
  - It typically manifests at a median of 5 days and leads to a cluster of clinical features, including fever, weight gain, leukocytosis, respiratory distress, interstitial infiltrates, and effusions.
  - Chest x-ray (CXR) demonstrates pulmonary edema manifesting as peribronchial cuffing, consolidation, nodules, air bronchograms, and pleural effusion. Episodic hypotension and acute renal failure may occur in some patients.
  - The syndrome typically responds well to high-dose corticosteroids and temporary discontinuation of ATRA.

Neurotoxicity

Chemotherapy-induced neurologic complications are a major source of morbidity in patients with cancer.

- Mechanisms
  - Direct neurotoxic effects
  - Indirect vascular, metabolic, infectious, or autoimmune effects
  - Blood-brain barrier (BBB) compromise from tumor-related endothelial damage or radiotherapy
  - Agents crossing BBB or direct intrathecal/intracerebral administration
  - Disruption of neurogenesis and white matter integrity
- Key agents and presentations
  - Ifosfamide: acute encephalopathy (15%-30%), onset hours to days, resolves in 48 to 72 hour after discontinuation.
  - Busulfan: high-dose causes seizures in up to 40% without prophylaxis.
  - Methotrexate: high-dose intravenous (IV) → acute encephalopathy, seizures; intrathecal → aseptic meningitis (~10%), headache, fever, nuchal rigidity; leukoencephalopathy (acute/subacute: 2.5%-15%, chronic: months-years) with stroke-like episodes or progressive dementia
  - ATRA: headache, possible idiopathic intracranial hypertension with papilledema

- Cytarabine: high-dose → acute cerebellar toxicity (10%-25%)
- L-Asparaginase: depletes coagulation/fibrinolysis proteins → venous sinus thrombosis (headache, acute mountain sickness [AMS], seizures)

- Management
  - Discontinue offending agent
  - Supportive care ± antiepileptics, steroids, anticoagulation (if thrombosis present)
  - Folinic acid for methotrexate toxicity
  - Anticoagulation for venous sinus thrombosis

Renal Toxicity

- Definition: renal and bladder injury due to urinary elimination of cytotoxic drugs
- Risk factors
  - Hypertension (HTN), diabetes mellitus (DM), hypovolemia, nephrotoxic co-medications, advanced age
- Key agents and effects
  - Cisplatin: proximal tubular injury → ↓ creatinine clearance (~15%), acute kidney injury (AKI) within 24 hours, electrolyte losses (Na, Ca, Mg); renal salt wasting syndrome (RSWS) possible within 12 hours, mimics syndrome of inappropriate antidiuretic hormone secretion (SIADH)
  - Ifosfamide/cyclophosphamide: acrolein metabolite → hemorrhagic cystitis; prevent with hydration + mesna
  - High-dose methotrexate: tubular precipitation → AKI; prevent with urine alkalinization and hydration; carboxypeptidase for severe toxicity
- Management
  - Hydration and electrolyte repletion
  - Hypertonic/isotonic saline for RSWS
  - Mesna for acrolein detoxification
  - Urine alkalinization for high-dose methotrexate

Gastrointestinal Toxicity

- Mucositis
  - Occurs in 5% to 40% of patients; dose-limiting; higher incidence with 5-FU, anthracyclines, taxanes, platinums, especially with concurrent radiation therapy (RT)
  - Pathophysiology: oxidative stress + inflammatory cytokine upregulation → mucosal ulceration
  - Management: hydration, topical anesthetics, systemic analgesia, total parenteral nutrition (TPN) in severe cases
- GI mucositis
  - Diarrhea possible → hypovolemia, electrolyte disturbances; octreotide if loperamide fails
- Nausea/vomiting
  - Up to 70% incidence; acute mediated by 5-HT3 receptor activation
  - High-risk drugs: cisplatin, high-dose cyclophosphamide, dacarbazine, procarbazine, dactinomycin, doxorubicin
  - Prophylaxis: aprepitant/fosaprepitant, ondansetron, olanzapine
- Other GI toxicities
  - Neutropenic enterocolitis (esp. in leukemia chemo) → diarrhea, pain, fever
  - Vinca alkaloids → ileus
  - Hepatotoxicity: veno-occlusive syndrome, cholestasis, transaminitis, steatosis, hepatitis B/hepatitis C (HBV/HCV) reactivation

Thrombotic Sequelae of Chemotherapy

- Epidemiology
  - Venous thromboembolism (VTE) in >50% of patients with cancer at autopsy
  - Tamoxifen → 2.4 × risk of deep venous thrombosis/ pulmonary embolism (DVT/PE)
  - Cisplatin → higher vascular complications (cardiovascular accident [CVA], arterial thrombosis, phlebitis, angina, DVT/PE)
- Thrombotic thrombocytopenic purpura (TTP)
  - Gemcitabine, cisplatin, mitomycin linked
  - Mechanism: endothelial dysfunction → immune complexes, platelet aggregates
  - Chemo-induced TTP: gradual onset, fewer neuro symptoms, less responsive to plasma exchange; often causes progressive renal failure

SUGGESTED READINGS

Amjad MT, Chidharla A, Kasi A. Cancer Chemotherapy. In: StatPearls. StatPearls Publishing; 2025. Accessed August 5, 2025. http://www.ncbi.nlm.nih.gov/books/NBK564367/

Basak D, Arrighi S, Darwiche Y, Deb S. Comparison of Anticancer Drug Toxicities: Paradigm Shift in Adverse Effect Profile. *Life (Basel)*. 2021;12(1):48.

Brianna, Lee SH. Chemotherapy: how to reduce its adverse effects while maintaining the potency? *Med Oncol*. 2023;40(3):1-13.

Dhamija E, Meena P, Ramalingam V, Sahoo R, Rastogi S, Thulkar S. Chemotherapy-induced pulmonary complications in cancer: Significance of clinicoradiological correlation. *Indian J Radiol Imaging*. 2020;30(1):20-26.

Herrmann J. Adverse cardiac effects of cancer therapies: cardiotoxicity and arrhythmia. Nat Rev Cardiol. 2020;17(8):474-502.

John E. Niederhuber, MD; James O. Armitage, MD; James H. Doroshow, MD; Michael B. Kastan, MD, PhD; Joel E. Tepper, MD. *Abeloff's Clinical Oncology*. 6th ed. Elsevier Inc; 2020. Accessed August 5, 2025. https://www.clinicalkey.com/#!/browse/book/3-s2.0-C20150054004

Karagiannis P, Klingler F, Arelin V, et al. Outcome of critically ill patients receiving systemic chemotherapy on the intensive care unit. *Front Oncol*. 2025;14.

Kumar V, Gupta N, Mishra S, eds. *Onco-Critical Care: An Evidence-Based Approach*. Springer Nature; 2022.

Lafarge A, Chean D, Whiting L, Clere-Jehl R. Management of hematological patients requiring emergency chemotherapy in the intensive care unit. *Intensive Care Med*. 2024;50(6):849-860.

Sebastian F. Winter MD, Jasmin Jo MD, David Schiff MD and Jorg Dietrich MD, PhD. Central Nervous System Complications Among Oncology Patients. *Hematology/Oncology Clinics of North America*. 2022;36(1):217-236.

Shimabukuro-Vornhagen A, Böll B, Kochanek M, Azoulay É, von Bergwelt-Baildon MS. Critical care of patients with cancer. *CA: A Cancer Journal for Clinicians*. 2016;66(6):496-517.

SECTION 7

Endocrine

Section Editor: Marvin G. Chang

7.1

General Neuroendocrine Axis

John A. Helmstetter and Richard M. Pino

Definition

- The neuroendocrine axis plays a central role in maintaining homeostasis and adapting to critical illness. It regulates metabolism, stress responses, fluid balance, and reproductive functions through interactions between the hypothalamus, pituitary gland, and effector organs.
  - Components and hormones associated
  - Pituitary
    - Anterior pituitary (adenohypophysis)
    - Thyroid-stimulating hormone (TSH) targets the thyroid gland, leading to the secretion of triiodothyronine (T3) and thyroxine (T4).
    - Follicle-stimulating hormone (FSH) targets the ovary to stimulate the release of estrogen and follicle growth, as well as the testis for sperm maturation.
    - Luteinizing hormone (LH) targets the ovary for ovulation, the corpus luteum for estrogen and progesterone synthesis, and the testis for the secretion of testosterone.
    - Adrenocorticotropic hormone (ACTH) targets the adrenal cortex for adrenal glucocorticoids.
    - Beta-lipotropin is released from the anterior pituitary as a precursor to beta-endorphin (an endogenous opioid); its direct effects on adipose tissue remain unclear.
    - Growth hormone (GH) targets most tissues for increase in height and weight, protein synthesis, fat utilization, inhibition of glucose utilization, and increases the production of IGH (insulin-like growth factor).
    - Prolactin targets mammary glands to increase growth and milk secretion.
    - Posterior pituitary (neurohypophysis)
    - Antidiuretic hormone (ADH/vasopressin)
    - ADH acts on V1 receptors via the phosphatidyl inositol/calcium/protein kinase C pathway to mediate vasoconstriction, notably during hemorrhage or other hypovolemic hemodynamic instability acts on V2 receptors (G protein-coupled) via the cyclic adenosine monophosphate (AMP)/protein kinase. A pathway to create aquaporin-2 water channels in the apical membrane of distal renal tubule and collecting duct, allowing water reentry from filtrate back into the bloodstream.
    - Oxytocin mediates uterine contraction and milk letdown reflex.
  - Hypothalamus
    - Chemical mediators act on the pituitary.
    - Corticotropin-releasing hormone (CRH) releases ACTH response to a variety of signals (cold, fever, infection, trauma, emotional distress, burns, inflammatory agents, pain, hypotension, exercise hemorrhage).
    - Somatotropin release–inhibiting factor (SRIF); somatostatin inhibits the secretion of GH.
    - Dopamine is the primary prolactin-inhibiting factor (PIF) and acts on the anterior pituitary to inhibit prolactin secretion.
    - Thyrotropin-releasing hormone (TRH) stimulates the release of TSH.
    - Excess TRH inhibits dopamine, which stimulates prolactin release from the adenohypophysis.
    - Gonadotropin-releasing hormone (GnRH) stimulates the release of FSH and LH.
    - Growth hormone–releasing hormone (GHRH) stimulates the release of GH.
    - GH-releasing peptide (ghrelin) improves GHRH response.
    - Dopamine inhibits prolactin release.
    - Other hypothalamic functions: temperature regulation, hunger, thirst, sleep, circadian cycles, heart rate control, vasoconstriction, sweating, digestion
    - The lateral hypothalamus projects to the lateral medulla that drives the autonomic nervous system.
    - Parasympathetic vagal nuclei and cells project to the sympathetic system in the spinal cord.
      - Primary critical care–related effector organs

- Thyroid gland
  - T4 is the primary thyroid hormone secreted by thyroid follicular cells, circulates as over 99% protein bound, and is metabolized by thyroid peroxidase (TPO) to T3.
  - T3 is 4 times as potent as T4. T4 is converted to T3 in peripheral tissues by deiodinases.
  - Both T3 and T4 increase temperature and basal metabolic rate; affect protein synthesis, neuron maturation, and the metabolism of protein, carbohydrate, fat, and vitamins; and enhance sensitivity to catecholamines.
  - Thyroid storm represents a severe manifestation of hyperthyroidism requiring intensive care unit (ICU)-level care for hemodynamic stabilization, temperature control, and reduction of thyroid hormone activity. Adrenal (Suprarenal gland) should be set at the same hierachy as Thyroid gland. It should read as follows.
    - Adrenal (suprarenal) gland
      - Cortex
        - Zona glomerulosa (mineralocorticoids)
          - aldosterone acts on the kidneys to increase blood pressure and volume and provide active reabsorption of sodium, passive reabsorption of water, secretion of potassium, and active secretion of protons via proton ATPases.
        - Zona fasciculata (glucocorticoids)
          - immune effects: upregulation of anti-inflammatory proteins, downregulation of pro-inflammatory proteins, role in the development of T-lymphocytes
          - metabolic effects: stimulation of gluconeogenesis, mobilization of amino acids from extrahepatic tissues, inhibition of glucose uptake in muscle and adipose tissue, stimulation of fat breakdown in adipose tissue
        - Zona reticularis (androgens and cortisol)
          - Cortisol is typically secreted in a diurnal pattern with a maximal circulatory level early in the morning, followed by a steady decrease throughout the day.
          - Negative feedback is exerted by cortisol at the level of both the hypothalamus and the pituitary to reduce secretion of both CRH and ACTH.
      - Medulla
        - Epinephrine (80%) increases heart rate, is a vasoconstrictor and a bronchodilator.
        - Norepinephrine (20%) increases heart rate, release of glucose from energy stores, and blood flow to skeletal muscle, and suppresses neuroinflammation.

SUGGESTED READINGS

Boonen E, Van den Berghe G. Endocrine responses to critical illness: novel insights and therapeutic implications. *J Clin Endocrinol Metab*. 2014;99:1569-1582.

Fowler C, Raoof N, Pastores SM. Sepsis and adrenal insufficiency. *J Intensive Care Med*. 2023;38:987-996.

Holt EH, Lupsa B, Lee GS, Bassyouni H, Peery HE, eds. Pituitary gland. In: *Goodman's Basic Medical Endocrinology*. 5th ed. Elsevier; 2021:43-73.

Téblick A, Gunst J, Van den Berghe GJ. Critical illness-induced corticosteroid insufficiency: what it is not and what it could be. *Clin Endocrinol Metab*. 2022;107:2057-2064.

7.2

Diabetes Mellitus

Sean Rajnic and Daniel W. Johnson

Hyperglycemia

- Common during critical illness in patients with and without a history of diabetes
- Associated with morbidity and mortality proportional to blood glucose levels

Type 1 Diabetes

- Marked insulin deficiency with hyperglycemia is usually due to immune-mediated destruction of pancreatic islet beta-cells
- 90% of diagnosed cases have one or more antibodies, and greater than two antibodies is highly predictive of developing type 1 diabetes within 5 years.
  - Glutamic acid decarboxylase (GAD65), pancreatic islet beta-cells (tyrosine phosphatase IA-2), and IA-2b zinc transporter (ZnT8), and/or insulin
- 5% to 10% of all diabetes cases, more commonly diagnosed in children or young adults of European ancestry
- Higher rates in children, ketosis, and is symptomatic at onset compared to type 2 diabetes

Type 2 Diabetes

- Progressive loss of beta-cell insulin secretion and decreased insulin sensitivity. Often asymptomatic and gradual onset
- Accounts for >90% of all diabetes cases, with genetic, socioeconomic, and environmental factors.

Etiologies of Hyperglycemia

- Undiagnosed type 1 diabetes mellitus (DM)/type 2 DM
- Stress hyperglycemia—transient hyperglycemia in the setting of acute illness
  - Cortisol release → gluconeogenesis and decreased glucose use
  - Catecholamines, inflammatory mediators → insulin resistance
- Disease of the exocrine pancreas includes
  - Pancreatitis, cystic fibrosis, neoplasm, hemochromatosis

- Endocrine disorders
  - Cushing syndrome, acromegaly, glucagonoma, pheochromocytoma, gestational diabetes
- Medication induced
  - Glucocorticoids, catecholamines, parenteral nutrition, nicotinic acid, thiazides, interferon-gamma, high-dose statins, atypical antipsychotics, immune checkpoint inhibitors, PI3 kinase inhibitors, tacrolimus, octreotide, estrogens, phenytoins
- Trauma
- Iatrogenic
  - Missed insulin dose, dextrose-containing fluids or medications

Sequela of Hyperglycemia

- Inflammation via production of cytokines (interleukin-6 [IL-6], IL-8, and tumor necrosis factor-alpha [TNFα]) and reactive oxygen species
- Impairment of neutrophil chemotaxis and bactericidal activity
- Increased tissue procoagulant activity, which may contribute to procoagulant state
- Osmotic diuresis and electrolyte derangements
- Microvascular and macrovascular complications due to endothelial glycocalyx dysfunction
- Hyperglycemic crises—diabetic ketoacidosis (DKA), hyperosmolar hyperglycemic state (HHS)

Diagnosis

- Hyperglycemia—blood glucose >140 mg/dL in hospitalized patients
- Diabetes
  - Fasting plasma glucose 125 mg/dL (post 8 hours overnight fast) or
  - Plasma glucose 200 mg/dL 2 hours post 75 g oral glucose after 8 8-hour fast
  - Symptoms of hyperglycemia (eg, polyuria, polydipsia, polyphagia) and
    - Random plasma glucose 200 mg/dL or hemoglobin A1C (HbA1C) level 6.5%, or
    - Plasma glucose ≥200 mg/dL on two separate occasions without symptoms
- HbA1C pitfalls for the diagnosis of diabetes
  - Conditions affecting blood cell maturity and survival
  - Impaired renal function
  - A1C levels may be higher in Blacks and Hispanics compared with Whites, despite equivalent levels of hyperglycemia in those with type 2 diabetes.

Treatment

- Correction of hyperglycemia can improve outcomes in morbidity and mortality.
- Circulating levels of cytokines, inflammatory markers, and cortisol return to normal levels after treatment with insulin

Therapeutic Targets

- Intensive targets of blood glucose 80 to 110 mg/dL have demonstrated a significantly higher risk of hypoglycemia and mortality.
- Insulin therapy and glycemic control protocols should be initiated in patients with two or more measures of blood glucose >180 mg/dL.
  - Titrate insulin to the goal blood sugar 140 to 180 mg/dL to avoid hypoglycemia.
- Intensive targets have not shown a difference in intensive care unit (ICU) length of care, 90-day ICU or hospital mortality, new infections, or mechanical ventilation duration.

Insulin Regimens and Monitoring

- Continuous intravenous (IV) insulin infusion
  - Insulin infusion is the most effective method for achieving glycemic targets in critically ill patients.
  - Dosing adjustments should be protocolized with predefined infusion rates based on glycemic fluctuations and the current insulin dose.
    - Should be validated for low risks of morbidity and hypoglycemia
    - Some computerized decision support protocols have been associated with lower rates of hypoglycemia compared to written protocols.
  - Point-of-care monitoring should be performed every 30 to 120 minutes.
    - More frequent with hypoglycemia or rapid changes in blood glucose
  - For patients receiving continuous parenteral nutrition, regular insulin can be added to the solution, particularly if >20 units have been used in the past 24 hours.
    - Start with 1 unit for every 10 g of dextrose and adjust daily.
    - Prevents hypoglycemia if nutrition is stopped
    - Should be combined and monitored with subcutaneous correctional insulin for hyperglycemia
  - Undesirable aspects of insulin infusion
    - Increased resource utilization, more frequent monitoring, higher nursing workload, more frequent hypoglycemic episodes
- Subcutaneous insulin
  - Consider when the condition stabilizes or transitions to a lower care level.
  - To transition from insulin infusion, calculate 24-hour infusion requirements.
  - 80% of the 24-hour insulin requirement is split between basal and bolus insulin.
    - ~20% to 30% basal insulin (eg, glargine)—peakless, lasts 24 hours
      - First dose should be 2 hours before the insulin drip is discontinued.
    - ~70% to 80% bolus insulin
      - Nutritional bolus
        - Rapid acting, dose based on projected carbohydrate intake
          - Taking regular diet or bolus tube feeds
            - Insulin scheduled 3 times daily (tid) with meals and every night at bedtime (qhs)
            - 1 unit for every 15 g carbohydrate
          - Continuous tube feeds or parenteral nutrition
            - Rapid insulin scheduled q4h, or regular Insulin scheduled q6h
      - Correctional bolus
        - Rapid acting (eg, lispro), dose based on glucose readings out of goal

- Glucocorticoid therapy
  - Intermediate-acting (eg, prednisone) plasma levels peak at 4 to 6 hours
  - Giving intermediate-acting NPH insulin with a peak action of 4 to 6 hours may be helpful.
  - For long-acting and frequently dosed glucocorticoids (eg, dexamethasone), basal insulin dose may help control blood glucose.
- Undesirable aspects of subcutaneous insulin
  - Nighttime awakening for dosing
  - More complex with multiple insulin types and a need to anticipate or react to changes in nutrition, medications, and clinical status
  - Subcutaneous edema can impair insulin absorption.

Monitoring

- Point-of-care glucose monitoring should match the insulin dosing strategy.
  - Continuous insulin infusion—every 30 minutes for rapid or significant insulin dose changes to every 120 minutes for stable requirements
  - Eating patients on subcutaneous insulin—prior to eating and at bedtime
  - Not eating or receiving continuous nutrition—q4 to q6h
  - Sources of error
    - Human factors—contamination from glucose on the skin
    - Environmental—enzymatic strips subject to change in temperature, oxygen partial pressure
    - Medications—acetaminophen overdose, icodextrin, ascorbic acid, mannitol, dopamine can result in falsely high measurements.
    - Physiologic factors—reduced perfusion (shock, pressors), hypertriglyceridemia can cause falsely low measurements
- Subcutaneous continuous glucose monitor (CGM)
  - Outpatients have demonstrated increased time in the glucose target range, improved A1C, decreased hypoglycemia, and severe hypoglycemia events.
  - Inpatient shows promise for detecting and reducing episodes of hypoglycemia and reducing resource utilization and workload.
  - Not U.S. Food and Drug Administration (FDA) approved for inpatient use due to accuracy concerns in states of hypovolemia, hypoperfusion, use of vasopressors

Hypoglycemia

- Blood glucose <70 m/dL
  - Level 1 <70—may be asymptomatic
  - Level 2 <54—needs immediate action, neurologic symptoms
    - Anxiety, palpitations, tremor, sweating, hunger, cognitive dysfunction
  - Level 3 <54 with severe altered mental or physical status that is life-threatening
    - Cognitive dysfunction, seizures, coma, death
- Etiology
  - In those with diabetes or hyperglycemia treatment
    - Iatrogenic/antidiabetic medication overdose, nutrition discontinuation, increased physical activity, increased alcohol intake
  - Not limited to diabetes or hyperglycemic treatment
    - Renal failure, liver failure, sepsis, adrenal insufficiency, myxedema coma, insulinoma and other rare tumors, starvation, medication overdose (eg, beta-blocker)
- Treatment
  - Able to swallow - Administer 15g oral glucose or juice
  - Unable to swallow - IV dextrose bolus 12.5 g for blood glucose 50 to 70, 25g for <50
  - If <70 following two doses, start a continuous dextrose infusion.
    - Higher concentration of dextrose risks venous sclerosis.
    - 5% and 10% safe for peripheral administration
    - Central access is recommended for continuous infusion of >10%.
    - Glucagon 1 mg IV or intramuscular (IM) can be considered drawbacks include:
      - May not work if glycogen stores are depleted
      - Nausea/vomiting side effects can impair oral intake.
      - 10 to 15 minutes to effect

Hyperglycemic Crises

- DKA
  - Mortality 2% to 5%, more common in type 1 diabetes
  - Initial presentation of disease in 20% of adult, 30% to 40% of children with type 1 diabetes
  - Onset <1 to 2 days
  - Pathogenesis
    - Hyperglycemia, metabolic acidosis, and elevated circulating total body ketone concentration
    - Insulin deficiency with elevated counterregulatory hormones (glucagon, catecholamines, cortisol, and growth hormones)
      - Stimulates gluconeogenesis, glycogenolysis, and lipolysis
      - Free fatty acids from lipolysis are oxidized to ketone bodies.
  - Precipitating factors
    - Poor adherence to treatment (40%-60%), new diagnosis of DM (20%), infection (15%)
  - Diagnosis
    - Signs and symptoms
      - Polyuria, polydipsia, weight loss, nausea, vomiting, abdominal pain, signs of dehydration, altered mental status, hypothermia, acetone scent on the patient's breath, Kussmaul respirations
    - Lab findings
      - Hyperglycemia—plasma glucose >250 mg/dL
      - Metabolic acidosis—pH 7.0 to 7.3
      - Hyperketonemia-beta-hydroxybutyrate
      - Hyperkalemia
      - Hyperphosphatemia
- HHS (hyperosmolar hyperglycemic nonketotic syndrome)
  - Mortality 15% (usually due to underlying cause rather than hyperglycemic metabolic changes)
  - Onset over several days → more severe hyperglycemia, dehydration, and hyperosmolarity compared to DKA
  - Pathogenesis
    - Relative insulin deficiency of insulin to maintain normoglycemia but adequate to prevent lipolysis and the generation of ketones

- Generally, fewer free fatty acids, cortisol, growth hormone, and glucagon compared to DKA
- Precipitating factors
  - Infection (30%-60%), poor adherence to treatment, cardiovascular accident (CVA), myocardial infarction (MI), trauma, new diabetes diagnosis (10%-15%)
- Diagnosis
  - Signs and symptoms
    - Same as DKA
    - 20% to 30% present with anion gap metabolic acidosis and ketoacidosis.
  - Lab findings
    - Hyperglycemia—plasma glucose >600 mg/dL
    - Arterial pH >7.30
    - Small serum and urine ketones
    - Effective serum osmolality (ESO) >320 mOsm/kg
      - ESO = 2[measured Na (mEq/L)] + glucose (mg/dL)/18

Treatment of Hyperglycemic Crises

- Due to similar pathogenesis, the treatment aims of DKA and HHS are similar.
- Fluid therapy
  - Initial goal is the correction of hypovolemia.
    - Water deficit in DKA ~100 mL/kg body weight, in HHS 100 to 200 mL/kg
    - 500 to 1,000 mL/h during the first 1 to 2 hours
    - Follow hemodynamics, input/output (I/O), examination, and lab values for volume status
  - Evaluate corrected serum sodium and hydration status.
    - Normal/high serum sodium—0.45% NaCl at 250 to 500 mL/h
    - Low serum sodium—0.9% NaCl at 250 to 500 mL/h
  - Should correct water deficit in the first 24 hours
  - Change fluids to 5% dextrose with 0.45 NaCl at 150 to 250 mL/h when:
    - Serum glucose reaches 200 mg/dL in DKA.
    - Serum glucose reaches 300 mg/dL in HHS.
  - Continue dextrose solution until ketoacidosis resolves.
- Insulin therapy
  - Bolus regular insulin 0.1 U/kg and start infusion 0.1 U/kg/h.
    - If glucose fails to fall by 10% in the first hour, repeat bolus.
  - DKA
    - At glucose 200 mg/dL, reduce infusion to 0.02 to 0.05 U/kg/h.
    - Keep glucose 150 to 200 mg/dL until DKA resolves.
  - HHS
    - At glucose 200 mg/dL, reduce infusion to 0.02 to 0.05 U/kg/h.
    - Keep glucose 200 to 300 mg/dL until the patient is mentally alert.
- Potassium replacement
  - Serum potassium labs demonstrate mild-to-moderate hyperkalemia despite total body potassium depletion and intracellular shift due to hypertonicity and acidosis.
  - Initiate potassium replacement at the upper limit of normal ~5.0 mEq/L.
    - Maintain a normal range of 4 to 5 mEq/L.
    - 20 to 30 mEq of potassium per liter of fluid
- Phosphate replacement
  - In DKA, serum phosphate is often normal or increased despite whole-body deficit.
    - Generally, replacement is not beneficial unless cardiac dysfunction, anemia, respiratory depression, or serum phosphate <1.0 mg/dL.

Bicarbonate Therapy

- It has not been shown to have a morbidity or mortality benefit in patients with pH 6.9 to 7.1.
- Severe acidosis can cause adverse cardiovascular effects, so guidelines recommend 1 to 2 amps in sterile water for pH <7.0.
- Bicarbonate should not be given in HHS as the acidosis is not severe, and sodium load can exacerbate the hyperosmolar state.

SUGGESTED READINGS

Alhatemi G, Aldiwani H, Alhatemi R, et al. Glycemic control in the critically ill: less is more. *Cleve Clin J Med*. 2022;89(4):191-199.

Blonde L, Umpierrez GE, Reddy SS, et al. American Association of Clinical Endocrinology clinical practice guideline: developing a diabetes mellitus comprehensive care plan—2022 update. *Endocr Pract*. 2022;28(10):923-1049.

ElSayed NA, Aleppo G, Aroda VR, et al. Diabetes care in the hospital: standards of care in diabetes—2023. *Diabetes Care*. 2022;46(supplement_1):S267-S278.

Falciglia M, Freyberg RW, Almenoff PL, et al. Hyperglycemia-related mortality in critically ill patients varies with admission diagnosis. *Crit Care Med*. 2009;37(12):3001-3009.

Finfer S, Chittock DR, Su SY, et al. Intensive versus conventional glucose control in critically ill patients. *N Engl J Med*. 2009;360(13):1283-1297.

Galicia-Garcia U, Benito-Vicente A, Jebari S, et al. Pathophysiology of type 2 diabetes mellitus. *Int J Mol Sci*. 2020;21(17):1-34.

Gunst J, Debaveye Y, Güiza F, et al. Tight blood-glucose control without early parenteral nutrition in the ICU. *N Engl J Med*. 2023;389(13):1180-1190.

Honarmand K, Sirimaturos M, Hirshberg EL, et al. Society of critical care medicine guidelines on glycemic control for critically ill children and adults 2024. *Crit Care Med*. 2024;52(4):e161-e181.

Kitabchi AE, Umpierrez GE, Miles JM, et al. Hyperglycemic crises in adult patients with diabetes. *Diabetes Care*. 2009;32(7):1335-1343.

Klonoff DC. Point-of-care blood glucose meter accuracy in the hospital setting. *Diabetes Spectr*. 2014;27(3):174-179.

McCall AL, Lieb DC, Gianchandani R, et al. Management of individuals with diabetes at high risk for hypoglycemia: an endocrine society clinical practice guideline. *J Clin Endocrinol Metab*. 2022;108(3):529-562.

Samson SL, Vellanki P, Blonde L, et al. American Association of Clinical Endocrinology consensus statement: comprehensive type 2 diabetes management algorithm—2023 update. *Endocr Pract*. 2023;29(5):305-340.

Stentz FB, Umpierrez GE, Cuervo R, et al. Proinflammatory cytokines, markers of cardiovascular risks, oxidative stress, and lipid peroxidation in patients with hyperglycemic crises. *Diabetes*. 2004;53(8):2079-2086.

Umpierrez G, Korytkowski M. Diabetic emergencies—ketoacidosis, hyperglycaemic hyperosmolar state and hypoglycaemia. *Nat Rev Endocrinol*. 2016;12(4):222-232.

Van den Berghe G, Wouters P, Weekers F, et al. Intensive insulin therapy in critically ill patients. *N Engl J Med*. 2001;345(19):1359-1367.

7.3

Adrenal Gland

Simona I. Lupu

Adrenal Insufficiency

Differential Diagnosis

- Primary/absolute
  - Rare; prevalence < 0.015% in the general population; incidence estimates range from ~4.4 to 6.2 new cases per million annually.
  - Multiple potential causes, of which isolated autoimmune adrenalitis is the most common (80%-90%) and is caused by anti-21-hydroxylase antibodies
  - Other causes include autoimmune syndrome (APS), infection, adrenal hemorrhage, infiltration with tumor, congenital adrenal hyperplasia, adrenoleukodystrophy, and/or secondary to drugs (such as etomidate, ketoconazole, checkpoint inhibitors, megestrol, or RU486).
  - Associated APSs include hypoparathyroidism, chronic mucocutaneous candidiasis, hyperthyroidism, premature ovarian failure, vitiligo, diabetes mellitus (DM) type 1, and pernicious anemia.
- Secondary adrenal insufficiency (AI)
  - Dysfunction of the hypothalamic-pituitary-adrenal (HPA) axis, leading to glucocorticoid deficiency with preserved mineralocorticoid production
  - Multiple potential causes including
    - Pituitary pathology: tumors (eg, craniopharyngioma, meningioma, ependymoma, or metastases), irradiation, traumatic brain injury, hemorrhage (eg, Sheehan), hypophysitis (eg, autoimmune, immune checkpoint inhibitor induced), infiltration (eg, tuberculosis [TB] or sarcoid)
    - Hypothalamic disease: rare (eg, corticotropin-releasing hormone [CRH] deficiency)
    - Chronic exogenous glucocorticoid therapy: risk of HPA axis suppression occurs after ≥3 to 4 weeks at daily doses equivalent to ≥15 to 25 mg hydrocortisone (4-6 mg prednisone, 3-5 mg methylprednisolone, or 0.25-0.5 mg dexamethasone), per 2024 European Society of Endocrinology and Endocrine Society (ESE/ES) Joint Clinical Guideline
    - Congenital disorders: proopiomelanocortin deficiency, combined pituitary hormone deficiency, congenitally absent adrenocorticotropic hormone (ACTH)
- Acute AI/adrenal crisis
  - Most typically in patients taking exogenous glucocorticoids who do not receive further supplementation during stress (infection, surgery), or those with sudden loss of adrenal function (hemorrhage, sepsis)
  - Combined glucocorticoid and mineralocorticoid deficiency can lead to hypovolemia and hypotension, which may progress to hypovolemic shock.
  - Clinical presentation includes severe hypotension, vomiting, abdominal pain (may mimic acute abdomen), altered mental status (may progress to stupor and coma), and fever (can be exaggerated by cortisol deficiency).
  - Ongoing illness or stress (eg, surgical) can precipitate an adrenal crisis with resultant profound and persistent hypotension.
  - Treatment should begin immediately, preferably with intravenous (IV) hydrocortisone 100 mg bolus + continuous 200 mg/d infusion or 50 mg IV q6h, all while ensuring adequate fluid resuscitation. Tapering of hydrocortisone can begin after clinical recovery, and in those with primary AI, fludrocortisone 100 μg/daily can start once hydrocortisone dose <50 mg/d.
- Relative AI/critical illness–related corticosteroid insufficiency (CIRCI)
  - Controversial concept in severely ill patients (typically those in intensive care units [ICUs]), characterized by inadequate cortisol response to severe stress
  - No official definition of laboratory results for diagnosis; however, per Society of Critical Care Medicine/European Society of Intensive Care Medicine (SCCM/ESICM) 2017 consensus, CIRCI can be considered if the change in cortisol is <9 μg/dL after administration of 250 mcg cosyntropin, or random plasma cortisol <10 μg/dL.
  - Since the possible benefits of corticosteroid therapy are not completely predicted by ACTH testing, current guidelines do not recommend using ACTH testing to guide the decision of whether or not to administer corticosteroids.

Signs and Symptoms

- Glucocorticoid deficiency
  - Fatigue, weight loss, anorexia, myalgias, fever (may reflect stress/infection), anemia, eosinophilia, hypoglycemia (more common in children), hyponatremia, postural hypotension, amenorrhea
- Mineralocorticoid deficiency (primary AI)
  - Abdominal pain, nausea, vomiting, dizziness, postural hypotension, hyponatremia, hyperkalemia, skin changes (hyperpigmentation and/or vitiligo in primary AI, alabaster pale skin in secondary AI)
- Adrenal androgen deficiency
  - Fatigue, pruritus, decreased libido, lack of axillary/pubic hair

Diagnosis

- Morning cortisol (8-9 AM)
  - <5 μg/dL: strongly suggests AI
  - 5 to 18 μg/dL: intermediate; perform ACTH stimulation test (cosyntropin test)
  - >18 μg/dL: AI unlikely
  - Note: cortisol-binding globulin (CBG) alterations (pregnancy, oral contraceptive pills [OCPs], liver disease) affect total cortisol; salivary/free cortisol test may be more useful in these settings.
- ACTH stimulation test (cosyntropin test) helps with confirmation.
  - 250 μg IV cosyntropin (ACTH1-24 peptide) with cortisol levels measured at baseline, 30, and 60 minutes. Hold hydrocortisone/prednisone for >24 hours before

testing; dexamethasone may be used if steroid is needed during evaluation.

- Normal response (negative test): >18 to 20 μg/dL (assay dependent)
- If test positive, primary versus secondary AI determined by ACTH
- Primary AI
  - Failure of the adrenal glands themselves to produce adequate cortisol (and usually aldosterone); ACTH rises due to loss of negative feedback.
  - ACTH high (>2× upper limit of normal); mineralocorticoid deficiency common (increased renin, decreased aldosterone, hyperkalemia)
- Central AI (secondary/tertiary)
  - Secondary AI: pituitary ACTH deficiency results in decreased cortisol.
  - Tertiary AI: hypothalamic/CRH suppression (most commonly from chronic exogenous glucocorticoids, revealed during withdrawal/stress) leads to decreased ACTH and results in decreased cortisol.
  - ACTH low or inappropriately normal; mineralocorticoid function usually preserved (intact renin-angiotensin-aldosterone system [RAAS])
- Controversy exists regarding the reliability of the cosyntropin test to diagnose relative AI/CIRCI.
- For critical illness (sepsis, acute respiratory distress syndrome [ARDS], community-acquired pneumonia [CAP]), the 2017 diagnostic criteria (eg, random cortisol <10 μg/dL or delta <9 μg/dL post-cosyntropin) are no longer recommended to guide therapy.
- According to 2024 SCCM/ESICM guidelines, the decision to treat is based on the clinical syndrome (eg, septic shock on any vasopressor) and not on ACTH stimulation testing, which does not reliably predict steroid responsiveness.

Management and Treatment

- Do not delay treatment to perform diagnostic tests if adrenal crisis is suspected based on symptoms (hypotension, dehydration, shock).
  - Primary AI: hormone replacement is the mainstay.
    - Hydrocortisone 15 to 25 mg/d with meals
      - Two-thirds of the dose in the morning, remainder in the midafternoon or 4 to 6 hours before bedtime
      - Dose titrated in 2.5 to 5 mg increments with goal being to alleviate symptoms
    - Fludrocortisone 0.05 to 0.1 mg daily orally (po), to replace aldosterone
    - Patient should also maintain good sodium intake of 3 to 4 g/d.
    - Females might need dehydroepiandrosterone (DHEA) po if measured to be low or if symptomatic.
    - Medical identification bracelets and patient education on stress dosing plans, emergency injection kits, and yearly osteoporosis screening
    - Treatment is monitored by blood pressure (BP) and electrolyte changes, and sometimes through plasma renin concentrations.
  - Secondary AI
    - Glucocorticoid therapy is the primary treatment, with doses similar to those for primary AI. No fludrocortisone needed as RAAS is intact.
  - Acute AI
    - Immediate rehydration with crystalloid infusion at initial rates of up to 1 L/h with continuous cardiac monitoring
    - Hydrocortisone 100 mg IV bolus immediately, then 100 to 200 mg daily by either continuous infusion or divided doses. Switch to po once stable.
    - Fludrocortisone administration if daily hydrocortisone <50 mg
    - Identify precipitant and treat concurrently.
  - Relative AI/CIRCI
    - 2024 SCCM/ESICM guidelines: treatment is based on the clinical syndrome, not on diagnostic testing (eg, ACTH stim test), which is no longer recommended to guide therapy in this setting.
      - Septic shock
        - Recommendation: "suggest" corticosteroids (conditional)
        - Key change: applies to patients on any vasopressor. (The previous 2017 guideline qualifier for "refractory shock" or moderate-/high-dose vasopressors is removed.)
        - Dose: typically IV hydrocortisone 200 mg/d (as continuous infusion or 50 mg q6h)
      - ARDS
        - Recommendation: "suggest" corticosteroids (conditional)
        - Key change: applies to all patients with ARDS (The previous 2017 guideline qualifier for "early moderate-to-severe" ARDS is removed.)
        - Dose: multiple regimens are acceptable (eg, dexamethasone 20 mg IV daily × 5d, then 10 mg daily × 5d; or methylprednisolone 1 mg/kg/d).
      - Severe CAP
        - Recommendation: "recommend" corticosteroids (strong)
        - Key change: this is a new strong recommendation for severe bacterial CAP. (No recommendation is made for less severe CAP.)
        - Dose: typically 5 to 7 days (eg, IV hydrocortisone 200 mg/d or IV methylprednisolone 0.5 mg/kg q12h)
        - See Table 7.3.1 for additional details.

TABLE 7.3.1 Corticosteroids for Septic Shock (2024 SCCM/ESICM Guideline)

- "Suggest" IV corticosteroids for adult patients with septic shock requiring any vasopressor (Conditional Recommendation). This removes the previous 2017 qualifier for "refractory" or "moderate-to high-dose" vasopressor therapy.
- Typical dose: IV hydrocortisone 200 mg/d (as a continuous infusion or 50 mg IV q6h), often for 5-7 d
- Tapering can be considered once vasopressors are no longer required.

ESICM, European Society of Intensive Care Medicine; IV, intravenous; q, every; SCCM, Society of Critical Care Medicine.

Pheochromocytoma—Tumor of Sympathoadrenal Chromaffin Cell Tumors

Differential Diagnosis

- Primary (sporadic), ~75% of cases
- Syndromic, ~25% of cases
  - Multiple endocrine neoplasia (MEN) 2A (medullary thyroid carcinoma, pheochromocytoma, hyperparathyroidism)
  - MEN 2B (medullary thyroid carcinoma, pheochromocytoma, mucosal neuromas, marfanoid habitus, developmental disorder)
  - von Hippel-Lindau syndrome (retinal and cerebellar hemangioblastomas, clear cell renal carcinomas, pancreatic islet cell tumors, endolymphatic sac tumors, pheochromocytoma, pancreatic, and/or renal cysts)
  - Neurofibromatosis type 1 (multiple neurofibromas, café-au-lait spots, axillary freckling, Lisch nodules, pheochromocytoma)

"Rule of 10s"

10% bilateral, 10% malignant, and 10% extraadrenal—percentages are higher in syndrome-associated pheochromocytomas.

Symptoms

- Hypertension (sustained or paroxysmal), plus the classic triad of episodic palpitations, headache, and sweating
- Typical ICU presentation: hypertensive crisis after angiography or during the perioperative period

Diagnosis

- Biochemical testing: plasma-free or 24-hour urinary fractionated metanephrines and catecholamines, collected supine after 30 minutes of rest. Clonidine suppression test if results are borderline
- Imaging: CT (risk of precipitating hypertensive crisis) or magnetic resonance imaging (MRI); 123-I-metaiodobenzylguanidine (MIBG) scan, octreotide scan, selective venous sampling, positron emission scan
- Genetic evaluation: recommended due to high frequency of hereditary forms

Management and Treatment

- Medical management of pheochromocytoma: alpha-blockade followed by beta-blockade
- Medical management
  - Acute control of hypertensive crisis
    - Phentolamine 2.5 to 5 mg IV every 5 minutes or sodium nitroprusside 0.5 to 10 μg/kg/min
  - Chronic control: start 7 to 14 days prior to planned surgery.
    - Phenoxybenzamine 10 mg po 2 times daily (bid) (increase gradually, max ~1 mg/kg/d) titrated to symptoms of orthostatic hypotension and/or high stool output
    - Ensure liberal salt and fluid intake to expand blood volume.
    - Add beta-blockers only after adequate alpha-blockade is established (evidenced by orthostatic symptoms, BP control, and heart rate response) to avoid unopposed alpha-adrenergic effects.
    - Other potential ancillary agents:
      - Prazosin: fewer side effects, shorter action, more cost-effective
      - Magnesium sulfate, calcium channel blockers, angiotensin-converting enzyme inhibitors: may stabilize BP when alpha-blockers are not enough
      - Metyrosine: started ~4 days pre-op for large/refractory tumors; tyrosine hydroxylase inhibitor, which can reduce catecholamine synthesis
- Surgical management
  - Elective surgery is recommended once medical optimization is complete to reduce perioperative morbidity and mortality.
  - Laparoscopic adrenalectomy is standard unless tumor is >6 cm, invasive, or malignant. Tumor manipulation during surgery may cause catecholamine surges and hypertensive crisis.
  - Perioperative ICU-related issues
    - Hypotension requiring vasopressors may persist until plasma catecholamine levels normalize.
    - Profound sudden hypotension may occur immediately after surgical occlusion of adrenal vein and may require vasopressor support and fluid resuscitation.
    - Persistent hypertension may indicate
      - Missed pheochromocytoma
      - Renal ischemia (surgical complication)
      - Underlying essential hypertension
    - Nonoptimized perioperative patients will require significant fluid resuscitation, likely with a dextrose-containing agent to combat hypoglycemia.
    - For bilateral adrenalectomy, patients may need steroid supplementation.
- Metastatic or inoperable disease
  - Possible treatment with iodine-123 MIBG therapy, peptide receptor radionuclide therapy, chemotherapy, and tyrosine kinase inhibitors

Acknowledgments

We gratefully acknowledge the contributions of previous edition authors, Ranjit Deshpande and Rebecca Aslakson, as portions of those chapters have been retained in this revision.

SUGGESTED READINGS

Annane D, Pastores SM, Rochwerg B, et al. Guidelines for the diagnosis and management of critical illness-related corticosteroid insufficiency (CIRCI) in critically ill patients (Part I): Society of Critical Care Medicine (SCCM) and European Society of Intensive Care Medicine (ESICM) 2017. *Crit Care Med.* 2017;45(12):2078-2088.

Artl W, Society for Endocrinology Clinical Committee. SOCIETY FOR ENDOCRINOLOGY ENDOCRINE EMERGENCY GUIDANCE: emergency management of acute adrenal insufficiency (adrenal crisis) in adult patients. *Endocr Connect.* 2016;5(5):G1-G3.

Beuschlein F, Else T, Bancos I, et al. European Society of Endocrinology and Endocrine Society joint clinical guideline: diagnosis and therapy of glucocorticoid-induced adrenal insufficiency. *J Clin Endocrinol Metab.* 2024;109(7):1657-1683.

Bornstein SR, Allolio B, Arlt W, et al. Diagnosis and treatment of primary adrenal insufficiency: an endocrine society clinical practice guideline. *J Clin Endocrinol Metab.* 101(1):364-389.

Chaudhuri D, Nei AM, Rochwerg B, et al. 2024 focused update: guidelines on the use of corticosteroids in sepsis, acute respiratory distress syndrome, and community-acquired pneumonia. *Crit Care Med.* 2024;52(5): e219-e233.

Dellinger RP, Levy MM, Carlet JM. Surviving Sepsis Campaign: international guidelines for management of severe sepsis and septic shock: 2008. *Crit Care Med.* 2008;36(1):296-327.

Hines RL, Marschall KE. *Stoelting's Anesthesia and Co-Existing Disease*. 5th ed. Elsevier Churchill Livingstone; 2008:1142-1144.

Lentschener C, Gaujoux S, Tesniere A, et al. Point of controversy: perioperative care of patients undergoing pheochromocytoma removal—time for reappraisal? *Eur J Endocrinol.* 2011;165:365-373.

Marik PE, Pastores SM, Annane D, et al. Recommendations for the diagnosis and management of corticosteroid insufficiency in critically ill adult patients: consensus statements from an international task force by the American College of Critical Care Medicine. *Crit Care Med.* 2008; 36:1937-1949.

Speckart PF, Nicoloff JT, Bethune JE. Screening for adrenocortical insufficiency with cosyntropin (synthetic ACTH). *Arch Intern Med.* 1971;128: 761-763.

Sprung CL, Annane D, Keh D, et al; CORTICUS Study Group. Hydrocortisone therapy for patients with septic shock. *N Engl J Med.* 2008;358(2):111-124.

7.4

Pituitary Hormone Disorders

Ilan Mizrahi

Syndrome of Inappropriate Antidiuretic Hormone Secretion

Excessive antidiuretic hormone (ADH) secretion leads to impaired water excretion, decreased urine output, and hyponatremia; isovolemic or hypervolemic volume status.

Differential Diagnosis and Causes

See Table 7.4.1.

Symptoms: Symptoms of Hyponatremia

- Mild: headache, impaired memory, difficulty concentrating, muscle cramps, and/or weakness
- Severe: confusion, hallucinations, seizures, coma, respiratory arrest

Diagnosis

- Criteria
  - Hyponatremia (Na <135 mEq/L)
  - Decreased serum osmolality (<275 mOsm/kg)
  - Increased urine osmolality (>100 mOsm/kg) with urine sodium >40 mEq/L (with normal sodium intake)
  - Clinical euvolemia
  - Normal thyroid and adrenal function
- No recent use of diuretic medications

Management and Treatment

- Treat underlying cause (resect tumor, stop medications, treat infections, etc).
  - Mild hyponatremia
    - Fluid restriction (~1-1.5 L/d)
    - Consider demeclocycline to inhibit the action of ADH.
  - Acute severe symptomatic hyponatremia
    - Calculate sodium deficit.

$$\text{Sodium deficit} = \text{TBW} \times ([\text{Na}]_{\text{normal}} - [\text{Na}]_{\text{current}})$$

(TBW = total body water. In males, TBW = 0.6 × lean body mass; females, TBW = 0.5 × lean body mass)

- Slow correction of serum sodium to avoid osmotic demyelination syndrome.
- Administer 3% hypertonic saline.

TABLE 7.4.1 Differential Diagnosis and Causes of Syndrome of Inappropriate ADH

Malignancies	Pulmonary Disorders	Neurologic Disorders	Medications	Others
Small cell lung carcinoma	Acute respiratory failure requiring mechanical ventilation	Encephalitis	Drugs that stimulate ADH	Major surgery (abdominal, thoracic)
Head and neck cancer	Pneumonia	Meningitis	Carbamazepine	Pain
Pancreatic carcinoma	Asthma	Brain abscess	Cyclophosphamide	Nausea
Gastric carcinoma	Cystic fibrosis	Brain tumor	SSRIs	Pituitary Resection
Prostate carcinoma	Tuberculosis	CVA	Tricyclic antidepressants	Stress
Thymoma		Subdural hematoma	3,4-methylenedioxymethamphetamine	Hereditary
Ewing sarcoma		Intracranial injury	NSAIDs	
		Multiple sclerosis	ADH analogs	
			Desmopressin	
			Oxytocin	
			Vasopressin	

ADH, antidiuretic hormone; CVA, cardiovascular accident; NSAIDs, nonsteroidal antiinflammatory drugs; SSRIs, selective serotonin reuptake inhibitors; MDMA, 3,4-methylenedioxymethamphetamine.

    - Target a rise of serum sodium no >1 mEq/L/h, with a maximum rise of serum sodium of ≤8 mEq/L in the first 24 hours. Maximum increase in serum sodium in the first 48 hours should be ≤20 mEq/L.
    - In severe hyponatremia with seizures or coma, an initial bolus of 100 mL of 3% hypertonic saline over 10 minutes can rapidly improve symptoms. Sodium levels must be carefully monitored to avoid overcorrection and the risk of osmotic demyelination syndrome.
    - During hypertonic saline administration, check serum sodium levels every 1 to 2 hours and adjust the rate to ensure a safe correction, halting the infusion once symptoms have resolved or target sodium levels are achieved.
  - Unknown duration of hyponatremia and moderate symptoms
    - 0.9% saline infusion, target increase of serum sodium of 1 mEq/L/h
    - Maximum rise of serum sodium should be <10 mEq/L in the first 24 hours.
    - Consider oral urea for aquaresis to eliminate excess body water.
  - Adverse effects include hypotension and hypokalemia.

Diabetes Insipidus

Polyuria (>3 L/d) due to either deficient secretion of ADH or ADH resistance in the kidneys, also leading to excessive thirst

Differential Diagnosis

- Central diabetes insipidus (DI) (neurogenic DI)
  - Deficient secretion of ADH
  - Most often idiopathic (25%)
  - Other causes include intracranial hemorrhage, traumatic brain injury, neurosurgical complication, intracranial lesions, and neurologic infections.
- Nephrogenic DI
  - ADH resistance in the distal tubules and collecting ducts of the kidneys
  - Multiple causes: lithium, demeclocycline, amphotericin hypercalcemia, severe hypokalemia, acute kidney injury, pregnancy

Diagnosis

- Fluid restriction test to rule out primary polydipsia
  - Patients with DI continue to produce large amounts of urine despite fluid restriction.
- Serum sodium sometimes helpful.
  - Usually low in primary polydipsia and high in DI
  - Normal serum sodium not helpful
- Urine osmolarity <300 mOsm/kg
- Desmopressin (DDAVP) can distinguish between central and nephrogenic DI. Central DI will respond to DDAVP with a significant increase in urine osmolality (>50%), whereas nephrogenic DI will not.
  - Central DI: urine osmolarity will increase by >50%
  - Nephrogenic DI: No change in urine osmolarity

Management and Treatment

- If DI is secondary to reversible causes, treat the underlying pathology.
- Central DI: DDAVP. Requires close monitoring to avoid hyponatremia. Less often used alternatives include carbamazepine, chlorpropamide, thiazides, and nonsteroidal antiinflammatory drugs (NSAIDs)
- Nephrogenic DI: reduce solute intake (low-sodium, low-protein diet) and provide free water to keep up with losses
- Thiazides and amiloride can decrease urine output by reducing sodium reabsorption in the kidneys, leading to a decrease in free water loss. Amiloride is particularly useful in lithium-induced nephrogenic DI.
- NSAIDs are beneficial in certain hereditary causes (Bartter and Gitelman syndromes) by inhibiting the production of prostaglandins, which are elevated in these conditions and contribute to renal salt wasting and polyuria.

Cerebral Salt Wasting

- Hypovolemic hyponatremia due to inappropriate urine sodium excretion
- Some debate as to whether cerebral salt wasting is a distinct condition or merely a form of syndrome of inappropriate antidiuretic hormone secretion (SIADH), as both share overlapping features such as hyponatremia and elevated urine sodium levels.

Causes

- Most commonly reported with subarachnoid hemorrhage
- Other causes include encephalitis, meningitis, central nervous system (CNS) tumors, and after neurologic surgery

Pathophysiology

Thought to be due to aldosterone deficiency and impaired sodium and water regulation

Diagnosis

- Hyponatremia (serum sodium <135 mEq/L)
- Volume depletion and evidence of hypovolemia from polyuria
- Low plasma osmolality (<285 mOsm/kg)
- Urine osmolality usually >100 mOsm/kg, with urine sodium usually >40 mEq/L

Management and Treatment

- Hyponatremia treated with 3% hypertonic saline, ensuring gradual correction to minimize the risk of osmotic demyelination syndrome
- Hypovolemia is managed with isotonic fluid and fludrocortisone to achieve euvolemia. Careful monitoring is necessary to prevent complications such as hypernatremia, fluid overload, or worsening cerebral edema, particularly in patients with underlying neurological conditions.

SUGGESTED READINGS

Adrogue HJ, Madias NE. The syndrome of inappropriate antidiuresis. *N Engl J Med*.2023;389:1499-1509.

Coussement J, Danguy C, Zouaoui-Boudjeltia K, et al. Treatment of the syndrome of inappropriate secretion of antidiuretic hormone with urea in critically ill patients. *Am J Nephrol*. 2012;35(3):265-270.

Lee P, Jones GRD, Center JR. Successful treatment of adult cerebral salt wasting with fludrocortisone. *Arch Intern Med*. 2008;168(3):325-326.

Lindner G, Funk GC. Hypernatremia in critically ill patients. *J Crit Care*. 2013;28(2):216.e11-216.e2.16E20.

Lopez-Garcia SC, Downie ML, Kim JS, et al. Treatment and long-term outcome in primary nephrogenic diabetes insipidus. *Nephrol Dial Transplant*. 2020;38(10):2120-2130.

Rondon-Berrios H. Diagnostic and therapeutic strategies to severe hyponatremia in the intensive care unit. *J Intensive Care Med*. 2023;39(11):1039-1054.

Spasovski G, Vanholder R, Allolio B, et al. Clinical practice guideline on diagnosis and treatment of hyponatremia. *Eur J Endocrinol*. 2014;170(3):G1-G47.

Sterns RH, Silver SM. Cerebral salt wasting versus SIADH: what difference. *J Am Soc Nephrol*. 2008;19(2):194-160.

Utiger R. Diabetes insipidus. *JAMA*. 1969;207(9):1699.

Verbalis JG. The curious story of cerebral salt wasting: fact or fiction? *Clin J Am Soc Nephrol*. 2020;15(11):1666-1668.

7.5

Thyroid Disorders

Samantha J. Stein and Diana Barragan-Bradford

Hyperthyroidism

Key Pathophysiology

- Results from an excess of thyroid hormone production, release, or extrathyroidal thyroid hormone availability, leading to a hypermetabolic state

Epidemiology

- Occurs more frequently among women than men, with a ratio of 5 to 1
- Occurs in 0.2% of men and 2% of women, though prevalence increases to 4% to 5% among older women
- *See Table 7.5.1 for differential diagnosis of hyperthyroidism.*

Symptoms

- Symptoms can be nonspecific and may manifest in patients with subclinical conditions while absent in those with obvious diseases, particularly in older adults.
- Symptoms include fatigue, weight loss, diaphoresis/heat intolerance, palpitations, insomnia, anxiety, restlessness, hair loss, diarrhea, and irregular menses. In older adults, hyperthyroidism may present atypically as apathetic hyperthyroidism, characterized by lethargy, weight loss, or depression, rather than the classic hypermetabolic symptoms.

TABLE 7.5.1 Differential Diagnosis of Hyperthyroidism
Graves disease
Thyroiditis
Toxic multinodular goiter
Solitary toxic adenoma
Amiodarone-induced thyrotoxicosis
Immune checkpoint inhibitor–induced thyrotoxicosis
Trophoblastic disease and germ cell tumors
Pituitary adenoma
Factitious (ingestion of thyroid hormone)

- Untreated hyperthyroidism can cause cardiac arrhythmias, heart failure, osteoporosis, and adverse pregnancy outcomes and is associated with increased mortality.

Diagnosis

- Suppressed thyroid-stimulating hormone (TSH) levels and elevated free thyroxine (T4) and triiodothyronine (T3) levels
- Subclinical hyperthyroidism will have low TSH but normal T4 and T3 levels.
- Graves disease → thyroid-stimulating immunoglobulin
- Hashimoto disease (autoimmune thyroiditis) → antithyroperoxidase and antithyroglobulin antibodies
- Radioactive iodine (RAI) uptake scanning may be helpful to elucidate the cause of hyperthyroidism when other tests are negative.

Management and Treatment

- Medical therapy aims at decreasing thyroid hormone synthesis with thionamides.
  - Methimazole and propylthiouracil (PTU) inhibit the organification of iodine and the coupling of iodothyronine.
  - Methimazole is typically the first-line treatment for hyperthyroidism, except during the first trimester of pregnancy or thyroid storm, where PTU is preferred due to safety considerations. PTU, however, carries a higher risk of hepatotoxicity, warranting caution in its use outside these specific indications.
  - Beta-blockers, particularly propranolol, are often used adjunctively to manage adrenergic symptoms and inhibit peripheral conversion of T4 to T3.
  - RAI is effective, but the effects are not immediate. In the first weeks after treatment, T4 and T3 concentrations can transiently increase. Of note, RAI is contraindicated in pregnancy and should be carefully considered in women of childbearing age. Additionally, RAI treatment may transiently worsen hyperthyroidism due to the release of preformed thyroid hormone. Beta-blockers or thionamides may be required as pretreatment to mitigate this effect.
- Surgical therapy can be considered as first-line treatment for toxic nodular goiter and as definitive treatment for Graves disease, particularly when other treatments are ineffective, not tolerated, or contraindicated.
- Thyroidectomy is also considered in patients with known malignancy, suspicious findings on fine-needle aspiration, history of neck irradiation, and patients with growing/nonfunctioning nodules.
- Radiofrequency ablation: minimally invasive alternative to surgery or RAI for the treatment of toxic nodules

Thyroid Storm

- Thought to be due to an inhibition of the binding of the thyroid hormone to thyroxin-binding globulin, therefore causing an acute rise in free hormone concentrations
  - Usually precipitated by a concurrent medical problem in a patient with partially treated hyperthyroidism, commonly a systemic infection (see Table 7.5.2)
  - Symptoms
    - Temperature >38.5 °C, tachycardia, atrial fibrillation, mental status changes, nausea, vomiting, diarrhea
    - Vascular collapse, shock, and multisystem organ failure
    - Coma and death can occur in 20% of patients.
      - Death is usually due to shock, dysrhythmias, congestive heart failure, or the precipitating illness.
  - Diagnosis: a clinical diagnosis, but also multiple lab abnormalities
    - Lab abnormalities
      - T3 > T4 concentrations, undetectable TSH
      - Elevated liver function tests (LFTs), elevated hematocrit (due to volume contraction), mild hyperglycemia, and hypercalcemia
      - The degree of hyperthyroidism (elevation of T4 and/or T3 and suppression of TSH) in patients with thyroid storm is, in general, comparable to that of patients with uncomplicated overt hyperthyroidism.
  - Management and treatment (Table 7.5.3)
    - Medical emergency requiring intensive care unit (ICU) admission
    - Thyroid-directed therapy is aimed at decreasing thyroid hormone production, conversion, and secretion and at blocking peripheral responses to thyroid hormone.
    - Supportive therapy, including temperature control, management of cardiovascular manifestations, and treating the precipitating cause
    - Thionamides: PTU is preferred in thyroid storm due to its dual action of blocking thyroid hormone synthesis and peripheral T4-to-T3 conversion. Methimazole can be used if PTU is unavailable or contraindicated.
    - Iodide therapy: administer iodide (eg, Lugol solution or saturated solution of potassium iodide [SSKI]) after thionamide therapy to block thyroid hormone release via the Wolff-Chaikoff effect. Administering iodide before thionamides may exacerbate thyroid hormone synthesis.

TABLE 7.5.2 Precipitating Factors for Thyroid Storm

TABLE 7.5.2 Precipitating Factors for Thyroid Storm
Surgery
Infections
Stress
Trauma
DKA
Labor
Cardiac disease
Iodinated contrast agents
Abrupt discontinuation of antithyroid medications (particularly in individuals with poorly controlled or severe hyperthyroidism)

DKA, diabetic ketoacidosis.

TABLE 7.5.3 Treatment of Thyroid Storm

Thyroid-directed therapy	*Inhibition of thyroid hormone synthesis*	Propylthiouracil 800 mg once, then 200-300 mg every 8 h or Methimazole 80 mg once, then 40-80 mg every 12 h
	Block release of thyroid hormone from the gland	Lugol solution 10 gtt every 8 h Or *SSKI* (saturated solution of potassium iodide) 5 gtt orally every 6 h
	Reduction of T4-to-T3 conversion	Hydrocortisone IV 300 mg load followed by 100 mg every 8 h
Supportive therapy	*Hyperthermia*	IV fluids Antipyretics Cooling blanket
	Hemodynamic	β-Blockers (propranolol, metoprolol, or esmolol) Vasopressors (for blood pressure support)
	Etiologic	Treat the underlying illness

IV, intravenous.

- Beta-blockers: beta-blockers, particularly propranolol, are used to control adrenergic symptoms (eg, tachycardia, hypertension) and inhibit peripheral T4-to-T3 conversion. Alternatives like esmolol or metoprolol may be used if propranolol is unavailable.
- Corticosteroids: hydrocortisone (300 mg intravenous [IV] bolus followed by 100 mg IV every 8 hours) should be administered to reduce T4-to-T3 conversion and treat potential concurrent adrenal insufficiency.

Hypothyroidism

Differential Diagnosis

- Can result from a defect anywhere along the hypothalamic-pituitary-adrenal (HPA) axis

Primary hypothyroidism (95% of cases): primary disease of the thyroid gland

- Most common cause of primary hypothyroidism is chronic autoimmune thyroiditis (Hashimoto).
- Other causes of primary disease include thyroidectomy, radioiodine therapy, iodine insufficiency, or external neck irradiation.
- Secondary and tertiary hypothyroidism are much less common and due to either hypothalamic (tertiary) or pituitary (secondary) dysfunction.
- Common medications that cause central (hypothalamic or pituitary) hypothyroidism include medications such as amiodarone, lithium, tyrosine kinase inhibitors, and immune checkpoint inhibitors.

Symptoms

- Fatigue, weakness, cold intolerance, dry skin, cognitive dysfunction, constipation, growth failure, pubertal delay, depression, weight gain, hair changes (dryness, thinning, loss), menstrual irregularities

Diagnosis

- Primary hypothyroidism: high TSH and low free T4
- Central hypothyroidism: inappropriately low or normal TSH despite low free T4
- Evaluating thyroid function in the inpatient setting is not recommended unless thyroid disease is strongly suspected since changes in thyroid hormones, binding proteins, and TSH concentrations can occur in severe nonthyroidal illness.

Management and Treatment

- Goals of therapy are to alleviate symptoms and normalize TSH.
- Treatment of choice is synthetic T4; nearly 80% is absorbed orally, with a half-life of 7 days
- Average replacement dose is 1.6 μg/kg once daily
- IV T4 replacement should be considered once without enteral access for >5 to 7 days at 80% of the oral daily dose.

Myxedema Coma

Epidemiology and Pathophysiology

- Severe manifestation of long-standing hypothyroidism
- Most commonly occurs in the older adults during the winter months
- Usually caused by a precipitating event in the partially treated hypothyroid patient

Sequelae

- Requires prompt intervention as mortality can exceed 60%

Symptoms

- Hypothermia (due to disordered thermoregulation)
- Altered mental status (lethargy, confusion, psychosis)
- Cardiac depression (bradycardia and hypotension)
- Gastrointestinal ileus
- Urinary retention
- Diffuse nonpitting edema

Diagnosis

- Similar to thyroid storm, this is a clinical diagnosis. Its symptoms often overlap with other critical illnesses, such as septic shock, hypothermia, or heart failure. A high index of suspicion is critical in differentiating these conditions.
- Associated laboratory values
  - Elevated TSH with low or undetectable T4 levels
  - Electrocardiogram (ECG) often demonstrates low-voltage and absent T-waves.
  - May also see hypoglycemia, hyponatremia, elevated lactate dehydrogenase (LDH), anemia, and acidosis

Treatment

- Supportive
  - Rewarming (active heating should be avoided to prevent further vasodilation and circulatory collapse)
  - Correction of metabolic abnormalities
  - Treatment of the precipitating incident
- Hydrocortisone 100 mg IV every 8 hours, given the 5% to 10 % incidence of concurrent adrenal insufficiency. It is important to give hydrocortisone before initiating thyroid hormone replacement to prevent adrenal crisis and ensure hemodynamic stability.
- Thyroid replacement: IV load of 200 to 400 μg of thyroxine followed by daily maintenance doses of 50 to 100 μg. Close monitoring for cardiovascular compromise is essential due to the risk of myocardial ischemia in patients with underlying coronary artery disease.
  - If no clinical response, then repeat dose.
  - Once clinically improved, then give 50 to 100 μg of thyroxine daily.
  - The TSH level should decrease by 50% per week with adequate treatment.
  - Long-term therapy includes thyroxine, titrated to normal T4 and serum TSH.

Nonthyroidal Illness Syndrome (Formerly Euthyroid Sick Syndrome)

Pathophysiology

- Secondary to severe underlying systemic illness
- Usually develops within 24 hours of critical illness
- Decreased peripheral conversion of T4 to T3 via deiodinase deficiency or inhibition
- Decreased production and function of thyroid-binding globulins
- Medications such as dopamine and steroids promote decreased TSH levels.

Sequelae

- 80% mortality occurs if T4 level drops to <2 μg/dL during the critical illness phase.
- Most patients recover as the acute illness resolves, though full recovery may take up to weeks to months.

Symptoms

- Patients are usually asymptomatic, with no overt thyroid-related symptoms.

Diagnosis

- The most common hormone pattern is a low total T3 level with low or normal T4 and TSH levels.
- Although total T4 and T3 levels are decreased and TSH levels are variable, free concentrations are usually normal; thus, the patients are clinically euthyroid.
- If the TSH level is >20 mU/mL, overt thyroid dysfunction, rather than nonthyroidal illness syndrome, should be strongly considered.

Management and Treatment

- Treatment and management of underlying medical illness is the main focus.
- Periodic monitoring of thyroid function should be done while the patient is in the hospital and no earlier than several weeks after discharge to confirm either overt thyroid dysfunction (persistent TSH abnormality) or nonthyroidal illness (normalization of TSH and T3). Nonthyroidal illness is transient and typically resolves as the acute illness subsides. Misdiagnosis of nonthyroidal illness as primary thyroid disease during the acute phase should be avoided to prevent unnecessary treatment or interventions.

- Treatment with thyroid hormone replacement therapy has NOT been shown to be of any benefit and may be harmful unless overt thyroid dysfunction is confirmed. Management should prioritize resolving the underlying critical illness.

SUGGESTED READINGS

Chaker L, Cooper DS, Walsh JP, Peeters RP. Hyperthyroidism. *Lancet*. 2024;403(10428):768-780.

Garber JR, Cobin RH, Gharib H, et al; American Association of Clinical Endocrinologists and American Thyroid Association Taskforce on Hypothyroidism in Adults. Clinical practice guidelines for hypothyroidism in adults [published correction appears in *Endocr Pract*. 2013;19(1):175]. *Endocr Pract*. 2012;18(6):988-1028.

Lee SY, Pearce EN. Hyperthyroidism: a review. *JAMA*. 2023;330(15): 1472-1483.

Wiersinga WM, Poppe KG, Effraimidis G. Hyperthyroidism: aetiology, pathogenesis, diagnosis, management, complications, and prognosis. *Lancet Diabetes Endocrinol*. 2023;11(4):282-298.

7.6

Pharmacologic Therapies for Endocrine Disorders

Gianna Lauren Casal and Jacqueline Lange

Steroids (Table 7.6.1)

- Glucocorticoids: primary effect on metabolism and inflammation
  - Cortisol, hydrocortisone, methylprednisolone, prednisone, prednisolone, dexamethasone
  - Common disease states
    - Autoimmune diseases, acute hypoxia, inflammation/airway edema, cytokine syndromes
  - Side effects: hyperglycemia, hypertension, immunosuppression, osteoporosis/necrosis, edema, adrenal atrophy, altered mental status
  - Pearls
    - Consider *Pneumocystis jirovecii* pneumonia (PJP) prophylaxis at doses >20 mg prednisone equivalents for >4 weeks. Sulfamethoxazole/trimethoprim is gold standard; can use atovaquone or pentamidine if unable.
    - In the cortisol stimulation test, acute administration of dexamethasone does not affect cortisol response to cosyntropin.
    - The stress dose steroid for adrenal insufficiency in septic shock is typically hydrocortisone, as it is the agent of choice based on current guidelines and evidence. Dose: 50 mg q6 or 100 mg q8.
- Mineralocorticoids primarily affect salt/water reabsorption and potassium excretion via distal convoluted tubules. Regulated by the renin-angiotensin-aldosterone system.
  - Aldosterone, fludrocortisone
  - Common disease states: adrenal insufficiency, orthostasis, hyponatremia, Addison disease, cerebral salt wasting, and vasogenic edema
  - Side effects: sodium and water retention, potassium excretion, Cushing syndrome

Antidiuretic Hormone (Vasopressin)

- Produced in the hypothalamus and secreted from the posterior pituitary in response to hyperosmolality or reduced blood volume, leading to stimulation of receptors:
  - V1: vasoconstriction via increased blood pressure and systemic vascular resistance
  - V2: reduces water excretion and increases water reabsorption to increase blood volume
  - Relative vasopressin deficiency in sepsis. It can be used as an adjunct vasopressor to reduce norepinephrine requirements. Generally, it does not induce tachycardia at 0.03 to 0.04 units/min.
  - It can also be used in diabetes insipidus to control polyuria.
- Desmopressin (DDAVP): antidiuretic hormone (ADH) analog
  - Longer duration of action allows for intermittent dosing (intravenous [IV], subcutaneous [SC]).
  - Commonly used for diabetes insipidus, prevention of overcorrecting hyponatremia, and uremic bleeding (0.3 µg/kg)
  - Generally, blood pressure is neutral.

Thyroid Disorders

- Hypothyroidism
  - Common etiologies: Hashimoto disease, thyroiditis, radiation
  - Levothyroxine: synthetic T4
    - Start at 1.6 µg/kg/d and titrate by 12 to 25 µg/d every 4 weeks.

TABLE 7.6.1 Steroid Comparison Chart and Relative Potencies

Class	Steroid	Equivalent Dose (mg)	Glucocorticoid Potency	Mineralocorticoid Potency
Glucocorticoid	Hydrocortisone (cortisol)	20	+	+
	Prednisone	5	++	–
	Methylprednisolone	4	++	–
Mineralocorticoid	Dexamethasone	0.75	+++++	–
Mineralocorticoid	Fludrocortisone	2	+++	+++++

- Increase by 20% to 30% as soon as pregnancy is detected.
- Half-life of enteral levothyroxine is ~7 days. Can wait at least 3 days to initiate IV therapy.
- IV:PO (oral) = 0.7:1
- While controversial, levothyroxine may be considered in organ donation candidates, particularly those with hemodynamic instability and cardiac collapse. Some guidelines and protocols recommend thyroid replacement therapy as part of a multimodal hormonal resuscitation strategy to stabilize hemodynamics and enhance organ procurement outcomes. More commonly used in candidates donating after brain death. Dose = 20 μg bolus followed by 10 μg/h infusion.

- Liothyronine: T3
  - Adjunct to levothyroxine in primary hypothyroidism if symptomatic with normal thyroid-stimulating hormone (TSH) after thyroidectomy/ablation or low T3
  - Dose: ~5% of the levothyroxine dose twice daily. Reduce levothyroxine by 80% if liothyronine is added. Ratio of levothyroxine:liothyronine should be about 13:1 to 16:1.

- Hyperthyroidism
  - Common etiologies: Graves disease, thyroiditis, toxic adenoma, toxic multimodal goiter, thyroid storm
  - Thionamides (methimazole): blocks synthesis of thyroid hormones via oxidation of iodine. Dose based on T4 levels
    - It may be combined with cholestyramine 4 g 4 times daily (qid) to enhance the enterohepatic excretion of thyroxine.
  - Glucocorticoids inhibit the conversion of peripheral T4 to T3.
  - Potassium iodide drops inhibit iodine organification, which reduces thyroid hormone synthesis. It also inhibits thyroglobulin proteolysis to inhibit the secretion of thyroid hormone.

TABLE 7.6.2 Insulin Comparison Chart

Insulin Types	Names	Frequency
Rapid	Aspart, glulisine, lispro	tid with meals
Short	Regular	q6
Intermediate	NPH	bid
Long	Detemir, glargine	q24

q, every; tid, 3 times daily.

  - Propranolol inhibits peripheral conversion of T4 to T3 and manages adrenergic symptoms. Administer IV for thyroid storm.
  - Propylthiouracil used to be recommended; however, concern for severe liver toxicity lowered its place in therapy, if at all.

Diabetes Mellitus

Insulin Therapy (Table 7.6.2)

- Increase glucose uptake by skeletal muscles and transport for glycogen synthesis
- Decreases gluconeogenesis
- Paracrine effects of suppressing glucagon secretion
- Intermediate- or long-acting insulin should be continued in type 1 diabetes, even when the patient is NPO.
- Regular insulin administered IV can be used to treat hyperkalemia. 10 units of IV regular insulin is typically administered in patients with normal renal function, while 5 units of IV regular insulin is recommended for patients at risk of hypoglycemia or with significant renal impairment. This is preceded by one ampule of D50W (50 mL of 50% dextrose) to prevent hypoglycemia.
- When utilizing enteral therapy, use a patient-centered approach when adding on agents of complementary mechanisms. Consider concomitant disease states as well as adherence.
- *See* Table 7.6.3 *for additional details.*

TABLE 7.6.3 Antihyperglycemics

Drug Class	Examples	Mechanism of Action	Weight Effect	Hypoglycemia Risk	Considerations
Secretagogues					
Sulfonylureas	Glipizide Glyburide Glimepiride	• Increased insulin secretion	↑	↑	• Hold if NPO.
Meglitinides	Repaglinide	• Increased insulin secretion	↑	↔	
GLP-1 agonist	Dulaglutide Exenatide Linaglutide Semaglutide	• Increase insulin secretion • Reduce glucagon secretion	↓	↔	• Hold peri-op can cause delayed gastric emptying or aspiration.
DPP4 inhibitor	Sitagliptin Saxagliptin	• Increase GLP-1, which increases insulin secretion	↔	↔	
Sensitizers					
Biguanides	Metformin	• Increase insulin sensitivity • Reduce gluconeogenesis	↓	↔	• Can cause lactic acidosis • Caution in renal dysfunction • Hold peri-op and with contrast administration.
Thiazolidinediones	Pioglitazone Rosiglitazone		↑	↔	

(continued)

TABLE 7.6.3 Antihyperglycemics (*continued*)

Drug Class	Examples	Mechanism of Action	Weight Effect	Hypoglycemia Risk	Considerations
Other					
SGLT-2 inhibitors	Empagliflozin Dapagliflozin Canagliflozin	• Decreased renal glucose reabsorption • Increased glucose excretion	↓	↔	• Hold peri-op, can cause euglycemic DKA. • Increasing patients given mortality benefit in HFrEF
α-Glucoside inhibitor	Acarbose	• Inhibit absorption of carbohydrates from small intestine	↓	↔	
Amylide analog	Pramlintide	• Mimics amylin to slow gastric emptying and increase satiety • Reduce glucagon secretion	↓	↔	

DKA, diabetic ketoacidosis; DPP4, dipeptidyl-peptidase-4; GLP-1, glucagon-like peptide-1; HFrEF, heart failure with reduced ejection fraction; NPO, nothing by mouth; SGLT-2, sodium-glucose cotransporter 2.

SUGGESTED READINGS

Achinger SG, Ayus JC. Use of desmopressin in hyponatremia: foe and friend. *Kidney Med*. 2019;1(2):65-70.

Alexandraki KI, Kaltsas GA, Chrousos GP. Adrenal suppression. In: Feingold KR, Anawalt B, Blackman MR, et al, eds. *Endotext* [Internet]. MDText.com, Inc; 2000. Accessed June 21, 2024. http://www.ncbi.nlm.nih.gov/books/NBK279047/

American Diabetes Association. 9. Pharmacologic approaches to glycemic treatment: *Standards of Medical Care in Diabetes—2020. Diabetes Care*. 2020;43(suppl 1):S98-S110.

Becker DE. Basic and clinical pharmacology of glucocorticosteroids. *Anesth Prog*. 2013;60(1):25-32.

Carroll R, Matfin G. Endocrine and metabolic emergencies: thyroid storm. *Ther Adv Endocrinol Metab*. 2010;1(3):139-145.

Dutta S, Kumar T, Singh S, Ambwani S, Charan J, Varthya SB. Euglycemic diabetic ketoacidosis associated with SGLT2 inhibitors: a systematic review and quantitative analysis. *J Fam Med Prim Care*. 2022;11(3):927-940.

Er C, Sule AA. Cholestyramine as monotherapy for Graves' hyperthyroidism. *Singapore Med J*. 2016;57(11):644-645.

Ericson-Neilsen W, Kaye AD. Steroids: pharmacology, complications, and practice delivery issues. *Ochsner J*. 2014;14(2):203-207.

Evans L, Rhodes A, Alhazzani W, et al. Surviving sepsis campaign: international guidelines for management of sepsis and septic shock 2021. *Crit Care Med*. 2021;49(11):e1063-e1143.

Nicolaides NC, Pavlaki AN, Maria Alexandra MA, Chrousos GP. Glucocorticoid therapy and adrenal suppression. In: Feingold KR, Anawalt B, Blackman MR, et al, eds. *Endotext* [Internet]. MDText.com, Inc; 2000. Accessed June 25, 2024. http://www.ncbi.nlm.nih.gov/books/NBK279156/

Petersen MC, Shulman GI. Mechanisms of insulin action and insulin resistance. *Physiol Rev*. 2018;98(4):2133-2223.

Russell JA, Walley KR, Singer J, et al. Vasopressin versus norepinephrine infusion in patients with septic shock. *N Engl J Med*. 2008;358(9):877-887.

Samson SL, Vellanki P, Blonde L, et al. American Association of Clinical Endocrinology consensus statement: comprehensive type 2 diabetes management algorithm—2023 update. *Endocr Pract*. 2023;29(5):305-340.

Sprung CL, Annane D, Keh D, et al. Hydrocortisone therapy for patients with septic shock. *N Engl J Med*. 2008;358(2):111-124.

Yasir M, Goyal A, Sonthalia S. Corticosteroid adverse effects. In: *StatPearls* [Internet]. StatPearls Publishing; 2024. Accessed June 21, 2024. http://www.ncbi.nlm.nih.gov/books/NBK531462/

SECTION 8

Neurology

Section Editors: Saef Izzy, Casey M. Luckhurst, and Edward A. Bittner

8.1

Coma, Encephalopathy, Delirium, and Other Altered States of Consciousness

Daniel S. Harrison and Eric S. Rosenthal

- Delirium is a neuropsychiatric syndrome characterized by:
  - A disturbance in attention (ie, reduced ability to direct, focus, sustain, and shift attention) and awareness (reduced orientation to the environment)
  - The disturbance develops over a short period of time (usually hours to days), represents a change from baseline attention and awareness, and tends to fluctuate during the day.
  - An additional disturbance in cognition (eg, memory deficit, disorientation, language, visuospatial ability, or perception)
  - The disturbances are not better explained by another preexisting, established, or evolving neurocognitive disorder and do not occur in the context of a severely reduced level of arousal, such as coma.
  - There is evidence from the history, physical examination, or laboratory findings that the disturbance is caused by the direct physiologic consequences of a general medical condition, substance intoxication or withdrawal (ie, due to drug abuse or a medication), or exposure to a toxin, or is due to multiple etiologies.
- The terms "encephalopathy" and "acute confusional state" are used interchangeably with delirium.
- Terms such as "intensive care unit (ICU) psychosis," "ICU syndrome," and "ICU delirium" are misnomers and should be avoided.
- "Altered mental status" (AMS) is a nonspecific term encompassing causes of impaired mental status, which may be either generalized (like delirium) or focal.
  - Focal neurologic deficits (including focal mental status deficits, such as aphasia) suggest against a generalized process and should prompt testing for a focal cause of altered mentation.
- Coma is a disorder of consciousness in which a patient is neither awake nor alert and cannot interact with the environment, including after noxious stimuli.
- Other disorders of consciousness in patients with widespread cerebral damage and prolonged impaired consciousness include:
  - Unresponsive wakefulness syndrome, in which spontaneous eye opening and sleep-wake cycles are present without awareness of self or the environment
  - Minimally conscious state, in which severe alteration of consciousness persists but purposeful behaviors, such as command following or visual tracking, are present

Delirium Pathophysiology

- Several complementary theories have been proposed to explain the multifactorial processes of delirium.
  - Neurotransmitter dysfunction with changes in cholinergic, dopaminergic, histaminergic, noradrenergic, gamma-aminobutyric acid (GABA), and serotonergic neurotransmission
  - Inflammatory response, potentially mediated via prostaglandins, tumor necrosis factor-alpha (TNF-α), interleukin-1 (IL-1) and IL-6 cytokines, interferons, pathogen-associated molecular patterns (PAMPs), and blood-brain barrier permeability to proteins and macrophages

TABLE 8.1.1 Selected Causes of Altered Mental Status

Common Etiologies	Life-Threatening Causes
Infection	*W*—Wernicke encephalopathy
Withdrawal	*H,H,H,H*—Hypoglycemia, Hypoxia, Hypotension, Hypertensive encephalopathy/PRES
Acute metabolic	*I*—Intracerebral hemorrhage
Trauma	*M,M*—Meningitis/encephalitis, Malignancy (brain tumor, paraneoplastic disorder, immune effector cell–associated neurotoxicity syndrome)
CNS pathology	*P*—Poisons (eg, anticholinergic excess)
Hypoxia	*S*—Seizures
Deficiencies	
Endocrine	
Acute vascular	
Toxins/drugs	
Heavy metals	

CNS, central nervous system; PRES, posterior reversible encephalopathy syndrome.

TABLE 8.1.2 Epidemiology of Delirium

Setting	Incidence of Delirium (%)
Hospitalized, medically ill patients with high-risk conditions and procedures	10-30
Hospitalized older patients	10-40
Hospitalized patients with cancer	25
Hospitalized patients infected with AIDS	30-40
Terminally ill patients	80
Surgical patients	25-50
Intensive care patients	20-80

  - Limbic-hypothalamic-pituitary-adrenal axis disturbances mediating changes in corticotropin-releasing hormone, adrenocorticotropic hormone (ACTH), cortisol, and vasopressin
  - Disruption to the basal-ganglia-thalamo-cortical circuit nodal points leading to increased vulnerability to the development of delirium
  - Oxidative stress initiated by disturbances in brain structures most vulnerable to insult (selective vulnerability) with the development of progression and dysfunction in other areas of the central nervous system (CNS) (progressive vulnerability)

Differential Diagnosis of Delirium

- Alcohol withdrawal—though patients with alcohol withdrawal may present with confusion, abrupt cessation of heavy and prolonged alcohol use combined with autonomic hyperactivity, increased tremor, insomnia, nausea, hallucinations, agitation, anxiety, or convulsions should increase suspicion for alcohol withdrawal.
- Dementia—dementia may be difficult to distinguish from delirium; however, collateral history of preexisting cognitive dysfunction with slow onset differentiates it from delirium, which develops over hours to days.
- Depression—hypoactive forms of delirium are often misdiagnosed as depression, given symptom overlap of psychomotor slowing, cognitive changes, sleep disturbances, irritability, and, in severe cases of depression, symptoms of psychosis and paranoia.
  - Attention and orientation are normal in patients who are depressed.
- Primary psychiatric disorders—symptoms of delirium may be caused by a primary psychotic disorder, or often in states of hyperactive delirium, these symptoms are thought to be due to underlying anxiety and, therefore, are erroneously treated with benzodiazepines.
  - Visual hallucinations are markedly rare in primary psychotic disorders, whereas auditory hallucinations are uncommon in delirium.
  - Furthermore, consciousness, attention, and cognition are generally not as impaired (if at all) in primary psychoses.
- Seizures—intermittent nonconvulsive seizures (NCSs) may present with a fluctuating level of arousal and may be present in up to 10% of general and 25% of neurologic critical care patients; on examination, intact command following is more suggestive of delirium than NCS. Continuous electroencephalography (cEEG) in patients with fluctuating level of arousal and impaired command following should be considered to evaluate for NCS.
- Posterior reversible encephalopathy syndrome (PRES)—likely due to breakdown of blood-brain barrier. Patients may present with confusion, depressed level of arousal, or seizure. Commonly associated with hypertension, acute or chronic kidney injury, connective tissue disorders, thrombotic microangiopathy, and selected immunomodulatory agents, such as tacrolimus. Head computed tomography (CT) classically shows predominantly subcortical white matter hypodensities, though the brainstem, cerebellum, and basal ganglia may be affected. Magnetic resonance imaging (MRI) shows T2 hyperintensities in these regions, possibly with hemorrhage, but typically without diffusion restriction.

Prevention

- Delirium may be prevented with strategies that facilitate normal orientation.
  - Promoting normal diurnal cycles
  - Stimulation of cognition and reorientation
  - Avoiding sensory deprivation (hearing aids, glasses)
  - Avoiding delirium-inducing medications

Delirium Monitoring and Management

- Definitive treatment involves quick and accurate identification of the underlying causes of delirium with the goal of correcting the underlying etiology(ies).
  - Confusion assessment method—ICU or the Intensive Care Delirium Screening Checklist (ICDSC) are both reasonable screening tools for the presence of delirium, and the ICDSC may also be used to track severity.
- Supportive care
  - Monitor vital signs, fluid intake and output, and oxygenation as indicated, taking care to discontinue unnecessary lines, tubes, drains, and monitors as soon as able
  - Provide frequent reorientation and behavioral de-escalation, as needed
  - Provide patient's glasses and hearing aids to minimize sensory deprivation
  - Treat dehydration, heart failure, and electrolyte disorders
  - Treat common infections: urinary, respiratory, soft tissue
  - Treat severe anemia, hypoxia, and hypotension
  - Identify and manage sources of pain
  - Maintain aspiration precautions
  - Discontinue deliriogenic medications
  - Assess and treat urinary retention and constipation
  - Anticipate and prevent immobility and falls
  - Avoid interruption of nighttime sleep if possible, maintain sleep-wake cycles
  - Mobilize with assistance and physical therapy as early as clinically feasible
- Pharmacologic strategies for agitation (second line after failure of nonpharmacologic de-escalation)
  - Dopamine antagonists
    - Haloperidol
      - Intravenous (IV) haloperidol is the first-line agent for the treatment of agitation in delirious patients in the ICU setting due to its minimal effects on

heart rate and blood pressure (BP). Dosing range is generally 0.5 to 20 mg IV.
            - Dose should be started at a lower dose and doubled every 15 minutes until the patient is calm (maximum single bolus 20 mg IV).
            - Avoid total daily doses of >30 mg.
        - Daily electrocardiogram (ECG) to monitor that QTc remains <550 ms in order to minimize theoretical risk for torsade de pointes.
            - Secondary analysis of 566 patients in the MIND trial did not reveal an association between haloperidol use and QTc interval prolongation.
        - Potassium and magnesium should be replete to high normal daily to assist in the minimization of QTc prolongation.
        - Relatively higher risk than atypical antipsychotics for extrapyramidal side effects (EPSs), including akathisia and acute dystonic reactions
    - Quetiapine
        - May be scheduled for patients with persistent hyperactive delirium
            - Less sedating with lower risk of EPS than typical antipsychotics like haloperidol
        - Dosing range is generally 12.5 to 200 mg 2 times daily/3 times daily (bid/tid) with a maximum of 400 mg/d.
        - In dopamine antagonist–naïve patients, doses >500 mg/d may cause anticholinergic excess (including decreased gastrointestinal motility and ileus), and this should be monitored for any patient on higher doses of quetiapine for >72 hours.
    - Olanzapine
        - Due to its anticholinergic properties, olanzapine has limited usefulness in the delirious agitated ICU patient at dosages >30 mg/d.
        - Dosing range is generally 2.5 to 15 mg and may be given every 4 hours as needed to a maximum daily dose of 30 mg.
        - Orally disintegrating tablet available, which is NOT absorbed orally, but rather is dissolved and swallowed, with absorption occurring in the stomach.
        - Avoid coadministration with IV/IM (intramuscular) benzodiazepine, given the possible association with increased mortality.
- Alpha agonists
    - Dexmedetomidine
        - Typical dosage range is 0.2 to 1.5 µg/kg/h, titrating by 0.2 µg/kg/h every 30 minutes.
        - Multiple studies have shown that dexmedetomidine is an effective agent for the control of agitation, including for the symptomatic management of alcohol withdrawal that develops in the ICU.
        - Loading doses generally should be avoided, given the potential for bradycardia and hypotension.
        - Bradycardia is a major dose-limiting side effect.
        - Hypotension may occur, particularly in association with hypovolemia, and once corrected, rechallenge may be considered.
        - Prophylactic therapy with dexmedetomidine has not shown a consistent benefit.
    - Clonidine
        - Clonidine may be used as a second- or third-line agent for the control of treatment-refractory agitation.
        - Its use may be higher yield in patients with GABA receptor withdrawal or autonomic storming from acute traumatic brain injury (TBI) with resulting diaphoresis, tachycardia, and hypertension.
- Other agents
    - Valproate
        - Valproate may be used as a second-line agent for the control of treatment-resistant agitation or for patients with prolonged QTc in whom the use of dopamine antagonists may be problematic
        - Typical starting dose of 250 mg PO tid or IV 4 times daily (qid), maximum dosage determined by serum level (total valproate 60-100 µg/mL, free valproate 5-15 µg/mL)
        - Monitor free and total valproate levels, as total valproate may not be reliable in critically ill patients.
        - Monitor for thrombocytopenia and hepatotoxicity (including isolated hyperammonemia).
    - Propranolol
        - Use of propranolol may be a reasonable second- or third-line agent for heart rate control in patients with treatment-resistant agitation.
        - It is commonly used for patients with TBI with autonomic storming and may be considered earlier in the treatment course.
        - Use of propranolol can cause AMS in certain patients.
    - Trazodone
        - Initial dose of 25 mg qHS, titrating up to 300 mg in 1 to 3 divided doses
        - May be used in patients with concomitant insomnia and agitation
        - Mild QTc prolongation has been reported in overdose.

Outcomes

- In older delirious patients:
    - Less than half of older hospital inpatients with delirium are fully recovered at the time of discharge.
    - 20% to 75% of older delirious patients die during hospitalization and 25% within 6 months of onset.
- In non-ICU patients, the development of delirium is associated with:
    - In-hospital mortality of 25% to 33%
    - Prolonged hospital stay
    - Three times increase in the chance of discharge to a nursing facility
- A prospective cohort study of mechanically ventilated patients ($n = 275$) demonstrated that patients who developed delirium had a 3-fold increase in 6-month mortality rates compared with those who did not.
- 10% increase in hazard of death (hazard ratio 1.10; 95% confidence interval, 1.02-1.18) up to 1 year after critical illness with each additional day of ICU stay.
- Delirium in the ICU is associated with longer hospital stays.
- ICU survivors may have long-term brain dysfunction (eg, functionally debilitating dementia–like illness), which appears to be predicted by delirium duration and is associated with increased rates of institutional placement.

SUGGESTED READINGS

American Psychiatric Association. *Diagnostic and Statistical Manual of Mental Disorders*. 5th ed. American Psychiatric Association; 2013.

American Psychiatric Association. Practice guideline for the treatment of patients with delirium. *Am J Psychiatry*. 1999;156:1-20.

Bamgbade OA. Dexmedetomidine for peri-operative sedation and analgesia in alcohol addiction. *Anaesthesia*. 2006;61:299-300.

Bergeron N, Dubois MJ, Dumont M, Dial S, Skrobik Y. Intensive care delirium screening checklist: evaluation of a new screening tool. *Intensive Care Med*. 2001;27:859-864.

Cassem NH, Murray GM, Lafayette JM, Stern TA. Delirious patients. In: Stern TA, Fricchione GL, Cassem NH, Jellinek MS, Rosenbaum JF, eds. *Massachusetts General Hospital Handbook of General Hospital Psychiatry*. Mosby; 2004:119-134.

Devlin JW, Roberts RJ, Fong JJ, et al. Efficacy and safety of quetiapine in critically ill patients with delirium: a prospective, multicenter, randomized, double-blind, placebo-controlled pilot study. *Crit Care Med*. 2010; 38:419-427.

Ely EW, Gautam S, Margolin R, et al. The impact of delirium in the intensive care unit on hospital length of stay. *Intensive Care Med*. 2001;27: 1892-1900.

Ely EW, Inouye SK, Bernard GR, et al. Delirium in mechanically ventilated patients: validity and reliability of the confusion assessment method for the intensive care unit (CAM-ICU). *JAMA*. 2001;286:2703-2710.

Ely EW, Shintani A, Truman B, et al. Delirium as a predictor of mortality in mechanically ventilated patients in the intensive care unit. *JAMA*. 2004;291:1753-1762.

Fann JR. The epidemiology of delirium: a review of studies and methodological issues. *Semin Clin Neuropsychiatry*. 2000;5:64-74.

Fricchione GL, Nejad SH, Esses JA, et al. Postoperative delirium. *Am J Psychiatry*. 2008;165:803-812.

Jackson JC, Gordon SM, Hart RP, Hopkins RO, Ely EW. The association between delirium and cognitive decline: a review of the empirical literature. *Neuropsychol Rev*. 2004;14:87-98.

Maclullich AM, Ferguson KJ, Miller T, de Rooij SE, Cunningham C. Unravelling the pathophysiology of delirium: a focus on the role of aberrant stress responses. *J Psychosom Res*. 2008;65(3):229-238.

Maldonado JR. Pathoetiological model of delirium: a comprehensive understanding of the neurobiology of delirium and an evidence-based approach to prevention and treatment. *Crit Care Clin*. 2008;24: 789-856; ix.

Pisani MA, Kong SY, Kasl SV, Murphy TE, Araujo KL, Van Ness PH. Days of delirium are associated with 1-year mortality in an older intensive care unit population. *Am J Respir Crit Care Med*. 2009;180:1092-1097.

Shehabi Y, Nakae H, Hammond N, Bass F, Nicholson L, Chen J. The effect of dexmedetomidine on agitation during weaning of mechanical ventilation in critically ill patients. *Anaesth Intensive Care*. 2010;38:82-90.

Skrobik YK, Bergeron N, Dumont M, Gottfried SB. Olanzapine vs haloperidol: treating delirium in a critical care setting. *Intensive Care Med*. 2004;30:444-449.

Tang JF, Chen PL, Tang EJ, May TA, Stiver SI. Dexmedetomidine controls agitation and facilitates reliable, serial neurological examinations in a non-intubated patient with traumatic brain injury. *Neurocritical Care*. 2011;15:175-181.

8.2

Status Epilepticus

Usaamah Khan and Sahar F. Zafar

Definitions

- Status epilepticus (SE) is a neurologic emergency characterized by prolonged seizure activity resulting from the failure of mechanisms that terminate seizures or from the initiation of mechanisms leading to sustained seizure activity. SE can result in irreversible neurologic injury or death if not promptly treated.
- Traditionally, SE has been defined as seizures lasting >5 minutes, or two seizures without a complete interictal recovery back to baseline.
- More recently, the working definition of SE is more nuanced and factors in seizure classification and duration. The definition is, therefore, specific to whether they are generalized convulsive or nonconvulsive seizures.
- The International League Against Epilepsy (ILAE) defines SE as 2 time points (t_1) and (t_2) to better understand the operational and contextual definition of SE and varies depending on the category of SE.
    - t_1: Duration after which seizure is abnormally prolonged from the failure of mechanisms responsible for terminating seizures or from the initiation of mechanisms that lead to abnormally prolonged seizures (treatment should begin)
    - t_2: Duration beyond which there is risk of long-term injury or death. These time points differ by seizure type:
    - *Convulsive SE*: continuous, prolonged seizure activity with prominent motor symptoms lasting at least 5 minutes (t_1 = 5 minutes). It is likely to cause long-term secondary neuronal damage if persistent for >30 minutes (t_2 = 30 minutes).
    - *Nonconvulsive status epilepticus (NCSE) or focal SE* requires at least 10 minutes of ongoing seizure activity (t_1 = 10 minutes), and it is speculated that long-term sequelae ensue at a t_2 of ~60 minutes.

Classification

Convulsive Status Epilepticus With Prominent Motor Symptoms

- The ILAE classified convulsive SE with prominent motor symptoms into various subtypes, including generalized convulsive SE, myoclonic SE, and focal motor SE.
- Generalized convulsive SE presents with continuous and prolonged seizure activity with prominent motor symptoms lasting at least 5 minutes and likely to cause long-term secondary neuronal damage if persists for >30 minutes.
- Convulsive activity is excessive abnormal muscle contractions that are usually bilateral and may be sustained or interrupted.
- Tonic flexion of the axial muscles, arms, and legs is followed by extension, clenching of teeth, forced expiration, upward or lateral eye deviation, and dilation of the pupils.
- The clonic phase is characterized by uninterrupted rhythmic jerking or muscle contractions.

    - Muscle contractions may become reduced with increased duration of the seizures, despite continued electrical seizure activity.
    - Generalized tonic-clonic SE is associated with high risk of major complications and requires aggressive treatment.
    - Generalized tonic-clonic SE carries a high mortality risk of up to 20%.
    - Generalized tonic-clonic SE is always associated with impairment in mentation.
    - Myoclonic SE presents as synchronous brief jerking of the limbs, face, or diaphragm with altered consciousness.
    - Myoclonic SE often occurs in the setting of global cerebral hypoxia (eg, postcardiac arrest, electrical injury, drug intoxication, or decompression sickness), and while it may be seizure related, it often reflects severe cortical injury with poor prognosis.
  - *SE without prominent motor symptoms (NCSE)*
    - NCSE refers to ongoing focal or generalized seizure activity without the prominent motor symptoms seen in convulsive SE.
    - Presentation can highly vary depending on whether there is generalized NCSE with or without coma, or focal NCSE with or without impairment of awareness.
    - Symptoms can range from mild confusion, an auditory, visual or gustatory aura, autonomic dysfunction, speech changes, or complete nonresponsiveness and coma.
    - NCSE is defined as at least 10 minutes of ongoing seizure activity; it is suggested that long-term sequelae in NCSE likely occur after 60 minutes of continuous seizure activity.
    - Unlike convulsive SE, NCSE diagnosis is more dependent on electroencephalogram (EEG) to identify electrographic seizures.
    - In patients on prolonged EEG monitoring, a total duration of >20% of any 60 minutes with seizure activity also meets criteria for NCSE.

Complications

- SE is a life-threatening condition that can result in a wide range of complications:
  - SE is a medical emergency and can result in irreversible neurologic injury, pyrexia and rhabdomyolysis, systemic inflammatory response, respiratory failure requiring ventilatory support, and circulatory collapse.
  - SE can result in cardiac injury due to massive catecholamine release, and an extreme metabolic stress associated with muscular convulsions can contribute to poor outcomes.
  - Prolonged seizure activity leads to internalization of GABA-A receptors and increased NMDA receptor expression, contributing to pharmacoresistance.

Common Causes to Remember

- Structural brain injury (tumor, stroke, subarachnoid hemorrhage)
- Metabolic and electrolyte abnormalities (hypoglycemia or hyperglycemia, uremia, hepatic encephalopathy, potassium or magnesium abnormalities)
- Central nervous system (CNS) infections (herpes simplex virus [HSV] encephalitis, bacterial/viral meningitis, HIV)
- Autoimmune or paraneoplastic encephalitides
- Withdrawal syndromes (alcohol, benzodiazepines, barbiturates)
- Antiseizure medication nonadherence
- Drugs that lower the seizure threshold (certain antibiotics including quinolones, metronidazole, and imipenem; tricyclic antidepressants; local anesthetics)

Epidemiology

- Affects 100 to 200,000 people in the United States per year
- Incidence is between 7 and 35 patients per intensive care unit (ICU) admission.
- Refractory to first- and second-line drug therapy in 30% to 43% of patients
- Associated mortality is 20% to 80% (higher after anoxic brain injury).

Key Pathophysiology

- The pathophysiology of SE is not well understood but can be divided into predispositions, that is, conditions that increase the likelihood of SE, and precipitants.
- Opening of ion channels that are coupled to excitatory amino acids (AMPA, NMDA, and metabotropic channels) can raise intracellular free calcium and lead to the generation of nitric oxide and oxygen free radicals, as well as phosphorylation of enzymes and receptor systems that result in an increased intracellular osmolality and neuronal swelling.
- Failure of adenosine triphosphate production and activation of immediate—early genes with the production of heat shock proteins have also been implicated.
- Hypersynchrony of neuronal circuits, increased density of synapses and gap junctions, and formation of sprouting and abnormal connections have been reported in temporal lobe epilepsy.
- The increased neuronal activity during SE elevates demand for oxygen and glucose, which can be partly compensated for through an increase in cerebral blood flow, but as energy supplies become exhausted, cellular ion pumps start to fail, initiating a cascade of events that can lead to irreversible neurologic injury.

Differential Diagnosis

- Hypoglycemia, hypoxia, or other metabolic or infectious encephalopathies
- Structural brain or brainstem injuries (eg, pontine lesions)
- Movement disorders (eg, tremors, dystonia)
- Psychogenic nonepileptic seizures: bilateral motor movements with preserved consciousness and normal EEG recordings. Creatinine kinase levels are not elevated.
- Syncope: impairment of arousal and loss of postural tone caused by vasovagal reaction, cardiac dysrhythmias, or neurologic and psychiatric disease. It is often self-limited and followed by complete recovery.
- Narcolepsy: a sleep disorder in which rapid eye movement sleep invades normal wakefulness

Management and Treatment

- Initial treatment includes airway control and support of respiration and circulation, as indicated.
- Generalized convulsive SE has a very high mortality rate of roughly 20% and, therefore, warrants prompt recognition and aggressive treatment.
- The algorithm below is largely applicable to the treatment and management of generalized convulsive SE.
- Thiamine (100 mg intravenous [IV]) and glucose (50 mL of 50% dextrose) should be administered when etiology is unknown, or if hypoglycemia or alcohol withdrawal is suspected.
- Correct obvious metabolic abnormalities (potassium, sodium, magnesium).
- Pharmacologic treatment options include benzodiazepines and antiseizure medications, such as levetiracetam, valproic acid, and phenytoin. For more refractory cases, escalation to the use of sedating anesthetics, such as propofol or midazolam infusions, is often used. Further escalation to use of agents such as ketamine infusion or barbiturates such as pentobarbital infusion may also be indicated for very refractory cases.
- Initial benzodiazepine treatment should ideally be administered IV or intramuscularly, but if formulation is not readily available, diazepam can be given through alternative routes (rectal, intranasal, or buccal mucosa).
- *First-line treatment*
    - Lorazepam is considered a first-line treatment for SE, despite its risk for respiratory depression.
    - It can be administered IV at the dose of −0.1 mg/kg (1-4 mg doses). Lack of response after 5 minutes should be considered a failure.
    - Midazolam is also an alternative agent and can be dosed at 10 mg bolus.
- *Second-line treatment*
    - Second-line antiseizure medication options include:
        - Levetiracetam at a loading dose of 60 mg/kg with a maximum dose of 4 g (in normal renal function)
        - Valproic acid at a loading dose of 40 mg/kg with a maximum dose of 3 g
        - Phenytoin at a loading dose of 20 mg/kg with a maximum dose of 1,500 mg

    Choice of antiseizure agent should be guided by comorbidities and possible drug-drug interactions for each patient.
    - In circumstances where seizure activity continues to occur, using a combination of the abovementioned medications in adjunct is also a reasonable escalation of treatment.
    - Electrocardiogram (ECG) should be continuously monitored for arrhythmias, including bradycardia and heart block.
    - Fosphenytoin, a water-soluble form of phenytoin, lacks the propylene glycol vehicle that has been implicated in the hypotension and arrhythmias associated with phenytoin administration.
- *Third-line treatment*
    - If seizure continues despite first- and second-line treatments, use of sedating anesthetics such as propofol or midazolam infusion should be utilized for seizure cessation. Airway should be promptly secured with intubation for ventilatory support, and the patient should be admitted to the ICU.
    - Prompt placement of a continuous EEG is imperative to assess for further electrographic seizure activity and the need for further escalation of therapy.
    - In refractory cases where seizures continue despite use of sedating medications such as propofol and midazolam, consideration for agents such ketamine (NMDA antagonist) or pentobarbital (barbiturate) should be considered.
    - If refractory seizures are secondary to a reversible structural etiology (eg, subdural hematoma), refractory seizures are an indication for urgent surgical evacuation.
    - In circumstances where refractory seizures are suspected in the setting of an inflammatory or autoimmune process, prompt treatment with high-dose steroids and immunotherapy such as IV immunoglobulin or plasmapheresis is considered an essential part of the treatment.
    - Lidocaine (3-4 mg/kg/h) stabilizes cell membranes and has been used with some success, but prolonged use has been associated with significant toxicity and exacerbation of seizures.
    - Therapeutic hypothermia may be considered to reduce cerebral metabolic rate oxygen demands and excitotoxic transmission; however, the evidence around this remains controversial. As per the HYBERNATUS trial, adverse effects associated with hypothermia may outweigh potential benefits. Acute use of neuromodulatory strategies such as vagal nerve or deep brain stimulation, responsive nerve stimulation, and transcranial magnetic stimulation has been investigated and remains an option at the provider's discretion.
- Treatment of complications
    - Hypervolemia and alkalinization of urine should be considered if rhabdomyolysis is suspected.
    - External cooling may be required to prevent hyperthermia if SE is not rapidly terminated.
    - Vasogenic cerebral edema may complicate SE and can lead to increased intracranial pressure, which may require aggressive pharmacologic management.

SUGGESTED READINGS

Bleck TP. Management approaches to prolonged seizures and status epilepticus. *Epilepsia*. 1999;40(suppl 1):S59-S63.

Bleck TP, Smith MC, Pierre-Louis JC, Jares JJ, Murray J, Hansen CA. Neurologic complications of critical medical illness. *Crit Care Med*. 1993;21:98-103.

Chen JW, Wasterlain CG. Status epilepticus: pathophysiology and management in adults. *Lancet Neurol*. 2006;5(3):246-256.

Dobesberger J, Ristić AJ, Walser G, et al. Duration of focal complex, secondarily generalized tonic–clonic, and primarily generalized tonic–clonic seizures—a video-EEG analysis. *Epilepsy Behav*. 2015;49:111-117.

Fountain NB, Lothman EW. Pathophysiology of status epilepticus. *J Clin Neurophysiol*. 1995;12:326-342.

Glauser T, Shinnar S, Gloss D, et al. Evidence-based guideline: treatment of convulsive status epilepticus in children and adults: report of the Guideline Committee of the American Epilepsy Society. *Epilepsy Curr*. 2016;16(1):48-61.

Hirsch LJ, Fong MWK, Leitinger M, et al. American Clinical Neurophysiology Society's standardized critical care EEG terminology: 2021 version. *J Clin Neurophysiol*. 2021;38(1):1-29.

Kaplan PW. Nonconvulsive status epilepticus. *Semin Neurol*. 1996;16:33-40.

Lorenzo RJ, Pellock JM, Towne AR, Boggs JG. Epidemiology of status epilepticus. *J Clin Neurophysiol*. 1995;12(4):316.

Privitera M, Hoffman M, Moore JL, Jester D. EEG detection of nontonic-clonic status epilepticus in patients with altered consciousness. *Epilepsy Res*. 1994;18(2):155.

Treiman DM. Generalized convulsive status epilepticus in the adult. *Epilepsia*. 1993;34(suppl 1):S2-S11.

Trieman DM, Meyers PD, Walton NY, et al; Veterans Affairs Status Epilepticus Cooperative Study Group. A comparison of four treatments for generalized convulsive status epilepticus. *N Engl J Med*. 1998;339(12):792-798.

Trinka E, Cock H, Hesdorffer D, et al. A definition and classification of status epilepticus—report of the ILAE task force on classification of status epilepticus. *Epilepsia*. 2015;56(10):1515-1523.

Trinka E, Rainer LJ, Granbichler CA, Zimmermann G, Leitinger M. Mortality, and life expectancy in epilepsy and status epilepticus—current trends and future aspects. *Front Epidemiol*. 2023;3:1081757.

Wijdicks EFM, Sharbrough FW. New-onset seizures in critically ill patients. *Neurology*. 1993;43:1042-1044.

8.3

Depressive Disorders

Karan S. Hingorani and Saef Izzy

Overview

There are four major types of mood episodes of which physicians should be aware when diagnosing mood disorders as defined by the *Diagnostic and Statistical Manual of Mental Disorders*, Fifth Edition. It is necessary to understand that these mood disorders are not attributable to a substance or another medical condition.

- Depressive
  - Characterized by depressed mood or anhedonia (the inability to experience pleasure) for most of the day, nearly every day, for at least 2 weeks and is accompanied by five or more of the following:
    - Alterations in sleep
    - Lack of interest
    - Excessive feelings of guilt or worthlessness
    - Low energy
    - Poor concentration
    - Change in appetite
    - Psychomotor agitation or retardation
    - Suicidal thoughts or behaviors
- Manic
  - Characterized by an elevated or irritable mood lasting for at least 1 week and accompanied by three or more (four or more if mood is only irritable) of the following:
    - Distractibility
    - Decreased need for sleep
    - Grandiosity or elevated self-esteem
    - Racing thoughts
    - Increased goal-directed activity or agitation
    - Talkativeness or pressured speech
    - Excessive engagement in pleasurable but risky activities
  - The symptoms lead to a marked disturbance in functioning or necessitate psychiatric hospitalization.
- Hypomanic
  - Characterized by an elevated or irritable mood lasting for at least 4 days and accompanied by three or more manic symptoms (four or more if mood is irritable and not elevated)
  - These symptoms indicate a definite change in functioning that is noticed by others but is not severe enough to cause a marked impairment in social or occupational functioning, does not necessitate hospitalization, and is not accompanied by psychotic symptoms.
- Manic or hypomanic episode with mixed features
  - Full criteria met for manic or hypomanic episode and at least three of the following symptoms are present during the majority of days of the manic/hypomanic episode:
  - Prominent dysphoria
  - Diminished interest/pleasure
  - Near-daily psychomotor retardation
  - Feelings of worthlessness/guilt
  - Recurrent thoughts of death/suicidal ideation with a plan
  - Fatigue

Definitions of Major Mood Disorders

- Major depressive disorder (MDD) is characterized by recurrent depressive episodes and by an absence of manic or hypomanic episodes.
- Bipolar I disorder is characterized by at least one manic episode with or without depressive episodes.
- Bipolar II disorder is characterized by at least one depressive episode, at least one hypomanic episode, and no manic episodes.

Definition of Persistent Depressive Disorder

- Depressed mood for most of the day for at least 2 years, accompanied by two or more: (1) changes in appetite, (2) changes in sleep, (3) low energy, (4) poor self-esteem, (5) poor concentration, or (6) hopelessness
- These patients have no history of depressive episodes (in the first 2 years of these symptoms) and have not been free from symptoms for >2 months during the 2-year period.

Definition of Adjustment Disorder

- Clinically significant, emotional, and behavioral symptoms in response to an *identifiable* stressor occurring within 3 months of the onset of the stressor
- These symptoms are out of proportion to what would be expected or significantly impact patient functioning and must resolve within 6 months of the termination of the stressor.
- The stress-related disturbance does not meet criteria for another mental disorder or an exacerbation of a previously known disorder or represent bereavement.

It is important to differentiate MDD from bipolar and adjustment disorders, as treatment and prognosis differ significantly among these disorders.

Other Affective States Frequently Seen in the Intensive Care Unit

- Apathy: indifference
- Abulia: a lack of motivation that is more severe than apathy
- These affective/motivational states can frequently be seen in patients with delirium or other medical disorders impacting psychiatric function.

Common Causes to Remember (Table 8.3.1)

TABLE 8.3.1 Common Causes of Affective States

• Normal reaction to trauma/illness
• Biologic/genetic factors (though no specific genes implicated)
• Substance induced
  • Alcohol
  • Cocaine
  • Stimulants
• Medications
  • Neurologic medications
  • Corticosteroids
  • HIV medications
• Interferon-alpha
	• General medical conditions
	  • Metabolic disturbances (hyponatremia, hypercalcemia)
	  • Cerebrovascular disease
	  • Neurodegenerative disorders (Parkinson, Huntington, multiple sclerosis)
	  • HIV/AIDS
	  • Nutritional deficiencies (B_{12}, folate)
	  • Malignancies
	  • Chronic illness (coronary artery disease, heart failure, end-stage renal disease, diabetes mellitus)

Epidemiology

- Lifetime prevalence of MDD in the general population: 13.3% to 17.1%
- Prevalence of depression in the intensive care unit (ICU) population
  - Very few studies have evaluated the prevalence of depression in patients admitted to the ICU, as many symptoms of depression are experienced in the setting of acute illness, even in the absence of a primary psychiatric disorder.
  - However, patients admitted to the ICU are at high risk for depression in the months following discharge.
  - Up to 28% of patients may suffer from clinically significant depressive symptoms by 1 month postdischarge, and some studies estimate 12% may have MDD at 1 year.
  - In-hospital psychosis and low levels of optimism have been correlated with postdischarge depression in some studies.

Key Pathophysiology

- The theories of MDD pathogenesis are multifactorial and invoke several hypotheses, including genetic anomalies, dysregulation of the hypothalamic-pituitary-adrenal (HPA) axis and monoaminergic pathways, inflammation, structural and functional brain remodeling, and environmental stressors.
  - Abnormalities in biogenic amines
    - Dysregulation of serotonin, norepinephrine, and dopamine has been implicated in the pathogenesis of some of the symptoms of MDD.
    - Medications that increase or enhance dopaminergic, serotonergic, and noradrenergic neurotransmission are frequently proposed to have antidepressant effects.
  - Abnormalities in the HPA axis
    - Hypersecretion of cortisol has been associated with MDD.
    - Evidence for this comes from findings that many patients with MDD fail to suppress cortisol production when given a dose of dexamethasone.
  - Structural and functional brain remodeling
    - Recent research has shown a link between decreased hippocampal neurogenesis and low levels of brain-derived neurotrophic factor (BDNF)—vital in neuronal plasticity and neuroprotection in the brains of depressed individuals.
    - Selective serotonin reuptake inhibitors (SSRIs) and ketamine are proposed to increase BDNF levels.

Differential Diagnosis for Major Depressive Disorder

- Bipolar disorder (see earlier)
- Dysthymic disorder (see earlier)
- Adjustment disorder (see earlier)
- Schizoaffective disorder—major depressive episode concurrent with schizophrenia criteria (delusions, hallucinations, disorganized speech, negative symptoms, disorganized behavior/catatonia for a significant portion in a 1-month period)
- Delirium
  - A disorder of disturbed attention and awareness with an acute change from baseline with fluctuation over the course of the day, and this disturbance is not better explained by an established neurologic disease affecting arousal or by medications or other drugs
    - Inattention
    - Perceptual disturbances
    - Cognitive changes (disorientation, memory deficits, language disturbance)
  - The patient's level of consciousness tends to fluctuate over the course of the day.
  - Delirium is the direct physiologic consequence of a medical illness but is not better explained by existing or evolving neurocognitive disorders or disorders causing a coma.
  - Patients with hypoactive delirium (ie, those patients without significant agitation but with greater degrees of withdrawal and sedation) are often mistaken for being depressed.
    - It is important to remember, however, that attention and orientation remain normal in depressed patients, distinguishing them from those with hypoactive delirium.
- Dementia
  - A disorder with a gradual onset and progressive course (months to years), which is characterized by
    - Memory impairment
    - Aphasia (language abnormalities)

- Apraxia (motor abnormalities)
- Agnosia (inability to recognize and identify objects)
- Executive dysfunction (poor planning, sequencing, etc)
- Differentiated from depression by its prominent cognitive deficits, its gradual onset, and its progressive as opposed to fluctuating course

- Substance-induced mood disorder
  - Common in patients who are intoxicated or withdrawing from substances; however, they can persist for several weeks after withdrawal is complete
  - Common causes of illicit drugs
    - Withdrawal from cocaine
    - Withdrawal from methamphetamine or other stimulants
    - Intoxication with or withdrawal from alcohol
    - Intoxication/withdrawal from opioid medications
  - Prescribed medications that have been associated with depression:
    - Neurologic medications: benzodiazepines, vigabatrin, topiramate, flunarizine
    - Corticosteroids
    - Antimalarial medications: mefloquine
    - Human immunodeficiency virus (HIV) medications: efavirenz
    - Hepatitis C virus medications: interferon-alpha
  - Correlation between depressive symptoms and the initiation or withdrawal of a medication/substance is useful to determine the likelihood that the depressive symptoms are related to the substance.
- Mood disorder secondary to a general medical condition
  - Endocrine disorders: hypothyroidism, adrenal disorders
  - Nutritional deficiencies (vitamin B_{12}, folate, niacin)
  - Metabolic abnormalities (hyponatremia, hypercalcemia)
  - Anemia
  - Chronic illness
    - Malignancy (eg, pancreatic cancer)
    - Cardiovascular disease (coronary artery disease [CAD], congestive heart failure)
    - Diabetes mellitus
    - End-stage renal disease
    - HIV
  - Neurologic disease
    - Cerebrovascular disease—most commonly involving the L hemisphere in the prefrontal cortex or basal ganglia
    - Parkinson disease
    - Huntington disease
    - Multiple sclerosis

Initial Laboratory Workup

- First line: basic metabolic panel, complete blood count, B_{12}, folate, thyroid-stimulating hormone (TSH)
- Second line: liver function tests, head imaging, HIV

Management and Treatment

- Supportive treatment
  - Utilized when
    - It is unclear if the diagnosis is delirium or depression (cannot make a new diagnosis of depression based on a patient's presentation when they are delirious).
    - Medical illness is so acute that pharmacologic treatments for depression would be potentially harmful to the patient.
- SSRIs
  - First-line treatment for MDD
  - In a large-scale, community-based study, citalopram (a representative SSRI) was shown to be moderately effective at ameliorating depressive symptoms, with a 47% response rate (reduction in symptoms by at least 50%) and a 30% remission rate (reduction of symptoms to below the level of MDD).
  - Typically well tolerated with few side effects (most commonly gastrointestinal [GI] upset and sexual side effects)
  - Potential serious side effects include induction of mania, worsening suicidal thoughts and behaviors, and hyponatremia (via syndrome of inappropriate antidiuretic hormone secretion [SIADH]).
  - Some benefits are usually apparent within 2 weeks, but the full effect can take 6 to 8 weeks.
  - All SSRIs are hepatically metabolized, and many can interact with other medications used in the critical care setting.
    - Citalopram is typically the least likely SSRI to interact with other medications and is, therefore, often utilized in the critical care population.
    - However, citalopram has been associated with QTc prolongation at doses >40 mg/d.
  - For patients who cannot swallow medications or have absorption problems, a liquid form of fluoxetine is available.
    - This is absorbed sublingually and, therefore, may be used in this population.
  - SSRI withdrawal
    - The abrupt discontinuation of SSRIs (especially those with a short half-life [most notably paroxetine]) can lead to withdrawal symptom, characterized by dizziness, nausea, nervousness, and electric shock-like sensations.
      - This is uncomfortable for the patient, but not dangerous.
    - Fluoxetine has the longest half-life of the SSRIs (fluoxetine half-life is 4-6 days, norfluoxetine half-life is 9 days) and, therefore, is the least likely to have a significant discontinuation/withdrawal syndrome.
    - If a patient has significant withdrawal symptoms, a 20-mg dose of fluoxetine can be given.
      - This will self-taper over the next several days and usually solves the problem.
- Serotonin-norepinephrine reuptake inhibitors (SNRIs)
  - Venlafaxine and duloxetine
  - Considered first line and are alternatives to SSRIs
  - Typically well tolerated when SSRIs have failed or when patients have concurrent neuropathic pain, as these medications have the added benefit of helping with neuropathic pain
  - Some benefits are usually apparent within 2 weeks, but the full effect can take 6 to 8 weeks.
  - Similar to SSRIs, these are fairly well tolerated, with the most common side effects being GI disturbance and sexual side effects.
  - They can also induce mania in patients with bipolar disorder and can worsen suicidal thoughts and behaviors.

  - Venlafaxine has been associated with mild increases in blood pressure and, therefore, should be used with caution in patients with significant autonomic hyperactivity or instability.
  - Venlafaxine has also been associated with a relatively benign but unpleasant withdrawal syndrome, which is related to its short half-life.
    - This is indistinguishable from the SSRI withdrawal syndrome described earlier.
- Dopamine-norepinephrine reuptake inhibitors
  - Most commonly used is bupropion
  - Considered first line and an alternative to SSRIs and SNRIs
  - Often used in patients with prominent anergia, as it can increase energy
  - It is also used in patients with poor response to SSRIs or in patients with SSRI-associated sexual side effects (bupropion typically does not cause sexual side effects and in fact can improve them in patients on concurrent SSRI therapy).
  - Some benefits are usually apparent within 2 weeks, but the full effect can take 6 to 8 weeks.
  - Can be activating and may lead to increased anxiety or jitteriness
  - Potential side effects
    - Anxiety, jitteriness, or restlessness
    - Induction of mania, worsening suicidal thoughts and behaviors
    - Seizures (particularly at higher doses and in patients with eating disorders)
    - Auditory and visual hallucinations (rare, but possible given its action of increasing dopamine neurotransmission)
- Tricyclic antidepressants
  - Can be useful for patients with depressive symptoms with comorbid neuropathic pain
  - However, should be considered second or third line in many critically ill patients, given the potential for cardiac conduction abnormalities (PR, QRS, and QTc prolongation)
  - Important side effects include orthostatic hypotension, arrhythmias, confusion (secondary to anticholinergic properties), induction of mania, and worsening suicidal thoughts and behaviors.
- Monoamine oxidase inhibitors (MAOIs)
  - Typically thought of as third line for the treatment of depression
    - However, they can be helpful in patients who have failed several other antidepressant trials in the past.
  - Patients taking these medications must comply with a tyramine-free diet, as the combination of an MAOI and tyramine can lead to hypertensive crisis.
  - The combination of an MAOI and stimulant can also lead to hypertensive crisis.
  - MAOIs can also interact with other antidepressants or antibiotics (especially SSRIs or linezolid) and can lead to serotonin syndrome.
  - Selegiline comes in a transdermal form that does not require the dietary restrictions at the 6 mg/d dose.
    - This may be useful for patients who are unable to take medications orally (po) or who have malabsorption syndromes.
- Stimulants
  - Most commonly used are methylphenidate and dextroamphetamine.
  - These medications have the benefit of increasing energy, interest, and appetite (in contrast to the effects of long-term amphetamine use or abuse, where they suppress appetite).
  - The effects of the medications are typically seen within 1 to 2 hours after a dose and usually last for 4 to 6 hours.
    - This means you can see the results quickly!
  - These medications can sometimes be used to target low energy and poor appetite in patients without an actual diagnosis of MDD and still can provide symptomatic improvement.
    - This is in contrast to SSRIs and other antidepressants, which are generally helpful only in patients with a true diagnosis of MDD.
  - For patients who cannot tolerate medications po or who have GI absorption problems, a transdermal form of methylphenidate is available.
  - Potential side effects
    - Increased heart rate and blood pressure (this can lead to increased myocardial demand and potentially ischemia in patients with severe CAD or decompensated heart failure)
    - Confusion, auditory, and visual hallucinations (these should be avoided in patients with delirium)
    - Suicidal thoughts and behaviors
    - Induction of mania
- Electroconvulsive therapy (ECT)
  - ECT is considered first-line treatment for depressed patients who:
    - Have failed multiple medication/psychotherapy trials
    - Have prominent psychotic symptoms or catatonia
    - Have an urgent need for response (eg, those who are acutely suicidal and try to harm themselves repeatedly in hospital, those who are refusing food and water)
    - Have had a good response to ECT in the past
    - Express a preference for ECT
  - It is useful because it can often help patients improve in a matter of days (as opposed to antidepressants, which can take several weeks to have an effect).
  - ECT has also been shown to be more effective than pharmacotherapy, with remission rates of up to 80%.
  - The most important side effects include cognitive impairment and cardiovascular side effects.
    - ECT causes an initial burst of parasympathetic activity (can lead to bradyarrhythmias), followed by significant sympathetic outflow (which can lead to hypertension, tachycardia, and, potentially, cardiac ischemia), followed by parasympathetic activity again.
- Sleep aides
  - Trazodone
    - An antidepressant in higher doses, this medication can be helpful at much lower doses (25-200 mg every night at bedtime [qhs]) for the treatment of insomnia.
    - A good choice initially as it often does not contribute to confusion/delirium and is fairly well tolerated
    - It has a long half-life, so it not only helps with initiation of sleep, but it also can assist with maintenance of sleep.

- The most notable side effects include sedation (which can linger into the morning), priapism, and the other typical side effects of antidepressants.
- Mirtazapine
  - An antidepressant that works by antagonizing 5-HT_2 and alpha-2 adrenergic receptors.
  - Commonly used in doses of 7.5 to 45 mg po qhs
    - Interestingly, lower doses are typically more helpful for insomnia than higher doses, while doses of 15 to 45 mg qhs are standard for the treatment of depression.
  - Often used for depression and insomnia in patients with poor sleep and low appetite, as mirtazapine typically stimulates appetite and is sedating
  - Potentially serious side effects include confusion or delirium, induction of mania, and worsening suicidal thoughts and behaviors.
- Atypical antipsychotics (quetiapine and olanzapine most commonly)
  - Olanzapine and quetiapine are often helpful for sleep and are less likely to cause confusion/delirium than other sleep aides available.
  - The most common side effects in the short term include restlessness, orthostatic hypotension, and sedation.
  - These are typically not optimal medications for the regulation of sleep in the long term, as they are associated with weight gain, hyperlipidemia, diabetes mellitus, tardive dyskinesia, and other side effects.
- Benzodiazepines (lorazepam most commonly)
  - Can be helpful for insomnia, especially when the insomnia is associated with significant anxiety
  - These medications are often avoided in the critically ill patient, as they can contribute to delirium and confusion.
  - Other potential side effects include tolerance, withdrawal symptoms, seizures (in long-term use and at higher doses), potential for abuse, dependency or diversion, falls (in the older adults), and interactions with other gamma-aminobutyric acid (GABA)-ergic agents.
- Anesthetics
  - Intranasal esketamine has shown promise and has received regulatory approval for refractory depression.
  - Proposed to work through glutamatergic neuromodulation to enhance the effects of SSRI and SNRIs
  - Most common side effects include nausea, dizziness, headache, and dissociation.
- Neuroactive steroids
  - Zuranolone has been approved specifically for postpartum depression in the United States.
  - Hypothesized to work by binding $GABA_A$ at an allosteric site, causing positive modulation and augmenting $GABA_A$ activity
  - Most common side effects include drowsiness, somnolence, fatigue, and urinary tract infections (UTIs).

Acknowledgments

We gratefully acknowledge the contributions of previous edition authors, Shamim H. Nejad and Christopher M. Celano, as portions of those chapters have been retained in this revision.

SUGGESTED READINGS

American Psychiatric Association. (2013). Diagnostic and statistical manual of mental disorders (5th ed.). https://doi.org/10.1176/appi.books.9780890425596.

Cui L, Li S, Wang S, et al. Major depressive disorder: hypothesis, mechanism, prevention and treatment. *Signal Transduct Target Ther*. 2024;9(1):30.

Cutler AJ, Mattingly GW, Maletic V. Understanding the mechanism of action and clinical effects of neuroactive steroids and GABAergic compounds in major depressive disorder. *Transl Psychiatry*. 2023;13(1):228.

Davydow DS, Gifford JM, Desai SV, Bienvenu OJ, Needham DM. Depression in general intensive care unit survivors: a systematic review. *Intensive Care Med*. 2009;35(5):796-809.

European Delirium Association; American Delirium Society. The DSM-5 criteria, level of arousal and delirium diagnosis: inclusiveness is safer. *BMC Med*. 2014;12(1):141.

Kennis M, Gerritsen L, van Dalen M, Williams A, Cuijpers P, Bockting C. Prospective biomarkers of major depressive disorder: a systematic review and meta-analysis. *Mol Psychiatry*. 2020;25(2):321-338.

Nikolin S, Rodgers A, Schwaab A, et al. Ketamine for the treatment of major depression: a systematic review and meta-analysis. *EClinicalMedicine*. 2023;62:102127.

Phillips C. Brain-derived neurotrophic factor, depression, and physical activity: making the neuroplastic connection. *Neural Plast*. 2017;2017(1):7260130.

Swainson J, Thomas RK, Archer S, et al. Esketamine for treatment resistant depression. *Expert Rev Neurother*. 2019;19(10):899-911

Yoo KH, Lee J, Oh J, et al. Depression or anxiety and long-term mortality among adult survivors of intensive care unit: a population-based cohort study. *Crit Care*. 2025;29(1):179.

8.4

Central Nervous System Infections

Amjad Elmashala and Nirupama Yechoor

- Infections of the central nervous system (CNS) can involve various anatomic structures, namely, the meninges resulting in meningitis, the brain parenchyma resulting in encephalitis or cerebral abscesses, or the spinal cord resulting in myelitis.
- They are associated with significant morbidity and mortality, partly due to diagnostic and therapeutic challenges.
- CNS infections are attributed to bacteria, viruses, fungi, parasites, and prions.
- A detailed history is key, including past medical and neurologic history, travel history, sick contacts, environmental exposures, immunocompetency, and history of neurosurgical procedures.
- Initial diagnostic workup includes a complete blood count, comprehensive metabolic panel, inflammatory markers, blood cultures, and lumbar puncture (LP) for cerebrospinal fluid (CSF) analysis.
- A multidisciplinary management approach is essential for the successful treatment of patients who are critically ill; this encompasses infectious disease, neurocritical care, and neurosurgery teams.

Meningitis

- Inflammation of the meninges, the tissues surrounding the brain and the spinal cord
- Meningoencephalitis refers to when the brain parenchyma is concurrently involved.
- Most commonly due to infections, but other etiologies include inflammatory diseases (autoimmune and rheumatologic), malignancy (leptomeningeal disease), and iatrogenic causes (medication side effects).
- Infectious etiologies are attributed to bacteria (including tuberculosis), viruses, fungi, and parasites.
- Classified by time course into acute (<4 weeks) and chronic (>4 weeks)
- Acute infectious meningitis is most commonly bacterial or viral, whereas chronic infectious meningitis is most commonly fungal or mycobacterial in etiology.
- Symptomatology is commonly characterized by fever, headache, neck stiffness, focal neurologic deficits, seizures, and altered mental status.
- CSF characteristics include pleocytosis (high white blood cell count) and elevated protein with or without low CSF glucose (Table 8.4.1).
- Magnetic resonance imaging (MRI) of the brain, which is the most sensitive imaging modality, can show inflammation of the meninges following contrast administration.
- MRI can identify signs of structural changes, increased intracranial pressure (ICP), and track disease progression.
- Definitive diagnosis is most often made by detecting pathogens via polymerase chain reaction (PCR), antigen tests, stains, or cultures.
- Patient with severe meningitis can suffer from increased ICP, which may impair cerebral perfusion, leading to ischemia, or cause herniation.
- There are no specific guidelines for ICP monitoring in meningitis; however, some experts suggest its use as an adjunct in management since its elevation has been shown to be a poor prognostic indicator.

Acute Bacterial Meningitis

- Most common pathogens implicated are *Streptococcus pneumoniae* (most common), *Neisseria meningitidis*, and *Haemophilus influenzae.*
- Source of acute bacterial meningitis (ABM) can be via direct spread from upper respiratory tract infections, otitis media, or sinusitis; via bacteremia from a distant source of infection; or via the introduction of pathogens following neurosurgical procedures.
- Blood cultures should be obtained as soon as possible and are positive in 70% of patients.
- Diagnostic tests (imaging and LP) should never delay initiation of treatment.
- Imaging prior to LP is indicated when there is concern for increased ICP due to the risk of worsening brain herniation with removal of CSF.

TABLE 8.4.1 Comparison of CSF Profiles for Bacterial, Tuberculous, Viral, and Fungal Meningitis

Category	Macroscopic Appearance	Cells	Protein (mg/dL)	Glucose (mg/dL)
Normal	Clear	<5 lymphocytes/mm^3	15-45	50-75
Bacterial meningitis	Cloudy or turbid	Increased (>200) Typically >90% PMNs	>100	<40
Tuberculous meningitis	Cloudy or turbid	Increased (100-400); PMNs early but converts to lymphocytic later	100-900	<40
Viral meningitis	Clear or opalescent	Increased; may have PMNs early but converts to lymphocytic type within 12-24 h	Usually <100	Normal
Fungal meningitis	Cloudy or turbid	Increased (100-400) with lymphocytic predominance	100-900	<40

CSF, cerebrospinal fluid; PMNs, polymorphonuclear cells.

- Infectious Disease Society of America guidelines recommend imaging if a patient has focal neurologic deficits, coma, new-onset seizures, papilledema, or an immunocompromised state.

Treatment

- Community-acquired meningitis: third-generation cephalosporins (ceftriaxone) to cover for *S. pneumoniae* and *N. meningitidis* and vancomycin to cover potentially ceftriaxone-resistant *S. pneumoniae* species.
- In patients who are immunocompromised or older than 50 years of age, ampicillin is added to the abovementioned regimen to cover for *Listeria monocytogenes*.
- Nosocomial meningitis (health care or recent neurosurgical procedure related): vancomycin and additional coverage for *Pseudomonas aeruginosa* is indicated with ceftazidime, cefepime, or meropenem.
- If meningoencephalitis is suspected, acyclovir is added empirically until herpes simplex virus (HSV) encephalitis is ruled out, given high morbidity and mortality.
- Steroids should be administered before or with the first dose of antibiotics, as they are associated with mortality benefits in adults with *S. pneumoniae* meningitis and reduce rates of hearing loss in children with *N. meningitidis*.
- Typical duration of treatment is 7 to 21 days depending on the etiology.

Viral Meningitis

- Viral infections can result in inflammation of the meninges (meningitis), the brain parenchyma (encephalitis), or both (meningoencephalitis).
- The most common pathogens implicated are herpesviruses (HSV-1, HSV-2, HHV-6, cytomegalovirus, varicella-zoster, and Epstein-Barr), non-polio enteroviruses, and arboviruses (St Louis, Powassan, Japanese, West Nile, and Eastern equine).
- Diagnosis remains challenging, with no definite etiology identified in ~50% of cases.

Treatment

- Most viral meningitis cases are benign, self-limited, and do not require any specific treatments, except for infections with herpesviruses (see section "Encephalitis").
- Empiric acyclovir is often initiated while awaiting a specific diagnosis.

Fungal Infections

- The most common pathogens implicated are *Cryptococcus*, *Histoplasma*, *Blastomyces*, *Coccidioides*, *Aspergillus*, and *Candida*.
- Specific factors including exposure history, immunocompromised state, and geographical location are key for diagnosis.
- Typical presentations are subacute to chronic in nature, unless patients develop acute vascular events or seizures.
- CSF shows lymphocytic pleocytosis, elevated protein, and low CSF glucose.
- Diagnosis is confirmed by the detection of CSF fungal antigen and culture.

Cryptococcal Meningitis

- *Cryptococcus* is the most common cause of fungal meningitis.
- Highly associated with increased ICP and hydrocephalus
- Most patients are immunocompromised, but up to 20% are immunocompetent.
- Delayed diagnosis and treatment are common among patients with cirrhosis as presentation mimics hepatic encephalopathy.
- CSF cryptococcal antigen is the most sensitive test for diagnosis; PCR can be supportive (52% sensitivity).
- India ink testing, demonstrating encapsulated yeasts, is insensitive.
- Culture and microscopy require expertise and are highly specific.

Treatment

- Three phases of treatment: induction, consolidation, and maintenance
- Induction treatment is with a combination of amphotericin B and flucytosine for 2 weeks, followed by consolidation treatment with high-dose oral fluconazole for 8 weeks, then maintenance treatment with low-dose oral fluconazole for 1 year.
- Patients with hydrocephalus may require serial LPs, temporary external ventricular drains, or permanent shunts to allow for CSF diversion as high ICP and delayed hydrocephalus are commonly observed despite adequate treatment.

Tuberculous Meningitis

- Most common form of CNS tuberculosis; other forms include intracranial tuberculoma and spinal manifestations.
- Caused by *Mycobacterium tuberculosis*, an acid-fast bacillus (AFB)
- Presentation is usually subacute to chronic; however, stroke is one of the most common complications leading to acute presentations.
- Symptoms include headache, fever, vomiting, neck stiffness, photophobia, and cranial nerve palsies.
- CSF shows lymphocytic pleocytosis, low glucose, and markedly elevated protein.
- Diagnosis relies on various tests, including AFB stains, *Mycobacterium* culture, and PCR.
- CSF culture is the gold standard test for definitive diagnosis.

Treatment

- Empiric treatment should be initiated early since cultures may take up to 4 weeks to become positive.
- Initial treatment is pursued with rifampicin, isoniazid, pyrazinamide, and ethambutol for 2 months, followed by rifampicin and isoniazid only for an additional 7 to 9 months.
- Steroids have been shown to reduce mortality, improve outcomes, and reduce relapse.
- Drug resistance is becoming increasingly common.

Encephalitis

- Inflammation of the brain parenchyma resulting in altered mental status, seizures, personality changes, and focal neurologic deficits
- Etiology can be infectious, autoimmune, or rheumatologic in nature.
- Infectious etiologies are most commonly viral; bacterial etiologies include *L. monocytogenes*, *Mycoplasma* species, and *Bartonella*.
- Most common infectious etiology overall is HSV.

Herpes Encephalitis

- Presentation varies and includes fever, altered mental status, seizures (temporal lobe symptomatic), focal neurologic deficits, and coma
- CSF most commonly shows a viral pattern of inflammation with lymphocytic pleocytosis and normal CSF glucose, though low CSF glucose has been reported.
- HSV is known for causing necrosis, edema, and hemorrhage in the brain parenchyma, which can be reflected by finding red blood cells on CSF analysis.
- Brain MRI is abnormal in nearly all patients and shows a predilection for involvement of the temporal, orbitofrontal, and insular regions.
- Electroencephalography is abnormal in 80% of patients, with findings including focal slowing, epileptiform discharges (particularly lateralized periodic discharges), or seizures.
- Diagnosis requires detection of HSV by PCR in the CSF, which is 96% sensitive and 99% specific.

Treatment

- Without acyclovir, mortality is as high as 70%.
- HSV may not be detected by PCR early in the course of illness; therefore, the continuation of acyclovir and repeat testing are warranted when clinical suspicion is present.
- The duration of treatment is typically 14 to 21 days.
- It is noteworthy that HSV encephalitis can trigger anti-*N*-methyl-D-aspartate (NMDA) receptor encephalitis, and patients may present with seizures and psychiatric disorders.

Parasitic Infections

- Parasites in some way live at the expense of other organisms (hosts).
- Divided into two categories: protozoa (unicellular organisms) and helminths (multicellular complex organisms)
- Most common parasitic infections of the CNS include toxoplasmosis, malaria, neurocysticercosis, and schistosomiasis.

Central Nervous System Toxoplasmosis

- Most common protozoan infection of the CNS
- Acquired through ingestion of cysts from contaminated food or water
- Toxoplasmosis is the most common opportunistic infection in patients infected with human immunodeficiency virus, especially when $CD4^+$ count is <100.
- Brain MRI shows characteristic single or multiple ring-enhancing lesions.
- LP is usually not performed given the risks of herniation, especially if multiple lesions with cerebral edema are present.
- Diagnosis is supported by the presence of immunoglobulin M (IgM) serology, rising IgG serology, or PCR.

Treatment

- Combination therapy of pyrimethamine-sulfadiazine or trimethoprim-sulfamethoxazole for 6 weeks
- Indefinite treatment might be required in patients who are immunosuppressed.
- Treatment of underlying immunodeficiency if present
- If there is no response to antimicrobial therapy, it is essential to reassess the diagnosis with lesion biopsy or nuclear imaging studies to rule out CNS lymphoma.

Neurocysticercosis

- Most common helminthic infection of the CNS
- Most common cause of acquired epilepsy worldwide, contributing to ~30% of cases of epilepsy
- Neurocysticercosis is caused by fecal-oral ingestion of the eggs of the pork tapeworm *Taenia solium*.
- Headaches and seizures are the most common symptoms; hydrocephalus and increased ICP carry worse prognosis.
- Brain MRI shows a multitude of findings depending on the stage of the infection.
- Diagnosis is often made by antigen or antibody detection.

Treatment

- This includes treatment of the infection and its complications.
- Antiparasitic treatment with albendazole is usually first line for 7 to 15 days; praziquantel may be added if multiple viable cysts are present.
- Treatment is contraindicated if ICP is uncontrollably elevated and may require the addition of steroids.
- Surgical management could be considered for the selected number of patients.

Cerebral Abscess

- A collection of pus in the brain parenchyma
- The most common microorganisms are *Streptococcus* and *Staphylococcus* species; up to 50% of cases are polymicrobial, involving aerobic, anaerobic, and fungal pathogens, especially in the immunocompromised.
- Abscesses occur through direct spread from nearby infection (eg, sinusitis, otitis, dental infection), hematogenous spread from a distant infectious source, or direct inoculation as a result of head trauma or neurosurgical procedures.
- Etiology is unknown in 25% to 30% of cases.
- Patients most commonly present with headaches (69%). Other features include fever, focal neurologic deficits, seizures, and altered mental status.
- Blood cultures are positive in < 50% of patients.
- Brain MRI shows a ring-enhancing lesion on T1 postcontrast imaging with high diffusion restriction signal centrally.

- CSF, if LP is not contraindicated, may show pleocytosis, elevated protein, and decreased glucose, but it can be normal in a significant proportion of patients.

Treatment

- Drainage (aspiration or surgical excision) and broad-spectrum intravenous (IV) antibiotic therapy with anaerobic coverage until identification of the inciting pathogen.
- Duration of treatment is usually 4 to 8 weeks but can be longer in patients who are immunocompromised.

Prion Disease

- Group of fatal neurodegenerative diseases, also known as "transmissible spongiform encephalopathies"
- Result from conversion of normal alpha-helical prion protein (PrP^C, "C" stands for cellular or normal) to an abnormal beta-pleated prion protein (PrP^{Sc}, "Sc" stands for scrapie)
- PrP^{Sc}, unlike PrP^C, is a protease-resistant protein; therefore, it cannot be degraded and accumulates in neurons, leading to neurotoxicity.
- Classification
  - Sporadic: sporadic Creutzfeldt-Jakob disease (sCJD) and sporadic fatal insomnia
  - Genetic: genetic CJD (gCJD) and fatal familial insomnia, due to mutations in the prion protein gene
  - Acquired: Kuru from human cannibalism, bovine spongiform encephalopathy; transmitted from infected cows, or iatrogenic from blood products, corneal transplants, dura mater grafts, and others

Sporadic Creutzfeldt-Jakob Disease

- Most common form of human prion disease, accounting for >90% of cases
- Neuropathology reveals neuronal loss, absence of inflammatory response, and small vacuoles within neurons producing a "spongiform" appearance of tissue.
- Patients present with rapidly progressive cognitive decline, personality changes, seizures, cerebellar signs, and pyramidal and extrapyramidal features.
- Pyramidal features result from upper motor neuron involvement and include weakness, spasticity, and hyperreflexia; while extrapyramidal features refer to those related to basal ganglia involvement, such as tremors, rigidity, dyskinesias (involuntary muscle movements), and dystonias (involuntary muscle contractions).
- Brain MRI shows abnormalities in the cerebral cortex and corpus striatum. One characteristic finding is "cortical ribboning" due to restricted diffusion of the affected gray matter with sparing of the underlying white matter.
- Electroencephalogram (EEG) may show classic bi- or triphasic periodic sharp wave complexes in at least two-thirds of patients.
- CSF is generally normal but may show mildly elevated protein. Markers useful as adjuncts include Tau and 14-3-3 proteins.
- CSF real-time quaking-induced conversion (RT-QuIC) test, which monitors formation of PrP^{Sc} aggregates in real time using fluorescent dyes, has 90% sensitivity and 98% to 100% specificity.
- Gold standard for diagnosis, however, remains pathologic via biopsy or autopsy, revealing vacuoles in neuronal cells.

Treatment

- No effective treatment to date
- Condition remains universally fatal, with a median disease duration of 6 months.

SUGGESTED READINGS

Aksamit AJ Jr, Berkowitz AL. Meningitis. *Continuum (Minneap Minn)*. 2021;27(4):836-854.

Berkowitz AL. Approach to neurologic infections. *Continuum (Minneap Minn)*. 2021;27(4):818-835.

Bradshaw MJ, Venkatesan A. Herpes simplex virus-1 encephalitis in adults: pathophysiology, diagnosis, and management. *Neurotherapeutics*. 2016;13(3):493-508.

Brouwer MC, Coutinho JM, van de Beek D. Clinical characteristics and outcome of brain abscess: systematic review and meta-analysis. *Neurology*. 2014;82(9):806-813.

Brouwer MC, McIntyre P, Prasad K, van de Beek D. Corticosteroids for acute bacterial meningitis. *Cochrane Database Syst Rev*. 2015;2015(9):Cd004405.

Del Brutto OH. Neurocysticercosis. *Continuum (Minneap Minn)*. 2012;18(6):1392-1416.

Foutz A, Appleby BS, Hamlin C, et al. Diagnostic and prognostic value of human prion detection in cerebrospinal fluid. *Ann Neurol*. 2017;81(1):79-92.

Garcia HH. Parasitic infections of the nervous system. *Continuum (Minneap Minn)*. 2021;27(4):943-962.

Hasbun R, Abrahams J, Jekel J, Quagliarello VJ. Computed tomography of the head before lumbar puncture in adults with suspected meningitis. *N Engl J Med*. 2001;345(24):1727-1733.

Kohil A, Jemmieh S, Smatti MK, Yassine HM. Viral meningitis: an overview. *Arch Virol*. 2021;166(2):335-345.

Puoti G, Bizzi A, Forloni G, Safar JG, Tagliavini F, Gambetti P. Sporadic human prion diseases: molecular insights and diagnosis. *Lancet Neurol*. 2012;11(7):618-628.

Saylor D. Neurologic complications of tuberculosis. *Continuum (Minneap Minn)*. 2021;27(4):992-1017.

Tunkel AR, Hartman BJ, Kaplan SL, et al. Practice guidelines for the management of bacterial meningitis. *Clin Infect Dis*. 2004;39(9):1267-1284.

Tunkel AR, Hasbun R, Bhimraj A, et al. 2017 Infectious Diseases Society of America's clinical practice guidelines for healthcare-associated ventriculitis and meningitis. *Clin Infect Dis*. 2017;64(6):e34-e65.

Venkatesan A. Encephalitis and brain abscess. *Continuum (Minneap Minn)*. 2021;27(4):855-886.

8.5

Acute Traumatic Brain Injury and Intracranial Hypertension

Helen S. Wei and Eric S. Rosenthal

Overview

- The general focus in the management of patients with acute traumatic brain injury (TBI) is to prevent secondary and delayed insults after the initial neurologic damage, promote neurologic recovery, and provide useful prognostic information.
- An improved outcome is attributed to the adoption of evidence-based clinical practice guidelines, that is, the Brain Trauma Foundation's "Guidelines for the management of severe traumatic brain injury."

Common Causes of Secondary Brain Injury After Traumatic Brain Injury

- Hypotension
- Hypoxia
- Cerebral edema, intracranial hypertension (elevated intracranial pressure [ICP])
- Seizure
- Cortical spreading depolarizations (measured using intracranial electroencephalogram [EEG])
- Electrolyte abnormalities
- Coagulopathy
- Traumatic vasospasm
- Delayed diffuse axonal injury
- Focal brain compression
- Thrombotic events following blunt cerebrovascular injury (BCVI) and dural venous thrombosis

Epidemiology

- Worldwide, an estimated 50 million people sustain TBI each year.
- In the United States, there were 214,110 TBI-related hospitalizations in 2020 and 69,473 TBI-related deaths in 2021.
- TBI is a contributing factor to 30% of all injury-related deaths in the United States.
- TBI is the leading cause of mortality in young adults.
- Medical costs and indirect costs, such as lost productivity after TBI, cost the global economy ~$400 billion annually.

Pathophysiology

- Primary injury is the immediate parenchymal damage (compressive, tensile, or shear injury) that occurs at the time of injury and can manifest as skull fractures, intracranial hematomas, contusions, and/or diffuse axonal injury.
- Secondary injury refers to potentially avoidable cellular damage from hypoxia, hypotension, hypercarbia, hyponatremia, and seizure that can occur after injury.
- Neurochemical mediators that are implicated in the pathophysiology of secondary injury include excitatory amino acids such as glutamate and aspartate that can cause an influx of chloride, sodium, and calcium ions, leading to acute neuronal swelling, deprivation of high-energy phosphate stores, and production of oxygen free radicals implicated in the destruction of cellular structures.
- Rapid deterioration after TBI is common. Patients who "talk and deteriorate," or "talk and die," comprise almost 15% of the TBI population.
  - These patients do not initially exhibit signs of significant brain injury but deteriorate in a delayed manner.
  - The majority (~75%) are the result of intracranial hematoma (epidural or subdural hematomas or contusions) expansion.

Stratification and Prognosis of Traumatic Brain Injury

- TBI is typically stratified based on the clinical indices of severity (eg, Glasgow Coma Scale [GCS] or the FOUR score), the pathoanatomic type of injury, or the physical mechanism and causative forces associated with the injury (blunt vs penetrating, low vs high velocity). The severity of the injury typically correlates with prognosis.
  - The most common system to categorize the severity of head trauma is based on the GCS score, with GCS 14 to 15 defined as mild, GCS 9 to 13 as moderate, and GCS 3 to 8 as severe.
  - The FOUR score is composed of eye response, motor response, brainstem reflexes, and respiration pattern and originated from Mayo Clinic.
  - The Marshall classification uses anatomy visualized on computed tomography (CT) scan to classify patients with TBI into six categories of increasing severity, based on the degree of edema (basal cistern compression and midline shift) and characteristics of intracranial blood.
  - The Rotterdam CT score classifies TBI severity into six categories based on CT imaging findings of basal cistern compression, midline shift, presence of epidural hematoma, and presence of intraventricular and/or subarachnoid blood.
- Diffuse axonal injury represents damage to the white matter and is graded based on the burden and anatomic distribution of the traumatic microlesions. Diffuse axonal injury may also occur in a delayed manner.
- BCVI can occur concurrently with TBI and contribute to worsening brain injury. Patients with trauma should be screened for BCVI based on the Denver Criteria, the Memphis Criteria, or clinical judgment.
- Prognostication after TBI is nuanced, and patients can continue to improve for up to 2 years after injury. Prognostic models such as IMPACT and CRASH were designed to predict outcomes at 6 months after TBI.
  - IMPACT prognostication includes the following variables: age, motor response, pupil reactivity, hypoxia, hypotension, Marshall classification, traumatic subarachnoid hemorrhage (tSAH), epidural hematoma, glucose, and hemoglobin (Hb).

- CRASH prognostication includes the following variables: high- versus middle-/low-income country, age, GCS, pupil reactivity, polytrauma, petechial hemorrhages on CT, appearance of ventricles/cisterns on CT, tSAH, midline shift, and nonevacuated hematoma.
- While the IMPACT and CRASH models are able to adequately predict unfavorable outcomes, they have limitations and may overestimate mortality.
- In the past decade, blood-based biomarkers for brain injury (glial fibrillary acidic protein [GFAP] for glial injury and ubiquitin C-terminal hydrolase L1 [UCH-L1] for neuronal injury) have been used to identify patients at risk for structural injury on head CT and are associated with brain injury severity. Incorporating biomarker data into prognostic models of long-term outcomes after TBI may help improve the accuracy of future models.

Management and Treatment

Immediate management of the patient with head-injured trauma should include:

- The ABCs of resuscitation: intubate any patient with concern for airway/breathing compromise or hypoxemia/hypercarbia, transfuse patients with significant blood loss, get control of ongoing bleeding, and prevent hypotension.
- Spine stability: use cervical collar and spine board until spinal stability is assessed.
- Seizure control: correct hyponatremia and hypoglycemia, administer antiepileptic drugs as indicated.
- Assess need for ICP monitoring and/or operative intervention.

The 2016 clinical practice guidelines by the Brain Trauma Foundation provide the following recommendations for the management of the head-injured patient:

- Avoid systolic blood pressure <100 mm Hg.
- Hyperventilation to a $Paco_2$ ≤25 mm Hg is *not* recommended.
- Cerebral perfusion pressure (CPP) should be maintained between 60 and 70 mm Hg.
- Jugular venous saturation, when measured, should be maintained >50%.
- Avoid prophylactic hypothermia.
- ICP monitoring should be considered for patients with GCS 3 to 8.
- ICP threshold for intervention is >22 mm Hg.
- Early cerebrospinal fluid (CSF) drainage to lower ICP may be considered if the initial GCS <6.
- Mannitol may be effective at a dose of 0.25 to 1 g/kg to reduce ICP. Hypertonic saline is an alternative and may be administered in concentrations such as 3%, 7.5%, 23.4%; balanced solutions with sodium acetate can be used to avoid hyperchloremia. There is no evidence that mannitol or hypertonic saline is superior to one another. Preference may relate to comorbid conditions (eg, hypervolemia, hypovolemia, congestive heart failure, renal failure).
- Barbiturates can help control elevated ICP refractory to maximum standard medical and surgical therapy.
- Steroids should not be used routinely in trauma due to the observed increase in mortality.
- Antiepileptic drugs should be administered prophylactically for the first 7 days after injury but should then be discontinued in patients without evidence of seizures or high risk for seizures.
- Surgical decompression should be considered for indications such as acute epidural hematoma with volume exceeding 30 mL or coma with anisocoria, subdural hematoma with thickness exceeding 10 mm, midline shift exceeding 5 mm, or neurologic deterioration, depressed skull fracture, large posterior fossa hematoma, or uncontrollable ICP.

General Care of Patients With Traumatic Brain Injury

- Admission to the intensive care unit (ICU) for patients with severe TBI
- Mechanical ventilation for patients with severe TBI
- Serial neurologic examinations, including pupillary examination
- HOB 30 °C to 45 °C
- Appropriate sedation
- Analgesia: important to control pain, particularly in patients with polytrauma
- Avoid fever >38 °C.
- Avoid hypercapnia $Paco_2$ >40 mm Hg.
- Avoid hyponatremia Na <135 mmol/L.
- Maintain CPP ≥60 mm Hg.
- Maintain Hb >7 g/dL.
- Maintain Spo_2 ≥94%.
- Avoid cerebral venous congestion (keep head midline, c-collars & tracheostomy collars should not be checked for effects on ICP, positive end-expiratory pressure [PEEP] levels of ≤10 cm water usually do not significantly increase ICP.)
- Seizure prophylaxis
- Nutrition: meeting caloric requirements by the fifth hospital day decreases mortality
- Deep vein thrombosis prophylaxis: mechanical compression devices should be employed as soon as possible.
  - Unless contraindicated (eg, presence of active bleeding or ongoing intracranial hemorrhage), prophylactic low-molecular-weight heparin or unfractionated heparin should be started within 6 to 48 hours.

Acute Intracranial Hypertension

- According to the Monro-Kellie doctrine, a change in the volume of one intracranial component (brain, CSF, or blood) results in a decrease of another component, or otherwise results in increased ICP.
- Normal range for ICP is <10 to 15 mm Hg for adults and between 3 and 7 mm Hg for children.
  - Intracranial hypertension in adults: ICP >22 mm Hg for >5 minutes
- The ICP waveform consists of three components:
  - P1—percussion wave: corresponds to cardiac systole
  - P2—tidal wave: reflects brain compliance
  - P3—dicrotic wave: corresponds to the dicrotic notch on the arterial pressure wave and closure of the aortic valve (Figure 8.5.1)
- Decreased brain compliance is associated with an increase in P2 amplitude.
- With increasing ICP, P2 and P3 amplitudes increase without a concomitant increase in P1.

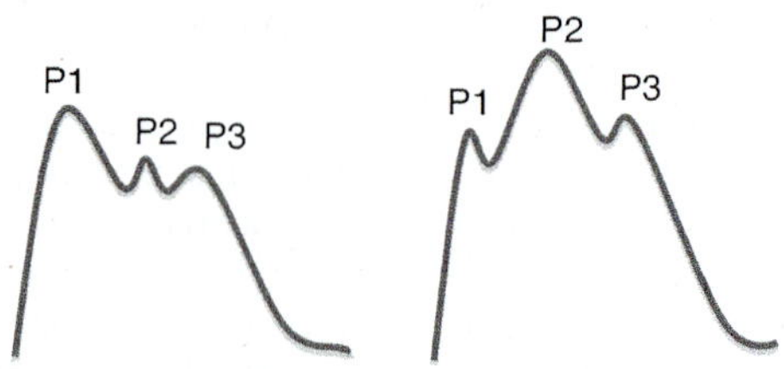

FIGURE 8.5.1 P3—dicrotic wave.

- The trend of the ICP over time can show plateau waves (Lundberg A waves) with decreasing brain compliance.
  - Sudden unpredictable increases in ICP to 50 to 100 mm Hg are recorded and may last for 5 to 20 minutes, before the pressure rapidly decreases.
  - Lundberg A waves are believed to be caused by a vasodilatory cascade and are always associated with intracranial pathology and a corresponding decrease in cerebral perfusion (Figure 8.5.2).
- Lundberg B waves are characterized by a rhythmic increase in the ICP (5-20 mm Hg) that lasts for 1 to 5 minutes and can represent vasomotor instability at the limits of autoregulation.
- Lundberg C waves are rhythmic changes in the ICP (<20 mm Hg) every 4 to 8 minutes that occur normally and are related to cardiac or respiratory cycles.
- Clinical symptoms associated with intracranial hypertension include:
  - Headache, nausea, and vomiting
  - Decreased arousal
  - Reflex hypertension, bradycardia, and respiratory irregularity (Cushing triad)
  - Visual symptoms such as upgaze paralysis with dorsal midbrain dysfunction and diplopia with cranial nerve (CN) VI palsy (false localizing sign)
  - Diabetes insipidus from pituitary apoplexy or shearing of the pituitary stalk
- Herniation syndromes
  - Uncal: ipsilateral CN III palsy with "blown" pupil and contralateral hemiplegia or posturing. With enough midline shift, the third ventricle can become compressed and obstructive hydrocephalus can develop.
  - Transtentorial: diencephalon gradually forced through the tentorial incisura, with unilateral or bilateral visual field deficits due to compression of the posterior cerebral artery or arteries.
  - Tonsillar: cerebellar tonsils "cone" through the foramen magnum, compressing the medulla oblongata, resulting in respiratory arrest.
  - Subfalcine: herniation beneath the falx cerebri, which can compress the anterior cerebral artery or arteries, causing contralateral leg weakness
  - If the herniation syndrome progresses, there is generally a rostral to caudal loss of brainstem reflexes, autonomic instability, central apnea, and ultimately brain death.

Management of Acute Intracranial Hypertension and Cerebral Edema

- General measures are reviewed in the "General Care of Patients With Traumatic Brain Injury" listed earlier.
- The period of highest risk for cerebral edema related to the primary injury is between days 3 and 5 postinjury.
- Brain tissue oxygenation is not currently routinely measured, but its use in guiding therapy is beginning to appear in TBI and intracranial hypertension management recommendations.
- Both prophylactic hyperosmolar therapy and prophylactic decompressive craniectomy (craniectomy in the absence of significant mass effect from a lesion, or prior to exhausting medical therapies in the absence of mass effect) have shown no benefit and may be harmful.
- Specific interventions for intracranial hypertension. Clinicians may consider three conditions: ICP elevated + brain tissue oxygenation normal; ICP normal + brain hypoxic; and ICP elevated + brain hypoxic. If no $Pbto_2$ is being measured via multimodality neuromonitoring, then the general condition will be considered "ICP elevated + brain tissue oxygenation normal."
  - First line (general)
    - Maintain CPP 60 to 70 mm Hg.
    - Increase analgesia and sedation to lower ICP.
    - Maintain $Paco_2$ at low normal (35-38 mm Hg).
    - Hyperosmolar therapy (discontinue when ICP normalizes)
      - Mannitol: intermittent 20% boluses dosed at 1.0 g/kg every 6 hours; if osmolar gap (measured − calculated serum osmolality) is >20 mOsm/L, avoid further mannitol due to the risk of renal

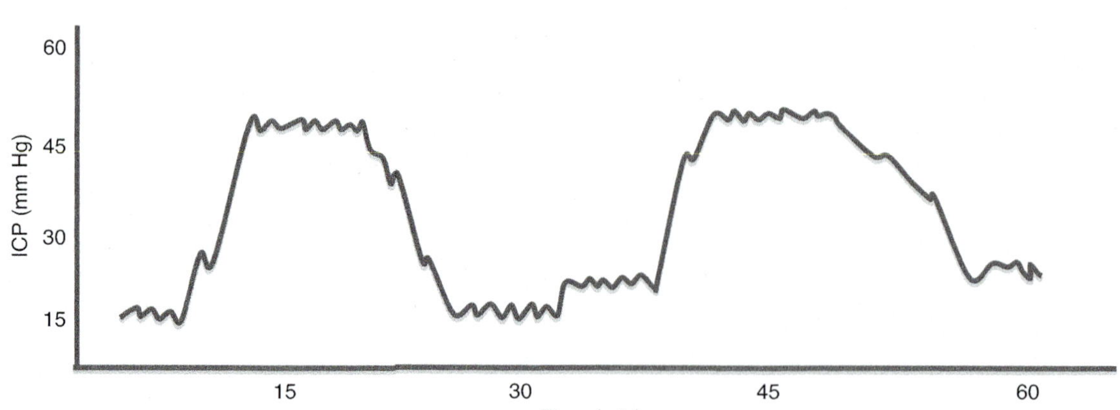

FIGURE 8.5.2 Lundberg A waves.

failure; mannitol is preferred to hypertonic saline in volume-overloaded patients
- Hypertonic saline: intermittent boluses every 6 hours, dosed as either 250 mL of 3%, 150 mL of 5%, or 30 mL of 23.4% solution over 10 minutes; repeat until serum sodium is 160 mEq/L

- CSF drainage via an intraventricular catheter, that is, an external ventricular drain (EVD)
- If "ICP normal + brain hypoxic," then consider:
  - Increase F_{IO_2}
- If "ICP elevated + brain hypoxic," then consider:
  - Increase F_{IO_2}

- Second line (general)
  - Mild hypocapnia (Pa_{CO_2} 32-35 mm Hg)
  - Neuromuscular paralysis: if a test dose is efficacious, then start an infusion; ensure adequate sedation; increases risk of critical illness myopathy.
  - Mean arterial pressure (MAP) challenge: in a controlled setting, use vasopressors to increase MAP by 10 mm Hg for ≤20 minutes, and assess the resultant ICP.
    - If autoregulation is intact (MAP ↑ leads to ICP ↓), leave the patient at the new higher MAP goal; otherwise, return to prior MAP goal.
  - If "ICP normal + brain hypoxic," then consider:
    - Increase Pa_{O_2} to 150 mm Hg via ventilator management
  - If "ICP elevated + brain hypoxic," then consider:
    - Increase Pa_{O_2} to 150 mm Hg via ventilator management
- Third line (general)
  - Barbiturate coma (believed to reduce cerebral metabolism and blood flow): trial a test dose, and if effective in lowering ICP, then titrate barbiturate dose to achieve burst suppression on EEG.
  - Hypocapnia to Pa_{CO_2} 30 to 32 mm Hg, particularly in the setting of preserved brain tissue oxygenation
  - Mild hypothermia to 35 °C to 36 °C
  - Secondary (salvage) decompressive craniectomy: decreases ICP and ICU length of stay, but long-term outcomes are poor (turns death into disability)
  - If "ICP normal + brain hypoxic," then consider:
    - No barbiturate coma
    - Increase Pa_{CO_2} to 45 to 50 mm Hg without increasing ICP
    - Normalizing Pa_{O_2} by treating pulmonary edema, atelectasis/collapse, pneumonia, etc
    - If Pbt_{O_2} remains <20 mm Hg, transfuse 1 u red blood cells (RBCs) if Hb <9 g/dL.
  - If "ICP elevated + brain hypoxic," then consider:
    - Normalizing Pa_{O_2} by treating pulmonary edema, atelectasis/collapse, pneumonia, etc
    - If Pbt_{O_2} remains <20 mm Hg, transfuse 1 u RBCs if Hb <9 g/dL.
    - Examining for seizure activity, including scalp-negative intracranial seizures

Monitoring for Secondary Brain Injury After Traumatic Brain Injury

- Transcranial Doppler (TCD): monitoring for traumatic cerebral vasospasm after TBI can be performed using TCD
- EEG: monitor for scalp-evident seizures. A 24-hour EEG (continuous EEG) is more sensitive than a routine 30-minute EEG.
- Invasive multimodality monitoring
  - Intracranial EEG: monitor for scalp-negative seizures. Intracranial electrodes increase sensitivity for detecting seizures from 15% to 25%.
  - ICP: monitor for elevation in ICP, elevation in PRx (pressure reactivity index, which is a measure of cerebral autoregulation), and facilitate CPP optimization.
  - Brain tissue oxygenation: facilitate prevention of brain tissue hypoxia.
  - Cerebral blood flow monitoring: facilitate optimization of cardiac output to avoid ischemia.
- CT imaging (focal or diffuse brain mass; hematoma expansion)
- Neurologic examinations

Treatment NOT Recommended for Management of Traumatic Brain Injury

- Hypertonic solution by nonbolus continuous intravenous infusion
- Scheduled hyperosmolar therapy rather than treatment in response to ICP elevations, brain tissue hypoxia, edema with mass effect, or other symptomatic edema
- Lumbar CSF drainage (as opposed to EVD), as it may encourage herniation
- Diuresis
- Routine use of steroids
- Routine administration of albumin for fluid resuscitation
- Routine use of therapeutic hypothermia to <35 °C
- High-dose propofol to attempt burst suppression
- Hypocapnia to Pa_{CO_2} <30 mm Hg
- Routinely increasing CPP >90 mm Hg

Delayed Neurologic Deterioration After Traumatic Brain Injury

- Patients with TBI are at risk for secondary injury and delayed neurologic deterioration. Preventing and recognizing secondary and delayed injuries are central to TBI management.
- Critical neurologic deterioration after TBI is defined as deterioration in clinical neurologic status such as:
  - Spontaneous sustained decrease in the GCS motor score ≥1 point
  - New decrease in pupillary reactivity
  - New pupillary asymmetry or bilateral mydriasis
  - New focal neurologic deficit
  - Herniation syndrome or Cushing triad
  - Deterioration in neuromonitoring parameters (Pbt_{O_2} <20 mm Hg, ICP >22 mm Hg) may also trigger treatment of neurologic deterioration.
- Response to critical neurologic deterioration after TBI
  - Emergent clinicoradiologic correlation, and evaluation of neuromonitoring to identify possible etiologies
  - If herniation or focal brain compression is suspected, begin empiric treatment (ie, transient hyperventilation and/or bolus of hyperosmolar therapy).
  - Escalate treatment quickly

- Differential diagnosis for neurologic deterioration after TBI
  - Expanding intracranial hematoma/lesion
  - Cerebral edema
  - Intracranial hypertension
  - Stroke
  - Seizure, convulsive and nonconvulsive
  - Tension pneumocephalus
  - Carotid or vertebral artery injury (BCVI) or embolism (including fat embolism)
  - Venous sinus thrombosis
  - Cerebral vasospasm
  - Systemic or central nervous system infections
  - Metabolic and electrolyte abnormalities (hypoxia, hypocapnia, hypercapnia, hyponatremia, hypoglycemia, hepatic encephalopathy, renal failure)
  - Hyper- or hypothermia
  - Medication effect

SUGGESTED READINGS

Carney N, Totten AM, O'Reilly C, et al. Brain trauma foundation guidelines for the management of severe traumatic brain injury, fourth edition. *Neurosurgery*. 2017;80(1):6-15.

Chesnut RM, Aguilera S, Buki A, et al. A management algorithm for adult patients with both brain oxygen and intracranial pressure monitoring: the Seattle International Severe Traumatic Brain Injury Consensus Conference (SIBICC). *Intensive Care Med*. 2020;46(5):919-929.

Chesnut RM, Marshall LF. Management of head injury—treatment of abnormal intracranial pressure. *Neurosurg Clin N Am*. 1991;2:267-284.

Choi DW. Ionic dependence of glutamate neurotoxicity. *J Neurosci*. 1987;7(2):369-379.

Cooper DJ, Rosenfeld JV, Murray L, et al. The DECRA trial investigators. Decompressive craniectomy in diffuse traumatic brain injury. *N Engl J Med*. 2011;364:1493-1502.

Czosnyka M, Smielewski P, Piechnik S, et al. Hemodynamic characterization of intracranial pressure plateau waves in head injury. *J Neurosurg*. 1999;91:11-19.

Eagle SR, Nwachuku E, Elmer J, Deng H, Okonkwo DO, Pease M. Performance of CRASH and IMPACT prognostic models for traumatic brain injury at 12 and 24 months post-injury. *Neurotrauma Rep*. 2023;4(1):118-123.

Edwards P, Arango M, Balica L, et al; CRASH Trial Collaborators. Final results of MRC CRASH, a randomised placebo-controlled trial of intravenous corticosteroid in adults with head injury-outcomes at 6 months. *Lancet*. 2005;365(9475):1957-1959.

Faul M, Xu L, Wald MM, Coronado VG. *Traumatic Brain Injury in the United States: Emergency Department Visits, Hospitalizations, and Deaths*. Centers for Disease Control and Prevention, National Center for Injury Prevention and Control; 2010.

Hawryluk GWJ, Rubiano AM, Totten AM, et al. Guidelines for the management of severe traumatic brain injury: 2020 update of the decompressive craniectomy recommendations. *Neurosurgery*. 2020;87(3):427-434.

Korley FK, Jain S, Sun X, et al; TRACK-TBI Study Investigators. Prognostic value of day-of-injury plasma GFAP and UCH-L1 concentrations for predicting functional recovery after traumatic brain injury in patients from the US TRACK-TBI cohort: an observational cohort study. *Lancet Neurol*. 2022;21(9):803-813.

Maas AIR, Menon DK, Adelson PD, et al; InTBIR Participants and Investigators. Traumatic brain injury: integrated approaches to improve prevention, clinical care, and research. *Lancet Neurol*. 2017;16(12):987-1048.

Saatman KE, Duhaime AC, Bullock R, et al. Classification of traumatic brain injury for targeted therapies. *J Neurotrauma*. 2008;25(7):719-738.

Vespa P, Tubi M, Claassen J, et al. Metabolic crisis occurs with seizures and periodic discharges after brain trauma. *Ann Neurol*. 2016;79(4):579-590.

Yue JK, Lee YM, Sun X, et al; The TRACK-TBI Investigators. Performance of the IMPACT and CRASH prognostic models for traumatic brain injury in a contemporary multicenter cohort: a TRACK-TBI study. *J Neurosurg*. 2024;141(2):417-429.

8.6

Spinal Cord Injury

Helen S. Wei and Cara Hannigan

Definition

- Neurologic outcome after spinal cord injury (SCI) is determined by:
  - Type of injury
  - Severity of the injury
  - Level of the injury
  - Nerve pathways involved
- The care of patients with SCI includes:
  - Stabilization of the vertebrae to prevent further injury
  - Prevention of cellular-level secondary damage (ischemia, inflammation, oxidative injury)
  - Correction of the cord compression and misalignments
- Have a higher suspicion for SCI in patients with trauma presenting with:
  - High energy mechanism
  - High injury burden
  - Loss of consciousness
  - Neck or back pain
  - Motor or sensory deficits
  - Autonomic dysfunction

Epidemiology

- The incidence of SCI in the United States is ~12,000 cases a year.
- The average age at injury is 40 years old.
- 80% of cases occur in males.

Etiology

- Mechanism of injury
  - Motor vehicle accidents, 48%
  - Falls, 16%
  - Violence, 12%
  - Sports-related injuries, 10%
  - Other, 14%

- The cervical spine is injured in 3% of patients with major trauma, most commonly in C1-C2 or C5-C7 regions.
- 20% of spinal fractures are at multiple levels.
- The major causes of death in patients with SCI are aspiration, circulatory failure, or shock.

Pathophysiology

- SCIs are a result of compression, contusion, or shear injuries, often in association with injuries to the vertebral column, such as fractures, dislocations, or ligamentous injuries.
- The initial insult is followed by a secondary progressive mechanism of cord injury, possibly involving mechanisms such as ischemia, inflammation, edema, excitotoxicity, and apoptosis, which evolve over several hours after injury.
- Spinal cord edema develops within hours of injury, reaching a peak after 3 to 6 days, and begins to recede after 9 days, when it is gradually replaced by a central hemorrhagic necrosis.
- *Classification*
  The severity of cord syndromes is classified using the American Spinal Injury Association (ASIA) Scale (Table 8.6.1).
- *Incomplete SCI syndromes* (Table 8.6.2)
- *SCI and neurogenic shock*
  - Higher level lesions are associated with the withdrawal of sympathetic neural outflow, particularly injuries at or above T6.
  - Unopposed parasympathetic neural output with hypotension, bradycardia, reflex vasodilation, and hypothermia, referred to as neurogenic shock
  - Sympathetic fibers originate in the thoracic and lumbar regions of the spinal cord (T1-L2).
  - Parasympathetic fibers originate in the cranial nerves and sacral spinal cord (S2-S4).
  - Autonomic function is transmitted in the anterior anteromedial tract of the spinal cord.
  - After a complete cervical SCI, 60% to 70% of patients demonstrate neurogenic shock, with bradycardia reported in 71% of patients and hypotension in 68% of patients.
  - Neurogenic shock is a separate entity from spinal shock.
    - Spinal shock is the temporary loss of spinal reflexes following SCI and can last for days to weeks.
    - Spinal shock is not associated with hypotension or bradycardia.
- See Table 8.6.3 for SCI and respiratory effects.

TABLE 8.6.1 ASIA Scale

Class	Type of Injury	Neurologic Findings
A	Complete	No motor or sensory function below the level of injury
B	Incomplete	Preserved sensory, but no motor function below the level of injury
C	Incomplete	Motor strength muscle grade <3 below the level of injury (no antigravity movement)
D	Incomplete	Motor strength muscle grade ≥3 below the level of injury (at least antigravity movement)
E	Normal	Preserved motor and sensory function

TABLE 8.6.2 Incomplete Spinal Cord Injury Syndromes

Syndrome	Associated Injury	Clinical Symptoms Below Level of Injury
Central cord injury Most common	Hyperextension	• Decreased or loss of motor function more pronounced in bilateral upper extremities than lower • Variable sensory loss • Preserved function of lower extremities
Brown-Séquard syndrome (hemisection injury)	Penetrating injury	• Ipsilateral loss of motor function, proprioception • Contralateral loss of pain and temperature sensation
Anterior cord syndrome	Flexion/ compression or vascular injury	• Bilateral loss of motor function • Bilateral loss of pain and temperature sensation • Preserved touch, vibration, and proprioception
Posterior cord syndrome	Rarely caused by trauma	• Loss of proprioception and vibration sense • Preserved motor function and pain/temp
Conus medullaris syndrome	Spinal fractures or disk herniation (T12-L2)	• Symmetric lower limb weakness • Early-onset bowel/bladder dysfunction • Saddle anesthesia
Cauda equina syndrome	Spinal fractures or disk herniation (L2 or lower)	• Asymmetric lower limb weakness • Severe radicular pain • Bowel/bladder dysfunction

TABLE 8.6.3 SCI Injury Level and Respiratory Effects

Injury Level	Respiratory Effects
C1-C2	Complete loss of phrenic nerve function
C3-C4	Partial loss of phrenic nerve function: shallow breathing, no voluntary cough
C5	Phrenic nerve dysfunction: weak cough, weak inspiration
C6-C7	Functional diaphragm but trunk and abdominal muscle paralysis
T1-T7	Partial paralysis of intercostal muscles: weak cough, weak deep inspiration
T8-T12	Partial paralysis of abdominal muscles: weak cough

SCI, spinal cord injury.

Differential Diagnosis

- Fracture of any part of the spine
  - Specific fracture patterns
    - Jefferson fracture—four-part fracture of C1 with bilateral fracture of the anterior and posterior arches, caused by axial load compression, such as a diving accident
    - Hangman fracture—bilateral pars interarticularis fracture of the C2 vertebral body with a variable degree of anterior subluxation, usually caused by hyperextension trauma
- Ligamentous injuries: subluxations may only be seen on dynamic studies (ie, flexion-extension films or magnetic resonance imaging [MRI]).
- Herniation of intervertebral disks
- Vascular injuries
  - Vascular malformation
  - Epidural hematoma
  - Spinal cord infarction: caused by vessel interruption, embolization, or hypoperfusion
  - Blunt cerebrovascular injury (BCVI): injury to carotid or vertebral arteries
    - BCVI has a strong association with cervical spine fractures, with or without neurologic deficits.
    - Consider screening for BCVI using computed tomographic (CT) angiography.
    - Early treatment with an antiplatelet agent or anticoagulation in BCVI reduces the risk of ischemic stroke, which is highest within 24 hours of injury.
- Subacute presentations unrelated to trauma
  - Infections (epidural abscess, bacterial diskitis, HIV myelopathy, syphilis)
  - Inflammatory disease (transverse myelitis, paraneoplastic syndrome)
  - Degenerative (amyotrophic lateral sclerosis, adrenomyeloneuropathy)
  - Neoplasm (metastases, intradural astrocytoma or ependymoma)
  - Metabolic or toxic (radiation myelopathy, B_{12} deficiency)

Medical Management of Spinal Cord Injury

- Initial management should follow the Advanced Trauma Life Support (ATLS) protocol.
- Spine movement should be minimized by placement of a rigid cervical collar, use of log-rolling, and a backboard for transfer.
- A neurologic examination should be completed as soon as possible.
- Involve spinal consultants as soon as SCI is suspected.
- Maintain adequate perfusion to the injured spinal cord to minimize secondary ischemic injury.
- Avoid hypotension, defined as systolic blood pressure <90 mm Hg.
- Consider placement of an indwelling urinary catheter for the prevention of bladder distension and for strict monitoring of urine output.
- Consider placement of a nasogastric tube as paralytic ileus is common.
- Obtain comprehensive imaging, including CT and MRI.
- Be mindful of patient positioning and bracing to prevent contracture and/or pressure injuries.
- Corticosteroids
  - Most guidelines recommend against the use of steroids in SCI.
  - Potential complications of steroid administration include increased risk of infections and sepsis, hyperglycemia, and acute corticosteroid myopathy.

Management of Hypotension

- Address all potential types of shock.
- Consider invasive monitoring of arterial, central venous, or pulmonary arterial pressures.
- Maintain a mean arterial blood pressure of at least 85 mm Hg for 7 days after injury using intravenous fluids and pharmacologic vasopressors if needed.
- Hypertonic saline has been suggested to improve spinal cord blood flow and preserve spinal cord function.
- Vasopressor selection
  - Norepinephrine is preferred due to its dual alpha- and beta-activity, effectively addressing hypotension and bradycardia.
  - Potent alpha-agonist agents (eg, phenylephrine) should be used with caution, as it may exacerbate bradycardia. Furthermore, a significant increase in the cardiac afterload in the setting of SCI may precipitate left ventricular failure and pulmonary edema.
- Despite the relative hypovolemia related to the vasodilation, many of these patients are prone to developing cardiogenic or noncardiogenic pulmonary edema. Prolonged hypoperfusion can adversely affect the neurologic outcome, but hypotension due to neurogenic shock is usually not associated with intestinal or renal ischemia or multiple organ dysfunction.

Management of Bradycardia

- All patients with complete cervical SCI exhibit some degree of bradycardia.
- Bradycardia is less common in patients with thoracic and lumbar lesions (specifically lesions below T6).
- Cardiac pauses with significant hemodynamic instability or even circulatory collapse can occur.
- Moderate bradycardia can be asymptomatic in many patients.
- Tracheal suctioning is a common trigger for bradycardia and often responds to vagolytic agents, such as atropine.
- Aminophylline, methylxanthines, and oral albuterol have been suggested to improve the heart rate and to prevent episodic bradyarrhythmia.
- A temporary or permanent pacemaker may be needed in those with prolonged and excessive bradycardia.
- Bradycardia often resolves within a few weeks to months.

Management of Poikilothermia

- Loss of sympathetic tone with vasoparalysis and lack of shivering can lead to poikilothermia.
- Maintain temperature control with external cooling and warming devices.
- Patients are prone to developing hypothermia in a cold environment, but vasogenic response and sympathetic control of the apocrine glands above the lesion are often enough to prevent hyperthermia.

Management of Neurogenic Pulmonary Edema

- Neurogenic pulmonary edema (NPE) is an increase in pulmonary interstitial and alveolar fluid within a few hours after a neurologic insult or SCI.
- It is characterized by marked pulmonary vascular congestion, extravasation of protein-rich edema fluid, and intra-alveolar hemorrhage.
- Treatment should focus on managing the underlying neurologic insult, which may include surgical options (decompression and stabilization of the SCI).
- Supportive care should be provided, including supplemental oxygen and mechanical ventilation as needed, diuretics, and optimization of cardiac output.
- NPE resolves within 48 to 72 hours in the majority of affected patients.

Management of Autonomic Hyperreflexia/Dysreflexia

- In patients with SCI at or above the T6 level, an exaggerated autonomic response may be triggered by normally innocuous stimuli, including bladder or bowel distension or manipulation of the urinary tract.
- Symptoms start to appear 2 to 3 weeks after SCI and include severe hypertension, bradycardia, pounding headache, flushing and sweating above the injury, cool and pale skin below the injury, nasal congestion, and anxiety.
- Pathophysiology: afferent impulses are transmitted along the pelvic, pudendal, and hypogastric nerves to the isolated spinal cord, triggering a massive sympathetic response from the adrenal medulla and sympathetic nervous system. There is vasoconstriction below the lesion and vasodilation above the lesion due to the reflex activity of the baroreceptors.
- Treatment includes immediate removal of the offending stimulus, patient positioning, and antihypertensive agents (nifedipine or sodium nitroprusside).
- Note that general and neuroaxial anesthesia are effective in preventing the reflex, but sedation and topical anesthesia do not consistently prevent the reflex.

Management of Deep Vein Thrombosis Prophylaxis

- The incidence of deep vein thrombosis (DVT) may be as high as 100% in patients with SCI, with an associated mortality of ~9%.
- The Spine section of the American Association of Neurological Surgeons/Central Nervous System (AANS/CNS) recommends that all patients with SCI with severe motor deficits be treated with DVT prophylaxis.
- Initiate chemoprophylaxis as early as medically possible, typically within 72 hours of injury, to reduce the risk of venous thromboembolism (VTE).
- Low-molecular-weight heparin (LMWH) is the most extensively studied, and it safely reduces VTE incidence without significantly increasing bleeding complications.
- Mechanical compression stockings should be used when anticoagulant therapy is contraindicated.
- Vena cava filters are recommended for patients who fail anticoagulation or who are not candidates for anticoagulation.

Surgical Management of Spinal Cord Injury

- Goals for surgical intervention in SCI include stabilization of the spine, as well as reduction of dislocations and decompression of neural elements.
- There are currently no evidence-based recommendations on the timing and method of vertebral decompression in acute SCI.
- Indications for cervical spine surgery include:
  - Significant cord compression with neurologic deficits
  - Progressive neurologic deficits
  - Deficits not responsive to closed reduction
  - Unstable vertebral fracture or dislocation
- Closed reduction is a treatment option for cervical spine fracture with subluxation.
  - Skull tongs or a halo headpiece is used to apply traction to the cervical spine.
  - An initial weight of 5 to 15 lb (3-5 lb per vertebral level) is applied, which is then increased in 5-lb increments.
  - Sedation, analgesia, and neuromuscular blockade may be used to facilitate reduction.
- Open decompression is a treatment for significant cord compression with neurologic deficits that are not amenable or do not respond to closed reduction, or an unstable vertebral fracture or dislocation.
  - Most clinicians also consider deteriorating neurologic function after incomplete SCI to be an indication to perform surgery.
  - In the absence of hemodynamic instability or significant coagulopathy, most surgeons prefer early decompression and stabilization of the spine.
  - Classification systems to identify patients who can benefit from surgery include:
    - The Thoracolumbar Injury Classification System (TLICS)
    - The Cervical Subaxial Injury Classification (SLIC)
    - The AOSpine Trauma Classification

Outcomes

- The mortality rate is as high as 20% after SCI, with the leading cause of death being complications such as pneumonia, pulmonary emboli, and sepsis.
- Patients with ASIA grade A injuries, higher calculated maximum spinal cord compression, and spinal cord hemorrhage and edema on the initial imaging have a worse neurologic outcome.
- Most recovery takes place within the first 3 to 6 months.
- Younger age and incomplete lesions are associated with better functional recovery.

Conclusions

- Effective management of SCIs requires early recognition to optimize neurologic outcomes and minimize complications.
- Initial care focuses on spine immobilization and hemodynamic support to prevent secondary spinal cord damage.
- Timely stabilization and decompression are critical in appropriate candidates.
- Long-term care involves rehabilitation and prevention of complications.

SUGGESTED READINGS

American College of Surgeons, Trauma Quality Programs. *Best Practices Guidelines—Spine Injury*. American College of Surgeons, Trauma Quality Programs; 2022. https://www.facs.org/media/k45gikqv/spine_injury_guidelines.pdf

Bracken MB, Shepard MJ, Collins WF, et al. A randomized, controlled trial of methylprednisolone or naloxone in the treatment of acute spinal-cord injury—results of the second national acute spinal cord injury study. *N Engl J Med*. 1990;322(20):1405-1411.

Bracken MB, Shepard MJ, Holford TR, et al; National Acute Spinal Cord Injury Study. Administration of methylprednisolone for 24 or 48 hours or tirilazad mesylate for 48 hours in the treatment of acute spinal cord injury: results of the third national acute spinal cord injury randomized controlled trial.. *JAMA*. 1997;277(20):1597-1604.

Fontes RB, Aguiar PH, Zanetti MV, et al. Acute neurogenic pulmonary edema: case reports and literature review. *J Neurosurg Anesthesiol*. 2003;15:144-150.

Geerts WH, Bergqvist D, Pineo GF, et al. Prevention of venous thromboembolism: American College of Chest Physicians evidence-based clinical practice guidelines (8th edition). *Chest*. 2008;133:S381-S483.

Grant GA, Mirza SK, Chapman JR, et al. Risk of early closed reduction in cervical spine subluxation injuries. *J Neurosurg*. 1999;90(1 suppl):13-18.

Guly HR, Bouamra O, Lecky FE. The incidence of neurogenic shock in patients with isolated spinal cord injury in the emergency department. *Resuscitation*. 2008;76:57-62.

Hadley MN, Walters BC, Grabb PA, et al. Blood pressure management after acute spinal cord injury. *Neurosurgery*. 2002;50(3 suppl):S58-S62.

Hadley MN, Walters BC, Grabb PA, et al. Clinical assessment after acute cervical spinal cord injury. *Neurosurgery*. 2002;50(3 suppl):S21-S29.

Huang YH, Yang TM, Lin WC, et al. The prognosis of acute blunt cervical spinal cord injury. *J Trauma*. 2009;66(5):1441-1445.

Janssen L, Hansebout RR. Pathogenesis of spinal cord injury and newer treatments: a review. *Spine*. 1989;14(1):23-32.

Kurnick NB. Autonomic hyperreflexia and its control in patients with spinal cord lesions. *Ann Intern Med*. 1956;44:678-686.

Kwon BK, Curt A, Belanger LM, et al. Intrathecal pressure monitoring and cerebrospinal fluid drainage in acute spinal cord injury: a prospective randomized trial. *J Neurosurg Spine*. 2009;10(3):181-193.

Levi L, Wolf A, Belzberg H. Hemodynamic parameters in patients with acute cervical cord trauma: description, intervention, and prediction of outcome. *Neurosurgery*. 1993;33(6):1007-1016.

Shea JD, Gioffre R, Carrion H, et al. Autonomic hyperreflexia in spinal cord injury. *South Med J*. 1973;66:869-872.

The National Spinal Cord Injury Statistical Center. *The UAB-SCIMS information network*. Accessed May 25, 2012. http://www.spinalcord.uab.edu

Ullery BW, Cheung AT, Fairman RM, et al. Risk factors, outcomes, and clinical manifestations of spinal cord ischemia following thoracic endovascular aortic repair. *J Vasc Surg*. 2011;54(3):677-684.

Urdaneta F, Layon AJ. Respiratory complications in patients with traumatic cervical spine injuries: case report and review of literature. *J Clin Anesth*. 2003;15:398-405.

Vaccaro AR, Zeiller SC, Hulbert RJ, et al. The thoracolumbar injury severity score: a proposed treatment algorithm. *J Spinal Disord Tech*. 2005;18(3):209-215.

Young WF, Rosenwasser RH, Vasthare US, et al. preservation of post-compression spinal cord function by infusion of hypertonic saline. *J Neurosurg Anesthesiol*. 1994;6:122-127.

8.7

Ischemic Stroke

Rashid A. Ahmed and Guy A. Rordorf

Definitions

- Stroke is defined as a sudden onset focal neurologic deficit due to vascular etiology, most commonly ischemia secondary to blood vessel occlusion.
- A slow progression of neurologic symptoms should make one consider alternative diagnoses.

Common Causes to Remember

- Internal carotid artery (ICA) atherosclerosis
- Atrial fibrillation
- Aortic arch atheroemboli
- Arterial dissection
- Intracranial stenosis
- Fat or air emboli
- Cerebral small vessel disease due to hypertension and/or diabetes mellitus
- Paradoxical emboli—venous thromboembolism causing arterial infarcts via intracardiac or pulmonary shunts, most commonly from patent foramen ovale (PFO)
- PFO relevant in younger patients with cryptogenic stroke, particularly with concomitant atrial septal aneurysm
- Watershed—infarction between major arterial territories due to global or regional hypoperfusion
- Hypercoagulable states (eg, cancer-associated thrombosis, antiphospholipid syndrome)

Common Stroke Syndromes

- See Table 8.7.1 for common large vessel stroke syndromes
- See Table 8.7.2 for common stroke syndromes associated with small vessels.

Epidemiology

- With an incidence of 795,000 per year, stroke is the leading cause of long-term disability and the fifth leading cause of death in the United States.
- Nearly 25% of all strokes occur in people under the age of 65.

Key Pathophysiology

- Nearly 80% of strokes are ischemic.
- Cardioembolic and atheroembolic events are the culprit in about 20% of ischemic strokes.
    - Large and small artery thromboses account for 40%, coagulopathy and low-flow states 10%, while 30% of ischemic strokes remain "cryptogenic."
- Cerebral blood flow is maintained via autoregulation within mean blood pressure (BP) of 60 to 150.
- Infarct core undergoes necrosis with a critical reduction in oxygen delivery.

TABLE 8.7.1 Stroke Syndromes: Large Vessel

Large Vessel	
Internal carotid artery occlusion	• Contralateral hemiparesis of the face and arm > leg due to middle cerebral artery involvement • Transient monocular blindness (amaurosis fugax) due to ophthalmic artery involvement • If dominant hemisphere involved, aphasia present. • Nondominant hemisphere causes neglect. • If poor collaterals, hemiplegia of face, arm, and leg with gaze deviation and decreased level of arousal
Middle cerebral artery	• Proximal occlusions result in contralateral hemiparesis of the face and arm more than the leg, as well as loss of cortico-sensory modalities. • Aphasia is present when the dominant hemisphere is involved, whereas involvement of the nondominant hemisphere can cause neglect.
Anterior cerebral artery	• Weakness of foot and leg more than arm or face
Posterior cerebral artery	• Presents with hemianopia, alexia without agraphia (dominant occipital lobe), or visual agnosias
Basilar Artery	
Top of the basilar	• Somnolence, small poorly reactive pupils, multiple gaze palsies • Involuntary movements of the extremities resembling convulsions, with or without hallucinations • Lesions affecting the ventral pons can result in quadriplegia and anarthria with preserved vertical eye movements and consciousness—termed the locked-in syndrome.
Pontine syndromes	• Bilateral or crossed findings and gaze palsies (ie, internuclear ophthalmoplegia) • Symptoms often fluctuate in the early stages.
Vertebral Artery	
Lateral medullary syndrome	• Vertigo, nystagmus. Ipsilateral facial sensory loss, pharyngeal paresis, and Horner syndrome (autonomic dysfunction) • Contralateral loss of pain/temperature to the body/limbs
Medial medullary syndrome	• Contralateral hemiparesis and posterior column dysfunction due to the medial lemniscus • Ipsilateral tongue paresis (rarely seen)
Cerebellar	
Posterior inferior cerebellar artery	• Vertigo, veering to ipsilateral side, ipsilateral limb ataxia, headache, and vomiting

- Area surrounding the core, or penumbra, undergoes apoptosis depending on the ability to maintain blood flow in the setting of impaired cerebral autoregulation.
- Cerebral autoregulation becomes dysfunctional during acute ischemia, particularly within the penumbra, leading to vulnerability to systemic BP fluctuations.
- ~10% of infarctions are space occupying, risking herniation and death due to a combination of vasogenic (increased blood-brain barrier permeability) and cytotoxic (failure of adenosine triphosphate–dependent pumps maintaining cellular gradients) edema.

TABLE 8.7.2 Stroke Syndromes: Small Vessel

Pure motor	• Face, arm, and leg all equally weak • No cognitive, sensory, or visual field loss (pons or internal capsule)
Pure sensory	• Numbness or paresthesias of face, arm, and leg without cognitive, motor, or visual field cut (medial or ventroposterolateral thalamus)
Dysarthria clumsy hand	• Contralateral hand clumsiness. Face/tongue weakness and slurred speech (pons)
Ataxic hemiparesis	• Contralateral ataxia and weakness without cognitive, sensory, or visual field cut (posterior limb of internal capsule or pons)

With brief central nervous system localization.

Differential Diagnosis

- Transient ischemic attack (TIA), seizure, and complicated migraine (Figure 8.7.1)
  - Stroke—generally produces a deficit that is sudden and maximal at onset
  - Seizure—progresses rapidly over a few seconds and may be associated with stereotyped motor movements and often impairment or loss of consciousness
  - Migraine—produces stereotypical visual, sensory, motor, or language symptoms in a predictable manner due to the presumed mechanism of "cortical spreading depression" from rising extracellular potassium levels occurring over minutes
  - TIA—same onset as stroke, but is a transient episode of neurologic dysfunction caused by focal brain, spinal cord, or retinal ischemia, without acute infarction
  - TIA should be treated with the same urgency and comprehensive evaluation as stroke, given studies showing a high risk of infarction in the early period following TIA.

Management and Treatment

Acute Management

- Intravenous (IV) thrombolysis
  - Establish the exact last known time that the patient was at their baseline.
  - Obtain immediate head computed tomography (CT) to rule out intracerebral hemorrhage.
  - IV thrombolysis can be given up to 4.5 hours after the patient was last seen well.
  - Best outcomes if thrombolysis given within ≤60 minutes
  - Tenecteplase is an alternative thrombolytic agent increasingly used in select centers due to ease of administration and noninferiority in early studies.

Contraindications to Intravenous Thrombolysis

- See Tables 8.7.3 and 8.7.4.

Mechanical Thrombectomy

- Patients generally must have more severe neurologic deficits (National Institutes of Health Stroke Score [NIHSS] >6) and arterial occlusion of ICA, M1 branch of MCA, M2 branch of MCA, and basilar artery.

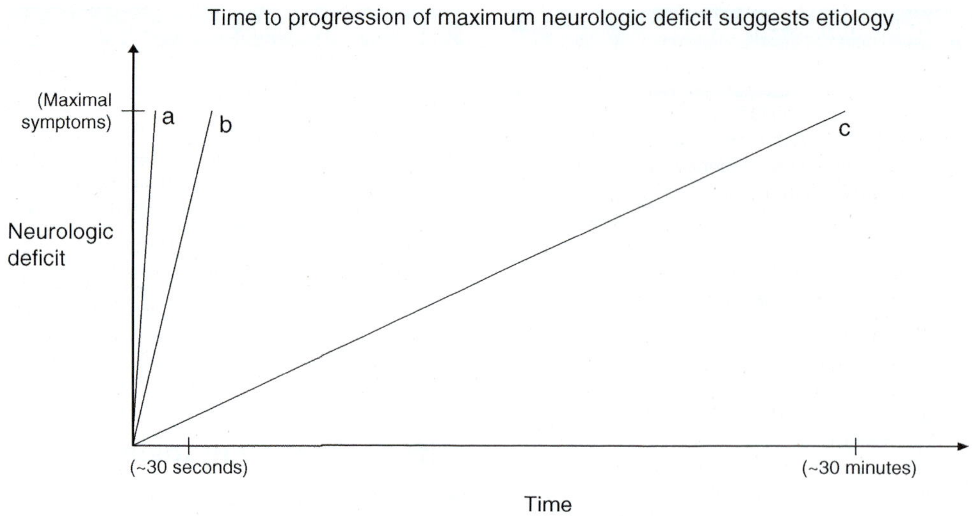

FIGURE 8.7.1 Stroke (a) and seizure (b) are characterized by sudden onset of symptoms. Migraine (c) related deficits have a slower pace of onset due to spreading cortical depression.

 - Mechanical thrombectomy is indicated up to 24 hours in select patients with perfusion-clinical mismatch, per DAWN/DEFUSE 3 trials.
 - IV thrombolysis is not a contraindication to catheter-based intervention.
- BP goals in acute ischemic stroke
 - Candidates for IV thrombolysis require BP <185/110 to start treatment, and BP should be maintained <180/105 for the first 24 hours after treatment.
 - Labetalol or nicardipine IV is the preferred agent.
 - Permissive hypertension should be considered, given that cerebral autoregulation is impaired in the penumbra.
 - Aggressive treatment of hypertension in acute stroke can result in worsening of stroke symptoms, with the risk of greater disability.
 - BP reduction occurs spontaneously outside the hyperacute period.
 - Optimum BP goals are influenced by baseline BP, pattern of cerebral collateral flow, and the degree of stenosis or occlusion of intracerebral arteries.
 - BPs as high as 220/120 are tolerated in the absence of other end-organ dysfunction (ie, cardiac or renal).
- Hemicraniectomy in space-occupying infarction
 - Space-occupying infarction is a very large stroke with >50% of MCA territory involved, or volume of >150 mL, and severe neurologic deficit.

TABLE 8.7.3 Absolute Contraindications to IV Thrombolysis

Hemorrhage or large infarction (>1/3 the arterial territory) on unenhanced head CT
Central nervous system lesion with a high likelihood of hemorrhage (tumor, vascular malformation, aneurysm, abscess, contusion)
Known infectious endocarditis
History of prior spontaneous intracerebral hemorrhage
INR >1.7 (or PT >15), PTT >40, platelet <100,000, glucose <50 mg/dL
Prior oral anticoagulant use
Previous stroke or serious head trauma within 3 mo

CT, computed tomography; INR, international normalized ratio; IV, intravenous; PT, prothrombin time; PTT, partial thromboplastin time.

 - There is a risk of death from cerebral edema and subsequent herniation.
 - Early decompressive hemicraniectomy may provide both functional and survival benefits when performed within 48 hours of stroke onset in persons under the age of 60.
 - Decisions should still be made on a case-by-case basis, given the significant risk of a poor prognosis.
- *Subacute management*
 - Evaluation for stroke etiology
   - Cerebral vessel imaging by computed tomographic angiography (CTA) or magnetic resonance angiography (MRA)
   - Carotid artery imaging by duplex ultrasound, CTA, or MRA
   - Echocardiogram for evaluating valvular function, atrial hypertrophy, intracardiac thrombus, ejection fraction, and the presence of a PFO.
   - Telemetry versus long-term Holter monitoring for atrial fibrillation
   - Fasting lipid profile, fasting blood glucose, HbA1C
   - Less common—homocysteine, Venereal Disease Research Laboratory (VDRL), antiphospholipid antibody syndrome panel
 - Stroke risk-factor modification
   - BP goal normotension (once outside the subacute period)
   - Optimize glycemic control if diabetic
   - Low-density lipoprotein (LDL) goal <70 mg/dL

TABLE 8.7.4 Relative Contraindications to IV Thrombolysis

Minor/rapidly improving symptoms
Seizure with postictal neurologic impairments
Major surgery within 14 d per minor surgery within 10 d
BP >185/110 (can correct with antihypertensive)
Pregnant or <10 d postpartum
Arterial puncture at noncompressible site in the previous 7 d
History of gastrointestinal or urinary tract hemorrhage within 21 d

BP, blood pressure; IV, intravenous.

- Tobacco use cessation
- Physical exercise and weight reduction through diet
- Secondary prevention strategies
  - Antiplatelet therapy remains the mainstay for treating large artery disease, small vessel disease, and cryptogenic stroke.
  - Dual-antiplatelet therapy (DAPT) for 21 days is indicated in minor stroke or high-risk TIA (eg, ABCD2 ≥4), based on CHANCE and POINT trials.
  - Atrial fibrillation, acute myocardial infarction complicated by left ventricular mural thrombus, mechanical prosthetic heart valves, and hypercoagulable disorders are the strongest indications for permanent anticoagulation for secondary prevention of ischemic stroke.
  - Short-duration anticoagulation of up to 3 months followed by antiplatelet therapy is often used in the setting of arterial dissection or with severe cardiomyopathy, although specific studies addressing these populations are limited.
  - Statins may have pleiotropic effects beyond LDL reduction and are commonly employed.

Outcomes

- Stroke mortality in the United States has been decreasing for the past 10 years.
- For every 100 patients treated with IV tissue plasminogen activator (tPA) within 3 hours of stroke onset, 32 will have a better and three will have a worse final global outcome.
- Despite a greater segment of the population aged >65, the improved survival is most likely attributable to a reduction in the severity of stroke, changing diagnostic criteria, and better stroke risk-factor control.

SUGGESTED READINGS

Amarenco P, Bogousslavsky J, Callahan A 3rd, et al; Stroke Prevention by Aggressive Reduction in Cholesterol Levels (SPARCL) Investigators. High-dose atorvastatin after stroke or transient ischemic attack. *N Engl J Med*. 2006;355(6):549-559.

Easton JD, Saver JL, Albers GW, et al. Definition and evaluation of transient ischemic attack: a scientific statement for healthcare professionals from the American Heart Association/American Stroke Association Stroke Council. *Stroke*. 2009;40(6):2276.

Hacke W, Kaste M, Bluhmki E, et al; ECASS Investigators. Thrombolysis with alteplase 3 to 4.5 hours after acute ischemic stroke. *N Engl J Med*. 2008;359(13):1317-1329.

National Institute of Neurological Disorders and Stroke rt-PA Stroke Study Group. Tissue plasminogen activator for acute ischemic stroke. *N Engl J Med*. 1995;333(24):1581-1587.

Nogueira RG, Jadhav AP, Haussen DC, et al. Thrombectomy 6 to 24 hours after stroke with a mismatch between deficit and infarct. *N Engl J Med*. 2018;378(1):11-21.

Powers WJ, Rabinstein AA, Ackerson T, et al. Guidelines for the early management of patients with acute ischemic stroke: 2019 update to the 2018 guidelines for the early management of acute ischemic stroke: a guideline for healthcare professionals from the American Heart Association/American Stroke. *Stroke*. 2019;50(12):e344-e418.

Roger VL, Go AS, Lloyd-Jones DM, et al; American Heart Association Statistics Committee and Stroke Statistics Subcommittee. Heart disease and stroke statistics—2011 update: a report from the American Heart Association. *Circulation*. 2011;123(4):e18.

Simard JM, Kent TA, Chen M, Tarasov KV, Gerzanich V. Brain oedema in focal ischaemia: molecular pathophysiology and theoretical implications. *Lancet Neurol*. 2007;6(3):258.

Stroke Prevention in Atrial Fibrillation Investigators. Warfarin versus aspirin for prevention of thromboembolism in atrial fibrillation. *Lancet*. 1994;343:687-691.

Vahedi K, Hofmeijer J, Juettler E, et al. Early decompressive surgery in malignant infarction of the middle cerebral artery: a pooled analysis of three randomised controlled trials. *Lancet Neurol*. 2007;6:215-222.

8.8

Intracerebral Hemorrhage

Jonathan A. Duskin and Jonathan Rosand

Background

- Intracerebral hemorrhage (ICH) accounts for ~10% to 20% of all strokes and is responsible for almost half of all stroke-related deaths and disability worldwide.

Common Causes to Remember

Primary	Secondary
Cerebral amyloid angiopathy (CAA) Hypertension (arteriolosclerosis) Coagulopathy	Hemorrhagic conversion of ischemic stroke Venous sinus thrombosis Vascular malformations Tumor, primary brain or metastatic

Epidemiology

- Annual incidence of ICH in the United States is ~42 cases per 100,000 person-years.
- Risk factors include hypertension, elevated body mass index, diabetes mellitus, smoking, older age, and male sex.

Key Pathophysiology

- Hypertension vasculopathy: arteriolosclerosis (aka lipohyalinosis) affecting the cerebral small vessels makes them more prone to rupture.
- CAA: abnormal protein deposition in vessel walls makes vessels fragile.
- Vascular malformations: abnormal flow dynamics and pressure lead to vessel rupture.
- Tumor: invades cerebral vascular and causes hemorrhage
- Hemorrhagic conversion: reperfusion of dead ischemic tissue leads to congestion and hemorrhage.
- Venous sinus thrombosis: venous thrombosis leads to venous congestion, capillary leakage, and hemorrhage.

Differential Diagnosis

- In primary ICH, the location of the ICH often reflects the likely underlying vasculopathy responsible for the vessel rupture

- Deep (basal ganglia, thalamus, cerebellum, pons): hypertensive vasculopathy, vascular malformations
- Lobar: CAA, hypertensive vasculopathy, primary brain tumor, metastatic cancer (most common: lung, breast, renal cell, thyroid, choriocarcinoma, melanoma), coagulopathy, vascular malformations
- Boston Criteria 2.0 for the diagnosis of CAA:
  - Definite CAA → requires full-brain postmortem examination
  - Probable CAA with supporting pathology → clinical data and pathologic tissue (eg, evacuated hematoma or cortical biopsy) demonstrating:
    - Spontaneous ICH, transient focal neurologic episodes, convexity subarachnoid hemorrhage, or cognitive impairment/dementia
    - CAA in specimen
    - Absence of other diagnostic lesions
  - Probable CAA → age 50 years and above, clinical and magnetic resonance imaging (MRI) data demonstrating:
    - Spontaneous ICH, transient focal neurologic episodes, or cognitive impairment/dementia
    - ≥2 of the following strictly lobar lesions on gradient-recalled echo (GRE) MRI (though MRI with susceptibility-weighted imaging [SWI] preferred in clinical practice): ICH, cerebral microbleeds, cortical superficial siderosis, or convexity subarachnoid hemorrhage
      OR
    - One lobar hemorrhagic lesion + one white matter feature (severe perivascular spaces in centrum semiovale or white matter hyperintensities in a multisport pattern)
    - Absence of any deep hemorrhagic lesions on GRE
    - Absence of other causes of hemorrhagic lesions
      - *Hemorrhagic lesion in cerebellum not counted as lobar or deep
  - Possible CAA → age 50 years and above, clinical and MRI data demonstrating:
    - Spontaneous ICH, transient focal neurologic episodes, or cognitive impairment/dementia
    - Absence of other causes of hemorrhage
    - One strictly lobar lesion on GRE MRI (though MRI with SWI) preferred in clinical practice): ICH, cerebral microbleeds, cortical superficial siderosis, or convexity subarachnoid hemorrhage
      OR
    - One white matter feature (severe perivascular spaces in centrum semiovale or white matter hyperintensities in a multisport pattern)
    - Absence of any deep hemorrhagic lesions on GRE
    - Absence of other causes of hemorrhagic lesions
      - *Hemorrhagic lesion in cerebellum not counted as lobar or deep

Acute Management

- Principles of acute management
  - Airway, breathing, circulation
  - Manage mass effect
  - Assess whether there is ongoing bleeding and arrest it.
- Imaging
  - Computed tomographic angiography (CTA) to rule out vascular malformation or aneurysm and assess for ongoing bleeding, mass effect, hydrocephalus
  - Stability CT within 6 hours of initial scan to evaluate for hematoma expansion or other complications (eg, hydrocephalus)
- Blood pressure (BP) management
  - Target systolic blood pressure (SBP) 140 mm Hg and maintain 130 to 150 within the first hour in patients, with mild-moderate severity ICH (Glasgow Coma Scale [GCS] >5, without massive hematoma) presenting with SBP 150 to 220
  - Avoid lowering SBP <130.
  - In patients with SBP >220, intensive lowering of BP could be harmful, thus target SBP 140 to 180.
  - Data are limited in patients with severe ICH or requiring surgical intervention, can consider SBP goals as above while maintaining cerebral perfusion pressure (CPP) >60 mm Hg.
  - Smooth and sustained control of BP is important and can be attained using intravenous (IV) pushes (eg, IV labetalol) and continuous infusions (eg, nicardipine).
  - Initiate short-acting enteral medications (eg, captopril) once BP is stabilized to facilitate transition off infusions.
- See Tables 8.8.1 and 8.8.2.
- Treatment of associated issues
  - Intubation and mechanical ventilation
    - Required if patient has a deteriorating or depressed consciousness (eg, GCS ≤8), suggesting an inability to protect airway
  - Elevated intracranial pressure (ICP)
    - Commonly measured with extraventricular drain (EVD) or intraparenchymal monitor
    - EVD indicated if hydrocephalus present
    - For mass effect or elevated ICP
      - Hyperosmolar therapy (hypertonic saline may be more effective than mannitol, and mannitol could lead to hematoma enlargement early after supratentorial ICH)
      - Sedation, paralysis, barbiturate coma, hypothermia
      - Hemicraniectomy (see table 8.8.2)

TABLE 8.8.1 Antiplatelet/Anticoagulant Reversal and Hemostasis

Aspirin/clopidogrel	• Consider desmopressin • Can also consider platelet transfusion *only* if plan for emergent neurosurgery (platelet transfusions otherwise potentially harmful in ICH)
Warfarin (INR >1.4)	• Prothrombin complex concentrate (Kcentra) + vitamin K
Apixaban/rivaroxaban	• Andexanet alfa (less hematoma expansion/more thrombotic events, including ischemic stroke, compared to Kcentra) vs Kcentra
Dabigatran	• Idarucizumab
Unfractionated or low-molecular-weight heparin	• Protamine
tPA	• Cryoprecipitate + tranexamic acid (TXA)
• Use of TXA as a hemostatic agent in spontaneous ICH not shown to improve functional outcome, but can be considered on a case-by-case basis, given reduction of hematoma expansion and early mortality.	

ICH, intracerebral hemorrhage; INR, international normalized ratio; tPA, tissue plasminogen activator.

TABLE 8.8.2 Neurosurgical Interventions

Minimally invasive trans-sulcal parafascicular intracerebral hemorrhage (ICH) evacuation	• Spontaneous lobar intraparenchymal hemorrhage (IPH), volume 30-80 mL, GCS 5-14, NIHSS >5, baseline mRS <2, last known well <24 h • Absence of culprit vascular malformation, venous sinus thrombosis (VST), or mass, or of irreversible coagulopathy
Extraventricular drain (EVD) placement	• Moderate-large intraventricular hemorrhage (IVH) or hydrocephalus with impaired level of consciousness
Decompressive hemicraniectomy ± hematoma evacuation	• Reduced mortality (no clear effect on functional outcome) in patients with supratentorial ICH who are in a coma, have significant mass effect, or have elevated intracranial pressure (ICP) refractory to medical management
Suboccipital craniectomy with hematoma evacuation	• Reduced mortality (no clear effect on functional outcome) in patients with cerebellar ICH and neurologic deterioration, brainstem compression, hydrocephalus, or ICH volume ≥15 mL
Treatment of underlying lesion	• ICH due to a vascular malformation (eg, arteriovenous malformation, dural arteriovenous fistula) can be a surgical emergency and requires urgent neurosurgical consultation. • ICH due to a mass requires multidisciplinary discussion on appropriate timing of resection.

GCS, Glasgow Coma Scale; NIHSS, National Institutes of Health Stroke Scale; mRS, modified Rankin Scale.

- Seizures
  - Much more common in lobar, rather than deep, ICH
  - Prophylactic antiseizure medications *not* recommended in spontaneous ICH
  - Antiseizure medications should be started in patients with clinical or electrographic seizures.
  - Continuous EEG (≥24 hours) should be done in patients with unexplained altered or fluctuating mental status.
- Deep venous thrombosis (DVT) and pulmonary embolism (PE) prophylaxis
  - Initiate intermittent pneumatic compression on arrival.
  - Begin prophylactic subcutaneous unfractionated heparin or low-molecular-weight heparin 48 hours after ICH stability unless contraindication (eg, coagulopathy, procedure, or continued bleeding as evidenced by radiographic ICH expansion).
- Glucose
  - Glucose should be monitored and treated if <60 or >180 mg/dL.
- Temperature
  - Fevers should be promptly treated with antipyretic medications and/or cooling devices.

- Special considerations
  - Intraventricular hemorrhage (IVH)
    - Digital subtraction angiography (DSA) is recommended for all cases of IVH without intraparenchymal hemorrhage (IPH).
    - Intraventricular tissue plasminogen activator (tPA) is safe and reduces mortality (but does not improve functional outcome) in patients with primary IVH or IVH extension from supratentorial ICH <30 mL, with EVD, and GCS >3.
  - Acute cerebral venous thrombosis
    - Anticoagulation with heparin (low-molecular-weight weakly recommended over unfractionated) is first-line therapy, even in the setting of ICH (see Chapter 8.7 for further details).
- Nutrition
  - Malnutrition is associated with poor functional outcome after ICH.
  - Hypocaloric enteral nutrition should be initiated within 48 hours of admission and increased to 80% to 100% of energy expenditure after day 3.

Subacute and Chronic Management

- MRI to help determine ICH etiology
  - Evidence of CAA, as described earlier
  - Additional lesions to suggest metastasis
  - Infarcts to suggest hemorrhagic conversion
  - May need to repeat MRI with contrast in 3 to 6 months to identify an underlying lesion
- Anticoagulation
  - The decision of how long after an ICH to wait to resume or initiate anticoagulation should be made by balancing the risk of ICH recurrence/expansion with initiation and of thromboembolism with delay.
  - Early resumption (within 2 weeks) could be considered in patients at high thromboembolic risk (eg, mechanical valve).
  - For patients with nonvalvular atrial fibrillation, can consider resuming anticoagulation around 7 to 8 weeks after ICH, though may need to wait longer or hold indefinitely in patients with evidence of CAA or other high-risk features (eg, uncontrolled hypertension).
- BP control
  - Prior to discharge, patients should be on a medication regimen that maintains BP <130/80 with minimal variability (ie, long-acting agents such as lisinopril and amlodipine) in order to reduce the risk of recurrent ICH.

Outcomes

- The ICH and FUNC scores are tools that can be used to help predict mortality and functional independence, respectively, after ICH. These tools should, however, be used with caution and only as an adjunct to clinical judgment as the ICH score, for example, has been shown to overpredict poor outcome.

SUGGESTED READINGS

Anderson CS, Heeley E, Huang Y, et al. Rapid blood-pressure lowering in patients with acute intracerebral hemorrhage. *N Engl J Med*. 2013;368: 2355-2365.

Biffi A, Anderson CD, Battey TW, et al. Association between blood pressure control and risk of recurrent intracerebral hemorrhage. *JAMA*. 2015; 314:904-912.

Castello JP, Teo KC, Abramson JR, et al. Long-term blood pressure variability and major adverse cardiovascular and cerebrovascular events after intracerebral hemorrhage. *J Am Heart Assoc*. 2022;11:e024158.

Charidimou A, Boulouis G, Frosch MP, et al. The Boston criteria version 2.0 for cerebral amyloid angiopathy: a multicentre, retrospective, MRI–neuropathology diagnostic accuracy study. *Lancet Neurol*. 2022;21:714-725.

Connolly SJ, Sharma M, Cohen AT, et al. Andexanet for factor Xa inhibitor–associated acute intracerebral hemorrhage. *N Engl J Med*. 2024;390: 1745-1755.

Cordonnier C, Demchuk A, Ziai W, et al. Intracerebral haemorrhage: current approaches to acute management. *Lancet*. 2018;392:1257-1268.

Duskin J, Yechoor N, Singh S, et al. Nutrition markers and discharge outcome in deep and lobar intracerebral hemorrhage. *Eur Stroke J*. 2024;9:1074-1082.

Feigin VL, Lawes CM, Bennett DA, et al. Stroke epidemiology: a review of population-based studies of incidence, prevalence, and case-fatality in the late 20th century. *Lancet Neurol*. 2003;2:43-53.

Ferro JM, Bousser MG, Canhão P, et al. European Stroke Organization guideline for the diagnosis and treatment of cerebral venous thrombosis—endorsed by the European Academy of Neurology. *Eur Stroke J*. 2017; 2:195-221.

GBD 2019 Stroke Collaborators. Global, regional, and national burden of stroke and its risk factors, 1990-2019: a systematic analysis for the Global Burden of Disease Study 2019. *Lancet Neurol*. 2021;20:795-820.

Greenberg SM, Ziai WC, Cordonnier C, et al. 2022 guideline for the management of patients with spontaneous intracerebral hemorrhage: a guideline from the American Heart Association/American Stroke Association. *Stroke*. 2022;53:e282-e361.

Gross BA, Jankowitz BT, Friedlander RM. Cerebral intraparenchymal hemorrhage: a review. *JAMA*. 2019;321:1295-1303.

Hanley DF, Lane K, McBee N, et al. Thrombolytic removal of intraventricular haemorrhage in treatment of severe stroke: results of the randomised, multicentre, multiregion, placebo-controlled CLEAR III trial. *Lancet*. 2017;389:603-611.

Hemphill JC, Bonovich DC, Besmertis L, et al. The ICH score. *Stroke*. 2001;32:891-897.

Kamel H, Navi BB, Nakagawa K, et al. Hypertonic saline versus mannitol for the treatment of elevated intracranial pressure: a meta-analysis of randomized clinical trials. *Crit Care Med*. 2011;39:554-559.

Kuramatsu JB, Biffi A, Gerner ST, et al. Association of surgical hematoma evacuation vs conservative treatment with functional outcome in patients with cerebellar intracerebral hemorrhage. *JAMA*. 2019;322: 1392-1403.

Li G, Lin Y, Yang J, et al. Intensive ambulance-delivered blood-pressure reduction in hyperacute stroke. *N Engl J Med*. 2024;390:1862-1872.

NICE-SUGAR Study Investigators; Finfer S, Chittock DR, et al. Intensive versus conventional glucose control in critically Ill patients. *N Engl J Med*. 2009;360:1283-1297.

O'Donnell MJ, Xavier D, Liu L, et al. Risk factors for ischaemic and intracerebral haemorrhagic stroke in 22 countries (the INTERSTROKE study): a case-control study. *Lancet*. 2010;376:112-123.

Poon MT, Fonville AF, Al-Shahi Salman R. Long-term prognosis after intracerebral haemorrhage: systematic review and meta-analysis. *J Neurol Neurosurg Psychiatry*. 2014;85:660-667.

Pradilla G, Ratcliff JJ, Hall AJ, et al. Trial of early minimally invasive removal of intracerebral hemorrhage. *N Engl J Med*. 2024;390:1277-1289.

Qureshi AI, Huang W, Lobanova I, et al. Outcomes of intensive systolic blood pressure reduction in patients with intracerebral hemorrhage and excessively high initial systolic blood pressure: post hoc analysis of a randomized clinical trial. *JAMA Neurology*. 2020;77:1355-1365.

Qureshi AI, Palesch YY, Barsan WG, et al. Intensive blood-pressure lowering in patients with acute cerebral hemorrhage. *N Engl J Med*. 2016;375: 1033-1043.

Rost NS, Smith EE, Chang Y, et al. Prediction of functional outcome in patients with primary intracerebral hemorrhage. *Stroke*. 2008;39:2304-2309.

Sembill JA, Gerner ST, Volbers B, et al. Severity assessment in maximally treated ICH patients: the max-ICH score. *Neurology*. 2017;89:423-431.

Sheikh ZB, Stretz C, Maciel CB, et al. Deep versus lobar intraparenchymal hemorrhage: seizures, hyperexcitable patterns, and clinical outcomes. *Crit Care Med*. 2020;48:e505-e513.

Shiga Y, Nezu T, Shimomura R, et al. Various effects of nutritional status on clinical outcomes after intracerebral hemorrhage. *Intern Emerg Med*. 2022;17:1043-1052.

Singer P, Blaser AR, Berger MM, et al. ESPEN guideline on clinical nutrition in the intensive care unit. *Clin Nutr*. 2019;38:48-79.

Sprigg N, Flaherty K, Appleton JP, et al. Tranexamic acid for hyperacute primary IntraCerebral Haemorrhage (TICH-2): an international randomised, placebo-controlled, phase 3 superiority trial. *Lancet*. 2018;391: 2107-2115.

Sun S, Li Y, Zhang H, et al. The effect of mannitol in the early stage of supratentorial hypertensive intracerebral hemorrhage: a systematic review and meta-analysis. *World Neurosurg*. 2019;124:386-396.

8.9

Subarachnoid Hemorrhage and Vascular Malformations

Nadia McMillan, Ali A. Alsarah, Robert W. Regenhardt, and Saef Izzy

Definition

- Aneurysms and vascular malformations can be associated with significant neurologic disability and intracranial hemorrhage (ICH).
- The clinical presentation, management, and hospital course of aneurysm versus vascular malformation rupture vary.

Common Disorders to Remember

- Aneurysm: focal saccular outpouching due to weakness in the arterial wall, most often at bifurcations. Rupture typically causes subarachnoid hemorrhage (SAH).
- Arteriovenous malformation (AVM): aberrant connection between arteries and veins without an intervening capillary bed, resulting in arteriovenous shunting
- Cavernous malformation (angioma): angiographically occult collection of dilated blood vessels (capillaries) prone to leakage, without a feeding artery or draining vein and no intervening brain tissue
- Developmental venous anomaly (DVA): congenital anomaly, rather than a malformation. Not associated with risk of bleeding but can be associated with cavernous malformations
- Dural arteriovenous fistula (DAVF): abnormal connection between a meningeal artery and a meningeal vein or a dural sinus. Can be associated with cortical venous reflux
- Capillary telangiectasia: incidentally found collection of dilated capillaries with intervening normal brain tissue, managed conservatively (not further discussed here)

Subarachnoid Hemorrhage

Clinical Presentation of Aneurysmal Subarachnoid Hemorrhage

- Heralded by sudden severe headache classically described as "worst headache of life" that peaks within minutes
- Other signs and symptoms: nausea, vomiting, nuchal rigidity, photophobia, loss or depressed level of consciousness, seizure, dilated pupil with complete or partial cranial nerve (CN) III palsy (suggests posterior communicating artery [PCOM] aneurysm), CN VI palsy (suggests elevated intracranial pressure [ICP]), focal neurologic deficits (due to parenchymal blood or ischemic stroke due to vasospasm), intraocular hemorrhage (Terson syndrome)
- Sentinel (warning) headaches may precede the onset in a subset of patients.
- Systemic signs: hypertension (HTN), hypoxemia, electrocardiogram (ECG) changes suggestive of myocardial infarction

Epidemiology

- Incidence of aneurysmal SAH (aSAH) in the United States is ~10 to 14/100,000 persons per year, highest in Finland and Japan, and accounts for 85% of all SAH.
- Prevalence of aneurysms is 0.4% to 3.6% based on autopsy studies, and 3.7% to 6.0% based on angiography studies; increases with age.
- 1:2 male-to-female ratio, mean age at presentation is 55 years, more common in men <40 years of age
- Frequent locations of aneurysms: anterior communicating artery (ACOM) (30%), PCOM (25%), middle cerebral artery (MCA) (20%), internal carotid artery (ICA) (7.5%), basilar tip (7%), and posterior inferior cerebellar artery (PICA) (3%)
- Risk of aneurysm rupture is 1% per year per the Unruptured Cerebral Aneurysm Study (UCAS) of Japan; size, location, and the presence of a daughter sac are important variables.
- PHASES score, derived from prospective cohorts, estimates 5-year rupture risk and includes factors such as population (Finnish/Japanese), age (>70), HTN, aneurysm size and site (anterior cerebral artery, PCOM, or posterior circulation as highest risk), and prior SAH.
- Case fatality rate is ~50%: 12.4% die before coming to medical attention, 10% to 12% within the first 24 hours, 19% to 45% at 1 week, and 25% to 60% at 3 months.
- Approximately one-third of the survivors become dependent needing long-term care.

Key Pathophysiology

- Saccular aneurysms are typically located in the circle of Willis at sites of bifurcation due to hemodynamic factors.
- Most aneurysms arise sporadically, but their development can be influenced by genetic and environmental factors including smoking, HTN, heavy alcohol use, cocaine and amphetamine use, pregnancy, oral contraceptive use, autosomal dominant form of polycystic kidney disease, connective tissue disease (Marfan, Ehlers-Danlos type IV, neurofibromatosis type 1 [NF-1], pseudoxanthoma elasticum, fibromuscular dysplasia), first-degree relative with SAH.
- Rupture often temporally associated with strenuous activities or Valsalva such as heavy lifting, straining, sexual activity, and physical exercise

Differential Diagnosis for Subarachnoid Hemorrhage (Table 8.9.1)

Diagnosis

Noncontrast Head Computed Tomography

- Highest sensitivity within the first 6 hours (98%-100%), drops to 90% at 24 hours, 85% after 5 days, 50% at 1 week, and 0% at 3 weeks.

Lumbar Puncture

- 3% of patients with SAH can have a sudden onset headache and a negative computed tomography (CT) within 12 hours of ictus.
- Lumbar puncture (LP) is needed to definitively rule out a SAH if CT scan is negative, especially if >6 hours from ictus.
  - Diagnostic yield for detecting xanthochromia in cerebrospinal fluid (CSF) is greater after 6 to 12 hours from symptom onset.

Magnetic Resonance Imaging

- Brain magnetic resonance imaging (MRI) may be less desirable as a first-line imaging modality due to longer acquisition time (difficult in the confused patient), and the highest sensitivity >24 hours from ictus.
- Vessel wall imaging may offer some guidance in equivocal cases.
- If noncontrast CT is equivocal and LP contraindicated, MRI fluid-attenuated inversion recovery (FLAIR) + susceptibility-weighted imaging (SWI) may help.
- If MRI is negative, LP is still recommended if the clinical suspicion for SAH is high.

Computed Tomographic Angiography

- Computed tomographic angiography (CTA) allows for visualization of the cerebral vessels and detection of aneurysms.
- The CTA sensitivity varies with aneurysm size, especially <3 mm (sensitivity of 30% for aneurysms <3 mm and 81.5% for 3-5 mm in size).
- CTA can also be helpful for procedural planning.

TABLE 8.9.1 Subarachnoid Hemorrhage Differential Diagnosis

• Ruptured intracranial aneurysm	• Trauma
• Angiogram-negative SAH	• Vasculitis
• AVMs	• Substance use (cocaine, amphetamines, etc)
• Carotid or vertebral artery dissection	• Coagulopathy (more often intraparenchymal or subdural)
• Spinal AVM	• Sickle cell disease
• Pituitary apoplexy	• Moyamoya disease
• Arteriovenous fistula	• Mycotic aneurysms

AVM, arteriovenous malformation; SAH, subarachnoid hemorrhage.

Digital Subtraction Angiography

- Considered the gold standard for aneurysm diagnosis; provides detailed anatomy of aneurysm morphology (including high-risk features), its relationship to other vessels aneurysm orientation, neck size, and presence of vasospasm
- If the first digital subtraction angiography (DSA) is negative, a follow-up DSA is often recommended in 7 to 14 days to exclude an aneurysm that may have been obscured by thrombosis or otherwise inadequately visualized.

Grading the Severity of Subarachnoid Hemorrhage (Table 8.9.2)

- Hunt-Hess Grade: clinical scale initially described to weigh the risks versus benefits of surgery and procedural planning
- World Federation of Neurological Surgeons (WFNS): clinical scale based on Glasgow Coma Scale (GCS)
- Fisher Scale: radiographic scale based on clot thickness on the initial CT scan; described as a predictor of vasospasm and delayed cerebral ischemia (DCI).

Aneurysms

Treatment

- Aims of critical care management include stabilization of the patient with ABCDE (airway, breathing, circulation, disability, exposure).
- If GCS <8, drop in score >2, or concern for airway protection, consider intubation.
- Avoid hypotension, monitor for arrhythmias, treat seizures, and prevent fever.
- Major goals of treatment included preventing rebleeding, controlling ICP, preventing and treating DCI/vasospasm, cardiopulmonary support, and preventing systemic complications.
- For ruptured aneurysms, definitive treatment is often with endovascular therapy > surgical clipping.

Prevention of Rebleeding

- Rebleeding is associated with a high morbidity and mortality.
- Risk factors for rebleeding include aneurysm size, worsening neurologic deficit, prior sentinel hemorrhage, loss of consciousness at ictus, treatment history of incomplete aneurysm occlusion, and delay to definitive treatment.
- Risk of rebleeding is as high as 25% within the first 24 hours, ~4% occurring in the first 24 hours.
- Initial systolic blood pressure (SBP) goal is typically <140 to 160, but this can be relaxed after the aneurysm is secured; a rapidly titratable medication is preferred for management.
- Consensus recommendations include *considering* a short course of antifibrinolytic therapy (<72 hours) until early definitive treatment of the aneurysm is achieved, weighed against the risk of ischemic events.

Surgical or Endovascular Treatment of Ruptured Aneurysm

- Most centers aim for definitive treatment within 48 hours to minimize the risk of rebleeding and permit safer use of hypertensive treatment in the event of vasospasm.
- International Subarachnoid Aneurysm Trial (ISAT), a randomized trial comparing clipping versus coiling of ruptured aneurysms, demonstrated a 7% absolute risk reduction in death or dependency with coiling over surgical clipping; benefit was sustained beyond 1 year.
- Endovascular coil embolization has been widely employed in the management of ruptured aneurysms and is now the favored treatment modality.
- Endovascular use of stents, including intravascular flow diverters, requires antiplatelet therapy, so use is typically restricted to specific situations, such as in the treatment of dissecting aneurysms or small aneurysms with wide necks.
- Factors that favor coiling include advanced age, significant comorbidities, surgically inaccessible location (eg, posterior circulation), small aneurysms, aneurysms with narrow necks.

TABLE 8.9.2 Grading the Severity of Subarachnoid Hemorrhage

Hunt-Hess Grade		WFNS Grade			Modified Fisher Scale[a]	
Grade	Findings	Grade	GCS	Findings	Grade	Subarachnoid Blood
I	No symptoms or mild headache	I	15	No motor symptoms	I	None
II	Moderate-severe headache, nuchal rigidity, ± cranial nerve deficits	II	14-13	No motor symptoms	II	Diffuse only, <1 mm
III	Confusion, lethargy, focal deficits	III	14-13	With motor symptoms	III	Clot, thick layer, ≥1 mm thick
IV	Stupor/hemiparesis	IV	12-7	± Motor symptoms	IV	Diffuse or none, with cerebral or ventricular blood
V	Comatose ± extensor posturing	V	6-3	± Motor symptoms		

DCI, delayed cerebral ischemia; GCS, Glasgow Coma Scale; IVH, intraventricular hemorrhage; WFNS, World Federation of Neurological Surgeons.
[a]Modified Fisher Scale: thick cisternal clot + IVH both strongly associated with DCI.

- Factors that favor clipping include surgically readily accessible location (eg, MCA), wide-neck aneurysms, incorporation of arterial branches in the aneurysm, SAH with parenchymal hemorrhage, and mass effect. However, intrasaccular flow diversion and other advances in device technology are expanding the endovascular options for aneurysms that were traditionally clipped.

Raised Intracranial Pressure/Acute Hydrocephalus

- ~20% of patients with aSAH have hydrocephalus at presentation and an additional 10% develop it by the first week; carries a poor prognosis and is associated with higher mortality.
- Clinically associated with impairment of consciousness and can be accompanied by downward gaze and/or small unreactive pupils
- CSF drainage is an established means to treat hydrocephalus and high ICP, typically with an external ventricular drain (EVD); however, to avoid rebleeding of an unsecured aneurysm, the drain should only be opened if the ICP >15 mm Hg until definitive aneurysm treatment.
- The EARLYDRAIN randomized trial demonstrated that early lumbar CSF drainage in aSAH significantly improved 6-month neurologic outcomes compared to standard care, likely due to more efficient clearance of subarachnoid blood. However, EVDs remain a standard and reasonable option, particularly in patients with hydrocephalus or elevated ICP.
- Protocols for both rapid and slow EVD wean exist. Permanent shunting may be needed in those who fail to wean from an EVD.

Vasospasm and Delayed Cerebral Ischemia

- Vasospasm, the radiographic narrowing of cerebral arteries, occurs in ~70% of aSAH as a result of oxyhemoglobin and free radical formation.
- Vasospasm peaks between days 3 and 14 postrupture.
- Vasospasm can be focal or diffuse and, when symptomatic, may result in DCI (~20%-30%). Additional elements such as microcirculatory dysfunction, loss of autoregulation, cortical spreading depolarization, and microthrombosis likely also contribute to the development of DCI.
- Vasospasm detection is routinely employed with daily transcranial Doppler (TCD) during the high-risk period, with the addition of CTA/CT perfusion (CTP) if worsening flow velocities (FVs) are noted on TCD.
- Mean FV >200 cm/s, increase in FV by ≥50 cm/s over 24 hours, or Lindegaard ratio ≥6 (FV in MCA/ipsilateral ICA) suggests severe vasospasm, correlates with angiographic vasospasm (gold standard), and usually precedes clinical deterioration.
- Nimodipine, an L-type calcium channel antagonist, has been shown to decrease the incidence of DCI and improve functional outcome at 3 months; it should be started as soon as possible or at least within 96 hours.
- "Triple-H" therapy (HTN, hypervolemia, hemodilution) is no longer routinely implemented to prevent vasospasm. The mainstay of treatment in symptomatic vasospasm is euvolemic-induced HTN, while the benefits of hypervolemia and hemodilution are controversial.
- Induced HTN for patients with DCI is recommended unless cardiac contraindications preclude the use of pressors.
- Intravenous (IV) milrinone, a phosphodiesterase III inhibitor with vasodilating and inotropic effects, is also often considered. Milrinone is increasingly used to treat vasospasm, though no randomized controlled trials (RCTs) exist.
- Endovascular spasmolysis with intra-arterial verapamil, milrinone, or nicardipine is typically first line for symptomatic vasospasm. For refractory and/or severe vasospasm in which the benefits outweigh the risks, balloon angioplasty and novel devices such as expandable stents are sometimes employed as rescue treatments.

Seizure

- Seizures can be seen in as many as ~26% of patients with SAH at presentation; however, this likely includes posturing, as well.
- Seizure at onset is not a risk factor for late seizures. Prophylactic antiepileptic drugs are conventionally used until an aneurysm is secured, given the repercussions of seizure in this scenario, although definitive evidence to support this practice is lacking.
- In-hospital seizures before aneurysm treatment are associated with rebleeding.
- The risk of nonconvulsive status epilepticus is ~8% in aSAH and is associated with worse outcomes; continuous electroencephalogram (EEG) monitoring should be employed in those with worse SAH grade and in coma.

Systemic Complications

- *Fevers*
  - Seen in 54% of patients with SAH, doubles the risk of poor outcome and should be aggressively treated
- *Pulmonary*
  - Over 20% of patients with aSAH have pulmonary complications, which account for 50% of nonneurologic causes of mortality.
  - The most common are aspiration and nosocomial pneumonia, congestive heart failure, and neurogenic pulmonary edema.
  - Treatment includes meticulous management of fluid status and antibiotics.
- *Cardiac*
- Troponin elevation (34%), arrhythmias (35%), and wall motion abnormalities on echocardiogram (28%) are common and thought to be secondary to catecholamine surge in aSAH.
- *Takotsubo* cardiomyopathy is a characteristic transient echocardiographic finding with left ventricular apical and midventricular ballooning and akinesis, accompanied by hemodynamic instability and pulmonary edema.
- Treatment of secondary cardiac complications focuses on cautious use of beta-blockers and inotropic support.
- Cardiac catheterization, anticoagulation, and permissive hypotension are generally not indicated.
- *Hyponatremia*
  - Most common electrolyte abnormality in aSAH, seen in 30% to 50% of cases between days 3 and 14 after rupture; associated with a higher incidence of DCI
  - Hypovolemic hyponatremia is the hallmark of cerebral salt wasting (CSW), whereas euvolemic or hypervolemic hyponatremia defines the syndrome of inappropriate antidiuretic hormone (SIADH).

- Fluid restriction, the traditional treatment for SIADH, would be dangerous in patients with aSAH with vasospasm.
- Hyponatremia is managed with volume repletion and with hypertonic saline +/− fludrocortisone in severe cases.

- *Hypoglycemia*
  - Hypoglycemia is associated with increased vasospasm and poor 3-month outcome; target blood glucose <200 mg/dL.
- *Anemia*
  - Higher hemoglobin is associated with lower risk of cerebral infarction, but the optimal transfusion threshold remains unclear.

Outcomes

- At 1 year, slightly >% of patients with aSAH survive.
- Over 50% are left with memory/cognitive deficits and personality changes, two-thirds of survivors resume work, but some with reduced responsibilities.
- 25% have reported complete neurologic recovery.

Arteriovenous Malformations

Epidemiology

- Prevalence of AVM is 15 to 18/100,000 adults; the typical age range at presentation is 20 to 50.
- Initial presentation is with ICH (45%), seizures (29%), headaches (13%), and focal deficits (7%); 30-day mortality is 18% after a hemorrhagic presentation. ICH may be accompanied by SAH.
- Rate of spontaneous hemorrhage is 1.5% to 4.0% per year.
- Recurrent rupture risk is 6% in the first year, thereafter 2% to 4% per year.
- Risk factors for AVM hemorrhage include prior hemorrhage, older age, nidus size, intranidal aneurysm, deep AVM location, and deep venous drainage.
- Ruptured AVM mortality rate is 12% to 29%, morbidity is 23%.

Key Pathophysiology

- AVMs are made up of feeding arteries, a dysplastic nidus, and draining veins.
- Lack of an intervening capillary bed to buffer the higher pressures seen by nidus and venous structures results in hemorrhage.
- 15% to 46% of AVMs are associated with aneurysms and have an increased rupture risk, especially if pre- or intranidally.

Differential Diagnosis

- Cavernoma
- Vascularized primary brain tumor
- DVA
- Moyamoya disease
- DAVF

Management and Treatment

- Cerebral angiography and MRI are modalities of choice for treatment decisions and technical procedural planning. Posttreatment angiography is used to demonstrate surgical efficacy.

TABLE 8.9.3 Spetzler-Martin Scale

Grade Feature	Points
Size	
Small (>3 cm)	1
Medium (3-6 cm)	2
Large (>6 cm)	3
Eloquence of adjacent brain	
Noneloquent	0
Eloquent	1
Pattern of venous drainage	
Superficial	0
Deep	1

- Surgical risk grading (Spetzler-Martin Scale) is based on nidus size (<3 cm, 3-6 cm, or >3 cm for 1, 2, or 3 points), involvement of eloquent area (motor/sensory cortex, language, visual areas, brainstem, hypothalamus, thalamus, cerebellar peduncles, 0 or 1 point), and involvement of deep venous drainage (0 or 1 point). (See Table 8.9.3 for additional details.)
  - AVM grades (sum of points) 1 to 2 are deemed lower surgical risk, and grade 3 is treated on a case-by-case basis.
  - AVM grades 4 to 5 are at risk for postsurgical neurologic deficits, and surgery is reserved for patients with recurrent hemorrhages or progressive deficits; however, these patients may be candidates for radiosurgery (if size <3 cm) or endovascular treatment (Table 8.9.4).
- Postoperative cerebral hemorrhage and/or edema are thought to be related to normal perfusion pressure breakthrough (NPPB) from loss of autoregulation of maximally dilated blood vessels surrounding the AVM and occlusive hyperemia from venous thrombosis or arterial stagnation.
- One strategy to limit hyperemia includes induced hypotension; the standard protocol is strict blood pressure control below baseline.
- Hypocarbia, steroids, hyperosmolar therapy, and burst suppression with barbiturates may be considered to prevent ischemia and promote neuroprotection in cases of hemorrhage and/or edema.
- Postoperative edema from thrombosis or stagnation may be cautiously managed with aspirin or low-dose heparin.

TABLE 8.9.4 Correlation of AVM grade with post-surgical outcomes

Grade (Sum of Points)	No Deficit (%)	Minor Deficit (%)	Major Deficit (%)
1	100	0	0
2	95	5	0
3	84	12	4
4	73	20	7
5	69	19	12

AVM, arteriovenous malformation.

- Seizure in the postoperative period due to hemodynamic changes, mass effect, or new postoperative hemorrhage warrants higher doses of anticonvulsants.
- *The ARUBA* (A Randomized trial of Unruptured Brain Arteriovenous malformations) trial concluded that medical management alone was superior to interventional therapy for unruptured AVMs in terms of stroke and death risk over a median follow-up of 33 months. However, the study has been widely criticized for short follow-up duration, limited generalizability, and selection bias, and its applicability remains controversial. Treatment decisions should be individualized based on hemorrhage risk and AVM characteristics.

Cavernous Malformations

Epidemiology

- Prevalence of ~0.5%, most commonly presents in the fourth decade, there is no clear gender predominance.
- Common presenting symptoms include seizures (37%), hemorrhage (36%), headaches (23%), and focal deficits (22%).
- Multiple cavernous malformations can be familial, with autosomal dominant inheritance, prominent in Hispanic Americans.
- Acquired forms reported after brain radiation and surgery
- Associated with DVAs (9%)
- Rupture rates of 0.25% to 2.4% per year, rebleeding rates per year range in the literature from 4.5% to 23%
- Risk factors for rebleeding include younger age, female, prior hemorrhage, presence of venous angioma, deep location, infratentorial location, familial disease, and incomplete resection.
- Morbidity and mortality are highest for brainstem lesions.

Key Pathophysiology

- Enlarge with rebleeding, accompanied by hemosiderin deposition from recurrent microhemorrhages and thrombosis
- Can be cortical, deep, intraventricular, spinal, and/or dural. Common locations include the cortex around the Rolandic fissure and temporal lobes, the brainstem, and the cerebellum.
- Familial form mapped to chromosomes 7q, 7p, and 3q

Differential Diagnosis

- Hemorrhagic metastasis, such as melanoma
- Low-grade glial tumors
- AVM
- Venous malformation

Management and Treatment

- Classically described as having a "popcorn" appearance on imaging; diagnosed on T2 and T2* (gradient recalled echo or GRE)-weighted MRI with T2 hypointense rim, variable T1 from different ages of blood products
- Expectant management for patients with minimal symptoms and those with cavernomatosis
- Surgery is considered for patients with recurrent hemorrhage, refractory seizures, and progressive deficits.
- High-risk cases may benefit from radiosurgery instead of open resection.
- Aspirin has been historically avoided due to a perceived bleeding risk, but some studies suggest lower risk of ICH with aspirin.

Developmental Venous Anomaly

Epidemiology

- Hemorrhage risk 0.2% per year
- Most frequently identified incidental vascular anomaly (0.5%-2.9%) in the fourth to fifth decades of life
- Can be found in 20% of patients with mucocutaneous venous malformations of the head and neck and can be associated with blue rubber bleb nevus syndrome and sinus pericrania (connection between the extracranial and intracranial) venous systems

Key Pathophysiology

- Radial array of dilated medullary veins ("caput medusa" appearance) that drain into a larger transcortical or subependymal vein and form part of normal venous outflow draining normal brain tissue
- Drainage can be cortical or deep, or into a dural sinus.
- Rebleeding uncommon
- DVAs are associated with cavernous malformations in 8%-33% of cases.

Differential Diagnosis

- Capillary telangiectasia
- Infiltrating glioma
- Cavernous malformation

Management and Treatment

- Most often clinically silent. When discovered, the initial presentation may include headaches, seizures, hemorrhage, and focal deficits.
- Commonly an incidental finding on MRI; on angiography, the caput medusa pattern is seen in the late venous phase.
- Conservative management is the standard of care since it drains normal brain tissue and surgical resection can result in venous infarction.
- In cases of hemorrhage, an alternative lesion should be excluded (eg, cavernous malformation or AVM).
- If associated with cavernous malformation for which surgery is pursued, care should be taken to preserve the DVA.

Dural Arteriovenous Fistulas

Epidemiology

- Rare but treatable cause of ICH can be acquired after trauma, previous neurosurgery, and most commonly after venous sinus/cortical vein thrombosis/thrombophlebitis.
- Incidence common to both genders, but clinically more aggressive in men. Men more commonly present with cortical venous reflux, while women more commonly present with a subtype involving the cavernous sinus, known as carotid-cavernous fistula (CCF).
- Risk of hemorrhage is 2% per year, most of which is attributable to cortical venous reflux, but other risk factors include location, flow dynamics, retrograde sinus drainage, presence of a venous varix, and drainage into the vein of Galen.
- Common sites of DAVFs are transverse/sigmoid sinus (39%), cavernous sinus (20%), and superior sagittal sinus (13%).

Key Pathophysiology

- Proposed pathophysiologic mechanisms include neovascularization following a previously occluded dural sinus; venous congestion/HTN results in dilated capillaries with eventual direct shunting between arteries and veins.
- Can result in intracerebral, subdural, and SAH, pulsatile tinnitus (particularly with transverse or sigmoid sinus involvement), diplopia, proptosis, chemosis, visual impairment (particularly with cavernous sinus lesions), intracranial HTN (especially with superior sagittal sinus involvement), seizures (often with cortical vein involvement), dementia, and rarely mass effect.
- Spinal DAVF presents with progressive myelopathy in 50% of cases.
- Based on the Cognard classification, there are five types of DAVF with escalating risk of hemorrhage or aggressive symptoms:
  - Type I—normal antegrade drainage into a sinus
  - Type II—antegrade drainage into a sinus but insufficient antegrade venous drainage (IIa—retrograde drainage into sinuses only; IIb—retrograde drainage into cortical veins only; IIa+IIb—retrograde drainage into sinuses and cortical veins)
  - Type III—drainage directly into cortical vein without venous ectasia
  - Type IV—drainage into cortical vein with venous ectasia >5 mm and 3 times larger than the draining vein
  - Type V—intracranial DAVF drains into spinal perimedullary veins.

Management and Treatment

- Rarity of the DAVF warrants high clinical suspicion to achieve the diagnosis. Importantly, it is a cause of reversible dementia.
- CT can identify a hemorrhage in an uncharacteristic location, particularly in younger patients; CTA may show accompanying dilated/congested veins.
- MRI with angiography or venography may more readily identify lesions.
- Catheter angiography (DSA) is the gold standard, given the greater spatial and temporal resolution, the latter of which can show arteriovenous shunting.
- Acute deterioration after an LP can occur due to unrecognized tonsillar herniation in cases of intracranial HTN.
- Intracranial HTN portends a poor prognosis in patients with DAVF.
- Spontaneous thrombosis of type 1 fistulas can result in resolution. These lesions are often treated conservatively unless symptoms are debilitating.
- For patients who present with type 2 or greater fistulas (cortical venous reflux or retrograde sinus reflux), treatment is indicated, particularly for those with a history of ICH, symptomatic cavernous sinus syndrome, or progressive disability.
- Treatment options include endovascular embolization, open surgical disconnection (often clipping the draining vein), radiosurgery, or a combined approach.
- Need long-term surveillance, given the potential for recurrence despite definitive treatment.

Acknowledgment

We gratefully acknowledge the contributions of previous edition author, Pankajavalli Ramakrishnan, as portions of those chapters have been retained in this revision.

SUGGESTED READINGS

Al-Shahi R, Fang JS, Lewis SC, Warlow CP. Prevalence of adults with brain arteriovenous malformations: a community based study in Scotland using capture-recapture analysis. *J Neurol Neurosurg Psychiatry.* 2002;73:547-551.

Anonymous. Report of world federation of neurological surgeons committee on a Universal Subarachnoid Hemorrhage Grading Scale. *J Neurosurg.* 1988;68:985-986.

Boukobza M, Enjolras O, Guichard JP, et al. Cerebral developmental venous anomalies associated with head and neck venous malformations. *AJNR Am J Neuroradiol.* 1996;17:987-994.

Brisman JL, Song JK, Newell DW. Cerebral aneurysms. *N Engl J Med.* 2006;355:928-939.

Brown RD Jr, Flemming KD, Meyer FB, Cloft HJ, Pollock BE, Link ML. Natural history, evaluation, and management of intracranial vascular malformations. *Mayo Clin Proc.* 2005;80:269-281.

Bruder N, Rabinstein A; Participants in the International Multi-Disciplinary Consensus Conference on the Critical Care Management of Subarachnoid Hemorrhage. Cardiovascular and pulmonary complications of aneurysmal subarachnoid hemorrhage. *Neurocrit Care.* 2011;15:257-269.

Byyny RL, Mower WR, Shum N, Gabayan GZ, Fang S, Baraff LJ. Sensitivity of noncontrast cranial computed tomography for the emergency department diagnosis of subarachnoid hemorrhage. *Ann Emerg Med.* 2008; 51:697-703.

Chaudhary MY, Sachdev VP, Cho SH, Weitzner I Jr, Puljic S, Huang YP. Dural arteriovenous malformation of the major venous sinuses: an acquired lesion. *AJNR Am J Neuroradiol.* 1982;3:13-19.

Cognard C, Casasco A, Toevi M, Houdart E, Chiras J, Merland JJ. Dural arteriovenous fistulas as a cause of intracranial hypertension due to impairment of cranial venous outflow. *J Neurol Neurosurg Psychiatry.* 1998;65:308-316.

Cognard C, Gobin YP, Pierot L, et al. Cerebral dural arteriovenous fistulas: clinical and angiographic correlation with a revised classification of venous drainage. *Radiology.* 1995;194:671-680.

Fisher CM, Kistler JP, Davis JM. Relation of cerebral vasospasm to subarachnoid hemorrhage visualized by computerized tomographic scanning. *Neurosurgery.* 1980;6:1-9.

Frontera, J. A. et al. Prediction of symptomatic vasospasm after subarachnoid hemorrhage: the modified fisher scale. *Neurosurgery* 59, 21-27; discussion 21-27 (2006). https://doi.org:10.1227/01.neu.0000243277.86222.6c

Gross BA, Lin N, Du R, Day AL. The natural history of intracranial cavernous malformations. *Neurosurg Focus.* 2011;30:E24.

Hackett ML, Anderson CS; The Australian Cooperative Research on Subarachnoid Hemorrhage Study Group. Health outcomes 1 year after subarachnoid hemorrhage: an international population-based study. *Neurology.* 2000;55:658-662.

Hasan D, Vermeulen M, Wijdicks EF, Hijdra A, van Gijn J. Management problems in acute hydrocephalus after subarachnoid hemorrhage. *Stroke.* 1989;20:747-753.

Hoh BL, Ko NU, Amin-Hanjani S, et al. 2023 guideline for the management of patients with aneurysmal subarachnoid hemorrhage: a guideline from the American Heart Association/American Stroke Association. *Stroke.* 2023;54:e314-e370.

Hop JW, Rinkel GJ, Algra A, van Gijn J. Case-fatality rates and functional outcome after subarachnoid hemorrhage: a systematic review. *Stroke.* 1997;28:660-664.

Hunt WE, Hess RM. Surgical risk as related to time of intervention in the repair of intracranial aneurysms. *J Neurosurg.* 1968;28:14-20.

Jafar JJ, Rezai AR. Acute surgical management of intracranial arteriovenous malformations. *Neurosurgery.* 1994;34:8-12; discussion 12-13.

Kassell NF, Sasaki T, Colohan AR, Nazar G. Cerebral vasospasm following aneurysmal subarachnoid hemorrhage. *Stroke.* 1985;16:562-572.

Lanzino G, D'Urso PI, Suarez J; Participants in the International Multi-Disciplinary Consensus Conference on the Critical Care Management of Subarachnoid Hemorrhage. Seizures and anticonvulsants after aneurysmal subarachnoid hemorrhage. *Neurocrit Care*. 2011;15:247-256.

Matsuda M, Watanabe K, Saito A, Matsumura K, Ichikawa M. Circumstances, activities, and events precipitating aneurysmal subarachnoid hemorrhage. *J Stroke Cerebrovasc Dis*. 2007;16:25-29.

McCormick WF. The pathology of vascular ("arteriovenous") malformations. *J Neurosurg*. 1966;24:807-816.

Molyneux A, Kerr R, Stratton I, et al. International Subarachnoid Aneurysm Trial (ISAT) of neurosurgical clipping versus endovascular coiling in 2143 patients with ruptured intracranial aneurysms: a randomised trial. *Lancet*. 2002;360:1267-1274.

Rammos SK, Maina R, Lanzino G. Developmental venous anomalies: current concepts and implications for management. *Neurosurgery*. 2009; 65:20-29; discussion 29-30.

Rastogi S, Liebeskind DS, Zager EL, Volpe NJ, Weigele JB, Hurst RW. Rapid cognitive decline following lumbar puncture in a patient with a duralarteriovenous fistula. *Surg Neurol*. 2004;62:341-345; discussion 345.

Rigamonti D, Hadley MN, Drayer BP, et al. Cerebral cavernous malformations. Incidence and familial occurrence. *N Engl J Med*. 1988;319:343-347.

Spetzler RF, Martin NA. A proposed grading system for arteriovenous malformations. *J Neurosurg*. 1986;65:476-483.

Stapf C, Mast H, Sciacca RR, et al. Predictors of hemorrhage in patients with untreated brain arteriovenous malformation. *Neurology*. 2006;66:1350-1355.

Starke RM, Connolly ES Jr; Participants in the International Multi-Disciplinary Consensus Conference on the Critical Care Management of Subarachnoid Hemorrhage. Rebleeding after aneurysmal subarachnoid hemorrhage. *Neurocrit Care*. 2011;15:241-246.

Suarez JI, Tarr RW, Selman WR. Aneurysmal subarachnoid hemorrhage. *N Engl J Med*. 2006;354:387-396.

Topper R, Jurgens E, Reul J, Thron A. Clinical significance of intracranial developmental venous anomalies. *J Neurol Neurosurg Psychiatry*. 1999; 67:234-238.

Treggiari MM, Rabinstein AA, Busl KM, et al. Guidelines for the neurocritical care management of aneurysmal subarachnoid hemorrhage. *Neurocrit Care*. 2023;39(1):1-28

van der Wee N, Rinkel GJ, Hasan D, van Gijn J. Detection of subarachnoid haemorrhage on early CT: is lumbar puncture still needed after a negative scan? *J Neurol Neurosurg Psychiatry*. 1995;58:357-359.

van Gijn J, Kerr RS, Rinkel GJ. Subarachnoid haemorrhage. *Lancet*. 2007; 369:306-318.

Wartenberg KE, Schmidt JM, Claassen J, et al. Impact of medical complications on outcome after subarachnoid hemorrhage. *Crit Care Med*. 2006; 34:617-623; quiz 624.

White PM, Wardlaw JM, Easton V. Can noninvasive imaging accurately depict intracranial aneurysms? *A Syst Rev Radiol*. 2000;217:361-370.

Wiebers DO, Whisnant JP, Huston J 3rd, et al. Unruptured intracranial aneurysms: natural history, clinical outcome, and risks of surgical and endovascular treatment. *Lancet*. 2003;362:103-110.

8.10

Cerebral Venous Thrombosis

Ali A. Alsarah, Nadia McMillan, Robert W. Regenhardt, and Saef Izzy

Definition

- Cerebral venous thrombosis (CVT) is a rare but potentially life-threatening cause of stroke, intracerebral hemorrhage, or isolated intracranial hypertension.
- Diagnosis is frequently delayed due to its wide range of clinical presentations. Therefore, maintaining a high clinical suspicion is key to diagnosis.
- Superior sagittal sinus is involved in 62% of presentations of CVT.

Epidemiology

- 12 cases per million per year.
- CVT accounts for 0.5% to 0.7% of all strokes, with an estimated female-to-male ratio of 3:1.
- 85% of the cases have an identifiable prothrombotic risk factor or proximal cause, and 44% of patients have more than one cause or predisposing factor for developing CVT.
- Peri- or postpartum risk of CVT is 12/100,000 deliveries.

Pathophysiology

- Hypercoagulability, hemostasis, vessel injury or inflammation, and venous outflow impairment are all risk factors.
- CVT can result in increased intracranial pressure through either increasing blood volume because of increased venous pressure or through increased cerebrospinal fluid volume due to impaired absorption.
- Venous infarction and cytotoxic/vasogenic edema act as contributors to neurologic deterioration.

Risk Factors

Transient Risk Factors

- Oral contraceptive (54%-71%)
- Pregnancy/postpartum (11%-59%)
- Hormone replacement therapy (4%)
- Head and neck infections (8%-11%)
- Dehydration (2%-19%)
- COVID-19 (7.6%)
- Head trauma (1%-3%)

Chronic Risk Factors

- Genetic thrombophilia (31%-41%): prothrombin G20210A mutation, factor V Leiden, protein C deficiency, protein S deficiency, and antithrombin III deficiency
- Antiphospholipid antibody syndrome (6%-17%)
- Other etiologies of hypercoagulability, including malignancy and autoimmune disease (eg, lupus)
- Intracranial hypotension post–lumbar puncture or shunt placement as a rare but reported risk

Clinical Presentation

- Common clinical manifestations of CVT include headache, which affects 90% of patients, while seizures occur in up to 40% at the time of presentation. Additional signs and symptoms related to increased intracranial pressure may include nausea, transient visual disturbances or vision loss (reported in 13%-27% of cases), papilledema, and diplopia (6%-14%).

- Other signs of CVT may involve dysfunction of cranial nerves III, IV, V1, V2, and VI, often accompanied by headache, fever, eye pain, oculomotor palsies, proptosis, and chemosis.
- Symptom onset may be subacute (days to weeks), unlike arterial strokes.
- Focal neurologic deficits (hemiparesis, aphasia) occur in 30% to 50%.

Workup and Treatment

- All patients with suspicion for CVT should undergo an initial noncontrast head computed tomography (CT) scan; this may show dense vessel sign within the sinuses. The traditional cord or string sign, a serpiginous or linear hyperdensity within a vein, or dense delta sign can be present up to 14 days after the onset of symptoms. Intracerebral hemorrhage can be seen in up to 40% of CVT cases.
- Noncontrast magnetic resonance imaging (MRI) with T1/T2 and susceptibility-weighted imaging (SWI) can reveal thrombus and hemorrhagic infarction.
- CT venography (CTV) and magnetic resonance venography (MRV) are the optimal tests to confirm a diagnosis of CVT.
  On CTV and MRV, thrombi present as filling defects ("empty delta sign" referred to the superior sagittal sinus). MRV can be performed with phase-contrast techniques or without contrast, with time of flight (TOF).
- Diagnostic angiograms are typically reserved, for instances, when endovascular treatment is considered, or the diagnosis is unclear with noninvasive imaging.
- Lab tests: complete blood count (CBC) with hematocrit, renal function test, pregnancy test for females, prothrombin time and activated partial thromboplastin time, erythrocyte sedimentation rate (ESR), D-dimer, iron studies, antiphospholipid panel, COVID-19 antigen, homocysteine, serum protein electrophoresis, and genetic studies for hypercoagulability if suspected
- Initial treatment of CVT includes anticoagulation, traditionally with parenteral heparin followed by a transition to oral vitamin K antagonists for 3 to 12 months, depending on the underlying cause, or indefinitely in the presence of thrombophilia or recurrent venous thromboembolism.
- Low-molecular-weight heparin (LMWH) is often preferred to unfractionated heparin in the acute treatment of CVT in patients with normal renal function due to the more predictable anticoagulation profile and less risk of thrombocytopenia.
- Direct oral anticoagulants (DOACs) are safe and effective options when compared to vitamin K antagonists. Recent studies RE-SPECT CVT, SECRET, and ACTION-CVT showed no significant CVT recurrence in patients treated with DOACs. Patients with malignancy and antiphospholipid syndrome were excluded from these studies.
- Endovascular treatment (EVT) includes mechanical thrombectomy (often with direct aspiration but stent retrievers can be helpful, sometimes with a balloon guide catheter to prevent pulmonary embolism), intrasinus thrombolysis, combination of mechanical thrombectomy and intrasinus thrombolysis, or intra-arterial thrombolysis. These approaches are considered if there is clinical or radiographic progression of thrombosis despite medical management or in patients with severe clinical deficits. The efficacy and safety profiles have not been robustly established.
- Decompressive hemicraniectomy is often offered as a lifesaving therapeutic approach in malignant CVT with midline shift or herniation.

Outcomes

- Early recognition and treatment are associated with a good prognosis.
- >80% of cases have a good outcome.
- Reports of mortality rate range from 3.4% within 30 days of presentation to as high as 15%.
- The most common cause of death during acute hospitalizations for CVT was cerebral herniation.
- Risk factors for poor outcome include coma, intracerebral hemorrhage on admission, thrombosis of the deep venous system, central nervous system infection, cancer, male gender, and age >37.
- Recurrent sinus thrombosis occurs in 2% and extracranial thrombosis in 4%.
- Risk of CVT recurrence in women during another pregnancy is low, but prophylaxis with LMWH is recommended.
- Recanalization rates of 84% to 85% after anticoagulation have been noted between 3 and 12 months.
- Some of the long-term sequelae include chronic headache, epilepsy, or cognitive dysfunction.

SUGGESTED READINGS

Ferro JM, Coutinho JM, Dentali F, et al. Safety and efficacy of dabigatran etexilate vs dose-adjusted warfarin in patients with cerebral venous thrombosis: a randomized clinical trial. *JAMA Neurol*. 2019;76(12):1457-1465.

Field TS, Dizonno V, Almekhlafi MA, et al. Study of rivaroxaban for cerebral venous thrombosis: a randomized controlled feasibility trial comparing anticoagulation with rivaroxaban to standard-of-care in symptomatic cerebral venous thrombosis. *Stroke*. 2023;54(11):2724-2736.

Payne AB, Adamski A, Abe K, et al. Epidemiology of cerebral venous sinus thrombosis and cerebral venous sinus thrombosis with thrombocytopenia in the United States, 2018 and 2019. *Res Pract Thromb Haemost*. 2022;6(2):e12682.

Saposnik G, Barinagarrementeria F, Brown RD Jr, et al. Diagnosis and management of cerebral venous thrombosis: a statement for healthcare professionals from the American Heart Association/American Stroke Association. *Stroke*. 2011;42(4):1158-1192.

Saposnik G, Bushnell C, Coutinho JM, et al. Diagnosis and management of cerebral venous thrombosis: a scientific statement from the American Heart Association. *Stroke*. 2024;55(3):e77-e90.

Yaghi S, Shu L, Bakradze E, et al. Direct oral anticoagulants versus warfarin in the treatment of cerebral venous thrombosis (ACTION-CVT): a Multicenter International Study. *Stroke*. 2022;53(3):728-738.

8.11

Autoimmune Encephalitis and Demyelinating Disease

Yasmin Aghajan and Giovanna S. Manzano

Autoimmune Encephalitis

- Patients with autoimmune encephalitis (AE) may require intensive care unit (ICU) care for the treatment of severely altered mental status, status epilepticus, elevated intracranial pressure, cerebral edema, and medical complications of disease, such as dysautonomia, aspiration, and respiratory failure.

Common Causes to Remember

- See Table 8.11.1.

TABLE 8.11.1 Autoimmune Encephalitis Clinical Presentation

Anti-NMDA receptor encephalitis	• More common in females, age 20-30s • Viral illness-like prodrome, with days to weeks of personality change (agitation, paranoia), short-term memory loss, and abnormal movements • Progresses to develop seizures, depressed level of consciousness, central hypoventilation, and dysautonomia • If related to malignancy, most likely associated with ovarian teratoma in women • CSF anti-NMDAR Ab testing is more sensitive than serum; thus, it is important to send autoimmune encephalopathy panels from *both* the serum and CSF.
Anti-LGI1 encephalitis	*Presentation* • More commonly in ages 60-80s • Presents with limbic encephalitis; short-term memory loss, faciobrachial dystonic seizures, epileptic seizures, and psychiatric symptoms with temporal lobe inflammation (eg, may be visualized using brain MRI demonstrating mesial temporal T2 FLAIR hyperintensities) • Dysautonomia and hyponatremia may also occur.

Ab, antibody; CSF, cerebrospinal fluid; FLAIR, Fluid Attenuated Inversion Recovery; MRI, magnetic resonance imaging.

Making the Diagnosis

- *Antibody (Ab) testing:* autoimmune encephalopathy autoantibodies require testing from both serum and cerebrospinal fluid (CSF) samples.
  - The sensitivity of serum and CSF autoantibody detection varies.
  - Serum testing is generally more sensitive for detecting anti-LGI1 Abs, while CSF testing is more sensitive for anti-NMDAR Abs. In fact, CSF Ab testing is often more sensitive in several AE syndromes, particularly those involving NMDAR.
  - Anti-LGI1 Abs can be found in both serum and CSF. These Abs are typically evaluated as part of a broader Autoimmune and Paraneoplastic Encephalopathy panel.
  - LGI1 encephalitis often lacks CSF inflammation, which may mislead clinicians.
- *CSF analysis*
  - Routine studies may show evidence of inflammation (eg, mild-to-moderate lymphocytic pleocytosis or elevated protein level), though these may not always be present.
  - It is necessary to appropriately exclude infectious pathogens via appropriate serum or CSF testing (eg, testing for herpes simplex virus [HSV] encephalitis via CSF HSV1/2 polymerase chain reaction [PCR]).
- *Electroencephalogram (EEG)*
  - May show temporal lobe slowing, epileptic discharges, or epileptic seizures
  - Aside from a pattern of extreme delta brush that may be seen in anti-NMDAR encephalitis, there are no other characteristic EEG findings to support the diagnosis.
- *Brain magnetic resonance imaging (MRI) with and without contrast*
  - May be normal (~60% normal in an NMDAR cohort)
  - Some cases of limbic AE may display FLAIR (Fluid Attenuated Inversion Recovery) hyperintensities involving the mesial temporal lobes.
  - GABA-A receptor AE has distinctive imaging features of confluent or patchy multifocal FLAIR hyperintensities throughout the brain parenchyma
- *Positron emission tomography (PET) of the* brain
  - Can be considered in the appropriate context for further supportive evidence
    - Anti-LGI1 typically demonstrates basal ganglia hypermetabolism.
    - NMDAR AE typically demonstrates parieto-occipital hypometabolism.
    - Mesial temporal lobe hypermetabolism may be seen in limbic AE.
- *Malignancy screening*
  - Evaluate for occult malignancy with cross-sectional imaging, and additionally gonadal ultrasound (ie, computed tomography [CT] of the chest/abdomen/pelvis and ovarian ultrasound or scrotal ultrasound as per sex of the patient).
  - Malignancy screening should be completed every ~2 years during the first 5 years from onset.
  - Screening schedule can be individualized by antibody subtype and initial tumor findings

Demyelinating Diseases

- Patients with aggressive forms of acute demyelinating diseases may require ICU care for the treatment of severely altered mental status, elevated intracranial pressure, cerebral edema, status epilepticus, or, in the case of high cervical cord lesions, respiratory failure.

Common Causes to Remember

- Tumefactive and aggressive demyelination
- Tumefactive demyelinating lesions are >2 cm on MRI and may resemble tumors radiographically.
- Acute inflammatory myelitis
- Acute disseminated encephalomyelitis (ADEM)
- Neuromyelitis optica spectrum disorder (NMOSD)
- Myelin oligodendrocyte glycoprotein antibody disease (MOGAD)

Tumefactive and Aggressive Demyelination

Presentation

- More common in female patients, average age of 35 to 45
- Presents with encephalopathy, seizures, and focal symptoms depending on lesion location

Making the Diagnosis

- Broad differential diagnosis: neoplasm, infection (abscess, progressive multifocal leukoencephalopathy "PML," toxoplasmosis, cryptococcosis), systemic (neurosarcoidosis, Behçet syndrome, rheumatologic disorders) and primary neurologic demyelinating disorders
- MRI features of demyelination: incomplete rim enhancement, mixed T2 iso- and hyperintensity, absence of mass effect, and absence of cortical involvement
- CSF analysis to evaluate for infectious and neoplastic etiologies, if safe to perform (caution in cerebral edema or mass effect)
  - CSF analysis often shows mild pleocytosis with normal or mildly elevated protein.
- Serial MRI and clinical monitoring to assess disease stability and treatment response
- Brain biopsy is reserved for atypical presentations, as it may be nondiagnostic, misleading, or high risk.

Acute Inflammatory Myelitis

Presentation

- Spinal cord inflammation manifesting as a subacute onset (hours to days) progression of focal neurologic symptoms as per the localization of inflammatory involvement
  - Symptoms may include weakness, sensory changes, bowel/bladder dysfunction, and, in cases of high cervical spine lesions, respiratory failure due to diaphragm weakness and potential dysautonomia.
- Lesion features: short segment or longitudinally extensive if spans ≥3 levels
  - Longitudinally extensive transverse myelitis (LETM) is more often seen in NMOSD or MOGAD, than multiple sclerosis.
  - LETM in sarcoidosis and systemic lupus erythematosus (SLE) can mimic NMOSD/MOGAD.

Making the Diagnosis

- *Neuroimaging:* MRIs of the brain, cervical and thoracic spine with and without contrast
  - Cord compression is absent (noncompressive myelopathy).
- *CSF analysis* to evaluate for infection, assess presence of inflammation, test for oligoclonal bands and pertinent autoantibody markers (ie, autoimmune myelopathy panel)
  - Due to high sensitivity of serum anti-aquaporin 4 (AQP4) for NMOSD, CSF testing for anti-AQP4 is not commonly practiced.
  - A critical diagnosis to exclude before initiating empiric treatment is spinal dural arteriovenous fistula, as steroid administration can lead to clinical worsening.

Acute Disseminated Encephalomyelitis

Presentation

- Acute to subacute demyelinating disease involving the central nervous system (CNS) with variable symptoms according to the localization of lesions. Key features include encephalopathy, fever, and focal neurologic deficit(s).
- Typically, monophasic and most commonly affects children (mean age of onset 5-8)
- Serum MOG-IgG (myelin oligodendrocyte glycoprotein immunoglobulin G) should be tested as ADEM is a clinical phenotype of MOGAD.
- May occur as a para- or postinfectious or postvaccination phenomenon
- Seizures may occur in 12% to 35%.

Making the Diagnosis

- Brain MRI and MRI of the cervical and thoracic spine with and without contrast:
  - Brain MRI commonly displays multiple bilateral, asymmetric FLAIR hyperintensities of different sizes, involving the supratentorium +/− infratentorium, with or without surrounding edema.
  - Lesions are often poorly marginated, "fluffy" appearing, and large.
  - Spinal cord is involved in up to one-third of patients.
- *CSF analysis* to exclude infectious etiologies and test for inflammation
  - CSF often shows mild pleocytosis, elevated protein, normal glucose, and elevated IgG index (not required for diagnosis).

Neuromyelitis Optica Spectrum Disorder and Myelin Oligodendrocyte Glycoprotein Antibody Disorders

Presentation

- NMOSD: longitudinally extensive (≥3 spinal segments) transverse myelitis, optic neuritis. Brain or brainstem lesions, especially near ventricles, periaqueductal region
- MOGAD: optic neuritis is the most common manifestation, followed by ADEM, myelitis, brainstem dysfunction, and cerebral cortical encephalitis (CCE).

TABLE 8.11.2 Initial Immunosuppressive Treatment for Acute Demyelinating Disorders and Autoimmune Encephalitis

First line	• IV methylprednisolone 1,000 mg daily for 3-5 d followed by an oral glucocorticosteroid taper	*Considerations while receiving oral steroid taper:* • Monitor for hyperglycemia and infections. • GI ulcer prophylaxis with H_2-blockers or PPI • Pneumocystis pneumonia prophylaxis with TMP-SMX or atovaquone • Osteoporosis prevention: vitamin D_3/calcium carbonate recommended
Second line	• Plasma exchange (5-7 cycles scheduled every other day) • IVIg in patients with contraindication to plasma exchange • *Loading dose: IVIg 2 g/kg IBW over 3-5 consecutive days* • Maintenance dosing: IVIg 1 g/kg IBW every 28 d	*Considerations:* • Concurrent plasma exchange with steroids as first line in severe cases in NMOSD (early plasma exchange associated with improved outcomes) • Give steroid dose after plasma exchange session to avoid clearance.
Third line	• Cyclophosphamide or rituximab	• In severe disease refractory to first- and second-line therapy, these medications can be used acutely. • Note cyclophosphamide or rituximab are commonly used as maintenance immunosuppressants for autoimmune encephalitis, foremost of these conditions reviewed.

GI, gastrointestinal; IBW, ideal body weight; IV, intravenous; IVIg, intravenous immunoglobulin; NMOSD, neuromyelitis optica spectrum disorder; PPI, proton pump inhibitor; TMP-SMX, trimethoprim-sulfamethoxazole.

Making the Diagnosis

- NMOSD: clinical characteristics with congruent neuroimaging (optic neuritis, myelitis, area postrema syndrome, acute brainstem syndrome, acute diencephalic syndrome, brain lesions) and positive serum test for anti-AQP4 IgG.
- MOGAD: monophasic or relapsing course with clinical syndrome (optic neuritis, myelitis, brainstem encephalitis, encephalitis) with congruent MRI findings of CNS demyelination and seropositivity for MOG-IgG

Management and Treatment

- See Table 8.11.2.

SUGGESTED READINGS

Abboud H, Probasco JC, Irani S, et al. Autoimmune encephalitis: proposed best practice recommendations for diagnosis and acute management. *J Neurol Neurosurg Psychiatry*. 2021;92(7):757-768.

Banwell B, Bennett JL, Marignier R, et al. Diagnosis of myelin oligodendrocyte glycoprotein antibody-associated disease: International MOGAD Panel proposed criteria. *Lancet Neurol*. 2023;22(3):268-282.

Czeisler BM. Emergent management of central nervous system demyelinating disorders. *Continuum (Minneap Minn)*. 2024;30(3, Neurocritical Care):781-817.

Deng B, Cai M, Qiu Y, et al. MRI characteristics of autoimmune encephalitis with autoantibodies to GABAA receptor: a case series [published correction appears in *Neurol Neuroimmunol Neuroinflamm*. 2022;9(6):e200040]. *Neurol Neuroimmunol Neuroinflamm*. 2022;9(3):e1158.

Diaz-Arias LA, Pardo CA, Probasco JC. Autoimmune encephalitis in the intensive care unit. *Neurointensive Care Unit*. 2019;249-263.

Frohman EM, Wingerchuk DM. Transverse myelitis. *N Engl J Med*. 2010;363:564-572.

Ropper AH, Brown RH. *Adams and Victor's Principles of Neurology*. 8th ed. McGraw-Hill; 2005:653-656, 778-793.

Zhao YY, Han B, Qin CH, et al. Brain magnetic resonance imaging predictors in anti-N-methyl-D-aspartate receptor encephalitis. *Ann Clin Transl Neurol*. 2022;9(12):1974-1984.

8.12

Neuromuscular Disorders

Sandro Marini and Sahar F. Zafar

Overview

- Neuromuscular disorders encountered in the intensive care unit (ICU) can present with a spectrum of symptoms ranging from generalized weakness to respiratory failure.
- Among the most common are critical illness–associated neuropathies and myopathies, which often develop secondary to prolonged hospitalization or systemic illness.

Critical Illness Neuropathy/Myopathy

- Critical illness neuropathy/myopathy, collectively termed *ICU-acquired weakness*, is a significant complication affecting hospitalized critically ill patients, characterized primarily by muscle weakness.
- The common weakness pattern is generalized, symmetric, proximal more than distal weakness. When severe, it affects the respiratory muscles but usually spares facial and ocular muscles. Deep tendon reflexes are reduced or absent.

Common Causes to Remember

- Risk factors: older age, premorbid disability/frailty, premorbid obesity, sepsis, use of vasopressors, aminoglycosides or corticosteroids, encephalopathy, hyperglycemia, hyperosmolality, hypoalbuminemia, renal replacement therapy

Epidemiology

- Incidence: 25% to 83% among ICU patients
- Diagnosis: simplified electrophysiologic assessment of peroneal motor nerve amplitude (>25% reduction in consecutive measurements has 94%-100% sensitivity in detecting ICU-acquired weakness)

Key Pathophysiology for Critical Illness Polyneuropathy

- A neurogenic disturbance more common in severe inflammatory states such as sepsis
- Clinically characterized by limb muscle weakness and atrophy and loss of peripheral sensation to light touch and pinprick
- Electromyography (EMG) and nerve conduction study (NCS) findings consistent with axonal motor and sensory polyneuropathy: amplitude reduction of motor and sensory action potentials and slowed conduction velocities
- Usually normal serum creatinine kinase levels

Key Pathophysiology for Critical Illness Myopathy

- The most common pathologic finding in critical illness myopathy (CIM) is selective loss of myosin.
- Sensation is normal if it can be tested reliably.
- EMG and NCS findings consistent with myopathy: compound muscle action potential <80% of normal, with normal sensory nerve action potential.
- Serum creatinine kinase levels may be mildly elevated.

Differential Diagnosis

- Bilateral or paramedian brain or brainstem lesions
- Spinal cord lesions (trauma, spinal cord infarction, myelopathies)
- Anterior horn cell disorders (amyotrophic lateral sclerosis [ALS])
- Polyradiculopathies (Guillain-Barré syndrome [GBS])
- Peripheral nerve disorders (paraneoplastic neuropathy, vasculitic neuropathy)
- Neuromuscular junction disorders (myasthenia gravis, Lambert-Eaton syndrome)
- Rhabdomyolysis
- Other myopathies (infectious, inflammatory, drug induced, congenital myopathies)
- Propofol infusion syndrome

Management and Treatment

- No specific treatment is available.
- Minimize the use of sedation and paralytics.
- Avoid prolonged use of vasopressors, aminoglycosides, or corticosteroids.
- Early mobilization and intensive rehabilitation
- Avoid malnutrition (though parenteral feeding was associated with worse outcome).
- Ensure glycemic control.
- Inconclusive evidence for passive electrical muscle stimulation (it may help with prevention)

Outcome

- Critical illness neuropathy/CIM is usually reversible over weeks to months, but overall carries an increased risk of mortality at 5 years.
- Up to 40% still required assistance in their daily routine at 12 months after discharge from the ICU.
- Patients with CIM have a generally better prognosis than patients with critical illness polyneuropathy (CIP), with greater chance of functional recovery.

Myasthenia Gravis

- In contrast to ICU-acquired weakness, some neuromuscular disorders are due to preexisting autoimmune conditions that may acutely worsen during hospitalization. Myasthenia gravis (MG) is one such disorder, often exacerbated by infection, medications, or changes in therapy, and it poses a unique challenge due to its potential for life-threatening respiratory crisis.
- Autoimmune disorder in which neuromuscular transmission is impaired by autoantibodies against postsynaptic protein (eg, acetylcholine receptor, muscle-specific tyrosine kinase)
- The classic findings are muscle weakness typically more proximal than distal limb weakness, ptosis, and diplopia. A subtype of MG affects only ocular muscles. Fatigability is the most classic feature of MG.
- Testing includes antibodies (see table), reversibility of weakness with short-acting anticholinesterase (pyridostigmine), and NCS (>15% decline in compound muscle action potential (CMAP) during 3-Hz repetitive stimulation).
- Crisis may lead to respiratory collapse and is usually precipitated by infections, certain medications, and modification of existing steroid therapy.
- Patients with generalized MG are at risk for myasthenic crisis, which is defined as significant worsening of weakness affecting respiratory function, necessitating mechanical ventilation.

Common Causes to Remember

Anti-acetylcholine receptor (AChR) immunoglobulin G (IgG)	80%-90% of generalized MG 40%-50% of ocular MG
Anti-MuSK	30%-40% of anti–AChR-negative patients
Anti-LRP4	13 % of seronegative patients
No identifiable antibody	~5%
Thymic hyperplasia	65% of patients with MG
Thymoma	10% of patients with MG

Remember to Assess for Offending/Inciting Agents

Paralytics	Rocuronium, succinylcholine
Antibiotics	Ciprofloxacin, gentamicin
Antiarrhythmics	Verapamil, quinine
Antiseizure medications	Phenytoin
Psychiatric	Lithium
Rheumatoid arthritis	D-penicillamine, chloroquine
Electrolytes	Magnesium intravenous (IV)
Antiinflammatory	Glucocorticoids

Epidemiology

- Annual incidence ~3 cases per 100,000 per year
- Prevalence 20 cases per 100,000 in the United States
- Biphasic peaks: young women and middle-aged men are most affected.
- Myasthenic crisis occurs in 15% to 30% of patients with MG and is the initial presentation in up to 20% of patients without a previous diagnosis of MG.

Key Pathophysiology

- T-cell–dependent autoimmune destruction of postsynaptic AChR: IgG antibodies may directly block AChR or activate complement cascade at the postsynaptic membrane.
- Repeated stimulation/activation promotes Ach depletion with subsequent progressive weakness.

Differential Diagnosis

- With ocular symptoms: brainstem and cranial nerve lesions, thyroid-related ophthalmopathy, oculopharyngeal muscular dystrophy, botulinum exposure
- With bulbar symptoms: skull base or nasal and oropharynx tumors, motor neuron disease
- With limb weakness: Lambert-Eaton syndrome, acute inflammatory demyelinating polyneuropathy (AIDP), motor neuron disease, inflammatory or toxic myopathies
- Others: organophosphate exposure, diphtheria, mitochondrial disorders

Management and Treatment

- Identify and manage underlying disease or triggering condition.
- Respiratory support: vital capacity <10 to 15 mL/kg and declining negative inspiratory force (worse than −20 cm H_2O) are helpful in assessing the need for mechanical ventilation.
- Cholinesterase inhibitors are used for symptom control (eg, pyridostigmine 0.5 mg IV every 3 hour).
- Pyridostigmine is typically held early in a crisis because of an increase in respiratory secretions and is resumed once a patient begins to show signs of improvement.
- Intravenous immunoglobulins (IVIGs) (2 g/kg IV in 2-5 divided daily doses) or plasma exchange (PE) for 5 days (preferred if the patient is at risk of thromboembolic events)
- Immunomodulatory drugs for disease suppression
  - Rituximab (effect onset after ~4 weeks)
  - Cyclosporine (effect onset after ~8 weeks)
  - Steroids: although an initial paradoxical deterioration is possible, IV methylprednisolone (eg, 2 g daily for 1-2 days) is generally used if the patient is on artificial ventilation Complement factor C5 inhibition and neonatal Fc receptor antagonism (e.g. Eculizumab, Efgartigimod).
- Thymoma resection

Outcome

- Mortality has improved over time and is now <5%.
- Highest mortality risk at 1 to 2 and 7 to 10 years after the diagnosis.
  - Poor outcomes factors are the presence of diaphragmatic failure and delay in treatment (IVIG or PE).
- Mortality and morbidity are usually due to respiratory failure or aspiration.

Acute Inflammatory Demyelinating Polyneuropathy (or Guillain-Barré Syndrome)

- Another important cause of acute neuromuscular weakness is GBS, the most common form of acute flaccid paralysis worldwide. Unlike ICU-acquired weakness or MG, GBS typically arises after an infectious trigger and requires prompt recognition due to its potential for rapid respiratory compromise.
- Acute onset of rapidly progressive and symmetric ascending weakness
- Dysesthesia of the feet and hands
- Cranial nerves: mainly affects facial and oropharyngeal muscles with sparing of ocular muscles
- Areflexia with loss of vibration and proprioception
- Possible autonomic instability
- Respiratory failure

Common Causes to Remember

Antecedent infection	*Campylobacter jejuni*, *Haemophilus influenzae*, *Mycoplasma pneumoniae*, cytomegalovirus, influenza A and B, COVID-19 virus
Vaccination	Influenza, rarer with recombinant zoster or meningococcus.

Epidemiology

- Incidence varies between 0.5 and 3 cases per 100,000 per year.
- Bimodal peak (children and >55 years)

Key Pathophysiology

- Autoimmunity (trigged by molecular mimicry) leading to demyelination or axonal injury of peripheral nerves
- Minority of the cases have identifiable antibodies: GM1, anti-GD1a, GQ1b, anti-GalNac-GD1a, and anti-GD1b (Miller Fisher variant).

- Cerebrospinal fluid demonstrates albumin-cytologic dissociation (elevated protein without pleocytosis, <50 nucleated cells).
  - Can be normal up to 33% in the first week of the disease

Differential Diagnosis

- Central causes (demyelination, bilateral strokes, cerebellar ataxia, and posterior fossa lesions)
- Spinal causes (compressive myelopathy, acute myelitis, anterior stroke, spinal epidural abscess)
- Peripheral nervous system causes (radiculitis, CIP, leptomeningeal malignancy, vasculitis, Lyme disease)
- Neuromuscular junction (botulism, MG, neuromuscular blocking agents)
- Metabolic myopathies (eg, hypokalemia, hyperkalemia)
- Toxic exposures (botulinum, organophosphates, thallium, arsenic)

Management and Treatment

- Supportive care
  - Consider intubation if vital capacity decreased to 20 mL/kg, maximal inspiratory pressure decreased to −30 cm H_2O, maximal expiratory pressure decreased to 40 cm H_2O or clinical respiratory distress.
  - Management of autonomic instability
  - Supportive nutrition (early enteral feeding)
- PE (4-6 treatments) or IVIG 2 g/kg over 2 to 5 days

Outcome

- 80% achieve full functional recovery.
  - Modified Erasmus global outcome score can help predict the ability to walk at 6 months.
- Mortality ~5%; the cause of death is usually pulmonary embolism, autonomic instability, or sepsis.
  - Poor prognostic factors are age >60 years, progression <7 days, distal CMAP <20%.

Amyotrophic Lateral Sclerosis

- While most neuromuscular disorders encountered in the ICU are acute or subacute in onset, it is essential to recognize chronic progressive conditions, such as ALS. Though rare, ALS may present as undifferentiated weakness or respiratory failure, and its diagnosis has important prognostic and management implications.
- ALS is a fatal neurodegenerative disorder affecting upper and lower motor neurons.
- The most common form presents with progressive, painless weakness without associated sensory loss. It typically spares the oculomotor muscles.
  - Bulbar onset is seen in 20% of patients and is characterized by a more rapid progression.
- Patients demonstrate diffuse fasciculations, atrophy, and hyperreflexia.
- ALS can be associated with frontotemporal dementia.

Common Causes to Remember

- *Sporadic (90%-95%)*: no clear genetic or environmental trigger
- *Familial (5%-10%)*: genetic mutations with autosomal dominant inheritance
- *SOD1*, *C9orf72*, *FUS*, and *TARDBP* are most commonly implicated genes.
- *Lifestyle factors*: smoking has been weakly associated with increased ALS risk.
- *Environmental exposures* (less established but under investigation)
- *Viral infections* (less established but under investigation)

Epidemiology

- Incidence of 2 to 4 per 100,000 person-years
- Usual age of onset is between 50 and 75 years of age.
- Among the young, men are more affected than women.

Key Pathophysiology

- Not well understood but believed to be mediated by glutamate toxicity, oxidative stress, mitochondrial dysfunction, and abnormal RNA processing

Differential Diagnosis

- AIDP (eg, multifocal motor neuropathy)
- Chronic inflammatory demyelinating polyneuropathy (CIDP)
- Paraneoplastic neuropathies
- Post-polio syndrome
- MG
- Myopathy (inclusion body myositis)
- Myelopathy (cervical compressive radiculopathy and myelopathy)
- Benign fasciculations
- Brainstem injury with myelopathy

Management and Treatment

- Disease-modifying therapies
  - Riluzole (glutamate release inhibitor)
  - Edaravone (free-radical scavenger)
- Avoid malnutrition and dysphagia management.
- Tracheostomy and gastrostomy surgeries and other supportive treatments

Outcome

- 50% mortality over 3 years and 70% mortality over 5 years

SUGGESTED READINGS

Crespo V, James ML. Neuromuscular disease in the neurointensive care unit. *Anesthesiol Clin*. 2016;34(3):601-619.

Damian MS, Wijdicks EFM. The clinical management of neuromuscular disorders in intensive care. *Neuromuscul Disord*. 2019;29(2):85-96.

Hauser SL, Josephson AS. *Harrison's Neurology in Clinical Medicine*. 2nd ed. McGraw-Hill; 2010.

Pincherle A, Jöhr J, Pancini L, et al. Intensive care admission and early neuro-rehabilitation. lessons for COVID-19? *Front Neurol*. 2020;11:880.

Ropper AH, Samuels MA. *Adams and Victor's Principles of Neurology*. 9th ed. McGraw-Hill; 2009.

Vanhorebeek I, Latronico N, Van den Berghe G. ICU-acquired weakness. *Intensive Care Med*. 2020;46(4):637-653.

Vincent JL, Abraham E, Kochanek PM, Moore FA. *Textbook of Critical Care: Expert Consult Premium Edition*. 6th ed. Elsevier; 2011.

8.13

Brain Death/Death by Neurologic Criteria

Amjad Elmashala and Ibrahim Migdady

Overview

- Brain death (BD) is the death of a person due to the permanent loss of brain function. This is defined by a catastrophic brain injury resulting in the permanent loss of the capacity for consciousness (ie, coma), brainstem reflexes, and the ability to breathe independently despite an adequate stimulus.
- The term *brain death/death by neurologic criteria* (BD/DNC) is preferably used in lieu of BD alone to emphasize that the death of the person, not only the brain, has occurred, similar to death by cardiopulmonary criteria.
- Publications by the World Brain Death Project (2020) and the American Academy of Neurology (AAN) in 2023 represent the most recent and comprehensive guidelines for BD/DNC determination at the time of writing. Because countries and states vary in the practice of determining BD/DNC, it is important to follow local institutional guidelines.
- BD/DNC determination is based on clinical assessment; ancillary testing is required only if the clinical assessment cannot be safely or fully completed, or confounders cannot be excluded or corrected. The complete clinical assessment of BD/DNC, including the apnea test, should be pursued to the fullest extent possible, even if there is a foreseeable need for an ancillary test.

Prerequisites for Brain Death/Death by Neurologic Criteria

- BD/DNC should only be considered in patients who are comatose, have absent brainstem reflexes, and are not breathing spontaneously (ie, not breathing above the set ventilator rate).
- Presence of an etiology as demonstrated by neuroimaging, the course and severity of which are known to cause irreversible neurologic injury leading to loss of capacity for consciousness and capable of causing BD/DNC. Common etiologies for BD/DNC are listed (Table 8.13.1).
- Exclusion of BD/DNC mimics: examples include fulminant Guillain-Barré syndrome, botulism, high cervical cord injuries, leptomeningeal carcinomatosis, and snake bites.
- Absence of confounders: severe acid-base disturbances, electrolyte derangements, hypothermia, and metabolic abnormalities. Practical thresholds for specific laboratory results based on consensus were provided by the AAN guideline in 2023 (Table 8.13.2).
- Negative toxicology evaluation (if indicated): see special circumstances below.
- Lack of neuromuscular blockade as demonstrated by train-of-four nerve stimulation in patients with recent or prolonged use of paralytics.
- Core body temperature ≥36 °C; if temperature was ≤35.5 °C, then clinicians should wait a minimum of 24 hours after rewarming to ≥36 °C before BD/DNC evaluation.
- Systolic blood pressure (SBP) ≥100 mm Hg and mean arterial pressure (MAP) ≥75 mm Hg; BP may be supported artificially with fluids, vasopressors, or inotropes as needed.

Clinical Examination for Brain Death/Death by Neurologic Criteria

- Clinicians must perform a minimum of one examination for BD/DNC; performance of two independent examinations may decrease the risk of a false-positive determination.
- Clinical examination encompasses three components: (1) coma, (2) brainstem areflexia, and (3) apnea in the setting of an adequate stimulus.
- Coma is defined by the absence of any responses to visual, auditory, and tactile stimulation.
- Cerebrally mediated motor responses to noxious stimulation to the head/face, neck, and extremities must be absent. Spinally mediated motor responses can be present and are sometimes difficult to distinguish from cerebrally mediated ones.
- Lack of brainstem reflexes
    - Pupils must be dilated between 4 and 9 mm in size and not reactive to light; small pupils should alert physicians but can be seen with pontine injuries and a history of ocular disease or surgery.
    - No oculocephalic reflexes (OCR) elicited bilaterally, that is, eyes remain fixed in the midline with lateral head movement; this is only tested when the integrity of the cervical spine and skull base is ensured.
    - No oculovestibular reflex (OVR) present with the caloric stimulation test. With the head of the bed elevated to 30 degrees, 30 to 50 mL of ice-cold water is irrigated in each ear while observing for any eye movements. The ears are tested 5 minutes apart. Lack of eye movements is consistent with BD.

TABLE 8.13.1 Common Etiologies of Brain Death/Death by Neurologic Criteria
Cerebrovascular disorders (ischemic/hemorrhagic stroke, subarachnoid hemorrhage)
Traumatic brain injury
Hypoxic-ischemic brain injury
Brain masses
Intracranial infections
Toxic ingestions
Metabolic disorders leading to malignant cerebral edema

TABLE 8.13.2 Suggested Thresholds for Specific Laboratory Results Based on Consensus Provided by the AAN 2023 Guideline

Laboratory Test	Value[a]
Ammonia	>75 μmol/L
Blood urea nitrogen	>75 mg/dL
Calcium (or ionized calcium)	<7 or >11 mg/dL (or <1 or >1.3 mmol/L)
Glucose	<70 or >300 mg/dL
Magnesium	<1.5 or >4 mg/dL
Potassium	<3 or >6 mmol/L
Sodium	<130 or >160 mmol/L
pH	<7.3 or >7.5
Total T4	<3 or >30 mg/dL
Free T4	≤0.4 or >5 ng/dL

AAN, American Academy of Neurology; BD/DNC, brain death/death by neurologic criteria.

[a]The thresholds for laboratory abnormalities affecting clinical evaluation are based on expert consensus only, and the precise values remain unknown. Some of the measurements are not necessary unless clinically indicated.

- If OCR cannot be tested, BD/DNC may still be diagnosed without ancillary testing, provided that OVR is absent bilaterally.
- No corneal reflex elicited by touching the cornea with a cotton swab
- No facial motor movement to noxious stimulation, for example, with supraorbital pressure, nasal stimulation with a Q-tip, or pressure at the level of the condyles
- No gag response to stimulation of the posterior pharynx with a tongue blade on each side
- No cough response to stimulation of the trachea with suctioning
- Accurate assessment of certain brainstem reflexes can be affected by corneal trauma, severe orbital or scleral edema or chemosis, ophthalmic surgery, anophthalmia, use of ocular or systemic anticholinergic medications, skull fracture, cervical spine fracture or high cervical cord injury, or a ruptured tympanic membrane, in which an ancillary test is needed.

Apnea Testing for Brain Death/Death by Neurologic Criteria

- Clinicians must perform at least one apnea test after the final BD/DNC neurologic examination in adults, if tolerated.
- Prerequisites (in addition to above-mentioned)
  - Eucapnia ($PaCO_2$ 35-45 mm Hg) and pH 7.35 to 7.45
    - For patients with chronic hypercarbia (eg, chronic obstructive pulmonary disease [COPD], severe obesity), the $Paco_2$ level before testing should be at the patient's chronic baseline level; if the level is unknown, then ancillary testing is needed in addition to a positive apnea test to declare BD/DNC.
  - Euvolemia
    - For patients requiring significant vasopressor support or having unstable cardiac arrhythmias and an apnea test is deemed unsafe, ancillary testing is needed.
- Preparation
  - Patients should be preoxygenated with 100% oxygen for at least 10 minutes to achieve PaO_2 >200 mm Hg.
  - Arterial blood gas (ABG) should be obtained after preoxygenation and before disconnecting the ventilator to determine baseline $PaCO_2$, $PaCO_2$, and pH levels.
- Procedure
  - The patient is disconnected from the ventilator and provided oxygen via a catheter at 4 to 6 L/min to the level of the carina. This is termed "apneic oxygenation."
  - Patient is watched closely for any respiratory movements.
  - Vital signs are monitored continuously; test is aborted if the patient develops hypoxemia (O_2 saturation <85%), hypotension (SBP <100 or MAP <75 mm Hg) despite fluid administration or vasopressor titration, cardiac arrhythmia with hemodynamic instability, or cardiac arrest.
  - An ABG is obtained after 8 to 10 minutes of apnea, but earlier measurements can be considered if there is a concern for hemodynamic stability. If the patient remains hemodynamically stable for 8 to 10 minutes, they can be kept off the ventilator until the arterial pH and $PaCO_2$ level criteria for BD/DNC determination are met.
  - If apnea test criteria for BD/DNC determination are not met (see later), ABG measurements can be checked every 2 minutes until BD/DNC is determined or the apnea test is aborted.
- Interpretation: apnea test is consistent with BD/DNC if *all of the following are met*:
  - No respirations occur throughout the apnea test
  - Arterial pH level <7.30
  - $Paco_2$ level criteria that are consistent with BD/DNC
    - In patients WITHOUT a known history of chronic hypercarbia, $PaCO_2$ ≥60 and ≥20 mm Hg above pretest $Paco_2$ baseline
    - In patients WITH a known history of chronic hypercarbia and known baseline $PaCO_2$, $PaCO_2$ ≥60 and ≥20 mm Hg above patient's known chronically elevated $PaCO_2$ baseline
    - In patients with SUSPECTED chronic hypercarbia and unknown baseline $PaCO_2$ level, $PaCO_2$ ≥60 and ≥20 mm Hg above pretest $PaCO_2$ baseline, AND ancillary testing must be performed.

Ancillary Testing for Brain Death/Death by Neurologic Criteria

- Ancillary testing is pursued when the clinical evaluation for BD/DNC determination is incomplete or inconclusive, or when confounders cannot be excluded or corrected.
- Ancillary tests are supportive of BD/DNC diagnosis and should never be used alone; none are 100% sensitive and specific.
- Examples of circumstances when ancillary testing is needed:
  - Extensive facial injuries or cervical spine injuries that limit adequate assessment of the cranial nerves, extremity movement, or spontaneous respirations
  - Inability to complete apnea testing due to the risks of cardiopulmonary decompensation or inability to interpret $Paco_2$ level in patients with suspected chronic hypercarbia and unknown baseline $Paco_2$ level
  - Difficulty with interpretation of whether limb movements are cerebrally or spinally mediated
  - Metabolic derangements that are difficult to adequately correct
- Modalities available test for electrophysiologic function or perfusion of the brain
  - Four-vessel catheter angiography: absence of filling in the internal carotid and vertebral arteries at the point where they enter the dura following contrast injection with the catheter positioned in the great vessels, leading to the brain. Although this has long been considered the gold standard test due to direct and dynamic assessment of intracranial flow, it is rarely performed due to the invasive and time-consuming nature of the procedure and requirement of an experienced neuroradiologist.
  - Nuclear imaging: no uptake of radionuclide isotopes with blood-brain barrier–crossing properties in the brain parenchyma on single-photon emission computed tomography (SPECT)
  - Transcranial Doppler (TCD) ultrasonography: oscillating flow or systolic spikes in the bilateral, anterior, and posterior proximal large intracranial arteries indicate cerebral circulatory arrest and are consistent with BD/DNC. Complete absence of flow is also consistent with BD/DNC, provided that the lack of flow is not due to technical reasons or inadequate windows (ie, a prior TCD confirming flow is necessary in such cases). This test is widely available but cannot be performed in ~10% of adults due to skull thickness precluding adequate insonation.
  - Neurophysiologic tests, including electroencephalography (EEG) and evoked potentials, are *no longer recommended* as ancillary tests since EEG assesses the function of the cerebral hemispheres and not the brainstem. The addition of evoked potentials cannot provide complete information about the entire brainstem.
  - Computed tomography (CT) and magnetic resonance (MR) angiography: these tests *not validated* and may yield false-positives—they should *not* be used as ancillary tests per the AAN guidelines.

Special Circumstances

- Intoxication
  - A toxicology screen, if clinically indicated, should be obtained to rule out any etiologies that could be confounding the BD/DNC determination.
  - If clinically indicated, confirmation of a negative toxicology (urine and blood) screen and blood alcohol level <80 mg/dL is advised.
  - If significant central nervous system (CNS)-depressing medications (eg, sedatives, narcotics, anticholinergics) or a positive toxicology screen is identified, then examination should be completed after at least five half-lives of the medication in question to allow for drug elimination or until levels are subtherapeutic.
  - Some medications may require longer than five half-lives clearance time in patients with renal or hepatic impairment, those who are obese, or those who were hypothermic.
  - If a history of pentobarbital exposure, then serum level must be <5 μg/mL.
  - If there is suspicion for an unknown or unmeasurable CNS-depressing medication, an ancillary test is needed.
- Extracorporeal membrane oxygenation (ECMO) patients
  - Prerequisites for BD/DNC evaluation do not change for patients on ECMO.
  - ECMO circuit can help in controlling the patient's temperature and BP before and during BD/DNC evaluation.
  - For venoarterial (VA) ECMO patients with limited native cardiac output, MAP, rather than SBP and diastolic BP, should be >75 mm Hg.
  - The clinical examination is unchanged; caution is advised to avoid displacing ECMO cannulas during the examination.
  - For apnea testing, lack of spontaneous breathing with hypercarbia and acidosis is consistent with BD/DNC.
  - Patients are preoxygenated using 100% oxygen on the ventilator and through the ECMO oxygenator.
  - To facilitate CO_2 accumulation in arterial blood, either exogenous CO_2 is titrated into the ECMO circuit or the rate of sweep gas flow is adjusted to 0.2 to 1 L/min.
  - ABG measurements of $Paco_2$ and pH should approximate values in the cerebral circulation:
    - For VA ECMO patients, ABG samples are obtained from both the patient's distal arterial line and the ECMO circuit postoxygenator.
      - If centrally cannulated (right carotid or right axillary arteries), distal arterial samples are obtained from the left upper extremity or lower extremity.
      - If cannulated through the femoral artery, distal arterial samples are obtained from the right upper extremity.
      - $Paco_2$ and pH values from both sample sites are required to meet BD/DNC criteria for the apnea test to be consistent with BD/DNC.
    - For venovenous (VV) ECMO, ABG samples are only obtained from the distal arterial line and tested against BD/DNC apnea testing criteria.
  - Hypotension during apnea testing on ECMO is managed with fluids or vasopressor/inotropic support.
- Hypothermia
  - Hypothermia is known to confound BD examination due to reversible brainstem areflexia and coma. There are a few case reports where BD/DNC was prematurely determined after rewarming from therapeutic hypothermia.
  - It is unknown how long hypothermia can affect the neurologic examination.
  - A core body temperature ≥36 °C is a prerequisite for BD/DNC evaluation.

- No specific guidance exists on the length of time necessary to delay BD/DNC evaluation in patients who are hypothermic after achieving normothermia, but a minimum of 24 hours after rewarming is complete or longer is usually advised.
- Temperature may be supported artificially with warming blankets, warmed fluids, or automated temperature regulation devices.
- Hypothermia can affect the pharmacokinetics and pharmacodynamics of certain medications, so a longer duration for clearance, that is, more than five half-lives, might be needed.

Ethical Consideration

- BD/DNC is medicolegally equivalent to death by cardiopulmonary criteria.
- There are many misperceptions surrounding BD; therefore, family should be approached and educated early and as soon as patients are believed to meet criteria for BD/DNC evaluation.
- Clinicians should always make reasonable efforts to inform family about the intent to perform BD/DNC evaluation; however, consent is not required unless required by the institution's policy or state laws or regulations.
- Families may object to the performance of BD/DNC evaluation or discontinuation of organ support for a variety of reasons (cultural, religious, guilt); therefore, objections must be handled in a consistent approach in conjunction with a multidisciplinary team involving the institution's ethics and legal teams.
- Death certificates require that the time of death be recorded. The process of reporting the time of death in patients who meet BD/DNC criteria should be consistent:
  - In patients who meet clinical criteria for BD/DNC, the time of death is the time during the final apnea test (if more than one test is performed) when the ABG results showed $Paco_2$ and pH levels consistent with BD/DNC.
  - In patients where ancillary testing was required, the time of death is the time an attending physician (nuclear medicine or angiographer) documents in the medical record that the ancillary test results are consistent with BD/DNC.
- Following the BD/DNC declaration, organ support is generally discontinued unless organ donation is considered.
- Organ support may be continued for a reasonable but limited amount of time following BD/DNC determination to provide family with a period of time with the deceased.
- Pregnancy is not a contraindication to BD/DNC evaluation. Following determination, clinicians (assisted by maternal-fetal medicine specialists, child neurologists, and neonatologists) should educate and discuss risks and benefits of continuing maternal organ support to the fetus with surrogate decision makers.

SUGGESTED READINGS

A definition of irreversible coma: report of the Ad Hoc Committee of the Harvard Medical School to examine the definition of brain death. *JAMA*. 1968;205(6):337-340.

Busl KM, Lewis A, Varelas PN. Apnea testing for the determination of brain death: a systematic scoping review. *Neurocrit Care*. 2021;34(2):608-620.

Chang JJ, Tsivgoulis G, Katsanos AH, Malkoff MD, Alexandrov AV. Diagnostic accuracy of transcranial Doppler for brain death confirmation: systematic review and meta-analysis. *AJNR Am J Neuroradiol*. 2016;37(3): 408-414.

Donohoe KJ, Agrawal G, Frey KA, et al. SNM practice guideline for brain death scintigraphy 2.0. *J Nucl Med Technol*. 2012;40(3):198-203.

Ducrocq X, Hassler W, Moritake K, et al. Consensus opinion on diagnosis of cerebral circulatory arrest using Doppler-sonography: Task Force Group on cerebral death of the Neurosonology Research Group of the World Federation of Neurology. *J Neurol Sci*. 1998;159(2):145-150.

Greer DM, Kirschen MP, Lewis A, et al. Pediatric and adult brain death/death by Neurologic Criteria Consensus Guideline. *Neurology*. 2023;101(24):1112-1132.

Greer DM, Shemie SD, Lewis A, et al. Determination of brain death/death by neurologic criteria: the World Brain Death Project. *JAMA*. 2020; 324(11):1078-1097.

Greer DM, Wang HH, Robinson JD, Varelas PN, Henderson GV, Wijdicks EF. Variability of brain death policies in the United States. *JAMA Neurol*. 2016;73(2):213-218.

Hoeper MM, Tudorache I, Kühn C, et al. Extracorporeal membrane oxygenation watershed. *Circulation*. 2014;130(10):864-865.

Kirschen MP, Lewis A, Greer DM. The 2023 American Academy of Neurology, American Academy of Pediatrics, Child Neurology Society, and Society of Critical Care Medicine Pediatric and Adult Brain Death/Death by Neurologic Criteria Determination Consensus Guidelines: what the critical care team needs to know. *Crit Care Med*. 2024;52(3):376-386.

Lewis A. An update on brain death/death by neurologic criteria since the World Brain Death Project. *Semin Neurol*. 2024;44(3):236-262.

Lewis A, Bakkar A, Kreiger-Benson E, et al. Determination of death by neurologic criteria around the world. *Neurology*. 2020;95(3):e299-e309.

Lewis A, Kirschen MP. Brain death/death by neurologic criteria determination. *Continuum (Minneap Minn)*. 2021;27(5):1444-1464.

Lewis A, Kirschen MP, Greer D. The 2023 AAN/AAP/CNS/SCCM Pediatric and Adult Brain Death/Death by Neurologic Criteria Consensus practice guideline: a comparison with the 2010 and 2011 guidelines. *Neurol Clin Pract*. 2023;13(6):e200189.

Lewis A, Liebman J, Kreiger-Benson E, et al. Ancillary testing for determination of death by neurologic criteria around the world. *Neurocrit Care*. 2021;34(2):473-484.

Migdady I, Stephens RS, Price C, Geocadin RG, Whitman G, Cho SM. The use of apnea test and brain death determination in patients on extracorporeal membrane oxygenation: a systematic review. *J Thorac Cardiovasc Surg*. 2021;162(3):867-877.e1.

Webb AC, Samuels OB. Reversible brain death after cardiopulmonary arrest and induced hypothermia. *Crit Care Med*. 2011;39(6):1538-1542.

Wieler H, Marohl K, Kaiser KP, Klawki P, Frössler H. Tc-99m HMPAO cerebral scintigraphy. A reliable, noninvasive method for determination of brain death. *Clin Nucl Med*. 1993;18(2):104-109.

Wijdicks EF. The diagnosis of brain death. *N Engl J Med*. 2001;344(16): 1215-1221.

Yee AH, Mandrekar J, Rabinstein AA, Wijdicks EF. Predictors of apnea test failure during brain death determination. *Neurocrit Care*. 2010;12(3): 352-325.

8.14

Anoxic Brain Injury, Temperature Control, and Neuroprognostication

Priya Srikanth and Guy A. Rordorf

Description

- Since the 1950s, moderate hypothermia has been employed for brain protection during cardiac arrest for certain cardiovascular surgeries.
- Multiple landmark trials investigating temperature management after cardiac arrest have driven an evolution in clinical practice:
  - Hypothermia to 33 °C was found to be superior to no targeted temperature management (TTM) for patients with out-of-hospital ventricular fibrillation or ventricular tachycardia arrest in two small, unblinded studies published in 2002.
  - The TTM1 trial, published in 2013, demonstrated that TTM to 36 °C was equivalent to 33 °C for patients with out-of-hospital cardiac arrest.
  - The HYPERION trial, published in 2019, studied the effects of TTM at 33 °C versus 37 °C in patients with nonshockable rhythms. There was an increase in favorable neurologic outcomes for patients treated to 33 °C. However, this finding is tempered by a fragility index of 1 (ie, if one patient had a different outcome, this finding would not have reached statistical significance), small effect size, and noted incomplete fever control in patients randomized to 37 °C.
  - TTM2, published in 2021, demonstrated that fever avoidance (treating ≥37.8 °C) was equivalent to 33 °C with respect to neurologic outcomes in patients after out-of-hospital cardiac arrest. Notably, patients in the 33 °C TTM group had longer ventilation times, increased cardiac arrhythmias causing hemodynamic instability, higher incidence of requiring paralysis, and an increased rate of serious adverse events.
  - TTM1 and TTM2 enrolled mostly patients who had shockable rhythms; nonshockable rhythms benefit less from TTM.
- International guidelines overall recommend temperature control, with variability in the specific target temperature and duration recommendations. The American Heart Association (AHA) guidelines recommend maintaining a temperature between 32 and 37.5 °C for at least 24 hours in patients who remain comatose after return of spontaneous circulation (ROSC). The European Resuscitation Council and International Liaison Committee on Resuscitation suggest temperature management targeting fever avoidance (<37.7 °C) for at least 72 hours.
- Given the results of the abovementioned studies, active fever prevention is a reasonable approach for comatose survivors of cardiac arrest. There may exist a subset of patients for whom therapeutic hypothermia would yield a benefit, but this remains unclear. Further studies [Influence of Cooling Duration on Efficacy in Cardiac Arrest Patients (ICECAP), TTM3, Sedation, Temperature and Pressure After Cardiac Arrest and Resuscitation (STEPCARE)] are ongoing and will hopefully further inform optimal target temperature, duration, and method of temperature management.
- Rapid passive or active rewarming (> 0.5 °C per hour) for patients with mild hypothermia should be avoided. While there are no large studies of rewarming rates, there is a potential risk of secondary injury with rapid temperature increase. Faster rewarming may be appropriate for patients with significant active bleeding or cardiac instability associated with profound hypothermia on arrival.
- Neuroprognostication for patients who are comatose after cardiac arrest should incorporate multiple diagnostic modalities and should occur no >72 hours after normothermia. Modalities to consider include neurologic examination, magnetic resonance imaging (MRI) of the brain, continuous electroencephalogram (EEG), neuron-specific enolase (NSE), and somatosensory evoked potentials (SSEPs). When uncertainty remains, prolonging observation and repeated testing are recommended rather than early withdrawal of life-sustaining therapy, given the risk of withdrawing care in patients who may have had a favorable neurologic outcome.

Temperature Control

- Recommended for
  - Adult patients who remain comatose after ROSC (ie, no meaningful response to verbal commands)
  - Patients in whom normotension can be maintained, with or without need for vasopressors or mechanical circulatory support

Management and Treatment

- Team should aim to initiate temperature control as soon as possible after ROSC, regardless of patient location.
- Goal temperature based on institutional protocols and clinician preference. Aggressive fever prevention with a target ≤37.5 °C for at least 72 hours is reasonable. If TTM with mild hypothermia (33-36 °C) is implemented, hypothermia should be maintained for 24 hours, followed by low rewarming to normothermia for an additional 48 hours (total 72 hours).
- Temperature control is often achieved using a surface cooling device, though methods and specific devices vary by institution. Intravenous cold saline infusion and/or ice packs may also be used to assist with achieving temperature control if needed.
- Relative exclusion criteria
  - No absolute contraindications exist for fever avoidance (≤37.5 °C).
  - For TTM with mild hypothermia (33-36 °C), a higher risk of adverse effects may be seen in patients with head trauma with intracerebral hemorrhage, recent major bleeding or active bleeding, major surgery within the last 2 weeks, or inability to maintain normotension despite the use of vasopressors.

- Monitoring
  - Continuous monitoring of temperature should be performed using two methods. Measurement of core temperature is preferred (eg, bladder or esophageal probe, pulmonary arterial [PA] catheter).
  - Administer standing acetaminophen to aid in fever avoidance in patients without contraindications (eg, acute liver failure, hepatic dysfunction).
  - Control shivering as needed with stepwise measures: skin counterwarming, magnesium infusion for goal Mg 3 to 4 mg/dL, sedation (dexmedetomidine, propofol, opioid infusion), and/or buspirone 30 mg every 8 hours. Paralysis with neuromuscular blockade should be used if all of the abovementioned therapies have failed or are contraindicated.
  - Hypothermia can increase the risk of bradycardia, hyperglycemia, hypokalemia, and coagulopathy.
  - Rewarming can be associated with hypotension, hypoglycemia, and hyperkalemia.

Neurologic Monitoring and Neuroprognostication

- Initial assessment
  - If there is concern for stroke or intracerebral hemorrhage, obtain a noncontrast head computed tomography (CT) when patient is clinically stable for imaging. Temperature control should not be delayed for head CT.
  - Pupillary reflexes should be monitored at least every 2 hours during temperature control.
  - Routine care should include continuous EEG monitoring within 12 hours if able, to evaluate for nonconvulsive seizures or status epilepticus.
- Diagnostic modalities for prognostication
  - No single diagnostic test can provide prognostic certainty, and a single test result should not be used to convey a likelihood of poor prognosis in isolation. Discussions regarding likely neurologic outcome should incorporate as many diagnostic modalities as possible and should occur ≥72 hours after ROSC or normothermia. In cases of diagnostic or prognostic uncertainty, consider allowing more time to allow for ongoing assessment of the patient's neurologic status.
  - Neurologic examination (≥72 hours after ROSC or normothermia): including level of arousal, awareness, brainstem reflexes, and extremity motor responses to noxious stimulation. Neurologic assessments are most informative when performed of all sedation and in the absence of confounding factors (severe metabolic encephalopathy and neuromuscular blockers). Bilateral absent pupillary light reflex is concerning for poor prognosis.
  - Continuous EEG (within 12 hours): patterns associated with poor prognosis include diffuse voltage attenuation, burst suppression, lack of reactivity, status epilepticus (including myoclonic status epilepticus), and epileptiform activity.
  - MRI brain (day 3-7 after ROSC): extensive diffusion restriction (affecting widespread bilateral cerebral cortex, basal ganglia) is associated with poor neurologic outcome. If unable to obtain MRI, a noncontrast head CT can be performed; diffuse hypodensity on CT at least 48 hours from ROSC is concerning for poor prognosis.
  - NSE: sent at 24, 48, and 72 hours after arrest. Although a single threshold value has not been validated in the literature, elevated (40-60 μg/L) and uptrending NSE (>90 μg/L) on serial measurements is associated with a lower likelihood of favorable neurologic outcome. Given variability in NSE cutoffs, interpretation should be cautious and NSE alone should not be considered a reliable predictor of poor functional outcome. NSE is also present in red blood cells (RBCs) and will be confounded in the presence of hemolysis.
  - SSEPs (≥48 hours after normothermia): bilateral absence of cortical N20 responses is highly suggestive of poor neurologic outcome.

SUGGESTED READINGS

Bernard S. Hypothermia after cardiac arrest: expanding the therapeutic scope. *Crit Care Med*. 2009;37:S277-S233.

Bernard SA, Gray TW, Buist MD, et al. Treatment of comatose survivors of out-of-hospital cardiac arrest with induced hypothermia. *N Engl J Med*. 2002;346(8):557-563.

Dankiewicz J, Cronberg T, Lilkja G, et al. Hypothermia versus normothermia after out-of-hospital cardiac arrest. *N Engl J Med*. 2021;384(24): 2283-2294.

Perman SM, Bartos JA, Del Rios M, et al. Temperature management for comatose adult survivors of cardiac arrest: a science advisory from the American Heart Association. *Circulation*. 2023;148(12):982-988.

Perman SM, Elmer J, Maciel CB, et al. 2023 American Heart Association Focused update on adult advanced cardiovascular life support: an update to the American Heart Association Guidelines for cardiopulmonary resuscitation and emergency cardiovascular care. *Circulation*. 2024; 149(5):e254-e273.

Rajajee V, Muehlschlegel S, Wartenberg KE, et al. Guidelines for neuroprognostication in comatose adult survivors of cardiac arrest. *Neurocrit Care*. 2023;38:533-563.

Sandroni C, Nolan JP, Andersen LW, et al. ERC-ESICM guidelines on temperature control after cardiac arrest in adults. *Intensive Care Med*. 2022;48(3):261-269.

8.15

Neurooncology

Kyle A. Lyman and Daniel B. Rubin

Primary Brain Tumors

- Primary central nervous system (CNS) tumors are broadly categorized as malignant (29.1%) and nonmalignant (70.9%). The 5-year survival rate for malignant CNS tumors is ~67%, while for nonmalignant tumors, it is significantly higher, around 92.1%.
  - Gliomas are tumors that arise from glial or precursor cells and include oligodendrogliomas, astrocytomas, and glioblastomas. The current World Health Organization (WHO) classification system incorporates genetic and histologic information in identifying a grade, with widely varying median survival.
    - Glioblastoma multiforme (GBM) is the most common primary CNS malignancy (49% of all malignant CNS tumors), with a median survival of 8 months.
    - GBM can be challenging to diagnose from imaging alone, with brain abscess, subacute stroke, and variants of multiple sclerosis as common mimics.
    - Extent of resection is associated with longer survival, although GBM invariably progresses.
    - Anticoagulation is not contraindicated in patients with GBM, but because of significant vascularity, GBM has an increased risk for hemorrhage.
    - Low-grade gliomas have an indolent course but have a high rate of epilepsy, over 85% in one series, compared to 49% in patients with GBM.
- Nonmalignant CNS tumors may cause substantial morbidity as there is limited room for growth, and compression can lead to significant symptoms.
  - Meningiomas are the most common nonmalignant tumor (39% of all CNS tumors) and are often noted incidentally. Serial imaging may be appropriate for some cases, but large meningiomas may cause symptomatic compression of the brain and vascular structures.
- While focal and generalized seizures are common in patients with primary brain tumors, current guidelines do not recommend starting antiseizure medications unless the patient has a seizure.
- Steroids are an effective treatment for vasogenic edema and restore the integrity of the blood-brain barrier. They typically begin to exert clinically significant benefits within hours, although days may be required before they reach maximum efficacy. Steroids should not be given for imaging findings alone (and may impact the diagnostic yield of biopsy for certain lesion subtypes), so they should be titrated to clinical benefit.

Brain Metastases

- Brain metastases are ~10× more common than primary CNS tumors. Primary malignancies with a high incidence of brain metastases include lung (small cell and non–small cell), renal cell carcinoma, melanoma, and breast.
  - The anatomic compartment involved is extremely important for management and prognostication. Parenchymal metastases are more easily seen on imaging and often come to attention because of seizure, hemorrhage, mass effect, or obstructive hydrocephalus.
    - Leptomeningeal spread refers to invasion of the arachnoid space and cerebrospinal fluid (CSF), discussed in the section that follows.
  - Communicating hydrocephalus often arises from leptomeningeal spread, while noncommunicating hydrocephalus (obstructive) typically results from parenchymal mass effect, especially in the posterior fossa.
- Patients with brain metastases from melanoma, renal cell carcinoma, thyroid carcinoma, and choriocarcinoma are regarded as having the highest risk of intracerebral hemorrhage, regardless of anticoagulation.
  - Meta-analyses of retrospective data suggest that anticoagulation is reasonable and should not be withheld if clinically indicated unless the patient has had a prior symptomatic intracerebral bleed.
  - Highly vascular lesions, especially melanoma, may appear bright on computed tomography (CT) imaging and be confused for an acute hemorrhage. Careful consideration of clinical context and prior imaging should guide subsequent clinical steps.
- Large, symptomatic lesions should be considered for resection, especially in the posterior fossa where compressive lesions may lead to noncommunicating hydrocephalus.
  - Steroids are often used to temporize patients prior to surgery for the management of symptomatic vasogenic edema.
  - Randomized trials have shown that stereotactic radiosurgery (SRS) for up to 10 metastases is as effective as SRS for patients with fewer metastases and should be considered. However, radiation is not effective acutely, and whole-brain radiation therapy (WBRT) may be considered an alternative if there are too many lesions.
- Brain metastases often lead to focal and generalized seizures, but antiseizure medications are not given prophylactically and should be reserved for diagnosed seizures.
- Metastases to the spinal cord or vertebral column can result in acute spinal cord dysfunction.
  - Emergent imaging is needed to assess if there has been vertebral collapse, malignant invasion of the cord, or acute hemorrhage producing symptoms. Magnetic resonance imaging (MRI) is the ideal modality, but CT is often performed first to assess vertebral integrity quickly.
  - Initial management involves high-dose steroids and neurosurgical consult.

Carcinomatous Meningitis

- Leptomeningeal disease (LMD)—also called carcinomatous meningitis or neoplastic meningitis—refers to the infiltration of malignant cells into the CSF and leptomeninges.
- LMD carries a very grave prognosis, regardless of the burden of malignancy elsewhere. Prognosis is often estimated at 8 to 16 weeks of survival from diagnosis of leptomeningeal involvement.

- Challenging to diagnose and requires a high index of suspicion. May be seen as contrast enhancement on MRI, although the gold standard is from cytology studies on lumbar puncture (LP). LP is only 50% to 70% sensitive, and serial LPs may be required.
  - MRI with and without contrast of the entire neuraxis can increase the likelihood of diagnosis.
  - May present with intractable headaches, communicating hydrocephalus, encephalopathy, cranial nerve deficits, spinal nerve root involvement (radicular pain and weakness), or cauda equina symptoms. Symptoms typically develop over days to weeks.
  - May cause plateau waves (also referred to as pressure waves and Lundberg A waves), which represent spikes of intracranial pressure (ICP) in the setting of limited intracranial compliance and preserved cerebral vasoregulation
    - Changes in position may provoke a drop in mean arterial pressure (MAP), leading to a rise in ICP as cerebral vasculature dilates to try and maintain cerebral perfusion pressure (CPP). The rise in ICP further limits CPP and perpetuates itself, leading to a minutes-long "wave" of high ICP during which cerebral perfusion is compromised.
    - Electroencephalography (EEG) may show moderate-severe slowing during the plateau wave. Perfusion imaging may reveal hypoperfusion during the wave, but head imaging may be unrevealing.
    - Individual plateau waves may be aborted by maintaining a high MAP, maximizing CSF drainage, and limiting provoking maneuvers.
    - LP or lumbar drain may temporize until permanent CSF diversion (via ventriculoperitoneal shunt or external ventricular drain placement), but opening pressures may be normal during non–plateau wave periods.
- Intrathecal chemotherapy and radiation can be considered for LMD, although the prognosis remains grave.
- *Complications of radiation therapy*: radiation may be to the whole brain (WBRT) in cases with innumerable metastases or SRS if a finite number of targetable metastases can be found (typically ≤10).
- Acute (days to weeks)
  - Fatigue, headaches, nausea/vomiting, fever, and encephalopathy are commonly seen.
  - Small increases in vasogenic edema can be seen, which are rarely associated with seizures or neurologic decline (2.2% of patients receiving SRS in one large series).
    - Steroids and supportive management would be indicated.
- Subacute (1-6 months)
  - *Pseudoprogression*: radiologic diagnosis made when MRI shows contrast enhancement and fluid-attenuated inversion recovery (FLAIR) hyperintensity at the site of prior irradiation and raising concern for progression of malignancy (typically distinguished retrospectively based on clinical course and serial imaging). Pseudoprogression is less commonly symptomatic, but symptoms can be managed with steroids and/or bevacizumab. See Figure 8.15.1 for additional details.
  - Lhermitte sign (movement eliciting electric sensation down the spine) can be seen if the radiation field involves the spinal cord. Typically resolves spontaneously

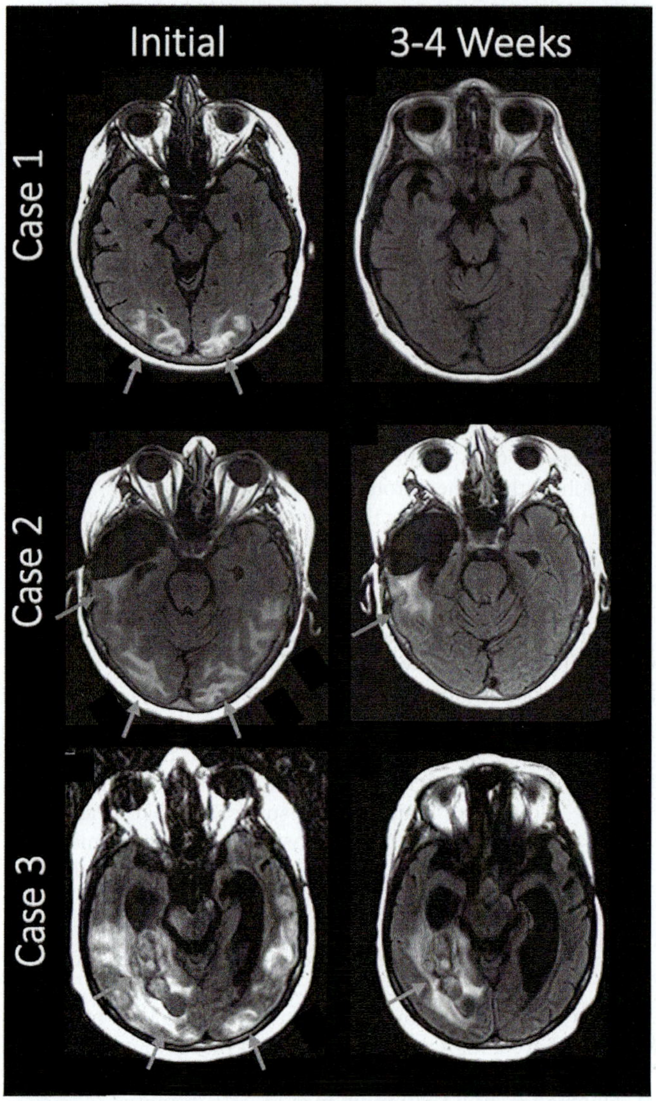

FIGURE 8.15.1 **Posterior reversible encephalopathy syndrome (PRES) is associated with fluid-attenuated inversion recovery (FLAIR) abnormalities that typically improve with time.** Three cases of PRES are presented, each with follow-up imaging 3–4 weeks later showing improvement in FLAIR abnormalities. Arrows show vasogenic edema that improves with time in case 1. Case 2 initially shows vasogenic edema that is attributable to PRES (resolves 3-4 weeks later) as well as vasogenic edema that persists at 3-4 weeks and is attributable to GBM adjacent to resection cavity. Case 3 similarly features vasogenic edema that resolves with arrow at 3-4 week time point highlighting GBM in situ. (From Kamiya-Matsuoka C, Cachia D, Olar A, Armstrong TS, Gilbert MR. Primary brain tumors and posterior reversible encephalopathy syndrome. Neurooncol Pract. 2014;1(4):184-190.)

- Chronic (>6 months)
  - Cognitive decline is common after WBRT but rarely seen after SRS, impairments can range from subtle deficits in short-term memory to profound dementia.
    - Memantine can be used prophylactically to try and limit excitotoxic damage, although evidence is inconclusive as to the benefit.

  - Delayed radiation toxicity occurs months to years after irradiation and can cause diffuse leukoencephalopathy with cortical atrophy.
- *SMART syndrome*: stroke-like migraine attacks, often years after radiation therapy
  - Presents with migraine-like headaches, focal neurologic deficits (which may be permanent), potentially seizures. MRI of the brain shows contrast enhancement in the previously irradiated cortex that resolves with time.
  - Steroids are often given with supportive management.
  - Deficits typically improve over weeks to months.
- *Radiation necrosis*: typically seen 1 to 3 years after radiation therapy and presenting as contrast enhancement on MRI, making it challenging to differentiate from progression of malignancy (reduced blood flow and reduced positron emission tomography [PET] uptake are consistent with necrosis, but not always diagnostic). Often requires biopsy to distinguish from tumor progression.
  - Bevacizumab is often used with steroids.
- Vascular changes
  - Radiation can cause acceleration of atherosclerotic changes in irradiated vessels (eg, extracranial carotid disease), which merits therapy directed at atherosclerosis. Small, sometimes asymptomatic, lacunar infarctions are also commonly seen.
  - Intracranial vasculopathy can also develop, causing focal narrowing and moyamoya physiology, which may cause ischemia (hypoperfusion) or hemorrhage (friable vessel proliferation).
  - Cavernomas are found more often after childhood brain radiation, although these lesions are seldom symptomatic and are typically associated with low-volume asymptomatic bleeding. Cerebral microhemorrhages and superficial siderosis have also been reported.
- *Optic neuropathy*: painless loss of vision can occur if the optic nerves are irradiated.
- Peripheral nerves are generally more resistant to the effect of radiation, but fibrotic scarring can cause entrapment neuropathies.
  - Painful peripheral neuropathies should elicit workup for malignant invasion of the nerve (especially brachial and lumbosacral plexus).
  - Electromyogram/nerve conduction study can help identify sequelae of radiation with characteristic "myokymia" pattern of discharges.
- Painless myelopathy (in contrast to the painful progression of malignancy) can be seen, thought to be secondary to myelin degeneration and neurotoxicity.
  - Imaging may reveal edematous changes and contrast enhancement, prompting consideration of bevacizumab or steroids for radiation necrosis as earlier.

Complications of Chemotherapy

- Bevacizumab (monoclonal antibody targeting vascular endothelial growth factor, VEGF): often used as a steroid-sparing agent for patients with CNS vasogenic edema
  - Often invoked as an etiology of intracerebral hemorrhage, although meta-analyses are not consistent with an increased hemorrhage risk (association confounded by increased risk of hemorrhage with CNS metastases and primary lesions)
    - Anticoagulation is not contraindicated by the use of bevacizumab.
  - Associated with delayed wound healing, proteinuria, and hypertension (HTN)
  - Lowers the threshold for PRES (posterior reversible encephalopathy syndrome), which may occur in the absence of HTN. PRES is a neurotoxic state characterized by vasogenic edema, commonly affecting posterior regions of the brain.
    - Steroids should not be used to treat PRES and are often implicated in precipitating PRES.
    - Less commonly, PRES is associated with tacrolimus, cyclophosphamide, cyclosporine, ifosfamide, and gemcitabine.
    - Presents with seizures, encephalopathy, new imaging findings showing vasogenic edema without an underlying mass lesion
    - Management: cessation of bevacizumab or other provoking agents. Lower blood pressure as for hypertensive urgency, supportive care with antiseizure medications if indicated. Serial imaging may show improvement in vasogenic edema.
- *Ifosfamide*: may cause encephalopathy and depressed mental status, rarely seizures, typically hours to days after administration
  - Intravenous thiamine and methylene blue have been used as treatment, but European guidelines recommend against this approach,
- *Methotrexate* (MTX): intrathecal administration can be used for LMD and acutely cause aseptic meningitis. The following comments are applicable to all modes of MTX administration.
  - Can acutely cause encephalopathy, seizures, focal MRI findings that are concerning for stroke (nonenhancing lesions that are diffusion-weighted imaging [DWI] bright but resolve spontaneously)
  - Months after administration, can cause leukoencephalopathy (injury to the white matter), PRES, cerebellar findings, lumbosacral radiculopathy, and, rarely, spinal cord injury
- Peripheral neuropathy is commonly seen with a range of agents (ie, taxanes, vincristine, platinum-containing compounds, bortezomib) and typically presents as length-dependent paresthesias with numbness and tingling but can also cause loss of distal reflexes (large fiber involvement) and deficits in proprioception.

Immunologic Complications of Cancer

- Paraneoplastic syndromes: complicate an estimated 1 in 300 cancer diagnoses and describes antibody production against a nervous system antigen in the context of aberrant antigen expression by the malignancy. (See Table 8.15.1)
  - Diagnosis is made on the basis of antibody detection in the appropriate clinical context matching the known syndrome. Differentiating a primary antibody-mediated disorder (eg, anti-LGI1, occurring outside the context of malignancy) from a paraneoplastic disorder (eg, anti-Yo antibodies, which are associated with rapidly progressive cerebellar syndrome and associated breast or

TABLE 8.15.1 Examples of Paraneoplastic Syndromes

Antibody Name	Syndromes Associated With Antibody Positivity	Frequency With Cancer, Usual Malignancy
Yo (PCA-1)	Rapidly progressive cerebellar syndrome with ataxia, nystagmus, MRI brain with cerebellar involvement	>90% are associated with breast or ovarian cancer. Rarely seen in men
Ma2 and/or Ma1	Limbic, diencephalic, and/or brainstem encephalitis. Seizures, MRI of the brain with hippocampal, thalamic, brainstem involvement	>75%, can be seen in testicular cancer or SCLC
P/Q voltage-gated calcium channel	Lambert-Eaton myasthenic syndrome (LEMS) featuring autonomic failure, proximal weakness beginning in the lower extremities. Also associated with a rapidly progressive cerebellar syndrome	~50% associated with SCLC. Note that LEMS can be caused by other antibodies as well, and the same antibody has been associated with multiple paraneoplastic syndromes.
Amphiphysin	Stiff person syndrome (axial stiffness and spasms), sensory neuronopathy (dorsal root ganglia are lost), encephalomyelitis	~80%, breast cancer
NMDA	Often progresses over days to weeks with psychotic symptoms, seizures, and profound alterations in awareness with movement disorders and autonomic instability	38%, most often ovarian teratomas but extraovarian teratomas and other malignancies have also been described

[a]Note: This list is not exhaustive, there are many more paraneoplastic syndromes that exist.

MRI, magnetic resonance imaging; SCLC, small cell lung cancer.

Adapted from Graus F, Vogrig A, Muñiz-Castrillo S, et al. Updated diagnostic criteria for paraneoplastic neurologic syndromes. Neurol Neuroimmunol Neuroinflamm. 2021;8(4):e1014.

ovarian cancer in over 90% of cases) relies on matching the antibody with clinical syndrome.

- Typically, paraneoplastic syndromes are diagnosed early in the course of the malignancy and often cause symptoms prior to the malignancy diagnosis.
- Scoring systems like the PNS-Care score can be used to diagnose a paraneoplastic syndrome.
- Key cancers with high rate of paraneoplastic disorders: non–small cell lung cancer, thymoma, ovarian (including teratomas), breast, testicular, and Hodgkin lymphoma
  - Small cell lung cancer has the highest incidence of paraneoplastic disorder (9.4% in one series with Lambert-Eaton myasthenic syndrome [LEMS]; 3.8%), sensory neuronopathy (1.9%), and limbic encephalitis (1.5%).
- Therapy is directed at the management of the underlying malignancy, although steroids, intravenous immune globulin (IVIG), and plasmapheresis are sometimes considered. Distinct paraneoplastic neurologic syndromes have different likelihoods of recovery based on the location of antigen expression, although most paraneoplastic-associated conditions cause irreversible neuronal loss.

- *Immune checkpoint inhibitors* (ICIs): cancer immunotherapy designed to increase T-cell activity against the malignancy but can provoke an autoimmune response to the nervous system
  - Lead to severe autoimmune response against the nervous system in 1% to 3% of cases, which can include exacerbation of preexisting disease (eg, myasthenia gravis) and de novo autoimmune syndromes
  - ICI autoimmune syndromes may mimic autoantibody syndromes, especially limbic encephalitis, but are often seronegative when antibody panels are used.
  - ICI may cause myasthenia gravis, Guillain-Barré syndrome, myelitis, and peripheral neuropathy.
    - Management of ICI-related neurologic complications includes discontinuation of checkpoint inhibitors and starting steroids (even for disease processes where steroids are not ordinarily used, as in the case of ICI-related Guillain-Barré syndrome).
- Immune effector cell–mediated neurotoxicity syndrome (ICANS) can be seen after chimeric antigen receptor T-cell (CAR-T) therapy.
  - ICANS most often occurs in parallel with cytokine release syndrome (CRS), a systemic inflammatory response seen after CAR-T infusion with fever, hypotension, and hypoxia, although ICANS can also occur after CRS has resolved.
    - ICANS is graded 0 to 4 based on the severity of deficits. Low-grade ICANS involves confusion, aphasia, myoclonus, and encephalopathy, but more severe involvement can lead to seizures, cerebral edema, and death.
    - Risk of ICANS varies with CAR-T product, extent of primary malignancy, and baseline neurologic status.
    - EEG is often used, but the absolute seizure risk for all patients receiving CAR-T is low (<10%). Higher grade ICANS carries an increased risk of nonconvulsive status epilepticus and merits EEG monitoring.
    - Focal findings on MRI have been described but are infrequently seen, except in high-grade ICANS. Common findings include diffuse cerebral edema, FLAIR abnormalities in the limbic structures, thalami, and brainstem, as well as leukoencephalopathy.
      - Imaging is always indicated for high grade ICANS to ensure there is no evidence of an alternative explanation for the change in mental status (eg, hemorrhage).
      - It can be challenging to distinguish the influence of fludarabine and cyclophosphamide used for

lymphodepletion prior to CAR-T infusion on subsequent MRI as these agents can also cause leukoencephalopathy.
  - Management of high-grade ICANS includes investigating for opportunistic infections and managing supportively to treat seizures and limit cerebral edema.
- Steroids and tocilizumab are often used to manage both CRS and ICANS, although there is a theoretical concern that tocilizumab, an interleukin-6 (IL-6) receptor antibody, may accelerate ICANS by increasing the free fraction of blood-brain barrier permeable IL-6.
  - Siltuximab, an antibody targeting IL-6 directly (as opposed to the IL-6 receptor), has been proposed as an alternative therapy for ICANS, although it has not been shown to be more efficacious for ICANS.
- Anakinra, an IL-1 receptor antagonist, has also been used for the treatment of ICANS.

SUGGESTED READINGS

Alvarado G, Noor R, Bassett R, et al. Risk of intracranial hemorrhage with anticoagulation therapy in melanoma patients with brain metastases. *Melanoma Res*. 2012;22(4):310-315.

Brown TJ, Brennan MC, Li M, et al. Association of the extent of resection with survival in glioblastoma: a systematic review and meta-analysis. *JAMA Oncol*. 2016;2(11):1460.

Burn S, Gunny R, Phipps K, Gaze M, Hayward R. Incidence of cavernoma development in children after radiotherapy for brain tumors. *J Neurosurg*. 2007;106(5):379-383.

Chin LS, Lazio BE, Biggins T, Amin P. Acute complications following gamma knife radiosurgery are rare. *Surg Neurol*. 2000;53(5):498-502.

Corn BW, Yousem DM, Scott CB, et al. White matter changes are correlated significantly with radiation dose. Observations from a randomized dose-escalation trial for malignant glioma (radiation therapy oncology group 83-02). *Cancer*. 1994;74(10):2828-2835.

Dalmau J, Graus F. Antibody-mediated encephalitis. *N Engl J Med*. 2018; 378(9):840-851.

de la Fuente MI. Adult-type diffuse gliomas. *Continuum (Minneap Minn)*. 2023;29(6):1662-1679.

Dietrich J. Neurotoxicity of cancer therapies. *Continuum (Minneap Minn)*. 2020;26(6):1646-1672.

Dominguez M, Malani R. Stroke-like migraine attacks after radiation therapy (SMART) syndrome: a comprehensive review. *Curr Pain Headache Rep*. 2021;25(5):33.

Donato J, Campigotto F, Uhlmann EJ, et al. Intracranial hemorrhage in patients with brain metastases treated with therapeutic enoxaparin: a matched cohort study. *Blood*. 2015;126(4):494-499.

Graus F, Dalmau J. Paraneoplastic neurological syndromes in the era of immune-checkpoint inhibitors. *Nat Rev Clin Oncol*. 2019;16(9):535-548.

Graus F, Vogrig A, Muñiz-Castrillo S, et al. Updated diagnostic criteria for paraneoplastic neurologic syndromes. *Neurol Neuroimmunol Neuroinflamm*. 2021;8(4):e1014.

Kamiya-Matsuoka C, Cachia D, Olar A, Armstrong TS, Gilbert MR. Primary brain tumors and posterior reversible encephalopathy syndrome. *Neurooncol Pract*. 2014;1(4):184-190.

Kumthekar P, Rhun EL. Brain metastases and leptomeningeal disease. *Continuum (Minneap Minn)*. 2023;29(6):1727-1751.

Lee A, Oley F, Lo M, et al. Direct oral anticoagulants or low-molecular-weight heparins for venous thromboembolism in patients with brain tumors. *Thromb Res*. 2021;208:148-155.

Lote K, Stenwig AE, Skullerud K, Hirschberg H. Prevalence and prognostic significance of epilepsy in patients with gliomas. *Eur J Cancer*. 1998;34(1):98-102.

Murphy ES, Xie H, Merchant TE, Yu JS, Chao ST, Suh JH. Review of cranial radiotherapy-induced vasculopathy. *J Neurooncol*. 2015;122(3): 421-429.

Nie EH, Ahmadian SS, Bharadwaj SN, et al. Multifocal demyelinating leukoencephalopathy and oligodendroglial lineage cell loss with immune effector cell-associated neurotoxicity syndrome (ICANS) following CD19 CAR T-cell therapy for mantle cell lymphoma. *J Neuropathol Exp Neurol*. 2023;82(2):160-168.

Nolan CP, DeAngelis LM. Neurologic complications of chemotherapy and radiation therapy. *Continuum (Minneap Minn)*. 2015;21(2 Neuro-oncology):429-451.

Ostrom QT, Cioffi G, Waite K, Kruchko C, Barnholtz-Sloan JS. CBTRUS statistical report: primary brain and other central nervous system tumors diagnosed in the United States in 2014-2018. *Neuro Oncol*. 2021;23(suppl 3):iii1-iii105.

Parikh NS, Schweitzer AD, Young RJ, et al. Corticosteroid therapy and severity of vasogenic edema in posterior reversible encephalopathy syndrome. *J Neurol Sci*. 2017;380:11-15.

Pelgrims J, Vos FD, Brande JV den, Schrijvers D, Prové A, Vermorken JB. Methylene blue in the treatment and prevention of ifosfamide-induced encephalopathy: report of 12 cases and a review of the literature. *Br J Cancer*. 2000;82(2):291-294.

Perrinjaquet C, Desbaillets N, Hottinger AF. Neurotoxicity associated with cancer immunotherapy: immune checkpoint inhibitors and chimeric antigen receptor T-cell therapy. *Curr Opin Neurol*. 2019;32(3):500-510.

Rubin DB, Danish HH, Ali AB, et al. Neurological toxicities associated with chimeric antigen receptor T-cell therapy. *Brain*. 2019;142(5): awz053.

Slawski D, Lyman KA, Thatikunta P, Gold CA, Albers GW. Cerebral perfusion imaging and plateau waves. *Stroke*. 2023;54(5):e224-e228.

Strati P, Nastoupil LJ, Westin J, et al. Clinical and radiologic correlates of neurotoxicity after axicabtagene ciloleucel in large B-cell lymphoma. *Blood Adv*. 2020;4(16):3943-3951.

Tanguturi SK, Alexander BM. Neurologic complications of radiation therapy. *Neurol Clin*. 2018;36(3):599-625.

Taylor JW. Neurologic complications of conventional chemotherapy and radiation therapy. *Continuum (Minneap Minn)*. 2023;29(6):1809-1826.

Welch MR. Management of complications in neuro-oncology patients. *Continuum (Minneap Minn)*. 2023;29(6):1844-1871.

Yang L, Chen CJ, Guo XL, et al. Bevacizumab and risk of intracranial hemorrhage in patients with brain metastases: a meta-analysis. *J Neurooncol*. 2018;137(1):49-56.

8.16

Analgesia, Sedation, Neuromuscular Blockade, and Other Pharmacologic Therapies for Neurologic Disorders

Dusan Hanidziar

Overview

- Management of sedation, analgesia, and neuromuscular blockade (NMB) is an essential aspect of care for mechanically ventilated patients in the intensive care unit (ICU).
- Goals include patient comfort, safety, ventilator synchrony, facilitation of procedures, and reduction of complications (eg, delirium, prolonged ventilation, immobility).
- Modern ICU practice emphasizes the ABCDEF (part of the ICU Liberation initiative) bundle, which integrates systematic pain assessment and management, light sedation, delirium prevention and monitoring, early mobility, and coordinated spontaneous awakening and breathing trials.
- To ensure optimal levels of sedation and analgesia, management needs to be individualized based on patient factors (eg, organ failure, encephalopathy), pharmacologic profiles of agents, and frequent clinical assessments.
- These strategies should follow evidence-based ICU bundles (eg, the ABCDEF bundle) and society guidelines (eg, the 2018 Society of Critical Care Medicine [SCCM] Prevention and Management of Pain, Agitation/Sedation, Delirium, Immobility, and Sleep Disruption [PADIS] recommendations for pain, agitation/sedation, and delirium).
- Bispectral index monitoring (BIS) or limited channel electroencephalography (EEG) should be used for sedation monitoring in specific situations: patients receiving NMB, those requiring deep sedation, or when titrating sedation for elevated intracranial pressure.
- BIS/EEG are NOT recommended for routine sedation assessment; clinical sedation scales (ie, RASS) remain the primary assessment tools per 2018 SCCM guidelines for the PADIS in adult patients in the ICU.

Analgesia in Critically Ill Mechanically Ventilated Patients

Adequate analgesia is essential to limit adverse consequences of pain, such as psychological stress, anxiety, insomnia, delirium, and sympathetic activation (tachycardia, hypertension, myocardial ischemia, hypermetabolism).

- Assessment
  - Encourage patients to self-report pain.
  - Utilize validated pain assessment tools (eg, numeric rating scale in communicative patients; Critical-Care Pain Observation Tool [CPOT] or Behavioral Pain Scale in noncommunicative patients).
- Preferred analgesia strategies
  - Analgesia-first approach as highlighted in ABCDEF bundle: optimize pain control before escalating sedative therapy; commonly used ICU sedatives and analgesics are summarized in Tables 8.16.1 and 8.16.2, respectively.

TABLE 8.16.1 Major sedatives used in the ICU

Agent	Mechanism	Kinetics	Major Considerations
Propofol	GABA-A receptor agonist	Onset: 30-45 s Duration: 3-10 min after single bolus Metabolism: hepatic and some extrahepatic	1. Hypotension 2. Hypertriglyceridemia (monitor triglycerides with prolonged high-dose infusions) 3. Propofol infusion syndrome (risk with high-dose, prolonged infusions)
Midazolam	Modulates GABA-ergic neurons at benzodiazepine-specific binding site	Onset: 2-3 min (IV) Duration: 2-6 h Metabolism: hepatic; metabolites renally excreted	1. Accumulation and prolonged sedation (especially with infusions, hepatic dysfunction; active metabolites accumulate in renal impairment) 2. Respiratory suppression 3. Delirium 4. Flumazenil is a competitive antagonist.
Lorazepam	Modulates GABA-ergic neurons at benzodiazepine-specific binding site	Onset: 5-20 min (IV) Duration: 6-10 h after single dose Metabolism: hepatic	1. Longer acting than midazolam 2. Propylene glycol toxicity risk with high-dose or prolonged IV lorazepam (high anion gap metabolic acidosis, elevated osmolar gap, hypotension, acute kidney injury); monitor osmolar gap 3. Delirium 4. Accumulation with prolonged use, especially in hepatic dysfunction and older patients
Dexmedetomidine	Selective alpha-2 adrenoreceptor agonist	Onset: 5-15 min (loading dose) Duration: 60-120 min Metabolism: hepatic	1. Bradycardia and hypotension 2. Infuse and titrate slowly 3. Tachyphylaxis with prolonged administration 4. Minimal respiratory depression

ICU, intensive care unit; IV, intravenous.

TABLE 8.16.2 Major Analgesics Used in the ICU

Agent	Mechanism	Kinetics	Major Considerations
Fentanyl	Mu-opioid receptor agonist	Onset: <1-2 min (IV) Duration: 30-60 min after single dose Metabolism: hepatic	1. Accumulation with prolonged infusion 2. Respiratory depression 3. Tolerance 4. Relatively minimal hemodynamic effects; often preferred in hemodynamic instability and renal failure
Hydromorphone	Mu-opioid receptor agonist	Onset: 5-10 min (IV) Duration: 3-4 h Metabolism: hepatic	1. Accumulation with prolonged infusion 2. Dose adjustment and close monitoring needed in patients with liver and renal failure 3. Respiratory depression 4. Tolerance 5. Less histamine release than morphine
Ketamine	NMDA receptor antagonist	Onset: <1 min (IV) Duration: 10-15 min Metabolism: hepatic	1. Preserves respiratory drive 2. Risk of psychomimetic effects (eg, hallucinations) 3. Low-dose infusion for opioid-sparing analgesia 4. May increase secretions
Morphine	Mu-opioid receptor agonist	Onset: 5-10 min (IV) Duration: 3-5 h Metabolism: hepatic glucuronidation to active metabolites; excretion: renal	1. Long duration 2. Active metabolites accumulate in renal dysfunction 3. Respiratory depression 4. Tolerance 5. Histamine release may cause hypotension.
Remifentanil	Mu-opioid receptor agonist	Onset: 1-3 min (IV) Duration: 3-10 min Metabolism: plasma esterases (organ independent)	1. Ultra-short acting 2. Useful for rapid awakening and neurologic assessments 3. Respiratory depression 4. Tolerance with prolonged use 5. No accumulation in organ failure 6. Risk of acute tolerance and opioid-induced hyperalgesia with prolonged use
Acetaminophen	Central prostaglandin inhibitor (exact mechanism unclear)	Onset: 15-30 min (IV); 30-60 min (PO) Duration: 4-6 h Metabolism: hepatic	1. Reduces opioid requirements 2. Hepatotoxicity with overdose (>4 g/d) 3. No antiinflammatory effects 4. Generally safe in renal impairment; primary concern is hepatotoxicity with cumulative dose >4 g/d.
NSAIDs (eg, ibuprofen, ketorolac)	COX-1/2 inhibitors	Onset: 15-30 min (IV ketorolac) Duration: 4-6 h Metabolism: hepatic; renally excreted	1. May be considered as adjuncts for inflammatory pain in carefully selected patients 2. Renal toxicity (avoid in significant AKI, advanced CKD, decompensated cirrhosis, or high bleeding risk) 3. Gastrointestinal bleeding risk 4. Platelet inhibition 5. Limit ketorolac to ≤5 d to minimize adverse effects
Gabapentinoids (eg, gabapentin, pregabalin)	Calcium channel modulators (alpha-2-delta subunit)	Onset: 1-2 h (oral) Duration: 6-8 h Eliminated unchanged by the kidney (minimal hepatic metabolism)	1. For neuropathic pain 2. Use cautiously in renal impairment (dose reduction) 3. Risk of delirium and sedation 4. Opioid-sparing effects 5. SCCM PADIS guidelines: strong recommendation (moderate evidence) with opioids for neuropathic pain; conditional, low-quality recommendation for ICU adults after cardiovascular surgery

AKI, acute kidney infection; CKD, chronic kidney infection; ICU, intensive care unit; IV, intravenous; NSAIDs, nonsteroidal antiinflammatory drugs; PADIS, Prevention and Management of Pain, Agitation/Sedation, Delirium, Immobility, and Sleep Disruption; SCCM, Society of Critical Care Medicine.

- Intravenous (IV) potent opioids (fentanyl, hydromorphone, morphine, remifentanil) administered intermittently or as continuous infusions titrated to effect are the most common initial strategy (Table 8.16.2).
- Consider multimodal analgesia including nonopioid adjuncts (eg, acetaminophen, nonsteroidal antiinflammatory drugs [NSAIDs], gabapentinoids, ketamine) when appropriate and not contraindicated (Table 8.16.2).

- Regional analgesia
  - Regional techniques (eg, nerve blocks, neuraxial anesthesia) can be considered in certain patients (eg, trauma, postoperative).

Sedation in Critically Ill Mechanically Ventilated Patients

Sedative agents typically need to be administered in addition to analgesics to alleviate anxiety and provide comfort for ventilated patients. Commonly used ICU sedatives (propofol, dexmedetomidine, midazolam, and lorazepam) and their key pharmacologic properties are summarized in Table 8.16.1. Although ketamine is categorized with analgesic agents in Table 8.16.2, it has important dose-dependent sedative/dissociative properties and is often used as an adjunctive sedative, particularly in hemodynamically unstable or opioid-tolerant patients.

- Sedation targets
  - Aim for light sedation (RASS −2 to 0), with RASS 0 to −1 generally preferred when feasible, unless there is a clear indication for deeper sedation targets (RASS −3 to −5) such as severe acute respiratory distress syndrome (ARDS) requiring prone positioning, refractory status epilepticus, elevated intracranial pressure, or therapeutic hypothermia. Contemporary practice increasingly targets the lightest possible sedation level (RASS −1 to 0) to minimize delirium and facilitate early mobilization.
- Assessment and monitoring Utilize standardized sedation scales (eg, RASS) for sedation assessment (performed at least every 2 hours) and ongoing titration of sedatives.
  - Screen for delirium at least once per nursing shift using a validated tool (eg, Confusion Assessment Method for the ICU [CAM-ICU] or Intensive Care Delirium Screening Checklist [ICDSC]) and address modifiable risk factors.
  - Limited channel EEG monitoring may be used to ensure that excessive depth of sedation (eg, burst suppression) is not unnecessarily maintained in patients.
- Preferred sedation strategies
  - First-line agents: nonbenzodiazepine sedatives (propofol or dexmedetomidine) are preferred.
    - Both are given as continuous infusions titrated to a defined sedation target (eg, RASS).
    - 2025 SCCM PADIS Focused Update: conditionally recommends dexmedetomidine over propofol when light sedation and delirium reduction are top priorities
    - Avoid benzodiazepines: benzodiazepine infusions (ie, midazolam, lorazepam, diazepam) are associated with higher delirium risk and longer ventilation time.
    - Interruptions of sedation, that is, spontaneous awakening trials (SATs), should be performed at least once daily and paired with spontaneous breathing trials (SBTs) to prevent oversedation and facilitate ventilator weaning. Assessments of delirium and pain should be performed during SATs.
    - Inhalational sedation with volatile anesthetics (isoflurane, sevoflurane) is an emerging, off-label practice in US ICUs for refractory cases (eg, status asthmaticus, ARDS) when IV sedatives fail.
    - Not included as a routine sedative in the SCCM PADIS guidelines
    - Needs dedicated delivery devices (eg, Sedaconda ACD-S) and scavenging systems
    - US Food and Drug Administration (FDA) status: investigational. Sedaconda (isoflurane) is not FDA approved but is available under an Early Access Program for difficult-to-sedate patients
    - INSPiRE-ICU trial: preliminary report of isoflurane noninferiority to propofol for time in target sedation
    - SESAR trial: trial stopped early after sevoflurane in patients with moderate-severe ARDS resulted in harm compared to propofol with fewer ventilator-free days and higher 90-day mortality

Neuromuscular Blockade in Critically Ill Mechanically Ventilated Patients

NMB is used selectively in mechanically ventilated patients when persistent patient-ventilator dyssynchrony or refractory hypoxemia cannot be managed with optimized sedation, lung-protective ventilation, and adjunctive measures (eg, prone positioning) or to facilitate procedures (eg, endotracheal intubation, percutaneous tracheostomy). Following the ROSE trial, routine early continuous NMB for ARDS is not recommended, as it did not improve mortality and was associated with more cardiovascular adverse events. In selected patients, NMB may still be considered, using the lowest effective dose and a short course (≤48 hours), and when feasible favoring brief or intermittent dosing rather than prolonged continuous infusions to limit cumulative exposure.

- NMB agents (Table 8.16.3)
  - Nondepolarizing: rocuronium, vecuronium (reduced dose with hepatic/renal dysfunction), cisatracurium (organ-independent elimination)
  - Depolarizing: succinylcholine usually avoided in critically ill patients. Prolonged illness, immobilization, or denervation causes a significant upregulation of acetylcholine receptors, which leads to life-threatening hyperkalemia when succinylcholine is given.
- Monitoring
  - Use peripheral nerve stimulation at the adductor pollicis with quantitative monitoring for titration to avoid excessive or prolonged paralysis in patients receiving continuous infusions.
- Protocols
  - Use only for clearly defined indications and discontinue as soon as possible.
  - The ROSE trial randomized patients with moderate-to-severe ARDS to early continuous cisatracurium versus usual care and found no difference in 90-day mortality, but more serious cardiovascular adverse events in the paralysis group. Current 2024 ATS guidelines give a conditional, low-certainty recommendation for NMB in early severe ARDS and do not specify a preferred bolus versus continuous strategy. The 2023 ARDS ESICM guidelines strongly recommend against routine continuous NMB agent infusions, reserving NMB for selected patients with refractory hypoxemia or severe ventilator dyssynchrony despite optimized lung-protective ventilation and sedation.
  - Ensure deep sedation (including EEG monitoring when available) prior to and during NMB to prevent awareness.
- Reversal of NMB
  - Sugammadex is a selective relaxant binding agent that rapidly reverses rocuronium- and vecuronium-induced NMB by encapsulating these agents.
  - Dosing: 2 mg/kg for moderate blockade (2 twitches on train of four [TOF]); 4 mg/kg for deep blockade (1-2 posttetanic counts); 16 mg/kg for immediate reversal (specific to rocuronium only)

TABLE 8.16.3 Neuromuscular Blocking Agents Used in the ICU

Agent/Dosage	Mechanism	Kinetics	Major Considerations
Succinylcholine (1-1.5 mg/kg IV)	A depolarizing neuromuscular blocking agent. Binds to postsynaptic acetylcholine receptor, resulting in stimulation (observed clinically as fasciculations), followed by paralysis	Onset: 45-60 s Duration: 5-20 min Metabolism: rapidly hydrolyzed by plasma pseudocholinesterase	1. Generally avoided in patients with denervating disease (stroke, spinal cord injury, neuromuscular disorders), major burns after 24-48 h, rhabdomyolysis, prolonged immobilization due to the risk for hyperkalemia 2. Contraindicated with personal or family history of malignant hyperthermia 3. Avoid in known or suspected pseudocholinesterase deficiency
Rocuronium (0.6-1.2 mg/kg IV)	Nondepolarizing neuromuscular blockade Inhibits depolarization at postsynaptic motor endplate	Onset: 45-60 s Duration: 40-150 min Metabolism: hepatic metabolism and biliary excretion; renal excretion, elimination half-life ~60 min	1. At higher doses (1.0-1.2 mg/kg) provides rapid intubating conditions comparable to succinylcholine 2. Commonly used for intubation in the ICU 3. Variable duration of action 4. Prolonged in hepatic and renal dysfunction 5. Can be reversed with sugammadex 6. Resistance in burn injury patients
Vecuronium (0.08-0.1 mg/kg IV bolus; infusion 0.8-1.2 mcg/kg/min)	Nondepolarizing neuromuscular blockade Inhibits depolarization at postsynaptic receptors	Onset: 2-3 min Duration: 30-60 min Metabolism: hepatic metabolism, biliary and renal excretion	1. Has active metabolite (3-desacetylvecuronium) that accumulates in renal failure causing prolonged paralysis 2. Prolonged effect in hepatic or renal dysfunction 3. Can be reversed with sugammadex 4. Resistance in burn injury patients
Cisatracurium (0.15-0.2 mg/kg IV bolus; infusion 1-3 mcg/kg/min)	Nondepolarizing neuromuscular blockade Inhibits depolarization at postsynaptic receptors	Onset: 2-3 min Duration: 20-60 min Metabolism: organ-independent Hofmann elimination and ester hydrolysis	1. Independent of renal and hepatic function 2. Often preferred in critical illness due to organ-independent elimination 3. No reversal agent 4. Resistance in burn injury patients

ICU, intensive care unit; IV, intravenous.

- Advantages: rapid reversal (2-3 min), predictable efficacy, no muscarinic side effects
- Considerations: does not reverse cisatracurium; use neostigmine with glycopyrrolate for alternative reversal

Special Pharmacologic Therapies in Neurocritically Ill Patients

Pharmacologic Management of Elevated Intracranial Pressure

- Hyperosmolar therapy
  - Hypertonic saline (bolus or infusion) or mannitol (bolus) is most used.
  - Monitor serum sodium, osmolality, and hemodynamic status during therapy.
- Corticosteroids
  - Indicated for vasogenic edema from brain tumors; contraindicated in traumatic brain injury and spontaneous intracerebral hemorrhage

Seizure Prophylaxis and Management

- Antiepileptic drugs (AEDs)
  - Levetiracetam and phenytoin are most commonly used; levetiracetam favored for ease of administration and minimal drug interactions.
- Refractory status epilepticus
  - May require continuous IV sedative infusions (propofol, midazolam, pentobarbital) with continuous EEG monitoring to ensure seizure suppression

Management of Hyponatremia

- Syndrome of inappropriate antidiuretic hormone (SIADH)
  - Managed primarily with free water restriction; vasopressin receptor antagonists for refractory cases
- Cerebral salt wasting
  - Managed with volume repletion and sodium replacement

Management of Coagulopathy in Intracranial Hemorrhage

- Rapid reversal of anticoagulation: critical for hematoma control
- Vitamin K together with prothrombin complex concentrate (PCC) or fresh frozen plasma (FFP) for warfarin reversal
- Protamine for heparin reversal
- Specific reversal agents (idarucizumab for dabigatran; andexanet alfa for factor Xa inhibitors) when appropriate

SUGGESTED READINGS

Badie S, Mahmud M, Williamson D, Burry L. Pharmacology of commonly used sedative agents. *Crit Care Clin.* 2025;41(4):625-639.

Bitar R, Khan UM, Rosenthal ES. Utility and rationale for continuous EEG monitoring: a primer for the general intensivist. *Crit Care.* 2024;28(1):244.

Boncyk C, Rolfsen ML, Richards D, et al. Management of pain and sedation in the intensive care unit. *BMJ.* 2024;387:e079789.

Chanques G, Constantin JM, Devlin JW, et al. Analgesia and sedation in patients with ARDS. *Intensive Care Med.* 2020;46(12):2342-2356.

Devlin JW, Skrobik Y, Gélinas C, et al. Clinical practice guidelines for the prevention and management of pain, agitation/sedation, delirium, immobility, and sleep disruption in adult patients in the ICU. *Crit Care Med*. 2018;46(9):e825-e873.

Hanidziar D, Westover MB. Monitoring of sedation in mechanically ventilated patients using remote technology. *Curr Opin Crit Care*. 2022; 28(3):360-366.

Jabaudon M, Quenot JP, Badie J, et al; SESAR Trial Investigators. Inhaled sedation in acute respiratory distress syndrome: the SESAR randomized clinical trial. *JAMA*. 2025;333(18):1608-1617.

Lam MSH, Luoma AMV, Reddy U. Acute perioperative neurological emergencies. *Int Anesthesiol Clin*. 2023;61(3):53-63.

Lewis K, Nunnally ME, Boncyk C, et al. A focused update to the clinical practice guidelines for the prevention and management of pain, anxiety, agitation/sedation, delirium, immobility, and sleep disruption in adult patients in the ICU. *Crit Care Med*. 2025;53(3):e711-e727.

Moss M, Huang DT, Brower RG, et al; National Heart, Lung, and Blood Institute PETAL Clinical Trials Network. Early neuromuscular blockade in the acute respiratory distress syndrome. *N Engl J Med*. 2019;380(21): 1997-2008.

Murray MJ, DeBlock H, Erstad B, et al. Clinical practice guidelines for sustained neuromuscular blockade in the adult critically ill patient. *Crit Care Med*. 2016;44(5):2079-2103.

Ouyang M, Allende MI, Anderson CS. Timely delivery of care in neurological emergencies: can standardized management protocols help? *Curr Opin Crit Care*. 2025;31(2):149-154.

Qadir N, Sahetya S, Munshi L, et al. An update on management of adult patients with acute respiratory distress syndrome: an official American Thoracic Society clinical practice guideline. *Am J Respir Crit Care Med*. 2024;209(1):24-36.

Rasulo FA, Hopkins P, Lobo FA, et al. Processed electroencephalogram-based monitoring to guide sedation in critically ill adult patients: recommendations from an international expert panel-based consensus. *Neurocrit Care*. 2023;38(2):296-311.

Yamamoto T, Kotani Y, Akutagawa K, et al. Volatile sedation in critically ill adults undergoing mechanical ventilation: a meta-analysis of randomized controlled trials. *Crit Care*. 2025;29(1):227.

8.17

Neurosurgical Management and Perioperative Complications

James Tanner McMahon, Adam C. Glaser, and Omar Arnaout

Seizures

- In the absence of a history of seizures, there is no evidence to support routine use of preoperative prophylactic antiepileptic drug in patients planned for neurosurgery consistent with the SNO–EANO guideline.
- There is no indication for postoperative seizure prophylaxis in patients undergoing *infratentorial*, as seizures cannot arise from this region.
- Although it is common practice to administer postoperative seizure prophylaxis in patients undergoing *supratentorial* neurosurgery, for example, 7 days of levetiracetam, a recent Cochrane review of 10 randomized controlled trials (RCTs) found this to lack evidence of benefit.
- Clinical or electrographic postoperative seizures should be managed in the typical manner as described in previous chapters.

Pneumocephalus

- Pneumocephalus (air within the intracranial space) is commonly seen after neurosurgery (Figure 8.17.1).
- Simple pneumocephalus can present with lethargy and altered mental status and tends to resolve over hours to days.

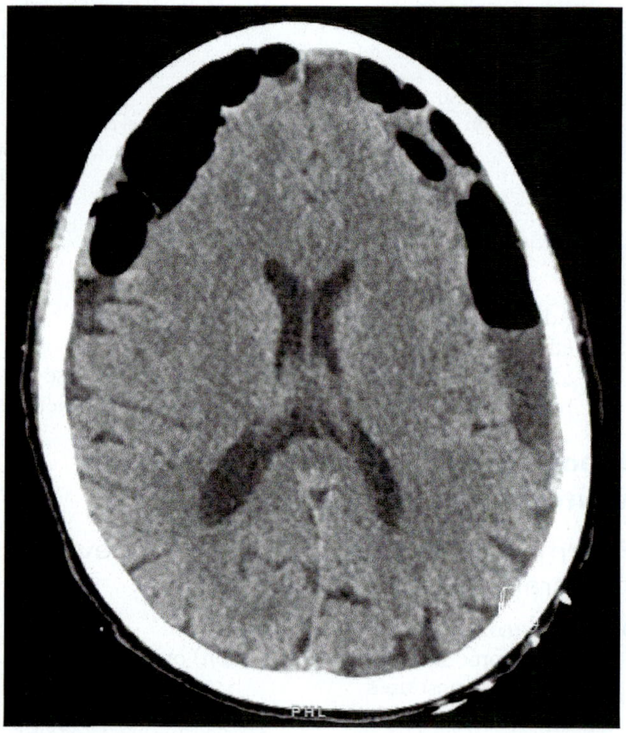

FIGURE 8.17.1 Postoperative pneumocephalus.

    - Supportive care entails laying the head of bed flat and administering 100% inspired F_{IO_2} via a nonrebreather mask for up to 24 to 48 hours, that is, normobaric oxygen therapy, which theoretically helps to encourage nitrogen gas resorption from the extra-axial space.
- Tension pneumocephalus is a very rare but life-threatening phenomenon in which a ball-valve mechanism allows ongoing air entry into the intracranial space, without a route for egress.
    - While the "Mount Fuji sign" (separation of the bilateral frontal lobes by air) is typically invoked as a sign of

tension pneumocephalus, this is not very specific and is seen frequently in nontension cases.
   - A clinical diagnosis is made with the picture of progressive neurologic decline in the absence of other etiologies.
   - Treatment entails emergent return to the operating room (OR) for removal of the bone flap and exploration of any ball-valve phenomenon.

Hemorrhage

- Postoperative hematoma is a common complication of neurosurgery.
- Hemorrhage can be located in the epidural, subdural, or intraparenchymal space.
- Notable risk factors for postoperative hematoma include preexisting medical comorbidities such as hypertension and coagulopathies, lesion pathologies such as high-grade gliomas, inadequate hemostasis, and uncontrolled postoperative hypertension.
   - It is common to target a systolic blood pressure goal of <140 mm Hg for at least the first 24 hours after craniotomy.
- Venous infarct and hemorrhage is a unique phenomenon in which a large draining vein or dural venous sinus is either sacrificed during surgery, or clots secondary to intraoperative factors, causing venous congestion and eventual hemorrhage.
   - Signs of this being the etiology of a postoperative intraparenchymal hematoma include proximity to major venous structures and significant perihematomal edema (from venous congestion) (Figure 8.17.2).
   - If suspected, this should be discussed with the neurosurgeon to identify any culprit veins.
   - If thrombosis is suspected, it is reasonable to consider anticoagulation.

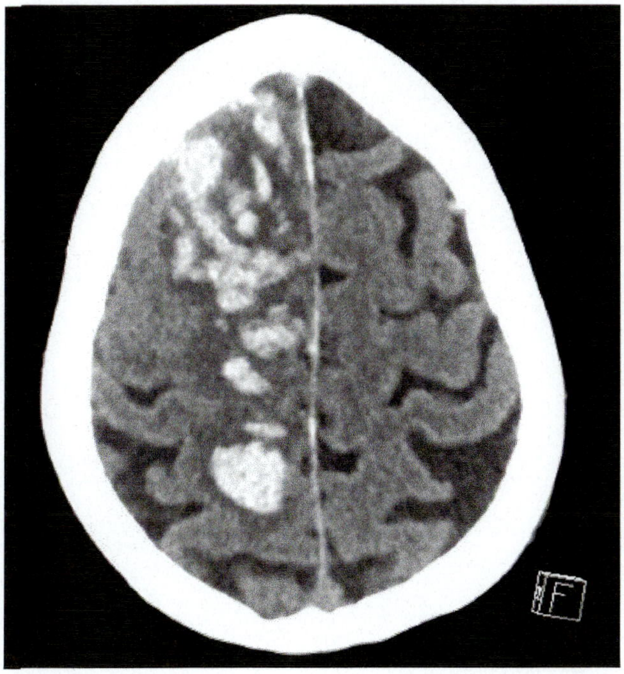

FIGURE 8.17.2 Venous infarction/hemorrhage. Computed tomographic venography demonstrated extensive thrombosis of the superior sagittal sinus.

Ischemia

- Most perioperative complications involving ischemia occur secondary to sacrifice or inadvertent occlusion of named arteries.
- Arteries at risk are in the vicinity of the surgical site and should be considered with an understanding of surgical anatomy and in discussion with the surgeon.
   - The recurrent artery of Heubner is classically at risk during clipping of anterior communicating (AComm) artery aneurysms.
      - Occlusion typically causes infarction of the head of the caudate.
      - Symptoms of occlusion include contralateral hemiplegia and dysarthria.
- Postoperative computed tomography (CT) angiogram, plus or minus CT perfusion, can be useful in identifying new vascular cutoffs and areas of ischemia in the postoperative period.

Infections

- The most common causative organism in postoperative wound infection and/or meningitis is *Staphylococcus aureus*.
   - A typical broad-spectrum regimen is vancomycin for methicillin-resistant *Staphylococcus aureus* (MRSA) coverage, with cefepime for Gram-negative coverage, including *Pseudomonas*.
- Ventriculoperitoneal (VP) shunt infection is a unique entity and can present in a delayed manner if infected with indolent organisms.
   - This can present with fever, altered mental status, and signs of shunt failure with worsening hydrocephalus.
   - Infected VP shunts should be removed and replaced with an external ventricular drain (EVD) while an antibiotic course is administered, typically for 2 weeks before reimplantation.

Cerebrospinal Fluid Leak

- Cerebrospinal fluid (CSF) leak occurs most commonly as a result of infratentorial surgery and spinal surgery, where the hydrostatic pressure of the fluid column (when the patient is upright) increases the risk of CSF egress from the surgical wound.
- CSF leak leads to intracranial hypotension, which presents with headaches and nausea/vomiting that are worse when upright, and can cause subdural hematoma formation.
- Posterior fossa CSF leak often requires revision surgery.
- Spinal CSF leak can sometimes be managed conservatively by keeping the patient flat.
- A lumbar drain (LD) can be considered in both cases to divert CSF from the egress tract.

External Ventricular Drain/Lumbar Drain Complications

- EVD placement is commonly performed for acute hydrocephalus, intracranial hypertension from diffuse cerebral edema, and/or significant intraventricular hemorrhage (IVH).

- Common EVD complications include misplacement, hemorrhage, infection, and clogging.
  - Bedside EVD placement is done with surface anatomic landmarks and thus misplacement is common. Replacement after an initial CT scan is standard.
  - Tract hemorrhage should be managed conservatively with blood pressure control and serial imaging.
  - EVDs can be antibiotic impregnated. If not, meningitis prophylaxis is recommended with either cefazolin or vancomycin + ceftriaxone, depending on institutional practice.
  - Clogging can occur due to proteinaceous CSF (eg, in the case of infection) or due to clotting from IVH.
    - Stepwise management includes flushing the drainage tubing distally, and/or the catheter proximally if that fails (which is riskier and must be done sterilely with 1-2 mL of saline).
    - Intraventricular administration of tissue plasminogen activator (tPA) to clear IVH has been investigated. It is unclear if these lead to better functional outcomes but seem to be effective in radiographic clearance of blood products.
- The most significant complications of LD are overdrainage and infection.
  - A typical LD goal is ~10 mL/h. Inadvertent overdrainage can cause sagging of the brain and eventual herniation, which can be life-threatening. This can be avoided with attentive nursing and self-limiting drainage systems. Sterile saline can be reinfused as an emergent intervention to reverse overdrainage.
  - Meningitis can occur from infection via the catheter. LD is typically not antibiotic impregnated, and thus prophylaxis (eg, cefazolin) is common.

Hyperperfusion

- Hyperperfusion syndrome can occur when a chronically ischemic region of the brain is suddenly revascularized, for example, after intracranial-extracranial bypass or carotid endarterectomy.
- Arterioles supplying this region are already maximally dilated and have lost the ability to autoregulate; thus, the brain receives more blood supply than it needs for.
- CT perfusion will reveal increased cerebral blood flow (CBF) and volume (CBV) with decreased mean transit time (MTT) and time to peak (TTP).
- Hyperperfusion typically presents with headache and can progress to altered mental status, seizures, and eventual intraparenchymal hemorrhage if not managed in a timely manner with blood pressure lowering.

SUGGESTED READINGS

Gore PA, Maan H, Chang S, Pitt AM, Spetzler RF, Nakaji P. Normobaric oxygen therapy strategies in the treatment of postcraniotomy pneumocephalus. *J Neurosurg*. 2008;108(5):926-929.

Greenhalgh J, Weston J, Dundar Y, Nevitt SJ, Marson AG. Antiepileptic drugs as prophylaxis for postcraniotomy seizures. *Cochrane Database Syst Rev*. 2018;5(5):Cd007286.

Hanley DF, Lane K, McBee N, et al. Thrombolytic removal of intraventricular haemorrhage in treatment of severe stroke: results of the randomised, multicentre, multiregion, placebo-controlled CLEAR III trial. *Lancet*. 2017;389(10069):603-611.

Seifman MA, Lewis PM, Rosenfeld JV, Hwang PY. Postoperative intracranial haemorrhage: a review. *Neurosurg Rev*. 2011;34(4):393-407.

van Mook WN, Rennenberg RJ, Schurink GW, et al. Cerebral hyperperfusion syndrome. *Lancet Neurol*. 2005;4(12):877-888.

Walbert T, Harrison RA, Schiff D, et al. SNO and EANO practice guideline update: anticonvulsant prophylaxis in patients with newly diagnosed brain tumors. *Neuro Oncol*. 2021;23(11):1835-1844.

SECTION 9

Infectious Disease and Virulence Factors

Section Editors: Raghu R. Chivukula and Marvin G. Chang

9.1

Infectious Disease and Virulence Factors

Simran Gupta and Lisa M. Bebell

Fever in the Intensive Care Unit

- Per the Society of Critical Care Medicine/Infectious Diseases Society of America (SCCM/IDSA), fever in the intensive care unit (ICU) is a single measurement ≥38.3 °C.
    - Consider a lower threshold if immunocompromised.
- Epidemiology
    - Incidence 26% to 88% depending on the type of ICU
    - Fever ≥39.5 °C associated with increased mortality (20% vs 12%)
    - Fever associated with increased length of stay and cost of care
- Common causes
    - Infectious
        - Ventilator-associated pneumonia (VAP)
        - Surgical site infection (SSI)
        - Central line–associated bloodstream infection (CLABSI)
        - Catheter-associated urinary tract infection (CAUTI)
        - *Clostridioides difficile* colitis
        - Candidemia
    - Noninfectious:
        - Drug fever
            - ~3% to 5% of febrile episodes in ICU
        - Postoperative fever
            - Common in the first 48 hours post-op
            - Usually due to an inflammatory response to surgery
        - Acalculous cholecystitis
            - ~1.5% of ICU patients
        - Venous thromboembolism (VTE)
            - Lower fever (~37.8 °C)
            - Prevalence of fever in VTE is 5% to 33%.
        - Cytokine-release syndrome
            - Consider specifically in chimeric antigen receptor T-cell (CAR-T) therapy patients
        - Ischemic bowel
        - Acute respiratory distress syndrome (ARDS)
            - Can occasionally cause noninfectious fever; ARDS is more commonly infectious (pneumonia or sepsis).
        - Pneumonitis (without pneumonia)
                - Immediate fever after the aspiration event
                - Fever should resolve in ~48 hours; if not, consider pneumonia.
            - Gastrointestinal (GI) bleed
                - Fever typically occurs with bowel perforation (gut translocation) or underlying infection/inflammatory condition.
- Less common causes
            - Transfusion reaction
            - Pulmonary infarction
            - Pancreatitis
            - Adrenal insufficiency
            - Thyroid storm
            - Acute myocardial infarction (MI)
                - Rare; mild fever due to inflammation
- Workup and treatment
    - Workup
        - Thorough physical examination and history for localizing symptoms
        - Prior to starting antimicrobials, obtain ≥2 sets of blood cultures from different sites, 1 to 2 from a central line (different lumens) if present.
            - Sensitivity of 1 blood culture 73% to 80%; 80% to 89% for 2
        - Chest x-ray (CXR)
        - Urinalysis, urine culture if >50 white blood cell/high-power field (WBC/hpf), and signs/symptoms of urinary tract infection (UTI)
        - Computed tomography (CT) of the chest and/or abdomen/pelvis if recent thoracic, abdominal, or pelvic surgery if no other obvious etiology
        - Abdominal ultrasound (U/S) if recent abdominal surgery and possible abdominal source (transaminitis, high alkaline phosphatase, or bilirubin)

- Endotracheal aspirate/sputum Gram stain/culture if respiratory signs/symptoms
- Procalcitonin and C-reactive protein (CRP)
  - CRP: acute-phase reactant, high in many inflammatory states = low specificity (~45%-70%) for sepsis, not a reliable indicator for the degree of inflammation—usually not helpful
  - Procalcitonin: better indicator of illness severity than CRP but also high in many noninfectious syndromes, including trauma, surgery, multiorgan failure = sensitivity 80% and specificity ~35% for bacterial infections—do not send routinely.

- Treatment
  - Fever reduction
    - Routine use of antipyretics for the specific purpose of reducing fever is controversial.
    - Use antipyretics over nonpharmacologic methods of reducing body temperature (ie, cooling blankets).
      - Cooling associated with hypermetabolism → increased O_2 consumption, high catecholamines
    - Generally recommended to control fever >40 °C
      - Especially in patients with neurologic injury—high antimicrobials
    - Start broad empiric antimicrobials early—if workup unrevealing, can begin de-escalating over 24 to 48 hours if clinical improvement.
    - Recommend initial coverage of both Gram-positive and Gram-negative organisms—de-escalate based on specific findings of workup.
    - Recommend against routine empiric antianaerobic antibiotics in ICU—recent data suggest increased adverse outcomes.

Select Infections (Not Covered Elsewhere)

Central Line–Associated Bloodstream Infections

- Definition
  - Centers for Disease Control and Prevention (CDC): primary bloodstream infection in the presence of a central venous catheter (CVC) or when CVC is present in the last 48 hours; not related to infection at another site
  - IDSA: isolation of the same organism from a quantitative blood culture drawn through CVC and peripheral vein with a single bacterial colony count >3-fold higher in the CVC versus peripheral culture
    - >2 hours shorter time to CVC versus peripheral culture positivity; also sensitive for diagnosis
- Epidemiology
  - Incidence 0.8/1,000 CVC days in the ICU
  - ~250,000 bloodstream infections annually, most related to intravascular devices
  - Mortality rate 12% to 15%; odds ratio of in-hospital death up to 2.75
  - Attributable CLABSI cost: $48,000/episode
  - Can increase hospital length of stay
- Risk factors
  - Prolonged catheterization, immunocompromised, comorbidities, inadequate hand hygiene, poor catheter insertion technique
- Common organisms
  - Gram-positives most common: coagulase-negative staphylococci (34%), enterococci (16%), *Staphylococcus aureus* (10%)
  - Gram-negatives: *Klebsiella* spp. (6%), *Enterobacter* spp. (4%), *Pseudomonas* (3%), *Escherichia coli* (3%), *Acinetobacter* (2%)
  - Others: *Candida* spp. (12%), others (11%)
- Clinical signs/symptoms
  - Fever is most common.
    - Rigors, chills, altered mental status, erythema, induration, tenderness, purulent discharge
- Management
  - If CLABSI is suspected, empiric antimicrobial therapy should target the most likely organism(s), considering host factors and clinical picture.
    - Short-term catheters
      - Uncomplicated CLABSI (fever resolves <72 hours in patient with no intravascular hardware, no evidence of endocarditis or suppurative thrombophlebitis [for *S. aureus*—no active malignancy or immunosuppression])
        - For infections caused by *S. aureus, Enterococcus,* Gram-negative bacilli, *Candida* spp.—remove catheter and treat with systemic antibiotics.
        - For infections caused by coagulase-negative staphylococci—can try catheter salvage with systemic antibiotics and lock therapy
      - Complicated CLABSI (suppurative thrombophlebitis, endocarditis, osteomyelitis, etc)
        - Remove catheter; treat with systemic antibiotics.
    - Long-term catheters/port
      - Uncomplicated infections
        - *S. aureus* and *Candida* spp.: remove catheter; treat with systemic antibiotics.
        - *Enterococcus*, Gram-negative bacilli, and coagulase-negative *Staphylococcus*—may trial catheter retention with systemic antibiotics and lock therapy
      - Complicated infections (tunnel infection, port abscess, septic thrombosis, endocarditis, osteomyelitis)
        - Remove catheter; treat with systemic antibiotics.
  - Prevention strategies during insertion
    - No difference in infection rate by insertion site (subclavian, internal jugular [IJ], femoral) if the operator complies with:
      - Aseptic technique
      - Hand hygiene
      - Maximal sterile barrier precautions, including full-body drape
      - 2% chlorhexidine skin prep
      - Dynamic U/S use during placement
      - Checklist completed
  - Prevention strategies during maintenance
    - Disinfect catheter hubs, injection ports, and connectors before accessing the catheter
    - Daily reassessment of CVC necessity

Necrotizing Soft Tissue Infections

- Infections characterized clinically by fulminant tissue destruction, systemic signs of toxicity, and high mortality

- Mortality 9% to 73%
  - Increased mortality: WBC >30, creatinine (Cr) >2, age >60, surgery delayed >24 hours, strep toxic shock, clostridial infection
- Necrotizing soft tissue infection (NSTI) characterized by the subtle and rapid onset of necrosis spreading from the fascia (due to poor blood supply) through muscles and subcutaneous fat tissue → necrosis of the adjacent skin
- Includes necrotizing forms of fasciitis, cellulitis, and myositis
- If localized to the perineum/scrotum, known as Fournier gangrene
- If localized to the submandibular space, known as Ludwig angina
- Epidemiology
  - Incidence 1.7 to 15.5 cases/100,000 persons-year
  - Up to 1.2% of ICU admissions
  - Predisposing factors: diabetes mellitus, immunocompromised, end-stage renal disease (ESRD), cirrhosis, obesity, peripheral vascular disease, malignancy, intradermal drug use (IDU)
- Microbiology
  - Polymicrobial (type I) infection: aerobic and anaerobic bacteria (55%-75%)
    - ≥1 anaerobe (*Bacteroides, Clostridium, Peptostreptococcus*), Enterobacteriaceae (*E. coli, Enterobacter, Klebsiella, Proteus*) and ≥1 facultative anaerobic streptococci (non–group A strep)
    - Fungi (*Candida*) uncommon, but can be isolated
    - In the head and neck, usually mouth anaerobes (*Fusobacterium*, anaerobic streptococci, *Bacteroides*)
- Monomicrobial (type II) infections
  - Typically group A strep or other beta-hemolytic streptococci
    - Often associated with toxins → cytokine production → shock, tissue destruction, and organ failure
  - Can also be caused by *S. aureus*
  - Less common: *Vibrio vulnificus, Aeromonas hydrophila* (traumatic injury associated with sea/fresh water, respectively)
- Necrotizing myositis typically group A strep and other beta-hemolytic strep—often preceded by skin abrasions, blunt trauma, or heavy exercise.
- Necrotizing cellulitis typically caused by anaerobic pathogens—clostridial (*Clostridium perfringens* or *Clostridium septicum*) versus nonclostridial
- Clinical manifestations
- Early stages are often not recognized.
- Crepitus (in 50%) and necrosis/bullae/ecchymosis (in 38%) often absent in early disease.
- Fever, tachycardia, malaise, and myalgias are common. Hypotension may be present initially or develop with progression.
- Elevated WBC with left shift, elevated creatine kinase [CK], aspartate aminotransferase (AST), prothrombin time (PT), or partial thromboplastin time (PTT); low albumin and serum Na may occur—nonspecific.
- Score-based diagnosis based on labs (such as LRINEC) is not recommended.
- Imaging (radiograph, CT, magnetic resonance imaging [MRI]) helpful—particularly if gas is present
- Careful history and physical examination are the most important—"pain out of proportion to examination" should prompt consideration of NSTI.
- Management and treatment
  - Surgical
    - NSTI is a surgical emergency—early and aggressive debridement of necrotic tissue is critical, even for unstable patients.
    - Extensive initial debridement and frequent reexploration are often required.
    - For severe extremity involvement, amputation may be necessary.
  - Antibiotics
    - Empiric therapy includes broad-spectrum antibiotics with activity against Gram-positives, Gram-negatives, and anaerobes.
    - Consider adding antibiotics to inhibit toxin (clindamycin, linezolid).
    - Start empiric therapy promptly after blood cultures are obtained.
    - Example of empiric therapy: carbapenem or piperacillin/tazobactam + anti-methicillin-resistant *S. aureus* (MRSA) agent (vancomycin/daptomycin) + clindamycin for antitoxin effect.
    - Linezolid can be used for both MRSA coverage and for antitoxin effect.
  - Adjunctive therapy
    - Aggressive fluid resuscitation and vasopressors may be required.
  - Hyperbaric oxygen and intravenous immunoglobulin (IVIg) controversial

Intra-Abdominal Infections

- Intra-abdominal infections (IAIs) typically occur secondary to GI tract disruption (surgical or spontaneous), less commonly genitourinary (GU) tract disruption, which allows normal GI/GU flora into the abdominal cavity.
- Usually polymicrobial
- Can result in a secondary peritonitis
  - Microbiology
    - Colonic flora common
      - *E. coli*, *Klebsiella* spp., *Proteus* spp., *Enterobacter* spp., enterococci, anaerobes (*Bacteroides fragilis*, *Clostridium* spp.) most common
      - *Candida* spp. can be a pathogen, especially when the proximal bowel/upper GI tract is disrupted.
      - Prior antimicrobial therapy, prolonged hospitalization associated with altered gut microbiome and *Pseudomonas*, vancomycin-resistant enterococci (VRE), *Candida* spp.
  - Management
    - Source control and antimicrobial therapy are key.
      - Source control: surgical washout and/or percutaneous drainage
      - Surgery may be needed to close an anatomic breach/leak.
      - Sterile procedures for source control also allow to collection of sterile specimens for microbiologic analysis.
    - Empiric antimicrobial therapy
      - Generally, unless a patient is septic or clinically unstable, collect samples for culture *before* starting antibiotics to increase culture yield (if collection delayed, can initiate antibiotics first).
      - Considerations when selecting empiric regimen: community-acquired versus health care–associated infection, patient history of multidrug-resistant

(MDR) organisms, specific patient features (frailty, older age, diabetes, immunocompromised)
- Community acquired
    - Gram-negatives + anaerobes (ie, piperacillin/tazobactam OR cephalosporin/fluoroquinolone + metronidazole)
        - Consider antipseudomonal cephalosporin (ie, cefepime) in patients with severe community-acquired IAIs or those at risk of worse outcomes.
    - Ampicillin/sulbactam not recommended as empiric therapy due to high rates of resistance among community-acquired *E. coli*
- Health care associated
    - High risk of antimicrobial resistance
    - Cover *Pseudomonas* and *Enterococcus,* and consider treating MDR Gram-negative bacilli.
    - Carbapenem alone or antipseudomonal cephalosporin + metronidazole + antienterococcal agent (vancomycin or ampicillin) or piperacillin/tazobactam are reasonable.
    - Use the patient's prior culture data (last 1-2 years) to guide the empiric regimen.
    - Consider empiric antifungal coverage with fluconazole or micafungin in patients with upper GI perforations, surgically treated pancreatitis, and those heavily colonized with *Candida.*

■ Targeted antimicrobial therapy
- Culture data obtained from sterile source control procedures should guide definitive/targeted antimicrobial therapy (do not use cultures from existing/old abdominopelvic drains/catheters to guide therapy).
- Consider early transition from intravenous (IV) → PO when clinically improving and source control achieved
- ID consult for complex cases with retained foreign material, difficult source control, and antimicrobial allergies

■ Duration of treatment
- When source control has been achieved and the patient is clinically improving, short courses of antibiotics (4-7 days) are appropriate (STOP-IT trial).
- Longer courses may be needed if source control is difficult to achieve (ie, undrained abscess, ongoing leak).

■ Clinical failure
- Typically due to inadequate source control rather than antimicrobial failure
- Consider reimaging and repeat intervention.

SUGGESTED READINGS

Bell T, O'Grady NP. Prevention of central line-associated bloodstream infections. *Infect Dis Clin North Am*. 2017;31(3):551-559.

Chanderraj R, Admon AJ, He Y, et al. Mortality of patients with sepsis administered piperacillin-tazobactam vs cefepime. *JAMA Intern Med*. 2024;184(7):e240581.

Hua C, Urbina T, Bosc R, et al. Necrotising soft-tissue infections. *Lancet Infect Dis*. 2023;23(3):e81-e94.

Laupland KB, Shahpori R, Kirkpatrick AW, Ross T, Gregson DB, Stelfox HT. Occurrence and outcome of fever in critically ill adults. *Crit Care Med*. 2008;36(5):1531-1535.

Mazuski JE, Tessier JM, May AK, et al. The Surgical Infection Society revised guidelines on the management of intra-abdominal infection. *Surg Infect (Larchmt)*. 2017;18(1):1-76.

Mermel LA, Allon M, Bouza E, et al. Clinical practice guidelines for the diagnosis and management of intravascular catheter-related infection: 2009 update by the Infectious Diseases Society of America. *Clin Infect Dis*. 2009;49(1):1-45.

O'Grady NP, Alexander E, Alhazzani W, et al. Society of Critical Care Medicine and the Infectious Diseases Society of America guidelines for evaluating new fever in adult patients in the ICU. *Crit Care Med*. 2023;51(11):1570-1586.

Peetermans M, de Prost N, Eckmann C, Norrby-Teglund A, Skrede S, De Waele JJ. Necrotizing skin and soft-tissue infections in the intensive care unit. *Clin Microbiol Infect*. 2020;26(1):8-17.

Sawyer RG, Claridge JA, Nathens AB, et al; STOP-IT Trial Investigators. Trial of short-course antimicrobial therapy for intraabdominal infection. *N Engl J Med*. 2015;372(21):1996-2005.

Stevens DL, Bisno AL, Chambers HF, et al; Infectious Diseases Society of America. Practice guidelines for the diagnosis and management of skin and soft tissue infections: 2014 update by the Infectious Diseases Society of America. *Clin Infect Dis*. 2014;59(2):e10-e52.

9.2

Antibiotic Therapy and Resistance

Simran Gupta, Tiffany Wu, and Lisa M. Bebell

Key Points

- Inappropriate use or overuse of antibiotics can lead to the development of resistant organisms.
- Use your hospital's antibiogram to guide empiric therapy selection.
- Don't treat colonization.
- Distinguish between community-acquired and hospital-acquired infections.
- Narrow antibiotics based on culture data.
- Source control is of utmost importance—appropriate antibiotics complement source control.
- *See* Table 9.2.1 *for additional details.*

Recognizing and Categorizing Infection

- Sepsis and septic shock
    - Updated definition published in 2016 (Sepsis-3)
        - Definitions
            - Sepsis: life-threatening organ dysfunction caused by a dysregulated host response to infection
            - Septic shock: sepsis with circulatory and cellular/metabolic abnormalities profound enough to substantially increase mortality

TABLE 9.2.1 Suggestions for Empiric Coverage

Infection	Organisms to Consider	Suggested Empiric Regimens
Sepsis, unknown source	Gram+ cocci Gram– bacilli MRSA PsA (if risk factors, see earlier)	Vancomycin + cefepime or piperacillin-tazobactam[a] OR Vancomycin + meropenem[a] OR Vancomycin + fluoroquinolone or Ceftriaxone + metronidazole[a] Empiric antianaerobic therapy for sepsis of unknown source may be associated with increased mortality and should be guided by the local antibiogram.
Pneumonia: CAP	Gram+ cocci Atypicals MRSA and/or PsA (based on risk factors)	Levofloxacin OR Ceftriaxone + azithromycin OR Vancomycin + cefepime/piperacillin-tazobactam + azithromycin (depending on patient risk factors)
Pneumonia: HCAP, VAP	Gram+ cocci MRSA Gram– bacilli PsA	Vancomycin + cefepime or piperacillin-tazobactam or meropenem
Intraabdominal	Gram+ cocci Gram– bacilli Anaerobes	Vancomycin + piperacillin-tazobactam OR Vancomycin + ceftriaxone or ciprofloxacin or cefepime + metronidazole
Endocarditis	Gram+ cocci	Vancomycin + ceftriaxone or ampicillin Consider aminoglycoside if resistant organisms.
Osteomyelitis	Gram+ cocci Gram– bacilli	Vancomycin + ceftriaxone or cefepime or fluoroquinolone
Septic arthritis	Gram+ cocci MRSA *Gonococcus*	Vancomycin + ceftriaxone
Cellulitis	Gram+ cocci MRSA	Cefazolin or ceftriaxone +/– vancomycin +/– Clindamycin or linezolid (if concern for NSTI)
Deep tissue, wound, gangrene	Gram+ cocci MRSA VRE *Enterococcus* Anaerobes	Vancomycin + meropenem/piperacillin-tazobactam +/– Clindamycin or linezolid (for toxin production)
UTI/pyelonephritis	Enteric Gram–bacilli	Ceftriaxone or cefepime OR fluoroquinolone or TMP-SMX
CNS (meningitis/encephalitis or abscess)	Gram+ and Gram– cocci Gram– bacilli Rickettsia Anaerobes Viral (West Nile, HSV) *Nocardia* (immunocompromised)	Vancomycin + ceftriaxone or cefepime + ampicillin for immunocompromised or older age + Acyclovir for some patients +/– Metronidazole in select cases *Nocardia*: carbapenem + TMP-SMX or linezolid
Clostridioides difficile colitis	*C. difficile*	PO (preferred) or PR (if no enteral access) vancomycin +/– IV metronidazole

CAP, community-acquired pneumonia; CNS, central nervous system; HCAP, health care–associated pneumonia; HSV, herpes simplex virus; IV, intravenous; MRSA, methicillin-resistant *Staphylococcus aureus*; NSTI, necrotizing soft tissue infections; PO, oral; PR, per rectum; PsA, *Pseudomonas aeruginosa*; TMP-SMX, trimethoprim-sulfamethoxazole; UTI, urinary tract infection; VAP, ventilator-associated pneumonia; VRE, vancomycin-resistant Enterobacterales.

Empiric antianaerobic therapy for sepsis of unknown source may be associated with increased mortality and should be guided by the local antibiogram.

- Clinical criteria
  - Sepsis: suspected/documented infection plus increase ≥2 in the Sequential Organ Failure Assessment (SOFA) score
  - Septic shock: sepsis + need for vasopressors to achieve mean arterial pressure (MAP) ≥65 mm Hg *and* lactate >2 mmol/L (18 mg/dL) after adequate fluid resuscitation
- Diagnostic workup
  - Complete blood count (CBC) with differential
  - Cultures (blood, sputum, urinalysis [with urine culture as appropriate])
    - ≥2 sets of blood cultures, ≥1 from a central venous catheter (CVC) if present
    - Ideally, obtain cultures before starting antibiotics, but do not delay antibiotics if cultures cannot be obtained immediately.
  - Consider additional testing based on symptoms/risk factors.
    - *Legionella* urinary Ag, acid-fast bacteria stain/cultures (mycobacteria), viral rapid diagnostics, cerebrospinal fluid (CSF), *Clostridioides difficile* testing
    - Sterile site cultures from wounds, chest tubes, surgical drains. Avoid sending cultures from nonsterile/existing sites unless ID consult involved—contamination risk is high.
  - Interpreting results
    - Contamination

- Coagulase-negative *Staphylococcus* spp in CVC or peripheral blood culture samples in only one or two culture bottles; especially if bottles turn positive after >24 hours and/or susceptibility patterns differ between isolates
- *Corynebacterium* spp, other pathogens on a case-by-case basis (discuss with ID consult)

- Colonization
  - Yeast or *Enterococcus* spp in urine or sputum—if cultured, change indwelling urinary catheter—*Enterococcus* in urine can occasionally be a pathogen.
  - <10K count of bacteria in urine
  - Positive cultures in the absence of signs/symptoms of infection
  - *Stenotrophomonas* spp are rarely virulent—when isolated from nonsterile or device sources (endotracheal tubes, catheters, drains), usually do not indicate infection. Exchange/remove urinary catheters when found.
    - If isolated from blood or other sterile site, treatment is likely indicated.
    - Consult ID if uncertain.
- *Staphylococcus aureus* or Gram-negative isolates from any source, or yeast from CVC, should generally be treated as a *real* infection even if only present in one culture bottle.
- Positive blood cultures from "thio broth only" may be contaminants; consider ID consult.

- Certain patient populations may not present with typical signs/symptoms of sepsis—have a high index of suspicion:
  - Older, immunocompromised (HIV, bone marrow disorders, chemotherapy, transplant patients, chronic corticosteroids)

Selecting Appropriate Antibiotics

- Considerations
  - Presence of end-organ dysfunction
  - Source (pneumonia, intraabdominal, skin and soft tissue, meningitis, etc)
  - Degree of illness/comorbidities (immunocompromised, diabetes, renal failure)
  - Likelihood of antimicrobial resistance:
    - Local prevalence, resistance patterns, and outbreaks (consult local antibiogram)
    - Recent patient exposure to broad-spectrum antibiotics (last 90 days)
    - Prior resistant organisms (last 1-2 years)
    - Setting where infection was acquired (community, hospital, other health care setting)
      - Infections acquired >48 hours after admission are considered hospital acquired (nosocomial).
      - Infections in patients admitted from nursing facilities/rehab, dialysis patients, and others with high health care contact are considered health care associated.
- Methicillin-resistant *Staphylococcus aureus* (MRSA) coverage and double *Pseudomonas aeruginosa* (PsA) coverage for ventilator-associated pneumonia (VAP):
  - Infectious Diseases Society of America (IDSA) recommends *considering* MRSA coverage and double antibiotic coverage for *Pseudomonas* in patients who:
    - Have risk factors for antimicrobial resistance
      - Intravenous (IV) antibiotic use in the last 90 days
      - Septic shock at the time of VAP
      - Acute respiratory distress syndrome (ARDS) preceding VAP
      - ≥5 days of hospitalization prior to VAP
      - Acute renal replacement therapy prior to VAP
    - Are being treated in patient-care units where >10% of Gram-negative isolates (ie, *Pseudomonas*) are resistant to the antibiotic being considered for monotherapy, or where >10% to 20% of *S. aureus* isolates are methicillin resistant (MRSA), or where local antimicrobial susceptibility rates are unknown (*Pseudomonas*, MRSA).
    - Have bronchiectasis or cystic fibrosis (*Pseudomonas*)
  - Utility of MRSA nasal swab
    - The negative predictive value (NPV) of MRSA nares screen is >95% and can be used to rule out MRSA pneumonia in most situations.
    - The positive predictive value of MRSA nares screen is 35% to 55% and should not be used to diagnose MRSA infections.
- Fungal coverage
  - Invasive candidiasis is associated with an in-hospital mortality rate ~30%.
  - Noncandidal fungal infections very rarely cause sepsis.
  - Current IDSA guidelines suggest the use of fluconazole, echinocandins, or liposomal amphotericin B in patients with suspected candidiasis. Echinocandin is preferred in hemodynamically unstable patients.
  - Fluconazole is the drug of choice for the treatment of *Candida* urinary tract infection (UTI)—other azoles and echinocandins do not reliably penetrate urine.
  - Considerations for empiric anticandidal coverage include:
    - Recent broad-spectrum antibiotic receipt for >72 hours
    - Presence of CVC or other intravascular devices
    - Receiving total parenteral nutrition
    - Current renal replacement therapy
    - Neutropenia
    - Immunosuppression
    - Abdominal surgery

Antibiotic Dosing Strategy

- For beta-lactams (eg, piperacillin/tazobactam), continuous or extended (eg, over 3 hours) infusion regimens should be used.
- Therapeutic drug monitoring (peak and trough) required for aminoglycosides
- Area under the curve (AUC)-guided vancomycin should be considered for confirmed MRSA systemic infections, whereas vancomycin trough monitoring alone may be adequate for other infections. In patients with renal failure or kidney disease, antibiotic doses may need to be adjusted to correlate with patient's renal function.

Adjunctive Management

- Early source control (<6 hours) associated with ~29% lower odds of mortality
  - Drain infected fluid collections/abscesses.
  - Remove infected hardware.
  - Exchange/remove infected CVCs and indwelling catheters.

- Remove unnecessary lines as soon as possible.
- Contact precautions for resistant/communicable organisms (MRSA, multidrug-resistant Gram-negatives, vancomycin-resistant Enterobacterales [VRE], some respiratory viruses).

Antimicrobial Duration

- Depends on the type of infection and extent of source control—usually combination IV/PO (oral)
  - ~7 days for VAP, culture-negative sepsis with patient improvement, uncomplicated Gram-negative bacteremia
  - 4 to 7 days for intraabdominal infections with source control (STOP-IT trial); longer if there is a lack of source control/residual abscess
  - 4 to 6 weeks for endocarditis, depending on organism
  - ~6 weeks for bacterial osteomyelitis; 3 to 6 months for fungal osteomyelitis
- If not improving in 48 to 72 hours, consider:
  - Broadening coverage for uncovered pathogens (*Candida*, resistant Gram-negatives), switching drug class
  - Inadequate source control
    - Perform or repeat advanced (computed tomography/magnetic resonance imaging [CT/MRI]).
    - Change CVCs, dialysis catheters.

Complications of Antimicrobial Therapy

- Monitor CBC with differential, electrolytes, renal, and liver function tests at least weekly.
- Nephrotoxicity common, especially with high doses or renal dysfunction
- Other serious complications occur with specific antibiotics (see Tables 9.2.2, 9.2.3, 9.2.24).
- Hypersensitivity reactions
  - If no prior anaphylaxis, may be able to use and treat hypersensitivity prophylactically
  - Most cephalosporins have low cross-reactivity with penicillins and can be used (except if prior anaphylaxis to penicillins).
  - Refer to penicillin and cephalosporin hypersensitivity pathways for advice.
    - Consider a test dose challenge for penicillins and cephalosporins when appropriate.
- Drug interactions: may modify drug metabolism via CYP450 pathways (see Tables 9.2.2, 9.2.3, 9.2.24)
- *C. difficile* infection—common with clindamycin, fluoroquinolones, but can occur with any antibiotic

Special Situations

- Hemodialysis (HD) and continuous renal replacement therapy (CRRT): difficult to predict drug clearance, dosing frequency may need to be reduced or increased
- Acute burns (>20% body surface area [BSA]): transient hypermetabolic state may require higher dosing.
- Extracorporeal membrane oxygenation (ECMO): altered volume of distribution alters drug clearance—very limited data on dose optimization and infectious clinical outcomes. Generally, use doses similar to other critically ill patients for hydrophilic antimicrobials (ie, beta-lactams).
- Central nervous system (CNS) infections: antibiotic and dose must cross blood-brain barrier (ie, piperacillin/tazobactam, cefazolin generally inadequate).
- Pregnancy and breastfeeding: consult individual drug labels for risks and recommendations.
- *See* Tables 9.2.3, 9.2.2 and 9.2.4 *for additional details.*

Clinically Important Organisms

- Gram-positive cocci
  - Skin flora
    - *Streptococcus* spp, *Staphylococcus epidermidis* (coagulase-negative *Staphylococcus*), *S. aureus* including MRSA
  - Gut flora
    - *Enterococcus faecalis* (usually ampicillin susceptible), *Enterococcus faecium* (often vancomycin resistant)
- Gram-negative cocci and *Mycoplasma* spp (atypicals)
  - *Neisseria meningitidis*, *Neisseria gonorrhoeae*, *Moraxella catarrhalis*, *Chlamydia pneumoniae*, *Mycoplasma pneumoniae*
- Gram-positive bacilli
  - Generally anaerobes or facultative anaerobes
  - *Clostridium perfringens* (gas gangrene), *C. difficile* (colitis), species of genera *Bacillus* (anthrax, food-borne), *Nocardia* (brain and other abscesses, usually in immunocompromised), *Corynebacterium* (often contaminants), *Listeria*, *Actinomyces*, *Lactobacillus*
- Gram-negative bacilli
  - Often part of normal enteric flora—*Escherichia coli*, *Klebsiella* spp; others include species of genera *Stenotrophomonas*, *Serratia*, *Pseudomonas*, *Acinetobacter*, *Citrobacter*, *Enterobacter*, *Legionella*, *Bacteroides*, *Prevotella*, *Fusobacterium*, *Proteus*; *Haemophilus influenzae* and *Helicobacter pylori*
- Mycobacteria
  - Detection requires acid-fast stain, specialized cultures, or antigen testing.
  - *Mycobacterium tuberculosis*: RIPE (Rifampicin, Isoniazid, Pyrazinamide, Ethambutol) +/− streptomycin (if resistance); isoniazid IV if unable to take PO
  - Other nontuberculous mycobacteria can cause disease—treat in consultation with ID/Pulm.
- Spirochetes and Rickettsiae
  - *Borrelia burgdorferi* (Lyme disease), *Treponema pallidum* (syphilis), *Rickettsia rickettsii* (Rocky Mountain spotted fever)
- Anaerobes
  - Often present in intraabdominal infections, abscesses, and deep tissue infections
  - *Clostridioides* spp and *Bacteroides* spp (intraabdominal), *Prevotella* spp and *Fusobacterium* spp (ENT/thoracic), *Propionibacterium* spp (upper extremity)
  - Metronidazole covers most anaerobes, including *C. difficile*.
  - Clindamycin has antianaerobic and antitoxin coverage.
- Enteric pathogens
  - Include both anaerobes and Gram-negatives, as earlier; *Enterococcus* spp also common
  - Cover enterics in intraabdominal infections, complicated UTI, some nosocomial infections
- AmpC beta-lactamase–producing Enterobacterales
  - Gram-negative organisms with inducible genes that produce AmpC beta-lactamase—can hydrolyze

TABLE 9.2.2 Antimicrobials by Class and Mechanism[a]

Drug and Initial Dosing	Use	Adverse Effects and Notes
Aminoglycosides Amikacin, 5 mg/kg IV q8h or 20-25 mg/kg/d Tobramycin, 2 mg/kg IV q8h or 8-10 mg/kg/d Gentamicin, 2 mg/kg IV q8h or 8-10 mg/kg/d	Gram-negative bacilli Gram-positive synergy NTM infections	• Nephro- and ototoxic • Must monitor peak and trough, start after second dose • Dose reduced needed for HD and low GFR • Rarely used as monotherapy • Synergistic with cell wall active second-generation agent for *Streptococcus* and *Enterococcus* endocarditis • Use adjusted body weight for >120% ideal body weight • Often needs pharmacy input for dosing/adjustments
Penicillinase-resistant penicillins Oxacillin, 2 g IV q4h Nafcillin, 2 g IV q4h	Methicillin-susceptible *Staphylococcus* (MSSA) and some *Streptococcus*	• High sodium load • No renal adjustment
Aminopenicillins Ampicillin 2 g IV q4-q6h Ampicillin-sulbactam[a], 3 g IV q6h	Gram+ cocci Enterococci Listeria Gram–bacilli[a] HACEK *Bacteroides* Oral flora	• Anaphylaxis, hypersensitivity reactions, pseudomembranous enterocolitis, SJS, thrombocytopenia, leukopenia relatively common • Renal dosing required • High sodium load • [a]Treats *Acinetobacter*, among others
β-Lactam—β-lactamase inhibitor extended-spectrum β-lactams Piperacillin/tazobactam, 3.375 g IV over 4h q6 or 4.5 g IV over 4h q6h for PsA	Same as ampicillin-sulbactam + PsA	• Synergistic with aminoglycosides • AmpC or ESBL *Klebsiella* and *Escherichia coli* may be resistant. • Time dependent; use prolonged infusion • Renal dosing required
Cephalosporins, first generation Cefazolin, 1-2 g IV q8h	Gram+ cocci (MSSA, some strep) Some *Proteus* and *E. coli*	• Cross-reactivity not common with penicillin hypersensitivities but possible • Avoid if history of anaphylaxis with penicillin • Utilize hypersensitivity pathways • Only third and fourth generations penetrate CNS. • Do not treat MRSA. • Ceftazidime is the only third-generation cephalosporin that covers PsA. • Cefiderocol only has Gram-negative coverage. • Enterococci intrinsically cephalosporin resistant
Cephalosporins, second generation Cefotetan, 2 g IV q12h Cefoxitin, 2 g IV q6h Cefuroxime, 1.5 g IV q6-8h	Gram+ cocci Some Gram–	
Cephalosporins, third generation Cefotaxime, 2 g IV q6h Ceftazidime, 2 g IV q8h Ceftriaxone, 1-2 g IV q24h (2 g q12h for CNS and for *Enterococcus* endocarditis if used in combination with ampicillin)	Gram+ cocci Gram+ bacilli Gram– bacilli Gram– cocci HACEK Lyme	
Cephalosporins, fourth generation Cefepime, 2 g IV q8h	Gram+ cocci Gram+ bacilli Gram– bacilli Gram– cocci	
Cephalosporins, fifth generation Ceftobiprole, 500 mg IV (over 2 h) q8h Ceftaroline, 600 mg IV q8h-q12h Cefiderocol 2 g IV q6	Gram+ including MRSA Gram–	
Carbapenems—extended-spectrum β-lactams Imipenem, 500 mg IV q6h Meropenem, 1 g IV q8h Ertapenem, 1 g IV q24h	Some Gram+ cocci Gram– bacilli PsA *Enterococcus*[a] Anaerobes	• Carbapenems not active against MRSA, *Enterococcus faecium* • Ertapenem does not cover PsA. • Imipenem has the highest risk of seizure (generally at higher doses or with renal failure).
Monobactams: narrow-spectrum β-lactams Aztreonam, 2 g IV q8h	Gram– only	• No cross-reactivity with other β-lactams (OK in penicillin hypersensitivity) • No activity against anaerobes or Gram+
Fluoroquinolones Ciprofloxacin, 400 mg IV q8h-q12h Levofloxacin, 750 mg IV q24h Moxifloxacin, 400 mg IV q24h	Gram+ cocci Gram+ bacilli Gram– bacilli Gram– cocci PsA (cipro/levo) TB *Stenotrophomonas*	• Hypersensitivity, tendonitis, QT prolongation, *Clostridioides difficile* colitis relatively common • Concentrate in prostate, lungs, and bile • Do not treat *C. difficile*. • Cipro not active against strep and anaerobes
Glycopeptides Vancomycin, 20 mg/kg load, then 15 mg/kg q8-q24h	Gram+ cocci *Enterococcus*	• Nephrotoxic, dose by trough levels, renal dose adjust • Not as effective as nafcillin/oxacillin/cefazolin for MSSA
Lincosamide Clindamycin, 600-900 mg IV q8h	Similar to macrolides plus anaerobes, *Staphylococcus pneumo*, malaria	• *C. difficile* colitis relatively common adverse effect • Does not penetrate CNS • Antitoxin/toxin-binding effect

TABLE 9.2.2 Antimicrobials by Class and Mechanism[a] (*continued*)

Drug and Initial Dosing	Use	Adverse Effects and Notes
Macrolides Azithromycin, 500 mg IV q24h Erythromycin, 250-500 mg IV q6h	Gram+ cocci (some) Gram– cocci *Treponema* *Helicobacter pylori*	• QT prolongation, GI cramping, hypermotility common
Oxazolidinones Linezolid, 600 mg IV q12h	Streptococci Staphylococci Enterococci (VRE) *Mycobacteria* *Nocardia*	• Monitor for serotonin syndrome with other MAOi/SSRis/TCAs (avoid if high dose or discuss with pharmacy). • Reversible myelosuppression (>2 wk' use) • Peripheral neuropathy, reversible optic neuropathy • Antitoxin/toxin-binding effect
Lipopeptides Daptomycin, 6-8 mg/kg IV q24h	Gram+ only	• Inactivated by pulmonary surfactant (do not use for PNA) • Can cause myopathy (monitor CK) and eosinophilic PNA • For isolates that are susceptible dose dependent (SDD) → may need higher doses (ie, 8-10 mg/kg IV q24 h) • For vanc-resistant *E. faecium* bacteremia, consider starting 10-12 mg/kg IV q24h.
Nitroimidazole Metronidazole, 500 mg IV q12h	*C. difficile* Obligate anaerobes *H. pylori* Protozoa (Amoeba, trichomonas, giardia)	• q8h only for CNS dosing or bloodstream infections • Adverse effects: GI upset, peripheral neuropathy, inhibits warfarin metabolism
Polymyxins (polypeptides) Colistin, 5 mg/kg IV load, then 1.5-5 mg/kg/d IV or inhaled in two or four divided doses Polymyxin-B 2.5-5 mg/kg/d load (optional), then 1.25-1.5 mg/kg q12h	Resistant Gram-negatives	• Nephrotoxicity common, adjust dose for renal function
Tetracyclines Tigecycline, 100 mg IV load × 1, then 50 mg IV q12h Minocycline, 200 mg IV/PO × 1, then 100 mg q12h	Gram+ including MRSA Resistant Gram– Anaerobes *Stenotrophomonas* (minocycline)	• Benign transaminitis common, rare hepatic dysfunction • Not active against PsA
Others Meropenem-vaborbactam, 4 g IV q8h Ceftolozane-tazobactam, 1.5-3 g IV q8h Cefiderocol, 2 g IV q6h Ceftazidime-avibactam, 2.5 g IV q8h Imipenem-relebactam, 1.25 g IV q6h	Resistant Gram-negatives (ie, CRE)	• Usually restricted, need ID consult/approval

CK, creatine kinase; CNS, central nervous system; CRE, carbapenem-resistant Enterobacterales; ESBL, extended-spectrum beta-lactamase; GFR, glomerular filtration rate; GI, gastrointestinal; HD, hemodialysis; IV, intravenous; MAOi, monoamine oxidase inhibitor; PNA, pneumonia; PO, oral; PsA, *Pseudomonas aeruginosa;* NTM, nontuberculous mycobacteria; q, every; SJS, Stevens-Johnson syndrome; SSRi, selective serotonin reuptake inhibitor; TB, tuberculosis; TCAs, tricyclic antidepressants.

[a]Discuss dosing with pharmacy colleagues. Dose by weight, kidney function, and serum level when necessary.

TABLE 9.2.3 Antifungals

Drug and Initial Dosing	Used For	Notes
Triazoles Fluconazole, 400 mg IV/PO q24h Voriconazole, load: 6 mg/kg IV/PO q12h for two doses, then 4 mg/kg IV/PO q12h Posaconazole, load 300 mg IV/PO q12h × 2 doses, then 300 mg IV/PO q24h Itraconazole, PO solution 200 mg q8h × 9 doses, then 200 q24h Isavuconazole, 372 mg IV/PO q8h × 6 doses, then 372 mg q24g	*Candida* Aspergillosis Fungemia Neutropenic fever Cryptococcal meningitis Other invasive fungal infection	• Fluconazole only treats *Candida* spp (and not all isolates) and *Cryptococcus*. • Monitor LFTs for QT prolongation (all azoles, except isavuconazole). • Itraconazole PO only • Azole antifungals interact with CYP450 isoenzymes (CYP3A4, CYP2c9, and CYP2C19), potentially altering the metabolism of concomitant medications and resulting in clinicaly important drug-drug interaactions
Echinocandins Micafungin, 100 mg IV q24h (150 mg q24h for fungal esophagitis, fungal endocarditis, BMI >40)	*Candida*, resistant candidal infections	• Do not penetrate urinary tract (do not use for UTI). • No renal adjustment • Monitor LFTs.
Amphotericins Liposomal amphotericin B, 3-5 mg /kg IV q24h	Mucormycosis Aspergillosis	• Infusion-related inflammatory response common (can pretreat with diphenhydramine, steroids, or APAP) • Nephrotoxicity, hypokalemia, hypomagnesemia common—give IVF with administration, monitor and replete electrolytes.

BMI, body mass index; IV, intravenous; IVF, in vitro fertilization; LFTs, liver function tests; PO, oral; q, every; UTI, urinary tract infection.

TABLE 9.2.4 Antivirals

Drug and Initial Dosing	Used For	Notes
Oseltamivir, 75 mg PO bid × 5 d	Influenza A and B	• Can extend to 10 d in immunocompromised
Acyclovir Encephalitis: 10 mg/kg IV q8h Other location: 5 mg/kg IV q8h	HSV, VZV	• Significant renal toxicity, needs dose adjustment for renal impairment, prehydrate, and give concurrent fluids to decrease renal toxicity • Can cause myelosuppression
Ganciclovir, 5 mg/kg IV q12h	HSV, VZV, CMV	• Can cause myelosuppression • Adjust dose for renal impairment.
Foscarnet, 60 mg/kg IV q8h	HSV, VZV, CMV, HHV-6	• Starting dose depends on specific virus, adjust for renal impairment. • Prehydration and concurrent fluid administration decrease renal toxicity. • Monitor Ca, K, Mg, and Phos and replete as necessary.

bid, twice daily; CMV, cytomegalovirus; HHV-6, human herpesvirus 6; HSV, herpes simplex virus; IV, intravenous; PO, oral; q, every; VZV, varicella zoster virus.

penicillins (ampicillin, piperacillin), first- (cefazolin) and third-generation (ceftriaxone, cefotaxime) cephalosporins, aztreonam
  - Can lead to resistance even if in vitro susceptibility testing shows susceptibility
  - Use cefepime or meropenem (PO fluoroquinolones if susceptible)
  - ECK organisms: commonly *Enterobacter cloacae*, *Citrobacter freundii*, *Klebsiella aerogenes*
- Extended-spectrum beta-lactamase (ESBL)-producing Enterobacterales
  - ESBLs inactivate most penicillins, cephalosporins, and aztreonam.
  - Any Gram-negative can become ESBL; *E. coli*, *Klebsiella* spp, *Proteus mirabilis* most common.
  - Ceftriaxone nonsusceptibility (ie, minimum inhibitory concentration [MIC] ≥2) often used as a proxy for ESBL
  - Treat with carbapenems.
- HACEK (endocarditis-specific Gram-negative bacilli)
  - *Haemophilus influenzae*, *Actinobacillus* spp, *Cardiobacterium* spp, *Eikenella* spp, *Kingella* spp
  - Treat with ampicillin/sulbactam, ceftriaxone, other third- or fourth-generation cephalosporins.

SUGGESTED READINGS

Berbari EF, Kanj SS, Kowalski TJ, et al; Infectious Diseases Society of America. 2015 Infectious Diseases Society of America (IDSA) clinical practice guidelines for the diagnosis and treatment of native vertebral osteomyelitis in adults. *Clin Infect Dis*. 2015;61(6):e26-e46.

Evans L, Rhodes A, Alhazzani W, et al. Surviving Sepsis Campaign: international guidelines for management of sepsis and septic shock 2021. *Crit Care Med*. 2021;49(11):e1063-e1143.

Fernando SM, Rochwerg B, Seely AJE. Clinical implications of the third international consensus definitions for sepsis and septic shock (Sepsis-3). *CMAJ*. 2018;190(36):E1058-E1059.

Harris PNA, Tambyah PA, Lye DC, et al. Effect of piperacillin-tazobactam vs meropenem on 30-day mortality for patients with *E. coli* or *Klebsiella pneumoniae* bloodstream infection and ceftriaxone resistance: a randomized clinical trial. *JAMA*. 2018;320(10):984-994.

Liu C, Bayer A, Cosgrove SE, et al. Clinical practice guidelines by the Infectious Diseases Society of America for the treatment of methicillin-resistant Staphylococcus aureus infections in adults and children: executive summary. *Clin Infect Dis*. 2011;52(3):285-292.

Mergenhagen KA, Starr KE, Wattengel BA, Lesse AJ, Sumon Z, Sellick JA. Determining the utility of methicillin-resistant Staphylococcus aureus nares screening in antimicrobial stewardship. *Clin Infect Dis*. 2020;71(5):1142-1148.

Metersky ML, Klompas M, Kalil AC. Less is more: a 7-day course of antibiotics is the evidence-based treatment for Pseudomonas aeruginosa ventilator-associated pneumonia. *Clin Infect Dis*. 2023;76(4):750-752.

Metlay JP, Waterer GW, Long AC, et al. Diagnosis and treatment of adults with community-acquired pneumonia. An Official Clinical Practice Guideline of the American Thoracic Society and Infectious Diseases Society of America. *Am J Respir Crit Care Med*. 2019;200(7):e45-e67.

Senneville É, Albalawi Z, van Asten SA, et al. IWGDF/IDSA guidelines on the diagnosis and treatment of diabetes-related foot infections (IWGDF/IDSA 2023). *Clin Infect Dis*. 2023:ciad527.

Singer M, Deutschman CS, Seymour CW, et al. The third international consensus definitions for sepsis and septic shock (Sepsis-3). *JAMA*. 2016;315(8):801-810.

Tamma PD, Aitken SL, Bonomo RA, Mathers AJ, van Duin D, Clancy CJ. Infectious Diseases Society of America 2023 guidance on the treatment of antimicrobial resistant gram-negative infections. *Clin Infect Dis*. 2023:ciad428.

SECTION 10

Immunology

Section Editor: Raghu R. Chivukula

10.1

The Immune System and Immunologic Disorders

Laura J. Yockey and Naomi J. Patel

The immune system (Table 10.1.1) is made up of multiple components that work together to protect against pathogens.

- *Ectoderm*
  - Surface barriers, such as enzymes and mucus and epithelial layers, have antimicrobial properties.
  - Any organism that breaks through this first barrier encounters the innate and acquired immune responses.
- *Innate (natural) responses*
  - Develops quickly (within hours to days) and is not specific to a given pathogen or antigen. It is triggered by conserved molecular patterns of pathogens and by damage signals produced by cells.
  - Composed of phagocytic cells (neutrophils, monocytes, and macrophages) that release inflammatory mediators (basophils, mast cells, and eosinophils) and cytotoxic natural killer cells
  - The molecular components of innate responses include complement, acute-phase proteins, and cytokines (eg, interferons, interleukins, and others).
  - There is close cross talk between cells and cytokines of the innate and adaptive immune responses.
- *Acquired (adaptive) responses*
  - Acquired responses involve the proliferation of antigen-specific B and T cells and occur when the surface receptors of these cells (B-cell receptors and T-cell receptors [TCRs]) bind to an antigen.
  - Specialized cells called antigen-presenting cells display the antigen to T lymphocytes and collaborate with them in the response to the antigen.
  - B cells contribute to humoral immunity. They can recognize proteins and polysaccharides in their native conformation. They secrete immunoglobulins that neutralize pathogens and target them for removal by complement and phagocytes.
  - T cells contribute to cellular immunity and are composed of cytotoxic and helper T cells.
    - T cells recognize peptides that are presented in major histocompatibility complexes (MHCs). Variable TCRs interact with unique MHC-peptide complexes.
    - Human leukocyte antigens (HLAs) are genes that make up the MHC and are common genes associated with differential susceptibility to autoimmune disease.
    - Cytotoxic (or CD8) T cells recognize peptides presented on MHC by non–antigen-presenting cells. They can directly interact with and kill infected cells.
    - Helper (or CD4) T cells recognize peptides that are presented on MHC by antigen-presenting cells (eg, dendritic cells and macrophages). They produce cytokines to coordinate immune responses with other immune cells (eg, B cells, phagocytic cells).

TABLE 10.1.1 Components of the Innate and Adaptive Immune Systems

	Innate System	Adaptive System
Stimulus	• Not antigen specific • Conserved molecular patterns and damage signals trigger response	• Specific for each different antigen • Initial exposure to an antigen produces memory cells.
Timing	• Provides a rapid response (hours to days) • The response does not improve with repeated exposure.	• Initial response takes time to develop (days to weeks). • Subsequent infections with the same antigen lead to a rapid and targeted response.
Cellular components	Monocytes/macrophage Neutrophils Eosinophils Basophils Mast cells Natural killer cells	B cells/plasma cells T cells
Secreted components	Complement Cytokines Lysozyme Acute-phase proteins Type I and III interferons	Antibodies Cytokines Interferons (particularly type II interferons)

- Lymph nodes, spleen, and mucosa-associated lymphoid tissue (eg, tonsils, adenoids) are all important structures for coordinating immune responses.
- In systemic autoimmune rheumatic diseases (SARDs), there are immune responses to self-antigens (ie, autoantigens) that can lead to inflammation and organ damage.
  - The pathogenesis of autoimmune diseases is complex.
  - Self-reactive T and B cells have been implicated in certain autoimmune diseases but can also be seen in healthy individuals.
- A combination of genetic and environmental factors predisposes individuals to SARDs.
- Autoinflammatory diseases (eg, periodic fever syndromes, adult-onset Still disease) are not antibody (Ab) mediated but are due to hyperactivation of the innate immune system.

Cytokines

- Cytokines are small, secreted proteins that act locally, via specific cell surface receptors, as part of both the innate and adaptive immune response.
- They have many effects, but in general, they stimulate the immune response through the growth, activation, and survival of various cells.

Systemic Autoimmune Rheumatic Diseases in the Intensive Care Unit

- 20% of individuals with SARDs admitted to the intensive care unit (ICU) receive their SARD diagnosis for the first time during the ICU admission.
- 10% to 25% of all individuals with SARDs visiting the emergency department require hospital admission, and up to one-third of the hospitalized patients need intensive care.
  - These patients form only a small percentage of all individuals admitted to the ICU.
- The main reason for admission to the ICU in individuals with SARDs is respiratory dysfunction or failure.
- Of those admitted to the ICU, systemic lupus erythematosus (SLE; 33.5% of reported patients), rheumatoid arthritis (RA; 25%), and systemic vasculitis (15%) were the most frequent SARDs.
- Mortality ranged from 17% to 55% in case series including those with a broad array of SARDs.
- Infection accounts for the most common reason for ICU admission, followed by flares of the underlying SARD, and then by unrelated acute illness or medication complications.
- In those admitted for acute illness unrelated to the SARD, the underlying SARD and its treatment may still influence the management and outcome of the acute illness.

Potential Critical Care Presentations Due to Underlying Systemic Autoimmune Rheumatic Disease

- Autoimmune diseases are a part of the differential diagnosis for many patients admitted to the ICU for respiratory failure and acute kidney injury (AKI), among other reasons.
- A thorough review of systems (Table 10.1.2) and selective testing of rheumatologic labs (Table 10.1.3) are helpful in assessing the overall concern for an underlying SARD.

TABLE 10.1.2 Rheumatologic Review of Systems

Organ System	Components
Constitutional	Fevers, chills, night sweats, weight loss, lymphadenopathy
Head, eyes, ears, nose, and throat	Hair loss, oral ulcers, vision changes, dry eyes, dry mouth, eye pain or redness, headaches, scalp tenderness, jaw claudication, parotid/submandibular gland swelling
Respiratory/cardiovascular	Shortness of breath, dyspnea, cough, palpitations, pleuritic chest pain, hemoptysis, epistaxis, nasal crusting
Gastrointestinal	Heartburn/reflux, dysphagia/difficulty swallowing, abdominal pain, nausea, melena/blood in stool
Genitourinary	Hematuria, foamy urine
Skin	Malar rash, photosensitivity, purpura, skin thickening of fingers/hands, Raynaud, fingertip ulcers/ischemia, other rashes
Musculoskeletal	Joint pain, joint swelling, morning stiffness (>1 h), proximal muscle weakness, limb claudication, edema
Neurologic	Weakness, numbness/tingling, seizures

Respiratory

Diffuse Alveolar Hemorrhage

- *Presentation*: hemoptysis, anemia, acute respiratory failure, diffuse pulmonary infiltrates on imaging. Hemoptysis may be absent in one-third of cases. Diagnosis is confirmed by serial bronchoalveolar lavage with progressive hemorrhage or by histopathology.
- *Associated diseases*
  - SARD-associated etiologies (often due to capillaritis): antineutrophil cytoplasmic antibody (ANCA)-associated vasculitis, SLE, antiphospholipid syndrome (APS), Goodpasture syndrome, other forms of vasculitis (Behçet, cryoglobulinemic vasculitis, immunoglobulin A [IgA] vasculitis), isolated pulmonary capillaritis
  - Nonrheumatologic etiologies: acute respiratory distress syndrome (ARDS), infection, malignancy, medications, anticoagulation, idiopathic pulmonary hemosiderosis, elevated pulmonary capillary wedge pressure (eg, mitral stenosis, veno-occlusive disease), lung transplant, or hematopoietic cell transplant
- *Evaluation*
  - Evaluate for extrapulmonary evidence of vasculitis (eg, glomerulonephritis, sinonasal involvement, palpable purpura, inflammatory arthritis)
  - Consider biopsy of extrapulmonary affected organ (eg, skin or kidney) or lung if diagnosis is unclear.
  - Antinuclear antigen (ANA), ANCA, urinalysis, rheumatoid factor (RF), cyclic citrullinated peptide (CCP), glomerular basement membrane (GBM) Ab, antiphospholipid antibodies (lupus anticoagulant, anticardiolipin, anti-beta-2 glycoprotein 1), cryoglobulins, complements

TABLE 10.1.3 Rheumatologic Lab Testing

Lab Test		Associated Disease(s)	Other Associations
Rheumatoid factor		Rheumatoid arthritis, Sjögren, cryoglobulinemia	Viral/bacterial Infection (high frequency with HCV, endocarditis), other SARD (eg, Sjögren), mixed cryoglobulinemia, PBC, cirrhosis
Cyclic citrullinated peptide (CCP)		Rheumatoid arthritis	Low titers associated with SLE, Sjögren syndrome, other SARDs
Antinuclear antibody (ANA; 1:160 or greater)		SLE, Sjögren syndrome, systemic sclerosis, polymyositis, juvenile arthritis	Common in healthy individuals, autoimmune thyroid disease, autoimmune hepatitis, PBC, infection (HBV, HCV, HIV, parvovirus), medications (eg, hydralazine, hydrochlorothiazide, minocycline, TNFi)
C3, C4		SLE (marker of disease activity when low)	Cryoglobulinemia, inherited disorder, infection (sepsis, endocarditis; particularly with isolated low C3), hepatic failure, severe malnutrition, acute pancreatitis, HUS/TTP
Extractable nuclear antigens (ENAs)	SS-A/Ro (Ro52 and Ro60) SS-B/La	Sjögren, SLE	SSc, dermatomyositis, IIM, MCTD, PBC, autoimmune liver disease, neonatal lupus, subacute cutaneous lupus, interstitial pneumonitis, myositis-associated ILD (worse outcomes)
	dsDNA	SLE (marker of disease activity when elevated/high titer)	TNF inhibitor use, viral infection (HIV, BK virus, parvovirus), myeloma
	Smith	SLE, MCTD	Highly specific for SLE but present in <30% of patients with SLE
	RNP	SLE, MCTD	Sjögren, SSc, polymyositis/dermatomyositis
	Scl70	Systemic sclerosis	In SSc, associated with diffuse disease and more severe ILD
Antiphospholipid antibodies (APLAs) • Cardiolipin IgG and IgM • β-2-glycoprotein-I IgG or IgM • Lupus anticoagulant		APS, SLE	Also associated with infections (eg, syphilis, Lyme, HCV, HIV, EBV, COVID-19) and medications (eg, procainamide, quinidine, phenytoin). Lupus anticoagulant can be falsely positive in patients on anticoagulation.
RNA polymerase III		Systemic sclerosis	In SSc, associated with diffuse disease and increased risk of scleroderma renal crisis
Th/TO		Systemic sclerosis	Associated with nucleolar staining on ANA assay. In SSc, associated with high rates of ILD and pulmonary hypertension
PR3 (typically C-ANCA)		Granulomatosis with polyangiitis (GPA) > microscopic polyangiitis (MPA), eosinophilic granulomatosis with polyangiitis (EGPA)	Drug-induced AAV (hydralazine, propylthiouracil, minocycline, cocaine/levamisole), endocarditis, bacteremia; ELISA-negative +ANCA associated with IBD, PBC, CF, other SARDs
MPO (typically P-ANCA)		MPA > GPA, EGPA, renal-limited vasculitis	
Jo-1, PL-7, PL-12, EJ, OJ, Ha/YRS, KS, Zo		Antisynthetase antibodies	PL-7 and PL-12 associated with severe ILD. Cytoplasmic staining can be seen on ANA assay.
MDA5		MDA5 dermatomyositis	Can be associated with rapidly progressive ILD. Considered to be a highly specific antibody (depending on assay used)
ARS, SAE, Mi2, NXP2, TIF1g		Dermatomyositis	NXP2, TIF1g are associated with malignancy.
HMGCR		Statin-associated immune-mediated necrotizing myopathy	Other inflammatory myopathies; can be cancer associated in a subset of patients. Often not included in standard myositis panel
SRP		Immune-mediated necrotizing myopathy, ILD	Polymyositis, dermatomyositis
NT5c1A		Inclusion body myositis	SLE, Sjögren
PM/SCl		Systemic sclerosis, polymyositis/dermatomyositis, and overlap syndromes	Associated with ILD and a more favorable prognosis compared to other SSc and polymyositis antibodies

AAV, ANCA-associated vasculitis; ANCA, antineutrophilic cytoplasmic antibody; APS, antiphospholipid syndrome; CF, cystic fibrosis; ELISA, enzyme linked immunosorbent assay; HBV, hepatitis B virus; HCV, hepatitis C virus; HIV, human immunodeficiency virus; HUS, hemolytic-uremic syndrome; IBD, inflammatory bowel disease; ILD, interstitial lung disease; MCTD, mixed connective tissue disease; PBC, primary biliary cirrhosis; SARD, systemic autoimmune rheumatic diseases; SLE, systemic lupus erythematosus; SSc, systemic sclerosis; TNFi, tumor necrosis factor inhibitor; TTP, thrombotic thrombocytopenic purpura.

Acute Interstitial Lung Disease

- *Presentation*: dyspnea, shortness of breath, hypoxemia, decline in forced vital capacity (FVC) or diffusing capacity of the lungs for carbon monoxide (DLCO) on pulmonary function tests (PFTs), pulmonary imaging showing characteristic changes (eg, ground-glass opacities, traction bronchiectasis, and honeycombing)
  - Rapidly progressive interstitial lung disease (ILD) is defined by the need for hospitalization for dyspnea requiring supplemental oxygen, high-resolution computed tomography (HRCT) with 20% involvement, decline in PFTs (FVC >10%, DLCO >15%) or arterial blood gas suggesting respiratory failure within 1 month of presentation.
- *Associated diseases:* polymyositis, dermatomyositis, systemic sclerosis (SSc), RA, mixed connective tissue disease (MCTD), Sjögren, SLE, ANCA-associated vasculitis, idiopathic interstitial pneumonia with autoimmune features (IPAFs)
- *Evaluation*
  - HRCT, PFTs to establish diagnosis
  - Consider lung biopsy if unclear.
  - Erythrocyte sedimentation rate (ESR), C-reactive protein (CRP), creatine kinase (CK), aldolase, ANA, RF, CCP, double-stranded DNA (dsDNA), Ro/SSA, La/SSB, Smith, ribonucleoprotein (RNP), Scl70, RNA polymerase III, myositis panel (to include Jo-1, PL-7, PL-12, PM-Scl, MDA5), ANCA

Renal

Scleroderma Renal Crisis

- *Presentation*: acute hypertension and AKI in a patient with SSc. Can rarely occur in patients who are normotensive. Other supporting features: microangiopathic hemolytic anemia (MAHA; new anemia, thrombocytopenia, schistocytes, hemolysis), evidence of end-organ damage (eg, headache, vision changes, pulmonary edema, seizures). Scleroderma renal crisis (SRC) can rarely be the first presenting symptom of SSc.
  - Risk factors: diffuse cutaneous disease, +RNA polymerase III, first 5 years of disease, recent high-dose glucocorticoids (particularly >15 mg of prednisone or equivalent daily)
- *Evaluation*
  - Complete metabolic panel (CMP), complete blood count (CBC) with differential, blood smear, lactate dehydrogenase (LDH), haptoglobin, urinalysis, urine protein/creatinine. Consider renal biopsy if diagnosis is unclear to rule out other etiologies. ANA, RNA polymerase III, Scl70 (if patient does not yet have a diagnosis of SSc).
- *Treatment:* first line: angiotensin-converting enzyme (ACE) inhibitor. Rapid control of blood pressure with intravenous (IV) vasodilators if systolic blood pressure >180 or diastolic blood pressure >110

Glomerulonephritis

- *Presentation:* hematuria (with urine microscopy/sediment showing dysmorphic red blood cells [RBCs] and/or RBC casts) and/or proteinuria (predominantly albuminuria). Can also have AKI, hypertension, edema, proteinuria, hypercoagulability
- *Associated diseases:* ANCA-associated vasculitis, SLE, infection (including *Streptococcus*, *Staphylococcus*, human immunodeficiency virus [HIV], hepatitis C virus [HCV], hepatitis B virus [HBV]), IgA vasculitis, cryoglobulinemia, primary membranous nephropathy
- *Evaluation*
  - Evaluate for evidence of systemic disease: rashes (especially palpable purpura), pulmonary nodules or infiltrates, fevers, weight loss, arthritis, recent infection.
  - CBC with differential (CBC with differential), 24-hour urine protein, urine microscopy, ANA, dsDNA, C3, C4, ANCA, GBM, serum protein electrophoresis (SPEP), serum free light chain (SFLC), HIV, HCV serologies, HBV serologies, blood cultures
  - Kidney biopsy (especially if declining kidney function or >500 mg urine protein/d)

Hematologic

Catastrophic Antiphospholipid Syndrome

- *Presentation:* multiorgan thrombosis (>3 sites, most commonly involves kidney, brain, lungs, heart, skin, liver, peripheral vessels, gastrointestinal [GI] tract) occurring over 1 week. There is typically evidence of both microvascular and large-vessel involvement. There is often evidence of MAHA (thrombocytopenia, schistocytes on smear). Can occur as first presentation of APS or in those with an established diagnosis of APS.
- *Associated diseases:* APS can be primary or associated with an underlying SARD. SLE is most common but can also be seen with RA and Sjögren.
- *Differential diagnosis of multiple thromboses*: SLE, ANCA-associated vasculitis, sepsis, disseminated intravascular coagulation (DIC), primary thrombotic microangiopathy (including thrombotic thrombocytopenic purpura [TTP], hemolytic-uremic syndrome [HUS], or hemolysis, elevated liver enzymes and low platelets syndrome [HELLP] in pregnant women)
- *Evaluation*
  - Imaging of the affected areas to confirm large-vessel thrombosis
  - Consider biopsy to confirm microvascular thrombosis.
  - Antiphospholipid Ab panel, ANA, dsDNA, Smith, RNP, C3, C4, CBC with differential, peripheral smear, CMP, reticulocytes, LDH, haptoglobin, C3, C4, ADAMTS13, PF4 if recent heparin exposure
- Treatment: therapeutic anticoagulation, glucocorticoids (typically IV methylprednisolone 0.5-1 g daily for 3 days followed by prednisone or equivalent of 1 mg/kg daily), IV immunoglobulin (IVIG) or plasma exchange, and consideration of further immunosuppression pending underlying etiology and course

Macrophage Activation Syndrome

- *Presentation:* persistent fevers, elevated CRP with low ESR, elevated ferritin, cytopenias, transaminitis, coagulopathy (low fibrinogen, elevated prothrombin time international normalized ratio [PT/INR]), splenomegaly, central nervous system (CNS) dysfunction
- *Associated diseases*
  - Macrophage activation syndrome (MAS) generally refers to a secondary form of hemophagocytic

lymphohistiocytosis (HLH) often associated with underlying autoimmunity
 - Rheumatologic: adult-onset Still disease, SLE, systemic juvenile arthritis
 - Nonrheumatologic: Infection, Epstein-Barr virus (EBV), malignancy, genetic predisposition
- *Evaluation:* CBC with differential, blood smear, CMP, ESR, CRP, ferritin, LDH, D-dimer, fibrinogen, PT/partial thromboplastin time (PTT), CXCL9, interleukin-18 (IL-18), sIL2R. Lumbar puncture if neurologic symptoms. Bone marrow biopsy often considered to confirm hemophagocytosis.
 - If etiology unclear, consider blood cultures, EBV, cytomegalovirus (CMV), adenovirus, respiratory virus testing, expedited genetic testing
- *Treatment:* depends on the underlying etiology
 - Initial treatment: supportive care, treatment directed toward underlying etiology (eg, empiric antimicrobial therapy, treatment of underlying SARD)
 - If persistent or severe: glucocorticoids, anakinra, IVIG are often first-line treatments. Etoposide is used in certain cases in discussion with hematology/oncology.

Neurologic

Central Nervous System Vasculitis

- *Presentation*: headaches, cognitive dysfunction, focal neurologic deficit, seizure, vision changes, multifocal cerebral infarcts (typically affecting different vascular territories), and/or angiography showing multifocal arterial narrowing and/or beading. Systemic symptoms (eg, fevers) or elevated ESR/CRP can be seen in various SARDs but are commonly absent in primarily CNS vasculitis.
- *Differential diagnosis:* atherosclerosis, embolic disease, infection (particularly viral, mycobacterial, or fungal infections), cerebral amyloid angiopathy, fibromuscular dysplasia, moyamoya disease, reversible cerebral vasoconstriction syndrome
- *Associated diseases:* primary angiitis of the CNS (if no underlying SARD), Behçet disease, polyarteritis nodosa (PAN), ANCA-associated vasculitis (very rarely), cryoglobulinemic vasculitis, SLE, Sjögren disease
 - Giant cell arteritis (GCA) and Takayasu arteritis can cause vasculitis of the large intracranial vessels. GCA typically affects the posterior circulation.
- *Evaluation:* dedicated vessel wall magnetic resonance imaging (MRI) (ie, "black blood" imaging), cerebrospinal fluid (CSF) studies
 - ESR, CRP, ANCA, ANA, SSA, SSB, tuberculosis (TB) testing, syphilis testing, HIV, HCV, cryoglobulins
 - Consider: brain biopsy, additional chest imaging, and large-vessel imaging (eg, CT angiogram of the chest/abdomen/pelvis)

Mononeuritis Multiplex

- *Presentation*: pain, weakness, and/or paresthesia affecting two or more peripheral nerve distributions. Affected areas can start simultaneously or sequentially. Mononeuritis can also affect a single nerve.
- *Associated diseases*
 - Rheumatologic: ANCA-associated vasculitis, PAN, SLE, Sjögren, RA
 - Nonrheumatologic: diabetes, amyloidosis, infection (eg, Lyme, HIV, leprosy)
- *Evaluation:* electromyography (EMG), CBC with differential, CMP, ESR, CRP, ANCA, consider sural nerve biopsy, skin biopsy if cutaneous findings are present.
 - Consider: Lyme testing, HIV, ANA, SSA/SSB, RF, CCP

Musculoskeletal

Acute Joint Pain and Swelling

- *Presentation:* warmth, swelling, effusion, erythema, and/or pain involving one or more joints
- *Differential diagnosis*
 - Monoarthritis: septic arthritis, gout, pseudogout (ie, calcium pyrophosphate deposition disease), spondyloarthropathy (eg, psoriatic arthritis), Lyme arthritis, gonococcal arthritis
 - Polyarthritis: RA, psoriatic arthritis, inflammatory bowel disease (IBD)-associated inflammatory arthritis, reactive arthritis, gout, pseudogout, palindromic rheumatism, systemic infection (eg, bacteremia), inflammatory arthritis associated with other SARD (including SLE, Sjögren, ANCA-associated vasculitis, SSc)
- *Evaluation*
 - Monoarthritis: x-ray of the affected joint, arthrocentesis (with Gram stain/culture, crystal analysis, cell count and differential of joint fluid), serum uric acid level
 - Polyarthritis: x-ray(s) of the affected joints, consider aspiration if feasible, uric acid, RF, CCP, ANA, SSA/SSB.
 - Consider: blood cultures, Lyme serologies, gonorrhea/chlamydia pending risk factors
- *Treatment*
 - Depends on etiology.
 - For acute treatment of gout or pseudogout: corticosteroid injection if monoarthritis or oligoarthritis, topical ice, nonsteroidal antiinflammatory drugs (NSAIDs) if not contraindicated, colchicine, systemic glucocorticoids, or anakinra if other medications are insufficient or contraindicated

Systemic Autoimmune Rheumatic Diseases

- SARDs, with the exception of RA, are rare, and collectively affect ~5% of the population in Western countries.

Inflammatory Arthritis

- RA
 - *Typical presentation:* chronic systemic progressive symmetrical polyarthritis that typically presents as joint pain, swelling, and stiffness, particularly in the morning, with improvement with activity. Small joints of hands and feet (eg, metacarpal joints [MCPs], proximal interphalangeal joints [PIPs], metatarsophalangeal joints [MTPs]) are often affected first, but large joints can also be commonly involved. Typical age of onset is 30 to 60 years, but half of patients can present at >60 years. Two-thirds of patients are women.
 - *Other complications:* ILD, pericarditis, pleuritis, episcleritis, scleritis, vasculitis (involving small > medium vessels in patients with severe, long-standing disease),

Felty syndrome (neutropenia and splenomegaly), tubulointerstitial or membranous nephritis, increased risk for coronary artery disease (CAD)
    - *Evaluation:* x-rays of the affected joints, RF, CCP. Consider joint aspiration, especially if oligoarthritis or monoarthritis, to rule out alternative etiologies.
    - *Treatment* (first line): methotrexate or tumor necrosis factor inhibitor (TNFi) for moderate-severe disease; hydroxychloroquine or sulfasalazine for mild disease
- *Spondyloarthropathies (ankylosing spondylitis, psoriatic arthritis, IBD-associated arthritis, reactive arthritis)*
    - *Typical presentation:* peripheral: asymmetric oligoarthritis or polyarthritis; distal interphalangeal (DIPs) often involved; enthesitis (eg, Achilles tendinitis, plantar fasciitis) and dactylitis are common. Axial: low back pain and stiffness, often worse at night with morning stiffness. Symptoms are worse with rest and relieved with activity. Patients with personal and family history of psoriasis and/or IBD are more likely to be affected.
    - *Other complications:* uveitis, conjunctivitis, IBD, cutaneous manifestations (psoriasis, keratoderma blennorrhagicum)
    - *Evaluation:* x-rays of the affected joints (particularly sacroiliac joint x-rays); if inflammatory low back pain, MRI of sacroiliac joints if x-ray negative. RF, CCP if peripheral involvement. Consider HLA-B27. Consider aspiration of the affected joint to rule out septic arthritis or crystalline arthritis, especially if monoarthritis.
    - *Treatment* (first line)
        - For peripheral arthritis: NSAIDs, sulfasalazine (if mild disease), methotrexate, TNFi
        - For axial involvement: NSAIDs, TNFi
        - If comorbid psoriasis or IBD, it is important to consider treatments that will target both diseases.

Connective Tissue Diseases

- *SLE*
    - *Typical presentation:* this chronic, multiorgan disease has a variable presentation. Common presenting symptoms/features are rashes (eg, malar rash, discoid lupus), photosensitivity, arthritis, oral ulcers, fever, fatigue, alopecia, Raynaud, pericarditis, pleuritis, cytopenias, and nephritis (with hematuria, proteinuria, AKI). Women are 9 times more likely to be affected than men. Patients commonly present at ages 17 to 35.
    - *Other complications:* thromboembolic disease, pulmonary (pneumonitis, ILD, pulmonary hypertension, diffuse alveolar hemorrhage [DAH]), other cardiac involvement (myocarditis, valvular abnormalities, increased risk of CAD), neurologic involvement (headaches, seizures, confusion), GI involvement (enteritis, esophageal dysmotility, mesenteric vasculitis, pancreatitis, hepatitis, enteritis)
    - *Evaluation*
        - For new diagnosis: ANA (ANA <1:80 makes SLE unlikely), C3/C4, dsDNA, Sm, RNP, SSA/SSB. Consider direct Coombs, APS antibodies. Check CMP, CBC with differential, urinalysis, and urine protein-to-creatine ratio (UPCR) in any patients with suspected SLE to evaluate for cytopenias and kidney involvement.
        - Cytopenias, hematuria, proteinuria, hypocomplementemia, positive dsDNA, and elevated inflammatory markers can help determine disease activity.
    - *Treatment:* hydroxychloroquine in most patients (reduces the risk of flare, mortality, and other complications). Additional treatment depends on organ involvement (mycophenolate, methotrexate, azathioprine, belimumab, anifrolumab, rituximab). Glucocorticoids are commonly used, especially in organ-threatening disease.
- *SSc*
    - *Typical presentation:* patients often present with Raynaud, skin thickening involving the fingers (sclerodactyly) that spreads proximally, telangiectasia, abnormal nail fold capillaries, calcinosis, gastroesophageal reflux (GER), and esophageal dysmotility. Many patients also develop ILD (typically nonspecific interstitial pneumonia [NSIP] > usual interstitial pneumonia [UIP] pattern) and pulmonary hypertension. Women are 4 times more likely than men to be affected. Typical presentation is between 30 and 50 years.
        - There are two forms:
            - (1) Limited: skin thickening is distal to the elbows/knees. The face can also be affected. This is associated with centromere antibodies. Patients have a higher risk of pulmonary hypertension and a lower risk of ILD.
            - (2) Diffuse: skin thickening extends proximal to the elbows/knees. This is associated with Scl70 or RNA polymerase III. Patients are at a higher risk of developing ILD (particularly if Scl70+) and SRC (particularly if RNA polymerase III+).
        - *Other complications*: digital ischemia, inflammatory arthritis, GI involvement (GER very common, esophageal dysmotility, constipation, diarrhea, malnutrition, small intestinal bacterial overgrowth [SIBO]), SRC
        - *Evaluation*
            - ANA, RNA polymerase III, Scl70, Th/To, ESR, CRP, CMP, CBC with differential
            - Physical examination to assess skin thickening, nail fold capillaroscopy, telangiectasias, digital pits, or ulcers
            - PFTs, HRCT, and transthoracic echocardiogram (TTE) to evaluate for ILD and pulmonary hypertension
            - Consider barium swallow and esophagogastroduodenoscopy (EGD) for refractory GER, esophageal manometry for esophageal dysmotility.
    - *Treatment:* targeted to specific disease manifestations
        - ILD: mycophenolate, tocilizumab (in early diffuse disease), antifibrotic (eg, nintedanib)
        - Skin thickening: mycophenolate or methotrexate
        - Raynaud/digital ischemia: calcium channel blockers, PDE5i

Sjögren Syndrome

- *Typical presentation:* xerostomia and xerophthalmia (sicca symptoms), dental carries, fatigue, parotid or submandibular swelling. Women are more likely to be affected (~90% of patients are women). Typical presentation is between ages 45 and 55 years. Sjögren can occur secondary to other SARDs (eg, RA, SLE).

- *Other complications:* arthritis, ILD (commonly NSIP, UIP, lymphoid interstitial pneumonia [LIP], or organizing pneumonia), cytopenias, cutaneous vasculitis, lymphoproliferative disorders, cryoglobulinemia, peripheral neuropathies (eg, dorsal root ganglionopathy, small fiber neuropathy, mononeuritis multiplex), tubulointerstitial nephritis
- *Evaluation:* ANA, SSA/SSB, RF, Schirmer test to assess ocular dryness, unstimulated whole saliva flow rate, minor salivary gland biopsy
- *Treatments:* targeted to specific disease manifestations
  - Sicca symptoms: artificial tears, mouth wash/spray, hydration, punctal plugs and other procedures in conjunction with ophthalmology management, muscarinic agonists (eg, cevimeline, pilocarpine), regular dental care (cleanings every 4 months)
  - Arthritis: hydroxychloroquine, methotrexate
  - Peripheral neuropathy: IVIG, rituximab, glucocorticoids

Idiopathic Inflammatory Myopathy

- *Typical presentation:* subacute proximal muscle weakness with elevated muscle enzymes. Dermatomyositis presents with characteristic dermatologic manifestations, including heliotrope rash, photosensitivity, shawl sign, Gottron papules, mechanic's hands, and pruritic scalp rash. Muscle edema on MRI. Polymyositis and dermatomyositis typically present with subacute, painless weakness in a proximal pattern. Inclusion body myositis typically presents with distal predominant weakness. Statin-associated necrotizing immune-mediated myopathy can present more acutely.
- *Other complications:* dysphagia, ILD (can be rapidly progressive), pulmonary hypertension, cardiac involvement (including myocarditis, conduction abnormalities), Raynaud, arthritis, calcinosis cutis, diffuse nonpitting edema (rare). Can be associated with malignancy
- *Differential diagnosis for CK/aldolase elevation*
  - Rheumatologic causes of CK/aldolase elevation due to inflammatory myopathy: polymyositis, dermatomyositis, inclusion body myositis, antisynthetase syndrome, immune-mediated necrotizing myopathy, myositis associated with underlying SARD (eg, SLE, Sjögren, SSc, sarcoidosis)
  - Nonrheumatologic etiologies of elevated CK/aldolase: viral infection, rhabdomyolysis, trauma, immobility, hyperkinetic state (eg, seizure), medications/toxins (eg, statin, colchicine, hydroxychloroquine, alcohol), hypo/hyperthyroidism, adrenal insufficiency, ischemia, electrolyte abnormalities
- *Evaluation*
  - Consider MRI of the affected muscle(s), EMG, muscle biopsy.
  - Myositis panel, ANA, SSA/SSB, HMGCR Ab
  - PFTs, HRCT, TTE (as screening for ILD, pulmonary hypertension)
  - Ensure patient is up to date on age-appropriate malignancy screening; consider enhanced malignancy screening with transvaginal ultrasound (TVUS), CT of the chest/abdomen/pelvis, and tumor markers in certain cases.
- *Treatment:* glucocorticoids, methotrexate, mycophenolate (if evidence of ILD), rituximab, IVIG, calcineurin inhibitor. Topical glucocorticoids for skin changes

Vasculitis

- Systemic vasculitides are characterized into those affecting the small, medium, and large vessels.

Giant Cell Arteritis

- *Typical presentation:* temporal headaches (though other locations are possible), scalp tenderness, jaw claudication, and painless vision changes or loss with elevated inflammatory markers in patients typically over 60. Patients may also have constitutional symptoms (eg, fever, fatigue, weight loss).
  - Patients with polymyalgia rheumatica (PMR) are at increased risk of developing GCA. PMR typically presents with shoulder and hip girdle pain, morning stiffness, and elevated inflammatory markers.
- *Other complications:* large-vessel vasculitis, aortic aneurysm and dissection (aortic arch and its branches and the thoracic aorta are most commonly involved), posterior circulation stroke, tongue or scalp necrosis, anemia
- *Evaluation:* vascular examination (including temporal artery pulses, peripheral pulses, and auscultating for bruits), temporal artery ultrasound, temporal artery biopsy, ophthalmology examination if visual symptoms, and large-vessel imaging (CT angiography, positron emission tomography [PET], or magnetic resonance angiography [MRA]) if diagnosis is confirmed or suspected. Temporal artery biopsy is the gold standard of diagnosis but has low sensitivity (~50%).
- *Treatments:* methylprednisolone 1 g IV daily for 3 days if visual symptoms, followed by prednisone taper. If no vision changes, prednisone 60 mg daily with taper over 6 to 12 months depending on whether glucocorticoid-sparing therapy (eg, tocilizumab) is used

Takayasu Arteritis

- *Typical presentation:* constitutional symptoms (eg, weight loss, fever), arthralgias, limb claudication, hypertension, elevated inflammatory markers. Imaging shows luminal narrowing and arterial wall thickening of the aorta and its branches consistent with large-vessel vasculitis. Women are primarily affected (80%-90% of patients). Typical onset before age 40.
- *Other complications:* angina and myocardial infarction, dyspnea (often related to pulmonary artery involvement), decreased cerebral perfusion (presenting with lightheadedness, syncope, vertigo, strokes), carotidynia, postprandial abdominal pain due to mesenteric artery involvement
- *Evaluation:* thorough vascular examination (including peripheral pulses, evaluation of bruits). Large-vessel imaging of the neck, chest, abdomen, and pelvis (MRA, CTA, or PET/CTA), ESR, CRP. Consider angiography, especially if considering revascularization.
- *Treatments:* glucocorticoids, TNFi, tocilizumab, methotrexate

Antineutrophil Cytoplasmic Antibody–Associated Vasculitis

- *Typical presentation:* upper respiratory (sinusitis, epistaxis, nasal crusting) and lower respiratory involvement (dyspnea, hemoptysis, lung nodules, DAH), glomerulonephritis, fevers, weight loss, arthritis (often migratory), dyspnea, palpable purpura, due to multisystem small-vessel vasculitis. Males and females are equally represented. Typical presentation age is between 40 and 60 years.
  - Granulomatosis with polyangiitis (GPA) and microscopic polyangiitis (MPA) are the two most common forms of ANCA-associated vasculitis and have similar organ involvement. GPA is defined by the presence of granulomas and is more likely to have destructive nasal disease and recurrent disease. 90% of patients are ANCA positive.
  - Eosinophilic granulomatosis with polyangiitis (EGPA): eosinophilia and long-standing asthma often precede vasculitis. Allergic rhinosinusitis, recurrent sinusitis, and nasal polyps are common. Cardiac involvement and peripheral neuropathy are more common than in other forms of ANCA-associated vasculitis. ANCA is positive in only 30% to 40% of cases.
- *Other manifestations:* ophthalmic and orbital involvement (uveitis, conjunctivitis, scleritis, optic neuropathy, retinal vasculitis), can rarely mimic GCA and cause temporal arteritis, subglottic and tracheal stenosis, gingivitis, neurologic involvement (mononeuritis multiplex, cranial nerve involvement, sensorineural hearing loss, meningeal disease, CNS vasculitis), cardiac involvement (pericarditis, myocarditis; most common with EGPA), rarely GI involvement
- *Evaluation:* CMP, CBC with differential, urinalysis, UPCR, ANCA, ANA, ESR, CRP, C3, C4, GBM antibodies (if lung or kidney involvement). Tissue biopsy of the affected organ when possible. CT of the chest for most individuals; imaging of other affected areas as indicated
- *Treatment:* pulsed-dose steroids (ie, 0.5-1 g IV methylprednisolone daily) for life- or organ-threatening disease, followed by high-dose prednisone (~1 mg/kg daily), often with rituximab with or without avacopan for severe disease, or methotrexate for mild or limited disease. Cyclophosphamide has similar efficacy to rituximab but has more potential toxicity. For nonsevere EGPA, can consider anti-IL-5 or IL-5R agents.

Prognosis

Higher illness severity scores at the time of admission are associated with worse outcomes among patients with SARDs admitted to the ICU.

- Greater comorbidity burden and glucocorticoid use prior to admission were associated with poor ICU outcomes.
- Patients with SSc have poorer outcomes than those with other SARDs.
- Most studies have shown that the ICU mortality rate is higher in individuals admitted for infections than for exacerbation of the underlying SARD.
- Overall ICU mortality rate in patients with systemic SARD ranges between 30% and 60% and has been shown to be higher than predicted using APACHE II scores.

Implications of Immunosuppression

- Differing degrees of immunosuppression warrant an individualized decision regarding prophylaxis against atypical infections.
- Level and duration of both neutropenia and lymphopenia can contribute to infectious risk.
- Parenchymal lung disease, glucocorticoid dose, and concomitant immunosuppression contribute to the risk of *Pneumocystis jirovecii* pneumonia. *P. jirovecii* pneumonia prophylaxis is typically recommended in patients who are expected to be on greater than prednisone 20 mg daily for at least 1 month.
- Certain medications (particularly Janus kinase [JAK] inhibitors, IL-6R inhibitors, and anifrolumab) increase the risk of varicella zoster infection.

Congenital (Primary)

- Affects 1 in 500 people
- Over 180 known types of primary immunodeficiency that affect B lymphocytes (X-linked agammaglobulinemia, Bruton), T lymphocytes (DiGeorge), combined B and T lymphocytes (severe combined immunodeficiency [SCID]), phagocytes (Kostmann syndrome), complement system, and others (Wiskott-Aldrich); B-cell deficiencies are the most common.
- Mostly genetic disorders are diagnosed before the first year of age, but milder forms may not be apparent until adulthood.
- Many patients also have inflammatory sequelae (including pulmonary disease, GI disease), atopic diseases, cytopenias, lymphoproliferative disorders, and other autoimmune diseases (eg, SLE, type 1 diabetes).
- *Diagnosis:* full blood count (lymphocyte and granulocyte) and immunoglobulin levels (IgG, IgA, and IgM)
  - Other tests depend on suspected disorders: CD counts, B lymphocytes, natural killer cells, delayed-type skin hypersensitivity (tests for T-cell function), antibodies to routine immunizations or commonly acquired infections (test for B-cell function), reduction of nitro blue tetrazolium chloride (tests for phagocytic function)
- *Management and treatment:* depends on the abnormality
  - This may include immunoglobulin replacement therapy in Ab deficiencies to hematopoietic stem cell transplantation for SCID and other severe deficiencies.
  - Genetic testing may reveal targeted therapy (eg, recombinant cytotoxic T-lymphocyte antigen 4 [CTLA4] in patients with CTLA4 mutations).
  - Prophylactic antimicrobials in an individualized manner. Treatment is targeted to specific defects.

Acquired (Secondary)

- Etiologies include HIV causing acquired immunodeficiency syndrome (AIDS), cytotoxic or immunosuppressive agents (eg, chemotherapy, glucocorticoids, biologic, targeted synthetic, or conventional synthetic disease-modifying antirheumatic drugs [csDMARDs]), malnutrition, increasing age, malignancy (eg, leukemia, lymphoma, multiple myeloma), chronic infections

Immunomodulatory Drugs

- Hematologic and hepatic toxicity are common with drugs used in the treatment of autoimmune disorders.
- Disease-modifying drugs have to be discontinued in 5% to 10% of patients because of blood dyscrasias and cytopenias.

General Considerations for Management of Immunosuppression in the Intensive Care Unit

- Most immunomodulatory drugs, except for hydroxychloroquine and sulfasalazine, should be held in the setting of infection or concern for infection.
  - If SARD is acutely organ or life-threatening, a multidisciplinary decision should be made regarding continuing versus holding immunosuppression.
- Glucocorticoids should not be stopped abruptly in patients who have been on therapy for >3 to 4 weeks as this could trigger an adrenal crisis; doses can often be reduced if needed.
- TB testing, HCV Ab, and HBV serologies (core Ab, surface Ab, surface antigen) should be performed prior to starting most immunosuppressive medications.

Glucocorticoids

- *Mechanism of action:* downregulate lymphocyte and macrophage function, upregulate collagenase function, interfere with inflammatory responses.
- *Acute effects*: infections (*P. jirovecii* pneumonia, molds, mycobacterial, CMV), poor wound healing, behavioral changes, gastritis/ulceration, bruising, hyperglycemia
- *Chronic effects*: atypical infections, osteoporosis, osteonecrosis, adrenal insufficiency, hypertension, skin thinning
- Adrenal insufficiency may present with severe hypotension, electrolyte disturbances, fevers, nausea, and vomiting.
  - At-risk patients: on <5 mg of prednisone who have been on prednisone for >3 weeks or patients with prolonged glucocorticoid exposure in the last year
  - Consider "sick dose" steroid dosing for patients with febrile illness or other stressor on <10 mg prednisone; consider increasing to 3 times typical dose for several days to prevent adrenal insufficiency. There are varying practice patterns.
  - For patients who are hypotensive or critically ill, consider "stress dose" steroids (eg, hydrocortisone 100 mg IV followed by 25-75 mg every 6 hours).
- To mitigate bruising and wound healing issues with steroid use postsurgically, can consider 25,000 units of vitamin A daily for 3 days, which downregulates the collagenase activation by steroids.
- *Clearance:* metabolized mainly in the liver

Conventional Synthetic Disease-Modifying Antirheumatic Drugs

Hydroxychloroquine

- *Mechanism of action*: originally an antimalarial drug. Blocks the activation of Toll-like receptors on plasmacytoid dendritic cells that reduce the activation of dendritic cells, therefore mitigating the inflammatory process
- *Common indications*: SLE, RA, Sjögren, and other SARDs. It reduces flares and complications and increases survival in patients with SLE.
- *Side effects:* nausea, diarrhea, skin rash, bone marrow suppression, agranulocytosis, retinopathy (requires an annual eye examination)
  - It can also worsen existing psoriasis and porphyria.
- *Clearance:* kidney
- *Typical dosing:* oral, daily to a maximum of 5 mg/kg

Methotrexate

- *Mechanism of action:* inhibits DNA synthesis; antiinflammatory component occurs by inhibition of T-cell activation.
- *Common indications*: first-line therapy for RA; used in inflammatory myositis/dermatomyositis, SLE, Takayasu arteritis, psoriasis, psoriatic arthritis, SSc
- *Side effects:* hepatotoxicity, cytopenias, pneumonitis, oral ulcers, hair thinning, GI upset
  - Absolutely contraindicated in pregnancy due to the risk of miscarriage and fetal malformation
- *Clearance:* biliary and renal
- *Typical dosing:* oral or subcutaneous injection, 15 to 25 mg once weekly; should be taken with folic acid 1 mg daily to limit toxicity

Mycophenolate Mofetil

- *Mechanism of action:* inhibits T- and B-cell proliferation by depletion of guanosine nucleotides
- *Common indications*: connective tissue disease (CTD)-associated ILD, SLE, inflammatory polymyositis/dermatomyositis, SSc
- *Side effects*: abdominal pain, diarrhea, nausea, cytopenias, rash
  - Mycophenolic acid is an alternative. Many patients tolerate this formulation with fewer GI side effects.
  - Absolutely contraindicated in pregnancy due to the risk of fetal malformation
- *Clearance:* hepatic
- *Typical dosing:* oral, titrate up to 2 to 3 g daily over a divided dose

Azathioprine

- *Mechanism of action*: purine analog (antimetabolite) that interferes with DNA synthesis
- *Common Indications*: SLE, inflammatory polymyositis/dermatomyositis, CTD-associated ILD
  - Can be used in pregnancy
- *Side effects:* nausea, vomiting, diarrhea, skin rashes, acute pancreatitis, hepatotoxicity, bone marrow suppression (can be life-threatening with genetic deficiency of thiopurine S-methyltransferase). A thiopurine methyltransferase (TPMT) level should be checked prior to initiation.
- *Clearance*: renal
- *Typical dosing*: oral, titrate up to 1 to 2.5 mg/kg daily

Sulfasalazine

- *Mechanism of action*: sulfasalazine and its metabolite 5-ASA are poorly absorbed in the gut.
  - *Common indications*: can be used in mild or oligoarticular arthritis or tenosynovitis in patients with RA and psoriatic arthritis

- *Side effects*: nausea, skin rash, thrombocytopenia, megaloblastic anemia, Stevens-Johnson syndrome, depression, reduced male fertility due to oligospermia, aplastic anemia, and neutropenia. A G6PD level should be checked prior to initiation.
  - Sulfasalazine is not thought to increase the risk of infection.
- *Clearance*: fecal
- *Typical dosing*: oral. Increase in 500 mg increments to 2 to 3 g/d in divided twice-daily dosing

Cyclophosphamide

- *Mechanism of action*: metabolite phosphoramide mustard forms DNA cross-links between and within DNA strands, which are irreversible and lead to apoptosis.
- *Common indications*: severe complications of SLE (neurologic or kidney disease), SSc, ANCA-associated vasculitis
- *Side effects:* acute myeloid leukemia, bladder cancer, permanent infertility, prompt fluid retention, severe hemorrhagic cystitis, cardiac toxicity, liver toxicity, and bone marrow toxicity
  - When administering IV, hydration and administration of mesna can help prevent the risk of hemorrhagic cystitis.
- *Clearance:* renal
- *Typical dosing:* IV or oral, dosing varies by indication and protocol.

Calcineurin Inhibitors (Tacrolimus [FK506], Cyclosporin, and Voclosporin)

- *Mechanism of action*: bind to the cytosolic protein cyclophilin of lymphocytes (especially T cells)
  - This cyclosporine/cyclophilin complex inhibits calcineurin, which is usually responsible for the activation of transcription of IL-2, which leads to inhibition of effector T cells.
  - *Common indications:* SLE nephritis, myositis-associated ILD
- *Side effects*: infections (viral, bacterial, and fungal), hirsutism, neurotoxicity, hyperkalemia, nephrotoxicity, hypertension, and tremors
- *clearance*: mainly in bile (fecal), some renal

Biologic Disease-Modifying Antirheumatic Drugs

Tumor Necrosis Factor-Alpha Inhibitors

- Includes etanercept, infliximab, adalimumab, certolizumab, and golimumab
- *Mechanism of action:* inhibit TNF-α, which is implicated in many forms of inflammation and is an end-stage product of the inflammatory cytokine cascade
- *Common indications:* RA, psoriatic arthritis, ankylosing spondylitis, Takayasu arteritis, sarcoidosis
- *Side effects*: neutropenia, heart failure, demyelinating disease, skin cancer, induction of drug-induced lupus, injection site reactions
  - These medications are associated with a higher occurrence of both typical and atypical infections, including reactivation of latent and miliary TB, listeriosis meningoencephalitis or septicemia, disseminated fungal disease, reactivation of hepatitis B, and herpes zoster infections
  - Live vaccination should be avoided.
- *Typical dosing*: depends on specific drug; IV and subcutaneous formulations dosed every 1 to 4 weeks depending on the medication

CD20 Inhibitors

- Includes rituximab, obinutuzumab, ocrelizumab
- *Mechanism of action:* a monoclonal Ab depletes CD20-expressing B cells
- *Common indications:* ANCA-associated vasculitis, IgG4-related disease, RA, CTD-associated ILD
- *Side effects:* infusion reaction, increased risk of infection (particularly severe coronavirus disease 2019 [COVID-19] infection, HBV reactivation), hypogammaglobulinemia, neutropenia
  - Patients have a blunted response to vaccination after rituximab, so it is important to administer all necessary vaccines 2 to 4 weeks before dosing rituximab when not urgent.
  - Consider preexposure prophylaxis for COVID-19 infection when available.
- *Typical dosing*: IV; loading dose: 1 g at 0 and 14 days followed by 1 g IV every 4 to 6 months, or weekly weight-based IV dosing

IL-6R Inhibitors

- Includes tocilizumab, sarilumab
- *Mechanism of action*: a monoclonal Ab inhibits IL-6R signaling
- *Common indications:* GCA, SSc ILD, RA, Takayasu arteritis
- *Side effects:* cytopenias, liver injury, rare increased risk of GI perforation, zoster infection
  - Patients with a history of diverticulitis should not be treated with tocilizumab due to rare risk of GI perforation.
- *Typical dosing*: subcutaneous injection (162 mg) weekly or every other week or IV monthly

SUGGESTED READINGS

Abbas AK, Lichtman AH, Pillai S. *Cellular and Molecular Immunology*. 10th ed. Elsevier; 2022.

Aggarwal R, Charles-Schoeman C, Schessl J, et al. Trial of intravenous immune globulin in dermatomyositis. *N Engl J Med*. 2022;387(14):1264-1278.

Auyezkhankyzy D, Izekenova A, Kocyigit BF. Emergencies in inflammatory rheumatic diseases. *Rheumatol Int*. 2024;44(9):1637-1646.

Boyle N, O'Callaghan M, Ataya A, et al. Pulmonary renal syndrome: a clinical review. *Breathe (Sheff)*. 2022;18(4):220208.

Dumas G, Arabi YM, Bartz R, et al. Diagnosis and management of autoimmune diseases in the ICU. *Intensive Care Med*. 2024;50(1):17-35.

Fraenkel L, Bathon JM, England BR, et al. 2021 American College of Rheumatology guideline for the treatment of rheumatoid arthritis. *Arthritis Rheumatol*. 2021;73(7):1108-1123.

Furie R, Rovin BH, Houssiau F, et al. Two-year, randomized, controlled trial of belimumab in lupus nephritis. *N Engl J Med*. 2020;383(12):1117-1128.

Gron KL, Arkema EV, Glintborg B, et al. Risk of serious infections in patients with rheumatoid arthritis treated in routine care with abatacept, rituximab and tocilizumab in Denmark and Sweden. *Ann Rheum Dis*. 2019;78(3):320-327.

Gutierrez-Gonzalez LA. Rheumatologic emergencies. *Clin Rheumatol*. 2015;34(12):2011-2019.

Janssen NM, Karnad DR, Guntupalli KK. Rheumatologic diseases in the intensive care unit: epidemiology, clinical approach, management, and outcome. *Crit Care Clin*. 2002;18(4):729-748.

Jayne DRW, Merkel PA, Schall TJ, Bekker P; ADVOCATE Study Group. Avacopan for the treatment of ANCA-associated vasculitis. *N Engl J Med*. 2021;384(7):599-609.

Johnson SR, Bernstein EJ, Bolster MB, et al. 2023 American College of Rheumatology (ACR)/American College of Chest Physicians (CHEST) guideline for the screening and monitoring of interstitial lung disease in people with systemic autoimmune rheumatic diseases. *Arthritis Care Res (Hoboken)*. 2024;76(8):1070-1082.

Johnson SR, Bernstein EJ, Bolster MB, et al. 2023 American College of Rheumatology (ACR)/American College of Chest Physicians (CHEST) guideline for the treatment of interstitial lung disease in people with systemic autoimmune rheumatic diseases. *Arthritis Rheumatol*. 2024; 76(8):1182-1200.

Khanna D, Lin CJF, Furst DE, et al. Tocilizumab in systemic sclerosis: a randomised, double-blind, placebo-controlled, phase 3 trial. *Lancet Respir Med*. 2020;8(10):963-974.

Lu X, Peng Q, Wang G. Anti-MDA5 antibody-positive dermatomyositis: pathogenesis and clinical progress. *Nat Rev Rheumatol*. 2024;20(1):48-62.

Martinez-Martinez MU, Oostdam DAH, Abud-Mendoza C. Diffuse alveolar hemorrhage in autoimmune diseases. *Curr Rheumatol Rep*. 2017;19(5):27.

Patel NJ, D'Silva KM, Hsu TY, et al. Coronavirus disease 2019 outcomes among recipients of anti-CD20 monoclonal antibodies for immune-mediated diseases: a comparative cohort study. *ACR Open Rheumatol*. 2022;4(3):238-246.

Rodriguez-Pinto I, Espinosa G, Erkan D, Shoenfeld Y, Cervera R; CAPS Registry Project Group. The effect of triple therapy on the mortality of catastrophic anti-phospholipid syndrome patients. *Rheumatology (Oxford)*. 2018;57(7):1264-1270.

Rovin BH, Teng YKO, Ginzler EM, et al. Efficacy and safety of voclosporin versus placebo for lupus nephritis (AURORA 1): a double-blind, randomised, multicentre, placebo-controlled, phase 3 trial. *Lancet*. 2021; 397(10289):2070-2080.

Schneeweiss-Gleixner M, Hillebrand C, Jaksits S, et al. Characteristics and outcome of critically ill patients with systemic rheumatic diseases referred to the intensive care unit. *RMD Open*. 2023;9(4):e003287.

Schwartz N, Stock AD, Putterman C. Neuropsychiatric lupus: new mechanistic insights and future treatment directions. *Nat Rev Rheumatol*. 2019; 15(3):137-152.

Shakoory B, Geerlinks A, Wilejto M, et al. The 2022 EULAR/ACR points to consider at the early stages of diagnosis and management of suspected haemophagocytic lymphohistiocytosis/macrophage activation syndrome (HLH/MAS). *Ann Rheum Dis*. 2023;82(10):1271-1285.

Stone JH, Tuckwell K, Dimonaco S, et al. Trial of tocilizumab in giant-cell arteritis. *N Engl J Med*. 2017;377(4):317-328.

Walsh M, Merkel PA, Peh CA, et al. Plasma exchange and glucocorticoids in severe ANCA-associated vasculitis. *N Engl J Med*. 2020;382(7):622-631.

Woodworth TG, Suliman YA, Li W, Furst DE, Clements P. Scleroderma renal crisis and renal involvement in systemic sclerosis. *Nat Rev Nephrol*. 2016;12(11):678-691.

SECTION 11

Dermatology

Section Editor: Edward A. Bittner

11.1

Dermatologic Conditions

John A. Helmstetter and Richard M. Pino

- Dermatologic conditions requiring intensive care are rare, representing 0.47% of all intensive care unit (ICU) admissions.
- Mortality is high, with a rate of 28.1% in the ICU and 40% overall in-hospital.
- Several dermatologic conditions, ranging from mild to life-threatening, should be recognizable and treatable by the ICU physician.

Stevens-Johnson Syndrome and Toxic Epidermal Necrolysis

Epidemiology

- Rare, affecting ~5 to 6/1,000,000 annually
- More common in females, 2:1 ratio

Key Pathophysiology

- Severe cutaneous drug reactions predominantly involving the skin and mucous membranes
- Stephens-Johnson syndrome (SJS) and toxic epidermal necrolysis (TEN) are two ends of a spectrum.
  - SJS <10% of body surface area (BSA) involved
  - SJS/TEN 10% to 30% BSA involved
  - TEN >30% BSA involved
- Characterized by mucocutaneous tenderness and typically hemorrhagic erosions, erythema, and epidermal detachment from the underlying dermis, presenting as blisters and denuded skin
- Several drugs are considered "high risk" for inducing SJS/TEN, including lamotrigine, allopurinol, aromatic anticonvulsants, sulfonamides, and COX-2 inhibitors.

Management and Treatment

- Treatment consists of supportive care.
- Debridement is unnecessary as blistered skin acts as a natural biologic dressing promoting reepithelialization.
- No specific drug therapy has shown efficacy in controlled clinical trials.
- Potential benefit from treatment with systemic corticosteroids, etanercept, cyclosporine, or a combination of intravenous immunoglobulin (IVIG) and systemic corticosteroids

Outcomes

- High risk of mortality: SJS 10%, TEN 30%.

Cellulitis

Key Pathophysiology

- Acute, spreading pyogenic inflammation of the dermis and subcutaneous tissue
- Due to rapidly progressive nature, can cause severe illness
- Area affected is usually tender, warm, erythematous, and swollen.
- Several anatomic and causal variants exist and must be determined to help guide accurate treatment.
- The likely bacterial causes include *Streptococcus*, *Staphylococcus aureus*, and *Enterococcus*; less often Enterobacteriaceae and *Haemophilus influenzae*.

Management and Treatment

- Initial empirical antibiotic treatment for severe nonpurulent infection consists of vancomycin plus piperacillin/tazobactam.
- Severe infections require surgical inspection/debridement.
- Mild infection can be treated with oral antibiotics, and moderate with IV penicillin, ceftriaxone, or clindamycin.

Necrotizing Soft Tissue Infections

Epidemiology

- Incidence of 8 to 10 per 1,000,000 annually

Key Pathophysiology

- Highly variable presentation, from skin/subcutaneous necrosis to septic shock
- Visible area of infection may not represent underlying necrosis in muscle and fascia. Infection type is categorized by either location, depth of involvement, or microbial source (most common).
- Type 1—polymicrobial, constitutes 55% to 75% of infections
  - Mix of aerobes and anaerobes, most commonly bacteroides, *Clostridium*, or peptostreptococcus in combination with *Escherichia coli*, *Enterobacter*, *Klebsiella*, or *Proteus*.
  - Risk factors include diabetes, vascular disease, obesity, renal insufficiency, HIV, alcohol abuse.
- Type 2—monobacterial, usually group A *Streptococcus* as well as beta-hemolytic streptococci. Less commonly *S. aureus*
  - Occurs in any age group and without predisposing conditions
  - Risk factors include trauma, intravenous drug use (IVDU), surgery, childbirth.
- Clostridial myonecrosis—gas gangrene that leads to life-threatening muscle infection, most commonly caused by *Clostridium perfringens* and *Clostridium septicum*
  - Occurs due to trauma or hematogenously from the gastrointestinal (GI) tract to muscle
  - *Clostridium* toxin release causes hemolysis, thrombosis, myonecrosis, and cardiovascular collapse.

Management and Treatment

- Surgical emergency, with early diagnosis critical, imaging studies should never delay surgical exploration.
- Broad-spectrum antibiotic therapy, including a carbapenem or piperacillin-tazobactam plus clindamycin as well as vancomycin
- Aggressive supportive care. May have high IV fluid and vasopressor requirements
- Hyperbaric oxygen therapy is controversial.

Outcomes

- Mortality rate ranges from 14% to 40%.

Other Skin Diseases

- *Contact dermatitis*
  - Red rash or bumps that can progress to fluid-filled blisters
  - Allergens include soaps, adhesives, rubber, and plant life (ie, poison ivy).
  - Diagnosed based on localized dermatitis in a patient with a history of exposure to irritants
  - Treatment consists of thoroughly washing with water, avoiding further contact with allergens, and the use of moisturizers and, occasionally, corticosteroid creams.
- *Atopic dermatitis*
  - Erythema, dry skin, excoriation, and severe pruritus
  - More commonly seen in young children but also seen in adults
  - Often appears in skin folds of elbows and behind knees.
  - Treatment is generally the same as for contact dermatitis.
- *Urticaria (hives)*
  - Itchy rash consisting of raised red bumps of various shapes and sizes
  - Acute urticaria is present for <6 weeks, may progress to chronic urticaria.
    - >2/3 acute cases are self-limited.
  - Often accompanied by angioedema: swelling of the lips, eyes, tongue, hands, and feet (CAUTION: possible airway compromise)
  - Pathogenesis is mast cell release of histamine and other cytokines, usually mediated through immunoglobulin E (IgE).
  - Most common causes include reactions to medications, foods, insect stings, and bites.
  - Treatment involves antihistamines, corticosteroids, and, if necessary, epinephrine, which not only provides cardiovascular support but also stabilizes mast cells.
- *Systemic lupus erythematosus (SLE)*
  - Long-term autoimmune disorder leading to inflammation of the skin, joints, kidneys, brain, and other organs
  - Characteristic "butterfly" rash over the cheeks and bridge of nose affects about half of the people with SLE.
  - Discoid skin rash and photosensitivity rash can also occur.
  - Cause of SLE is unknown, with increased risk after exposure to some medications.
    - High-risk drugs include procainamide and hydralazine.
    - Moderate-risk drugs include quinidine.
    - Low-risk drugs include methyldopa, isoniazid, and many others.
  - Treatment consists of hydroxychloroquine, oral steroids, and corticosteroid creams.
- *Scleroderma*
  - Autoimmune connective tissue disease with progressive fibrosis of internal organs and skin as well as vascular dysfunction
  - Skin manifestations include Raynaud phenomenon, hair loss, skin hardness, and thickening of skin around fingers, hands, and forearms, among others.
  - Treatment includes systemic immunosuppressive therapy, topical emollients, antihistamines, and topical capsaicin.

SUGGESTED READINGS

Bruun T, Rath E, Madsen MB, et al; INFECT Study Group. Risk factors and predictors of mortality in streptococcal necrotizing soft-tissue infections: a multicenter prospective study. *Clin Infect Dis*. 2021;72:293-300.

Charlton OA, Harris V, Phan K, Mewton E, Jackson C, Cooper A. Toxic epidermal necrolysis and Steven-Johnson syndrome: a comprehensive review. *Adv Wound Care*. 2020;9:426-439.

May AK, Talisa VB, Wilfret DA, et al. Estimating the impact of necrotizing soft tissue infections in the United States: incidence and re-admissions. *Surg Infect*. 2021;22:509-515.

Shields BE, Wanat KA, Chiu YE. Undiagnosed and rare diseases in critical care: severe mucocutaneous medication reactions. *Crit Care Clin*. 2022;38:243-269.

Soutor C, Hordinsky M. *Clinical Dermatology: Diagnosis and Management of Common Disorders*. 2nd ed. McGraw Hill; 2022.

Stevens DL, Bisno AL, Chambers HF, et al. Practice guidelines for the diagnosis and management of skin and soft tissue infections: 2014 update by the Infectious Diseases Society of America. *Clin Infect Dis*. 2014;59:147-159.

SECTION 12

Thermoregulation

Section Editor: Edward A. Bittner

12.1

Fever

Jay Saggu and Christoph G.S. Nabzdyk

Definition

- Fever or pyrexia is a phylogenetically preserved response to a variety of infectious and noninfectious triggers, which induce an upregulation of the thermostatic set point, resulting in an elevated body temperature.
- Hyperthermia, in contrast to fever, occurs when heat production or absorption overwhelms the body's ability to dissipate heat, resulting in an elevated temperature. Hyperthermic syndromes include thyroid storm, neuroleptic malignant syndrome, malignant hyperthermia, serotonin syndrome, and heat stroke.
- The Society of Critical Care Medicine and the Infectious Disease Society of America define fever as a temperature ≥38.3 °C and >39.5 °C as high fever. Lower temperature thresholds are applied in immunocompromised, neutropenic, or older patients; patients on scheduled antipyretics; or patients on extracorporeal membranous oxygenation (ECMO) or continuous renal replacement therapy (CRRT) devices.
- The incidence of fever in the intensive care unit (ICU) ranges from 23% to 70% with an infectious etiology in 40% to 50% of cases and is associated with significant morbidity and mortality. In a retrospective cohort of 24,204 ICU patients, high fevers defined as temperatures >39.5 °C were associated with a significantly increased risk of death (20.3% vs. 12%, $P < .0001$).
- In patients who are neutropenic, defined as an absolute neutrophil count of <500 cells/μL, temperature threshold ≥38.0 °C sustained over 1 hour or recurrent over 12 hours or a single temperature >38.3 °C is generally accepted as fever. In the absence of a definitive noninfectious cause, this should be regarded as a sign of infection and treated accordingly.
- Maximum temperature and pattern of temperature changes can yield valuable information. Temperatures >41 °C are less commonly infectious and concerning for hyperthermic syndromes.
- Central temperature measurements (pulmonary artery catheters thermistor, esophageal temperature probes, and bladder thermistors) are preferred to axillary, surface, or chemical dot thermometers. Oral or rectal measurements can be used when central measurements are unavailable.

Pathophysiology

- Several different mechanisms likely result in the febrile response. Classically, in infection-triggered fever, pathogen-associated molecular patterns (PAMPs) stimulate leukocytes to produce cytokines, including interleukin-1 (IL-1), tumor necrosis factor-alpha, and IL-6, which function as endogenous pyrogens. Endogenous pyrogens activate the febrile response by inducing prostaglandin E2 (PGE2) synthesis in the organum vasculosum of the lamina terminalis surrounded by the medial and lateral preoptic hypothalamic nuclei. PGE2 production alters temperature-sensitive neuron firing, resulting in higher body temperature. Table 12.1.1 lists some common infectious causes of ICU fever.

TABLE 12.1.1 Common Infectious Etiology

Cardiovascular: Endocarditis, pacemaker infections, viral pericarditis or myocarditis	**Renal:** Urinary tract infection, cystitis, pyelonephritis	**Gastrointestinal:** Viral hepatitis, colitis, biliary infection, abdominal abscess, diverticulitis, cholecystitis, ischemic colitis, cholangitis, abscess
Respiratory: Pneumonia, empyema, sinusitis, tracheobronchitis	**Skin:** Cellulitis, decubitus ulcer infection, surgical site or wound infection, abscess	**CNS:** Discitis, meningitis, encephalitis, abscess
Musculoskeletal: Osteomyelitis, septic arthritis, necrotizing soft tissue infections, gangrene	**Heme:** Catheter-related bloodstream infection, bacteremia	

CNS, central nervous system.

- Trauma and sterile inflammation can lead to the occurrence of damage-associated molecular patterns (DAMPs), a heterogeneous group of molecules (eg, DNA, RNA, histones, ATP), which are from damaged cells. DAMPs, like PAMPs, can trigger a systemic inflammatory response, including fever. Table 12.1.2 lists some common noninfectious causes of ICU fever.
- Certain medications can trigger a fever. Table 12.1.3 lists medications associated with a fever response.
- This rise in temperature is balanced by cryogens, such as IL-10, alpha-melanocyte–stimulating hormone, corticotropin, neuropeptide Y, and bombesin. Cryogens increase heat loss and inhibit the heat-generating response.
- Fever is recognized as a component of the host response to infection, leading to reduced bacterial growth, enhanced synthesis of antibodies and cytokines, and activation of neutrophils, macrophages, and T lymphocytes.
- Fever increases metabolic rate, minute ventilation, and oxygen consumption and may exacerbate tissue hypoxia in patients with poor cardiopulmonary reserve and in patients with neurologic insults.
- The effect of hyperthermia and fever has been widely studied in the literature with evolving evidence in postcardiac arrest hypoxic ischemic brain injury. Fever or hyperthermia in this setting may exacerbate local neural injury by disrupting the blood-brain barrier, increasing cerebral metabolism, increasing intracellular calcium influx, augmenting neuronal excitotoxicity, increasing free radical species, reducing cytoskeletal stability, and disrupting cerebral autoregulation. These changes may exacerbate cerebral edema through impaired cerebral perfusion and worsened ischemic injury. In comparison to earlier clinical trials, which investigated therapeutic hypothermia, recent trials have focused on maintaining normothermia in postcardiac arrest patients. The recent Targeted Temperature Management 2 (TTM2) Trial randomized 1,850 patients with coma after out-of-hospital cardiac arrest to targeted hypothermia (33 °C) or normothermia (≤37.5 °C). The investigators found no difference at 6 months in mortality or modified Rankin Scale ≥4 between the two groups. Most current guidelines recommend avoiding hyperthermia and maintaining temperatures <37.5 °C to 37.7 °C postcardiac arrest for at least 72 hours after return of spontaneous circulation.

TABLE 12.1.3 Common Medications Associated With Fever

Type	Medication
Antibiotics	Beta-lactams, sulfonamides, nitrofurantoin
Antiarrhythmics	Procainamide, quinidine
Antiepileptics	Phenytoin, carbamazepine
Sedatives	Dexmedetomidine, barbiturates
Sulfa containing	Loop diuretics, stool softeners

- Patients with other forms of neurologic injury, including subarachnoid hemorrhage (SAH), intracerebral hemorrhage (ICH), acute ischemic stroke (AIS), traumatic brain injury (TBI), and global ischemic injury, can be negatively impacted by fever or hyperthermia. Maintenance of normothermia and aggressive correction of fever or hyperthermia is recommended. Experts agree to target a temperature around 37.0 °C ± 0.5 °C for patients with ICH, SAH, or AIS who develop neurogenic fever. For patients with severe TBI, hyperthermia and fever should be avoided with targeted normothermia 36.0 °C to 37.5 °C as a goal unless hypothermia is required for intracranial pressure management.

Workup of Fever in the Intensive Care Unit

- Workup of a new fever includes a focused history and physical as well as laboratory, microbiologic, and imaging studies. Both noninfectious and infectious causes should be considered. In the critically ill patient with fever, infectious etiologies should be ruled out as early treatment is associated with improved outcomes.
- Commonly observed infections in the ICU include urinary tract infection (UTI), respiratory tract infections, septicemia, skin and soft tissue infections (SSTIs), vascular catheter-associated bloodstream infections, and wound infections.
- Underlying conditions of the patient, including their procedural history, presence of invasive intravascular lines and monitors, indwelling Foley catheters and immunocompetence, should be thoroughly investigated.

TABLE 12.1.2 Noninfectious Causes of Fever in the ICU Patients

Malignancy: Lymphoma, hepatocellular cancer, renal cell carcinoma	**Noninfectious pulmonary inflammation:** Fibroproliferative ARDS, organizing pneumonia, aspiration pneumonitis	**Neurogenic Fever:** Intracranial hemorrhage, traumatic brain injury, stroke, anti-NMDA receptor encephalitis	**Withdrawal:** Substances include alcohol, opiates, barbiturates, benzodiazepines
Cardiac: Acute myocardial infarction, pericarditis	**Rheumatologic:** Gout, vasculitis, systemic lupus erythematosus, rheumatoid arthritis, Goodpasture syndrome	Venous thrombosis, fat emboli	Acute postoperative state
Pulmonary: Atelectasis, pulmonary embolism, ARDS	**Hepatobiliary and gastrointestinal:** Acalculous cholecystitis, acute pancreatitis, active Crohn disease, toxic megacolon, alcoholic hepatitis, pancreatitis	**Endocrine:** Hyperthyroidism, adrenal insufficiency, pheochromocytoma	**Immune system:** Immune reconstitution inflammatory syndrome, Tumor lysis syndrome, transplant rejection
Medications: Drug fever	Nonconvulsive status epilepticus	**Heme:** Blood production transfusion	

ARDS, acute respiratory distress syndrome; ICU, intensive care unit.

- Postoperative patients are at risk for SSTIs, *Clostridium difficile* colitis, intravascular line–associated bloodstream infections, and catheter-associated urinary tract infections(CAUTI). Postoperative neurosurgical patients are additionally at risk for ventriculitis and meningitis. Importantly, arterial vascular catheters are often an underrecognized source of infections and should be evaluated regularly.
- Presence of diarrhea, abdominal tenderness, purulent drainage, and standard markers of inflammation (rubor, tumor, calor, and dolor) can aid the clinician in evaluating sources of infection. Respiratory dynamics, gas exchange, secretion burden, imaging, and physical lung examination are vital in evaluating for a respiratory tract infection. In postsurgical patients, it is essential to examine surgical sites for signs of infection. Additionally, a thorough evaluation of decubitus ulcers is crucial, as they may serve as a potential source of infection.
- Laboratory studies such as complete blood counts, markers of inflammation (procalcitonin, erythrocyte sedimentation rate, C-reactive protein), and organ function (creatinine, electrolytes, blood urea, liver function tests, alkaline phosphatase) can yield valuable diagnostic information. Depending on the risk factors, thyroid and adrenal function tests and hemolysis studies can be considered. Lumbar puncture and neuroimaging should be considered for at-risk patients (eg, neurosurgical) with signs and symptoms of central nervous system infections.
- For patients who have recently had thoracic, abdominal, or pelvic surgery, computed tomography (CT) scans are recommended if the initial assessment does not reveal the cause of the fever. Additional imaging studies like chest radiographs, abdominal, thoracic, and extremity ultrasounds can assist in pinpointing the origin and may be indicated based on the patient's history and physical examination. If workup remains inconclusive, advanced imaging studies such as 18F-fluorodeoxyglucose positron emission tomography/CT may be considered.
- Microbiologic investigations are often necessary and should be guided by history and evaluation of the patient as false-positive rates can be high. Investigations include respiratory cultures, blood cultures, and urine cultures. Two sets of blood cultures from two different sites collected consecutively, of at least 60 mL total, yield the most reasonable data. In patients with pyuria with suspected UTI and an indwelling Foley catheter, the catheter should be replaced, and urine analysis and reflex culture sent from the new Foley catheter. Testing for viral pathogens using viral nucleic acid amplification tests should be considered for patients with new respiratory symptoms alongside standard Gram stain and culture. Certain pathogens, such as severe acute respiratory syndrome coronavirus 2 (SARS-CoV-2) and influenza, may only be detected in samples from the lower respiratory tract.
- *Escherichia coli*, *Staphylococcus aureus,* and *Streptococcus pneumoniae* are common pathogens in patients admitted to the ICU with community-acquired bloodstream infections. *S. aureus, E. coli,* and *Enterococcus faecalis* are important pathogens in hospital-acquired bloodstream infections. Coagulase-negative staphylococci are most associated with catheter-related bloodstream infections; however, *S. aureus*, Enterobacteriaceae, and enterococcal have also been implicated.
- SSTIs encompass a wide range from more benign infections like impetigo to potentially fatal necrotizing SSTIs. *S. aureus* and streptococci are most implicated in SSTIs. Burn patients are at a high risk for *Pseudomonas* spp. infections. Bacteremia caused by *S. aureus*, group A streptococci, *Neisseria meningitidis*, and *Pseudomonas aeruginosa* may have cutaneous manifestations. *Candida*, herpes simplex, and zoster infection; impetigo; and folliculitis are common in transplant recipients. Necrotizing soft tissue infections (NSTIs) have high morbidity and mortality and often require emergent surgical debridement. *Streptococcus pyogenes* and *S. aureus* are implicated in monomicrobial infections, type II NSTI. The etiology of polymicrobial NSTIs, type I NSTI, varies anatomically, with *E. coli, Pseudomonas* spp., and *Bacteroides* spp. being frequently implicated. *Vibrio* spp. are common in type III, Gram-negative monomicrobial NSTI. Type IV NSTI, or fungal NSTI, pathogens include *Candida* as well as *Mucor* and *Rhizopus* spp. In a multicenter retrospective cohort study of patients admitted for surgically confirmed NSTI, *Streptococcal* spp., *Staphylococcus* spp., *Pseudomonas* spp., and *E. coli* were the most frequently cultured species. In a similar study of 41 consecutive Fournier gangrene cases, *Bacteroides* spp., *E. coli,* and *Prevotella* spp. were the most common pathogens cultured.
- Central nervous system infections carry a mortality rate of around 30% and frequently result in long-lasting neurologic impairments. Meningitis in adults is often caused by *S. pneumoniae* and *N. meningitidis*. *Listeria monocytogenes* is more prevalent among adults aged 60 years and above. Herpes simplex virus (HSV) and varicella zoster virus (VZV) are common viral culprits of meningitis and encephalitis. In individuals with human immunodeficiency virus (HIV) infection, conditions such as HIV encephalitis, cerebral toxoplasmosis, tuberculous meningitis, cryptococcal meningitis, and progressive multifocal leukoencephalopathy (PML) should additionally be considered.
- Organisms commonly associated with community-acquired pneumonia include *S. pneumoniae*, *Haemophilus influenzae*, *Mycoplasma pneumoniae*, *Legionella* spp., *Chlamydia pneumoniae*, and *Moraxella catarrhalis*. Risk factors for health care–associated pneumonia encompass recent hospitalization, residency in a health care facility, hemodialysis, recent intravenous antibiotic therapy, chemotherapy, or wound care. Polymicrobial pneumonia often involves methicillin-sensitive *Staphylococcus aureus*, *H. influenzae*, and various Enterobacteriaceae. For all cases of ventilator-associated pneumonia, empiric treatment should include coverage for Gram-positive bacteria, including *S. aureus*, and Gram-negative bacteria, including *P. aeruginosa*. As mentioned earlier, microbiologic testing should include viral nucleic acid amplification tests with influenza, SARS-CoV-2, respiratory syncytial virus, and human metapneumovirus commonly implicated. As mentioned earlier, microbiologic testing should include viral nucleic acid amplification tests with influenza, SARS-CoV-2, respiratory syncytial virus, and human metapneumovirus commonly implicated.
- Nosocomial UTIs are one of the most common types of hospital-acquired infection, constituting 20% to 30% of all nosocomial infections in medical or surgical ICUs.

The presence of an indwelling catheter and duration of catheterization are the most cited risk factors for nosocomial UTIs. Organisms responsible vary; however, they commonly include *E. coli, Klebsiella* spp, *Enterococcus* spp., and *Pseudomonas* spp. Other risk factors include an age over 50 years, diabetes, or an immunocompromised status. Due to frequent need for monitoring, ICU patients with indwelling Foley catheters are at a high risk for CAUTI and urosepsis.

- Fungal infections with *Candida* spp. are most common. Fungal etiologies should be evaluated in all patients undergoing an infection workup. Risk factors for *Candida* infections include sepsis, impaired immune system, recent surgeries, parenteral nutrition, and recent broad-spectrum antibiotics.

Management

- Management of fever and hyperthermia is focused on identifying the underlying cause.
- Briefly, in hyperthermic syndromes, cooling, hydration, and discontinuing the offending agent are essential. Complications of severe hyperthermia include rhabdomyolysis, disseminated intravascular coagulation, renal and liver failure, and severe metabolic derangements, including hypoglycemia, lactic acidosis, and hyperkalemia. In all cases, supportive care is essential. Benzodiazepines, dantrolene, and bromocriptine can be considered in neuroleptic malignant syndrome. Dantrolene is also recommended in malignant hyperthermia. Benzodiazepine and cyproheptadine may be beneficial in serotonin syndrome.
- Routine use of antipyretics is not recommended in critically ill patients for the sole purpose of reducing nonlethal fever. Acetaminophen administration has not been shown to decrease morbidity. For symptomatic control, pharmacologic methods are recommended over nonpharmacologic methods.
- In rapidly deteriorating or immunocompromised patients with a likely infectious cause, broad-spectrum empiric antibiotics are vital, which can be narrowed per culture data.

Conclusion

- Fever is common in the ICU with a broad differential, including both infectious and noninfectious etiologies, and is distinct from hyperthermic syndromes.
- Infectious and noninfectious causes should be thoroughly investigated based on a focused history and physical, laboratory, imaging, and microbiologic studies.
- Due to the high risk of delaying treatment in infection cases, obtaining culture data and early empiric antibiotics should be considered in high-risk patients with signs of organ dysfunction.
- Hyperthermic syndromes are distinct from fever and need to be considered and treated in the patient context.

SUGGESTED READING

Andrews PJD, Verma V, Healy M, et al. Targeted temperature management in patients with intracerebral haemorrhage, subarachnoid haemorrhage, or acute ischaemic stroke: consensus recommendations. *Br J Anaesth*. 2018; 121:768-775.

Dankiewicz J, Cronberg T, Lilja G, et al. Hypothermia versus normothermia after out-of-hospital cardiac arrest. *N Engl J Med*. 2021;384, 2283-2294.

Fernandez Hernandez S, Barlow B, Pertsovskaya V, Maciel CB. Temperature control after cardiac arrest: a narrative review. *Adv Ther*. 2023;40: 2097-2115.

Greer DM, Funk SE, Reaven NL, Ouzounelli M, Uman GC. Impact of fever on outcome in patients with stroke and neurologic injury: a comprehensive meta-analysis. *Stroke*. 2008;39:3029-3035.

Keck JM, Wingler MJB, Cretella DA, et al. Approach to fever in patients with neutropenia: a review of diagnosis and management. *Ther Adv Infect Dis*. 2022;9:20499361221138346.

Launey Y, Nesseler N, Mallédant Y, Seguin P. Clinical review: fever in septic ICU patients—friend or foe? *Crit Care*. 2011;15:222.

Laupland KB, Shahpori R, Kirkpatrick AW, et al. Occurrence and outcome of fever in critically ill adults. *Crit Care Med*. 2008;36:1531-1535.

Lavinio A, Coles JP, Robba C, et al. Targeted temperature control following traumatic brain injury: ESICM/NACCS best practice consensus recommendations. *Crit Care*. 2024;28:1-14.

Lee BH, Inui D, Suh GY, et al. Association of body temperature and antipyretic treatments with mortality of critically ill patients with and without sepsis: multi-centered prospective observational study. *Crit Care*. 2012;16:R33.

Marik PE. Fever in the ICU. *Chest*. 2000;117, 855-869.

McMahon A, Conrick-Martin I. Commonly encountered central nervous system infections in the intensive care unit. *BJA Educ*. 2023;23:212-220.

Moffarah AS, Al Mohajer M, Hurwitz BL, Armstrong DG. Skin and soft tissue infections. *Microbiol Spectr*. 2016;4.

Morgan MS. Diagnosis and management of necrotising fasciitis: a multiparametric approach. *J Hosp Infect*. 2010;75:249-257.

Niven DJ, Laupland KB. Pyrexia: aetiology in the ICU. *Crit Care*. 2016; 20:247.

Nohra E, Appelbaum RD, Farrell MS, et al. Fever and infections in surgical intensive care: an American Association for the Surgery of Trauma Critical Care Committee clinical consensus document. *Trauma Surg Acute Care Open*. 2024;9:e001303.

Nolan JP, Sandroni C, Böttiger BW, et al. European Resuscitation Council and European Society of Intensive Care Medicine guidelines 2021: post-resuscitation care. *Resuscitation*. 2021;161:220-269.

O'Grady NP, Alexander E, Alhazzani W, et al. Society of Critical Care Medicine and the Infectious Diseases Society of America guidelines for evaluating new fever in adult patients in the ICU. *Crit Care Med*. 2023;51:1570-1586.

Ogoina D. Fever, fever patterns and diseases called 'fever'—a review. *J Infect Public Health*. 2011;4:108-124.

Panchal AR, Bartos JA, Cabañas JG, et al. Part 3: adult basic and advanced life support: 2020 American Heart Association guidelines for cardiopulmonary resuscitation and emergency cardiovascular care. *Circulation*. 2020;142:S366-S468.

Pradhan A, Caplivski D. Fever in the ICU. In: Oropello JM, Pastores SM, Kvetan VK, eds. *Critical Care*. McGraw-Hill Education. 2017.

12.2

Malignant Hyperthermia

Kyle Sanchez and Ryan J. Horvath

- A genetic disorder of skeletal muscle triggered in most instances by volatile anesthetics and/or succinylcholine, resulting in hypermetabolism, rhabdomyolysis, hyperthermia, and death if untreated
- Prior safe exposure to triggering agents does not preclude future development of malignant hyperthermia (MH).

Key Points

- Unexplained hypercapnia resistant to increasing minute ventilation
- Hyperthermia is a late sign of MH.
- Common triggering agents—volatile anesthetics (sevoflurane, desflurane, isoflurane) and succinylcholine
- Discontinue all triggering agents if MH is suspected.
- Control airway and ventilation.
- Call for help, MH cart, and Malignant Hyperthermia Association of the United States (MHAUS) Hotline.
- Administer dantrolene or Ryanodex.
- Manage/monitor postexposure in the intensive care unit (ICU) setting.

Common Symptoms to Remember

Early Signs	Late Signs
• Increased CO_2 production (S) • Sinus tachycardia (NS) • Masseter muscle rigidity (NS) • Muscle rigidity (S) • Myoglobinuria (NS)	• Rhabdomyolysis (S) • Hyperthermia (S) • Tachypnea (NS) • Hyperkalemia/ electrocardiogram (ECG) changes (NS) • Acidosis—metabolic/ respiratory (NS)

Epidemiology

- Children: 1:15,000 general anesthetics
- Adults: 1:30,000 when general inhalational anesthetics and succinylcholine are used or 1:220,000 when general inhalation anesthetics are used only

Key Pathophysiology

- MH is an autosomal dominant disease with variable penetrance characterized by a mutation in ryanodine receptor type 1 (RYR1).
- This condition leads to an excessive and sometimes sustained release of calcium from the sarcoplasmic reticulum, causing persistent skeletal muscle contraction in the presence of triggering anesthetic agents.
- Sustained muscle contraction via accelerated aerobic and anaerobic metabolism leads to cellular acidosis, hypercarbia, hyperthermia, and, eventually, rhabdomyolysis.
- Susceptibility testing can be completed through genetic testing for RYR1 mutations and muscle biopsy contracture testing, where the patient's muscle biopsy specimen is exposed to triggering agents in vitro.

Differential Diagnosis

- Any condition that impairs the elimination of carbon dioxide
  - Hypoventilation
  - Pneumothorax
  - Bronchial obstruction
- Intracranial bleed
- Traumatic brain injury
- Hypoxic encephalopathy
- Thyrotoxicosis
- Pheochromocytoma
- Sepsis
- Heat stroke
- Serotonin syndrome
- Neuroleptic malignant syndrome
- Drugs of abuse (eg, cocaine, methamphetamines)
- CO_2 absorption during laparoscopy
- Exhausted CO_2 absorbent
- Genetic conditions associated with MH
  - Central core myopathy—very high risk associated with MH
  - King-Denborough syndrome
  - Multicore myopathy
  - STAC3 myopathy

Management and Treatment

- Proceed with MH treatment while excluding other causes of hypercarbia and muscle rigidity.
- Communication
  - Call for the MH cart and additional help.
  - Notify surgeon/complete operation if applicable, arrange for post-op care in the ICU setting.
  - Call MHAUS Hotline: 1-800-644-9737.
- Discontinue offending agents.
  - Inhalational agents and succinylcholine
- 100% oxygenation with controlled hyperventilation
- Administer dantrolene or Ryanodex.
  - Older formulations of dantrolene (Dantrium, Renovo, generic dantrolene sodium) have the same chemical structure and mechanism of action as the newest formulation (Ryanodex), antagonism of RYR1 and indirect inhibition of calcium release from sarcoplasmic reticulum.
  - Common side effects include venous irritation and thrombosis, nausea, malaise, and lightheadedness. Chronic oral dantrolene therapy is associated with hepatotoxicity.

Old Formulations (Dantrium, Renovo, dantrolene sodium)	New Formulation (Ryanodex)
• Challenging to dissolve and many vials are required for treatment. • Each 20 mg vial is reconstituted with 60 mL of sterile water. • Dose: 2.5 *mg/kg bolus* through large-bore intravenous (IV), repeat until a decrease in end-tidal CO_2 ($EtCO_2$), muscle rigidity, and decreased heart rate. May require redosing up to 10 mg/kg • Example: 80-kg patient receiving 10 mg/kg would require *40 vials of dantrolene and 2.4 L of water*.	• Easier to dissolve and 150× the concentration of dantrolene • Each 250 mg vial is reconstituted with 5 mL of sterile water. • Dose: 2.5 *mg/kg bolus* through large-bore IV, repeat until a decrease in $EtCO_2$, muscle rigidity, or decreased heart rate. May require redosing up to 10 mg/kg • Example: 80-kg patient receiving 10 mg/kg would require *4 vials of Ryanodex and 20 mL of water*.

- Laboratory values
  - Assess electrolytes, $ETCO_2$, blood gases, creatine phosphokinase, serum myoglobin, core temperature, urine output, and color and coagulation studies.
- Hyperkalemia
  - Treat with calcium, insulin, glucose, albuterol, bicarbonate, sodium zirconium silicate, and furosemide.
- Cardiac arrhythmias
  - Resolves with the treatment of acidosis and hyperkalemia
  - Typical antiarrhythmics may be used if arrhythmias persist, but calcium channel blockers are contraindicated because they can worsen hyperkalemia and result in cardiac collapse.
- Cool the patient.
  - Target euthermia with temperature goal of <38.5 °C (101.3 °F).
- Treat rhabdomyolysis.
  - Target urine output >1 mL/kg/h through IV fluids and diuresis.
- Continuous monitoring and support of respiratory, cardiovascular, and renal function in the ICU.
- Recurrence of the signs and symptoms of MH can occur in up to 25% patients after initial treatment.
- Dantrolene should be continued at 1 mg/kg IV every 4 to 6 hours for at least 24 hours. If all signs and symptoms are improving after 24 hours, the dosing interval can be increased to every 8 or 12 hours until the following conditions are met: metabolic stability for 24 hours, euthermia without active cooling, creatine kinase (CK) decreasing with no evidence of myoglobinuria, no muscle rigidity.

Outcomes

- Mortality is estimated at 1% to 20%.
- Development of disseminated intravascular coagulation—greater risk for cardiac arrest and death
- Susceptible individuals should avoid anesthesia with triggering agents.
- Family and relatives should be informed, and the susceptibility of MH should be discussed.

SUGGESTED READINGS

Burkman JM, Posner KL, Domino KB. Analysis of the clinical variables associated with recrudescence after malignant hyperthermia reactions. *Anesthesiology*. 2007;106:901-906.

Cong Z, Wan T, Wang J, et al. Epidemiological and clinical features of malignant hyperthermia: a scoping review. *Clin Genet*. 2024;105:233-242.

D'Arcy CE, Bjorksten A, Yiu EM, et al. King-Denborough syndrome caused by a novel mutation in the ryanodine receptor gene. *Neurology*. 2008;71:776-777.

Hopkins PM, Girard T, Dalay S, et al. Malignant hyperthermia 2020: guideline from the Association of Anaesthetists. *Anaesthesia*. 2021;76(5):655-664.

Larach MG, Gronert GA, Allen GC, et al. Clinical presentation, treatment, and complications of malignant hyperthermia in North America from 1987 to 2006. *Anesth Analg*. 2010;110:498.

Malignant Hyperthermia Association of the United States. http://www.mhaus.org/

Pinyavat T, Riazi S, Deng J, et al. Malignant hyperthermia. *Crit Care Med*. 2024;52(12):1934-1940.

Rotto D, Joyner R. Dantrolene. In: *StatPearls*. Statpearls Publishing; 2024.

12.3

Neuroleptic Malignant Syndrome

Cristina Mietto and Lorenzo Berra

- The neuroleptic malignant syndrome (NMS) is an idiosyncratic, rare but potentially life-threatening complication of treatment with antipsychotic medication. It is a medical emergency.
- NMS is associated with the use of dopamine antagonist medications (antipsychotics, antiemetics, etc), commonly used in critical care medicine.
- All antipsychotic medications have been associated with NMS.
- Characterized by administration of D2-blocking drugs and early development of hyperthermia, muscle rigidity, mental status changes, and autonomic instability (hypertension or hypotension, tachycardia, tachypnea, and diaphoresis). Other drug-induced, systemic, or other neuropsychiatric illnesses should be excluded before making a diagnosis of NMS.
- Risk factors
  - History of NMS or catatonia
  - Preexisting organic brain disease, especially involving diminished central brain dopamine activity or receptor function (eg, Parkinson disease, traumatic brain injury)
  - Use of high-potency antipsychotics
  - Dehydration

- Patients with significant fluid shifts (ie, postpartum women)
- Agitated men under the age of 40 years
- Genetic susceptibility (reports of incidence among certain families)

- Clinical characteristics: NMS presents as a classic tetrad in the setting of antipsychotic use.
  - Fever
  - Rigidity (lead pipe)
  - Autonomic instability
  - Altered mental status
- Early signs include unexpected mental status changes and muscle rigidity developing over the course of a few days (range: hours to weeks) in association with the introduction of D2 blockade or removal of dopamine potentiation.
  - Mental status changes are nonspecific and typically include confusion, delirium, clouding of consciousness, and stupor, with ~50% having abnormal electroencephalograms (EEGs).
  - Muscle rigidity can develop acutely or be characterized by worsening of preexisting rigidity. Lead-pipe or generalized rigidity can be associated with tremor, dystonia, trismus, myoclonus, dysarthria, and dysphagia.
  - Hyperthermia usually develops late. Diaphoresis or flushing are signs of thermoregulation abnormalities.
  - Autonomic dysfunction may develop at any point and be characterized by liable hypertension, tachycardia, tachypnea, and urinary incontinence.
- Laboratory abnormalities
  - Elevated creatine phosphokinase (CPK; up to 95% of patients)
  - Leukocytosis is common, but not specific.
  - Acute renal failure (16%-25% of patients) may occur secondary to myoglobinuria from muscle necrosis (poor prognostic sign).
  - Metabolic acidosis
- A common mnemonic is FALTER:
  - *F*—Fever
  - *A*—Autonomic instability
  - *L*—Leukocytosis
  - *T*—Tremor
  - *E*—Elevated enzymes (elevated CPK generally >2,000, although this will be less specific in surgical patients with recent operations)
  - *R*—Rigidity of muscles (lead pipe)

Common Causes to Remember

• Dopamine antagonists	Antipsychotics (haloperidol, chlorpromazine, risperidone, olanzapine, quetiapine, etc); antiemetics (metoclopramide, prochlorperazine); amoxapine, reserpine
• Discontinuation of dopamine agonists	L-DOPA, amantadine, bromocriptine, ropinirole, pramipexole

Epidemiology

- Affects 0.02% to 3% of patients treated with dopamine receptor antagonists
- Most commonly occurs within 1 week of dopamine antagonist initiation
- Historically, associated mortality was reported to be 12% to 20%, usually from cardiorespiratory failure. Literature reports a declining trend in mortality of around 5% to 9% after the year 2000s.
- A meta-analysis reported that respiratory difficulties, hyperthermia severity, and older age are associated with increased mortality.

Key Pathophysiology

- Clinical signs of NMS are thought to be due to an acute reduction in brain dopamine activity. Specifically, drug-induced dopamine D2-receptor blockade leads to decreased dopamine activity within the basal ganglia-thalamocortical circuits.
- Decreased dopamine in motor circuits leads to muscle rigidity. Decreased dopamine in the anterior-cingulate-medial orbitofrontal circuit leads to diminished arousal, mutism, and akinesia. Decreased dopamine transmission from the anterior-cingulate-medial orbitofrontal cortex to the lateral hypothalamus leads to hyperthermia and autonomic dysfunction. Other neurotransmitters (serotonin, GABA, and glutamate) may also play a role in NMS pathogenesis.
- A similar syndrome may occur in Parkinson disease in the context of withdrawal of dopamine agonist medications.

Differential Diagnosis

- Other systemic hypermetabolic syndromes present with fever that mimics NMS:
  - Serotonin syndrome—multiple signs and symptoms overlap with NMS (mental status changes, neuromuscular symptoms, and autonomic instability). Rigidity is typical of NMS, whereas hyperreflexia and myoclonus are typical findings in serotonin syndrome. Serotonin syndrome develops rapidly in association with high levels of serotonergic drugs (overdose or combinations of multiple serotonergic agents).
  - Malignant catatonia—can present nearly identically to NMS. Some experts consider NMS a neuroleptic-induced malignant catatonia. Temporal association with dopamine-blocking agents helps to differentiate the two syndromes.
  - Malignant hyperthermia (MH)—a drug-induced hypermetabolic syndrome associated with the administration of anesthetic gases and succinylcholine during anesthesia. Most cases are due to a mutation of the ryanodine receptor (type 1), located on the sarcoplasmic reticulum.
  - Encephalopathy/sepsis—also presents with confusion, clouding of consciousness, hypermetabolism, with tachycardia and autonomic instability
  - Heat stroke—occurs during prolonged exposure to high ambient temperatures, rapid onset. Diaphoresis and muscle rigidity are not present.

Management and Treatment

- Early recognition is the key to preventing morbidity and mortality.
- Prompt cessation of offending dopamine-blocking agents, or (re)starting dopamine agonists (depending on the cause), as soon as the NMS is suspected.

- Supportive treatment—fluid replacement and cooling measures are important. Monitor patients for cardiorespiratory failure (may require intubation and ventilatory support), aspiration pneumonia, thromboembolism, and renal failure. Fluid therapy is essential in case of rhabdomyolysis in an attempt to prevent acute kidney injury.
- Physical cooling measures must be implemented to treat hyperthermia, as antipyretic medications have limited efficacy.
- Benzodiazepines—clinical overlap between NMS and malignant catatonia has prompted the use of benzodiazepines for the management of NMS. A trial of intravenous (IV) lorazepam can help determine whether benzodiazepines will be helpful. Dose range 6 to 20 mg/d, in divided doses (ie, 1-2 mg IV 3 times daily [tid]).
- Dopamine agonists—may reverse the acute dopamine deficit implicated in NMS and facilitate resolution of the syndrome. Amantadine has been shown to be an effective treatment, in the range of 200 to 400 mg/d given orally in divided doses. Bromocriptine can also expedite resolution of the syndrome, in dosages up to 45 mg/d (divided).
- Anticholinergic medications—generally not recommended; anticholinergic medications can further impair heat loss (via inhibition of sweating) and worsen hyperthermia.
- Dantrolene—has been used successfully in the treatment of NMS, MH, and other hyperthermic conditions by inhibiting skeletal muscle contraction, thereby decreasing peripheral heat production. Unlike MH, its use in NMS has been controversial and reportedly less effective.
- Electroconvulsive therapy (ECT)—evidence suggests that ECT can be used acutely or if pharmacologic strategies have failed. Most patients respond within 72 hours. Use of ECT should not be delayed past 5 days, given increased morbidity and mortality with prolonged duration of illness. If significant rhabdomyolysis is present, succinylcholine use (for paralysis for ECT) should be avoided, and alternative agents should be used.

Outcomes

- With supportive treatment alone, the mean recovery time after cessation of dopamine antagonists has been shown to be ~10 days.
- The mortality of NMS has declined over time, possibly due to increased awareness of the syndrome along with early recognition and management.

SUGGESTED READINGS

Addonizio G, Susman VL, Roth SD. Neuroleptic malignant syndrome: review and analysis of 115 cases. *Biol Psychiatry*. 1987;22(8):1004-1020.

Bellamy CJ, Kane-Gill SL, Falcione BA, et al. Neuroleptic malignant syndrome in traumatic brain injury patients treated with haloperidol. *J Trauma*. 2009;66(3):954-958.

Fricchione G, Mann SC, Caroff SN. Catatonia, lethal catatonia and neuroleptic malignant syndrome. *Psychiatr Ann*. 2000;30:347-355.

Modi S, Dharaiya D, Schultz L, Varelas P. Neuroleptic malignant syndrome: complications, outcomes, and mortality. *Neurocrit Care*. 2016;24:97-103.

Sato I, Onishi H, Kawanishi C, Yamada S, Ishida M, Kawakami K. Neuroleptic malignant syndrome in patients with cancer: a systematic review. *BMJ Support Palliat Care*. 2020;10:265-270.

12.4

Serotonin Syndrome

Cristina Mietto

Definition

- Serotonin syndrome is a drug-induced syndrome characterized by symptoms associated with increased serotonin (5-hydroxytryptamine, 5-HT) levels (central and peripheral).
- Classic triad of symptoms include altered mental status, neuromuscular hyperactivity, and autonomic dysregulation.
- Symptom severity can progress from mild to life-threatening, worsening with the progression of increased serotonin levels.
- The diagnosis is clinical, requiring the presence of a serotonergic drug and symptoms associated with serotonin toxicity. Not all cases present with the classic triad of symptoms.
- Toxicity can develop after new use or increased dose of a single agent, or in the presence of coadministration of multiple agents, even if within therapeutic doses.

Key Pathophysiology

- No single serotonin receptor has been clearly linked to the syndrome, but evidence suggests a major role played by postsynaptic 5-HT1A and 5-HT2A receptors.
- Monoamine oxidase inhibitor (MAOi), selective serotonin reuptake inhibitors (SSRIs), serotonin-norepinephrine reuptake inhibitors (SNRIs), and drug-drug interactions are more commonly present in cases of moderate and severe symptoms.
- Common triggers include new therapy, an increase in therapeutic dose, and an unintentional effect in the presence of multiple medications or overdose.

Risk Factors

- Use of serotonergic drugs. Table 12.4.1 shows the medications most often involved in serotonin syndrome.
- Caution must be used in patients on polypharmaceutical therapy, especially in the older patients.
- Literature reports that more severe reactions are often associated with the use of MAOi.

Epidemiology

- The true incidence of serotonin syndrome is difficult to estimate, especially since mild cases can be easily misinterpreted, especially in the older patients.

TABLE 12.4.1 Drugs Associated With Serotonin Syndrome

Mechanism	Agent
Decreased serotonin breakdown	MAOi: phenelzine, tranylcypromine, isocarboxazid, moclobemide, selegiline, rasagiline Antibiotics: linezolid Others: methylene blue, procarbazine, Syrian rue
Increased serotonin precursors or agonists	Antidepressants: Selective serotonin reuptake inhibitors Serotonin-norepinephrine reuptake inhibitors: venlafaxine, duloxetine, milnacipran Tricyclic antidepressants: clomipramine, imipramine St. John wort Opioids: meperidine, buprenorphine, tramadol, tapentadol, dextromethorphan Antiepileptics: valproate, carbamazepine Antiemetics: ondansetron, granisetron, metoclopramide
Increased serotonin precursors or agonists	Tryptophan, lithium, fentanyl, lysergic acid diethylamide
Increased serotonin release	Central nervous system stimulants: amphetamines Anorectics: fenfluramine, dexfenfluramine, phentermine Drugs of abuse: methylenedioxymethamphetamine (ecstasy), cocaine
CYP2D6 and CYP3A4 inhibitors	Antibiotics: erythromycin, ciprofloxacin Antifungal: fluconazole Antiretroviral: ritonavir

MAOi, monoamine oxidase inhibitor.

- SSRIs are widely prescribed and are the medications most commonly associated with serotonin syndrome.
- Moderate serotonin syndrome is reported to occur in 15% of SSRI overdoses.
- Severe serotonin syndrome is more commonly associated with MAOi and SNRIs treatment.
- Early diagnosis and treatment are the key factors to ensure good outcomes, even in severe cases that can be otherwise evolve in multiorgan failure and death.

Clinical Presentation

- Classic presentation is characterized by the acute (usually within hours) onset of:
  - Neuromuscular excitation (hyperreflexia, clonus, inducible spontaneous, ocular, myoclonus, rigidity), most marked in the lower extremities and easily elicited with ankle dorsiflexion. In severe cases, it can evolve into muscle rigidity and hyperthermia.
  - Altered mental status with agitation and confusion due to increased central nervous system serotonin levels, affecting attention, behavior, and alertness
  - Autonomic nervous system dysregulation and development of tachycardia, pressure lability, increased gastrointestinal motility, and bronchoconstriction

TABLE 12.4.2 The Hunter Criteria for Serotonin Syndrome

Presence of a serotonergic agent	Must be confirmed
Plus one of the following:	
Spontaneous clonus	Rhythmic, involuntary muscle contractions
Inducible clonus plus agitation or diaphoresis	Muscle contractions elicited by examiner, along with agitation or excessive sweating
Ocular clonus plus agitation or diaphoresis	Rapid, involuntary eye movements with agitation or excessive sweating
Tremor plus hyperreflexia	Trembling and overactive reflexes
Hypertonia plus temperature > 38°C PLUS ocular or inducible clonus	Muscle rigidity and high body temperature with eye muscle contractions or inducible clonus

Diagnosis

- The Hunter criteria, the most widely used diagnostic tool reported in the literature (Table 12.4.2), requires the presence of a serotonergic agent and one of the following symptoms:
  - Spontaneous clonus
  - Inducible clonus plus agitation or diaphoresis
  - Ocular clonus plus agitation or diaphoresis
  - Tremor plus hyperreflexia
  - Hypertonia plus temperature above 38 °C plus ocular or inducible clonus
- The Sternbach criteria are a different clinical tool proposed in the literature but showed lower sensitivity and specificity.
- No specific laboratory tests are required for diagnosis, but they are useful to monitor complications and evaluate alternative diagnoses.
- Timing of presentation is usually acute, most often within 6 to 24 hours from the introduction of a new medication or change in dose.

Differential Diagnosis

- Neuroleptic syndrome: idiosyncratic reaction to antipsychotic medications usually with subacute onset over days to weeks, slower resolution over days, characterized by rigidity and bradyreflexia. Leukocytosis, elevated creatine phosphokinase, elevated hepatic transaminases, and metabolic acidosis may be present in both conditions.
- Malignant hyperthermia: associated with halogenated volatile anesthetics or depolarizing muscle relaxants, presenting with increased end-tidal carbon dioxide, muscle rigidity, tachycardia, hyperthermia, and metabolic acidosis
- Anticholinergic poisoning: presents with mydriasis, dry mucous membranes, urinary retention, and decreased bowel motility, with normal muscle tone and reflexes

Management and Treatment

- Treatment depends on the severity of symptoms.
- The main interventions are to discontinue the medication and provide supportive therapy.
- Mild-to-moderate symptoms usually resolve within one to a few days after the discontinuation of the serotonergic agent, though longer recovery times may be needed with MAOi or SNRIs.

- Mild cases: characterized by anxiety, restlessness, hyperreflexia, tremor or myoclonus, diaphoresis, mydriasis, and tachycardia.
- Moderate cases: may exhibit autonomic instability, agitation, clonus, opsoclonus, hypertension, diarrhea, nausea/vomiting, and hyperthermia
  - Main interventions are the discontinuation of the medication, supportive therapy, and sedation.
  - Benzodiazepines are the preferred agent to control agitation.
- Severe cases are a medical emergency: characterized by confusion, delirium, coma, seizures, rigidity, labile blood pressure, and hyperthermia
  - These patients require close monitoring of vitals, hemodynamic support, possible neuromuscular paralysis, and tracheal intubation.
  - Management of autonomic instability may be difficult; short-acting agents are preferable to treat hypertension and tachycardia.
  - Physical cooling measures are necessary, as hyperthermia is due to increased muscular activity and does not respond to antipyretics. Control of temperature can prevent the development of complications, such as rhabdomyolysis, disseminated intravascular coagulation, arrhythmia, and metabolic acidosis.

Antidote

- Cyproheptadine is a histamine-1 receptor antagonist with potent nonspecific 5-HT1A and 5-HT2A antagonistic properties.
- No strong data to support its efficacy
- The most common side effect is hypotension, due to the reversal of serotonin-mediated increases in vascular tone.
- Chlorpromazine is another 5-HT receptor antagonist, with its use is less frequently reported in the literature due to side effects such as hypotension, dystonic reactions, and neuroleptic malignant syndrome.

Prevention

- Awareness of drugs with potent serotonergic effects
- Avoidance of drug-drug interactions
- Monitoring after new medication initiation or an increase in dosage
- Ensuring correct washout periods after a change in therapy

SUGGESTED READINGS

Chiew AL, Buckley NA. The serotonin toxidrome: shortfalls of current diagnostic criteria for related syndromes. *Clin Toxicol (Phila)*. 2022;60(2):143-158.

Francescangeli J, Karamchandani K, Powell M, Bonavia A. The serotonin syndrome: from molecular mechanisms to clinical practice. *Int J Mol Sci*. 2019;20(9):2288.

Mikkelsen N, Damkier P, Pedersen SA. Serotonin syndrome—a focused review. *Basic Clin Pharmacol Toxicol*. 2023;133(2):124-129.

Pedavally S, Fugate JE, Rabinstein AA. Serotonin syndrome in the intensive care unit: clinical presentations and precipitating medications. *Neurocrit Care*. 2014;21(1):108-113.

Prakash S, Shah CS, Prakash A. Serotonin syndrome controversies: a need for consensus. *World J Crit Care Med*. 2024;13(2):94707.

12.5

Heat Stroke

Gamonmas Ekkapat and Lorenzo Berra

Heat Stroke

- Elevated core temperature ≥40 °C or 104 °F
- Central nervous system (CNS) dysfunction
- Severe environmental heat exposure

Key Points

- Heat stroke occurs when the body's cooling mechanisms are overwhelmed by heat and humidity, leading to a rapid rise in body temperature.
- Heat stroke is a life-threatening medical emergency, carrying a high mortality risk without prompt recognition and treatment.
- The primary goal of treatment is to rapidly lower the core body temperature to prevent organ damage and death.
- Heat-related deaths and illnesses are preventable.

Epidemiology

- ~1,220 people in the United States die from extreme heat every year.
- Between 2019 and 2023, heat stroke incidence among Active Component Members of the US Armed Forces decreased by 15.6%, while heat exhaustion incidence rate increased by 4.6%. In 2023, the rate was down to 31.7 cases per 100,000 person-years, reflecting a successful heat illness prevention effort.

Two Types of Heat Stroke

- Nonexertional (classic) heat stroke
  - Occur in individuals exposed to high environmental heat with decreased thermoregulatory capacity
  - Common among vulnerable populations, such as the older, children, and infants
  - Epidemic during heat waves
- Exertional heat stroke
  - Typically affect individuals engaging in strenuous exercise during periods of high temperature and humidity
  - Commonly observed in athletes and military recruits undergoing basic training
  - Occur sporadically throughout the year

Key Pathophysiology

- Thermoregulation is maintained by balancing heat production (metabolism and environment) with heat loss.
- To dissipate heat when the core temperature rises, the preoptic nucleus in the anterior hypothalamus activates the autonomic nervous system, promoting sweating and increasing blood flow to the skin (cutaneous vasodilation).
- Heat loss in hot environment:
    - Evaporation: principal mechanism to cool down, but ineffective when the relative humidity gets too high (>75%).
    - Radiation, conduction, convection: less effective when environment is warmer than skin.
- Heat stroke occurs when the thermoregulatory mechanisms fail due to overwhelming heat and humidity, leading to core temperature rise, cessation of sweating, and an inability to dissipate heat.
- Physiologic effects of heat stroke
    - Increased metabolic rate and oxygen consumption
    - Systemic inflammation and heat-shock protein production
    - Blood flow shift to skin and muscles, potentially harming gut function (ischemia, increased permeability)
    - Organ damage, with liver, blood vessels, and brain most susceptible
    - Risk of multiorgan failure and disseminated intravascular coagulation (DIC) in severe cases
    - Enzyme dysfunction and breakdown of cellular processes such as uncoupling of oxidative phosphorylation >42 °C (108 °F)

Differential Diagnosis (Table 12.5.1)

Management and Treatment

- Early diagnosis and rapid cooling are critical.
    - Prompt recognition and aggressive cooling measures are essential for improving outcomes.

TABLE 12.5.1 Differential Diagnosis

Causes	Considerations
Infections	Overwhelming infections such as sepsis
Endocrine	Pheochromocytoma, thyroid storm
Central nervous system insults	Catatonia, traumatic brain injury, hypothalamic stroke, status epilepticus
Toxic etiologies	Salicylate, lithium, sympathomimetic, anticholinergic overdoses
Neuroleptic malignant syndrome	Antipsychotic medications and rarely from withdrawal of anti-Parkinson medications. Symptoms include hyperthermia, lead-pipe muscle rigidity, altered mental status, choreoathetosis, and autonomic instability.
Serotonin syndrome	Any medication or combination that increases serotonin levels in the brain (eg, antidepressants, illicit drugs). Typically onset of symptoms within 24 h of exposure to a new drug, or change in dosage. Symptoms include hyperthermia, myoclonus, altered mental status, and autonomic instability.
Malignant hyperthermia	A rare autosomal dominant disorder that causes muscle rigidity, tachycardia, hypercarbia, and hyperthermia, typically after receiving succinylcholine and/or an inhaled anesthetic.

- Goal temperature
    - Aim for a core body temperature of 38 °C to 39 °C (100.4 °F-102.2 °F) to prevent iatrogenic hypothermia
    - Sustain target temperature for at least 24 hours
- Prehospital care
    - Early detection: look for hyperthermia with altered consciousness (confusion, dizziness, seizure)
    - Avoidance: immediate removal from heat source
    - Immediate cooling measures
    - Transportation: continue cooling measures while transporting the person to the hospital
- Supportive care measures
    - Airway and breathing
        - Tracheal intubation and ventilation may be needed for patients with compromised airway or breathing.
    - Hemodynamic support
        - Intravenous fluids are used to address dehydration and hypotension.
        - Avoid alpha-adrenergic agonists as they can hinder heat dissipation because of the vasoconstrictive effect.
        - Vasopressors like norepinephrine might be used in severe cases.
    - Electrolyte replacement
        - Correct electrolyte imbalances caused by sweating and dehydration.
    - Consider the following monitoring devices:
        - Central venous pressure monitoring and urinary catheter for volume status
        - Continuous core body temperature monitoring by either rectal, esophageal, or Foley catheter
    - Consider the following diagnostic tests:
        - Chest x-ray, electrocardiogram
        - Complete blood count, serum electrolytes including renal function, urinalysis
        - Liver function, coagulation profile, serum creatine kinase
        - Toxicology screen
        - Computed tomography scan of the head and lumbar puncture to assess for CNS etiologies
    - Cooling methods
        - No single cooling method proven best for heat stroke. Choose based on patient and resources (Table 12.5.2)
        - Cooling precautions: avoid alcohol sponge baths due to potential toxicity and cold gastric lavage due to the risk of water intoxication
    - Pharmacologic therapy
        - Not routinely used
        - Antipyretics (acetaminophen, aspirin) are ineffective and can worsen complications such as hepatic injury and coagulopathy.
        - Dantrolene is not helpful for heat stroke.
        - Antibiotics may be considered if infection is suspected.

Complications

Many patients develop some form of multiorgan dysfunction, including respiratory dysfunction, seizures, rhabdomyolysis, kidney injury, hepatic injury, and disseminated intravascular coagulopathy.

TABLE 12.5.2 Cooling Methods

External Cooling Methods	Descriptions
Ice pack, ice sheet, cool, wet clothes	Apply to the groin, armpits, neck, and head
Cold water/ice submersion	Either immerse the patient or pour ice water onto the patient. Avoid in the older and severely brain-injured patients. There is a possible increase in mortality when used in these two groups.
Evaporative and convective cooling	Fan the person to promote air circulation. Encourage gentle misting with lukewarm water or removing clothing if safe.
Cooling blankets	
Tepid sponge bath	
Environmental cooling	Move to a cool, shaded area, decrease room temperature.
Internal Cooling Methods	**Descriptions**
Intravenous (IV) cold crystalloid fluids	Total fluid intake should not exceed 4 L/d unless prescribed by a doctor
Endovascular cooling	Requires specialized medical equipment and expertise
Cold thoracic/peritoneal lavage	For extreme situations, consider cold thoracic and peritoneal lavages. Avoid cold gastric lavage as it causes water intoxication.

Outcomes

- Patients with heat stroke have a high mortality ranging from 21% to 63%.
- Risk factors for mortality include the following:
  - Higher degree of temperature elevation
  - Longer time to initiation of cooling
  - Number of organ systems affected
  - Taking antihypertensive medications
  - Lack of access to air conditioning
  - Social isolation
  - Inability to care for self

Keywords

Heat-related illness, heat stroke, thermoregulation, cooling methods

SUGGESTED READINGS

Bouchama A, Dehbi M, Chaves-Carballo E. Cooling and hemodynamic management in heatstroke: practical recommendations. *Crit Care*. 2007;11(3):R54.

Epstein Y, Yanovich R. Heatstroke. *N Engl J Med*. 2019;380(25):2449-2459.

Hifumi T, Kondo Y, Shimizu K, Miyake Y. Heat stroke. *J Intensive Care*. 2018;6:30.

Maule AL, Scatliffe-Carrion KD, Kotas KS, Smith JD, Ambrose JF. Heat exhaustion and heat stroke among active component members of the U.S. Armed Forces, 2019-2023. *MSMR*. 2024;31(4):3-8.

Sorensen C, Hess J. Treatment and prevention of heat-related illness. *N Engl J Med*. 2022;387(15):1404-1413.

12.6

Hypothermia

Yasmine Tameze

Three types of hypothermia: accidental (this section), metabolic/secondary (sepsis, hypo-endocrine states), and therapeutic (targeted temperature management [TTM] discussed elsewhere)

Definitions

Accidental: unintentional drop in core temperature to <35 °C, ideally measured in the lower third of the esophagus in the unconscious patient. In the conscious patient, temperature can be estimated by clinical signs (Table 12.6.1).

TABLE 12.6.1 Hypothermia Scale and Clinical Findings

Stage	Core Temperature	Clinical Signs
Mild	32-°C35 °C	• Confusion, not able to care for self • Increase in metabolism via shivering, increase ventilation, and MAP and cardiac output • "Cold diuresis"
Moderate	28-°C32 °C	• Altered consciousness/lethargy • Reduced shivering • Rewarming with addition of exogenous heat
Severe	<25 °C-28 °C	• Obtunded/coma • Dilated and fixed pupil (not a sign of brain death)—reverse with warming • Oliguria, generalized edema • Bradycardia • No shivering • Apnea and high risk of VF systole

MAP, mean arterial pressure; VF, ventricular fibrillation.

Key Pathophysiology

- Result of net heat loss from the body via evaporation, radiation, conduction, and convection: convection (to cold air) and conduction (to water) are the most common mechanisms of accidental hypothermia.
- Physiologic effects of hypothermia:
  - Initial stages of cooling: secondary responses predominate until about 32 °C:
    - Shivering thermogenesis → ↑ metabolism, ↑ ventilation, ↑ cardiac output (CO), and ↑ mean arterial pressure (MAP)
    - Brain: starts declining at core temperature of about 34 °C → irritability eventually to coma. Decreases cerebral oxygen requirements → protection during anoxic conditions, such as cold-water drowning
  - Once the core temperature reaches ~32 °C
    - Metabolism, ventilation, and CO begin declining. Shivering is less effective.
    - Bradycardia occurs in addition to other abnormalities in cardiac electrical conduction. <28 °C high risk of ventricular fibrillation (VF) (acidosis, hypoxia).
    - Shivering stops below ~30 °C.
- The hypothalamus controls thermoregulation and uses autonomic mechanisms to maintain core temperature at ~37 °C.
  - In response to heat: vasodilation/sweating (heat loss)
  - In response to cold: vasoconstriction (heat retention)/shivering (heat production), increased thyroid, catecholamine, and adrenal activity (more effective for mild hypothermia)

Risk Factors/Epidemiology for Accidental Hypothermia

- Hypothalamus response to cold effective for mild hypothermia; therefore, the prevention of hypothermia mainly depends on behavior (ie, clothing and shelter).
  - Hypothermia pronounced when these responses are impaired, such as
    - Intoxication/ethanol use
    - Homelessness
    - Psychiatric diseases
    - Wilderness/cold winters
    - Older age: impaired reserve, social isolation
- Trauma population at increased risk
  - Laparotomy and opening of body cavities
  - Administration of a large volume of unwarned fluids and blood products
  - Exposure to water/drowning
  - Burns

Laboratory/Imaging Findings

- Inhibition of the enzymes of the coagulation cascade: partial thromboplastin time (PTT) and prothrombin time (PT) are always reported at 37 °C and might be reported as normal, but they are coagulopathic in vivo.
- Oxygenation: a pulse oximeter placed on the ear or forehead might be less affected by peripheral vasoconstriction.
- Arterial blood gas (ABG): reported by the laboratory at 37 °C. While gas tension changes with temperature, using the uncorrected value (ie, one at 37 °C given by the laboratory, alpha-stat strategy) to guide therapy is better for prognostication.

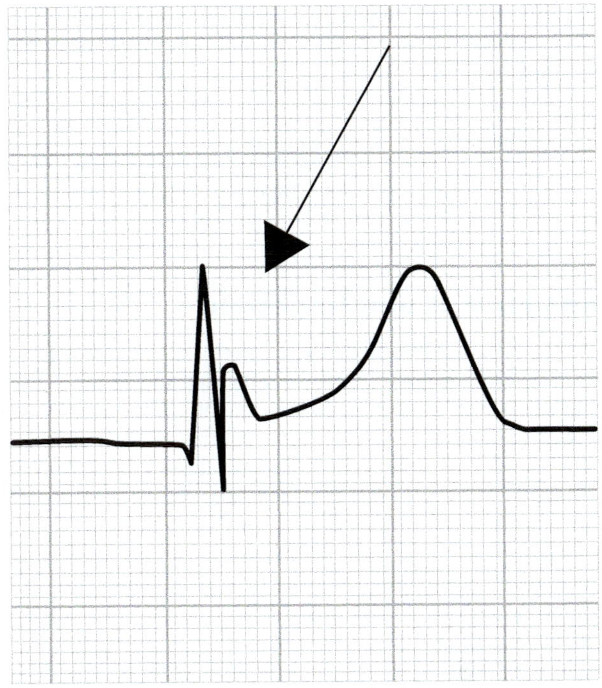

FIGURE 12.6.1 Osborn wave.

- White blood cells and platelet counts: decreased secondary to splenic sequestration
- Hemoglobin/hematocrit: elevated secondary to hemoconcentration. Hematocrit increased 2% per 1 °C drop in temperature.
- Lipase: might be elevated because of hypothermia-induced pancreatitis
- Electrolytes: no consistent abnormality
- Electrocardiogram (ECG): slow impulse conduction through K channels: prolongs all intervals (RR, PR, QRS, QT). J or Osborn wave—elevation of the J point in the presence of normal ST segment (Figure 12.6.1). T-wave inversions. Arrhythmias

Differential Diagnosis

Table 12.6.2.

Physical Examination

- Very sensitive to movement: heart prone to arrhythmias with movement
- Total body survey: to assess trauma and local cold-related injuries (ie, Frostbite)

TABLE 12.6.2 Causes of Hypothermia

Causes of Hypothermia	
• Environmental exposures • Drugs (alcohol, β-blockers, general anesthesia, anxiolytics, oral antihyperglycemic) • Skin impairment (burns)	• Endocrine (hypothyroidism, adrenal insufficiency, diabetes) • Sepsis • Massive volume resuscitation • Cold fluid infusion

- Temperature measurement
  - Esophageal temperature is the gold standard, especially in severe hypothermia with an intubated patient.
  - Rectal: reasonable for conscious patients (not accurate during peritoneal lavage)
  - Bladder: adequate for mild-to-moderate hypothermia
  - Both rectal and bladder temperatures should not be used during rewarming as the temperature lags the core temperature.

Management and Treatment

- Advanced Cardiovascular Life Support (ACLS): making sure patient is rewarming at the same rate and shock at the highest power, since defibrillation might be less effective at low temperatures (<30 °C). Low end-tidal carbon dioxide ($Etco_2$) values are the result of low basal metabolic rates (BMRs), not hypoperfusion, in patients who are hypothermic and should not prompt stopping resuscitation efforts.
- Arrhythmias: will resolve with rewarming. Bradycardia is physiologic in hypothermia and does not require pacing unless associated with severe hypotension or perseveres after rewarming.
- Hypotension: from dehydration and fluid shifts. Treat with warm intravenous fluids and vasopressors if needed. *Rewarming:* remove wet clothing. Aim for rewarming rate of ~0.5 °C to 2 °C an hour.
- Prevention: prehospital passive rewarming
- Passive external rewarming
  - Cover with insulating material in a warm environment.
  - Usually adequate for mild hypothermia
  - Keep room temperature ~28 °C. Relies on the ability of the patient to increase heat production (ie, shivering)
  - If rate <0.5 °C per hour, add active rewarming, consider other etiology of hypothermia.
- Active external rewarming (rate ~2 °C per hour)
  - Involves applying heat directly to the skin from any of several sources (heating pads, forced air, heat lamps)
  - Watch for "rewarming shock" (peripheral vasodilation in the setting of intravascular hypovolemia).
    - Trunk should be warmed before the extremities to minimize core temperature drop due to vasodilation. If both are warmed simultaneously:
      - The cold acidic peripheral blood returns to the core, causing a drop in core temperature and pH.
      - Removal from cold environment causes peripheral vasodilation → hypotension.
      - Both can lead to poor coronary perfusion and arrhythmias during rewarming.
- Active core rewarming
  - Used in moderate-to-severe hypothermia, when the patient is still maintaining adequate perfusion
  - Can rewarm via vascular (warm fluids 40 °C-42 °C) or pulmonary (warm humidified air) routes
  - Lavage of various cavities (thoracic, peritoneal, urinary bladder) can also be used but is risky and only marginally effective.
- Cardiopulmonary bypass can be used for severe hypothermia with circulatory arrest.
- Watch for hyperkalemia with rewarming.
- Failure to rewarm: consider alternative and concurrent diagnosis, such as sepsis, endocrine (myxedema coma/adrenal insufficiency).

SUGGESTED READINGS

Bjertnæs LJ, Næsheim TO, Reierth E, et al. Physiological changes in subjects exposed to accidental hypothermia: an update. *Front Med (Lausanne)*. 2022;9:824395.

Brown DJ, Brugger H, Boyd J, Paal P. Accidental hypothermia. *N Engl J Med*. 2012;367(20):1930-1938.

Darocha T, Debaty G, Ageron FX, et al. Hypothermia is associated with a low ETCO2 and low pH-stat $Paco_2$ in refractory cardiac arrest. *Resuscitation*. 2022;174:83-90.

Dow J, Giesbrecht GG, Danzl DF, et al. Wilderness Medical Society Clinical Practice Guidelines for the out-of-hospital evaluation and treatment of accidental hypothermia: 2019 update. *Wilderness Environ Med*. 2019;30(4 suppl):S47-S69.

Duong H, Patel G. Hypothermia. In: *StatPearls* [Internet]. StatPearls Publishing; 2024.

Savioli G, Ceresa IF, Bavestrello Piccini G, et al. Hypothermia: beyond the narrative review-the point of view of emergency physicians and medico-legal considerations. *J Pers Med*. 2023;13(12):1690.

SECTION 13

Obstetrics

Section Editor: Marvin G. Chang

13.1

Preeclampsia/Eclampsia and HELLP Syndrome

Christine Zachek and Marvin G. Chang

Normal Physiologic Changes in Pregnancy (Table 13.1.1)

Hypertensive Disorders of Pregnancy

Definitions

- A progressive multisystem, pregnancy-specific condition defined as new-onset hypertension after 20 weeks of gestation with evidence of end-organ dysfunction
- Typical onset in the third trimester; however, early-onset and de novo postpartum preeclampsia are increasingly recognized.
- HELLP (hemolysis, elevated liver enzymes, and low platelets) syndrome can have atypical presentations, with 15% of patients lacking hypertension or proteinuria.
- Although no longer part of the diagnostic criteria, peripheral edema, oliguria, and hemoconcentration are frequently observed because of vasospasm and capillary leak. (See Table 13.1.2.)

Epidemiology

- Hypertensive disorders of pregnancy complicate 2% to 8% of all pregnancies.
- Eclampsia and HELLP syndrome occur more rarely (~2%-3% and 1%, respectively, of pregnancies with pre-eclampsia with severe features who did not receive seizure prophylaxis) but have high rates of morbidity and mortality.

Risk Factors

- Nulliparity
- History of preeclampsia, particularly preterm preeclampsia

TABLE 13.1.1 Normal Physiologic Changes in Pregnancy

Cardiovascular	Respiratory	GI	Renal	Hematologic	Endocrine
↑ Cardiac output (30%-50%)	↓ Functional residual capacity	↓ Lower esophageal sphincter tone	↑ Renal blood flow (35%-60%)	↑ Red cell mass (but only 20%-30% vs blood volume 40%-50%), leading to dilutional anemia	↑ Insulin resistance
↑ Blood volume (40%-50%)	↑ Minute ventilation	↑ Alkaline phosphatase (placental production)	↑ Glomerular filtration rate (40%-50%)	↑ Clotting factors, including fibrinogen (hypercoagulable state)	↑ Prolactin
↓ BP and systemic vascular resistance (second trimester)	↑ O_2 consumption	↓ Total protein and albumin	↓ Creatinine		Transient hyperthyroidism (first trimester)
↑ Heart rate (20%)	Compensated respiratory alkalosis		Physiologic hydronephrosis from ureteral relaxation		
Unchanged central venous pressure					

BP, blood pressure; GI, gastrointestinal.

TABLE 13.1.2 Diagnostic Criteria

Preeclampsia[a]	Preeclampsia With Severe Features	Eclampsia	HELLP[b]

• Blood pressure ≥140 systolic or 90 diastolic on two occasions at least 4 h apart after 20 wk of gestation
• 300 mg protein in a 24-h urine sample or protein/creatinine ratio of ≥0.3
In the absence of proteinuria, new-onset hypertension plus any of the following are diagnostic for preeclampsia:
• Platelet count <100
• Serum creatinine >1.1 mg/dL or double baseline creatinine
• Liver function tests 2 × upper limit of normal
• Pulmonary edema
• New neurologic symptoms: blurred vision, headache nonresponsive to medications
• Severe right upper quadrant or epigastric pain (not explained by other diagnoses)
	• Blood pressure of 160 mm Hg systolic or higher or 110 mm Hg diastolic or higher on two occasions at least 4 h apart (unless antihypertensive therapy is initiated before this time)
	• Platelet count <100
	• Serum creatinine >1.1 mg/dL or double baseline creatinine
	• Liver function tests 2 × upper limit of normal
	• Pulmonary edema
	• New neurologic symptoms: blurred vision, headache nonresponsive to medications
	• Severe right upper quadrant or epigastric pain (not explained by other diagnoses)
		• New-onset tonic-clonic, focal, or multifocal seizures in the setting of pregnancy-associated hypertension without an alternative cause	• Hemolysis:
			  • Schistocytes or burr cells on peripheral blood smear
			  • Bilirubin ≥1.2 mg/dL
			  • Haptoglobin ≤25 mg/dL or LDH ≥600 IU/L
			  • Hgb <8-10 g/dL without evidence of blood loss
			• AST/ALT elevated 2× upper limit of normal
			• Platelet count <100

ALT, alanine aminotransferase; AST, aspartate aminotransferase; HELLP, hemolysis, elevated liver enzymes, and low platelets; Hgb, hemoglobin; LDH, lactate dehydrogenase.
[a]International organizations also include markers of uteroplacental dysfunction (ie, fetal growth restriction, stillbirth) as part of the diagnostic criteria.
[b]There is no consensus definition for HELLP syndrome; the abovementioned laboratory criteria are helpful in establishing the diagnosis.

- Maternal age ≥35
- Diabetes (preexisting and gestational)
- Obesity
- Multiple gestations
- Chronic hypertension
- Autoimmune disease (eg, lupus, antiphospholipid syndrome, rheumatoid arthritis)
- Kidney disease
- Assisted reproductive technology
- Obstructive sleep apnea
- Thrombophilia

Differential Diagnosis

- Drug-induced hepatotoxicity (acetaminophen)
- Acute fatty liver of pregnancy
- Viral hepatitis
- Chronic or gestational hypertension
- Thrombotic thrombocytopenic purpura (TTP)
- Hemolytic uremic syndrome
- Lupus exacerbation

Eclampsia Differential Diagnosis

- Epilepsy
- Intracranial hemorrhage or infarction
- Toxic metabolic encephalopathy
- Local anesthetic systemic toxicity

Pathophysiology

- Pathogenesis is incompletely characterized but is thought to originate from abnormal development of placental vasculature:
  - Abnormal placental artery remodeling during implantation → uteroplacental ischemia → overexpression of angiogenic factors → angiogenic factors bind to and decrease mediators of endothelial function → systemic endothelial dysfunction → vasoconstriction, microemboli, oxidative stress
- Immune dysregulation, genetic susceptibility, and preexisting cardiovascular dysfunction are also implicated in preeclampsia development.

Management and Treatment

- Daily low-dose aspirin for the prevention of preeclampsia is recommended starting at 12 weeks for patients at high risk.
- Limited options for the physician to control the extent of the preeclampsia other than delivery of the fetus and placenta
- Delivery decisions are complex and involve assessing the severity of preeclampsia, gestational age of the fetus (weighing the risks of prematurity against maternal risks), and assessing fetal status. Expert consultation with high-risk obstetrics and neonatology, if premature, for decisions around delivery timing and mode of delivery is warranted.
- Patients with high-risk complications like HELLP, eclampsia, stroke, and myocardial infarction should proceed to delivery immediately after maternal stabilization, regardless of gestational age.

Acute Treatment

- Principles of acute management include: (1) rapid blood pressure (BP) control to reduce stroke risk, (2) initiation of magnesium infusion for seizure prophylaxis, (3) delivery consideration, and (4) close monitoring for complications.
  - Serious complications include hemorrhagic stroke (the leading cause of maternal mortality in preeclampsia),

posterior reversible encephalopathy syndrome (PRES), retinal detachment/cortical blindness, myocardial infarction, heart failure, pulmonary edema, hepatic rupture, acute kidney injury, placental abruption, disseminated intravascular coagulation (DIC), and maternal and fetal death.
  - Eclamptic seizures can lead to severe hypoxia, trauma, and aspiration pneumonia.
- Management of hypertensive emergency
  - Considered ≥160 or 110 diastolic, persistent over 15 minutes
  - Intravenous (IV) labetalol 20 mg, IV hydralazine 5 to 10 mg, and immediate-release oral (PO) nifedipine 10 mg are most commonly used; frequent and escalating redosing is often needed to achieve BP control.
  - Transfer to an intensive care unit for continuous infusions may be indicated in refractory cases; avoid nitroprusside, given the association with fetal cyanide toxicity, except as the last option for BP control.
  - Prompt treatment helps prevent maternal stroke and placental abruption.
  - Aim for BP 140/90; avoid drastic drops in BP that may result in placental and maternal hypoperfusion.
- Magnesium sulfate infusion to decrease the risk of eclamptic seizure
  - Administer for preeclampsia with severe features, eclampsia, and HELLP at diagnosis until 24 hours postpartum.
  - 4 to 6 g loading dose followed by 1 to 2 g/h infusion
  - Aim for a magnesium level between 4 and 8 mEq/L.
  - Monitor for magnesium toxicity.
    - Renally cleared; consider dose reduction and/or monitoring serial magnesium levels for patients with renal impairment.
    - Contraindicated in patients with myasthenia gravis
    - Monitor respiratory status, urine output, creatinine clearance, and deep tendon reflexes.
    - Magnesium levels >9 mg/dL are associated with loss of deep tendon reflexes; respiratory depression and cardiac arrest can occur at levels ≥12 mg/dL.
    - Antidote: 1 g calcium gluconate IV push over 5 minutes
- Management of eclampsia
  - Stabilize patient; implement aspiration and fall precautions.
  - Eclamptic seizures are generally self-limited and have a short postictal phase (10-20 minutes).
  - Administer magnesium as above to prevent seizure recurrence; intramuscular (IM) bolus (5 mg IM × 2 buttocks) can be used for patients without IV access.
  - Benzodiazepines can be used for prolonged seizure activity, similar to nonpregnant adults.
  - Consider alternate causes of seizure and pursue neurologic imaging, toxic/metabolic, and infectious workup (particularly if seizures occur <20 weeks of gestation or for persistent focal neurologic deficits).
- Management of HELLP
  - Monitor for evidence of DIC and support with blood product transfusion, as necessary.
  - Treat severe hypertension.
  - Seizure prophylaxis with magnesium sulfate
  - Delivery is generally recommended after maternal stabilization to prevent maternal and fetal complications.
  - Consider hepatic imaging for persistent, severe right upper quadrant/epigastric pain due to the risk of hematoma and rupture.
  - Most laboratory abnormalities peak around 48 hours and normalize within 7 days after delivery.

Outcomes

- Responsible for 14% of maternal deaths worldwide, with cerebral hemorrhage representing the leading cause of maternal death
- Impaired placental perfusion increases the risk of stillbirth, fetal growth restriction, and premature delivery.
- Increased risk of preeclampsia in future pregnancies, and maternal cardiovascular and end-stage renal disease later in life

SUGGESTED READINGS

Altman D, Carroli G, Duley L, et al; Magpie Trial Collaboration Group. Do women with pre-eclampsia, and their babies, benefit from magnesium sulphate? The Magpie Trial: a randomised placebo-controlled trial. *Lancet*. 2002;359(9321):1877-1890.

American College of Obstetrics and Gynecology. Gestational hypertension and preeclampsia: ACOG Practice Bulletin, Number 222. *Obstet Gynecol*. 2020;135(6):e237-e260.

Ives CW, Sinkey R, Rajapreyar I, Tita ATN, Oparil S. Preeclampsia-pathophysiology and clinical presentations: JACC state-of-the-art review. *J Am Coll Cardiol*. 2020;76(14):1690-1702.

Magee LA, Brown MA, Hall DR, et al. The 2021 International Society for the Study of Hypertension in Pregnancy classification, diagnosis & management recommendations for international practice. *Pregnancy Hypertens*. 2022;27:148-169.

13.2

Acute Fatty Liver of Pregnancy

Christine Zachek and Marvin G. Chang

Acute Fatty Liver of Pregnancy

Definition

- Acute fatty liver of pregnancy (AFLP) is characterized by microvesicular fatty infiltration of hepatocytes, resulting in liver insufficiency, coagulopathy, and electrolyte abnormalities.

Epidemiology

- Estimated prevalence 1 to 3 cases per 10,000 deliveries
- Occurs typically in the third trimester or early postpartum period

Risk Factors

- Multiple gestations
- Male fetus
- Fetal fatty acid oxidation defects, such as long-chain 3-hydroxyacyl-coenzyme A dehydrogenase (LCHAD) deficiency
- Underlying metabolic and hepatic disorders (obesity, diabetes, intrahepatic cholestasis, metabolic dysfunction–associated steatotic liver disease)

Differential Diagnosis

- Drug-induced hepatotoxicity (acetaminophen)
- Hemolysis, elevated liver enzymes, and low platelets (HELLP) syndrome
- Thrombotic thrombocytopenic purpura (TTP)
- Viral hepatitis
- Alcoholic liver disease
- Autoimmune hepatitis
- Preeclampsia
- Budd-Chiari syndrome
- Intrahepatic cholestasis of pregnancy

Pathophysiology

- Exact pathophysiology of AFLP is unclear, but it is strongly associated with genetic defects in fatty acid metabolism, particularly in the fetus.
- Fetal LCHAD deficiency is most strongly linked to acute fatty liver. This enzyme deficiency impairs the fetus's ability to metabolize long-chain fatty acids, leading to the accumulation of hepatotoxic fatty acids that can cross into the maternal circulation and overwhelm mitochondrial function, resulting in microvesicular fatty infiltration of hepatocytes, oxidative stress, and activation of inflammatory pathways.
- The accumulation of fatty acids metabolites in the maternal liver → microvesicular fatty infiltration and reactive oxygen species generation → activation of inflammatory pathways → hepatocellular damage
- Fatty acid oxidation disorders such as LCHAD deficiency have autosomal recessive inheritance. The mother is usually a carrier and able to metabolize fatty acids under normal conditions, but may be unable to effectively metabolize the overwhelming burden of free fatty acids contributed by the fetus during pregnancy, leading to the development of AFLP.

Diagnosis

- The Swansea criteria have been validated for diagnosing AFLP and require six or more of the following features, in the absence of another identifiable cause (Table 13.2.1):
- Other common symptoms include:
  - Hypertension
  - Jaundice
  - Gastrointestinal bleeding
  - Pruritis
- Distinguishing between HELLP syndrome and AFLP can be challenging due to overlapping clinical features; however, severe hypoglycemia, a hallmark of AFLP, along with coagulopathy and encephalopathy are more characteristic of AFLP and reflect its generally more profound hepatic dysfunction compared to HELLP.
- Radiographic imaging may demonstrate ascites or increased echogenicity on ultrasound. While it may be useful for ruling out alternative diagnoses, imaging has low sensitivity for detecting AFLP.
- Antithrombin activity is often reduced compared to normal pregnancy values; however, this test may not be readily available.

TABLE 13.2.1 Swansea Criteria

Clinical Features
• Nausea/vomiting
• Abdominal pain
• Polydipsia/polyuria
• Encephalopathy
Laboratory Findings
• Hypoglycemia
• Hyperbilirubinemia
• Transaminitis
• Hyperammonemia
• Acute renal failure
• Coagulopathy
• Leukocytosis
• Elevated uric acid
Imaging
• Ascites or echogenic liver on ultrasound
Pathology
• Microvesicular steatosis on liver biopsy

Management and Treatment

- No specific medical treatment
- Prompt delivery of the fetus once the diagnosis is confirmed or strongly suspected.
- Mode of delivery is dependent on the fetal status, maternal coagulation status, and likelihood of successful vaginal delivery with induction of labor.
- Possible use of plasma exchange, continuous renal replacement therapy (CRRT), or molecular adsorbent recirculating system (MARS) to treat severe cases
- Initiate transfer to a tertiary care center capable of liver transplantation in cases of acute liver failure
- Because the early diagnosis of LCHAD deficiency in the newborn can be lifesaving, all women with AFLP and their newborns should undergo molecular testing for LCHAD.
- Closely monitor for and treat complications:
  - Hypoglycemia: most require 5% dextrose intravenous fluids
  - Supportive care of maternal coagulopathy with blood products, guided by clinical context and laboratory results
  - Cerebral edema and elevated intracranial pressures (ICPs) may require directed therapy and/or invasive monitoring.
  - Closely monitor fluid balance, as patients may develop pulmonary edema due to low plasma oncotic pressures.
  - Pancreatitis may be present (~15%); some experts recommend trending amylase/lipase and obtaining imaging, if abnormal.
  - Infectious complications and poor wound healing are common in the setting of critical illness and weakened immune function.

Outcomes

- High maternal and neonatal morbidity and mortality if not diagnosed and treated promptly
- Maternal mortality rates have decreased dramatically from 70% to 90% reported in the 1980s to more recent data estimating 2% to 13%.
- Neonatal mortality rate of ~10% to 20%
- Most patients experience clinical recovery 3 to 4 days after delivery, but laboratory abnormalities can persist for several days to weeks after delivery.

SUGGESTED READINGS

Liu J, Ghaziani TT, Wolf JL. Acute fatty liver disease of pregnancy: updates in pathogenesis, diagnosis, and management. *Am J Gastroenterol*. 2017;112(6):838-846.

Naoum EE, Leffert LR, Chitilian HV, Gray KJ, Bateman BT. Acute fatty liver of pregnancy: pathophysiology, anesthetic implications, and obstetrical management. *Anesthesiology*. 2019;130(3):446-461.

Nelson DB, Byrne JJ, Cunningham FG. Acute fatty liver of pregnancy. *Obstet Gynecol*. 2021;137(3):535-546.

13.3

Amniotic Fluid Embolism

Christine Zachek and Marvin G. Chang

Definition

- Amniotic fluid embolism (AFE), formerly known as anaphylactoid syndrome of pregnancy, is a rare and catastrophic obstetric emergency characterized by a pathologic pro-inflammatory maternal response triggered by the entry of amniotic fluid, fetal cells, or other fetal material into the maternal circulation
- Unpredictable and carries high mortality rate up to 60%
- Most occur during delivery but can present after trauma, amniocentesis, and termination procedures
- Typical presentation is a classic triad of sudden hypoxia and hypotension, followed by coagulopathy; however, atypical presentations may also occur

Epidemiology

- Rare, with a reported frequency of 1.9 to 6.1 per 100,000 live births.
- Incidence and outcomes vary globally, with higher maternal mortality reported in resource-limited settings due to delayed recognition and lack of advanced critical care resources.

Risk Factors

- Placenta previa, abruption, or accreta spectrum
- Polyhydramnios
- Multiple gestation
- Cesarean section and operative vaginal delivery
- Cervical laceration/uterine rupture
- Advanced maternal age
- Hypertensive disorders (eg, preeclampsia, chronic hypertension)
- Chorioamnionitis

Differential Diagnosis

- Eclampsia
- Stroke
- Aortic dissection
- Spinal anesthesia or local anesthetic toxicity
- Pulmonary embolism/air embolism
- Anaphylaxis
- Septic shock
- Aspiration
- Myocardial infarction
- Obstetric hemorrhagic shock

Key Pathophysiology

- Amniotic fluid, fetal cells, or other fetal material enters maternal circulation with pathologic release of inflammatory mediators, resulting in severe cardiovascular, pulmonary, and hematologic dysfunction.
- The systemic release of cytokines and vasoactive substances contributes to widespread endothelial injury and organ dysfunction.

TABLE 13.3.1 Phases of Amniotic Fluid Embolism

Phase I	Pulmonary artery vasospasm and release of vasoconstrictors → pulmonary hypertension → severe V̇/Q̇ mismatching and elevated right ventricular (RV) pressure → hypoxemic respiratory failure and RV failure
Phase II	RV failure, possible myocardial ischemia → left ventricle (LV) failure → noncardiogenic pulmonary edema, systemic hypotension
Phase III	Amniotic fluid activates factor VII and inflammatory response further activates clotting cascade → DIC → massive hemorrhage → hemodynamic instability, end-organ ischemia

DIC, disseminated intravascular coagulation.

- AFE is a diagnosis of exclusion, and the clinical presentation requires prompt evaluation and management to address life-threatening complications and exclude differential diagnoses.
- Diagnosis is clinical, and the work-up should include a broad investigation of obstetric and non-obstetric causes of cardiorespiratory compromise.
  - Patients may initially complain of a sense of doom, agitation, chest pain, or nausea/vomiting
  - Sudden onset of dyspnea and hypotension
  - Patients may progress rapidly to cardiovascular collapse
  - Neurologic manifestations can also include altered mental status or seizures
  - Massive disseminated intravascular coagulation (DIC)-associated hemorrhage
  - See Table 13.3.1 for phases of amniotic fluid embolism

Management and Treatment

- No specific treatment—supportive interventions to improve hemodynamics, support right ventricular (RV) and left ventricular (LV) failure, and correct coagulopathy
- Follow Advanced Cardiac Life Support (ACLS) protocols for pregnancy in the event of cardiac arrest (Table 13.3.2).
- Arterial line and central venous catheter placement to assist with hemodynamic monitoring and medications
- Pulmonary artery catheters may provide useful information in patients with shock, pulmonary edema, and uncertain intravascular volume status, but treatment should not be delayed for placement.

TABLE 13.3.2 Pregnancy-Specific Considerations for Management of Cardiac Arrest

- Maintain continuous manual left-lateral uterine displacement to relieve inferior vena cava compression.
- Establish IV access above the diaphragm to avoid obstruction from the gravid uterus.
- Anticipate a difficult airway; intubations should be performed by an experienced provider.
- ACLS medications, dosages, and defibrillation protocols are the same as a nonpregnant patient.
- Perform a resuscitative hysterotomy if return of spontaneous circulation (ROSC) is not achieved within ~4 min.

ACLS, Advanced Cardiac Life Support; IV, intravenous.

- Transthoracic or transesophageal echocardiogram can provide early identification of RV failure and narrow the differential diagnosis.
- Timing and mode of delivery are considered on a case-by-case basis; but in general, delivery of a viable fetus (>23 weeks of gestation) is recommended in cases of maternal cardiac arrest to improve hemodynamics.
- Reduce RV afterload and improve cardiac contractility
  - Avoid hypoxemia, hypercapnia, and acidosis to limit increases in pulmonary vascular resistance.
  - Avoid excessive fluids and preferentially use vasopressors for hypotension.
  - Pulmonary vasodilators (eg, inhaled nitric oxide, sildenafil, epoprostenol)
  - Inotropes such as dobutamine, milrinone, or epinephrine
- Anticipate DIC and prepare for massive transfusion of blood products.
  - Balanced transfusion, guided by clinical context and laboratory results
  - Medical management of uterine atony with uterotonics and/or surgical intervention may also be required, depending on the etiology of bleeding.
- Extracorporeal membrane oxygenation (ECMO) can be considered for cases with persistent hemodynamic instability refractory to medical management.

Outcomes

- Maternal mortality rate 11% to 60%
- Neonatal mortality rate ~40%
- Survivors may have neurologic injury due to cerebral hypoxia; however, prompt recognition and aggressive management may improve survival rates and reduce the risk of long-term neurologic deficits.
- Advancements in resuscitation techniques, such as massive transfusion protocols, mechanical circulatory support (eg, ECMO), and enhanced hemodynamic monitoring, may contribute to improved survival rates and reduced complications.

SUGGESTED READINGS

Jeejeebhoy FM, Zelop CM, Lipman S, et al; American Heart Association Emergency Cardiovascular Care Committee, Council on Cardiopulmonary, Critical Care, Perioperative and Resuscitation, Council on Cardiovascular Diseases in the Young, and Council on Clinical Cardiology. Cardiac arrest in pregnancy: a scientific statement from the American Heart Association. *Circulation*. 2015;132(18):1747-1773.

McDonnell NJ, Percival V, Paech MJ. Amniotic fluid embolism: a leading cause of maternal death yet still a medical conundrum. *Int J Obstet Anesth*. 2013;22(4):329-336.

Pacheco LD, Clark SL, Klassen M, Hankins GDV. Amniotic fluid embolism: principles of early clinical management. *Am J Obstet Gynecol*. 2020;222(1):48-52.

Pacheco LD, Saade GR, Costantine MM, Clark SL, Hankins GD. An update on the use of massive transfusion protocols in obstetrics. *Am J Obstet Gynecol*. 2016;214(3):340-344.

Society for Maternal-Fetal Medicine; Pacheco LD, Saade G, Hankins GD, Clark SL. Amniotic fluid embolism: diagnosis and management. *Am J Obstet Gynecol*. 2016;215:B16-B24.

Sultan P, Seligman K, Carvalho B. Amniotic fluid embolism: update and review. *Curr Opin Anaesthesiol*. 2016;29(3):288-296.

13.4

Postpartum Hemorrhage

Christine Zachek and Marvin G. Chang

Definition

- *Primary:* cumulative blood loss ≥1,000 mL within the first 24 hours of delivery, regardless of mode of delivery, with or without signs or symptoms of hypovolemia
- *Secondary:* excessive bleeding after the first 24 hours and up to 12 weeks postpartum

Epidemiology

- The leading preventable cause of maternal morbidity and mortality worldwide
- A full-term uterus requires 600 mL of blood per minute to support a pregnancy.
- A pregnant woman can fully compensate for 15% to 20% blood volume loss due to a physiologic increase in plasma volume during pregnancy—even subtle vital sign changes can indicate early decompensation and rapid progression to hypovolemic shock.

Risk Factors

- Prior postpartum hemorrhage
- Previous cesarean or other uterine surgery
- Abnormal placentation (placenta accreta spectrum, placenta previa)
- Uterine fibroids
- Rapid or prolonged labor
- Grand multiparity (>4 prior deliveries)
- Uterine overdistention
    - Multiple gestation
    - Polyhydramnios (excess amniotic fluid)
    - Estimated fetal weight >4,000 g
- Thrombocytopenia or known coagulation defect
- Chorioamnionitis
- Preeclampsia
- Medications (anticoagulation, magnesium sulfate, general anesthesia, prolonged oxytocin use, terbutaline, nitroglycerine)
- Intrauterine fetal demise

Causes of Postpartum Hemorrhage

- Uterine atony (70%)
- Cervical or vaginal lacerations
- Retained placenta
- Uterine inversion or uterine rupture
- Placental abruption
- Disseminated intravascular coagulation (DIC)

Management and Treatment

- Recognize risk factors and prepare for hemorrhage control.
    - Ensure adequate intravenous access, consider central access.
    - Crossmatch blood products in the blood bank.
    - Alert appropriate multidisciplinary teams: obstetrics, anesthesia, intensive care, nursing, transfusion medicine, and, possibly, interventional radiology.
- Evaluate for the etiology.
    - Ultrasound for retained products of conception, intra-abdominal bleeding, and uterine abnormalities (ie, uterine rupture, inversion)
    - Careful inspection of cervix and perineum for lacerations or hematomas
    - Complete blood count and coagulation studies—fibrinogen values are typically elevated in pregnancy, and <200 can signal risk for progression to severe hemorrhage.
- Medical Management
    - Bimanual uterine massage
    - Intravenous (IV) fluid resuscitation
    - Balanced blood product transfusion, guided by clinical context and laboratory results
    - Place a urinary catheter to aid in uterine contraction and monitor urine output.
    - Warming blankets to maintain normothermia
    - Uterotonic agents (Table 13.4.1)
    - Early administration of tranexamic acid (TXA 1 g IV) as soon as possible after the onset of postpartum hemorrhage and within 3 hours of delivery reduces mortality due to bleeding, as demonstrated by the WOMAN trial and recommended by the World Health Organization (WHO).
        - It does not affect overall mortality or rate of hysterectomy.
        - Caution is advised in patients with known thrombophilia or active thromboembolic disease, and decisions should be based on individual risk-benefit assessments.

TABLE 13.4.1 Uterotonic Agents for Postpartum Hemorrhage

Drug	Dose/Route	Frequency	Contraindications/Notes
Oxytocin (Pitocin)	10 units IM or up to 40 units in 1 L NS or lactated Ringer	Continuous drip or IM up to 4 doses	Excessive (>60 units) may lead to hyponatremia; rapid bolus may cause hypotension.
Methylergonovine (Methergine)	0.2 mg IM	q2-4h up to 5 doses	Avoid in hypertension, cardiovascular disease
15-Methyl $PGF_{2\alpha}$ (Hemabate)	250 μg IM	Every 15 min up to 8 doses	Avoid in asthmatics; relatively contraindicated in hepatic, renal, and cardiac disease
Misoprostol (Cytotec)	600-1,000 μg oral, sublingual, or rectal	One time	Can cause GI disturbance and transient fever; questionable efficacy

GI, gastrointestinal; IM, intramuscular; NS, normal saline; q, every.

      - A second dose may be given if bleeding continues after 30 minutes or restarts within 24 hours.
      - TXA should be slowly administered over 10 minutes to reduce the risk of transient hypotension.
   - For hemodynamically stable patients unresponsive to medical management, uterine artery embolization can be considered at centers with specialized expertise. In hemodynamically unstable patients, surgical management, including possibly hysterectomy, may be necessary if bleeding cannot be controlled by other means. Management should be tailored to the patient's condition and available resources.
- Surgical Management
   - Intrauterine tamponade balloon
   - Suture repair of lacerations and possible vaginal packing for hematomas
   - Dilation and curettage to remove retained products of conception
   - Laparotomy
      - Uterine artery ligation sutures to decrease the pulse pressure to the uterus
      - B-Lynch uterine compression sutures
      - Repair of uterine rupture
      - Hysterectomy is the definitive intervention when all other measures have failed to control a life-threatening hemorrhage.

Outcomes

- Postpartum hemorrhage is responsible for ~8% of maternal deaths in developed countries and 20% in developing countries.
- Complications can include coagulopathy, acute renal failure, hepatic dysfunction, transfusion-related complications, and infertility from interventions to control massive blood loss.
- Early identification of high-risk patients, treatment of anemia, prophylactic oxytocin, and prompt, aggressive treatments can reduce severe maternal morbidity and mortality.

SUGGESTED READINGS

Bienstock JL, Eke AC, Hueppchen NA. Postpartum hemorrhage. *N Engl J Med*. 2021;384(17):1635-1645.

Committee on Practice Bulletins-Obstetrics. Practice Bulletin No. 183: postpartum hemorrhage. *Obstet Gynecol*. 2017;130(4):e168-e186.

Gallos I, Devall A, Martin J, et al. Randomized trial of early detection and treatment of postpartum hemorrhage. *N Engl J Med*. 2023;389(1):11-21.

Rigouzzo A, Froissant PA, Louvet N. Changing hemostatic management in post-partum hemorrhage. *Am J Hematol*. 2024;99(suppl 1):S13-S18.

WOMAN Trial Collaborators. Effect of early tranexamic acid administration on mortality, hysterectomy, and other morbidities in women with post-partum haemorrhage (WOMAN): an international, randomised, double-blind, placebo-controlled trial. *Lancet*. 2017;389(10084):2105-2116.

13.5

Peripartum Cardiomyopathy

Kait Brennan and Christina Anne Jelly

Definition

- Peripartum cardiomyopathy (PPCM) or pregnancy-associated cardiomyopathy is a rare, mostly dilated form of cardiomyopathy marked by left ventricular (LV) systolic dysfunction (left ventricular ejection fraction [LVEF] <45%).
- Affects women late in pregnancy or in the early postpartum (PP) period.

Key Points

- Occurs in the late third trimester or the early PP period
- Delayed diagnosis is common.
- Likely due to a combination of genetic risk factors and pregnancy specific cytokines
- May require urgent delivery if cardiogenic shock is present
- LVEF <35% confers a high risk of LV thrombus, warranting strong consideration for therapeutic anticoagulation.
- High rate of recovery, usually in the first 6 months PP

Epidemiology

- Affects women from all ethnicities worldwide, but women with Black ancestry are at the highest risk. Incidence in women of Nigerian or Haitian descent is as high as 1:100 to 1:300 compared to 1:1,000 to 4,000 in the United States.
- Cardiovascular disease is a leading cause of maternal morbidity in the United States, with PPCM accounting for a substantial amount of maternal cardiovascular morbidity.
- Known risk factors include preeclampsia, advanced maternal age (>30 years), African ancestry, multiparity, multiple gestation pregnancies, maternal cocaine use, autoimmune disease, and maternal cardiovascular risk factors.

Key Pathophysiology

- Complete pathogenesis of PPCM is unknown, but research has suggested a "two hit" model where a vascular insult caused by impaired antivascular and hormonal effects in women with a genetic predisposition leads to a final common pathway resulting in increased oxidative stress, abnormal prolactin processing, and impaired vascular endothelial signaling.
- Other biologic factors include genetic predisposition, abnormal inflammatory cytokine signaling, and infectious and environmental factors given that myocarditis has been attributed as a possible cause of PPCM.

Clinical Manifestations

- Unlikely to present before 36 weeks of gestation and most commonly presents during the first month postpartum. Symptoms can mimic pregnancy; as a result, delayed diagnosis is common. Providers should maintain a high index of suspicion for PPCM in patients presenting with unexplained dyspnea, edema, or fatigue in the late third trimester or postpartum period (PP), especially those with risk factors.

- Patients present with symptoms consistent with congestion in systolic heart failure (HF), such as dyspnea, orthopnea, paroxysmal nocturnal dyspnea, and peripheral edema. Signs typically found include those consistent with left- or right-sided HF, such as pulmonary rales, raised jugular venous pressure, and peripheral edema.

Diagnosis and Differential Diagnoses

- Diagnosis is based on the three clinical criteria:
  - Development of HF toward the end of pregnancy
  - Absence of another identifiable cause of HF
  - LV systolic dysfunction with an LVEF generally <45%
- Diagnostic testing usually includes electrocardiogram (ECG), echocardiogram, BNP or pro-BNP levels, and may include cardiac magnetic resonance imaging (MRI), cardiac catheterization, endomyocardial biopsy, and/or genetic testing as the diagnosis of PPCM is one of exclusion.
- Echocardiography may demonstrate right ventricular (RV) dilation and dysfunction, pulmonary hypertension, left atrial or biatrial enlargement, functional mitral and tricuspid regurgitation, and intracardiac thrombus.
- Differential diagnoses include preexisting cardiomyopathies, valvular disease or undiagnosed congenital heart disease, pulmonary arterial hypertension, myocardial infarction, and hypertensive heart disease.
- Point-of-care ultrasound (POCUS) can facilitate the rapid identification of cardiac dysfunction and assist in ruling out other potential causes of dyspnea, including pulmonary embolism, pneumonia, pneumothorax, asthma or chronic obstructive pulmonary disease (COPD) exacerbation, pericardial effusion, pleural effusion, as well as cardiogenic and noncardiogenic pulmonary edema.

Management and Treatment

- HF medications safe in pregnancy include beta-blockers, hydralazine, loop diuretics, digoxin, and isosorbide. Angiotensin-converting enzyme inhibitor/angiotensin receptor blockers (ACEI/ARBs) should be avoided in pregnancy.
- Early delivery should be considered if cardiogenic shock is present. Management, including delivery timing and mode of delivery, should be coordinated by a specialized cardio-obstetric team.
- LVEF <35% should prompt therapeutic anticoagulation, as LV thrombus is a common complication of PPCM, occurring in 10% to 20% of patients with PPCM.
- ACEI (enalapril and captopril) and ARBs are safe medications to use in breastfeeding patients. There are currently data to guide treatment with sacubitril-valsartan and ivabradine, and most cardio-obstetric specialists avoid these medications in breastfeeding patients.
- Bromocriptine may confer a survival benefit in PPCM, potentially via inhibition of prolactin secretion that contributes to disease pathophysiology. However, its use must be carefully weighed against the associated risk of thromboembolism, often necessitating concurrent anticoagulation. While international studies have been inconclusive, a large US & Canadian trial (REBIRTH) is currently underway to clarify its potential benefits and establish evidence-based guidelines for its use in PPCM.

Prognosis and Outcomes

- More than half of the women affected recover systolic function. Recovery usually occurs within 3 to 6 months but can occur up to 2 years after diagnosis.
- Poor prognostic factors include LVEF <30%, presence of LV thrombus, RV dysfunction, and African American race.
- Implantable therapies, including left ventricular assist device (LVAD) and implantable cardioverter-defibrillator (ICD), should be delayed for 6 months PP to allow for possible recovery.
- Contraception counseling should include the risk of worsening PPCM in subsequent pregnancies, especially if LVEF is not fully recovered.
- Medication therapy may be discontinued in a stepwise manner if LVEF recovers fully. Subsequent pregnancies carry a significant risk of recurrence, particularly if LVEF does not normalize. Patients should receive preconception counseling from a cardio-obstetric specialist.

SUGGESTED READINGS

Arany Z. Peripartum cardiomyopathy. *N Engl J Med*. 2024;390(2):154-164.

Bauersachs J, Arrigo M, Hilfiker-Kleiner D, et al. Current management of patients with severe acute peripartum cardiomyopathy: practical guidelines from the Heart Failure Association of the European Society of Cardiology Study Group on peripartum cardiomyopathy. *Eur J Heart Fail*. 2016;18:1096.

Davis MB, Arany Z, McNamara DM, Goland S, Elkayam U. Peripartum cardiomyopathy: JACC state-of-the-art review. *J Am Coll Cardiol*. 2020;75(2):207-221.

Honigberg MC, Givertz MM. Peripartum cardiomyopathy a state of the art review. *BMJ*. 2019;364:k5287.

McNamara DM, Elkayam U, Alharethi R, et al; IPAC Investigators. Clinical outcomes for peripartum cardiomyopathy in North America: results of the IPAC study (Investigations of Pregnancy-Associated Cardiomyopathy). *J Am Coll Cardiol*. 2015;66(8):905-914.

Regitz-Zagrosek V, Roos-Hesselin JW, Bauersachs J, et al. 2018 ESC guidelines for the management of cardiovascular diseases during pregnancy. *Kardiol Pol*. 2019;77:245.

13.6

Peripartum Infections

Scott A. Harvey, Ulrich H. Schmidt, and Angela Meier

Definition

- According to the World Health Organization, maternal sepsis refers to sepsis that results "from infection during pregnancy, childbirth, post-abortion, or the postpartum period [42 days]."
- The U.S. Centers for Disease Control and Prevention (CDC) defines a pregnancy-related death as "the death of a woman while pregnant or within one year of pregnancy, regardless of the outcome, duration, or site of pregnancy—from any cause related to or aggravated by the pregnancy or its management, but not from accidental or incidental causes." These data are contributed to the CDC by state Maternal Review Boards, where careful examination of each maternal death is assessed by a multidisciplinary committee.

Epidemiology

- Maternal infections are a significant contributor to maternal mortality, accounting for ~14% to 28% of maternal deaths in the United States. They consistently rank among the top 2 to 5 leading causes of maternal mortality, reflecting their serious impact on maternal health. This equates to roughly 290,000 deaths worldwide per year.
- Extensive reviews by maternal mortality review boards in the United States deem 63% of maternal deaths from sepsis may be prevented, citing concerns over recognition and management.

Common Pitfalls Interfering With Timely and Effective Treatment of Maternal Sepsis

- Delays in diagnosis due to normal maternal physiology mimicking sepsis, such as a higher heart rate, relatively elevated white blood cell count, and vasodilation from estrogen, leading to slight reductions of systemic vascular resistance and blood pressure
- Underdosing due to the fact that pregnant patients may require higher dosing of antibiotics due to higher volume of distribution and increased hepatorenal metabolism in pregnancy, such as in antibiotics that require dose-level monitoring (ie, vancomycin, gentamicin, etc)

Immunology

- While the prevailing concept of immunodeficiency in pregnancy is now understood to be a far more complex interplay between tolerance and defense as opposed to a mere suppression or deficiency, there are numerous changes to the immune system during healthy pregnancy that leave mother and child at risk for infection and its consequences.
- During pregnancy, the immune system adapts to tolerate the semiallogeneic fetus (which is genetically distinct from the mother due to the paternal genetic contribution). This adaptation involves a shift from a proinflammatory to an antiinflammatory immune state, particularly in the second and third trimesters.
- Pregnancy is furthermore characterized by changes in the populations and functions of various immune cells, such as an increase in regulatory T cells (Tregs), which help suppress maternal immune responses against fetal antigens.
- Cytokine production during pregnancy is modulated to favor a Th2-type response (antiinflammatory) over a Th1-type response (proinflammatory). This shift helps prevent fetal rejection and supports fetal growth, but it can also make pregnant women more susceptible to certain infections and reduce their ability to respond to some pathogens effectively.
- Despite this, studies have shown an exaggerated proinflammatory response of monocytes and plasmacytoid dendritic cells response to influenza in pregnancy, yet the mortality of influenza is increased in pregnant women compared to nonpregnant women.
- For practical purposes, it is of note that demarginalization of white blood cell counts up to 15 mm^3/dL is considered normal.

Diagnosis

- The leading obstetric societies in the United States (American College of Obstetrics & Gynecology and the Society of Maternal Fetal Medicine) endorse Sepsis 3 definitions to classify sepsis in pregnancy, which relies upon Sequential Organ Failure Assessment (SOFA) increasing by two points due to an infectious etiology. See *Table 13.6.1*.
    - In suspected sepsis, obtaining laboratory and biometric data to calculate a SOFA score is essential. The baseline values and thresholds for the SOFA score remain consistent for pregnant and nonpregnant patients.
- Many hospitals and Centers for Medicare/Medicaid still rely upon Sepsis 2 criteria (Systemic Inflammatory Response Syndrome due to infection) because of its simplicity and sensitivity in identifying early sepsis, particularly in pregnant patients. However, these criteria lack specificity, which can lead to overdiagnosis in cases where physiologic changes of pregnancy mimic systemic inflammatory response syndrome (SIRS).
    - The California Maternal Quality Care Collaborative (CMQCC) and United Kingdom Obstetric Surveillance System (UKOSS) both use early warning tools and diagnostic criteria for sepsis in patients >20 weeks pregnant based on Sepsis 2 criteria. These tools are highly sensitive, improving early detection of sepsis, but their reduced specificity may contribute to overdiagnosis in some cases. See Table 13.6.2.
    - CMQCC Maternal Sepsis has two steps:
        - Step 1: initial sepsis screen (two or more triggers evaluation)
            - Oral temperature <36 °C or >38 °C
            - Heart rate >110 beats per minute
            - Respiratory rate >24 breaths per minute
            - White blood cell (WBC count) >15,000/mm^3 or <4,000/mm^3, or >10% bands

TABLE 13.6.1 Criteria for End-Organ Injury for Diagnosis of Maternal Sepsis[a]

Organ System	Parameter	0	1	2	3	4
Respiratory	Pao_2/Fio_2 (mm Hg)	≥400	<400	<300	<200 (with resp support)	< 100 (with resp support)
Coagulation	Platelets (×10³/μL)	≥150	<150	<100	<50	< 20
Liver	Bilirubin (mg/dL)	<1.2	1.2–1.9	2.0–5.9	6.0–11.9	≥ 12.0
Cardiovascular	MAP (mm Hg) or vasopressor requirement	MAP ≥70 mm Hg	MAP<70	Dopamine ≤5 or dobutamine (any dose)	Dopamine >5 or epi/ norepi ≤ 0.1 μg/kg/min	Dopamine > 15 or epi/ norepi > 0.1 μg/kg/min
CNS	Glasgow Coma Scale (GCS)	15	13–14	10–12	6–9	< 6
Renal	Creatinine (mg/dL) or urine output (UO)	<1.2	1.2–1.9	2.0–3.4	3.5–4.9 or UO <500 mL/d	≥ 5.0 or UO <200 mL/d

CNS, central nervous system; Fio_2, fraction of inspired oxygen; MAP, mean arterial pressure; Pao_2, partial pressure of oxygen in the alveoli.
[a]Only one criterion is sufficient for diagnosis. End organs are the same as for Sepsis 3.

- Step 2: sepsis confirmed one or more is present.
  - Respiratory: new need for mechanical ventilation of Pao_2/Fio_2 <300 mm Hg
  - Coagulation platelets <100,000/L, or international normalized ratio (INR) >1.5, or partial thromboplastin time (PTT) >60 s
  - Liver: bilirubin >2 mg/dL
  - Cardiovascular: systolic blood pressure (SBP) <85 mm Hg or mean arterial pressure (MAP) <65 mm Hg or >40 mm Hg drop in systolic blood pressure after intravenous (IV) fluid hydration
  - Renal: creatinine ≥1.2 mg/dL or doubling of creatinine or urine output <0.5 mL/kg/h × 2 hours
  - Mental status: agitated, confused, or unresponsive
  - Lactic acid: >2 mmol/L in the absence of labor
- Septic shock diagnosed with MAP <65 mm Hg after 30 mL/kg IV fluids administered. See Table 13.6.3.

- Maternal sepsis occurs ~20% antepartum, 50% postpartum, and 30% intrapartum. The most common sources of sepsis are chorioamnionitis, pneumonia, and pyelonephritis.
- Most maternal sepsis deaths are from nonreproductive sources, most commonly pulmonary or urinary in origin.

Management

- Surviving Sepsis Campaign management techniques for pregnant patients are similar to those for nonpregnant patients.
  - Urgent assessment for diagnosis, including labs (complete blood count, liver enzymes, electrolytes, lactic acid, blood cultures, targeted organ cultures) and appropriate imaging. Aside from an expected WBC count up to 15,000 mm³, elevated alkaline phosphatase, and reduced albumin, most laboratory values generally remain unchanged in pregnancy.
  - Early administration of antibiotics after attaining cultures, 30 mL/kg (current total body weight) of isotonic crystalloids for hypotension or lactic acidemia. Patients in labor may have lactic acidemia due to elevated metabolic activity, but typically, it is <4 mmol/dL and resolves after delivery.

TABLE 13.6.2 Initial Sepsis Screen for All Patients With Suspected Infection[a]

- Oral temperature <36 °C (96.8 °F) or ≥38 °C (100.4 °F)
- Heart rate >110 beats per minute and sustained for 15 min
- Respiratory rate >24 breaths per minute and sustained for 15 min
- White blood cell count >15,000/mm³ or <4,000/mm³ or >10% immature neutrophils (bands)

[a]POSITIVE if two or more criteria are met.

TABLE 13.6.3 Confirmation of Sepsis Test to Evaluate End-Organ Injury Laboratory Values

- Complete blood count (including % immature neutrophils [bands], platelets)
- Coagulation status (prothrombin time/international normalized ratio [INR]/partial thromboplastin time [PTT])
- Comprehensive metabolic panel (specifically include bilirubin and creatinine)
- Venous lactic acid bedside assessment
- Urine output (place Foley catheter with urometer)
- Pulse oximetry
  - See Table 13.6.1 for Criteria for End-Organ Injury
  - Measure of End-Organ Injury Criteria (one criterion is sufficient for diagnosis)

Respiratory function
- Acute respiratory failure as evidenced by acute need for invasive or noninvasive mechanical ventilation, OR
- Pao_2/Fio_2 <300

Coagulation status
- Platelets <100 × 109/L, OR
- INR >1.5, OR
- PTT >60 s

Liver function
- Bilirubin >2 mg/dL

Cardiovascular function
- Persistent hypotension after fluid administration:
  - SBP <85 mm Hg, OR
  - MAP <65 mm Hg, OR
  - > 40 mm Hg decrease in SBP

Renal function
- Creatinine >1.2 mg/dL, OR
- Doubling of creatinine, OR
- Urine output <0.5 mL/kg/h (for 2 hours)

Mental status assessment
- Agitation, confusion, or unresponsiveness

Lactic acid
- 2 mmol/L in the absence of labor (Lactic acid is not used for diagnosis in labor but remains important for treatment.)

Fio_2, fraction of inspired oxygen; MAP, mean arterial pressure; Pao_2, partial pressure of oxygen in the alveoli; SBP, systolic blood pressure.

- Maternal and fetal monitoring if ≥23 to 24 weeks gestation, with frequent maternal assessments
- Medical Therapy
  - **Neurological:** Usual pain management and sedation techniques can be used with caution, given that sedatives cross the placenta and sedate the fetus. Muscle relaxants do not cross the placenta. Some medications may be contraindicated in pregnancy (eg, nonsteroidal antiinflammatory drugs [NSAIDs] and gabapentin). See Table 13.6.4.
  - **Cardiovascular**
    - Central venous pressure and pulmonary artery occlusion pressure are like nonpregnant patients. Systemic and pulmonary vascular resistance may be reduced.
    - Increased blood volume by about 1.5 L by the third trimester. Increased preload, decreased afterload, and cardiac hypertrophy lead to increased cardiac output.
    - Fetal heart monitoring is generally performed once the fetus is considered viable (gestational age ≥23 weeks) to assess uteroplacental perfusion and identify signs of fetal distress, which may guide management decisions.
    - Goals for MAP >65 mm Hg, with consideration to decrease to >60 mm Hg if there are normal maternal perfusion parameters and reactive fetal heart rate
    - Norepinephrine is the first-line vasopressor for managing hypotension in sepsis during pregnancy, as it maintains maternal perfusion and supports uteroplacental blood flow. Phenylephrine and

TABLE 13.6.4 Common Medications Used in the Intensive Care Unit and Their Safety in Pregnancy

System	Medication	Notes
Neurologic—pain		
	Acetaminophen	Generally safe in pregnancy
	Nonsteroidal antiinflammatory drugs (NSAIDs)	Avoided in pregnancy as they may cause fetal renal complications and prematurely close the ductus arteriosus, rarely used for a limited period to stop preterm labor
	Gabapentin	Generally avoided and reports suggestion may cause teratogenic risk to fetus
	Lidocaine/ketamine	When given intermittently, it is not suggestive of congenital anomalies. When used chronically, may cause congenital defects in brain, liver, and kidney.
Neurologic—agitation		
	Propofol	Generally safe in pregnancy in monitored circumstances, crosses placenta, and sedates the fetus. Acute use during delivery may cause respiratory depression in neonate.
	Benzodiazepines	Generally safe when used in acute situations such as in anesthesia and ICU sedation, generally avoided due to potential risks of congenital malformations, withdrawal symptoms in the newborn, and neonatal flaccidity. If necessary, use should be limited to the lowest effective dose and shortest duration possible.
	Dexmedetomidine	May affect uterine contractions
	Barbiturates	Generally avoided due to risks of congenital malformations, neonatal withdrawal, and potential long-term neurodevelopmental effects
	Nonbenzodiazepine hypnotics	Limited data, but generally considered safer than benzodiazepines. However, caution is still advised, especially during the first trimester.
	Histamine-1 blockers	Generally safe in pregnancy for short-term use during pregnancy. Often used to treat nausea and insomnia in pregnant women
	Trazodone/mirtazapine	Trazodone and mirtazapine are sometimes used for their sedative effects. Risks and benefits should be carefully weighed, and these medications should be used under close supervision by a health care provider.
Neurologic—delirium		
	Quetiapine	May increase risk for gestational diabetes, low birth weight, and delayed behavioral development when used chronically through pregnancy
	Valproic acid	May increase risk of congenital malformations such as spina bifida, open neurotube defects, delayed development, behavior/social skills, and cardiac defects—supplement with 4 mg of folic acid daily if using
Cardiovascular		
	Amiodarone	May affect the fetal thyroid, monitoring in the neonatal ICU is recommended after delivery
	Beta-blockers	Generally safe, avoid atenolol as it may cause fetal growth restriction. Labetalol and metoprolol are preferred.
	Calcium channel blockers	Generally safe in pregnancy
	Norepinephrine	Generally safe and first-line pressor in sepsis and shock

TABLE 13.6.4 Common Medications Used in the Intensive Care Unit and Their Safety in Pregnancy (*continued*)

System	Medication	Notes
	Phenylephrine	Generally safe and used for neurogenic shock
	Vasopressin	Generally avoided as it will induce uterine contractions
	Epinephrine	Use if necessary but will cause uterine ischemia.
Pulmonary		
	Albuterol	Generally safe in pregnancy
	Ipratropium	Generally safe in pregnancy
	Inhaled corticosteroids	Generally safe in pregnancy
Gastrointestinal		
	Histamine-2 blockers	Generally safe in pregnancy: famotidine best studied for safety
	Proton pump inhibitors	Omeprazole and esomeprazole have been used safely during pregnancy.
	Ursodiol	Generally safe in pregnancy
Renal		
	ACE inhibitors and angiotensin receptor blockers	Crosses placenta and may cause fetal renal failure
	Bicarbonate	Generally safe in pregnancy
	Hydrochlorothiazide/furosemide	Generally safe in pregnancy
Hematologic		
	Intravenous and oral iron	Safe in pregnancy
	Folic acid and B_{12}	Recommended in pregnancy
	Heparin and Enoxaparin	Safe in pregnancy, does not cross placenta
	Warfarin	Generally avoided in pregnancy, especially in the first trimester for congenital defects. It has indicated use for mechanical heart valves in the second and third trimesters.
	Xa inhibitors	Contraindicated in pregnancy, crosses placenta and may cause fetal intracranial hemorrhage and congenital defects
	Vitamins	Recommended in pregnancy
	Aspirin <163 mg	Generally safe in pregnancy
Infectious disease		
	Penicillin class	Generally considered safe during all trimesters, except for amoxicillin/clavulanic acid
	Cephalosporins	Generally considered safe during all trimesters
	Macrolides	Erythromycin is generally considered safe; however, certain formulations, such as erythromycin estolate should be avoided due to risk of hepatotoxicity. Azithromycin is also considered relatively safe.
	Clindamycin	Considered safe during pregnancy and is often used as an alternative in penicillin-allergic patients
	Sulfonamides	Generally avoided, especially during the first trimester and near term, due to potential risks of birth defects and neonatal jaundice
	Tetracyclines	Contraindicated during pregnancy due to risks of teeth discoloration and inhibition of bone growth in the fetus
	Fluoroquinolones	Generally avoided due to concerns about potential adverse effects on fetal cartilage development
	Aminoglycosides	Generally avoided due to potential risks of ototoxicity and nephrotoxicity to the fetus
	Nitrofurans	Generally considered safe, but some concerns exist about use near term due to potential risk of hemolytic anemia in the newborn
	Metronidazole	Generally considered safe, although some controversy exists regarding use in the first trimester
	Aminoglycosides	Generally avoided due to potential risks of ototoxicity and nephrotoxicity to the fetus
	Remdesivir	Generally safe for the treatment of severe COVID-19 during pregnancy

(*continued*)

TABLE 13.6.4 Common Medications Used in the Intensive Care Unit and Their Safety in Pregnancy (*continued*)

System	Medication	Notes
Endocrine		
	Metformin	Generally safe in pregnancy
	Insulin	Generally safe in pregnancy
	GLP-1 agonists	Avoid in pregnancy
	Alpha-glucosidase inhibitors	Avoid in pregnancy
	Sulfonylureas	Generally safe in pregnancy
	Levothyroxine	Generally safe in pregnancy
	Betamethasone/dexamethasone	Used in pregnancy for fetal maturation, short-term use is encouraged as chronic use may lead to craniosynostosis and developmental delay
	Methylprednisolone, hydrocortisone, fludrocortisone, prednisone	Generally safe in pregnancy, does not cross the placenta
Pregnancy		
	Magnesium	Generally safe in pregnancy
	Terbutaline	Generally safe in pregnancy
	Misoprostol	Contraindicated in pregnancy, unless used to attempt delivery or induce abortion
	Oxytocin	Used to induce and augment labor

ACE, angiotensin-converting enzyme; ICU, intensive care unit.

dopamine are safe. Vasopressin has a theoretical risk of inducing uterine contractions and is generally avoided. Due to high splanchnic vasoconstriction with the use of IV epinephrine, high doses may lead to uterine ischemia and fetal death.
- It is recommended to avoid delivery for the sole indication of maternal sepsis; consider delivering the fetus if ≥23 weeks gestation for usual fetal indications.

Respiratory
- Increased minute ventilation in pregnancy decreases $Paco_2$ and increases pH.
- Normal arterial blood gas (ABG) in pregnancy >12 weeks gestation: pH >7.43, $Paco_2$ 28 to 32 mm Hg, Pao_2 100 mm Hg (acceptable if >70 mm Hg), HCO_3^- 18 to 22 mEq/dL.
- High-risk airway with laryngeal edema, pretracheal fat, and aspiration risk due to gastric compression and a looser lower esophageal sphincter
- Risk for rapid desaturation due to decreased functional residual capacity and higher oxygen consumption
- Fetus may not tolerate acidemia and hypoxia, potentially inducing preterm labor. The most experienced provider should intubate with a smaller endotracheal tube (ETT) of 6.0 to 6.5 mm. Early intubation is recommended as continuous positive airway pressure/bilevel positive airway pressure (CPAP/BIPAP) may lead to aspiration.

Gastrointestinal
- Supplement with an extra 300 kcal/d during pregnancy and an additional 500 kcal/d if breastfeeding postpartum
- Postpyloric feeding in intubated patients to prevent aspiration. Peptic ulcer prophylaxis is safe in pregnancy. Constipation is common; patients should be given a stool regimen if critically ill.

Renal
- Increased kidney metabolism leads to high rates of acute renal injury in the setting of underperfusion. Increased glomerular filtration rate (GFR) leads to increased clearance of medications.

Hematologic
- Physiologic anemia due to hemodilution in pregnancy (normal hemoglobin [Hb] >11.0 g/dL in the first and third trimesters, 10.5 in the second trimester). Increased WBC count from demarginalization. Platelet counts remain unchanged. Higher synthesis of coagulation factors leads to a prothrombotic state; consider deep venous thrombosis (DVT) prophylaxis.

Endocrine
- Insulin is safe to use during pregnancy.
- Placental factors lead to increased insulin resistance, often necessitating higher doses of insulin to achieve glycemic control in pregnant patients.
- Slight increase in thyroid metabolism during pregnancy
- Hydrocortisone, prednisone, and methylprednisolone do not cross the placenta; dexamethasone and betamethasone do and may be used for fetal maturation in preterm birth.

Infectious disease
- Most antibiotics are safe in pregnancy. Higher dosing may be required due to increased volume of distribution and enhanced metabolism. Any patient with chorioamnionitis should be promptly delivered. Encourage early surgical source control, especially in appendicitis and cholecystitis. See Table 13.6.4.

Obstetric
- Fetal monitoring may provide useful data on maternal perfusion if ≥23 weeks gestation. Consider delivery for usual obstetric indications, but not for the sole indication of maternal sepsis.

- Patients 23 weeks 0 days to 36 weeks 6 days should be considered for antenatal corticosteroids for fetal maturation if delivery is anticipated.
- Patients 23 weeks 0 days to 31 weeks 6 days should receive a 4 to 6-gram bolus of magnesium if delivery is anticipated within 12 hours to prevent cerebral palsy.

Antepartum Infections

- **Intraamniotic infection and inflammation (III)**
  - III is a diagnosis of infection of amniotic fluid, placenta, fetus, amniotic membranes, or uterine decidua; typically polymicrobial during ongoing pregnancy and may be diagnosed objectively or clinically.
    - Objective diagnosis with amniotic fluid Gram stain or culture, or biochemical analysis, typically collected by amniocentesis
    - Clinical diagnosis made by:
      - Maternal fever of >39 °C
        OR
      - >38 °C to 39 °C and with one of the following: maternal leukocytosis, purulent cervical drainage, or fetal tachycardia
      - >38 °C to 39 °C that is persistent over 30 minutes
        AND
      - Not due to another suspected infectious process
  - III complicates 2% to 5% of term deliveries but may occur anytime during pregnancy from ascending rectovaginal bacteria (high risk with premature rupture of membranes), hematologic spread of bacterial sepsis, and occasionally after intrauterine procedures (eg, fetal surgery or amniocentesis).
  - Chorioamnionitis and funisitis is a histologic diagnosis that confirms III.
  - III is associated with significant maternal morbidity (dysfunctional labor, postpartum atony, hemorrhage, endometritis, sepsis, acute renal distress syndrome [ARDS]) and fetal/neonatal sepsis, cerebral palsy, meningitis, pneumonia, long-term disabilities, and death.
  - Treatment includes delivery, regardless of gestational age. Antibiotics such as IV ampicillin and gentamicin, or alternatives depending on allergy profile, should be given, and the patient may deliver vaginally or by cesarean delivery based on usual obstetric criteria.
  - Diagnosis during labor may be particularly challenging due to overlapping symptoms, including fever from epidural anesthesia or medications such as misoprostol, hypotension potentially caused by epidural anesthesia or other medications, and elevated lactic acid from increased metabolic activity during uterine contractions.
- **Urinary tract infections**
  - **Pyelonephritis:** High rate of pulmonary compromise. Consider renal ultrasound if not improving after 24 hours of antibiotics. Recommended treatment with a third-generation cephalosporin and 14 days of antibiotics, followed by urinary antibiotic prophylaxis for the remainder of the pregnancy.
  - **Asymptomatic bacteriuria or cystitis:** Encourage a full course of antibiotics to prevent pyelonephritis, preterm labor, and preterm delivery.
- **Pneumonia**
  - Higher risk for respiratory failure due to respiratory physiology in pregnancy
  - First-line treatment with third-generation cephalosporin and azithromycin. Avoid amoxicillin/clavulanic acid if anticipating delivery soon.
  - Antivirals such as oseltamivir and nirmatrelvir/ritonavir are safe.
- **Cholecystitis:** perform cholecystectomy or cholecystostomy tube placement after IV fluids, antibiotics, and observation, regardless of trimester.
- **Pancreatitis:** treatment is like nonpregnant patients. Encourage postpyloric feeding to prevent aspiration.
- **Appendicitis:** surgical management is encouraged to prevent an increased risk of fetal death from rupture. Imaging starts with ultrasound, then MRI, and computed tomography (CT) if other imaging is not available.
- **Skin/soft tissue infections:** appropriate antibiotics and debridement during pregnancy. Use penicillin-class medications and methicillin-resistant *Staphylococcus aureus* (MRSA) coverage in endemic regions.
- **Atypical infections:** involve maternal-fetal medicine and infectious disease specialists for disseminated fungal, mold, or parasite infections.

Postpartum Infections

- **Endometritis:** first-line therapy with gentamicin and clindamycin. Consider piperacillin-tazobactam and ampicillin-sulbactam.
- **Wound infections:** perineal and cesarean incisions carry a small risk. Necrotizing fasciitis requires emergent surgical debridement.

SUGGESTED READINGS

Albright CM, Ali TN, Lopes V, Rouse DJ, Anderson BL. The Sepsis in Obstetrics Score: a model to identify risk of morbidity from sepsis in pregnancy. *Am J Obstet Gynecol*. 2014;211(1):39.e1-39.e8.

American College of Obstetricians and Gynecologists. Intrapartum management of intraamniotic infection. Committee Opinion No. 712. *Obstet Gynecol*. 2017;130:e95-e101.

American College of Obstetricians and Gynecologists. Use of prophylactic antibiotics in labor and delivery. ACOG Practice bulletin no. 120. *Obstet Gynecol*. 2011;117(6):1472-1483.

Bauer ME, Fuller M, Kovacheva V, et al. Performance characteristics of sepsis screening tools during antepartum and postpartum admissions. *Obstet Gynecol*. 2024;143:336-335.

Bauer ME, Housey M, Bauer ST, et al. Risk factors, etiologies, and screening tools for sepsis in pregnant women: a multicenter case-control study. *Anesth Analg*. 2019;129:1613-1620.

Brioschi Dos Santos AP, Vicente CR, Cola JP, et al. The impact of COVID-19 on maternal death and fetal death, a cohort study in Brazil. *PLoS One*. 2023;18:e0290343.

California Department of Public Health. *The California Pregnancy-Associated Mortality Review. Report from 2002-2007 Maternal Death Reviews*. California Department of Public Health, Maternal, Child and Adolescent Health Division; 2017. https://www.cdph.ca.gov/Programs/CFH/DMCAH/CDPH%20Document%20Library/PAMR/CA-PAMR-Report-1.pdf

Centers for Disease Control and Prevention. Data from the pregnancy mortality surveillance system. Maternal Mortality Prevention. 2024. https://www.cdc.gov/maternal-mortality/php/pregnancy-mortality-surveillance/index.html

Centers for Disease Control and Prevention. Pregnancy-related deaths: data from maternal mortality review committees in 36 U.S. States, 2017–2019. 2022. https://www.cdc.gov/maternal-mortality/media/pdfs/Pregnancy-Related-Deaths-Data-MMRCs-2017-2019-H.pdf

Gibbs R, Bauer M, Olvera L, Sakowski C, Cape V, Main E. *Improving Diagnosis and Treatment of Maternal Sepsis: A Quality Improvement Toolkit*. California Maternal Quality Care Collaborative; 2020. https://www.cmqcc.org/sites/default/files/Sepsis%20Toolkit_FINAL.2_Errata_7.1.22.pdf

Institute of Medicine (US) and National Research Council (US) Committee to Reexamine IOM Pregnancy Weight Guidelines. *Weight Gain During Pregnancy: Reexamining the Guidelines*. The National Academies Press; 2009.

Le Gars M, Kay AW, Bayless NL, et al. Increased proinflammatory responses of monocytes and plasmacytoid dendritic cells to influenza A virus infection during pregnancy. *J Infect Dis*. 2016;214:1666-1671.

Main EK, Fuller M, Kovacheva VP, et al. Performance characteristics of sepsis screening tools during delivery admissions. *Obstet Gynecol*. 2024; 143:326-335.

MBRRACE-UK. *Saving Lives, Improving Mothers' Care: Lessons Learned to Inform Future Maternity Care from the UK and Ireland Confidential Inquiries Into Maternal Deaths and Morbidity 2009-2012*. National Perinatal Epidemiology Unit (NPEU), University of Oxford; 2015.

Mor G, Cardenas I. The immune system in pregnancy: a unique complexity. *Am J Reprod Immunol*. 2010;63:425-433.

MotherToBaby. Worrying for two? 2024. https://mothertobaby.org

National Institutes of Health, Office of Research on Women's Health. Maternal morbidity and mortality: what do we know? How are we addressing it? https://orwh.od.nih.gov/sites/orwh/files/docs/ORWH_MMM_Booklet_93020_508c.pdf

Plante LA, Pacheco LD, Louis JM, Society for Maternal-Fetal Medicine (SMFM). SMFM Consult Series# 47: Sepsis during pregnancy and the puerperium. *Am J Obstet Gynecol*. 2019;220(4):B2-B10.

Saito S, Nakashima A, Shima T, Ito M. Th1/Th2/Th17 and regulatory T-cell paradigm in pregnancy. *Am J Reprod Immunol*. 2010;63:601-610.

Sepsis Alliance. Pregnancy & childbirth. 2023. https://www.sepsis.org/sepsisand/pregnancy-childbirth/

Silverman MD, Turrentine MA. Urinary tract infections in pregnant individuals. *Obstet Gynecol*. 2023;142(2):435-445.

Society for Maternal-Fetal Medicine (SMFM); Shields AD, Plante LA, Pacheco LD, Louis JM; SMFM Publications Committee. Electronic address: pubs@smfm.org. Society for Maternal-Fetal Medicine Consult Series #67: Maternal sepsis. *Am J Obstet Gynecol*. 2023;229(3):B2-B19.

Society for Maternal-Fetal Medicine. Electronic address: pubs@smfm.org; Plante LA, Pacheco LD, Louis JM. SMFM Consult Series #47: sepsis during pregnancy and the puerperium. *Am J Obstet Gynecol*. 2019;220:B2-B10.

World Health Organization. Maternal sepsis. https://www.who.int/teams/sexual-and-reproductive-health-and-research-(srh)/areas-of-work/maternal-and-perinatal-health/maternal-sepsis#:~:text=Maternal%20sepsis%20is%20the%20third,abortion%20or%20the%20postpartum%20period

13.7

Posterior Reversible Encephalopathy Syndrome

Spandan Rajuri and Jose L. Diaz-Gomez

Background

- Posterior reversible encephalopathy syndrome (PRES) is a clinicoradiologic diagnosis that is based on a combination of typical clinical features and risk factors and supported by radiologic findings. Although PRES may develop at any age from infants to the older adults, it most frequently affects young or middle-aged adults, with a mean age of 45 years. There appears to be a female predominance, even after excluding patients with eclampsia.
- Among adults, PRES is present in up to 98% of patients with eclampsia, in 2.7% to 25% of patients following bone marrow transplantation, in 0.4% to 6% of patients following solid organ transplantation, and, less commonly, (0.4%-0.8%) in end-stage renal disease or systemic lupus erythematosus.

Pathophysiology

- The cerebral circulation normally maintains a constant cerebral blood flow, despite changes in cerebral perfusion pressure that is within the range of about 50 to 150 mm Hg by a process called cerebral autoregulation.
- Despite various etiologic theories proposed for PRES, a rapid hypertension exceeding the upper limit of autoregulation prevails as the main theory. When the blood pressure rise is rapid and severe, the autoregulatory response might be insufficient, hyperperfusion can occur, and the blood-brain barrier breaks down, allowing the interstitial extravasation of plasma and macromolecules.
- The posterior brain regions are particularly susceptible to hyperperfusion due to their relatively lower sympathetic innervation.
- However, 15% to 20% of patients with PRES are normotensive or hypotensive and, even among patients who are hypertensive, >50% have a documented mean arterial pressure above the characterized upper limit of cerebral blood flow autoregulation (≥140-150 mm Hg). In this set of patients, pronounced fluctuations of blood pressure, rather than absolute blood pressure increase, might precede the syndrome.
- Other proposed mechanisms include the cytotoxic, immunogenic, and the neuropeptide theories.

Risk Factors

See Table 13.7.1.

TABLE 13.7.1 Conditions Associated With Development of PRES

Preeclampsia and eclampsia
Solid and bone marrow transplantation
Acute kidney injury (independent factor)
Hypertension
Sepsis
Autoimmune disorders
Cytotoxic and immunosuppressive medications

PRES, posterior reversible encephalopathy syndrome.

Clinical Presentation

- PRES often presents nonspecifically with symptoms manifesting over several hours or days.
- The incidence of PRES is higher after 36 weeks of pregnancy and postpartum. Further, PRES is most associated with eclampsia than preeclampsia.
- Headaches occur in up to half of patients with PRES and are typically dull, diffuse, and gradual in onset, unlike thunderclap headaches in reversible cerebral vasoconstriction syndrome (RCVS) or subarachnoid hemorrhage.
- Encephalopathy develops in 28% to 94% of patients and ranges from mild confusion and cognitive deficits to stupor and sometimes coma.
- Seizures affect up to 74% to 87% of patients and typically occur within 24 to 48 hours of presentation. In a minority of cases (3%-17%), seizures may evolve into status epilepticus, and rarely this is the presenting symptom.
- Despite PRES often affecting the occipital regions, only 39% of patients have visual symptoms, including reduced visual acuity, diplopia, visual field deficits, cortical blindness, color vision abnormalities, and visual hallucinations.
- Focal neurologic deficits such as aphasia and hemiparesis occur in 19% of patients.

Differential Diagnosis (Table 13.7.2)

TABLE 13.7.2 Differential Diagnosis

Vascular
Cerebral ischemia (ie, posterior stroke)
Cerebral venous sinus thrombosis
Intracerebral hemorrhage
Subcortical leukoaraiosis
CNS vasculitis
Reversible cerebral vasoconstriction syndrome
Degenerative/Autoimmune
Acute demyelinating encephalomyelitis
Multiple sclerosis/acute disseminated encephalomyelitis
Other autoimmune encephalitis (eg, limbic encephalitis, Hashimoto, Rasmussen, systemic lupus erythematosus [SLE], Behçet)
Cerebral autosomal dominant arteriopathy with subcortical infarcts and leukoencephalopathy (CADASIL)
Mitochondrial encephalopathy, lactic acidosis, and stroke-like episodes (MELAS)
Creutzfeldt-Jakob disease
Infectious
Herpes simplex encephalitis
Other infectious encephalitis
Progressive multifocal leukoencephalopathy
Cancer-Related
Malignancy or tumor (lymphoma, gliomatosis cerebri, metastatic disease)
Paraneoplastic encephalitis
Chemotherapy-related demyelinating disorder
Radiation necrosis
Metabolic
Metabolic encephalopathy
Osmotic demyelinating syndrome (central pontine myelinolysis)
Toxic leukoencephalopathy

CNS, central nervous system.

Diagnosis

- Computed tomography (CT) is often the initial imaging modality due to speed and availability, but its sensitivity is low; magnetic resonance imaging (MRI) is the gold standard for diagnosing PRES.
- The typical CT and MRI features of PRES include symmetrical hemispheric vasogenic edema affecting subcortical white matter and often extending to the overlying cortex, which is best recognized on MRI with fluid-attenuation inversion recovery (FLAIR) sequences. MRI diffusion-weighted imaging usually confirms vasogenic edema with the absence of restricted diffusion.
- Brain imaging shows bilateral cortical-subcortical vasogenic edema that falls into three anatomic patterns seen in about 70% of patients: (a) dominant parieto-occipital pattern (22%), (b) holohemispheric watershed pattern (23%), and (c) superior frontal sulcus pattern (27%). A central-variant (brainstem) pattern has also been identified, affecting the brainstem, basal ganglia, posterior limb of the internal capsule, cerebellum, and periventricular regions, but has no cortical or subcortical involvement.
- PRES and RCVS are well known to overlap and so cerebral CT or MR angiography is recommended to help distinguish them. In RCVS, vessel wall MR angiography shows arterial wall thickening but without arterial wall enhancement, consistent with transient vasoconstriction. However, PRES occurs in 9% to 38% of RCVS cases and 87% of PRES cases have angiographic changes consistent with RCVS, such as diffuse vasoconstriction, focal vasculopathy, or vessel pruning. Therefore, it is conceivable that PRES and RCVS are divergent phenotypical manifestations of a shared pathophysiology.
- Digital subtraction angiography is worth considering in patients with PRES with possible RCVS or those in whom CT or MR angiography shows a possible intracranial arteriopathy. Digital subtraction angiography may identify typical features of RCVS or of cerebral vasculitis, leading to specific therapies for each, including calcium channel blockers for RCVS or immune therapy for cerebral vasculitis.
- *See* Table 13.7.3 *for additional details.*

TABLE 13.7.3 Diagnosis Criteria for Posterior Reversible Encephalopathy Syndrome

New Onset of Neurologic Symptoms (>1)	Risk Factors (>1)	Brain Imaging Findings
Seizures Encephalopathy or confusion Headache Visual disturbances	Severe hypertension/ blood pressure fluctuations Renal failure Immunosuppressant therapy or chemotherapy Eclampsia Autoimmune disorder	Bilateral vasogenic edema (posterior > anterior) Cytotoxic edema with pattern of PRES Imaging may be normal early in disease.
Absence of an alternative diagnosis → PRES		

PRES, posterior reversible encephalopathy syndrome.

Adapted from Fugate JE, Rabinstein AA. Posterior reversible encephalopathy syndrome: clinical and radiological manifestations, pathophysiology, and outstanding questions. *Lancet Neurol.* 2015;14:914-925.

Management

- The acute management of PRES is supportive and includes removing or reversing precipitating factor—for example, correcting hypertension and avoiding significant blood pressure fluctuations with invasive blood pressure monitoring, early delivery in pregnancy, or discontinuing any offending chemotherapy or immunosuppressive agents.
- In pregnancy, immediate blood pressure control, magnesium sulfate infusion administration, and timely delivery are associated with favorable outcomes. Most effective antihypertensive agents include nicardipine, nimodipine, hydralazine, and labetalol. Moreover, cerebral vasodilatory medications like sodium nitroprusside and nitroglycerine should be avoided. Additionally, angiotensin-converting enzyme (ACE) inhibitors should be avoided due to their toxic effects on the fetal kidney.
- Except in the setting of eclampsia (as magnesium sulfate is given as first line), most patients with PRES and seizures are treated with antiseizure medications. When seizures are documented or strongly suspected, an antiseizure medication can be given as an intravenous bolus followed by maintenance.
- Malignant PRES is defined based on clinical criteria consisting of a Glasgow Coma Scale (GCS) score of <8 and clinical decline despite standard medical management for intracranial hypertension. In addition, there must be radiologic evidence of edema or intracerebral hemorrhage exerting mass effect, such as effacement of basal cisterns, trans tentorial, tonsillar, or uncal herniation.
- Malignant PRES requires aggressive supportive care that may include airway protection with endotracheal intubation, passive mechanical ventilation support, transfusion of blood products for reversal of coagulopathy, and corticosteroids for those with autoimmune disorders. Patients with PRES whose GCS score is ≤ 8 should have intracranial pressure monitoring whenever possible. Various interventions undertaken in patients with intracranial hypertension include osmotherapy, cerebrospinal fluid (CSF) drainage by external ventricular drain, craniectomy, and evacuation of hematomas. These are reported to reduce mortality rates in comparison to historic reports. Patients with acute obstructive hydrocephalus may require an external ventricular drain.

Prognosis

- In most cases, PRES has a good short- and long-term prognosis if treated timely and adequately, especially if MRI findings and clinical symptoms are reversible after several hours or days. Studies have reported complete resolution of edema and clinical recovery in 70% to 90% of cases. However, cerebral hemorrhage or ischemia and irreversible neurologic deficits or death can occur.
- Factors associated with poor outcomes include severe encephalopathy, a hypertensive or neoplastic cause, a longer time to control the causative factor, the presence of multiple comorbidities, hyperglycemia, elevated C-reactive protein levels, low CSF glucose levels, and coagulopathy. Furthermore, various imaging features associated with poor outcome include corpus callosum involvement, extensive cerebral edema or worsening imaging severity, intracerebral hemorrhage, subarachnoid hemorrhage, and restrictive diffusion on imaging.

SUGGESTED READINGS

Bartynski WS. Posterior reversible encephalopathy syndrome, part 1: fundamental imaging and clinical features. *AJNR Am J Neuroradiol*. 2008;29:1036-1042.

Brewer J, Owens MY, Wallace K, et al. Posterior reversible encephalopathy syndrome in 46 of 47 patients with eclampsia. *Am J Obstet Gynecol*. 2013;208:468.e1-468.e6.

Fugate JE, Rabinstein AA. Posterior reversible encephalopathy syndrome: clinical and radiological manifestations, pathophysiology, and outstanding questions. *Lancet Neurol*. 2015;14:914-925.

Hinchey J, Chaves C, Appignani B, et al. A reversible posterior leukoencephalopathy syndrome. *N Engl J Med*. 1996;334:494-500.

Lee VH, Wijdicks EFM, Manno EM, et al. Clinical spectrum of reversible posterior leukoencephalopathy syndrome. *Arch Neurol*. 2008;65:205-210.

Liman TG, Siebert E, Endres M, et al. Posterior reversible encephalopathy syndrome. *Curr Opin Neurol*. 2019;32:25-35.

Schweitzer AD, Parikh NS, Askin G, et al. Imaging characteristics associated with clinical outcomes in posterior reversible encephalopathy syndrome. *Neuroradiology*. 2017;59:379-386.

Staykov D, Schwab S. Posterior reversible encephalopathy syndrome. *J Intensive Care Med*. 2012;27:11-24.

Triplett JD, Kutlubaev MA, Kermode AG, Hardy T. Posterior reversible encephalopathy syndrome (PRES): diagnosis and management. *Pract Neurol*. 2022;22(3):183-189.

13.8

Other Obstetric Emergencies

Emma Heubner and Michael Wolfe

Advanced Cardiovascular Life Support Considerations in the Pregnant Patient

Epidemiology

- Cardiac arrest occurs in 1 in 10,000 to 30,000 pregnancies.
- Causes vary and include obstetric (preeclampsia, hemorrhage, amniotic fluid embolism) and nonobstetric (drug reaction, trauma, sepsis, cardiogenic) causes

Management and Treatment

- Table 13.8.1 shows key points for Advanced Cardiovascular Life Support (ACLS) in pregnancy.
- Perform continuous manual left uterine displacement if >20 weeks estimated gestational age, paired with high-quality cardiopulmonary resuscitation (CPR).
- Defibrillation should not be delayed, if indicated, with no modifications.
- Medication doses do not require alteration.
- No medication should be withheld due to concerns about teratogenicity.
- Medications and fluid should preferably be given via upper extremity access, as the gravid uterus may restrict venous return.
- Fetal assessment should not be performed during resuscitation.
- Fetal monitors should be removed or detached as soon as possible to facilitate resuscitative hysterotomy (RH)—also known as perimortem cesarean delivery (PMCD)—if this intervention is needed.
- RH/PMCD
  - Required in ~1 in 53,000 pregnancies
  - If the pregnant patient (with a fundus height at or above the umbilicus) has not achieved return of spontaneous circulation (ROSC) after 4 minutes, RH should be strongly considered.
    - 5-4 Rule; infant delivery should occur within the fifth minute following 4 minutes of maternal CPR.
    - Shorter times from collapse to delivery may improve both maternal and infant outcomes.
    - Optimal timing of an RH depends on multiple factors: the cause of the arrest, maternal pathology and cardiac function, fetal gestational age, and resources.
    - If maternal viability is not possible, RH should be started immediately.
    - RH should optimally occur at the site of the arrest.
- May consider extracorporeal membrane oxygenation (ECMO) for refractory arrest
  - Target higher flow rates due to increased maternal cardiac output (5-6 L/min)
  - Goal Pao$_2$ >70 mm Hg, pH >7.40, Paco$_2$ 28 to 32 mm Hg, HCO$_3$ 18 to 21 mmol/L
  - Maternal acidosis, hypercapnia, and hypocapnia are poorly tolerated by the fetus.

TABLE 13.8.1 Key Points for ACLS in Pregnancy

- Manual left uterine displacement once fundus ≥umbilicus (≈≥20 wk)
- Defibrillation: standard pad placement/doses; do not delay
- Drugs: standard dosing; none withheld for teratogenicity during arrest
- Access: upper extremity preferred (gravid uterus may impede return)
- Fetal monitors off to enable CPR/RH/ECMO cannulation
- RH: 4-min no ROSC → deliver by 5 min
- Consider ECMO for refractory arrest; target flows 5-6 L/min; maternal ABG goals: Pao$_2$ >70, pH >7.40, Paco$_2$ 28-32, HCO$_3$ 18-21

ABG, arterial blood gas; ACLS; Advanced Cardiovascular Life Support; CPR, cardiopulmonary resuscitation; ECMO, extracorporeal membrane oxygenation; RH, resuscitative hysterotomy; ROSC, return of spontaneous circulation.

Outcomes

- Survival to hospital discharge ≥50%; outcomes vary by etiology, time to RH/ECMO, and system factors.

Trauma in the Pregnant Patient

Epidemiology

- Trauma is the leading nonobstetric cause of maternal death and affects about 1 in 12 pregnancies in the United States.
- Injuries from motor vehicle collisions account for about half of trauma during pregnancy, and >80% of trauma-related fetal demise.

Assessment, Management, and Treatment

- Similar to the nonpregnant patients with trauma: airway, breathing, circulation
- Airway + breathing
  - Emphasize adequate preoxygenation
  - Combination of decreased functional residual capacity and higher oxygen consumption results in rapid desaturation.
  - Use small tracheal tubes (6.0-6.5 mm internal diameter).
  - Higher proportion of Mallampati IV airways
  - Soft tissue edema due to vascular engorgement may lead to increased friability of the tissues and airway bleeding that can obscure laryngoscope views and may reduce the size of the glottic opening.
  - Strongly consider rapid sequence intubation, especially after 18 to 20 weeks.
    - Increased risk of aspiration due to decreased lower esophageal sphincter tone and cephalad displacement of the stomach by the gravid uterus
    - Succinylcholine and rocuronium are unlikely to cross the placenta and are safe to use in pregnancy.
  - Alterations to mechanical ventilation settings
    - Target normal Paco$_2$ range for pregnancy (27-34 mm Hg)
    - If a spontaneously breathing pregnant patient with trauma in later stages of pregnancy has a Paco$_2$ level nearing normal adult levels (~40 mm Hg), this may herald impending hypercarbic respiratory failure.

Circulation

- The first sign of hypovolemia may be a nonreassuring fetal heart rate (FHR) pattern caused by a reduction in uterine blood flow.
  - Increased intravascular volume allows for more blood loss to occur before signs of shock are evident.
  - Prevent compression of the inferior vena cava (IVC) by the gravid uterus by placing the patient in a left lateral tilt of 30 degrees
  - If chest compressions are necessary, perform two-handed manual left uterine displacement.
  - Vasopressors can be used in the setting of traumatic shock, if necessary, to maintain normotension, until euvolemia can be restored.
  - Vascular access should be obtained above the level of the diaphragm to ensure that intravenous (IV) therapy is not obstructed by the gravid uterus.
  - Hemorrhage management in pregnant patients with trauma
    - 1:1:1 ratio plasma:red blood cell (RBC):platelet (similar to nonobstetric trauma)
    - Higher threshold for administration of cryoprecipitate: <200 mg/dL
- Anti-D immunoglobulin G (IgG) should be administered within 72 hours to all Rh-negative mothers who present to the hospital after trauma.
  - Kleihauer-Betke (KB) test: used to detect fetal cells in the maternal circulation

Outcomes

- Penetrating trauma has a high rate of fetal mortality.
- Penetrating trauma may have less maternal morbidity and mortality compared with the nonpregnant patient, due to shielding of maternal organs by the gravid uterus; outcomes depend on injury trajectory, velocity, and gestational age.
- Blunt trauma leads to high rates of fetal mortality.

Nonobstetric Surgical Urgencies and Emergencies

Epidemiology

- Incidence 0.5% to 2%
- ~5% rate of major postoperative complications
- Most common indications for surgery include appendicitis, acute cholecystitis, gynecologic surgery, and surgery for trauma.
- Other emergent pathologies include bowel obstruction, bowel perforation, mesenteric ischemia, severe soft tissue infections, and aortic dissection.

Evaluation

- Ultrasound and magnetic resonance imaging (MRI) are preferred when possible because they do not use radiation and are not associated with risk to the fetus.
- Gadolinium-based contrast agents: avoid routine use; use only when benefits clearly outweigh risks and critical for diagnosis (crosses placenta, unknown duration of fetal exposure, theoretical toxicity concerns).
- There is a negligible risk to the fetus for radiation doses <50 mGy.
  - A computed tomography (CT) of the abdomen and pelvis provides a fetal dose of 10 to 50 mGy (protocol dependent; higher with multiphase/older protocols).
  - Do not withhold CT or iodinated contrast when clinically indicated; the diagnostic benefit to the mother outweighs the negligible fetal risk.
  - Studies are additive and can exceed that threshold of 50 mGy if multiple ionizing studies are necessary; optimize protocols and avoid unnecessary multiphase scans.

Management

- No emergent surgery should be delayed for fear of anesthetic or procedural risk to the pregnant patient and fetus.
- Medications
  - Studies have not found an increased risk of major birth defects associated with nonobstetric surgery, nor have retrospective analyses found increased risk of cognitive or behavioral deficits in children exposed to antenatal anesthetics.
  - Historical association of benzodiazepine use and increased incidence of cleft palate and cardiac anomalies has been refuted in more recent studies.
  - Increased risk of spontaneous abortion and low birth weight in retrospective studies
    - Possible confounding: underlying maternal pathophysiology (rather than anesthetic exposure)
  - Sugammadex: per Society for Obstetric Anesthesia and Perinatology (SOAP), avoid in early pregnancy due to insufficient data and theoretical progesterone-binding risk (critical for pregnancy maintenance; potential 34% reduction in unbound levels); avoid or use with caution at term/near term due to unknown effects on lactation (appears safe for maternal reversal but use judiciously with shared decision-making and prefer traditional agents).
  - To reduce any theoretical risk of anesthesia-related maternal and fetal effects, regional anesthesia is preferred to general anesthesia in the appropriate clinical context.
    - Eliminates need for maternal airway manipulation and decreases risk of fetal hypoxia
    - Prolonged reductions in uteroplacental perfusion because of anesthetic-induced hypotension significantly increase the risk of hypoxemia, acidosis, and potentially fetal demise
    - Almost all anesthetics have been observed to transfer across the placenta (except neuromuscular-blocking agents), but the exact effects of these drugs on fetal well-being are poorly understood.
  - Consider perioperative corticosteroid administration to patients with viable fetus of premature gestational ages due to the risk of preterm delivery.

Intraoperative Fetal Monitoring

- Per American College of Obstetricians and Gynecologists (ACOG), the decision to use FHR monitoring should be individualized for pregnant patients undergoing surgery.
  - Previable (<22 weeks): obtaining FHR by Doppler before and after surgery is generally sufficient.
  - Viable (≥22 weeks): at minimum, electronic FHR and contraction monitoring before and after the procedure to

assess fetal well-being and absence of contractions; intraoperative monitoring may be appropriate when the fetus is viable, physically possible to perform, and an obstetric provider with cesarean privileges is readily available.
    - FHR monitoring may assist in maternal positioning and cardiorespiratory management.
    - Loss of FHR variability may be an expected physiologic reaction in response to the effects of general anesthesia on the fetal autonomic nervous system.
    - Intraoperative fetal bradycardia is more concerning as it may suggest prolonged fetal hypoxemia and developing acidosis.
- If premature labor occurs, tocolytic therapy will be necessary to preserve the pregnancy.
  - If tocolytics are not immediately available, adjunctive measures to achieve uterine relaxation include high-concentration volatile anesthetics and IV nitroglycerin.
    - Large degree of placental metabolization of nitroglycerin; therefore, minimal effects are observed on the fetus
- Consideration of cesarean section in viable fetus with severe signs of fetal distress

Acute Cardiovascular Complications and Cardiac Surgery During Pregnancy

Background and Epidemiology

- Cardiovascular diseases are the most common cause of nonobstetric death during pregnancy, and mortality rates among hospitalized cardiac patients during pregnancy reach 5%.

Arrhythmias

- Supraventricular arrhythmias
  - New-onset or recurrent supraventricular tachyarrhythmias are not uncommon in those with structural heart disease or advanced age.
  - Ventricular arrhythmias and symptomatic bradycardia are rare.
  - Supraventricular tachycardias in women with congenital heart disease (CHD) and paroxysmal atrial fibrillation are associated with increased maternal morbidity/mortality.
  - In hemodynamically unstable patients or with fetal compromise, synchronized electrical cardioversion should be performed as soon as feasible.
    - Cardioversion is generally well tolerated with minimal fetal risk.
  - Hemodynamically stable atrioventricular (AV) node-dependent arrhythmias such as supraventricular tachycardia (SVT) can be terminated using vagal maneuvers, adenosine, or beta-blockers.
  - Class I antiarrhythmic medications can be considered after consultation with a cardiac electrophysiologist.
  - Amiodarone should be avoided, or reserved as a last resort for refractory cases, as it can cause adverse fetal effects such as thyroid abnormalities.
  - Anticoagulation
    - Short-term systemic anticoagulation with low-molecular-weight heparin (LMWH) should be considered in pregnant patients with atrial fibrillation or atrial flutter.
    - Direct oral anticoagulants (DOACs) are contraindicated in pregnancy.
  - Catheter ablation of supraventricular arrhythmias during pregnancy is feasible and can be performed with low risk to the mother and the fetus, but it is reserved for recurrent arrhythmias refractory to medication, usually after the first trimester.
    - Expect varying amounts of fetal radiation exposure
- Ventricular arrhythmias
  - Without a history of heart disease, consider cardiomyopathy, right ventricular infundibular tachycardia (the most common type of ventricular tachycardia in young pregnant women with structurally normal hearts), and inherited arrhythmogenic syndromes (eg, long QT syndrome, Brugada syndrome).
  - Sustained ventricular arrhythmias typically require cardioversion, especially if there are signs of maternal or fetal compromise

Acute Heart Failure in Pregnancy

- Background
  - Causes include preexisting cardiomyopathy, CHD, peripartum cardiomyopathy (PPCM) (discussed in separate chapter), stress/toxic cardiomyopathy, valvular disease, ischemia due to spontaneous coronary artery dissection (SCAD), or atherosclerosis.
  - Delivery and postpartum period are sensitive due to rapid volume shifts, hormonal changes, and increased ventricular afterload.
  - Potential for delayed diagnosis due to overlapping symptoms with late-term pregnancy (dyspnea, orthopnea, fatigue, tachycardia, lower extremity edema, S3 gallop on auscultation)
- Treatment and management
  - Medications
    - Avoid teratogenic medications.
      - Include angiotensin-converting enzyme inhibitors, aldosterone antagonists, neprilysin inhibitors, sodium-glucose co-transporter 2 inhibitors.
    - Loop diuretics, such as furosemide, are considered safe in pregnancy and should be initiated early for symptomatic control and the prevention of volume overload.

Acute Aortic Events in Pregnancy

- Background and epidemiology
  - Acute aortic events, such as aortic dissection or rupture, are relatively more common in pregnant women compared to age-matched nonpregnant controls and are associated with significant morbidity and mortality.
  - Risk factors: inherited connective tissue and vascular disorders, bicuspid aortic valve with severe ascending aortic dilatation, uncontrolled hypertension, and aortic coarctation
- Evaluation
  - In the presence of high clinical suspicion, the diagnostic test of choice is an emergency CT scan.
  - Cardiac MRI may be used as an alternative to avoid radiation in stable cases, if promptly available.
- Management
  - In hemodynamically stable patients, blood pressure control can be achieved using a beta-blocker,

nitroglycerine, or nitroprusside (only for short periods due to the risk of fetal cyanide toxicity) and adequate pain management, with continuous fetal monitoring.
- Type A aortic dissection is a surgical emergency.
  - Associated maternal mortality rate is similar to the general population.
  - Significant 30% to 40% risk of fetal loss
- Decision on whether to perform emergent cesarean delivery before surgery requires multidisciplinary team discussion with the patient.
- The decision for delivery is based on the type and extent of the dissection, presence of hemodynamic instability, gestational age, and evidence of fetal compromise.

Acute Coronary Syndromes in Pregnancy

- Background and epidemiology
  - Acute coronary syndromes (ACSs) are overall rare (1.7-6.2/100,000).
  - Responsible for ~20% of cardiovascular mortality during pregnancy
  - There is increased risk of nonatherosclerotic causes of coronary artery disease (CAD) (eg, SCAD) in pregnancy
    - SCAD: risk of coronary dissection peaks at the end of pregnancy and postpartum.
    - Typically involves the left coronary artery territory, but on occasion may be multivessel
    - Cause is unclear, typically involves exacerbation of an underlying vascular predisposition, such as connective tissue disorders or vasospasm.
  - Other potential causes of CAD in the pregnant population include coronary embolism, vasospasm, thrombus due to a hypercoagulable state, or atherosclerosis.
- Management
  - Similar to the treatment of ACS as in nonpregnant patients
  - IV unfractionated heparin (UFH) and oral/sublingual aspirin are safe during pregnancy.
  - Clopidogrel is also considered safe to use if dual-antiplatelet therapy (DAPT) is required; however, the shortest duration possible is recommended.
    - Note antiplatelet agents used and time of discontinuation prior to neuraxial interventions for delivery.
  - Very limited safety and efficacy data exist on bivalirudin, prasugrel, ticagrelor, and glycoprotein IIb/IIIa inhibitors, which are not usually used during pregnancy
  - Beta-blockers are advised and safe to use during pregnancy, though may have effects on fetal growth.
  - Revascularization
    - Similar indications for acute revascularization as in nonpregnant patients
    - Periprocedural anticoagulation, while associated with increased risk for bleeding, is recommended for use.
    - Ionizing radiation risk should not limit access to revascularization procedures.
    - Stenting is considered only in case of ongoing symptoms or with hemodynamic instability with a flow-limiting lesion.
  - Systemic thrombolysis is rarely performed due to limited effectiveness, the high risk of maternal bleeding, and fetal mortality.

SUGGESTED READINGS

ACOG Committee Opinion No. 775: Nonobstetric surgery during pregnancy. *Obstet Gynecol*. 2019;133(4):e285-e286.

Aftab N, Halalmeh DR, Vrana A, et al. Enhancing maternal survival in traumatic cardiovascular collapse during pregnancy: a case series on resuscitative hysterotomy (RH) from a level 1 trauma center. *Injury*. 2025; 56(1):111923.

April MD, Long B. Trauma in pregnancy: a narrative review of the current literature. *Am J Emerg Med*. 2024;81:53-61.

Assenza GE, Dimopoulos K, Budts W, et al. Management of acute cardiovascular complications in pregnancy. *Eur Heart J*. 2021;42(41): 4224-4240.

Elassy SMR, Elmidany AA, Elbawab HY. Urgent cardiac surgery during pregnancy: a continuous challenge. *Ann Thorac Surg*. 2014;97(5): 1624-1629.

Jain C. ACOG Committee Opinion No. 723: guidelines for diagnostic imaging during pregnancy and lactation. *Obstet Gynecol*. 2019;133(1):186.

Lankford AS, Chow JH, Jackson AM, et al. Clinical outcomes of pregnant and postpartum extracorporeal membrane oxygenation patients. *Anesth Analg*. 2021;132(3):777-787.

Mhyre JM, Tsen LC, Einav S, Kuklina EV, Leffert LR, Bateman BT. Cardiac arrest during hospitalization for delivery in the United States, 1998-2011. *Anesthesiology*. 2014;120(4):810-818.

Panchal AR, Bartos JA, Cabañas JG, et al. Part 3: adult basic and advanced life support: 2020 American Heart Association guidelines for cardiopulmonary resuscitation and emergency cardiovascular care. *Circulation*. 2020;142(16_suppl_2):S366-S468.

Society for Obstetric Anesthesia and Perinatology. Statement on sugammadex during pregnancy and lactation. *Society for Obstetric Anesthesia and Perinatology*. 2019. Accessed November 1, 2025. https://www.soap.org/assets/docs/SOAP_Statement_Sugammadex_During_Pregnancy_Lactation_APPROVED.pdf

Traweek R, Phan V, Griesbach C, Hall C. General surgery during pregnancy and gynecologic emergencies. *Surg Clin North Am*. 2023;103(6): 1217-1229.

13.9

Obstetric Imaging Modalities

Minhazur Sarker, Scott A. Harvey, and Ulrich H. Schmidt

Definition

- Organogenesis for the fetus occurs primarily in the early portions of the first trimester (4-10 weeks gestational age), and there is a 2% to 3% baseline risk for congenital abnormalities.
- Risks to the developing fetus from radiation significantly decrease after the first trimester, and thus, elective imaging should be deferred.
- Radiation exposure from radiography, computed tomography (CT), or nuclear medicine imaging is a dose much lower than exposure associated with fetal harm. These imaging modalities should only be used when clinically indicated, with careful consideration of the risks and benefits to both the mother and the fetus.
    - Extremely high doses of radiation exposure (>1 Gy) in early embryogenesis may be lethal to the developing embryo.
    - Radiation in the first 4 weeks of gestation has an "all or none" phenomenon, where there are no congenital defects associated with radiation exposure but may cause an embryonic demise.
- Lateral decubitus positioning during imaging may be beneficial if a prolonged time for evaluation is expected, if the patient is >20 weeks of gestation.
- Plain film radiography (x-ray)
    - Generally avoided in the first trimester given fetal organogenesis, has very low radiation exposure, and near-zero risk of congenital malformations
- Ultrasound (US)
    - No ionizing radiation and not associated with significant fetal risk
    - Initial imaging modality of choice for most pathology in obstetrics and some nonobstetric conditions due to its safety profile and lack of ionizing radiation
- CT scan
    - Use of CT scan and associated contrast agents should not be withheld if clinically indicated, as the benefits of accurate diagnosis and timely management outweigh the theoretical risks to the fetus.
    - Benefit from early and accurate diagnosis of maternal pathology outweighs the theoretical risk to the fetus.
    - Oral and intravenous (IV) contrast agents are considered safe and acceptable in pregnancy if clinically indicated (contrast may cross the placenta but has not been associated with any fetal harm).
        - There is a modest increase in childhood cancers with high radiation exposure during pregnancy.
    - Lactation may be continued after exposure to iodinated contrast from CT scans.
- Nuclear medicine imaging
    - Fetal risk associated with nuclear medicine imaging depends on the properties of the radioisotope used.
    - Technetium 99m is well tolerated in pregnancy.
    - Radioactive iodine (iodine-131) can affect the fetal thyroid and thus should not be used in pregnancy.

TABLE 13.9.1 Imaging for Common Acute Pathology in Pregnancy

	Imaging Modality	Notes
Pulmonary embolism (PE)	• Chest x-ray • Compression venous Doppler • Echocardiogram • CT angiography • V̇/Q̇scan (if chest x-ray normal and pretest probability remains high)	• If deep venous thrombosis present, symptoms can diagnose a presumed PE. • CT scan should not be withheld if clinical suspicion is high. • CT angiography has lower radiation than V̇/Q̇ scan.
Stroke (hemorrhagic or thrombotic)	• CT of the head with or without contrast • MRI of the brain with or without contrast	• Benefits of early imaging and diagnosis significantly outweigh risks.
Appendicitis	• Abdominal US has high specificity but variable sensitivity (66%-100%). • CT scan has high sensitivity and specificity. • MRI also has high sensitivity and specificity.	• No role for x-ray unless concerning for bowel obstruction or perforation • Consider CT scan if unclear diagnosis or the appendix not seen on US. • Awaiting MRI to avoid radiation may delay diagnosis.
Cholecystitis or cholelithiasis	• Abdominal US (high accuracy) • Magnetic resonance cholangiopancreatography (extraductal stones) • Endoscopic retrograde cholangiopancreatography (ERCP)	
Pancreatitis	• Upper abdominal US is safe and sensitive. • MRI provides further characterization.	• If clinical suspicion high, low threshold to proceed with MRI
Nephrolithiasis or pyelonephritis	• KUB (kidney-ureter-bladder) x-ray • Renal US (characterizes kidneys but NOT needed for diagnosis) • Noncontrast CT scan	• X-ray only identifies radiopaque stones. • Renal US may be used to assess kidneys but not needed for diagnosis of either. • Asymptomatic hydronephrosis is common after the second trimester (almost 90% of patients) due to mechanical obstruction by gravid uterus.

CT, computed tomography; MRI, magnetic resonance imaging; US, ultrasound.

- Magnetic resonance imaging (MRI)
  - No ionizing radiation and not associated with fetal risk
  - Established role in obstetrics for placenta accreta spectrum, certain maternal disorders, and further characterization of fetal anomalies
  - Should be performed and interpreted by clinicians with expertise in obstetric MRIs and be strongly correlated to clinical history to limit bias from nonspecific findings
  - Should only be considered if additional information will affect pregnancy management (prenatally or postnatally)
  - Gadolinium-based MRI contrast crosses the placenta into fetal circulation, and its effects on the fetus remain uncertain, particularly due to unclear duration of exposure; its use should be avoided unless under consultation with maternal-fetal medicine specialists.
  - Written consent is NO LONGER necessary.
- Common acute pathology warranting imaging (see Table 13.9.1)

SUGGESTED READINGS

Albakri AA, Alzahrani MM, Alghamdi SH. Medical imaging in pregnancy: safety, appropriate utilization, and alternative modalities for imaging pregnant patients. *Cureus*. 2024;16(2):e54346.

Alsadery HA, Bamalan OA, Aljubran HJ, Albaish LJ, Al Ghanim BZ. Non-obstetric acute abdomen in pregnancy: a review of literature. *Med Arch*. 2023;77(4):293-298.

American College of Obstetricians and Gynecologists. Committee Opinion No. 723: guidelines for diagnostic imaging during pregnancy and lactation [published correction appears in *Obstet Gynecol*. 2018;132(3):786]. *Obstet Gynecol*. 2017;130(4):e210-e216.

Anne Kennedy, MBBCH, and Paula J. Woodward, MD. Role of magnetic resonance imaging in obstetric imaging. In: Lockwood CJ, Copel J, Resnik R, Silver RM, Moore T, eds. *Creasy and Resnik's Maternal-Fetal Medicine: Principles and Practice*. 9th ed. Elsevier. 2022; 272-282.

Chen MM, Coakley FV, Kaimal A, Laros RK Jr. Guidelines for computed tomography and magnetic resonance imaging use during pregnancy and lactation. *Obstet Gynecol*. 2008;112(2 Pt 1):333-340.

Expert Panel on MR Safety; Kanal E, Barkovich AJ, Bell C, et al. ACR guidance document on MR safe practices: 2013. *J Magn Reson Imaging*. 2013;37(3):501-530.

Gjelsteen AC, Ching BH, Meyermann MW, et al. CT, MRI, PET, PET/CT, and ultrasound in the evaluation of obstetric and gynecologic patients. *Surg Clin North Am*. 2008;88(2):361-390, vii.

Groen RS, Bae JY, Lim KJ. Fear of the unknown: ionizing radiation exposure during pregnancy. *Am J Obstet Gynecol*. 2012;206(6):456-462.

Long SS, Long C, Lai H, Macura KJ. Imaging strategies for right lower quadrant pain in pregnancy. *AJR Am J Roentgenol*. 2011;196(1):4-12.

Odedra D, Mellnick VM, Patlas MN. Imaging of trauma in pregnancy. *Radiol Clin North Am*. 2023;61(1):129-139.

Patel SJ, Reede DL, Katz DS, Subramaniam R, Amorosa JK. Imaging the pregnant patient for nonobstetric conditions: algorithms and radiation dose considerations. *Radiographics*. 2007;27(6):1705-1722.

Sachs HC; Committee on Drugs. The transfer of drugs and therapeutics into human breast milk: an update on selected topics. *Pediatrics*. 2013; 132(3):e796-e809.

Theilen LH, Mellnick VM, Longman RE, et al. Utility of magnetic resonance imaging for suspected appendicitis in pregnant women. *Am J Obstet Gynecol*. 2015;212(3):345.e1-345.e3456.

Tremblay E, Thérasse E, Thomassin-Naggara I, Trop I. Quality initiatives: guidelines for use of medical imaging during pregnancy and lactation. *Radiographics*. 2012;32(3):897-911.

Webb JA, Thomsen HS, Morcos SK; Members of Contrast Media Safety Committee of European Society of Urogenital Radiology. The use of iodinated and gadolinium contrast media during pregnancy and lactation. *Eur Radiol*. 2005;15(6):1234-1240.

SECTION 14

Fluid Management

Section Editor: Marvin G. Chang

14.1

Fluid Management

Lukas H. Matern

Types of Fluid Therapies

- Prescribed fluids have varying properties with respect to electrolyte balance, solute content, tonicity, and pH (see Table 14.1.1).
  - Hypotonic fluids, such as 5% dextrose in water (D5W), are given to replete insensible losses, to replace free water deficits, or to carry dextrose.
  - Isotonic fluids, such as normal (0.9%) saline, are given chiefly to expand or replace body fluid volume.
  - Hypertonic fluids, such as 3% saline, are given to lower intracranial pressure and to replace sodium.
- Intravenous (IV) fluids are categorized into crystalloids, which consist primarily of electrolyte solutions, and colloids, which contain suspended proteins or starch molecules.
  - Crystalloids are divided into saline solutions and "balanced" fluids, such as lactated Ringer (LR) solution and Plasma-Lyte, which more closely approximate human plasma electrolyte concentrations.
  - Colloids can be derived from human blood (eg, 5% albumin) or manufactured as synthetic starches, dextrans, and gelatins (eg, hetastarch).

Indications and Dosing

- IV fluids should be administered for targeted indications with the same care and attention as drugs.
  - Clinically significant adverse changes in body fluid composition, such as volume overload, electrolyte derangements, and acid-base imbalances, may result when fluids are given inappropriately or in excess.
  - IV fluids can cause the destruction of red blood cells if the tonicity of the fluid leads to rapid osmotic shifts into or out of the cells.
- Most critically ill patients will receive IV fluids, but patients with an inability to tolerate enteral intake and those with high fluid losses will be more dependent on fluid therapy.
- Targeted replacement of fluid deficits and losses varies with the patient's clinical condition and the etiology of fluid loss.
  - Sepsis and diabetic ketoacidosis may require large volumes of IV fluids.

TABLE 14.1.1 Characteristics of Selected Intravenous Fluids

Name	Na^+	Cl^-	K^+	pH	Osm	Notes
5% dextrose in water (D5W)	0	0	0	~4	252	Usually given to replace free water
5% dextrose in 0.45% normal saline (D5-½NS)	77	77	0	~4	406	Common "maintenance" fluid, sometimes with 20 mEq/L KCl added
0.9% NS	154	154	0	~5.5	308	
Lactated Ringer (LR)	130	109	4	~6.5	274	Also contains calcium and lactate
Plasma-Lyte	140	98	5	~7.4	294	Also contains magnesium, acetate, and gluconate
3% saline	513	513	0	~5.0	1,026	Typically given to treat intracranial hypertension
5% albumin	145	145	0	~6.9	~300	Colloid consisting of pooled, pasteurized human plasma albumin in an isotonic fluid
Starches and gelatins	Varies	Varies	0	Varies	Varies	Synthetic colloids with various formulations per package labels

- How about: The 2021 Surviving Sepsis Campaign guidelines suggest that at least 30 mL/kg of IV crystalloid fluid be given within the first 3 hours of resuscitation, and that balanced crystalloids be used instead of normal saline for resuscitation.
  - Pancreatitis, large open wounds, and diffuse burns initially require large fluid resuscitation due to massive losses of intravascular volume.
  - Gastrointestinal losses of fluids, including diarrhea, nasogastric suction, and enterocutaneous fistulae, may require extensive replacement.
  - Inappropriate urine production, as in diabetes insipidus, postobstructive diuresis, or the recovery phase of acute tubular necrosis, may require volume replacement.
  - While hypovolemia from trauma and acute hemorrhage was traditionally treated with large volumes of IV fluids, current Advanced Trauma Life Support (ATLS) guidelines recommend early blood product transfusion with limited crystalloid resuscitation.
- Daily maintenance fluid requirements in adults depend on the patient's size and comorbidities.
  - 1 to 1.5 mL/kg/h is a commonly used range for continuous administration of adult maintenance fluids.
- Pediatric maintenance fluids are typically dosed according to formulae such as the 4-2-1 or BSA rules.
  - The "4-2-1 rule" prescribes fluid rates based on weight: 4 mL/kg for the first 10 kg, 2 mL/kg for the next 10 kg, and 1 mL/kg for every kilogram >20 kg/h.
- IV fluids should be administered to replace insensible and measurable fluid losses.
  - Baseline insensible losses may total 400 to 500 mL/d.
  - In febrile patients, each 1 °C over 38 °C can increase insensible losses by 500 mL/d.
  - Insensible losses may be greatly increased in the setting of burned skin, open wounds, and elevated minute ventilation.

Management Considerations

- If a patient is clinically hypovolemic, resuscitation with IV fluids to restore circulating volume may aid in restoring hemodynamic stability and end-organ perfusion.
- Assessing a patient's volume status, while sometimes difficult, is essential in guiding fluid therapy.
  - The physical examination, in addition to physiologic monitoring data (eg, central venous pressure) and diagnostic tests such as bedside ultrasonography or brain natriuretic peptide (BNP) levels, can be used to assess volume status and help determine the need for fluid therapy.
  - Dynamic measures such as passive leg raising with continuous cardiac output or stroke volume monitoring (for example, LVOT VTI by echocardiography or pulse contour analysis) and pulse pressure variation (PPV) and stroke volume variation (SVV) predict fluid responsiveness better than static measures such as central venous pressure; PPV and SVV are reliable only with controlled ventilation, regular rhythm, and adequate tidal volume. Targeting capillary refill time in personalized protocols may improve outcomes in septic shock.
  - Repeating volume status assessments over time allows for tailored fluid management in response to therapy.
- It is generally appropriate to withhold IV fluid from patients exhibiting evidence of volume overload or intolerance, such as those with decompensated congestive heart failure.
  - In the setting of acute respiratory distress syndrome, withholding excess fluid may also improve lung function and shorten the intensive care unit (ICU) length of stay, and does not affect mortality, incidence of shock, or need for dialysis (FACTT trial).

Special Considerations

- There are insufficient data to guide the precise use of IV fluids in most clinical situations, and the optimal choice of fluid to administer in various clinical scenarios remains a topic of expert debate.
  - Balanced crystalloids are often preferred over 0.9% saline for many critically ill and non-critically ill hospitalized patients due to lower chloride content and associations with fewer major adverse kidney events (composite of death, dialysis, or persistent renal dysfunction) in some studies (the SMART and SALT-ED trials); however, large randomized trials in ICU patients showed no clear difference in 90-day mortality or AKI (PLUS and BaSICS trials), and a hospital-wide crossover trial found no difference in the composite of death or readmission (FLUID trial).
- Albumin may produce equivalent outcomes compared to balanced crystalloids in most patient populations, with no consistent evidence of mortality benefit (SAFE and ALBIOS trials)
  - Administration of concentrated albumin solutions to patients with sepsis and hypoalbuminemia (serum albumin <3.0 g/dL) may reduce the duration of shock, though it does not confer a mortality benefit.

    Albumin worsens morbidity and mortality in patients with severe traumatic brain injury due to increased cerebral edema in the presence of a dysregulated blood-brain barrier permeability.
- While hypovolemia from trauma and acute hemorrhage was traditionally treated with large volumes of IV fluids, current Advanced Trauma Life Support (ATLS) guidelines recommend early blood product transfusion with limited crystalloid resuscitation.

SUGGESTED READINGS

American College of Surgeons Committee on Trauma. ATLS® Student Course Manual. 10th ed. Chicago, IL: American College of Surgeons; 2018.

ANDROMEDA-SHOCK-2 Investigators for the ANDROMEDA Research Network, Spanish Society of Anesthesiology, Reanimation and Pain Therapy (SEDAR), and Latin American Intensive Care Network (LIVEN); Hernandez G, Ospina-Tascón GA, Kattan E, Ibarra-Estrada M, Ramasco F, Orozco N, Ramos K, Aldana JL, Ferri G, Hamzaoui O, De Backer D, Teboul JL, Vieillard-Baron A, Petri Damiani L, García-Gallardo GA, Morales S, Carmona Garcia P, Mendez R, Hernandez-Gilsoul T, Pérez-Nieto OR, Olea Vielba C, Ramos S, Dominguez D, Bruna M, David S, Wendel-Garcia PD, Galiana-Ivars M, Myatra SN, Messina A, Cecconi M, Pozo M, Amthauer M, Higuera E, Al Duhalib Z, Rico-Feijoo J, Ferrer-Gómez C, Pérez-Carbonell A, Martinez-Castro S, Redondo Calvo FJ, Vives M, Sanchez HF, Bilbao I, Fernandez P, Al-Fares A, Benitez-Cano A, Gonzalez C, Reyes LF, Rodriguez-Guillen JH, Cristino AV, Pendino JC, Ortiz G, Alonso-Gonzalez MC, Murias G, Aguirre-Ávalos G, Hernández L, Calderón Barajas ZA, Zarragoikoetxea I, Monnet X,

Goury A, Mendonça Dos Santos T, Vallecilla L, Martins de Lima L, Sady E, Alegria L, Ostermann M, Bakker J, Biasi Cavalcanti A. Personalized Hemodynamic Resuscitation Targeting Capillary Refill Time in Early Septic Shock: The ANDROMEDA-SHOCK-2 Randomized Clinical Trial. JAMA. 2025 Oct 29:e2520402.

Brunkhorst FM, Engel C, Bloos F, Meier-Hellmann A, Ragaller M, Weiler N, Moerer O, Gruendling M, Oppert M, Grond S, Olthoff D, Jaschinski U, John S, Rossaint R, Welte T, Schaefer M, Kern P, Kuhnt E, Kiehntopf M, Hartog C, Natanson C, Loeffler M, Reinhart K; German Competence Network Sepsis (SepNet). Intensive insulin therapy and pentastarch resuscitation in severe sepsis. N Engl J Med. 2008 Jan 10;358(2):125-39.

Finfer S, Micallef S, Hammond N, Navarra L, Bellomo R, Billot L, Delaney A, Gallagher M, Gattas D, Li Q, Mackle D, Mysore J, Saxena M, Taylor C, Young P, Myburgh J; PLUS Study Investigators and the Australian New Zealand Intensive Care Society Clinical Trials Group. Balanced Multielectrolyte Solution versus Saline in Critically Ill Adults. N Engl J Med. 2022 Mar 3;386(9):815-826. doi: 10.1056/NEJMoa2114464. Epub 2022 Jan 18.

McIntyre L, Fergusson D, McArdle T, English S, Cook DJ, Fox-Robichaud AE, Martin C, Marshall J, Pugliese M, Menon K, Thavorn K, Graham ID, Hawken S, Iyengar A, Kyeremanteng K, Saginur R, Seely AJE, Stiell IG, Bainbridge D, Weijer C, Taljaard M; Canadian Critical Care Trials Group. A Crossover Trial of Hospital-Wide Lactated Ringer's Solution versus Normal Saline. N Engl J Med. 2025 Aug 14;393(7):660-670. doi: 10.1056/NEJMoa2416761. Epub 2025 Jun 12.

Myburgh JA, Finfer S, Bellomo R, Billot L, Cass A, Gattas D, Glass P, Lipman J, Liu B, McArthur C, McGuinness S, Rajbhandari D, Taylor CB, Webb SA; CHEST Investigators; Australian and New Zealand Intensive Care Society Clinical Trials Group. Hydroxyethyl starch or saline for fluid resuscitation in intensive care. N Engl J Med. 2012 Nov 15;367(20):1901-11. doi: 10.1056/NEJMoa1209759. Epub 2012 Oct 17. Erratum in: N Engl J Med. 2016 Mar 31;374(13):1298.

National Heart, Lung, and Blood Institute Acute Respiratory Distress Syndrome (ARDS) Clinical Trials Network; Wiedemann HP, Wheeler AP, Bernard GR, Thompson BT, Hayden D, deBoisblanc B, Connors AF Jr, Hite RD, Harabin AL. Comparison of two fluid-management strategies in acute lung injury. N Engl J Med. 2006 Jun 15;354(24):2564-75.

Perner A, Haase N, Guttormsen AB, Tenhunen J, Klemenzson G, Åneman A, Madsen KR, Møller MH, Elkjær JM, Poulsen LM, Bendtsen A, Winding R, Steensen M, Berezowicz P, Søe-Jensen P, Bestle M, Strand K, Wiis J, White JO, Thornberg KJ, Quist L, Nielsen J, Andersen LH, Holst LB, Thormar K, Kjældgaard AL, Fabritius ML, Mondrup F, Pott FC, Møller TP, Winkel P, Wetterslev J; 6S Trial Group; Scandinavian Critical Care Trials Group. Hydroxyethyl starch 130/0.42 versus Ringer's acetate in severe sepsis. N Engl J Med. 2012 Jul 12;367(2):124-34.

Zampieri FG, Machado FR, Biondi RS, Freitas FGR, Veiga VC, Figueiredo RC, Lovato WJ, Amêndola CP, Serpa-Neto A, Paranhos JLR, Guedes MAV, Lúcio EA, Oliveira-Júnior LC, Lisboa TC, Lacerda FH, Maia IS, Grion CMC, Assunção MSC, Manoel ALO, Silva-Junior JM, Duarte P, Soares RM, Miranda TA, de Lima LM, Gurgel RM, Paisani DM, Corrêa TD, Azevedo LCP, Kellum JA, Damiani LP, Brandão da Silva N, Cavalcanti AB; BaSICS investigators and the BRICNet members. Effect of Intravenous Fluid Treatment With a Balanced Solution vs 0.9% Saline Solution on Mortality in Critically Ill Patients: The BaSICS Randomized Clinical Trial. JAMA. 2021 Aug 10;326(9):1–12.

14.2

Sodium and Chloride Balance

Alice Nova and Lorenzo Berra

Disorders of Water Homeostasis

- Hyponatremia and hypernatremia reflect disorders of water homeostasis, as changes in sodium levels are commonly caused by changes in the amount of body water rather than by low or high salt intake.
- Sodium is the most plentiful plasma ion and is regulated in the range of 135 to 145 mEq/L. Calculated serum osmolarity, which normally ranges between 275 and 290 mOsm/L, is closely related to twice the sodium concentration, with minimal contributions from glucose and blood urea nitrogen (BUN) in the absence of hyperglycemia or marked uremia. Serum osmolarity can be estimated using the following formula:

$$\text{Osm} = (2\ [\text{sodium}] + [\text{glucose}]/18 + [\text{BUN}]/2.8)$$

Hyponatremia

- Hyponatremia is common in critically ill patients, ranging from 13% to 15% in intensive care unit (ICU) admission, depending on the definition.

Pathophysiology and Differential Diagnosis

Hyponatremia may coexist with normal, high, or low plasma osmolality and with different volume statuses. Therefore, the diagnostic algorithm for hyponatremia should take into account plasma osmolality, clinical history, and physical examination with volume status assessment (Figure 14.2.1).

- Isotonic hyponatremia (serum osmolarity between 280 and 295 mOsm/L) is also known as pseudohyponatremia. It is a laboratory artifact that occurs in the presence of marked hypertriglyceridemia or hyperproteinemia, as seen in multiple myeloma. If pseudohyponatremia is suspected, using direct potentiometry, which employs an ion-selective electrode in undiluted plasma, can avoid this artifact.
- Hypertonic hyponatremia (serum osmolarity >295 mOsm/L) results from the presence of abnormal solutes other than sodium (eg, glucose, mannitol, or glycerol) in the extracellular fluid (ECF). These solutes exert osmotic pressure, leading to the redistribution of water from the intracellular fluid (ICF) to the ECF, causing cellular dehydration. This condition occurs in the very acute phase of diabetic ketoacidosis (DKA).

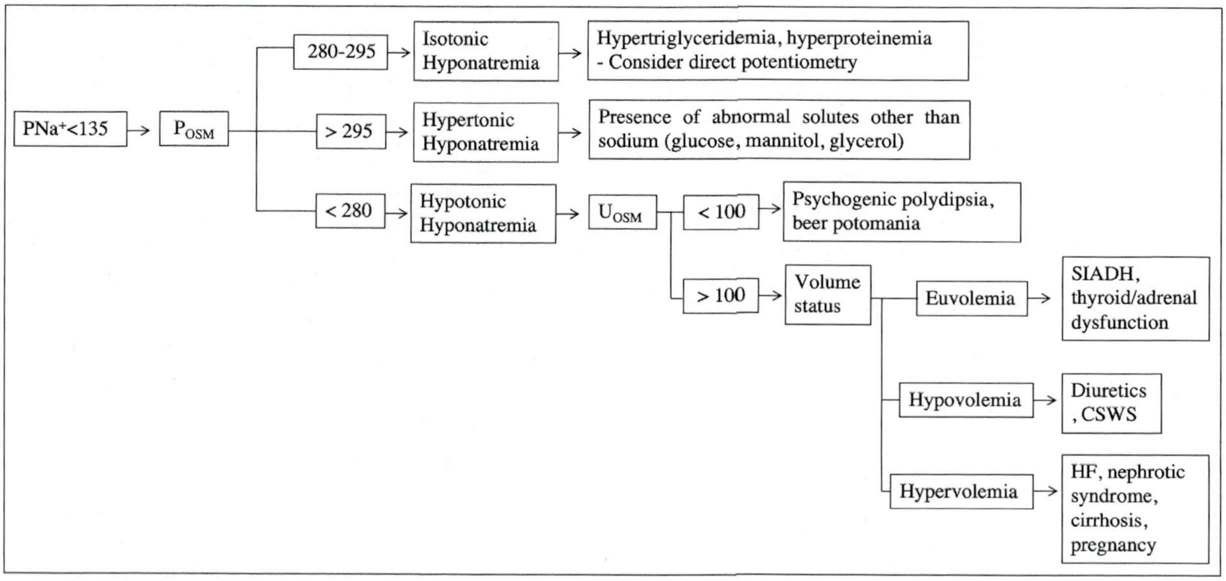

FIGURE 14.2.1 Diagnostic flowchart for hyponatremia. CSWS, cerebral salt-wasting syndrome; HF, heart failure; PNa^+, plasma sodium concentration (mmol/L); P_{OSM}, plasma osmolality (mOsm/L); SIADH, syndrome of inappropriate antidiuretic hormone secretion; U_{OSM}, urine osmolality (mOsm/kg).

- Hypotonic hyponatremia (serum osmolarity <280 mOsm/L) is caused by the inability of the kidney to excrete sufficient electrolyte-free water to match water intake. Measuring the urine osmolarity is useful for the differential diagnosis:
  - Urine osmolality <100 mOsm/kg: the normal diluting capacity of the kidney is overwhelmed by excessive water intake. This occurs in cases of psychogenic polydipsia or a diet deficient in protein and salt (beer potomania). In both of these cases, the patient appears clinically euvolemic.
  - Urine osmolality >100 mOsm/kg: the diluting capacity of the kidney is impaired. This condition may be associated with normal, decreased, or increased extracellular volume:
    - Euvolemic hyponatremia: the excess water distributes throughout the total body water space (only one-third of the total body water is ECF, and only 20% of ECF is intravascular water). The paradigm of euvolemic hyponatremia with concentrated urine is the syndrome of inappropriate antidiuretic hormone (SIADH). Additionally, hypothyroidism and glucocorticoid insufficiency may impair urinary dilution, leading to euvolemic hyponatremia.
    - Hypovolemic hyponatremia: a state of volume contraction stimulates antidiuretic hormone (ADH) release, leading to water retention. When the cause of the volume contraction is unknown, the urine sodium concentration (UNa^+) can be helpful in distinguishing between renal (eg, diuretic medications, cerebral salt-wasting syndrome [CSWS]—UNa^+ >30 mEq/L) and extrarenal solute losses (eg, hemorrhage, vomiting, diarrhea—UNa^+ <30 mEq/L). CSWS, typically seen in patients with brain injury, is associated with hypovolemia, inappropriate sodium excretion despite volume depletion, and low total body sodium. In contrast, SIADH usually presents with euvolemia, inappropriate water retention, and low serum sodium due to excessive ADH activity.
    - Hypervolemic hyponatremia: in disorders characterized by reduced effective circulating volume, the renal ability to eliminate water and sodium is compromised due to perceived intravascular volume depletion. This is the case of heart failure, nephrotic syndrome, cirrhosis, or pregnancy.

Clinical Manifestation and Treatment

- The clinical manifestations of hyponatremia are largely attributed to cerebral edema resulting from intracellular volume expansion, which occurs only when hyponatremia is associated with hypotonicity. Mild neurologic symptoms (eg, anorexia, nausea, and malaise) typically occur for plasma sodium concentrations between 125 and 120 mEq/L. Headache, lethargy, confusion, agitation, and obtundation may be seen for plasma sodium concentrations between 120 and 110 mEq/L. More severe symptoms, such as seizures and coma, may occur when plasma levels fall <110 mEq/L.
- Although symptoms generally resolve with correction of the hypotonicity, profound hypotonicity developing over < 24 hours may lead to severe cerebral edema, carry a high mortality rate (up to 50% in some cases), and may result in residual neurologic deficits.
- Hyponatremia is best treated by finding the underlying causes and developing an appropriate plan of care. The rate of correction must be carefully regulated, especially in chronic hyponatremia, where cellular volume adaptations may be complete. In this case, rapid correction can lead to the development of osmotic demyelination syndrome (ODS). Hyponatremia per se requires treatment only when it is associated with hypotonicity. The therapy of hypotonic hyponatremia should be titrated on the patient's symptoms and the duration of the disorder:

- Acute (<24 hours) and symptomatic hyponatremia should be treated as an emergency to reduce intracranial pressure. An intravenous bolus of 100 mL of 3% saline infused over 10 minutes is recommended. Repeat boluses may be considered every 10 minutes until symptoms improve or a target sodium increase of 4 to 6 mEq/L is achieved within the first 6 hours. Careful monitoring of serum sodium levels is essential to avoid overcorrection, which can lead to ODS.
- In cases of chronic (>48 hours) or unknown duration and symptomatic hyponatremia, plasma sodium concentration should be raised by no > 1 mmol/L per hour in the first 6 hours, after which the increase should be halted.
- The treatment of chronic asymptomatic hypotonicity should be directed at correcting the underlying pathophysiologic mechanisms involved, with care to avoid rapid sodium correction which risks ODS.

Hypernatremia

- Sustained hypernatremia develops in patients whose water output exceeds their input. It commonly occurs in patients who have impaired thirst sensation, those who cannot access water, or those unable to express their need for water (eg, infants, patients with neurologic impairments, critically ill patients).
- Hypernatremia presents in about 9% of patients at ICU admission and develops during the course of the ICU stay in 6% of patients.

Pathophysiology and Differential Diagnosis

Hypernatremia can result from pure water loss, hyponatremic fluid loss, or sodium or hypernatremic fluid gain. It is always associated with increased serum osmolality and may be associated with various volume statuses (Figure 14.2.2).

- Euvolemic hypernatremia is caused by pure water loss. The patient appears euvolemic because the water is lost proportionately from both the ECF and ICF. Pure water can be lost through the skin and respiratory tract (uncompensated insensible losses) or through urine (compensated diabetes insipidus, DI). DI causes filtration of plasma without water retention. DI can originate from a "central" cause due to a lack of ADH release from the pituitary gland or a "nephrogenic" cause, which involves dysfunction of the renal aquaporin channels.
- Hypovolemic hypernatremia occurs due to loss of both sodium and water, with greater water loss compared to sodium. Common causes include gastrointestinal (GI) fluid loss (most GI fluids have lower sodium concentration than plasma), osmotic or medication-induced diuresis (eg, from loop diuretics), excessive sweating, or severe uncompensated DI.
- Hypervolemic hypernatremia, often iatrogenic, primarily results from the administration of hypertonic sodium solutions (eg, for cerebral edema treatment or hyponatremia correction with hyperosmolar therapy) or excessive sodium intake in patients with restricted access to water.

Clinical Manifestation and Treatment

- The clinical manifestations of hypernatremia are proportional to the magnitude and rate of rise of the plasma sodium concentration and are primarily due to intracellular volume contraction.
- Chronic progressive hypernatremia typically presents with fewer and milder symptoms compared to acute and severe hypernatremia, which can cause weakness, lethargy, and confusion. Seizures and coma may occur, especially in children.
- The initial treatment of the patient with hypernatremia depends on the volume status. For euvolemic and hypovolemic hypernatremia, the therapy aims to reduce the ongoing water losses and to replace the existing water deficit. The water deficit can be calculated as follows:

$$\text{Water deficit} = ((0.6_{\text{ for men}}) \text{ or } (0.5_{\text{ for women}}) \times \text{weight (kg)} \times ((\text{measured sodium}/140) - 1)$$

- This calculation assumes a euvolemic baseline and may not account for concurrent volume abnormalities such as hypovolemia or hypervolemia, which require additional assessment for appropriate fluid replacement.
- One should aim to lower the plasma sodium concentration by no >10 mmol/L per day. Water is best administered enterally. If the oral route is unavailable, 5% dextrose in water (D5W) may be used intravenously to provide free water without adding sodium.

Chloride Balance

- After sodium, chloride is the most abundant electrolyte in serum, with a normal range between 97 and 110 mmol/L.
- Chloride has a key role in the regulation of body fluids, electrolyte balance, preservation of electrical neutrality, and acid-base status.

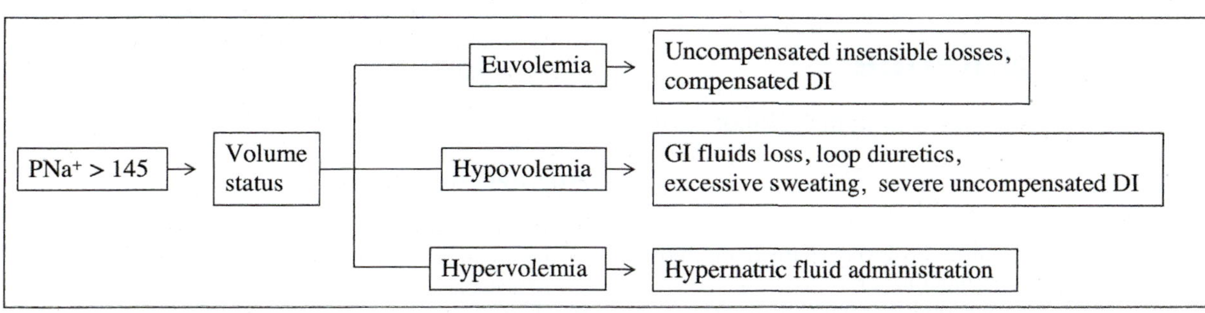

FIGURE 14.2.2 Diagnostic flowchart for hypernatremia. DI, diabetes insipidus, PNa^+, plasma sodium concentration (mmol/L).

- Abnormal chloride levels alone usually signify a more serious underlying metabolic disorder, such as metabolic acidosis or alkalosis.
- Both hypochloremia and hyperchloremia manifest through nonspecific symptoms, primarily noticeable due to acid-base status impairment and the underlying cause.

Hypochloremia

Three main mechanisms may lead to hypochloremia:

- Chloride loss: this can occur through the GI tract (eg, massive vomiting, high-output fistula, villous intestinal adenomas) or the kidneys (eg, loop or thiazide diuretics, Bartter syndrome).
- Expansion of the extracellular space by a fluid with low or zero chloride content: this occurs in conditions such as advanced heart failure, SIADH, or excessive infusion of hypotonic solutions, which dilutes chloride levels.

  In these cases, chloride concentration correlates inversely with bicarbonate concentration. Decreased chloride levels stimulate renal bicarbonate reabsorption rates, contributing to or exacerbating metabolic alkalosis.
- Chronic respiratory failure: increased chloride losses occur through the kidney as a result of compensatory bicarbonate reabsorption in response to chronic respiratory acidosis.

Hyperchloremia

By etiology, hyperchloremia can be divided into three types:

- Dilutional hyperchloremia: iatrogenic fluid therapy with chloride-rich solutions may cause hyperchloremia associated with metabolic acidosis due to the decrease in the strong ion difference (SID).
- Loss of pure water or higher loss of water compared to chlorides: this can occur from renal causes (eg, DI, diuretic medications, polyuric phase of renal failure) or extrarenal causes (eg, fever, hypermetabolism, diarrhea, burns).
- Increased renal chloride reabsorption: this can be due to conditions such as renal tubular acidosis, renal failure, acetazolamide use, and posthypocapnia states.

SUGGESTED READINGS

Adrogué HJ, Madias NE. Hypernatremia. *N Engl J Med*. 2000;342(20):1493-1499.

Alshayeb HM, Showkat A, Babar F, Mangold T, Wall BM. Severe hypernatremia correction rate and mortality in hospitalized patients. *Am J Med Sci*. 2011;341(5):356-360.

Astapenko D, Navratil P, Pouska J, Cerny V. Clinical physiology aspects of chloremia in fluid therapy: a systematic review. *Perioper Med (Lond)*. 2020;9(1):40.

Ayus JC, Arieff AI. Pulmonary complications of hyponatremic encephalopathy: noncardiogenic pulmonary edema and hypercapnic respiratory failure. *Chest*. 1995;107(2):517-521.

Berend K, van Hulsteijn LH, Gans RO. Chloride: the queen of electrolytes? *Eur J Intern Med*. 2012;23(3):203-211.

Funk GC, Lindner G, Druml W, et al. Incidence and prognosis of dysnatremias present on ICU admission. *Intensive Care Med*. 2010;36(2):304-311.

Garibaldi BT, Cameron SJ, Choi M. Pseudohyponatremia in a patient with HIV and hepatitis C coinfection. *J Gen Intern Med*. 2008;23(2):202-205.

Kaplan LJ, Kellum JA. Fluids, pH, ions and electrolytes. *Curr Opin Crit Care*. 2010;16(4):323-331.

Kellum JA, Elbers PWG. *Stewart's Textbook of Acid-Base*. 2nd ed. Lulu Enterprises; 2009.

Kraft MD, Btaiche IF, Sacks GS, Kudsk KA. Treatment of electrolyte disorders in adult patients in the intensive care unit. *Am J Health Syst Pharm*. 2005;62(16):1663-1682.

Kumar S, Berl T. Sodium. *Lancet*. 1998;352(9123):220-228.

Lindner G, Funk GC, Schwarz C, et al. Hypernatremia in the critically ill is an independent risk factor for mortality. *Am J Kidney Dis*. 2007;50(6):952-957.

Martin RJ. Central pontine and extrapontine myelinolysis: the osmotic demyelination syndromes. *J Neurol Neurosurg Psychiatry*. 2004;75 suppl 3(suppl 3):iii22-iii28.

Silversides JA, Quinn LD, Parker MJ, Austin SJ. Is the cause of hypernatraemia in critically ill patients more obvious than we think? *Anaesthesia*. 2010;65(1):87-88.

Sterns RH. Severe symptomatic hyponatremia: treatment and outcome: a study of 64 cases. *Ann Intern Med*. 1987;107(5):656-664.

Sterns RH. The management of symptomatic hyponatremia. *Semin Nephrol*. 1990;10(6):503-514.

Verbalis JG, Berl T. Disorders of water balance. In: Brenner B, ed. *Brenner & Rector's the Kidney*. 8th ed. Saunders; 2007.

Weiss-Guillet EM, Takala J, Jakob SM. Diagnosis and management of electrolyte emergencies. *Best Pract Res Clin Endocrinol Metab*. 2003;17(4):623-651.

14.3

Potassium Balance

Mariana L. Laporta Miranda and Juan G. Ripoll Sanz

Definition

- Potassium is the most plentiful positively charged ion in the body and the major intracellular cation.
- Of the 3,500 mEq that constitute the total content of potassium in the body, nearly 98% is intracellular at concentrations of 140 to 150 mEq/L.
- Membrane ion pumps actively transport potassium into cells so that only ~2% of the total potassium is found in the extracellular space.
- Plasma potassium is regulated in the range of 3.5 to 5 mEq/L by the Na^+/K^+/ATPase pump.
- Potassium balance is crucial for the proper functioning of nerve and muscle tissues, so disorders of potassium can be life-threatening.

Hyperkalemia

- Hyperkalemia can produce life-threatening dysrhythmias, even in patients without preexisting cardiac disease.
- Levels >5.5 mEq/L may produce symptoms.
- Levels >6.5 mEq/L are more likely to be life-threatening and deserve immediate treatment.

Hyperkalemia produces electrocardiogram (ECG) changes that become more pronounced as the condition becomes more life-threatening.

- The sequence of ECG changes in hyperkalemia typically includes (1) symmetric peaking of T waves, (2) reduced P-wave voltage and widened QRS complex, (3) sinusoidal-shaped wave, and (4) ventricular tachycardia, ventricular fibrillation, or asystole.

Toxicity from hyperkalemia can vary depending on patient factors, such as hypocalcemia, preexisting structural heart disease, and metabolic acidosis.

Causes of Hyperkalemia

- Acidemia can shift potassium out of cells, causing acute hyperkalemia.
- Rapid transfusion of stored red blood cells can produce hyperkalemia, especially if the blood is nearing the end of its storage life.
- Many drugs in the intensive care unit can contribute to hyperkalemia. Examples include:
  - Potassium supplements
  - Potassium-sparing diuretics (ie, triamterene, spironolactone, amiloride)
  - Beta-blockers
  - Digoxin
  - Succinylcholine
  - Angiotensin-converting enzyme inhibitors or angiotensin receptor blockers
  - Cyclosporine
  - Tacrolimus

Hypokalemia

- Mild hypokalemia is usually not serious unless there is concurrent intoxication or cardiac ischemia that produces a susceptibility to dysrhythmia.
- Rapidly acquired hypokalemia or severe hypokalemia with plasma values <2 mEq/L can cause life-threatening complications such as neurologic weakness and, in rare cases, rhabdomyolysis.
- The most common cause of hypokalemia is the use of diuretics, especially loop diuretics.
- Multiple drugs can contribute to hypokalemia. Examples include:
  - Antimicrobials (eg, aminoglycosides, amphotericin B, penicillin)
  - Inotropes and pressors with beta-2 adrenergic activity (eg, epinephrine, isoproterenol)
  - Inhaled beta-2 receptor agonists (eg, albuterol, salmeterol)
  - Insulin
  - Methylxanthines (eg, theophylline)
  - Diuretics (eg, thiazide diuretics, loop diuretics, carbonic-anhydrase inhibitors)
  - Laxatives

Common Causes to Remember (Table 14.3.1)

TABLE 14.3.1 Common Causes of Hyperkalemia and Hypokalemia

Hyperkalemia	Hypokalemia
Acidosis—especially metabolic	Diuretic use, especially loop diuretics
Adrenal insufficiency	Alkalosis—especially acute metabolic alkalosis
Tissue injury, burns, crush injuries, compartment syndromes, stored blood	Hyperaldosteronism
Increased tissue catabolism, fever, shivering, tumor lysis syndrome, intense exercise	Excess renal losses of potassium
Renal failure	Hypomagnesemia
Exuberant potassium ingestion	Low potassium intake
β-Blocker therapy	Gastrointestinal (GI) losses: diarrhea, gastric fluid suction, vomiting
Hyperglycemia and hyperosmolar states	Antibiotic effects on the kidney, especially penicillin, aminoglycosides, and amphotericin
Reperfusion following local ischemia	Hypothermia

Epidemiology

- Hyperkalemia and hypokalemia are the most common electrolyte abnormalities in hospitalized patients, with a high incidence in the intensive care unit.

Key Pathophysiology

- Hydrogen ions, with their positive charge, can displace potassium ions from the intracellular space, raising the extracellular potassium levels.
- Shifting potassium from the intracellular space to the extracellular space produces the majority of hyperkalemia.
  - Fortunately, shifting the potassium back into the cells is usually possible with medical intervention.
- Typical daily potassium intake is usually balanced with renal and gastrointestinal (GI) losses.
- Changes in the balance of intake and loss can lead to hyperkalemia or hypokalemia over time.

Management and Treatment

- *Treatment of hyperkalemia*
  - Acute treatment includes shifting potassium to the intracellular space, elimination therapy, and/or stabilization of the cardiomyocyte membranes to prevent the cardiac myocyte's arrhythmogenic effects.
  - Intracellular shift:
    - Intravenous (IV) insulin and dextrose: usually 10 units of regular insulin IV and 12.5 to 25 g of IV dextrose (eg, 500 mL of 10% or 50 mL of 50% dextrose). The effects begin within 5 minutes, peak around 60 minutes, and last several hours.
    - Inhaled beta-2 agonists like salmeterol or albuterol can also be used.
    - Administration of sodium bicarbonate raises the pH and helps to shift potassium intracellularly.
  - Elimination therapy

Potassium can be eliminated by:

- The kidneys, with the help of diuretics, most commonly loop diuretics or thiazides

- The GI system, with the help of cation exchange resin, such as sodium polystyrene (or Kayexalate)
  - Kayexalate produces an osmotic load that can lead to tissue ischemia if gut perfusion is threatened. Constipation is a common side effect that would also decrease the efficacy of the binding resin.
  - AVOID in patients with shock or recent (<1 week) GI surgery
- Mechanically through dialysis
  - Severe hyperkalemia that is refractory to medical treatment is an urgent indication for dialysis.
- Stabilization of the cardiomyocyte membranes:
  - IV calcium can be used to treat hyperkalemia, particularly in patients with ECG changes, by antagonizing the effects of potassium on the threshold potential and the speed of impulse propagation at the cellular level, thus transiently stabilizing the cardiomyocytes' membranes.
  - This therapy mitigates the risk of arrhythmias and reverses the ECG changes. However, it does not lower serum potassium levels and should be combined with other therapies to lower serum potassium.
  - The effect of this intervention is fast but short-lived.
- IV calcium is administered either as 10 mL of 10% calcium gluconate over 2 minutes or as 10% calcium chloride, which contains 3 times the amount of calcium per 10 mL dose, preferably administered via central access.

Treatment of Hypokalemia

- Hypokalemia usually responds to oral or IV supplementation of potassium.
  - Potassium deficit: if mild and asymptomatic, usually replete between 40 and 80 mEq orally daily. If profound or symptomatic, more aggressive repletion is possible with strict monitoring. Peripheral potassium infusion should not be more concentrated than 50 to 60 mmol/L (equivalent to 50-60 mEq/L) to minimize the risk for phlebitis. The maximum infusion rate for potassium should generally not exceed 10 mEq/h for peripheral administration and 20 mEq/h for central administration, with appropriate cardiac and laboratory monitoring.
  - Consider concurrent hypomagnesemia.
    - Hypomagnesemia worsens renal potassium losses, so replenishing magnesium is sometimes necessary for effective potassium replacement.

Outcomes

- If appropriate medical attention is provided, mortality from potassium disturbances usually depends on the underlying cause.
- Untreated hyperkalemia can be rapidly fatal, but dialysis is an effective treatment.

SUGGESTED READINGS

Kraft MD, Btaiche IF, Sacks GS, et al. Treatment of electrolyte disorders in adult patients in the intensive care unit. *Am J Health Syst Pharm.* 2005;62:1663-1682.

Mahoney BA, Smith WA, Lo DS, et al. Emergency interventions for hyperkalaemia. *Cochrane Database Syst Rev.* 2005;2005(2):CD003235.

Mandal AK. Hypokalemia and hyperkalemia. *Med Clin North Am.* 1997; 81:611-639.

Vraets A, Lin Y, Callum JL. Transfusion-associated hyperkalemia. *Transfus Med Rev.* 2011;25:184.

14.4

Calcium, Magnesium, and Phosphorus Balance

Marvin G. Chang and Edward A. Bittner

Overview

- Normal Values
  - Calcium
    - Total calcium: 8.5 to 10.5 mg/dL (2.1-2.6 mmol/L)
    - Ionized calcium: 1.1 to 1.3 mmol/L (4.5-5.3 mg/dL)
  - Magnesium: 1.7 to 2.2 mg/dL (0.7-0.9 mmol/L)
  - Phosphorus: 2.5 to 4.5 mg/dL (0.8-1.5 mmol/L)
- Calcium
  - Plays critical roles in cellular activity, important to both electrical and mechanical muscular contraction
  - A very small fraction of total body calcium is dissolved.
  - Most of the calcium is stored in bone.
  - A key contributor to the proper function of the clotting cascade (once known as factor IV in the clotting cascade)
  - Binds to albumin and plasma proteins
    - Corrected Ca (mg/dL) = measured Ca + 0.8 × (4 − albumin [g/dL])
      - Often unreliable in critically ill due to protein binding shifts with pH, citrate (massive transfusion), and acute-phase inflammatory changes
    - Measuring ionized calcium is preferred.
  - One gram of calcium gluconate provides about 93 mg of elemental calcium; can be given peripherally.
  - One gram of calcium chloride provides about 273 mg of elemental calcium.
    - Calcium chloride is a sclerotic vein irritant and is best administered through a central line.
- *Magnesium*
  - The second most common intracellular positive ion behind potassium
  - An important cofactor in many enzymatic processes
- Phosphorous
  - The third most common inorganic anion in the plasma (after chloride and bicarbonate), yet the vast majority of the phosphorus in the body (~85%) is stored in bone and soft tissue.

- A crucial factor in energy storage and utilization at the cellular level
- An important component of nucleic acids and soft tissue proteins

Epidemiology

- Prevalence of these disorders varies with the patient population and is difficult to quantify.
- States of deficiency are more common in the intensive care unit (ICU) than states of excess, unless concurrent renal failure is present.
- States of excess
  - Hypercalcemia sometimes causes patients to seek medical attention, particularly if associated with malignancy.
    - Hypercalcemia is relatively uncommon in critically ill patients (2%-15% overall; <1% severe), typically malignancy or iatrogenic related, whereas hypocalcemia occurs in up to 88% of ICU patients and is more prevalent with greater illness severity.
  - Hypermagnesemia is very uncommon and is usually due to an iatrogenic administration of magnesium, or ingestion of high magnesium-containing laxatives.
  - Hyperphosphatemia is seen in renal failure and is commonly seen in patients with renal failure.
    - For patients with mild renal dysfunction, hyperphosphatemia can occur after ingestion of concentrated phosphorus compounds (eg, phospho-soda laxatives).
    - Tissue destruction states can precipitate hyperphosphatemia during tumor lysis syndrome or compartment syndrome.
    - Rhabdomyolysis releases intracellular phosphate, potassium, and myoglobin and frequently causes hyperphosphatemia—particularly when accompanied by acute kidney injury, which impairs renal phosphate excretion.
    - Hyperphosphatemia frequently accompanies propofol infusion syndrome (PRIS) due to rhabdomyolysis (phosphate release from damaged muscle) and acute kidney injury (impaired renal excretion) but is not a defining diagnostic criterion.
- States of deficiency
  - 15% to 88% of hospitalized patients have hypocalcemia, depending on the method of measurement and patient population studied.
    - Very common after parathyroidectomy
  - Hypomagnesemia and hypophosphatemia are seen regularly in the ICU.

Key Pathophysiology

- **Hypercalcemia**
  - Hyperparathyroidism is the most common cause of hypercalcemia, but its severity is usually modest.
  - Severe hypercalcemia can be caused by metastatic cancers that could increase calcium through bone lysis and/or parathyroid hormone (PTH)–related peptide (PTHrP).
  - Granulomatous diseases, including sarcoidosis, can cause hypercalcemia.
  - Exuberant ingestion of calcium, particularly associated with concurrent ingestion of basic materials, can produce hypercalcemia.
  - Iatrogenic hypercalcemia can be seen after rapid intravenous (IV) administration.
  - QTc shortening can be seen.
  - Symptoms of hypercalcemia include fatigue, weakness, confusion, constipation, polyuria, polydipsia, nephrolithiasis, and cardiac arrhythmias, with severity correlating to the degree and rapidity of calcium elevation.
- *Hypocalcemia*
  - The body has tremendous stores of calcium in bone, but only about 1% of the body calcium can equilibrate with the extracellular fluid.
    - Much of the plasma calcium is protein bound.
  - Can be seen with massive transfusion of blood products (due to citrate binding circulating calcium ion), hypoparathyroidism (ie, after parathyroidectomy or thyroidectomy), and with hypomagnesemia (impairs secretion of PTH)
  - Hypocalcemia can cause hypotension due to both vascular smooth muscle dysfunction and loss of cardiac inotropy.
  - Chronic severe hypocalcemia is uncommon due to the large calcium reserves in the bone.
  - Hypoparathyroidism can lead to acute or chronic hypocalcemia.
  - Trousseau and Chvostek signs are seen on physical examination.
    - Trousseau sign: carpal spasm when blood pressure cuff inflated above systolic pressure for 3 minutes
    - Chvostek sign: facial muscle twitching when facial nerve tapped anterior to ear
    - Both have low sensitivity/specificity.
  - QTc prolongation can be seen.
- **Hypermagnesemia**
  - Usually iatrogenic or due to over-ingestion of magnesium (potentially through magnesium-containing laxatives), particularly with renal failure
  - Hypermagnesemia can lead to nerve dysfunction, muscle weakness, hyporeflexia, and mental status changes.
- **Hypomagnesemia**
  - Common in the critically ill, and commonly seen after large volumes of IV fluids
  - Hypomagnesemia can cause torsades de pointes and other ventricular arrhythmias, increase atrial fibrillation susceptibility, and prevent correction of coexisting hypokalemia (via loss of potassium channel inhibition) and hypocalcemia (via impaired PTH secretion and end-organ resistance).
- *Hyperphosphatemia*
  - Excess phosphate binds to calcium, forming calcium-phosphate precipitation, which can lead to acute kidney injury (tubular deposition/nephrocalcinosis) and symptomatic hypocalcemia (decreases ionized calcium).
- *Hypophosphatemia*
  - Develops through transcellular shifts (refeeding syndrome, respiratory alkalosis, insulin), impaired absorption (aluminum- or calcium-based antacids), increased losses or consumption (sepsis, alcohol use), or dilution from large-volume IV fluid resuscitation
  - Severe hypophosphatemia (<1.0 mg/dL) can cause respiratory failure from diaphragmatic weakness, impaired oxygen delivery due to decreased 2,3-DPG, rhabdomyolysis, hemolysis, and cardiac dysfunction.
  - Severe hypophosphatemia is a hallmark of refeeding syndrome and can be life-threatening.

Management and Treatment

- States of electrolyte excess are typically more difficult to manage than states of electrolyte deficiency.
- Supplementation of the low electrolyte, with IV or oral replacement is usually all that is needed to correct a deficiency state.
- Hypercalcemia
  - First-line therapy:
    - Discontinue inciting factors (eg, thiazides, lithium, calcium/vitamin D supplements)
    - IV isotonic crystalloid
      - Traditionally, 0.9% normal saline is recommended because sodium delivery (not chloride) drives calciuresis by competitively inhibiting calcium reabsorption in the thick ascending limb; balanced crystalloids such as Plasma-Lyte may be preferred to avoid hyperchloremic acidosis.
      - Corrects volume depletion, restores glomerular filtration rate (GFR), and enhances renal calcium excretion through increased glomerular filtration and natriuresis
    - Note: furosemide is no longer routinely recommended and is reserved for volume overload after adequate hydration.
  - Pharmacologic treatments (for moderate-severe or symptomatic hypercalcemia)
    - Calcitonin
      - Inhibits osteoclast-mediated bone resorption and increases renal calcium excretion; fastest onset (hours) but limited by tachyphylaxis after 24 to 48 hours
      - Used as bridge therapy while awaiting bisphosphonate effect
    - Bisphosphonates (mainstay)
      - Inhibit osteoclast activity providing sustained calcium reduction
      - Delayed onset (days) but prolonged duration (weeks)
      - Zoledronic acid preferred to pamidronate because more potent, has faster and more sustained calcium-lowering effects, and is easier to administer (shorter infusion time).
      - Use with caution/avoid in significant renal impairment
    - Glucocorticoids
      - Reduce calcitriol production; effective for granulomatous disease, vitamin D toxicity, and hematologic malignancies; not effective for most solid tumors
    - Denosumab
      - Monoclonal antibody that blocks receptor activator of nuclear factor kappa-B ligand (RANKL), a key cytokine required for osteoclast formation/activation and prevents osteoclast-mediated bone resorption
      - Used for refractory hypercalcemia or when bisphosphonates are contraindicated (eg, severe renal failure)
    - Cinacalcet
      - A calcimimetic that suppresses PTH secretion that is used specifically for PTH-driven hypercalcemia, such as in parathyroid carcinoma or in primary hyperparathyroidism when surgery is not an option
      - Not effective for malignancy-related hypercalcemia from PTHrP or other mechanisms
  - Dialysis may be considered for severe refractory hypercalcemia unresponsive to medical therapy or when aggressive IV hydration is contraindicated (life-threatening Ca, renal failure/volume overload, or contraindications to meds).
- **Hypocalcemia**
  - Typically responds to calcium supplementation
  - It is important to check and correct coexisting hypomagnesemia.
- **Hypermagnesemia**
  - Supportive therapy is typically all that is needed.
  - Dialysis is an option for severe hypermagnesemia.
- **Hypomagnesemia**
  - Responds to IV supplementation
    - Rapid IV magnesium administration can produce profound hypotension; slow infusion is recommended.
  - Enteral supplementation may eventually lead to correction of hypomagnesemia, but diarrhea is commonly seen with generous magnesium supplementation.
  - Magnesium should be corrected before treating coexisting hypokalemia or hypocalcemia, as these electrolyte abnormalities are often refractory to replacement therapy until magnesium is repleted.
- **Hyperphosphatemia**
  - Typically associated with renal failure
  - Low-phosphorus diets are poorly tolerated.
  - Phosphorus binders can be given with food to lower the absorbed phosphorus.
  - Dialysis may be needed for acute hyperphosphatemia.
- **Hypophosphatemia**
  - Responds to supplementation
  - During refeeding syndrome, nutrition should be withheld or advanced slowly until hypophosphatemia is corrected.

Outcomes

- The outcomes of these electrolyte imbalances typically depend on the patient's underlying condition.
- Hypercalcemia: mortality is primarily driven by the underlying malignancy. Severe hypercalcemia (>14 mg/dL) or the presence of neurologic symptoms indicates a need for urgent treatment and carries a high hospital mortality.
- Hypocalcemia: ionized calcium <0.9 mmol/L is associated with increased ICU mortality.
- Hypomagnesemia: prognosis is worsened if associated refractory hypokalemia/hypocalcemia are not recognized and treated.
- Hyperphosphatemia: in renal failure, chronic hyperphosphatemia is a major driver of long-term cardiovascular mortality.
- Hypophosphatemia: severe hypophosphatemia, especially during refeeding syndrome, can be fatal if unrecognized and untreated.

Acknowledgments

We gratefully acknowledge the contributions of the previous edition author, Jonathan Charnin, as portions of those chapters have been retained in this revision.

SUGGESTED READINGS

Aberegg SK. Ionized calcium in the ICU: should it be measured and corrected? *Chest*. 2016;149(3):846-855.

Ehrenpreis ED, Jarrouj G, Meader R, Wagner C, Ellis M. A comprehensive review of hypomagnesemia. *Dis Mon*. 2022;68(2):101285.

Fernandes C, Pereira L. Hypocalcemia in critical care settings, from its clinical relevance to its treatment: a narrative review. *Anaesth Crit Care Pain Med*. 2024;43(6):101438.

Maier JD, Levine SN. Hypercalcemia in the intensive care unit: a review of pathophysiology, diagnosis, and modern therapy. *J Intensive Care Med*. 2015;30(5):235-252.

Major P, Lortholary A, Hon J, et al. Zoledronic acid is superior to pamidronate in the treatment of hypercalcemia of malignancy: a pooled analysis of two randomized, controlled clinical trials. *J Clin Oncol*. 2001;19(2): 558-567.

Reintam Blaser A, Gunst J, Ichai C, et al. Hypophosphatemia in critically ill adults and children—a systematic review. *Clin Nutr*. 2021;40(4): 1744-1754.

Van Laecke S. Hypomagnesemia and hypermagnesemia. *Acta Clin Belg*. 2019;74(1):41-47.

Zheng WH, Yao Y, Zhou H, Xu Y, Huang HB. Hyperphosphatemia and outcomes in critically ill patients: a systematic review and meta-analysis. *Front Med (Lausanne)*. 2022;9:870637.

Zivin JR, Gooley T, Zager RA, Ryan MJ. Hypocalcemia: a pervasive metabolic abnormality in the critically ill. *Am J Kidney Dis*. 2001;37(4): 689-698.

SECTION 15

Nutrition

Section Editor: Casey M. Luckhurst

15.1

Basal and Stress Energy Requirements

Caroline H. Jensen and Jamie L. Sparling

Indications for Nutritional Support

- The first step in the initiation of nutrition is to determine which patients will benefit, when they will benefit from supplemental enteral or parenteral nutrition, and how much nutrition they need.
- The following are the broad groups of patients who may benefit from supplemental nutrition.
  - Those with preexisting malnourishment or weight loss (>5%-20%)
    - Examples include the older, patients with advanced cancer, malignancies that result in decreased oral intake (eg, oropharyngeal cancer, esophageal cancer), or chronic inflammatory states like Crohn disease.
  - Those subjected to significant inflammatory injury such as severe trauma, burns >20% total body surface area (TBSA), pancreatitis, and infection/sepsis
  - Those who will be or have been without nutrition for ≥7 days, or those who have had reduced intake or moderate malabsorption/gastrointestinal (GI) symptoms for >2 weeks
  - Patients unable to take any nutrition independently (eg, intubated patients), who are not anticipated to do so within 24 to 72 hours
  - Those with significant chronic disease
  - Interestingly, body mass index (BMI) is often not the best predictor of malnutrition, as fluid resuscitation, routine diuresis, and rapid muscle wasting impact daily weight measurements.

Determining Nutritional Requirements

- Once a patient has been deemed appropriate for nutritional supplementation, the nutritional needs must be calculated.
- *Calculating basal energy expenditure (BEE)*
  - The best tool for determining energy requirements is indirect calorimetry (IC).
  - However, when IC is not available, ASPEN guidelines suggest a weight-based calculation to measure the BEE.
  - BEE = 25 kcal/kg × wt (kg) per day
  - Alternatively, there are predictive equations such as the Harrison-Benedict equation that calculate energy requirements for men and women by weight, height, and age.
    - Men = 66.5 + (13.7 × wt) + (5.0 × ht) − (6.76 × age)
    - Women = 65.5 + (9.6 × wt) + (1.85 × ht) − (4.68 × age)
  - Resting energy expenditure (REE) can be calculated with IC by measuring the subject's oxygen uptake, CO_2 production, and applying the following formula:
    - REE = $(3.9 \times \dot{V}O_2) + (1.1 \times \dot{V}CO_2) - 61$
- Increasingly, new devices for IC are becoming more accessible, and IC is now considered the standard of care for objective determination of intensive care unit (ICU) energy needs. Limitations of IC include the need for specialized equipment and specially trained personnel, and the need for an FIO_2 <50%.
- Caloric requirements are higher with stress, and stress factors have historically been used in tandem with calculating basal energy requirements. Current evidence suggests most accurate determination of energy requirements is made with IC rather than the utilization of a stress factor in calculations.
- *Sources of calories*
  - In addition to calculating the total number of calories, it is important to ensure that patients receive these calories from appropriate sources, namely, carbohydrates, lipids, and protein.
  - Each gram of carbohydrate contains 3.4 kcal/g of energy, lipids have 9 kcal/g, and proteins comprise 4 kcal/g.
  - *Protein*: protein requirements typically start at 0.8 to 1.0 g/kg/d.
    - *Protein is regarded as the most important macronutrient, as it impacts wound healing, immune function, and lean body mass.*
      - Protein requirements can be quantitatively determined by measuring the nitrogen balance, though this method is limited in the ICU setting.
      - Measuring the nitrogen balance requires measuring the quantity of protein that the patient

is receiving per day and measuring the nitrogen loss using a 24-hour urine collection.
- *Lipid*: the lipid content in enteral formulas is usually limited to ≤30% because at higher levels, it can promote diarrhea.
- *Carbohydrate*: the remaining calories should be composed of carbohydrate.
  - This typically consists of 40% to 50% of total calories.
- Other components of nutritional support, such as vitamin deficiencies and immunonutrition, are discussed in the sections Feeding and Deficiency States.
- Determining the formulation of a feeding solution requires the utilization of the methods described in this section. More information on different modes of feeding (ie, enteral vs parenteral) and when to use them is available in the Section 16.4: Nutrition Support.
  - First, the total calories are calculated, followed by total protein requirements, both in grams/day and calories/day.
  - The protein calories are subtracted from the total calories, leaving the combined total carbohydrate and lipid calories.
  - Typically, these remaining calories are split, with 70% of the non-protein calories being carbohydrates and ≤30% as lipids.
  - It is important to consider lipid and carbohydrate sources from medications (such as propofol and citrate) and account for them in these calculations.
- Below is an example illustrating these calculations in an 80-kg patient with severe septic shock:
  - Determine total calories: 25 kcal/kg/d × 80 kg = 2,000 kcal/d
  - REE based on IC = 3,000 kcal/d
  - Calculate total protein:
    - Calories from protein (using 1.5 g for ease of calculation):
      - 80 kg × 1.5 g/kg/d = 120 g protein daily
      - 120 g protein × 4 kcal/g = 480 protein calories
  - Calculate carbohydrate and lipid calories:
    - Subtract protein from total calories:
      - 3,000 kcal −480 kcal= 2,520 kcal carbohydrates + lipids
    - Carbohydrate calories:
      - 2,520 × 0.7 = 1,764 kcal proteins
    - Lipid calories:
      - 2,520−1,764 = 736 kcal lipids
    - Calculate grams of carbohydrate and lipids:
      - Carbohydrate: 1,764 kcal/3.4 kcal/g = 518.8 g carbohydrates daily
      - Lipids: 746 kcal × 9 kcal/g = 82.8 g lipids daily
- Therefore, this patient would require a total of 120 g of protein, 518.8 g of carbohydrates, and 82.8 g of lipid each day for total nutritional support.
- These goals are accomplished using standard concentrations of carbohydrates, lipids, and proteins.

Considerations During the Initiation of Nutrition

- *Aspiration*
  - There are some important issues that may arise during the initiation of feeding.
  - One of the most common concerns with enteral nutrition is aspiration.
  - In addition to assuring proper tube placement, other steps taken to reduce that risk may include elevating the head of bed 30 to 45 degrees, distal placement of the feeding tube (beyond the ligament of Treitz), delivering continuous enteral feeding, and adding promotility agents.
  - Such agents include prokinetic substances like metoclopramide and erythromycin or narcotic antagonists like alvimopan and naltrexone.
- *Refeeding*
  - Refeeding syndrome can occur when severely malnourished patients begin to receive nutritional supplementation.
  - See Section 15.5: Refeeding Syndrome.
- *Overfeeding*
  - Overfeeding can increase CO_2 production and increase respiratory demands for patients, potentially resulting in intubation or contributing to difficulty weaning from the ventilator.
  - Overfeeding of carbohydrates or lipids for prolonged periods of time can result in fatty deposition in the liver and hepatic failure.
    - This can be monitored by checking liver function tests.
  - Significantly elevated protein delivery can result in elevated blood urea nitrogen (BUN), especially when BUN levels rise to >30% of baseline.
    - At extreme levels, this can pose challenges in balancing protein needs with the potential for dialysis.

Assessment of Nutritional Support

- After initiation of feeding, the next important consideration is to assess the adequacy of nutritional support.
- One simple approach is to weigh the patient daily or weekly.
  - While simple, this approach has limited use in the ICU, given the potential for large fluid shifts, and patients' inability to stand on scales, forcing reliance on bed weights that may not be precise.
  - Weight trends may be more useful to trend than the absolute value of the measurement on a given day.
- While there are laboratory assessments that can be considered in overall nutritional assessment, none has been validated as predictive in critically ill patients.
  - Serum albumin is a good surrogate measure of outpatient nutritional status and preoperative hypoalbuminemia is strongly associated with postoperative complications and mortality, but albumin takes 21 days to turnover in the body, and serum levels may be affected (lowered) by acute inflammation.
    - Prealbumin (transthyretin) can be considered because its turnover in the body occurs every 4 to 7 days. However, serum prealbumin levels are also lowered by acute inflammation, and some authors recommend sending C-reactive protein levels at the same time as prealbumin assessment to attempt to account for this.
    - Retinol-binding protein is another biomarker that can more quickly reflect response to nutritional therapy (half-life is ~12 hours), either alone or in conjunction

with prealbumin; however, it is likewise affected by inflammation and infection.
- Nutritional risk scores (NRSs) exist to help characterize the nutritional risk of a patient and can guide the initiation of nutrition.
  - NRS 2002 (>5 high nutritional risk)
  - NUTRIC score (>5 high nutritional risk, >6 if interleukin-6 [IL-6] available)
- In addition to laboratory values, another way to assess the adequacy of nutritional therapy is through IC measuring both REE and the respiratory quotient (RQ).
- The RQ is calculated through IC and is obtained with the following equation:
  - RQ = (CO_2 eliminated)/(O_2 produced)
- The ideal RQ is 1.
- When patients are being overfed, it is >1.
- For pure protein metabolism, the RQ = 0.8, and with fat metabolism alone, the RQ = 0.7.
- When the RQ is <0.7, the patient is undergoing starvation.
- RQ values between these ranges represent combined metabolism.
- For example, a value of 0.9 is a combination of carbohydrate and protein metabolism.

Acknowledgments

We gratefully acknowledge the contributions of previous edition authors, Jonathon Friedstat and Molly Moore, as portions of those chapters have been retained in this revision.

SUGGESTED READINGS

Casaer MP, Mesotten D, Hermans G, et al. Early versus late parenteral nutrition in critically ill adults. *N Engl J Med.* 2011;365(6):506-517.

Deane A, Chapman MJ, Fraser RJ, Horowitz M. Bench-to-bedside review: the gut as an endocrine organ in the critically ill. *Crit Care.* 2010;14(5):228.

Dickerson RN, Pitts SL, Maish GO 3rd, et al. A reappraisal of nitrogen requirements for patients with critical illness and trauma. *J Trauma Acute Care Surg.* 2012;73(3):549-557.

Gibbs J, Cull W, Henderson W, Daley J, Hur K, Khuri SF. Preoperative serum albumin level as a predictor of operative mortality and morbidity: results from the National VA Surgical Risk Study. *Arch Surg.* 1999;134(1):36-42.

Heyland DK, Dhaliwal R, Jiang X, Day AG. Identifying critically ill patients who benefit the most from nutrition therapy: the development and initial validation of a novel risk assessment tool. *Crit Care.* 2011;15(6):R268.

Khan LU, Ahmed J, Khan S, Macfie J. Refeeding syndrome: a literature review. *Gastroenterol Res Pract.* 2011;pii:410971.

Marik PE, Zaloga GP. Immunonutrition in critically ill patients: a systematic review and analysis of the literature. *Intensive Care Med.* 2008;34:1980-1990.

Marino PL. *The ICU Book.* 4th ed. Lippincott Williams & Wilkins. Chapters 47-49. 2013.

McClave SA, Taylor BE, Martindale RG, et al; Society of Critical Care Medicine; American Society for Parenteral and Enteral Nutrition. Guidelines for the provision and assessment of nutrition support therapy in the adult critically ill patient: Society of Critical Care Medicine (SCCM) and American Society for Parenteral and Enteral Nutrition (A.S.P.E.N.). *JPEN J Parenter Enteral Nutr.* 2016;40(2):159-211.

NICE-SUGAR Study Investigators; Finfer S, Chittock DR, et al. Intensive versus conventional glucose control in critically ill patients. *N Engl J Med.* 2009;360(13):1283-1297.

Norbury WB, Herndon DN. Modulation of the hypermetabolic response after burn injury. In: Herndon DN, ed. *Total Burn Care.* 3rd ed. Saunders; 2007:420-433.

Pontes-Arruda A, Aragão AMA, Albuquerque JD. Effects of enteral feeding with eicosapentaenoic acid, [gamma]-linolenic acid, and antioxidants in mechanically ventilated patients with severe sepsis and septic shock. *Crit Care Med.* 2006;34(9):2325-2333.

Saffle JR, Graves C. Nutritional support of the burned patient. In: Herndon DN, ed. *Total Burn Care.* 3rd ed. Saunders; 2007:398-419.

Schlein KM, Coulter SP. Best practices for determining resting energy expenditure in critically ill adults. *Nutr Clin Pract.* 2014;29(1):44-55.

Stucky CC, Moncure M, Hise M, Gossage CM, Northrop D. How accurate are resting energy expenditure prediction equations in obese trauma and burn patients? *JPEN J Parenter Enteral Nutr.* 2008;32(4):420-426.

Yeh DD, Johnson E, Harrison T, et al. Serum levels of albumin and prealbumin do not correlate with nutrient delivery in surgical intensive care unit patients. *Nutr Clin Prac.* 2018;33(3):419-425.

15.2

Stress Hormone Response

Jeremy Goverman and Paul B. Comish

Definition

- Definition of stress: a variety of conditions or insults whose common denominators include:
  - Distortion of the body's homeostasis
  - Threat to the body's safety and well-being
  - Increase in the demands placed on the body's metabolic machinery
- Examples: trauma, surgery, sepsis, burns, prolonged starvation, strenuous exercise, hypotension, and critical illness (eg, acute myocardial infarction, diabetic ketoacidosis)
- The body's response to stress is multisystem, including metabolic, immunologic, cardiovascular, respiratory, and neurologic.
- The increased metabolic response is aimed at providing the body with adequate energy to cope with the stress.
- The degree of hypermetabolism is roughly proportional to the severity of the stress.
- The metabolic responses are largely hormone mediated, with contributions from the immunologic and neural systems.

Metabolic Response to Stress

Carbohydrate Metabolism

- Hyperglycemia is one of the classic responses to stress.

- It results from increased hepatic glycogenolysis, increased hepatic gluconeogenesis, and decreased peripheral utilization of glucose.
- The hyperglycemic response is mediated by the counterregulatory and counter-insulin hormones: cortisol, glucagon, and catecholamines.
- Tight blood glucose monitoring increases the risk of hypoglycemia; therefore, blood glucose goals should be <180 mg/dL in critically ill patients.

Protein Metabolism

- In general, stressful conditions are characterized by increased protein breakdown, resulting in increased release of amino acids into the bloodstream, increased urinary nitrogen loss, and a negative nitrogen balance.
- However, hepatic synthesis of acute-phase proteins is increased.
- Tissues with large obligate glucose needs (eg, brain, healing tissues) drive rapid protein breakdown, resulting in dramatic muscle loss during periods of acute stress.
- Skeletal muscle is the major victim of this protein hypercatabolism.
- There is loss of visceral/carrier proteins (albumin, globulin, and various binding proteins) and proteins involved in immunologic functions (eg, immunoglobulins).
- Glucocorticoids, tumor necrosis factor, and interleukin-1 are the primary mediators of protein catabolism in stress.

Lipid Metabolism

- During stress, lipolysis (the breakdown of adipose tissue triglycerides into fatty acids and glycerol) is increased.
- This is due to the action of the counterregulatory hormones, which activate hormone-sensitive lipase.
- Fatty acids are oxidized in the liver via beta-oxidation and the citric acid cycle to yield energy.
- Fatty acids can also be converted to ketone bodies, which serve as an alternate source of fuel for the brain, sparing other proteins from being broken down.
- Glycerol from lipid breakdown is used as a substrate for gluconeogenesis.
  - Glycerol by itself is not sufficient to fulfill the glucose needs.
  - The presence of fatty stores does not protect patients against protein breakdown during stress.
- Lipids are the major source of energy after trauma.

Electrolyte and Water Metabolism

- Changes in electrolyte and water metabolism are particularly prominent when stress produces a drop in blood pressure, such as in severe hemorrhage.
- These changes include increased renal retention of water in excess of solute, leading to an increase in extracellular fluid volume and a net decrease in plasma osmolality.
- This effect is one of the adaptive responses to increase the arterial blood pressure and is mediated by the antidiuretic hormone (vasopressin).
- The sympathetic response that accompanies most stressful stimuli also stimulates the release of renin from the juxtaglomerular cells of the kidney.
  - Renin stimulates angiotensin II production.
  - Angiotensin II releases aldosterone from the zona glomerulosa of the adrenal cortex, leading to sodium and water retention via the kidneys.

Hormonal Mediators of the Metabolic Response to Stress

- The metabolic response to stress is mediated by a number of hormones, including:
  - Counterregulatory hormones (cortisol, glucagon, catecholamines)
  - Growth hormone
  - Thyroid hormones (triiodothyronine, T3, and thyroxine, T4)
  - Vasopressin

Cortisol

- Cortisol, a corticosteroid, is the major stress hormone with increased secretion during stress.
- It is secreted by the adrenal cortex.
- Secretion is stimulated by adrenocorticotropic hormone (ACTH).
- Its metabolic actions include stimulation of gluconeogenesis and proteolysis, as well as inhibition of insulin action in the peripheral tissues, leading to an increase in blood glucose level.
- Cortisol also increases the production of ketone bodies and potentiates the gluconeogenic actions of glucagon and the catecholamines.

Glucagon

- Glucagon is a peptide hormone secreted mainly by the alpha cells of the pancreatic islets.
- Secretion is stimulated by exercise, infections, other stressors, and glucocorticoids.
- Acts through multiple molecular pathways, including the cyclic adenosine monophosphate (AMP) and phospholipase C pathways, to promote gluconeogenesis, glycogenolysis, lipolysis, and ketogenesis
- Also exhibits an anti-insulin action

Catecholamines

- Epinephrine and norepinephrine are the two catecholamines involved in the stress response.
- Whereas epinephrine is secreted mainly by the adrenal medulla, the major source of plasma norepinephrine is diffusion from the sympathetic nerve endings after being released as part of the "fight-or-flight response."
- The catecholamines promote hepatic gluconeogenesis and lipolysis, in addition to inhibiting both insulin release and the peripheral actions of insulin.

Growth Hormone

- Growth hormone is produced and secreted by the anterior pituitary gland.
- Its secretion is under the control of growth hormone–releasing hormone and somatostatin, which exhibit stimulatory and inhibitory effects, respectively.
- Growth hormone secretion increases during acute stress but is reduced when the stress becomes chronic.
- Metabolic actions include ketogenesis, decreased peripheral uptake of glucose, and increased hepatic glucose output, leading to hyperglycemia.

Thyroid Hormones

- The thyroid hormones, T3 and T4, are produced by the thyroid gland, and under normal physiologic conditions, they promote carbohydrate absorption from the gut and potentiate the actions of the catecholamines.
- The concentrations of total and free T3 decrease during stressful conditions, an action that may be related to the thyroid hormone–suppressing action of cortisol, as the latter is increased by stressors.

Renin, Angiotensin II, Aldosterone, and Antidiuretic Hormone

- The sources and actions of these hormones have already been described (see section "Electrolyte and Water Metabolism").

Clinical Significance

Inadequate Stress Hormone Response

- Individuals with a deficient endogenous glucocorticoid production may be unable to mount an adequate response to various forms of stress and become susceptible to the negative effects of the stressors.
- Patients with Addison disease and those on chronic glucocorticoid therapy fall in this category.
- *Critical illness–related corticosteroid insufficiency* (CIRCI) refers to relative adrenal failure after prolonged critical illness secondary to suppression of ACTH by elevated peripheral cortisol

Excessive Stress Hormone Response

- Excessive stress response has been implicated in various diseases.
- Examples include anxiety, depression, angina pectoris, myocardial infarction, hypertension, stroke, gastric ulcer, and inflammatory bowel disease.

Modulating the Metabolic Response to Stress

- The metabolic responses to stress, if excessive or chronic, can have negative consequences for the individual.
- For the critically ill patients, modulating these responses may have a beneficial effect.
- Modulation can be in the form of nutritional support, choice of anesthetic agents, hormonal therapy, or pharmacologic therapy.
  - Aside from nutritional therapy and anesthesia that have unequivocal benefits, the other two remain controversial.
  - Beta-blockade, typically with propranolol, is a commonly used medication to treat the catabolic muscle wasting in extreme hypermetabolic states, such as a major burn.
- Early feeding in critically ill patients provides an alternative source of energy and attenuates the use of body proteins and fat for energy production.
- There is some evidence that regional anesthesia with local anesthetic agents attenuates the stress response to surgery, with beneficial postoperative outcomes.

SUGGESTED READINGS

Cheema SA, Ahmed UT, Nasir H, Dogar SR, Mustafa Z. Effects of propranolol in accelerating wound healing and attenuation of hypermetabolism in adult burn patients. *J Coll Physicians Surg Pak*. 2020;30(1):46-50.

Corwin, EJ. Homeostasis and the stress response. In: *Handbook of Pathophysiology*. 3rd ed. Lippincott Williams & Wilkins; 2008;160-171.

Cuesta JM, Singer M. The stress response and critical illness: a review. *Crit Care Med*. 2012;40:3283-3289.

Desborough JP. The stress response to trauma and surgery. *Br J Anaesth*. 2000;85:109-117.

Ganong WF. *Review of Medical Physiology*. 22nd ed. The McGraw-Hill Companies, Inc; 2005.

Straub RH, Pongratz G, Hirvonen H, Pohjolainen T, Mikkelsson M, Leirisalo-Repo M. Acute cold stress in rheumatoid arthritis inadequately activates stress responses and induces an increase of interleukin 6. *Ann Rheum Dis*. 2009;68:572-578.

Téblick A, Peeters B, Langouche L, Van den Berghe G. Adrenal function and dysfunction in critically ill patients. *Nat Rev Endocrinol*. 2019;15(7):417-427.

Welssman C. The metabolic response to stress: an overview and update. *Anesthesiology*. 1990;73:308-327.

Wray CJ, Mammen JMV, Hasselgren P. Catabolic response to stress and potential benefits of nutrition support. *Nutrition*. 2002;18:971-977.

15.3

Nutritional Deficiency States

Jeremy Goverman and Paul B. Comish

Overview

- Intensive care unit (ICU) patients with poor nutritional status are at risk for:
  - Immune dysfunction and increased infectious morbidity
  - Respiratory and peripheral muscle weakness
  - Reduced tolerance to enteral feeds
  - Poor wound healing
- ICU patients typically experience catabolic stress, which can exacerbate a suboptimal baseline nutritional status or result in rapidly worsening caloric deficit.
- Current evidence suggests that there is value to shifting away from the traditional "supportive nutrition" approach to a more "therapeutic nutrition" approach in critically ill patients.

Common Causes to Remember

- Macronutrient deficiency (protein, fat, and carbohydrates)
- Micronutrient deficiency (trace elements and vitamins)
- Electrolyte derangements
- Altered basal metabolic demand

Epidemiology

- Nutritional deficiencies may be observed in >50% of all ICU patients.

- Associated with ↑ risk of undesirable outcomes
  - Infections
  - Pressure ulcers
  - Wound healing
  - Hospital length of stay (LOS)
  - Health care costs
  - Morbidity and mortality
- Key barriers to adequate nutritional support include:
  - Delivered protein and calories may not be tailored to meet the *specific* needs of the patient.
  - Commercially available enteral nutrition (EN) formulas vary substantially in terms of calories, protein content, fiber, tonicity, and cost.
  - Whereas aspiration and absorption of EN may be influenced by the location of the feeding tube, placement of dedicated intravenous (IV) access for parenteral nutrition (PN) has its own challenges.
  - Factors such as line placement (IV vs alimentary), radiographic confirmation, and selection of the appropriate nutritional support may all influence the time to initiation of feeds.
  - Institutional culture, provider preferences, and unique patient characteristics can strongly determine how quickly prescribed goal nutritional support is achieved.
  - Placing feeds on hold for tests, procedures, and during travel away from the ICU may result in significant ↓ in feeding time.
  - Age, sex, baseline nutritional status, severity of illness, and need for mechanical ventilation (MV) all heavily influence individual patient caloric needs.
  - Significant opportunity for education of health care providers exists as nutritional status is often overshadowed by more acute critical issues.

Key Pathophysiology

- The combination of ↑ resting energy expenditure (REE) and ↓ nutritional delivery contributes to the ↑ risk of malnutrition in critically ill patients.
- Up to 60% of ICU patients may develop gastrointestinal dysfunction, which may exacerbate total caloric deficit and expedite the loss of lean body mass.
- Although EN is typically initiated within 24 to 48 hours following ICU admission in appropriate patients, meeting adequate caloric and protein requirements is often challenging.
- Emerging evidence suggests that supplementation with PN may be beneficial in patients who are:
  - Malnourished at baseline (body mass index [BMI] <25 or ≥ 35 kg/m^2)
  - In a high mortality risk group
  - Expected to require prolonged ICU care
  - Expected to require prolonged MV
- Overfeeding is associated with harm (↑ risk of infections).

Differential Diagnosis

- Reduced macro/micronutrient absorption can be seen in chronic conditions, such as diabetes, or after certain surgical procedures, such as gastric bypass.
- Albumin, a negative acute-phase reactant, may be falsely low in inflammatory conditions.

Management and Treatment

- Suboptimal caloric intake
  - Typical starting point is 25 kcal/kg/d.
  - Formulas to predict REE are not accurate in critically ill patients.
  - Indirect calorimetry remains the gold standard for objective calibration of prescribed calories.
- Suboptimal protein intake
  - Typical starting point is 1.3 to 2.0 g/kg/d.
  - Higher protein formulations are associated with better outcomes.
  - Nitrogen balance remains the gold standard for objective titration of protein content in the nutritional plan for ICU patients.
  - Glutamine (free amino acid) at doses between 0.3 and 0.5 g/kg/d is associated with ↓ risk of mortality, infection, and LOS in all ICU patients.
  - Arginine (free amino acid) at doses between 12 and 15 g/d is associated with ↓ risk of mortality, infection, and LOS in the perioperative setting; the role of arginine in patients with trauma and those who are septic remains controversial.
- Suboptimal lipid/fatty acid intake
  - Lipid infusions should not exceed 110 mg/kg/h.
  - Lipids allow for significant ↓ in exogenous glucose administration while still meeting caloric needs.
  - Commercial lipid preparations in the United States typically contain long-chain triglycerides, which provide omega-6 fatty acids (linoleic acid); however, these may promote inflammatory mediators.
  - Fish oils contain omega-3 fatty acids (linolenic acid), which may suppress inflammatory mediators; strong theoretical benefit has not been validated in limited clinical studies.
  - Hypertriglyceridemia can occur in up to one-third of ICU patients on continuous highly lipid-soluble sedatives, such as propofol; triglycerides should be monitored accordingly.
- Suboptimal micronutrient intake
  - Micronutrients are essential for optimal utilization of macronutrients.
  - Micronutrient supplementation is associated with ↓ risk of infectious complications and LOS.
  - Circulating micronutrient levels are affected by systemic inflammatory responses, and as such, exact dosing in critical illness has been difficult to establish.
  - Suggested daily IV dosing ranges during the early stage of critical illness (3-5 days) are as follows:
    - Copper: 2 to 4 mg
    - Zinc: 10 to 30 mg
    - Selenium: 100 to 500 μg
    - Ascorbic acid (vitamin C): 500 to 3,000 mg
    - Thiamine (vitamin B_1): 100 to 300 mg
  - Increased use of vitamin C in ICU patients does not reduce mortality and is not routinely recommended as it may cause calcium oxalate nephropathy.
  - Routine vitamin E supplementation is controversial, since doses >150 IU/d are associated with increased all-cause mortality in the general population.
  - Increasing number of studies demonstrate an association between low 25-hydroxyvitamin D (25(OH)D) levels

and mortality in critically ill patients; while there are no current recommendations for routine vitamin D supplementation in the ICU, maintaining 25(OH)D levels between 20 and 50 ng/mL is likely to be of benefit.
  - Iron supplementation in critical illness is very controversial, given strong theoretical evidence that it may induce oxidative stress and promote bacterial growth; a limited number of prospective studies suggest a modest benefit or no harm with enteral or IV supplementation.
- Inadequate electrolyte repletion
  - Several anabolic processes depend on adequate electrolyte stores.
  - Negative nitrogen balance is more likely in the setting of low potassium, magnesium, and/or phosphate.
  - Suggested serum target concentrations during critical illness:
    - Potassium: 4.0 to 4.5 mEq/L
    - Magnesium: 2.0 to 2.5 mg/dL
    - Phosphorus: 3.0 to 4.0 mg/dL
- Excessive metabolic demand
  - Optimize analgesia and anxiolysis.
  - Following appropriate diagnostic workup for fever, consider adding acetaminophen and/or cooling to therapeutic regimen.
  - Avoid overfeeding.
  - Initiate early goal-directed therapy.

Outcomes

- The majority of current evidence related to nutrition and critical illness is derived from observational studies.
  - Vasopressor-dependent patients given EN within the first 48 hours have a significant survival advantage versus those whose feeding is delayed.
  - Even though early EN is favored for most ICU patients, caloric and protein needs are often not met.
  - Increased intake of calories and proteins is associated with ↓ mortality rates and ↓ duration of MV in patients with body mass index (BMI) <25 and ≥35 kg/m^2.
  - Each 30 g/d increment of protein is associated with ↓ mortality rate.
  - Use of lipids as an energy source ↓ the amount of glucose infused, resulting in ↓ risk of hyperglycemia and ↓ insulin requirements; compared with a purely glucose-based PN strategy, there is ↓ negative protein balance and ↓ CO_2 production.
  - Overfeeding is associated with hyperglycemia, fatty liver, and ↑ risk of bloodstream infections.
  - Vitamin D deficiency at initiation of ICU care is associated with ↑ 30, 60, and 90-day mortality, in-hospital mortality, 1-year mortality, as well as risk of infection.
  - There is a great need for high-quality randomized clinical trials (RCTs) to better understand the impact of nutrition on critical illness.
  - Early versus late parenteral nutrition in critically ill adults (EPaNIC) trial
    - Large (n = 4,640), single-center, RCT
    - Comparing patients on EN who had early (<48 hours) versus late (≥8 days) PN supplementation after ICU admission
    - Patients in the late PN group had a significant ↓ in ICU and inpatient mortality rate.
    - Patients in the late PN also had significantly ↓ ICU infections, ↓ duration of MV, and ↓ course of renal replacement therapy.
    - Patients with chronic malnutrition were excluded from the study.
    - Patients did not receive any immunomodulating agents in their PN formulation (eg, glutamine).
    - The investigators did not control for the presence of immunomodulating agents in the EN that patients received.
    - Patients in the trial received low protein delivery (median dose of 0.8 g/kg/d after day 3).
    - Only low mortality risk and low severity of illness patient groups were included in the trial.
  - The tight calorie control study (TICACOS)
    - Small (n = 130), single-center, RCT
    - Comparing patients on EN receiving supplementation with PN targeted to a goal of 25 kcal/kg/d versus repeat indirect calorimetry assessments.
    - Patients randomized to energy targets based on repeated indirect calorimetry had ↓ 60-day mortality rate despite ↑ length of MV and ↑ ICU LOS.
    - Patients randomized to energy targets based on repeated indirect calorimetry also had ↑ caloric and protein intake.
    - Only high mortality risk and high severity of illness patients were included in the study.
  - Four level 1 and 13 level 2 RCTs in critically ill patients (n = 900) demonstrate that glutamine-supplemented PN is associated with a significant ↓ in mortality rate, infections, and LOS.
  - Meta-analysis of all glutamine-related RCTs (EN and PN) indicates a significant ↓ in mortality rate in ICU patients of all types (21 studies with >1,500 patients).

SUGGESTED READINGS

Corrado MJ, Kovacevic MP, Dube KM, Lupi KE, Szumita PM, DeGrado JR. The incidence of propofol-induced hypertriglyceridemia and identification of associated risk factors. *Crit Care Explor*. 2020;2(12):e0282.

Haugen HA, Chan LN, Li F. Indirect calorimetry: a practical guide for clinicians. *Nutr Clin Pract*. 2007;22(4):377-388.

Hegazi RA, Wischmeyer PE. Clinical review: optimizing enteral nutrition for critically ill patients—a simple data-driven formula. *Crit Care*. 2011;15(6):234.

Heming N, Montravers P, Lasocki S. Iron deficiency in critically ill patients: highlighting the role of hepcidin. *Crit Care*. 2011;15(2):210.

Jeejeebhoy KN. Parenteral nutrition in the intensive care unit. *Nutr Rev*. 2012;70(11):623-630.

Konstantinides FN. Nitrogen balance studies in clinical nutrition. *Nutr Clin Pract*. 1992;7(5):231-238.

Manzanares W, Hardy G. Thiamine supplementation in the critically ill. *Curr Opin Clin Nutr Metab Care*. 2011;14(6):610-617.

Nair P, Venkatesh B. Vitamin D in the ICU: anything new under the sun? *Crit Care Resusc*. 2012;14(4):268-273.

Visser J, Labadarios D, Blaauw R. Micronutrient supplementation for critically ill adults: a systematic review and meta-analysis. *Nutrition*. 2011;27(7-8):745-758.

Wacker DA, Burton SL, Berger JP, et al. Evaluating vitamin C in septic shock: a randomized controlled trial of vitamin C monotherapy. *Crit Care Med*. 2022;50(5):e458-e467.

15.4

Nutrition Support

Caroline H. Jensen and Jamie L. Sparling

Definitions

- Malnutrition is a major challenge in critically ill patients, impacting morbidity, mortality, and intensive care unit (ICU) length of stay.
- All ICU patients should be considered at risk of malnutrition, and initiation of early nutrition is critically important to patient outcomes.
  - Low body mass index (BMI) is an independent predictor of mortality in cases of multiorgan failure.
  - Medical ICU patients who receive <25% of caloric requirements have higher risk of nosocomial bloodstream infections.
- Methods of nutritional support
  - The first important consideration is the method by which nutrition is provided. There are two major methods: enteral or parenteral feeding.
  - Enteral nutrition formulations may vary in order to address a patient's underlying condition.
  - Examples include:
    - Lowering carbohydrate levels so as to decrease CO_2 in the setting of pulmonary disease
    - Lowering protein and electrolyte levels and total volume in renal failure
    - Lowering carbohydrate levels in diabetes
    - Lowering protein and high-level branched-chain amino acid levels to avoid encephalopathy in liver failure
    - Elemental formulations for small bowel feeding
    - Others vary the amount of protein, quantity of fiber, or osmolarity.
  - Enteral feeding can be delivered via several methods.
    - A common way is via a nasoenteric route through a weighted feeding tube.
    - Usually, this tube terminates in the stomach, but its distal end may be varied based on the underlying condition or injury.
    - Prokinetic agents can be trialed in the case of gastric feeding intolerance prior to placement of a postpyloric feeding tube. Intravenous (IV) erythromycin should be trialed as the first-line prokinetic agent, followed by IV metoclopramide or combination therapy.
    - Postpyloric enteric access can be considered in patients after gastrointestinal (GI) surgery, where some degree of gastric emptying is expected.
  - Awaiting placement of a postpyloric tube can delay initiation of enteral nutrition, and postpyloric tubes are typically not necessary unless the patient is at very high risk of aspiration or has undergone surgery on the foregut.
- *Parenteral nutrition (PN)*
  - In cases where the GI tract cannot be used, IV nutrition is indicated.
    - Peripheral PN provides a small number of total calories but can be given through a peripheral vein.
    - More commonly utilized is total parenteral nutrition (TPN), which can provide total caloric requirements.
    - TPN requires a central venous catheter since its high osmolality can result in venous sclerosis, especially of smaller peripheral veins.
- When TPN is started, it usually begins at half the total goal so as to reduce the risk of infusion complications.
- The infusion is advanced to total calorie goals over the subsequent few days.
- Daily electrolytes should be monitored, and TPN composition modified for any specific requirements.
- One of the benefits of enteral nutrition is maintaining the integrity of the gut; there are infectious risks in the setting of disuse, which are attributed to bacterial translocation.
- For critically ill patients without a contraindication, enteral nutrition should be used rather than PN. Patients receiving nutritional support from TPN should be transitioned to enteral feeding whenever possible.
- Guidelines for initiating nutrition support
  - Enteral nutrition should be initiated early after admission to the ICU. Starting enteral nutrition at the time of admission reduces ICU length of stay and ventilator time, as well as reduces infectious morbidity in ICU patients.
    - Advance to goal over the next 48 to 72 hours while monitoring for refeeding syndrome.
    - Critically ill patients are at risk for protein-calorie malnutrition, secondary to hypermetabolism.
  - In patients with contraindications to enteral nutrition (see later), initiate TPN in the following circumstances:
    - For high nutrition risk patients, PN should be started as soon as possible following ICU admission.
    - For lower nutrition risk patients, PN should be initiated after 7 days of poor or absent intake.
    - For patients who are unable to meet >60% of their energy and protein requirements by enteral nutrition, supplemental PN should be considered after 7 to 10 days.
    - Preexisting malnourishment or severe weight loss (>10% of body weight)
  - In severely malnourished patients, electrolytes may need to be corrected before initiating nutritional support to avoid refeeding syndrome.

Enteral Nutrition Versus Total Parenteral Nutrition

- Enteral feeding is preferred to parenteral whenever feasible.
- Negative effects of TPN
  - Infectious complications
    - Line sepsis
    - Bacterial translocation secondary to intestinal mucosal atrophy
  - Cholestasis
  - Immune suppression
    - Hyperglycemia inhibits neutrophil chemotaxis and phagocytosis.

- Benefits of enteral nutrition
  - Exerts a protective effect on the gut mucosa
    - Provides immunocompetent barrier to endogenous gut bacteria
  - Cost-effective
  - Improves wound healing
- If TPN is the primary source of nutrition, consider giving trophic tube feeds (TFs) (10-20 mL/h) to maintain GI mucosal integrity and immune function.

Contraindications to Enteral Feeds

Enteral nutrition should be avoided in the case of:

- Uncontrolled shock
- Uncontrolled hypoxemia and acidosis
- Uncontrolled GI bleeding
- Bowel ischemia
- Bowel obstruction
- Abdominal compartment syndrome
- High-output fistula

Determination of Requirements

- Calculate daily caloric needs—see Section 16.1: Basic Pharmacokinetics and Pharmacodynamics.
- More recently, research has emerged suggesting that there are faster recovery times, lower rates of vomiting, diarrhea, and bowel ischemia for patients receiving early, low-calorie and low-protein targets relative to standard calorie and protein targets.

Formulas

- Basic rules when selecting formulas:
  - Patients with renal failure
    - Predialysis
      - Low volume
      - High calorie
      - Low protein
      - Low electrolytes
    - On dialysis
      - Increased protein requirement
  - Patients with liver failure
    - Low protein
    - High-level branched-chain amino acids to limit encephalopathy
  - Patients with respiratory failure
    - High calorie
    - High fat, low carbohydrate to limit CO_2 accumulation
- Specific formulas
  - Jevity
    - Standard formula, isotonic
  - Osmolite
    - Isotonic, elemental
  - Vital HN
    - Isotonic, elemental, low fat
    - Useful in pancreatitis, pancreatic insufficiency, malabsorption syndromes
  - Nepro
    - Low volume
    - Low in Na and K
    - Dialysis patients
    - Increased protein
  - Promote
    - High protein
    - Patients with burn and trauma (hypercatabolic)
- Notes on terminology:
  - Elemental formulas are known to be easier on the digestive system, enhancing both digestion and absorption; they are preferred in patients with concerns for malabsorption.
  - Isotonic formulas have a physiologic osmolality and thus minimize problems with GI intolerance. Formulas with higher tonicity may lead to osmotically induced diarrhea.
  - The numeric value associated with a TF formula (eg, Osmolite 1.5) is the caloric concentration in kcal/mL.

Tube Feed Tolerance

- Residuals for gastric feeds
  - Gastric residuals should not be routinely checked.
  - However, if they are checked as a part of hospital protocols, current guidelines recommend to hold feeds for volumes >500 mL.
    - Residuals do not predict aspiration risk, and holding for residuals in the absence of other signs of intolerance can hinder nutritional goals.
- Watch for distension, diarrhea, and bloating.
  - Change to more elemental formula if this occurs, or dilute TFs.
  - Add fiber to the formula in the event of diarrhea.
    - Soluble fiber only
    - Avoid fiber in patients at high risk for bowel ischemia or severe dysmotility.
  - In the ICU setting, neither bowel sounds nor bowel movements are required to initiate feeding.
- Practice aspiration precautions.
  - Head of bed 30 to 45 degrees
  - Initiate promotility drugs (metoclopramide, erythromycin) or narcotic antagonists (naltrexone) for slow motility when feasible.
  - Chlorhexidine mouthwash twice daily to reduce the risk of ventilator-associated pneumonia (VAP)
- Hold enteral feeds in the setting of severe hemodynamic compromise until patient is stable or fully resuscitated. Enteral nutrition can be started in patients requiring low- to moderate-dose vasopressors (<0.3 μg/kg/min norepinephrine equivalents), with gradual advancement while monitoring for signs and symptoms of intolerance. Similarly, patients receiving neuromuscular blockade may safely receive enteral nutrition as neuromuscular blockers do not affect the smooth muscle of the GI tract.

Immunonutrition

- Randomized controlled trials have demonstrated reduced infectious complications in surgical and burn patients; however, benefits in all critically ill patients are less certain.
  - Studies and formulas used are too heterogeneous to make definitive recommendations.
- Glutamine
  - Protective effects on the GI mucosa
  - Data suggest decreased infections and length of stay when administered to burn patients.

- Arginine
  - In animal models, improves microcirculatory perfusion in sepsis
  - Supplementation may be associated with increased mortality in patients with severe sepsis.
  - No clear benefit in clinical trials
- Fish oil
  - Modulates membrane phospholipid composition, with a shift toward a less inflammatory pattern
  - Diets rich in fish oil have been shown to improve outcomes (mortality, secondary infections, length of stay) in medical ICU patients with systemic inflammatory response syndrome (SIRS), sepsis, and adult respiratory distress syndrome (ARDS).

Acknowledgments

We gratefully acknowledge the contributions of previous edition author, Kathryn L. Butler, as portions of those chapters have been retained in this revision.

SUGGESTED READINGS

Bongers T, Griffiths RD. Are there any real differences between enteral feed formulations used in the critically ill? *Curr Opin Crit Care*. 2006;12:131-135.

Braga M, Gionotti L, Nespoli L. Nutritional approach in malnourished surgical patients: a prospective randomized study. *Arch Surg*. 2002;137:174-180.

Braunschweig CL, Levy P, Sheean PM, Wang X. Enteral compared with parenteral nutrition: a meta-analysis. *Am J Clin Nutr*. 2001;74:534-542.

Casaer MP, Mesotten D, Hermans G, et al. Early versus late parenteral nutrition in critically ill adults. *N Engl J Med*. 2011;365(6):506-517.

Marik PE, Zaloga GP. Immunonutrition in critically ill patients: a systematic review and analysis of the literature. *Intensive Care Med*. 2008;34:1980-1990.

McClave SA, Lukan JK, Stefater JA. Poor validity of residual volumes as a marker for risk of aspiration in critically ill patients. *Crit Care Med*. 2005;33:324-330.

McClave SA, Taylor BE, Martindale RG, et al; Society of Critical Care Medicine; American Society for Parenteral and Enteral Nutrition. Guidelines for the provision and assessment of nutrition support therapy in the adult critically ill patient: Society of Critical Care Medicine (SCCM) and American Society for Parenteral and Enteral Nutrition (A.S.P.E.N.). *JPEN J Parenter Enteral Nutr*. 2016;40(2):159-211.

Mulherin DW, Cogle SV. Updates in nutrition support for critically ill adult patients. *Hosp Pharm*. 2017;52(1):17-26.

Özkan AE, Koca N, Tekeli AH. Assessment of nutritional status and clinical outcomes: a comprehensive retrospective analysis of critically ill patients. *Medicine*. 2023;102(44):e36018.

Peres IT, Hamacher S, Oliveira FLC, Thomé AMT, Bozza FA. What factors predict length of stay in the intensive care unit? Systematic review and meta-analysis. *J Crit Care*. 2020;60:183-194.

Reignier J, Mercier E, Le Gouge A, et al. Effect of not monitoring residual gastric volume on risk of ventilator-associated pneumonia in adults receiving mechanical ventilation and early enteral feeding: a randomized controlled trial. *JAMA*. 2013;309(3):249-256.

Singer P, Blaser AR, Berger MM, et al. ESPEN guideline on clinical nutrition in the intensive care unit. *Clin Nutr*. 2019;38(1):48-79.

15.5

Refeeding Syndrome

Spencer Lord

Definitions

- A potential life-threatening complication of initiating nutritional support in malnourished patients, whether orally, enterally, or parenterally that is characterized by (Table 15.5.1):
  - Occurs within 5 days of initiation of feeding
  - Electrolyte depletion
    - Characteristically hypophosphatemia
    - Hypokalemia
    - Hypomagnesemia
  - Volume overload
  - Organ dysfunction
  - Can be accompanied by thiamine deficiency

TABLE 15.5.1 Common Causes and Risk Factors to Remember

Social	Medical	Surgical
Chronic alcoholism Homelessness Incarceration	ICU patients BMI <16 kg/m^2 Anorexia nervosa Older age Diseases of high catabolic states (cancer, COPD, inflammatory diseases) Dementia Chronic malabsorption >10%-15% body weight loss Prolonged convalescence Hypophosphatemia Hypomagnesemia Hypokalemia HIV	Abdominal surgery Prolonged NPO status Head, neck, and gastrointestinal cancer Patients with trauma and burn Hepatic resection

BMI, body mass index; COPD, chronic obstructive pulmonary disease; HIV, human immunodeficiency virus; ICU, intensive care unit; NPO, nil per os.

Epidemiology

- The true incidence of refeeding syndrome varies by patient population.
- Approximately one-third of at-risk intensive care unit (ICU) patients develop significant hypophosphatemia during refeeding.
- Incidence of at-risk ICU patients can increase to two-thirds in patients receiving an initial caloric intake of > 20 kcal/kg/d.
- Patients on total parenteral nutrition have hypophosphatemia despite supplementation.
- A significant number of critically ill patients are at risk for metabolic complications during nutritional support.

Key Pathophysiology

- Normal phosphate metabolism
  - The majority of nonmineral phosphate is intracellular, where it is the primary anion.
  - It is required for a diverse range of critical cellular components, including nucleotides, phospholipids, and adenosine triphosphate (ATP).
  - Required for key processes such as enzyme regulation, energy transactions, intracellular acid-base buffering, and oxygen delivery
  - Normal serum phosphate concentrations are 2.6 to 4.9 mg/dL, with severe hypophosphatemia occurring at levels <1.0 mg/dL.
- Refeeding metabolism
  - Refeeding after a period of starvation and nutrient depletion results in a shift from catabolic to anabolic metabolism.
  - This increases phosphate utilization for ATP generation and cellular processes and results in cellular uptake of phosphate, magnesium, thiamine, and other nutrients.
  - Increased levels of insulin stimulate sodium-potassium transporter activity, leading to rapid intracellular absorption of potassium, magnesium, and phosphate, leading to hypokalemia, hypomagnesemia, and hypophosphatemia.
  - Osmotic fluid shifts and renal sodium and water reabsorption lead to fluid retention and hypervolemia.
- Refeeding syndrome
  - Refeeding syndrome is a potential complication of initiating nutritional support in malnourished patients and may occur with oral, enteral, or parenteral nutrition.
  - Aggressive initiation of nutritional support in at-risk patients results in rapid nutrient depletion due to baseline deficiency and cellular uptake, leading to potentially severely low serum levels.
  - Hypophosphatemia is the hallmark component of refeeding syndrome, which may be exacerbated by hypomagnesemia, hypokalemia, and/or thiamine depletion.
  - Organ dysfunction may be complicated by volume overload, contributing to cardiopulmonary complications.
  - Manifestation of symptom onset is within the first 72 to 96 hours of refeeding.
  - Symptom onset occurs more rapidly in those with more severe risk factors.
  - Manifestations of refeeding syndrome include:
    - Neurologic: delirium, encephalopathy, seizures
    - Pulmonary: respiratory insufficiency from diaphragm weakness, pulmonary edema
    - Cardiac: dysrhythmia, heart failure, cardiac arrest
    - Muscular: weakness, fatigue, rhabdomyolysis
    - Hematologic: hemolysis, impaired oxygen delivery from decreased 2,3-DPG

Differential Diagnosis

- Other potential causes of severe hypophosphatemia include:
  - Primary renal tubular dysfunction
  - Intestinal malabsorption
  - Hyperglycemia
  - Thiamine deficiency
  - Gram-negative bacterial sepsis
  - Cirrhosis
  - Acute pancreatitis
  - Steroid therapy
  - Insulin therapy

Management and Treatment

- Prevention
  - At-risk patients should be identified prior to initiation of nutritional support, and preexisting electrolyte abnormalities should be corrected if possible.
  - Empiric thiamine, folate, and multivitamin supplements should be considered in all at-risk patients prior to initiation of nutrition for 5 to ≥7 days.
- Feeding at-risk patients
  - For patients with risk factors for refeeding syndrome, nutritional support should be started at 5 to 10 kcal/kg/d and increased incrementally to full support over the course of 4 to 10 days.
  - If electrolytes become difficult to correct or drop rapidly, reduce caloric intake by 50% and advance by roughly one-third of goal every 1 to 2 days.
  - Phosphorus, magnesium, calcium, and potassium levels should be monitored and repleted every 12 hours for the first 3 days to maintain normal serum concentrations.
  - High-risk patients should be monitored with cardiac telemetry and followed up by a trained dietician.
  - Recovery is defined as no requirement for electrolyte supplementation for 2 days, meeting the goal caloric intake, and treatment of underlying causes.

SUGGESTED READINGS

Adika E, Jia R, Li J, Seres D, Freedberg DE. Evaluation of the ASPEN guidelines for refeeding syndrome among hospitalized patients receiving enteral nutrition: a retrospective cohort study. *J Parenter Enteral Nutr*. 2022;46(8):1859-1866.

Cioffi I, Ponzo V, Pellegrini M, et al. The incidence of the refeeding syndrome. A systematic review and meta-analyses of literature. *Clin Nutr*. 2021;40(6):3688-3701.

Da Silva J, Seres D, Sabino K, et al. ASPEN consensus recommendations for refeeding syndrome. *Nutr Clin Pract*. 2020;35(2):178-195.

Friedli N, Stanga Z, Culkin A, et al. Management and prevention of refeeding syndrome in medical inpatients: an evidence-based and consensus-supported algorithm. *Nutrition*. 2018;47:13-20.

Friedli N, Stanga Z, Sobotka L, et al. Revisiting the refeeding syndrome: results of a systematic review. *Nutrition*. 2017;35:151-160.

Fuentebella J, Kerner J. Refeeding syndrome. *Pediatr Clin North Am*. 2009;56(5):1201-1210.

Lo Gullo A, Rifici C, Caliri S, et al. Refeeding syndrome in a woman with pancreatitis: a case report. *J Int Med Res*. 2021;49(2):300060520986675.

Nunes G, Brito M, Santos C, Fonseca J. Refeeding syndrome in the gastroenterology practice: how concerned should we be? *Eur J Gastroenterol Hepatol*. 2018;30(11):1270-1276.

Olthof L, Koekkoek W, van Setten C, et al. Impact of caloric intake in critically ill patients with, and without, refeeding syndrome: a retrospective study. *Clin Nutr*. 2018;37(5):1609-1617.

Ponzo V, Pellegrini M, Cioffi I, Scaglione L, Bo S. The refeeding syndrome: a neglected but potentially serious condition for inpatients. A narrative review. *Intern Emerg Med*. 2021;16(1):49-60.

Pourhassan M, Cuvelier I, Gehrke I, et al. Prevalence of risk factors for the refeeding syndrome in older hospitalized patients. *J Nutr Health Aging*. 2018;22(3):321-327.

Runde J, Rivera-Rivera E, Pompeii-Wolfe C, Clardy C, Sentongo T. Hypophosphatemia in a malnourished child: when renal Fanconi syndrome does not stand for refeeding syndrome. *J Parenter Enteral Nutr*. 2019;43(1):166-169.

Skipper A. Refeeding syndrome or refeeding hypophosphatemia: a systematic review of cases. *Nutr Clin Pract*. 2012;27(1):34-40.

Tongyoo S, Rawangban P, Naorungroj T. Prevalence, predictive factors and outcomes of refeeding syndrome among medically critically ill patients: a retrospective cohort study. *Nutr Clin Pract*. 2025;40(1):125-133.

SECTION 16

Pharmacology and Toxicology

Section Editor: Edward A. Bittner

16.1

Basic Pharmacokinetics and Pharmacodynamics

Matthew G. Tung and Edward A. Bittner

Pharmacokinetics

- *Definition:* study of the absorption, distribution, metabolism, and excretion of drugs in the body
- Absorption
  - Drugs administered extravascularly must be absorbed across biologic membranes to reach systemic circulation.
  - Extent and rate of drug absorption are determined by physicochemical properties, formulation, and route of administration.
  - Nonintravenous administration may result in reduced absorption.
    - Enteral absorption may be reduced due to gut hypomotility, hypoperfusion, changes in gastrointestinal (GI) pH, and enteral feeding.
    - Subcutaneous/intramuscular/transdermal absorption may be reduced due to hypoperfusion of muscles, skin, and splanchnic organs.
  - Bioavailability (F)—the fraction of unchanged drug that reaches systemic circulation following administration
    - Drugs given intravenously have 100% bioavailability.
    - Drugs administered orally have reduced bioavailability primarily due to incomplete absorption and first-pass elimination.
  - First-pass elimination—drug removed from the blood or plasma via GI and hepatic enzymes following absorption from the GI tract, prior to reaching the systemic circulation
    - Significantly reduces oral bioavailability
    - Bypassed by buccal administration and partially bypassed by rectal administration
    - Examples: diltiazem, labetalol, lidocaine, metoprolol, morphine, nitroglycerin, verapamil, propranolol
- *Distribution*
  - The passage of drug molecules from the blood into tissues and organs
  - Volume of distribution (V_d) is the relationship between the total amount of drug in the body and the plasma drug concentration (C_p):

$$V_d(\text{mL}) = \frac{\text{Amount of drug in the body (mg)}}{C_p\left(\frac{\text{mg}}{\text{mL}}\right)}$$

  - V_d is affected by extravascular accumulation, protein binding, and organ function.
  - Table 16.1.1 describes the pharmacokinetic factors that influence C_p and V_d.
  - Drugs tend to have an increased C_p and decreased V_d if they have low lipid solubility, increased plasma protein binding, or decreased tissue binding.
- *Clearance*
  - Clearance—volume of serum from which a drug is completely removed per unit time
  - At steady state, the clearance of a drug is determined by its metabolism and excretion.
- *Metabolism*
  - Metabolism—chemical conversion of a drug molecule into a different form, typically via an enzymatic reaction
  - The liver is the primary site of drug metabolism.
  - ~50% of drugs undergo some form of hepatic metabolism.
  - Cytochrome P450 (CYP450) enzymes are responsible for the majority of hepatic drug metabolism.
    - Two of the most important CYP enzymes for drug metabolism are 3A4 and 2D6.
    - CYP 3A4 and CYP 2D6 metabolize ~60% and 25% of all prescribed drugs.
    - Table 16.1.2 provides an abbreviated list of common intensive care unit (ICU) drug interactions for these two enzymes.
    - Drugs that are ≥60% metabolized by the liver will require dosage adjustments in liver disease.

TABLE 16.1.1 Volume of Distribution

Pharmacokinetic Factors			Effect on V_d
Extravascular accumulation	Lipophilic drugs	• Better able to cross lipid layers, so accumulate outside vasculature, resulting in fewer drug molecules remaining in the plasma • Examples: diazepam, lorazepam, midazolam, fentanyl, ciprofloxacin, levofloxacin	Increased
	Hydrophilic drugs	• Less likely to pass through lipid layers, so remain more within the plasma • Examples: aminoglycosides, β-lactams, daptomycin, vancomycin, morphine, hydromorphone	Decreased
	"Third spacing"	• Increased extravascular fluid accumulation results in greater movement of drug molecules out of vasculature, independent of hydrophobicity. • Examples: pancreatitis, burns, hypoalbuminemia	Increased
Protein binding	Increased acute-phase reactant proteins (eg, α_1-acid glycoprotein)	• Basic drugs are highly bound to α-1-acid glycoprotein, causing decreased unbound (active) fraction of drug. • Only unbound drug can distribute out of the plasma. • Increased α-1-acid glycoprotein concentrations cause increased binding and decreased V_d of basic drugs. • Examples: amitriptyline, chlorpromazine, lidocaine, nortriptyline, propranolol, quinidine, phenobarbital	Decreased
	Hypoalbuminemia	• Acidic and neutral drugs are highly bound to albumin, causing decreased unbound (active) fraction of drug. • Decreased albumin concentrations cause decreased binding and increased V_d of acidic and neutral drugs. • Examples: phenytoin, diazepam, warfarin, midazolam, valproic acid	Increased
Organ function	Impaired hepatic and renal clearance	• Hypoperfusion of these organs reduces clearance of drugs and increases C_p.	Decreased

- There is no endogenous marker that can be used to estimate the hepatic clearance of drugs.
- The Child-Pugh score can be used to guide dosing.
  - Score of 8 to 9: decrease initial daily dose by ~25% and titrate to response.
  - Score ≥10: decrease initial daily dose by ~50% and titrate to response.
- Clinical response is the most important factor when adjusting doses.

❍ Hepatic drug clearance is determined by blood flow to the liver, free fraction of the drug in blood, the liver's intrinsic clearance, and hepatic extraction.

❍ High hepatic extraction drugs undergo ≥60% extraction during the first pass through the liver, and approximate bioavailability is ≤40%.
- In hepatic failure, high-extraction drugs display increased bioavailability and decreased hepatic clearance due to decreased hepatic blood flow.
- Examples—lidocaine, beta-blockers, morphine, midazolam, promethazine, sertraline, venlafaxine, lovastatin, fluvastatin

● *Excretion*

❍ Excretion—irreversible removal of drug molecules from the body

TABLE 16.1.2 Common ICU Drug Interactions

Enzyme	Substrate	Inhibitor	Inducer	Enzyme	Substrate	Inhibitor
3A4	Amlodipine Amiodarone Carvedilol Diltiazem Dexamethasone Fentanyl Losartan Methadone Midazolam Sildenafil Simvastatin Tacrolimus Ondansetron Verapamil Voriconazole	Amiodarone Clarithromycin Ciprofloxacin Diltiazem Erythromycin Fluconazole Ketoconazole Ritonavir Verapamil Voriconazole	Carbamazepine Phenytoin Phenobarbital Rifampin St John wort	*2D6*	Carvedilol Codeine Flecainide Fluoxetine Haloperidol Hydrocodone Lidocaine Metoclopramide Metoprolol Ondansetron Oxycodone Propranolol Tramadol Trazodone Venlafaxine	Amiodarone Bupropion Cannabidiol Cinacalcet Fluoxetine Haloperidol Metoclopramide Paroxetine Quinidine Ritonavir Sertraline

ICU, intensive care unit.

- The kidneys are responsible for the excretion of most drugs.
- Excretion can also occur via the biliary system and, to a lesser degree, via bowel, saliva, sweat, lungs, and breast milk.

- *Medication dosing*
  - *Loading dose*
    - The loading dose of a medication depends on its volume of distribution, bioavailability, and the plasma concentration for the desired effect (see section "Pharmacodynamics"):

$$\text{Loading dose (mg)} = \frac{\text{Desired } C_p\left(\frac{\text{mg}}{\text{mL}}\right) * V_d(\text{mL})}{\text{F (dimensionless)}}$$

  - *Maintenance dose*
    - The maintenance dose of a medication depends on its clearance, bioavailability, and the plasma concentration for the desired effect:

$$\text{Maintenance dose (mg/min)} = \frac{\textit{Desired } C_p\left(\frac{\text{mg}}{\text{mL}}\right) * \text{Cl (mL/min)}}{F \text{ (dimensionless)}}$$

    - Medications can be maintained by continuous infusion or intermittent doses.

Pharmacodynamics

- *Definition:* relationship between drug concentration at its site of action and an observable effect
- Terminology
  - Emax—the largest effect that a drug can produce
  - EC50—the concentration of the drug (at steady state) that produces half of Emax
  - Potency—the inverse of EC50 (more potent drugs achieve an effect at lower concentrations)
  - Direct effects—those that result from the drug interacting with its target (eg, fentanyl and analgesia) and often occur soon after drug administration
  - Indirect effects—those that result further "downstream" from a drug-target interaction (eg, warfarin and prothrombin time) and often have a delayed response
  - Reversible effects—those that terminate after drug dissociates from its binding target
  - Irreversible effects—those that persist until the binding target is replaced in the body
- Most drugs used in the ICU are examples of drugs that produce a direct and reversible response (eg, sedatives, opioids, vasopressors).
- Antimicrobials, antiplatelets, and antineoplastics are examples of drugs that produce an irreversible response.
  - Antimicrobials are classified as concentration or time dependent (see Table 16.1.3 for select antibiotics):
    - *Concentration dependent*: bactericidal effect correlates with the ratio of peak serum concentrations to the pathogen's minimum inhibitory concentration (MIC).
    - *Time dependent*: bactericidal effect correlates with the time that serum concentration is greater than the pathogen's MIC.

TABLE 16.1.3 Efficacy of Select Antibiotics Based on Pharmacodynamic Properties

Bactericidal Parameter	Concentration Dependent	Time Dependent
	Amikacin	Ampicillin
	Ciprofloxacin[a]	Aztreonam
	Daptomycin	Cefazolin
	Gentamicin	Cefepime
	Levofloxacin[a]	Cefotaxime
	Metronidazole	Ceftriaxone
	Tobramycin	Clindamycin
		Imipenem
		Linezolid
		Meropenem
		Nafcillin
		Oxacillin
		Piperacillin
		Vancomycin[a]

[a]Dependent on both concentration and time.

SUGGESTED READINGS

Bauer LA. *Applied Clinical Pharmacokinetics*. 3rd ed. McGraw Hill Medical; 2014.

Bauer LA. Clinical pharmacokinetics and pharmacodynamics. In: Dipiro JT, Talbert RL, Yee GC, et al, eds. *Pharmacotherapy: A Pathophysiologic Approach*. 7th ed. Appleton and Lange; 2008:42-63.

Devlin JW, Barletta JF. Principles of drug dosing in critically ill patients. In: Parillo JE, Dellinger JE, eds. *Critical Care Medicine: Principles of Diagnosis and Management in the Adult*. 3rd ed. Elsevier; 2008:1343-1376.

Lodise TP, Drusano GL. Pharmacokinetics and pharmacodynamics: optimal antimicrobial therapy in the intensive care unit. *Crit Care Clin*. 2011; 27:1-18.

Morales Castro D, Dresser L, Granton J, Fan E. Pharmacokinetic alterations associated with critical illness. *Clin Pharmacokinet*. 2023;62(2): 209-220.

Phe K, Heil EL, Tam VH. Optimizing pharmacokinetics-pharmacodynamics of antimicrobial management in patients with sepsis: a review. *J Infect Dis*. 2020;222(suppl 2):S132-S141.

Porter RS, Kaplan JL, eds. Overview of pharmacokinetics and pharmacodynamics. In: *The Merck Manual of Diagnosis and Therapy*. 19th ed. Merck and Co; 2011:chap 318-319:3354-3364.

Roger C. Understanding antimicrobial pharmacokinetics in critically ill patients to optimize antimicrobial therapy: a narrative review. *J Intensive Med*. 2024;4(3):287-298.

Weersink RA, Burger DM, Hayward KL, Taxis K, Drenth JPH, Borgsteede SD. Safe use of medication in patients with cirrhosis: pharmacokinetic and pharmacodynamic considerations. *Expert Opin Drug Metab Toxicol*. 2020;16(1):45-57.

Zhou SF, Liu JP, Lai XS. Substrate specificity, inhibitors and regulation of human cytochrome P450 2D6 and implications in drug development. *Curr Med Chem*. 2009;16(21):2661-2805.

16.2

Drug-Drug Interactions

Gianna Lauren Casal and Jacqueline Lange

Overview

- Drug-drug interactions may cause unnecessary harm and could be preventable.
- Drug-drug interactions require many risk/benefit analyses if drug interactions are unavoidable.
- Infinite interactions exist by innumerable mechanisms, but this chapter focuses on discussing the most common drug-drug interactions.

Drug-Food Interactions

- Medication absorption may be increased or decreased when taken with nutrition.
- Cations, chelators, and proteins in nutrition and supplements can lead to reduced drug concentrations (levothyroxine, mycophenolate, phenytoin, antibiotics).
- Alternatively, meals high in fat can increase absorption of lipophilic medications.
- Some medications may be advised to take with food to combat potential adverse effects as opposed to a pharmacokinetic interaction.
- Warfarin effects can be influenced by vitamin K–rich "greens" such as broccoli, lettuce, spinach, kale, and Brussels sprouts, leading to increased warfarin requirements. Patients on warfarin can eat these foods as long as they eat them in consistent amounts.
- Grapefruit juice yields strong cytochrome (CYP)3A4 inhibition.

Gastric Acid–Reducing Drug Interactions

- Antacids, proton pump inhibitors (PPIs) and histamine$_2$ receptor antagonists (H2RAs) increase gastric pH, which can significantly alter absorption of many other medications, such as antiretroviral therapy, mycophenolate, azole antifungals, phenytoin, and tyrosine kinase inhibitors.
- Acid-reducing agents can also cause drug-drug interactions via altering absorption by chelation, dosage form dissolution, CYP450 and transporter modulation, and urine alkalization.

Hematology

- Utilization of CYP450/P-gp (P-glycoprotein) inducers of oral anticoagulants (rifampin, carbamazepine, phenytoin) can lead to insufficient anticoagulation with certain oral anticoagulants.
- Utilization of CYP450 inhibitors that interfere with the metabolism of warfarin (amiodarone, ciprofloxacin, sulfamethoxazole/trimethoprim, voriconazole) can lead to supratherapeutic concentrations of anticoagulation.
- Consider alternatives, such as enoxaparin, if the medications interacting with oral anticoagulants cannot be changed or discontinued.

Infectious Disease

- Carbapenems will immediately reduce concentrations of valproic acid and have been used for valproic acid toxicity. While the interaction with valproic acid occurs rapidly, the effect may persist for up to 14 days after discontinuation of carbapenem therapy. This interaction is clinically significant for patients on valproic acid for seizures, but patients on valproic acid for mood disorder can be managed with alternative therapies.
- Ciprofloxacin inhibits the metabolism of tizanidine and has led to increased hypotension and sedation when used in combination.

Synergistic QTc Prolongation (Table 16.2.1)

- QTc prolongation increases the risk of the lethal arrhythmia torsades de pointes (TdP).
- Many medications can cause QTc prolongation, and the risk is increased when combining multiple (≥2) QTc-prolonging medications.

TABLE 16.2.1 QTc-Prolonging Medications

Neurology	Cardiology	GI	Infectious Disease	Hematology/Immunology
Antipsychotics Methadone Hydroxyzine Propofol SSRIs SNRIs TCAs	Antiarrhythmics Cilostazol	5-HT3 antagonists Metoclopramide	Azole antifungals[a] Macrolides Fluoroquinolones Pentamidine	Arsenic trioxide Hydroxychloroquine

GI, gastrointestinal; SNRIs, serotonin-norepinephrine reuptake inhibitors; SSRIs, selective serotonin reuptake inhibitors; TCAs, tricyclic antidepressants.
[a]Except isavuconazole.
From Thompson JL, Crossman RR. Drug-induced QT prolongation. Uspharmacist.com. February 20, 2007. Accessed June 25, 2024. https://www.uspharmacist.com/article/drug-induced-qt-prolongation

TABLE 16.2.2 CYP450 and P-gp Inhibitors

System	1A2	2C9	2C19	2D6	3A4	P-gp
Neuro	Fluvoxamine		Cenobamate Felbamate Fluvoxamine	Bupropion Citalopram Clobazam Duloxetine Escitalopram Fluoxetine Paroxetine Sertraline	Nefazodone	
Cardio	Mexiletine	Amiodarone		Amiodarone	Amiodarone Diltiazem Dronedarone Verapamil	Amiodarone Dronedarone Propafenone Quinidine Ranolazine Verapamil
GI	Cimetidine		Omeprazole	Cimetidine	Cimetidine Erythromycin Grapefruit juice	
ID	Ciprofloxacin Efavirenz Rifampin	Efavirenz Fluconazole Isoniazid Metronidazole Rifampin Sulfamethoxazole/ trimethoprim Voriconazole	Fluconazole Isoniazid Rifampin Voriconazole	Cobicistat Ritonavir	Ciprofloxacin Clarithromycin Cobicistat Fluconazole Isavuconazole Itraconazole Posaconazole Ritonavir Voriconazole	Azithromycin Cobicistat Erythromycin Isavuconazole Itraconazole Ketoconazole Posaconazole

P-gp, P-glycoprotein.
From Clinical Pharmacology, School of Medicine. Drug interactions. Accessed June 25, 2024. https://drug-interactions.medicine.iu.edu/

- Routine electrocardiogram (ECG) monitoring should be completed for patients on QTc-prolonging medications. Prolonged QTc is defined as >460 ms in males and >470 ms in females; however, the majority of documented TdP cases occur with preceding QTc >500 ms.

Cytochrome P450 and P-Glycoprotein

CYP450 are enzymes used for drug metabolism in phase I oxidation, and P-gps are responsible for the efflux of medications from inside cells.

- Drugs can be substrates, inhibitors, and/or inducers of CYP450 enzymes or P-gls.
- Combination of substrate + inhibitor → increased concentrations of substrate and potential adverse effects.
- Combination of substrate + inducer → reduced concentrations of substrate and potential subtherapeutic effects.

Onset of CYP 450 and P-gp Interactions (Tables 16.2.2-16.2.4)

- The onset of interactions can be dependent on half-life, but generally, inhibition occurs more rapidly than induction.
- Maximum induction can take up to 2 weeks, whereas inhibition can be maximal within 2 days.

TABLE 16.2.3 Inducers

System	1A2	2C9	2C19	3A4	P-gp
Neuro	Carbamazepine	Carbamazepine Phenobarbital		Carbamazepine Modafinil Phenobarbital Phenytoin St John wart	Carbamazepine Fosphenytoin Phenytoin St John wart
Infectious Disease	Rifampin	Rifampin	Rifampin	Rifampin	Rifampin
Hematology/Immunology		Enzalutamide	Enzalutamide	Enzalutamide	Cyclosporine

P-gp, P-glycoprotein.
From Clinical Pharmacology, School of Medicine. Drug interactions. Accessed June 25, 2024. https://drug-interactions.medicine.iu.edu/

TABLE 16.2.4 Substrates

System	1A2	2C9	2C19	3A4	P-gp
Neuro	Cyclobenzaprine Clozapine Duloxetine Haloperidol Imipramine Naproxen Olanzapine Tizanidine	Amitriptyline Fluoxetine Meloxicam Phenytoin Valproic acid Venlafaxine	Amitriptyline Brivaracetam Clobazam Diazepam Escitalopram Phenytoin Valproic acid Venlafaxine	Aripiprazole Carbamazepine Citalopram Escitalopram Fentanyl Haloperidol Methadone Quetiapine Risperidone Suvorexant	
Cardio	Propranolol Theophylline Triamterene Verapamil	Clopidogrel Losartan Torsemide	Clopidogrel Labetalol Propranolol	Amiodarone Amlodipine Atorvastatin Cilostazol Diltiazem Dronedarone Ticagrelor	Digoxin Diltiazem Quinidine
GI	Ondansetron		Esomeprazole Omeprazole Pantoprazole	Aprepitant Omeprazole Ondansetron	Loperamide
ID		Voriconazole	Voriconazole	Clarithromycin Dapsone Isavuconazole Voriconazole	
Hematology/ Immunology	Warfarin	Capecitabine Warfarin		Apixaban Colchicine Dexamethasone Sirolimus Rivaroxaban	Colchicine Dabigatran Edoxaban Vinblastine
	Tyrosine kinase inhibitors are often CYP450 substrates; see package insert for interactions.				

GI, gastrointestinal; P-gp, P-glycoprotein.

From Drug interactions. Clinical Pharmacology, School of Medicine. Accessed June 25, 2024. https://drug-interactions.medicine.iu.edu/

SUGGESTED READINGS

Al-Quteimat O, Laila A. Valproate interaction with carbapenems: review and recommendations. *Hosp Pharm*. 2020;55(3):181-187.

Bushra R, Aslam N, Khan AY. Food-drug interactions. *Oman Med J*. 2011; 26(2):77-83.

Choi JH, Ko CM. Food and drug interactions. *J Lifestyle Med*. 2017;7(1):1-9.

Deodhar M, Al Rihani SB, Arwood MJ, et al. Mechanisms of CYP450 inhibition: understanding drug-drug interactions due to mechanism-based inhibition in clinical practice. *Pharmaceutics*. 2020;12(9):846.

Fernandes FM, Silva EP, Martins RR, Oliveira AG. QTc interval prolongation in critically ill patients: prevalence, risk factors and associated medications. *PLoS One*. 2018;13(6):e0199028.

Granfors MT, Backman JT, Neuvonen M, Neuvonen PJ. Ciprofloxacin greatly increases concentrations and hypotensive effect of tizanidine by inhibiting its cytochrome P450 1A2-mediated presystemic metabolism. *Clin Pharmacol Ther*. 2004;76(6):598-606.

Koziolek M, Alcaro S, Augustijns P, et al. The mechanisms of pharmacokinetic food-drug interactions—a perspective from the UNGAP group. *Eur J Pharm Sci*. 2019;134:31-59.

McDonnell AM, Dang CH. Basic review of the cytochrome p450 system. *J Adv Pract Oncol*. 2013;4(4):263-268.

Patel D, Bertz R, Ren S, Boulton DW, Någård M. A systematic review of gastric acid-reducing agent-mediated drug-drug interactions with orally administered medications. *Clin Pharmacokinet*. 2020;59(4):447-462.

Zeltser D, Justo D, Halkin A, Prokhorov V, Heller K, Viskin S. Torsade de Pointes due to noncardiac drugs: most patients have easily identifiable risk factors. *Medicine (Baltimore)*. 2003;82(4):282-290.

16.3

Toxicology, Drug Overdose, and Poisoning

Matthew Mueller and Christopher Tainter

Topics Covered in Other Chapters

- Malignant Hyperthermia (12.2)
- Neuroleptic Malignant Syndrome (NMS) (12.3)
- Serotonin Syndrome (12.4)
- Heat Stroke (12.5)
- Hypothermia (12.6)
- Basic Pharmacokinetics and Pharmacodynamics (16.1)
- Drug-Drug Interactions (16.2)
- Adverse Effects of Drugs (16.3)
- Burns and Thermal Injury (23.1)
- Nuclear, Radiologic, Chemical, and Biologic Exposures (24.2)
- Drowning (24.3)
- Altitude Injury (24.5)

General Approach to Poisoning and Overdose

- Definitions
  - Poison: any substance that can harm the body
  - Toxicity: the ability of a substance to cause harm to the body
  - The approach to the poisoned patient should be methodical and thorough. A comprehensive history and physical examination will help identify the toxin, possible co-ingestions, timing of ingestion, severity of illness, and whether the poisoning was intentional.
  - The clinician should ensure a safe environment for the patient and staff, which may require patient and/or environmental decontamination, chemical or physical restraints, and prompt intervention.
  - Co-ingestions are very common. Clinicians should have a high index of suspicion to evaluate for and treat co-ingestions.
- Physical examination
  - Characteristic odors (Table 16.3.3)
  - Mental status (e.g., central nervous system [CNS] depression, agitation)
  - Pupils (e.g., myosis, mydriasis, nystagmus)
  - Neuromuscular (e.g., seizures, myoclonus, weakness, paralysis)
  - Temperature (e.g., hypothermia, hyperthermia)
  - Heart rate (e.g., tachycardia, bradycardia)
  - Blood pressure (e.g., hypertension, hypotension)
  - Respiratory rate (e.g., tachypnea, bradypnea, hyperpnea, hypopnea)
  - Skin (e.g., dry, diaphoretic, cyanotic)
- Evaluation of the poisoned patient
  - Electrocardiogram (ECG) to screen for arrhythmias and interval prolongation
  - Point-of-care (POC) glucose
  - Acetaminophen, salicylate, and ethanol levels (to evaluate for co-ingestions)
  - Qualitative pregnancy test (in appropriate patients)
  - Urine drug screen (UDS) is unlikely helpful in most patients, given the cross-reactivity with many common medications, the half-life of some drugs of abuse, and the limited drug panel (i.e., fentanyl is not routinely tested).
- Consultation
  - Consultation with a toxicologist or an expert in toxicology can help identify the etiology of poisoning and guide management.
  - Mental health evaluation following intentional poisonings
- Poison control centers
  - Poison control centers offer advice and resources to the public and medical professionals. Management of toxic ingestions should be guided by a poison control center or a topic expert (e.g., clinical toxicologist), when available.
  - The United States
    - 55 regional poison control centers
    - Phone: 1-800-222-1222
    - Web: www.poisonhelp.org
  - International
    - World directory of poison centers can be found on the World Health Organization's website.
    - www.who.int/data/gho/data/themes/topics/indicator-groups/poison-control-and-unintentional-poisoning
- Decontamination and elimination
  - Induced emesis
    - The American Association of Poison Control Centers discourages induced emesis due to low efficacy and increased risk for aspiration.
  - Gastric lavage
    - Placement of an orogastric or nasogastric tube and administration of aliquots and subsequent aspiration of small volumes of fluid
    - Not routinely recommended
  - Activated charcoal (AC), multidose-activated charcoal (MDAC)
    - Mechanism
      - Adsorbs toxic substances to reduce/inhibit absorption
      - MDAC reduces enterohepatic and enteroenteric circulation of some toxins.
    - Indications
      - Should only be considered if the timing of ingestion is recent (i.e., toxin within stomach) and toxin is readily adsorbed by AC
      - MDAC mnemonic
        - **T**hese **P**eople **D**rink **C**harcoal **Q**uickly
          - **T**heophylline
          - **P**henobarbital
          - **D**apsone
          - **C**arbamazepine
          - **Q**uinine
    - Contraindications
      - Timing from ingestion is >1 to 2 hours as toxin is likely no longer within the stomach.

- Toxins that are poorly adsorbed by AC.
  - Heavy metals, inorganic ions, corrosives, alcohols
- Depressed mental state (i.e., unable to protect airway)
- Need for endoscopy
- Intestinal obstruction
- Dose
  - Single
    - 10:1 charcoal-to-toxin ratio
    - Children ≤12 years
      - 0.5 to 1.0 g/kg (max dose 50 g)
    - Adolescents and adults ≥13 years
      - If toxin dose is unknown, 25 to 100 g
  - MDAC: 50 to 100 g, then 25 to 50 g every 4 hours
- Whole-bowel irrigation (WBI)
  - Mechanism
    - Administration of polyethylene glycol electrolyte solution to induce stool output. Continue WBI until rectal effluent is clear.
  - Indication
    - Ingestion of toxic dose of enteric-coated and extended-release medications, or ingestion of drug packets
  - Contraindication
    - Ileus, bowel obstruction, bowel perforation, gastrointestinal (GI) hemorrhage
  - Dose
    - Children aged 9 months to 6 years: 500 mL/h
    - Children aged 6 to 12 years: 1,000 mL/h
    - Adolescents and adults ≥13 years: 1,500 to 2,000 mL/h
- Urinary alkalization
  - Mechanism
    - Increasing urinary pH enhances conversion of weak organic acids (HA) into lipid-insoluble charged ions (H^+ or A^-) within the renal tubular lumen that cannot easily be reabsorbed. This results in increased toxin excretion in the urine.
    - $HA \leftrightarrow H^+ + A^-$
  - Indications
    - Clearance of toxins that are weak organic acids (e.g., aspirin, methotrexate, phenobarbital, sulfonamides)
  - Contraindications
    - Toxins not renally cleared
    - Toxins that are not weak acids
  - Dose
    - 150 mEq $NaHCO_3$ in 1 L D_5W, administer at 1.5 to 2 × maintenance rate
- Hemodialysis (HD)
  - Mechanism
    - Directly removes toxins from the plasma
  - Indications
    - Toxin should have low molecular weight (<500 Da), low plasma protein binding, small volume of distribution (<1 L/kg), and poor endogenous clearance (<4 mL/min/kg).
    - Dialyzable toxins mnemonic
      - **I STUMBLED**
        - **I**soniazid, **I**sopropyl alcohol
        - **S**alicylates
        - **T**ylenol, **T**heophylline
        - **U**remia
        - **M**ethanol
        - **B**arbiturates
        - **L**ithium
        - **E**thylene glycol
        - **D**epakote
    - Severe acidosis, even if the toxin is not readily dialyzable
  - Contraindications
    - Does not meet criteria listed earlier
- Continuous renal replacement therapy (CRRT)
  - Mechanism
    - Directly removes toxins from the plasma, similar to HD, albeit at a slower rate
  - Indications
    - CRRT may be an acceptable alternative to HD in patients who are unable to tolerate high-flow rates (i.e., hemodynamically unstable).
    - Indications for CRRT are the same as for HD. However, larger toxins, up to 50,000 Da (depending on pore size), may be removed with CVVH (as opposed to CVVHD).
  - Contraindications
    - Same as for HD

- Anion gap (AG)
  - Defined as the concentration of measured cations minus the concentration of measured anions
  - The most abundantly measured serum cations are sodium (Na^+) and potassium (K^+), while the most abundantly measured serum anions are chloride (Cl^-) and bicarbonate (HCO_3^-). Other cations and anions (i.e., not Na^+, K^+, Cl^-, or HCO_3^-) are considered unmeasured.
  - Calculations

$$AG = Na^+ - (Cl^- + HCO_3^-)$$

$$AG = (Na^+ + K^+) - (Cl^- + HCO_3^-)$$

  - Under physiologic circumstances, an AG exists and is defined as 4 to 12 when potassium is not included in the equation, or 8 to 16 when potassium is included. Normal AG may differ depending on the analyzer used.
  - Albumin is the primary unmeasured anion contributing to the AG.
  - High AG
    - Defined as an AG >12 or >16, depending on if potassium is included in the AG calculation
    - The AG will increase if the concentration of unmeasured anions increases and/or the unmeasured cations decrease.
    - Elevated in the presence of an unmeasured anion (e.g., ketoacids, sulfates from uremia, salicylates)
  - Low AG
    - Defined as an AG <3 mEq/L
    - The AG will decrease if the concentration of unmeasured anions decreases and/or the unmeasured cations increase.
    - May be seen in lithium toxicity, bromide toxicity, monoclonal immunoglobulin G (IgG) gammopathy, and hypoalbuminemia, among other causes
- Osmolar gap
  - Osmolality (Osm) is defined as the number of moles (mol) of dissolved particles per kilogram (mol/kg) of

solvent (e.g., water), whereas osmolarity is defined as the number of dissolved particles per liter (mol/L) of solution.
- In clinical applications, osmolality and osmolarity tend to be interchangeable. However, direct measurements refer to osmolality, while calculated measurements refer to osmolality.
- Solutes that contribute most to serum osmolality are sodium, chloride, bicarbonate, glucose, and urea, measured as blood urea nitrogen (BUN). Alcohol (ETOH) should be accounted for, if present.
- Calculations
  - Osmolar gap = measured osmolality − calculated osmolality

    Serum osmolality =

    $$(2 \times [Na]) + \left(\frac{[Glucose]}{18}\right) + \left(\frac{[BUN]}{2.8}\right) + \left(\frac{[ETOH]}{2.8}\right)$$

    - where Na is measured in mmol/L, glucose measured in mg/dL, BUN measured in mg/dL, and ETOH measured in mg/dL.

    Serum osmolality =

    $$(2 \times [Na]) + [Glucose] + [BUN] + [ETOH]$$

    - where Na, glucose, and BUN are measured as mmol/L.
- Elevated osmolar gap
  - Normal serum osmolality is 285 mmol/kg (275-295 mmol/kg).
  - An osmolar gap exists if the calculated osmolality is greater than the measured osmolarity by >10 mmol/kg.
  - An Elevated osmolar gap suggests the presence of an unmeasured, osmotically active substance (e.g., ethanol, methanol, ethylene glycol).
  - An elevated osmolar gap can help detect uncharged substances (e.g., methanol prior to its conversion to formic acid) in serum.

- Toxicologic clinical syndromes (Table 16.3.1)
- Antidotes (Table 16.3.2)
- Characteristic odors (Table 16.3.3)
- ECG findings (Table 16.3.3)

TABLE 16.3.1 Toxidromes

Toxidrome	Agents	Clinical Presentation	Treatment
Anticholinergic	Diphenhydramine Atropine	Altered mental status Mydriasis Flushed skin Anhidrosis Dry mucus membranes Urinary retention Constipation	Physostigmine
Cholinergic	Organophosphates Carbamates Nerve agents	**Muscarinic symptoms** SLUDGE Salivation Lacrimation Urination Diaphoresis, diarrhea Gastrointestinal distress Emesis DUMBBELLSS Diarrhea Urination Miosis Bradycardia Bronchospasm Emesis Lacrimation Lethargy Salivation Seizures **Nicotinic symptoms** Muscle weakness Fasciculations Paralysis	Atropine, 2-PAM
Sympathomimetic	Amphetamine Cocaine Ephedrine	Tachycardia Tachypnea Hypertension Mydriasis Diaphoresis Hyperthermia	Benzodiazepines Sodium bicarbonate
Opioid	Morphine Heroin Fentanyl	Miosis Respiratory depression CNS depression	Naloxone

(*continued*)

TABLE 16.3.1 Toxidromes (*continued*)

Toxidrome	Agents	Clinical Presentation	Treatment
Sedative hypnotic	Barbiturates Benzodiazepines Nonbenzodiazepine Benzodiazepine receptor agonist	Hypotension Bradycardia Respiratory depression	Supportive care Flumazenil (benzodiazepine toxicity)
Serotonin syndrome	SSRI SNRI MAOI TCA Dextromethorphan Meperidine	Agitation, delirium Tachycardia Hypertension Tachypnea Mydriasis Diaphoresis Diarrhea Hyperreflexia, clonus, ocular clonus	Cyproheptadine

CNS, central nervous system; MAOI, monoamine oxidase inhibitor; SNRI, serotonin-norepinephrine reuptake inhibitor; SSRI, selective serotonin reuptake inhibitor; TCA, tricyclic antidepressant.

TABLE 16.3.2 Antidotes

Toxin	Antidote
Acetaminophen	*N*-Acetylcysteine
Amphetamines	Benzodiazepines
Anticholinergics	Physostigmine
Arsenic, mercury, gold	Dimercaprol/BAL
Beta antagonist	Calcium, glucagon, high-dose insulin, lipid emulsion, pacing
Bath salts	Benzodiazepines
Benzodiazepines	Flumazenil
Calcium channel antagonist	Calcium, glucagon, high-dose insulin, lipid emulsion, pacing
Carbon monoxide	100% oxygen, hyperbaric oxygen
Cholinergics	Atropine
Cocaine	Benzodiazepines
Copper	Penicillamine
Coumadin	Vitamin K, FFP, PCC
Cyanide	Sodium nitrite and sodium thiosulfate, hydroxocobalamin
Cyclic antidepressants (TCAs)	Blood alkalinization
Dabigatran	Idarucizumab
Digoxin	Digoxin immune Fab
Ethylene glycol	Ethanol, fomepizole
Factor Xa inhibitors (e.g., rivaroxaban, apixaban)	Andexanet alfa, PCC
Heparin	Protamine
Hydrogen fluoride	Calcium gluconate/calcium chloride
Iron	Deferoxamine
Isoniazid	Pyridoxine
Lithium	Hemodialysis
Lead	Succimer/DMSA, dimercaprol/BAL, EDTA
Local anesthetics	Lipid emulsion
Metformin	Hemodialysis
Methanol	Ethanol, fomepizole
Methemoglobin	Methylene blue
Nitrates/nitrites	Methylene blue
Opioids	Naloxone
Oral hypoglycemic agents, insulin	Dextrose, octreotide
Organophosphates, carbamates	Atropine, pralidoxime
Salicylates	Urinary alkalinization, hemodialysis
Synthetic cannabinoids	Benzodiazepines
Theophylline	MDAC, hemodialysis

BAL, British anti-Lewisite; FFP, fresh frozen plasma; MDAC, multidose-activated charcoal; PCC, prothrombin complex concentrate; TCAs, tricyclic antidepressants.

TABLE 16.3.3 Characteristic Odors

Odor	Agent(s)
Acetone/fruity	Ethanol, isopropyl alcohol, salicylates
Bitter almonds	Cyanide
Garlic	Arsenic, organophosphates, phosphorous
Mothballs	Naphthalene, camphor
Freshly mown hay	Phosgene
Rotten eggs	Hydrogen sulfide, sulfur dioxide
Wintergreen	Methyl salicylate

TABLE 16.3.4 ECG Findings in Poisoning

ECG Findings	Drug Classes
Tachycardia/tachyarrhythmia	Sympathomimetics Anticholinergics
Bradycardia/bradyarrhythmia	Alpha$_2$-adrenergic antagonists Beta-adrenergic antagonists Calcium channel antagonists Cardiac glycosides Antiarrhythmics not listed above
Ischemic changes	Sympathomimetics
QTc prolongation	Antidepressants Antiarrhythmics Antipsychotics Hydrofluoric acid
QRS prolongation	Tricyclic antidepressant Quinidine Cocaine Antihistamines Other Na^+ channel antagonists
Agent	**ECG Findings**
Digoxin	Digoxin effect seen in therapeutic use and toxicity Scooped ST depression with slurred appearance Flattened, inverted, or biphasic T waves Shortened QT interval
Tricyclic antidepressant	Rightward axis of QRS Terminal R wave in aVR QRS prolongation

ECG, electrocardiogram.

Over-the-Counter Medications

- Acetaminophen (*N*-acetyl-*p*-aminophenol [APAP], paracetamol)
  - Therapeutic dose
    - Children
      - 10 to 15 mg/kg/dose, every 4 to 6 hours
      - Maximum daily dose: 80 mg/kg
    - Adults
      - 325 to 1,000 mg/dose, every 4 to 6 hours
      - Maximum daily dose: 4 g
  - Acute ingestion of toxic dose within an 8-hour period
    - Children: >150 mg/kg
    - Adults: >7.5 g
  - Mechanism and toxicity
    - Acetaminophen is primarily metabolized in the liver and, to a lesser extent, via the kidney and intestine.
    - At therapeutic doses
      - Acetaminophen is conjugated with glucuronide or sulfate to pharmacologically inactive metabolites, APAP-glucuronide and APAP-sulfate, respectively, by hepatic cytochrome P450 (CYP2E1, CYP1A2, CYP3A4) (Figure 16.3.1).
      - ~5% is oxidized to *N*-acetyl-*p*-benzoquinone imine (NAPQI), a toxic metabolite.
      - Glutathione (GSH) binds NAPQI to form nontoxic metabolites that are ultimately excreted in the urine.
    - At toxic doses
      - Glucuronide and sulfate conjugation are overwhelmed, leading to increasing amounts of APAP being oxidized to NAPQI.
      - GSH stores are eventually depleted, leading to free NAPQI irreversibly binding cellular proteins (e.g., mitochondrial proteins and ion channels), resulting in hepatocellular centrilobular (zone III) necrosis.
  - Clinical features
    - Stage I—preclinical
      - 0.5 to 24 hours following acute ingestion
      - Typically, asymptomatic
      - May have nausea, vomiting, and/or malaise
      - Laboratory values are typically normal.
    - Stage II—onset of hepatic injury
      - 24 to 72 hours following acute ingestion
      - Stage I symptoms resolve, but patient will develop right upper quadrant pain and tenderness as stage 2 progresses.
      - Aminotransferase elevation

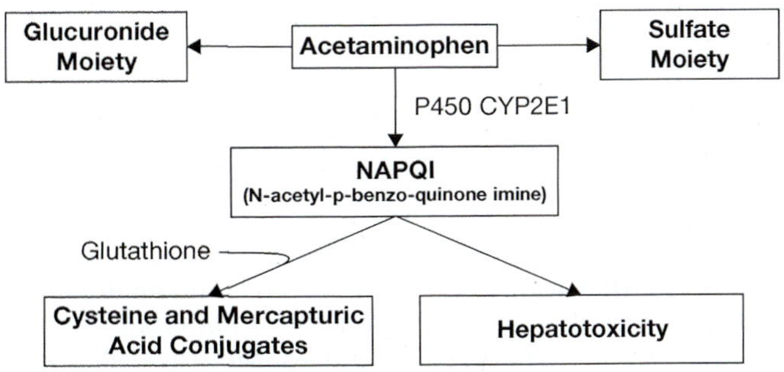

FIGURE 16.3.1 **Acetaminophen metabolism.**

- Stage III—hepatotoxicity
    - 72 to 96 hours following acute ingestion
    - Significant elevation in aminotransferases, aspartate aminotransferase (AST) and alanine aminotransferase (ALT) may be >10,000 IU/L.
    - Prolonged prothrombin time/international normalized ratio (PT/INR) and partial thromboplastin time (PTT), elevated lactate and bilirubin, hypoglycemia
    - Renal dysfunction (10%-25%)
    - Confusion, jaundice, hemorrhage, acute respiratory distress syndrome (ARDS)
    - Death occurs during stage 3, commonly from multiorgan system failure.
- Stage IV—recovery
    - 4 days to 2 weeks
    - Patients who survive stage 3 enter the recovery phase.
    - Lab values normalize over several weeks.
    - Hepatic regeneration over weeks to months

○ Diagnosis
- Acute ingestion
    - Obtain a serum acetaminophen level at 4 to 24 hours following ingestion and plot on the Rumack-Matthew normogram (Figure 16.3.2).
    - ≥150 μg/mL at 4 hours postingestion is considered toxic and should be treated.
    - >10 μg/mL, obtain repeat concentration 4 to 6 hours after the first measurement.

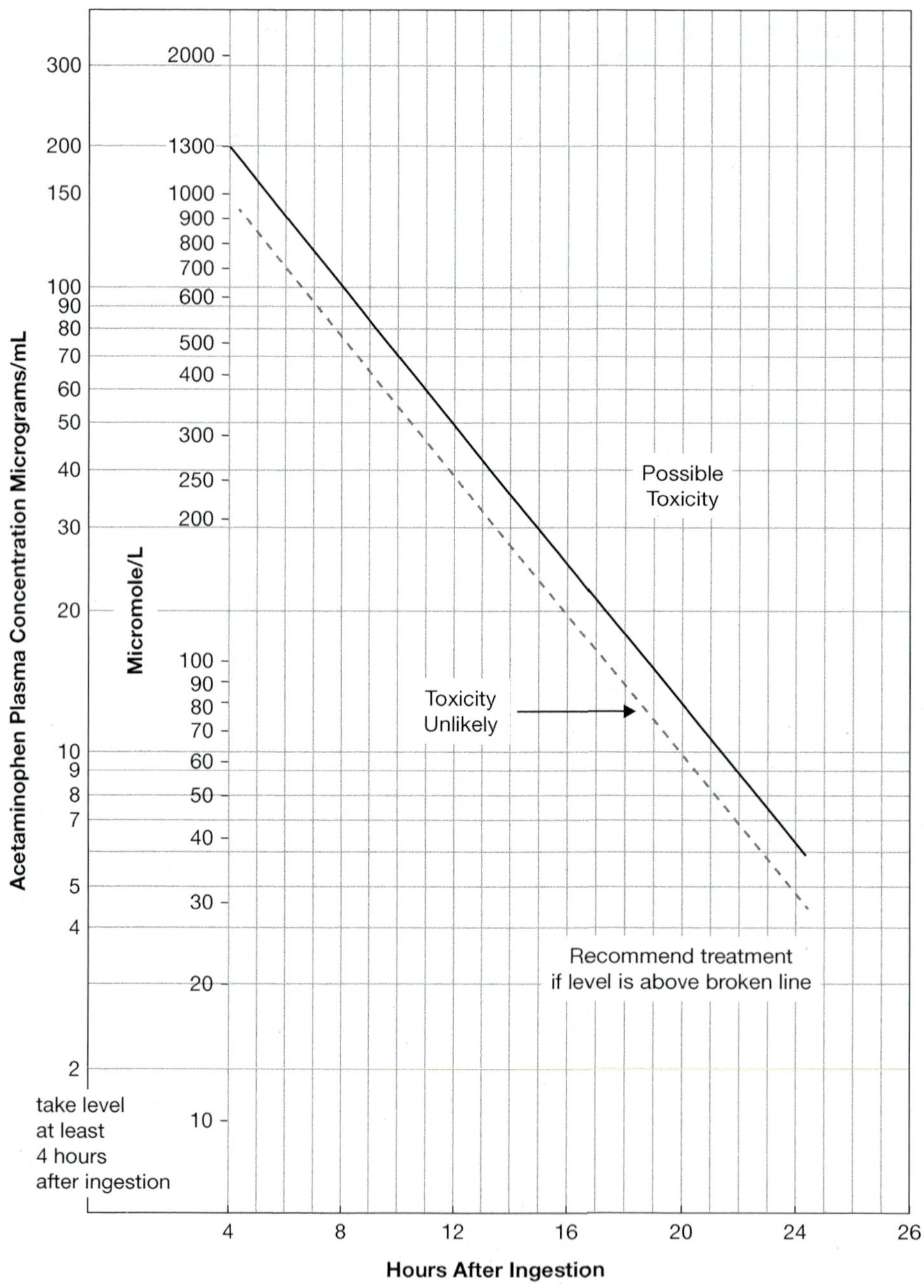

FIGURE 16.3.2 **Rumack-Matthew nomogram.** (From Tintinalli JE, Ma OJ, Yealy DM, Meckler GD, et al. Acetaminophen. In: *Tintinalli's Emergency Medicine: A Comprehensive Study Guide.* 9th ed. McGraw-Hill Education; 2020:chapter 190.)

- Chronic ingestion
  - Do not plot on the Rumack-Matthew nomogram.
  - Treat if >20 μg/mL and/or elevations in AST and ALT.
- Treatment
  - Supportive therapy
  - AC *may* be considered if <2 hours from ingestion.
  - Antidote
    - *N*-Acetylcysteine (NAC)
      - Should be administered as soon as the need for treatment is identified
      - Treatment regimen
        - Multiple regimens available, but all are administered over 20 to 24 hours.
        - NAC stopping criteria
          - Acetaminophen <10 μg/mL
          - INR <2.0
          - AST/ALT normal for the patient or have decreased by 25% to 50% from peak
          - The patient is clinically well appearing.
        - If NAC stopping criteria are not met
          - Continue NAC.
          - Measure acetaminophen concentration, AST, ALT, and PT/INR every 12 to 24 hours.
          - Reassess NAC stopping criteria.
        - Treatment regimen example
          - Load: 150 mg/kg over 1 hour, then
          - 12.5 mg/kg/h × 4 hours, then
          - 6.25 mg/kg/h × 16 hours
      - Oral (PO) versus intravenous (IV)
        - Formulations are equally efficacious.
        - PO formulation undergoes significant first-pass metabolism.
        - IV formulation should be used in pregnant women due to significant first-pass metabolism with oral formulation.
        - IV formulation may cause anaphylactoid reactions.
  - HD
    - Recommended when the acetaminophen concentration is ≥900 μg/mL, acidosis, or altered level of consciousness (LOC)
  - Liver transplantation
    - Consultation with a liver transplant team should be considered in case of acetaminophen toxicity and hepatic injury.
    - King's College Criteria can be used to guide who should be immediately referred for liver transplantation.
      - pH <7.3 after resuscitation, or
      - INR >6.5, creatinine >3.4 mg/dL, and grade 3 or 4 encephalopathy

- Salicylates
  - Found either alone or in combination with other drugs in a variety of over-the-counter (OTC) medications, including analgesics (e.g., aspirin), antidiarrheals (e.g., bismuth salicylate), cold medicines, decongestants, antihistamines, and topical oils and ointments
  - Mechanism
    - Salicylates irreversibly inhibit cyclooxygenase-1 (COX-1) and COX-2, leading to reduced prostaglandin, prostacyclin, and thromboxane synthesis, and thus reduced platelet aggregation.
    - At physiologic pH, ionized salicylates do not cross the blood-brain barrier and are not readily reabsorbed in the renal tubules. Acidemia reduces ionization, enabling the nonionized form to cross the blood-brain barrier and be reabsorbed in the kidneys.
  - Toxicity
    - Uncouples oxidative phosphorylation, resulting in anaerobic metabolism, metabolic acidosis, hyperthermia, and fluid loss
    - Stimulates the medullary chemoreceptor trigger zone, causing nausea and vomiting
    - Stimulates medullary respiratory center, resulting in tachypnea and respiratory alkalosis
    - Inhibits COX-1 and COX-2, leading to reduced platelet aggregation and gastric mucosal injury
    - Impairs gluconeogenesis and depletes glycogen stores, leading to hypoglycemia
    - Directly irritates the gastric mucosa, leading to ulceration and GI hemorrhage
    - Damages cochlear hair cells and afferent fibers of the eighth cranial nerve, leading to tinnitus and hearing loss
  - Clinical features
    - Acute toxicity
      - Early symptoms (within hours)
        - Nausea, vomiting, tinnitus
      - Symptom progression
        - Nausea, vomiting, tinnitus, tachypnea, hyperpnea, hyperthermia
        - Mixed metabolic high AG metabolic acidosis and respiratory alkalosis
      - Severe toxicity
        - Metabolic acidosis, hyperthermia, encephalopathy, cerebral edema, seizure, noncardiogenic pulmonary edema, hypoglycemia
        - Sinus tachycardia may devolved into ventricular dysrhythmias from electrolyte shifts.
        - Vasodilation and distributive shock
        - Leukocytosis, thrombocytopenia, and hemorrhage may occur rarely.
    - Chronic toxicity
      - Similar to acute toxicity, but the onset is more insidious.
  - Diagnosis
    - History and physical examination
    - Clinical symptoms proceed serum concentrations
    - Laboratory tests
      - Salicylate concentration: >30 mg/dL
      - Arterial blood gas (ABG), basic metabolic panel (BMP)
        - Early: high AG metabolic acidosis and respiratory alkalosis
        - Late: high AG metabolic acidosis
  - Treatment
    - Treatment should not be delayed while awaiting a serum concentration if salicylate toxicity is presumed.
    - Supportive care
      - Airway: avoid endotracheal intubation unless the patient is hypoventilating or not protecting their airway.

- Breathing: hyperventilation is a compensatory mechanism for metabolic acidosis. If the patient is intubated, maintain a high minute ventilation for compensation.
- Circulation: fluid resuscitation is essential as these patients may be profoundly hypovolemic.
- Decontamination: AC *may* be considered.
- Antidote
  - Urine alkalinization to maintain urine pH 7.5 to 8.0
    - Goal of treatment: maintain salicylate in the ionized form
    - Bolus: 1 to 2 mEq/kg $NaHCO_3$
    - Infusion: 1.5 to 2 × maintenance fluid rate
  - Electrolyte repletion
    - Hypokalemia reduces the effectiveness of urinary alkalinization via sodium bicarbonate infusion. Aggressive repletion necessary
- HD
  - Clinical indications
    - Encephalopathy, seizure, cerebral and/or pulmonary edema, acidosis (pH <7.3) despite resuscitation, fluid overload that limits aggressive resuscitation and bicarbonate infusion, acute kidney injury (AKI) or chronic kidney disease (CKD) resulting in unchanged salicylate concentration despite bicarbonate infusion
  - Indications based on serum concentration
    - >100 mg/dL: acute toxicity and normal renal function
    - >90 mg/dL: acute toxicity and impaired kidney function
    - >60 mg/dL: chronic toxicity
- Monitoring
  - Frequently assess salicylate concentration and electrolytes
- End of treatment: when salicylate concentration is below the upper limit of therapeutic window, the patient is asymptomatic, and the acid-base status has normalized.

- Nonsteroidal antiinflammatory drugs (NSAIDs)
  - NSAIDs are taken by millions of people worldwide to treat pain and fever.
  - Mechanism
    - Competitively inhibit COX-1 and COX-2 to prevent prostaglandin and thromboxane synthesis
    - NSAIDs are weak acids that are almost exclusively protein bound with a small volume of distribution.
    - Metabolized in the liver and excreted in the urine
    - Half-life is dependent on the specific drug.
  - Toxicity
    - <100 mg/kg: unlikely to cause significant toxicity
    - >200 mg/kg: toxic ingestion
    - >400 mg/kg (child) or >6 g (adult) is considered a massive ingestion.
  - Clinical features
    - Acid-base: high AG metabolic acidosis
    - Renal: reduced renal perfusion leads to renal papillary necrosis. Patients may have hematuria and renal colic.
    - CNS: cerebral edema, seizures, coma
    - Cardiovascular: hypotension and cardiovascular collapse associated with massive overdose
    - Hematologic: aplastic anemia, agranulocytosis, and coagulopathy. Associated with indomethacin and phenylbutazone
  - Diagnosis
    - Diagnosis is based on history and physical examination.
    - NSAID concentrations may not correlate with clinical symptoms and should not be used to guide diagnosis or management.
  - Treatment
    - Supportive care
    - Decontamination
      - AC may be used within 2 hours of acute ingestion.
      - MDAC may be useful in massive overdoses of sustained-release formulations.
    - HD ineffective due to the high degree of protein binding
- Iron
  - Iron is taken as a supplement, alone, or in multivitamins. Oral iron is much more likely to result in toxicity than IV formulations.
  - Toxicity
    - Toxic dose is determined by the iron formulation and route of exposure. Toxicity is more likely with oral formulation.
    - Toxic dose: >20 mg/kg elemental iron
    - Unbound ferric iron (Fe^{3+}) is directly toxic and results in tissue damage from free-radical production and lipid peroxidation. This leads to uncoupling of oxidative phosphorylation and organ failure.
  - Clinical features
    - Phase 1—GI phase
      - 30 minutes to 6 hours following ingestion
      - Direct mucosal injury leads to nausea, vomiting, diarrhea, hematemesis, and melena.
      - Vomiting suggests severe toxicity.
      - Most patients with mild or moderate toxicity do not progress to phase 2. Symptoms resolve in 4 to 6 hours.
    - Phase 2—latent phase
      - 6 to 24 hours following ingestion
      - Period of clinical improvement
      - May not occur in severe toxicity
    - Phase 3—shock phase
      - 6 to 72 hours following ingestion
      - Nausea, vomiting, and diarrhea return
      - Shock, may be hypovolemic, distributive, and/or cardiogenic
      - Multisystem organ failure: ARDS, GI hemorrhage, coagulopathy, renal dysfunction, encephalopathy
      - High AG metabolic acidosis
    - Phase 4—fulminant hepatic failure
      - 12 to 96 hours following ingestion
      - Hepatocellular necrosis from oxidative injury
      - Liver failure is the second most common cause of death from iron poisoning.
    - Phase 5—delayed sequelae and bowel obstruction
      - 2 to 8 weeks following ingestion
      - GI scarring can lead to bowel obstruction, commonly at gastric outlet.
  - Diagnosis
    - History and physical examination
      - History of ingestion with nausea, vomiting, and/or diarrhea, or more severe symptoms described earlier

- Patients at risk for severe toxicity
  - ≥60 mg/kg of elemental iron ingested
  - Peak serum iron concentration ≥500 µg/dL
  - Persistent, serious, and/or systemic symptoms
- Laboratory findings
  - High AG metabolic acidosis and elevated lactate
  - Elevated transaminases, bilirubin, and coagulation time seen in more severe disease
  - Obtain peak serum iron concentrations.
    - Regular formulation: 4 to 6 hours following ingestion
    - Extended-release formulation: 8 hours following ingestion
  - Degree of toxicity
    - <350 µg/dL: minimal toxicity
    - 350 to 500 µg/dL: mild-to-moderate toxicity
    - ≥500 µg/dL: severe toxicity
    - >1,000 µg/dL: increased mortality risk
- Abdominal radiograph
  - Obtain in all patients with symptoms of toxicity, large ingestions (>40 mg/kg), or intentional ingestion.
  - Presence of radiopaque pills in a patient with suspected iron ingestion confirms ingestion, but lack of this finding does not rule out ingestion.

- Treatment
  - Supportive care
  - Decontamination
    - AC will not adsorb iron.
    - WBI may be considered in large ingestions and/or if radiopaque pills are observed on abdominal radiograph.
  - Antidote
    - Deferoxamine chelates ferric iron to form ferrioxamine, which is excreted in the urine. May cause urine to appear pink or red in color "vin-rose"
    - Indications
      - Peak concentration ≥500 µg/dL
      - Estimated ingestion ≥60 mg/kg elemental iron
      - High AG metabolic acidosis
      - Moderate-to-severe symptoms including persistent vomiting, shock, lethargy, encephalopathy, and/or coma

- Diphenhydramine
  - First-generation antihistamine with anticholinergic properties that can cross the blood-brain barrier
  - Mechanism
    - H_1-receptor antagonism, muscarinic receptor antagonism, and Na^+ channel antagonism
  - Toxicity
    - Anticholinergic agents like diphenhydramine competitively inhibit acetylcholine (ACh) from binding muscarine ACh receptors in the CNS, heart, smooth muscle, secretory glands, and ciliary body of the eye.
  - Clinical features
    - Anticholinergic toxidrome (Table 16.3.1)
      - Mnemonic
        - Mad as a hatter (encephalopathy)
        - Blind as a bat (mydriasis)
        - Red as a beat (flushed skin, vasodilation)
        - Hot as a hare (anhidrosis)
        - Dry as a bone (dry mucous membranes)
        - Full as a flask (urinary retention)
        - Stuffed as a pepper (constipation)
    - H_1-receptor antagonism causes sedation and CNS depression.
    - Na^+ channel antagonism causes QRS prolongation and seizure
  - Diagnosis
    - Clinical diagnosis is based on history and physical examination.
    - Obtain an ECG in all patients suspected of diphenhydramine toxicity to evaluate for QRS prolongation and dysrhythmias.
    - Laboratory tests
      - If rhabdomyolysis is suspected, obtain a creatinine kinase and BMP.
  - Treatment
    - Supportive care
      - Benzodiazepines for agitation and seizures
      - IV sodium bicarbonate for QRS prolongation
    - Antidote: physostigmine for severe central anticholinergic toxicity

- Dextromethorphan
  - Found in many OTC cough medications and may also be used recreationally
  - Dextromethorphan is the D-isomer of levorphanol, a synthetic opioid.
  - Mechanism
    - The active metabolite, dextrorphan, binds medullary sigma opioid receptors and inhibits *N*-methyl-D-aspartate (NMDA) receptors. Dextrorphan does not bind mu or delta opioid receptors.
    - Inhibits serotonin reuptake
  - Toxicity
    - Toxicity is dose dependent and occurs at doses ≥1.5 mg/kg.
  - Clinical features
    - Euphoria and hallucinations may progress to agitation, ataxia, and dissociation.
    - Tachycardia, diaphoresis, mydriasis, nystagmus
    - Coma and respiratory depression may be seen in severe toxicity. Severe agitation may lead to hyperthermia and rhabdomyolysis.
    - Serotonin syndrome may occur with co-ingestion of serotonergic agents (e.g., selective serotonin reuptake inhibitor [SSRI], serotonin-norepinephrine reuptake inhibitor [SNRI], monoamine oxidase inhibitor MAOI, linezolid).
  - Diagnosis
    - Clinical diagnosis based on history and physical examination
  - Treatment
    - Supportive care

Prescription Medications (Psychotropic medications)

- Tricyclic antidepressants (TCAs)
  - TCAs and tetracyclic antidepressants are used to treat depression, generalized anxiety disorder, posttraumatic stress syndrome, bulimia nervosa, smoking cessation, headaches, neuropathy, and sleep disorders.

- Examples include amitriptyline, amoxapine, clomipramine, desipramine, doxepin, and nortriptyline.
- Mechanism and toxicity
  - Serotonin and norepinephrine reuptake inhibition
  - Fast sodium channel inhibition: widened QRS complex
  - Muscarinic ACh receptor antagonism: anticholinergic toxidrome (Table 16.3.1)
  - $Alpha_1$-adrenergic receptor antagonism: hypotension, vasodilation
  - Histamine (H_1) receptor antagonism: sedation
  - $GABA_A$ receptor antagonism: seizures
- Clinical features
  - Cardiovascular: hypotension and reflex tachycardia, ventricular tachycardia, ventricular fibrillation, QRS prolongation
  - Neurologic: decreased LOC, delirium, seizures
  - Anticholinergic effects: hyperthermia, flushing, mydriasis
- Diagnosis
  - Clinical diagnosis based on history and physical examination
  - Classic ECG findings (Figure 16.3.3)
    - Terminal R wave >3 mm in aVR
    - RVS ratio 0.7 in aVR
    - QRS >100 milliseconds
- Treatment
  - Supportive care
    - Benzodiazepines for seizures and agitation, avoid sodium channel blocking agents such as phenytoin.
    - Lidocaine is a class IB antidysrhythmic that can be considered for arrhythmia treatment in cases refractory to sodium bicarbonate.
    - Extracorporeal membrane oxygenation (ECMO) can be considered in patients with refractory hypotension.
  - Decontamination
    - AC may be considered within 2 hours of ingestion.
  - Antidote
    - Sodium bicarbonate
      - Should be given if the QRS is >100 milliseconds or if arrhythmias are present
      - 1 to 2 mEq/kg until QRS narrows
    - Intralipid
      - 20% lipid emulsion can be considered in unstable patients due to TCAs' lipophilicity.

- SSRIs and SNRIs
  - Commonly prescribed medication, either alone or in combination, for the treatment of major depressive disorder, anxiety, sleep disorders, posttraumatic stress disorder, and chronic pain, among others
  - Mechanism
    - SSRI
      - Toxicity risk is dependent on the specific drug. SSRIs may exist as a single isomer (e.g., sertraline, paroxetine) or racemic mixtures of two isomers (e.g., fluoxetine, citalopram).
      - Inhibit presynaptic serotonin reuptake, resulting in increased postsynaptic serotonin receptor agonism
      - Over time, increased serotonin concentration and receptor binding can lead to an upregulation of serotonin receptors.
    - SNRI
      - Inhibit serotonin and norepinephrine reuptake. May lead to increased sympathetic response
  - Toxicity
    - Serotonergic toxicity (serotonin syndrome) occurs because of increased serotonin concentration within the CNS.
    - Most SSRIs have a wide therapeutic window, and toxicity (i.e., serotonin syndrome) may not occur unless >50 times the daily recommended dose is consumed.
    - Significant toxicity is more likely when very large doses (>150 times the daily dose) are consumed with co-ingestion of ethanol and/or benzodiazepines.
    - Citalopram has the greatest potential for toxicity of the SSRIs due to its unique chemical structure.
    - SNRIs are contraindicated within 2 weeks of taking an MAOI due to increased risk for serotonin syndrome and hypertensive crisis.
  - Clinical features (Table 16.3.1)
    - Neurologic:
      - Agitation, delirium, confusion
      - Tremor, hyperreflexia, clonus, ocular clonus, rigidity, seizures
    - Cardiovascular: tachycardia, hypertension; may develop QTc prolongation
    - Respiratory: tachypnea
    - Pupils: mydriasis
    - Skin: diaphoresis, warm, flushed
    - GI: nausea, diarrhea
  - Diagnosis
    - Clinical diagnosis
  - Treatment
    - Supportive care
      - Careful monitoring for QTc prolongation and arrhythmias may be required.
    - Decontamination
      - AC if ingestion occurred within 2 hours may be considered.
    - Antidote
      - Cyproheptadine is a serotonin antagonist and antihistamine that can be used in conjunction with supportive care for the treatment of serotonin syndrome. Oral formulation (i.e., no IV formulation) is currently available.

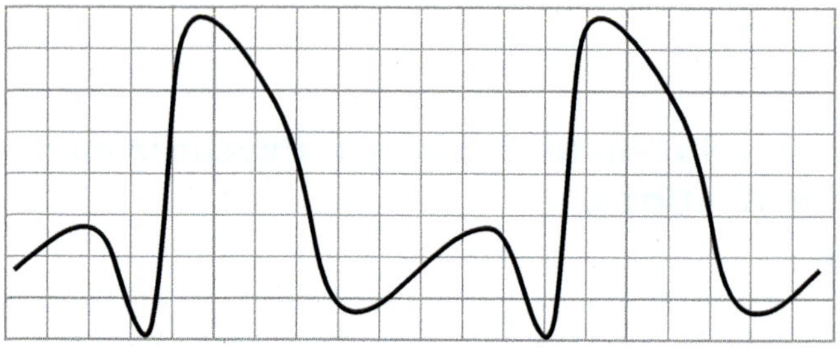

FIGURE 16.3.3 Electrocardiogram findings in tricyclic antidepressant toxicity.

- MAOI
  - Primarily used to treat major depressive disorder and Parkinson disease, but their toxicity limits their

utility when much safer medications are available (e.g., SSRIs). As a result, MAOIs are often not first-line medications.
- Examples include isocarboxazid, phenelzine, tranylcypromine, and selegiline.
- Mechanism
  - MAOIs have varied chemical structures that influence whether they reversibly or irreversibly inhibit monoamine oxidase A (MAO-A), monoamine oxidase B (MAO-B), or both.
  - MAOs metabolize endogenous amines like dopamine, norepinephrine, serotonin, and exogenous amines like tyramine.
  - Inhibition of MAOs results in increased concentrations of circulating bioactive amines.
- Toxicity
  - Toxicity can result from MAOIs, either alone or when used in combination with serotonergic agents, thus causing serotonin syndrome.
  - Monoamine oxidase may take weeks to regenerate after discontinuing MAOI use. Initiating an SSRI or SNRI should only occur at least 2 weeks after discontinuing an MAOI.
  - Consuming tyramine-rich foods (e.g., red wine, cheese) can precipitate toxicity, even at therapeutic MAOI dosing.
- Clinical features
  - Signs or symptoms may be delayed up to 12 hours following MAOI overdose.
  - Serotonin syndrome (Table 16.3.1)
  - Hypertensive emergency
- Diagnosis
  - Clinical diagnosis
- Treatment
  - Supportive care
    - Benzodiazepines are effective for seizures.
    - Aggressive treatment for agitation, rigidity, and hyperthermia to prevent rhabdomyolysis
  - Antidote
    - Cyproheptadine for the treatment of serotonin syndrome

- Anticonvulsants
  - Developed for the treatment of seizures but are also used for mood disorders, headaches/migraines, and chronic pain. Benzodiazepines and barbiturates will be discussed later. Some examples of anticonvulsants and their indicated uses other than seizure include:
    - Pain: carbamazepine, gabapentin, pregabalin, phenytoin
    - Mood disorders: valproic acid (VPA), lamotrigine, topiramate, carbamazepine
    - Migraines: VPA, topiramate
    - Tremor: primidone
  - Mechanism
    - Anticonvulsants can be categorized by the primary mechanism of action. Although some anticonvulsants rely on multiple mechanisms, or the precise mechanism of action may not be known.
    - Voltage-dependent sodium channel inhibition:
      - carbamazepine, lacosamide, lamotrigine, oxcarbazepine, phenytoin, topiramate, and VPA, among others.
    - Calcium channel inhibition
      - Ethosuximide, gabapentin, pregabalin, VPA
    - GABA receptor agonism
      - Benzodiazepines, phenobarbital
    - Glutamate receptor modulation
      - Topiramate, perampanel
    - Synaptic vesicle protein SV2A modulation
      - Levetiracetam
  - Toxicity
    - Toxicity can occur at therapeutic doses or supratherapeutic doses.
    - CNS depression
      - Present in all anticonvulsant overdoses
    - Valproate-induced hyperammonemic encephalopathy
      - A metabolite of VPA inhibits carbamoyl phosphate synthetase I, ultimately leading to hyperammonemia. A relative carnitine deficiency can also contribute to elevated ammonia levels.
      - Hyperammonemia is associated with nausea, vomiting, encephalopathy, and seizures and, in rare cases, can cause death.
      - Toxicity can occur in acute overdose or in chronic therapy.
    - Drug reaction with eosinophilia and systemic symptoms (DRESS)
      - Severe drug reaction with extensive rash and associated lymphadenopathy, eosinophilia, lymphocytosis, and organ involvement
      - Associated with aromatic anticonvulsants, including lamotrigine, phenytoin, carbamazepine, oxcarbazepine, primidone, felbamate, zonisamide, and phenobarbital
    - Stevens-Johnson syndrome (SJS)/toxic epidermal necrolysis (TEN)
      - Severe cutaneous reaction characterized by extensive epidermal necrosis. Commonly involves mucus membranes
      - Associated with aromatic anticonvulsants
    - Bone marrow suppression and aplastic anemia
      - Associated with carbamazepine, VPA, phenytoin, and felbamate use. Aplastic anemia is more common within the first few months after initiation.
    - Gingival hyperplasia observed with phenytoin use
    - Cardiovascular
      - Cardiac arrest can occur as a result of rapid IV infusion of phenytoin due to its dilution in propylene glycol.
      - QRS prolongation, ventricular arrhythmias
    - Hepatotoxicity
      - Direct liver injury as a result of VPA and other anticonvulsants
    - Renal tubular acidosis (RTA)
      - Topiramate and zonisamide have carbonic anhydrase activity that can cause urinary bicarbonate loss and subsequent non-AG metabolic acidosis.
  - Clinical features
    - Neurologic
      - CNS depression is common to all anticonvulsant overdoses.
      - Ataxia, stupor, coma, seizures, hallucinations
    - Cardiovascular: bradycardia, hypotension
    - GI: nausea, vomiting

- Diagnosis
  - Clinical diagnosis supported by drug concentrations
  - Laboratory findings
    - Drug concentrations can be measured for some anticonvulsants (e.g., levetiracetam, phenytoin, VPA, carbamazepine)
    - Ammonia level should be measured in patients taking VPA.
- Treatment
  - Supportive care
    - Valproate-induced hepatic encephalopathy
      - L-carnitine will help facilitate enhanced ammonia clearance.
    - Naloxone has been shown to reverse CNS depression.
  - Decontamination
    - AC can be trialed in patients with acute overdose.
    - MDAC is recommended for carbamazepine and phenobarbital.
  - HD may be effective for phenobarbital and VPA toxicity.

- Antipsychotics
  - Broad class of medications used to treat schizophrenia, bipolar disorder, major depressive disorder, psychosis, agitation, and nausea, among other uses. They can be classified into first-generation (typical antipsychotics) and second-generation (atypical antipsychotics).
  - First-generation antipsychotics (FGA)
    - Fluphenazine, thorazine, loxapine, haloperidol, molindone, perphenazine, thioridazine, chlorpromazine
  - Second-generation antipsychotics (SGA)
    - Aripiprazole, clozapine, lurasidone, olanzapine, paliperidone, quetiapine, risperidone, ziprasidone
  - Mechanism
    - FGA
      - Postsynaptic dopamine-2 (D2) receptor antagonism
      - Other receptor interaction is drug dependent and includes serotonin 5-HT2a, alpha-1, histamine-1, and muscarinic receptors. Can also inhibit sodium and potassium channels
      - Lipophilic, protein bound, large volume of distribution, and hepatically metabolized
    - SGA
      - Similar receptor and ion channel interaction as with FGAs
      - Some SGAs may be D2 receptor partial agonists (e.g., aripiprazole) and/or may interact with the D3 receptor (e.g., cariprazine).
      - Most SGAs have a higher affinity for 5HT2 receptors than FGAs.
  - Toxicity and clinical features
    - Extrapyramidal symptoms (EPSs)
      - Occurs due to an imbalance in dopamine and ACh
      - More likely in patients taking high-potency FGA (e.g., fluphenazine, haloperidol, loxapine)
      - Acute dystonia
        - Sustained or repetitive muscle contractions that result in repetitive or fixed postures
      - Parkinsonism
        - Masked facies, cogwheel rigidity, tremor, bradykinesia
      - Akathisia
        - Most common
        - Motor restlessness, inability to sit still
      - Tardive dyskinesia
        - Hyperkinetic, involuntary movement disorder characterized by orofacial dyskinesia, athetosis, dystonia, chorea, and tics
        - Can persist for several months after discontinuing antipsychotic use or may be permanent
    - NMS
      - Encephalopathy, hyperthermia, muscular rigidity, and autonomic instability
      - NMS can lead to elevated serum creatinine kinase levels and rhabdomyolysis.
    - Encephalopathy
      - Result of histamine and muscarinic receptor interactions
      - Symptoms include agitated delirium, somnolence, and coma.
    - Cardiovascular
      - QT prolongation (K^+ channel)
      - Tachycardia (alpha-1 receptor, muscarinic receptor)
      - Hypotension (alpha-1 receptor)
    - Hematologic dyscrasias
      - Clozapine can cause agranulocytosis, leukopenia, and neutropenia.
    - Hyperprolactinemia
      - Most FGAs and a few SGAs can cause increased prolactin levels, which can lead to galactorrhea, sexual dysfunction, and gynecomastia.
    - Seizures
      - Can occur with most antipsychotics, likely dose dependent
    - Anticholinergic toxidrome (Table 16.3.1)
  - Diagnosis
    - Clinical diagnosis based on history and physical examination
    - Consider in patients prescribed antipsychotics, medications with similar mechanisms, and/or medications with known interactions.
  - Treatment
    - Supportive care
      - Discontinuation of offending agent
      - IV fluids, antiemetics, vasopressors as needed
      - Benzodiazepines are effective in treating seizures.
      - Aggressive sedation and cooling for NMS
      - EPS
        - Benztropine: anticholinergic to counteract ACh excess
        - Diphenhydramine
        - Propranolol: used to treat motor symptoms
      - NMS
        - Benzodiazepines: for agitation
        - Bromocriptine and amantadine: dopamine agonists that may be useful in restoring dopamine levels
        - Dantrolene: skeletal muscle relaxant for severe cases
    - Decontamination
      - AC if within the first 2 hours following a large ingestion

Sedative Hypnotics

- Barbiturates
  - Used as sedatives, anesthetics, seizures, and psychiatric disease
  - Mechanism and toxicity
    - Binds $GABA_A$ chloride channel to increase the duration of channel opening, leading to hyperpolarization of postsynaptic cell membranes and neuronal firing suppression
    - Depresses medullary respiratory centers
    - Duration of action is drug dependent
      - Short-acting: pentobarbital, thiopental, methohexital
      - Intermediate-acting: butalbital
      - Long-acting: phenobarbital
    - Metabolism: hepatic
    - Elimination: renal
  - Clinical features
    - Neurologic: ataxia, myosis, lethargy, sedation, coma, suppression of brainstem reflex
    - Cardiovascular: hypotension, bradycardia
    - Respiratory: respiratory depression
    - GI: phenobarbital can cause liver injury.
    - Skin: bullae
    - Other clinical features
      - Phenobarbital can cause SJS and TEN.
      - DRESS
      - Pentobarbital and phenobarbital may be diluted in propylene glycol and are associated with propylene glycol toxicity.
  - Diagnosis
    - Clinical diagnosis based on history and physical examination
    - Obtain serum phenobarbital level, if suspected.
  - Treatment
    - Supportive care
      - Urinary alkalinization may be useful for phenobarbital toxicity.
    - Decontamination
      - MDAC for phenobarbital
    - HD for severe phenobarbital toxicity
- Benzodiazepines
  - Used as sedatives, anesthetics, and to treat seizures
  - Mechanism
    - Binds $GABA_A$ chloride channel to increase the frequency of channel opening, thus hyperpolarizing postsynaptic cell membranes and suppressing neuronal firing
    - Rapidly absorbed in GI tract, most are lipophilic and protein bound
    - Duration of action is drug dependent.
      - Short-acting: midazolam
      - Intermediate-acting: alprazolam, lorazepam
      - Long-acting: diazepam, chlordiazepoxide, clonazepam
    - Metabolism: hepatic, majority by CYP enzymes
      - Oxazepam, temazepam, and lorazepam are directly conjugated to inactive metabolites. Metabolism is not altered in hepatic impairment.
  - Clinical features
    - Neurologic: ataxia, myosis, lethargy, sedation, coma
    - Respiratory: respiratory depression
    - Diazepam and lorazepam may be diluted in propylene glycol and are associated with propylene glycol toxicity.
  - Diagnosis
    - Clinical diagnosis based on history and physical examination
    - UDS has poor sensitivity and specificity and does not confirm acute exposure. A UDS positive for benzodiazepines may suggest recent use.
  - Treatment
    - Supportive care
    - Antidote
      - Flumazenil
        - Competitive benzodiazepine receptor antagonist
        - Indicated for severe toxicity in patients who do not regularly use benzodiazepines
        - May induce seizures in patients who chronically use benzodiazepines and is not recommended
- Lithium
  - Mood stabilizer used to treat bipolar disorder, major depressive disorder, and psychosis
  - Mechanism
    - The mechanism of action is not fully understood.
    - Lithium salts (e.g., lithium carbonate) alter cation transport across cell membranes in neurons and myocytes, influence serotonin and norepinephrine neurotransmission, and alter inositol monophosphate and glycogen synthase kinase-3 signaling pathways.
    - Near-complete bioavailability, rapidly absorbed, low volume of distribution, no protein binding
    - Peak concentration
      - Immediate-release:1 to 2 hours
      - Sustained-release: 4 to 6 hours
    - Half-life: ~27 hours (children), 18 to 36 hours (adults)
    - Elimination: renal, similar mechanism to sodium elimination
  - Toxicity and clinical features
    - Toxicity may occur at therapeutic doses, but toxic ingestions are defined as a single ingestion >2,400 mg (adults) or >30 mg/kg (children).
    - Time to peak concentration may take ≥12 hours in acute overdose.
    - Signs and symptoms may differ in their severity or timing of onset dependent if toxicity is acute, acute on chronic, or chronic.
    - Neurologic
      - Appear first (i.e., before GI symptoms) in chronic toxicity
      - Ataxia, confusion, agitation, fasciculations, myoclonus
      - Tremors: fine tremors are common at therapeutic levels, but coarse tremors may predominate at toxic levels.
      - Coma, seizures, nonconvulsive status epilepticus, and encephalopathy
    - GI
      - Appear first (i.e., before neurologic symptoms) in acute toxicity
      - Nausea, vomiting, diarrhea
    - Syndrome of Irreversible Lithium-Effectuated Neurotoxicity (SILENT)
      - Can occur following lithium overdose/toxicity despite fully clearing lithium from the body

        - Symptoms include cerebellar dysfunction (i.e., ataxia), EPS, brainstem dysfunction, and dementia.
      - Cardiovascular
        - QTc prolongation and bradycardia, arrhythmias are rare.
      - Arginine vasopressin resistance (aka nephrogenic diabetes insipidus)
        - Chronic lithium use can lead to alcohol dehydrogenase (ADH) resistance, causing polyuria and polydipsia, which may be irreversible.
      - CKD
        - Chronic lithium use associated with CKD that can progress to end-stage renal disease
        - Lithium can cause chronic interstitial nephritis. The degree of fibrosis correlates with the duration and cumulative lithium dose.
      - RTA
        - Distal tubular defects caused by lithium can reduce the ability to acidify the urine, resulting in RTA type 1.
    - Diagnosis
      - History and physical examination consistent with lithium use and/or toxicity
      - Laboratory findings
        - Serum lithium concentration
          - Acute toxicity: serum concentrations do not correlate to CNS lithium concentration and thus do not correlate with symptoms.
          - Chronic toxicity: serum concentrations more closely correlate with symptoms.
          - Lithium level should be obtained every 4 to 6 hours until peak.
          - Therapeutic: 0.8 to 1.2 mEq/L
          - Mild toxicity: 1.2 to 2.5 mEq/L
          - Moderate-to-severe toxicity: >2.5 mEq/L
    - Treatment
      - Supportive care
        - Fluid resuscitation to achieve and maintain euvolemia
      - Decontamination
        - WBI is recommended after a large ingestion.
        - Immediate-release: WBI within 1 hour
        - Sustained-release: WBI within 4 hours
      - Antidote
        - HD is the treatment of choice for lithium toxicity.
        - Indications for HD differ depending on the source. It is recommended to follow local protocols.
        - After HD cessation
          - Obtain lithium level immediately following HD and again 6 hours following.
          - Rebound effect may occur after cessation of HD when intracellular lithium moves into the extracellular space.
          - Repeat HD session may be required.

Cardioactive Medications

- Antidysrhythmics and antihypertensives
  - Specific antidysrhythmics and antihypertensive toxicities are discussed later. Additional antihypertensives and their effects are listed in Table 16.3.5.

TABLE 16.3.5 Additional Antihypertensive Agents

Agent	Mechanism	Clinical Syndrome
Doxazosin Prazosin Terazosin	$Alpha_1$ receptor antagonist	Hypotension Tachycardia Syncope
Hydralazine	Direct-acting vasodilator	Hypotension Tachycardia
Methyldopa	Central $alpha_2$ agonist	Hypotension Miosis Sedation Respiratory depression
Minoxidil	Direct-acting arteriodilator	Hypotension Tachycardia
Nitroprusside Nitroglycerine	Direct-acting venodilator	Hypotension Tachycardia Cyanide toxicity (nitroprusside) Methemoglobinemia (nitroglycerin)

- $Alpha_2$-adrenergic agonist
  - Clonidine is an imidazoline antihypertensive, and its chemical structure is related to other imidazoline medications, including tizanidine, guanfacine, dexmedetomidine, and xylazine.
  - Clonidine is also used for opioid detoxification, as an adjunct to sedation, spinal anesthesia, smoking cessation, glaucoma, and is used for sleep disorders.
  - methyldopa is a centrally acting antihypertensive that is structurally different from clonidine (i.e., not an imidazoline).
  - Mechanism
    - Central $alpha_2$ agonism results in decreased sympathetic tone and leads to hypotension and bradycardia. These agents also interact with GABA, opioid, and serotonin pathways, resulting in sedation.
    - Peripheral $alpha_2$ agonism leads to vasoconstriction and transient hypertension.
    - Topical $alpha_2$ agonists are less likely to enter the CNS.
    - Absorption, distribution, and elimination are influenced by formulation.
      - PO clonidine
        - Bioavailability: up to 100%
        - Peak concentration: 2 hours
        - Half-life: 12 to 16 hours
        - Elimination: renal
      - Transdermal clonidine
        - Absorption: constant over 7 days
        - Half-life: up to 55 hours
  - Toxicity and clinical features
    - Profound effects can occur at very low doses in some patients.
    - Neurologic: sedation, coma
    - Pupils: miosis
    - Cardiovascular: transient hypertension, then hypotension and bradycardia
    - Respiratory: respiratory depression
    - Other: hypothermia, dry mouth

- Diagnosis
    - Clinical diagnosis based on history and physical examination
    - Ask about access to alpha$_2$ agonists and possible co-ingestions, including illicit drug use. Xylazine may be used either alone or as an adulterant in illicit drugs, commonly in fentanyl and heroin.
- Treatment
    - Supportive care
        - Naloxone may reverse the sedative effects of alpha$_2$ agonists.
        - Atropine may be useful in symptomatic bradycardia, but longer acting agents may be necessary (e.g., dopamine, epinephrine).
        - Hypotension usually resolves with chronotropic restoration or improved mental status. Some patients may require continued vasopressor support.
    - Decontamination
        - Remove topical applications if present.
        - AC may be useful within 1 hour after ingestion of clonidine tablets or within 30 minutes following liquid formulation.
        - WBI is suggested following transdermal patch ingestion.

- Beta-adrenergic antagonists
    - Also known as beta-blockers or Class II antidysrhythmics, this class of medications includes medications indicated for hypertension, rate control in atrial fibrillation, and as part of goal-directed therapy for heart failure. Some beta-blockers also possess alpha-adrenergic antagonistic properties (e.g., carvedilol, labetalol).
    - Mechanism and toxicity
        - Beta antagonism results in a reduction of cyclic adenosine 3′,5′-monophosphate (cAMP). This mechanism reduces free calcium ions necessary for myocyte contraction.
        - Beta antagonists competitively inhibit the beta-1, beta-2, and/or beta-3 receptors. Specific receptor activity is medication specific.
            - Beta$_1$
                - Primarily found in cardiac myocytes, but also found in the eyes and kidneys
                - Activation causes increased heart rate, contractility, and atrioventricular (AV) nodal conduction in the heart.
                - Eye: increased aqueous humor production
                - Kidney: increased renin production
            - Beta$_2$
                - Found in cardiac myocytes, bronchial and peripheral vascular smooth muscle
                - Activation causes smooth muscle relaxation and vasodilation.
            - Beta$_3$
                - Found in cardiac and adipose tissue
                - Activation leads to lipolysis and may influence thermogenesis and contractility.
        - Intrinsic sympathomimetic activity
            - Some beta antagonists exert partial beta agonism, which leads to reduced frequency of hypotension, bradycardia, and/or bronchoconstriction at toxic doses (e.g., labetalol, acebutolol).
        - Lipophilicity
            - Some beta antagonists readily enter the CNS due to their high degree of lipid solubility (e.g., propranolol, carvedilol). This may result in altered mentation, coma, or seizures.
        - Membrane stabilizing activity
            - Some beta antagonists inhibit myocardial fast sodium channels, leading to QRS prolongation (e.g., carvedilol, propranolol).
        - Half-life: drug dependent; 3 minutes (esmolol), >20 hours (metoprolol succinate, nadolol)
        - Elimination: drug specific
            - Hepatic: most beta antagonists
            - Renal: atenolol, nadolol, sotalol
            - Erythrocyte esterase: esmolol
            - Mixed hepatic and renal: acebutolol, bisoprolol, pindolol, timolol
    - Clinical features
        - Neurologic: encephalopathy, coma, seizures
            - Neurologic symptoms more likely with lipophilic medications
        - Cardiovascular: bradycardia, hypotension, cardiogenic shock
            - ECG: PR prolongation, or any bradyarrhythmia; some may cause QRS prolongation (propranolol, carvedilol).
        - Respiratory: respiratory depression, bronchoconstriction
        - Skin: cold extremities
        - Laboratory findings: hypoglycemia, hyperkalemia
    - Diagnosis
        - History and physical examination consistent with beta-adrenergic antagonism use. The patient or their family members may have a prescription for this medication. Toxicity can occur from accidental or intentional overdose.
        - Beta-blocker toxicity should always be considered in patients with bradycardia and hypotension.
    - Treatment
        - Supportive care
            - Atropine, initially, for symptomatic bradycardia while treating with additional agents
            - Cardiac pacing can be trialed concurrently with treatment.
            - ECMO can be considered in refractory cases.
        - Decontamination
            - AC if administered within 2 hours of ingestion
            - WBI in large ingestions of extended-release formulations
        - Antidote
            - IV glucagon
                - Activates adenylate cyclase to increase intracellular cAMP and thus increase contractility and blood pressure. Occurs at a site independent from beta antagonist activity
            - IV calcium
            - Vasopressors (e.g., epinephrine or norepinephrine)
            - High-dose insulin
                - Bolus: 1 U/kg IV regular insulin
                - Infusion: start at 0.5 to 1 U/kg, titrate to hemodynamic improvement
            - IV lipid emulsion (20%)

- Calcium channel antagonists
  - Also known as calcium channel blockers (CCBs) or class IV antidysrhythmics, they can be divided into two categories based on their mechanism (e.g., dihydropyridines and nondihydropyridines).
  - Mechanism and toxicity
    - Dihydropyridines
      - Amlodipine, felodipine, isradipine, nicardipine, nifedipine
      - Antagonize L-type calcium channels in peripheral vasculature
      - Cause vasodilation
      - At supratherapeutic doses, will cause hypotension and reflex tachycardia
      - At toxic doses, will cause bradycardia, reduced inotropy, and hypotension
    - Nondihydropyridines
      - Verapamil, diltiazem
      - Selectively antagonize L-type calcium channels in the myocardium
      - Result in reduced contractility, weak vasodilators
      - At toxic doses, will cause bradycardia, reduced inotropy, and hypotension
    - Highly protein bound, large volume of distribution
    - Duration of action: increases with increasing doses
    - Elimination: hepatic
  - Clinical features
    - Neurologic: may deteriorate when perfusion is diminished
    - Cardiovascular: bradycardia (verapamil, diltiazem, and severe dihydropyridine toxicity), hypotension, heart failure, cardiogenic shock
      - ECG: PR prolongation or bradyarrhythmia
    - Respiratory: pulmonary edema (from heart failure)
    - Skin: warm extremities
    - Laboratory findings: hyperglycemia (insulin release is calcium mediated)
  - Diagnosis
    - Clinical diagnosis, consider in patients who are bradycardic, hypotensive, and hyperglycemic.
  - Treatment
    - Supportive care
      - Atropine, initially, while treating with additional agents
      - Cardiac pacing can be trialed concurrently with treatment.
      - ECMO can be considered in refractory cases
    - Decontamination
      - AC within 2 hours of ingestion
      - WBI in large ingestions of extended-release formulations
    - Antidote
      - IV glucagon
      - IV calcium
      - Vasopressors (e.g., epinephrine or norepinephrine)
      - High-dose insulin
      - IV lipid emulsion (20%)
- Digoxin
  - Digoxin is a cardiac glycoside used for rate control in atrial fibrillation and for improving inotropy in heart failure. Naturally occurring cardiac glycosides include foxglove, lily of the valley, oleander, squill, dogbane, wallflower, and cane toad venom.
  - Mechanism
    - Reversibly inhibits sodium-potassium ATPase in cardiac myocytes, leading to increased intracellular sodium and decreased intracellular potassium. This ultimately leads to calcium influx and increased contractility and automaticity.
    - Direct AV nodal suppression increases effective refractory period.
    - Large volume of distribution
    - Duration of action: 3 to 4 days
    - Peak concentration: 1 to 3 hours
    - Elimination
      - Age and renal function dependent
      - 36 to 48 hours (adults), 18 to 36 hours (children)
  - Toxicity
    - Digoxin has a narrow therapeutic window.
    - Inhibiting sodium-potassium ATPase results in increased extracellular potassium to potentially toxic levels.
      - Acute toxicity: degree of hyperkalemia correlates with mortality.
      - Chronic toxicity: hypokalemia may increase susceptibility to toxicity.
    - Excessive intracellular calcium because of sodium-potassium ATPase inhibition can increase the risk of arrhythmias.
    - Chronic toxicity can occur because of reduced renal function or hypokalemia at unchanged digoxin doses.
    - Medications that inhibit or reduce p-glycoprotein activity can increase serum digoxin concentrations (e.g., amiodarone, verapamil, diltiazem).
    - Serum concentrations do not necessarily correlate with toxicity.
  - Clinical features
    - Chronic toxicity may have a more insidious onset than acute toxicity. Symptoms of chronic toxicity may occur over days to weeks. Neurologic symptoms and ventricular arrhythmias are more common in chronic toxicity.
    - Neurologic: visual changes (e.g., xanthopsia, diplopia, photophobia, scotomas), headaches, weakness, delirium, altered mental state
    - Cardiovascular: bradycardia, premature ventricular contractions, interventricular conduction delay and block, ventricular arrhythmias
      - ECG: digitalis effect indicates digoxin use, not toxicity.
    - GI: nausea, vomiting, anorexia
  - Diagnosis
    - Clinical diagnosis supported with characteristic ECG findings and elevated serum concentration
    - ECG findings—digitalis effect (Figure 16.3.4)
      - Downsloping ST depression with slurred upstroke, also described as scooped ST segment with ST depression (Salvador Dali Mustache)
      - Flattened, inverted, or biphasic T waves
      - Shortened QT interval
    - Laboratory findings
      - Serum digoxin concentration
        - Obtain at presentation and again in 6 hours.
        - Therapeutic: 0.5 to 0.8 ng/mL

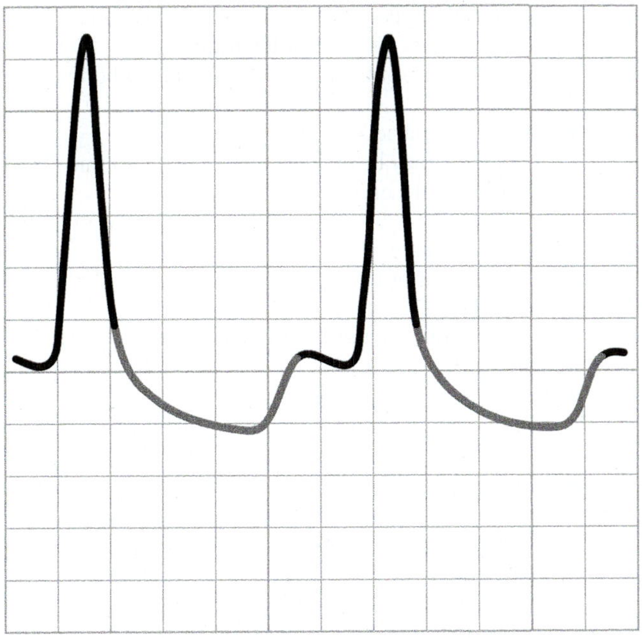

FIGURE 16.3.4 **Electrocardiogram findings in digoxin toxicity.**

- Potassium
  - Hyperkalemia common in acute toxicity
  - Hypokalemia may occur in chronic toxicity from polypharmacy (e.g., loop diuretics).
- Creatinine clearance
  - Renal function should be assessed as it is a common culprit in chronic toxicity.

- Treatment
  - Supportive care
    - Treat hyperkalemia and arrhythmias if applicable.
  - Decontamination
    - AC within 2 hours of ingestion
    - Mixed evidence for MDAC
  - Antidote
    - Digoxin-specific fragment antibody (digoxin immune Fab)
      - Empiric dose: 10 vials
      - Known ingestion:

$$\# \text{ vials} = \frac{\text{weight (kg)} \times \text{concentration} \left(\frac{\text{ng}}{\text{mL}}\right)}{100}$$

- Nitrates
  - Nitroglycerin is used in patients with acute coronary syndrome, acute decompensated heart failure, and hypertension, among other uses.
  - Sodium nitroprusside is approved for use in patients with hypertensive emergency, acute aortic syndromes, and acute decompensated heart failure, but has fallen out of favor due to its toxicity.
  - Mechanism and toxicity
    - Nitrates form nitric oxide that activate guanylate cyclase, leading to increased cGMP and smooth muscle relaxation.
    - Vasodilatory effect more pronounced in veins than in arteries
    - Nitroprusside contains five cyanide groups per molecule. Cyanide toxicity occurs after prolonged infusion, high doses, and in patients with renal failure.
    - Methemoglobinemia can occur after prolonged infusions or high doses of nitroglycerin.
  - Clinical features
    - Hypotension and tachycardia
    - Signs and symptoms of cyanide toxicity (nitroprusside) or methemoglobinemia (nitroglycerin)
  - Diagnosis
    - History and physical examination consistent with nitrate use
    - Laboratory evaluation as needed for cyanide toxicity and methemoglobinemia
  - Treatment
    - Supportive care
      - Stop offending agent.
      - Hypotension associated with nitrate use is relatively short-lived, given the short half-life of these medications. Vasopressors (e.g., norepinephrine) may be briefly required.
    - Antidote
      - Methylene blue (methemoglobinemia)
      - Hydroxocobalamin or sodium nitrite and sodium thiosulfate (cyanide toxicity)
    - HD may be considered in patients with cyanide toxicity.

Antihyperglycemics

- Broad group of medications intended to lower blood glucose levels, and some (not all) may result in hypoglycemia.
- Symptoms of hypoglycemia include confusion, agitation, tachycardia, diaphoresis, and nausea and can lead to seizures.
- The mainstay of treatment for hypoglycemic patients is to increase plasma glucose levels, whether through oral intake, intramuscular (IM) glucagon, and/or IV dextrose solutions.
- Many of the medications in this group do not have excessive toxicity and are not reviewed. If there is concern for unintentional ingestion or overdose of an antihyperglycemic agent, assess for hypoglycemia and treat as necessary. Specific diabetic medications and their unique characteristics are listed as follows:
- Biguanides
  - Oral agents, including metformin, are unlikely to cause hypoglycemia, even in an overdose. Hypoglycemia is likely due to co-ingestion.
  - Mechanism
    - Decreases hepatic glucose production and intestinal glucose absorption
    - Increases peripheral glucose use
    - Half-life: ~5 hours
    - Elimination: renal
  - Toxicity
    - Lactic acidosis
      - Metformin promotes glucose to lactate conversion.
      - Metformin inhibits mitochondrial respiratory chain complex 1, which results in reduced hepatic gluconeogenesis.
      - Symptoms: nausea and abdominal pain

- Signs: tachycardia, hypotension, tachypnea, altered mentation
- Diagnosis
  - History and physical examination consistent with metformin ingestion
  - Laboratory findings: lactic acidosis
- Treatment
  - Supportive care
  - Decontamination
    - AC may be used in acute ingestion.
  - Antidote
    - HD recommended in patient with severe toxicity from acute overdose or chronic use
      - Lactate >20 mmol/L
      - pH ≤7.0
      - Failure to improve with supportive care within 2 to 4 hours

- Sulfonylurea
  - Long-acting oral agents used in the treatment of diabetes mellitus, including chlorpropamide, glipizide, glyburide, glimepiride, and others.
  - Unintentional ingestion of even a single sulfonylurea pill can result in hypoglycemia, especially in children.
  - Mechanism and toxicity
    - Inhibit adenosine triphosphate (ATP)-sensitive potassium channels in pancreatic beta cells that ultimately leads to endogenous insulin release. When taken appropriately, intended to result in euglycemia, but overdose leads to hypoglycemia.
    - Kinetics are drug specific, but in general, sulfonylureas have a long duration of action (up to 24 hours) and may be even longer in acute overdose.
    - Metabolism: hepatic, but some form active metabolites that are renally cleared.
  - Diagnosis
    - History and physical examination consistent with sulfonylurea ingestion
    - Due to the long duration of action, serial testing of serum glucose is likely necessary to monitor for hypoglycemia.
  - Treatment
    - Supportive care
    - Decontamination
      - AC within the first 2 hours following ingestion
    - Antidote
      - Octreotide recommended for symptomatic hypoglycemia
- Sodium-glucose cotransporter-2 (SGLT2) inhibitor
  - SGLT2 inhibitors are not first-line therapy for patients with diabetes mellitus but are often prescribed after trialing other therapies or due to comorbid conditions (e.g., heart failure).
  - SGLT2 inhibitors include empagliflozin, dapagliflozin, and canagliflozin.
  - Mechanism
    - SGLT2 is expressed in the proximal renal tubule, and inhibition results in increased renal excretion of glucose with a modest reduction in serum glucose. Also results in osmotic diuresis.
  - Toxicity
    - Hypoglycemia rarely occurs with SGLT2 inhibitors.
    - Increased risk of genitourinary tract infection
    - Orthostatic hypotension as a result of osmotic diuresis, particularly in older adults
    - Increased risk of fractures due to lowered bone density
    - Diabetic ketoacidosis (DKA)
      - Patients may be euglycemic (i.e., euglycemic DKA) or hyperglycemic.
  - Treatment
    - Supportive care
      - Treatment of DKA discussed in Chapter 7.2
- Isoniazid (INH)
  - INH is an antibiotic used to treat tuberculosis (TB).
  - Mechanism
    - Selective for mycobacteria
    - Inhibits mycolic acid synthesis to disrupt cell wall synthesis
    - Inhibits pyridoxine phosphokinase, thus preventing conversion of pyridoxine to its active form, pyridoxal 5′ phosphate, an important cofactor for metabolic processes
    - Inhibits glutamate decarboxylase, preventing conversion of glutamate to GABA. Results in ↑ glutamate and ↓ GABA
    - Low volume of distribution, low protein binding
    - Bioavailability: 90%
    - Peak concentration: 2 hours
    - Half-life: dependent upon acetylation rate, 1 to 4 hours
    - Elimination: renal
  - Toxicity
    - Peripheral neuropathy likely occurs due to pyridoxine deficiency.
    - Seizures are a result of GABA deficiency.
    - INH metabolites cause direct hepatocellular toxicity.
  - Clinical features
    - Acute toxicity
      - Neurologic: encephalopathy, seizures
      - Cardiovascular: tachycardia
      - Respiratory: tachypnea
      - Renal: metabolic acidosis and rhabdomyolysis due to seizures
      - Other: hyperthermia
    - Chronic toxicity
      - Hepatotoxicity
      - Peripheral neuropathy
      - Neurologic: ataxia and nystagmus are rare.
  - Diagnosis
    - Clinical diagnosis
    - Suspect in patients presenting with seizures who are being treated for TB
  - Treatment
    - Supportive care
      - Benzodiazepines and barbiturates for seizures if unable to administer pyridoxine rapidly. Phenytoin and fosphenytoin are unlikely to be effective.
    - Decontamination
      - AC within 2 hours of ingestion
    - Antidote
      - Pyridoxine binds to INH, restores pyridoxine levels, and helps to restore GABA production.
    - HD
      - INH is dialyzable, may be beneficial in massive overdose.

- Local anesthetic
  - Classes
    - Esters: tetracaine, procaine, benzocaine
    - Amides: bupivacaine, lidocaine, mepivacaine, ropivacaine
  - Mechanism
    - Reversible sodium channel inhibition
    - Regional anesthesia and nerve blocks contribute to the majority of local anesthetic poisonings.
    - Topical applications have a higher risk of leading to toxicity when applied to mucus membranes.
  - Toxicity
    - Local toxicity may result in prolonged anesthetic effects and respiratory arrest if respiratory muscles are anesthetized.
    - Local anesthetic systemic toxicity (LAST) can occur when local anesthetics are administered at supratherapeutic doses
  - Clinical features
    - Confusion, anxiety, sense of impending doom, headache, drowsiness, lightheadedness, tremors, tinnitus, oral numbness
    - May progress to seizures and hemodynamic collapse
    - Sodium channel antagonism may lead to PR interval prolongation, QRS complex widening, ventricular tachycardia, ventricular fibrillation, and asystole.
    - Methemoglobinemia can result from benzocaine and prilocaine.
  - Treatment
    - Supportive care
    - Antidote
      - IV intralipid
        - 20% lipid emulsion bolus followed by a continuous infusion. Dosing may vary per local policy.
        - Acts as a lipid sink by forming micelles around anesthetic, thus preventing it from the site of activity
        - Recommended for patients with seizures, cardiovascular collapse, or signs of impending seizures and/or cardiovascular collapse

Anticoagulants

- Warfarin
  - Warfarin is an oral anticoagulant used for stroke prevention in patients with atrial fibrillation, venous thromboembolism (VTE), clotting disorders, mechanical heart valves, and with long-term left ventricular assist devices (LVADs), among other uses.
  - Warfarin and warfarin-like products are common rodenticides (e.g., brodifacoum), many of which are considered "superwarfarins" due to their potency and long half-lives.
  - Mechanism
    - Competitively inhibits vitamin K epoxide reductase complex 1 (VKORC1) to prevent vitamin K activation. This results in reduced synthesis of vitamin K–dependent clotting factors, II, VII, IX, X, and proteins C and S.
  - Toxicity
    - Toxicity may be delayed until activated clotting factors are depleted (≥15 hours).
    - Warfarin's duration of action may be up to 6 days, while warfarin-like rodenticides may be much longer.
    - Dietary vitamin K influences warfarin efficacy. Patients with low vitamin K levels are more likely to develop supratherapeutic anticoagulation levels.
    - Inhibition of CYP2C9 results in decreased warfarin metabolism, which may occur due to many medications.
    - Toxic ingestion: >1 mg or unknown dose
  - Clinical features
    - Bruising, hematomas, joint effusions, and bleeding
    - Clinical findings may be spontaneous or related to trauma, and may occur at therapeutic or supratherapeutic dosing.
  - Diagnosis
    - History and physical examination notable for warfarin (or warfarin-based rodenticide) consumption and signs of coagulopathy and/or bleeding
    - Laboratory findings
      - Elevated PT/INR
  - Treatment
    - Supportive care
      - Blood product transfusions may be needed in cases of significant bleeding.
      - Hold warfarin dose if supratherapeutic INR is identified and the patient is prescribed warfarin.
    - Decontamination
      - AC may be used for recent ingestions.
    - Antidote
      - Coagulopathy, no bleeding
        - INR <4.5: no reversal necessary in most patients
        - INR 4.5 to 10: vitamin K (1-2.5 mg) may be administered in patients with an increased risk of bleeding.
        - INR >10: vitamin K (2.5-5 mg) may be administered in patients with increased risk of bleeding.
      - Serious or life-threatening bleeding
        - Full reversal recommended
        - Vitamin K: 10 mg IV
        - 4-Factor prothrombin complex concentrate (PCC): follow institutional protocols for dosing.
        - Fresh frozen plasma (FFP): used as an alternative to PCC, when PCC is not available, and/or as a component of massive transfusion
      - Rodenticides
        - Long-acting and high-potency warfarin-like compounds may require large and repeated vitamin K dosing.
- Heparin
  - Heparin products include unfractionated heparin, low-molecular-weight heparin (LMWH), and fondaparinux and are three of the most commonly used anticoagulants.
  - Mechanism
    - Binds antithrombin (AT) to induce a conformational change and inactivate factors IIa (thrombin), IXa, Xa, XIa, and XIIa
    - Fondaparinux only inactivates factor Xa.
  - Toxicity
    - Bruising, hematomas, joint effusions, and bleeding
    - Clinical findings may be spontaneous or related to trauma and may occur at therapeutic or supratherapeutic dosing.

- Heparin products may also induce heparin-induced thrombocytopenia (HIT), which is discussed elsewhere.
- Diagnosis
  - History and physical examination notable for heparin use and signs of coagulopathy and/or bleeding
  - Laboratory findings
    - Elevated activated PTT (aPTT) or Xa
- Treatment
  - Supportive care
    - Blood product transfusions may be needed in cases of significant bleeding.
  - Antidote
    - Protamine sulfate
      - Recommended in cases of severe or life-threatening bleeding in patients receiving unfractionated heparin and LMWH. However, protamine is ineffective against fondaparinux
  - Additional therapies
    - PCC and FFP may be considered to reverse the anticoagulant effect of all heparin products, including fondaparinux.
    - Tranexamic acid (TXA)
    - Aminocaproic acid

- Direct thrombin inhibitors (DTIs)
  - DTIs are an alternative class of anticoagulant, including dabigatran, argatroban, and bivalirudin. They are indicated for the prophylaxis and treatment of VTE, for stroke prevention in patients with atrial fibrillation, and in patients with HIT.
  - Mechanism and toxicity
    - DTIs inactivate free and fibrin-bound factor IIa.
    - Bleeding can occur at therapeutic and supratherapeutic doses.
  - Diagnosis
    - History and physical examination consistent with DTI use
    - Laboratory findings
      - Prolonged aPTT
    - Anticoagulation status can be assessed based on time since last dose. A patient is no longer considered anticoagulated after five half-lives have elapsed.
      - Half-life: 12 to 17 hours
      - Five half-lives: 2.5 to 3.5 days
  - Treatment
    - Supportive care
      - Blood product transfusions may be needed in cases of significant bleeding.
    - Decontamination
      - AC within the first 2 hours following ingestion
    - Antidote
      - Idarucizumab is an anti-dabigatran monoclonal antibody fragment that is used for dabigatran reversal in life-threatening bleeding.
      - PCC or FFP.

- Direct oral anticoagulants (DOACs)
  - DOACs directly inhibit factor Xa and include apixaban, rivaroxaban, and edoxaban.
  - Approved for VTE prophylaxis and treatment, for stroke prevention in patients with atrial fibrillation, HIT, and for the treatment and prevention of left ventricular thrombus.
  - Mechanism and toxicity
    - DOACs inactivate circulating and fibrin-bound Xa.
    - Bleeding can occur at therapeutic and supratherapeutic doses
  - Diagnosis
    - History and physical examination consistent with DOAC use
    - PT/INR and aPTT may be prolonged, factor Xa activity may be increased. Thromboelastography (TEG) may demonstrate prolonged clotting time.
    - Anticoagulation status can be assessed based on time since last dose. A patient is no longer considered anticoagulated after five half-lives have elapsed. However, elimination is dependent on renal and hepatic function.
      - Apixaban
        - Half-life: 8 to 15 hours
        - Five half-lives: 1.5 to 3 days
      - Edoxaban
        - Half-life: 6 to 11 hours
        - Five half-lives: 1.2 to 2 days
      - Rivaroxaban
        - Half-life: 5 to 9 hours
        - Five half-lives: 1 to 2 days
  - Treatment
    - Supportive care
      - Blood product transfusions may be needed in cases of significant bleeding.
    - Decontamination
      - AC may be considered if last dose is within 2 hours.
    - Antidote
      - Andexanet alfa is a recombinant human factor Xa that acts as a decoy. The decoy molecule binds to and sequesters factor Xa inhibitors, neutralizing their effect.
      - Andexanet alfa is recommended for patients with life-threatening bleeding who take rivaroxaban or apixiban.
    - Additional therapies
      - PCC, TXA, aminocaproic acid

- Methylxanthines
  - Methylxanthines include caffeine, theophylline, and theobromine.
    - Caffeine is the most commonly used drug in the world.
    - Theophylline is used for asthma and chronic obstructive pulmonary disease and for apnea and bradycardia of prematurity.
    - Theobromine is found in chocolate and teas.
  - Mechanism
    - Methylxanthines are adenosine receptor antagonists that lead to increased catecholamine release.
    - Theophylline also induces bronchodilation by inhibition of phosphodiesterases.
  - Toxicity
    - Toxic dose: >150 mg/kg
  - Clinical features
    - Neurologic: elevated mood, nervousness, agitation, seizures
    - GI: nausea, vomiting

- Cardiovascular: tachycardia, hypertension, arrhythmias; hypotension may develop due to vasodilation.
- Respiratory: tachypnea, respiratory alkalosis
- Metabolic: hypokalemia, hyperglycemia
- Diagnosis
  - Clinical diagnosis
  - If theophylline toxicity is suspected, serum theophylline concentration should be obtained.
- Treatment
  - Supportive care
    - Arrhythmias can be treated with beta-blockade (e.g., esmolol, metoprolol).
  - Decontamination
    - MDAC
    - WBI may be reasonable for large ingestion of sustained-release formulations.
  - HD recommended in severe toxicity.

- Neuromuscular blocking agents (NMBAs)
  - Used to facilitate intubation, during surgical procedures, and sometimes used in the intensive care unit in specific scenarios (e.g. refractory ARDS, status asthmaticus).
  - Mechanism
    - Depolarizing NMBA
      - Succinylcholine (SCh) is an ACh analog that binds postsynaptic ACh receptors to cause continuous stimulation, fasciculations, and muscle paralysis.
    - Nondepolarizing NMBAs
      - Competitively inhibit postsynaptic Ach receptors to prevent depolarization and induce paralysis. These agents do not cause membrane depolarization.
      - Agents include rocuronium, vecuronium, pancuronium, and cisatracurium.
  - Toxicity
    - SCh can cause hyperkalemia, malignant hyperthermia, and trismus and may increase intraocular pressure.
      - SCh may raise serum potassium by ~0.5 mEq/L.
      - Disease states that upregulate ACh receptors (e.g., burns, crush injuries, rhabdomyolysis) may cause a clinically significant increase in potassium.
  - Treatment
    - Supportive care
    - Antidote
      - Sugammadex
        - Binds steroidal NMBAs (e.g., rocuronium, vecuronium, pancuronium), resulting in rapid reversal of muscle relaxant
      - Neostigmine
        - Acetylcholinesterase (AChE) inhibitor can be used when ~40% of neuromuscular function is restored. Facilitates ACh stimulation at neuromuscular junction to outcompete nondepolarizing NMBA
- Drugs of abuse (Table 16.3.6)

TABLE 16.3.6 Drugs of Abuse

Class	Examples	Symptoms	Treatment
Cannabinoids			
Cannabis (marijuana)	Cannabis Delta-8 THC Delta-9 THC Delta-10 THC	Euphoria Tachycardia Hypertension or hypotension Tachypnea Dry mouth Increased appetite Nystagmus Conjunctival injection Slurred speech Ataxia Lethargy Children may exhibit lethargy, nausea, vomiting, ataxia	Supportive Evaluate for co-ingestion if severe symptoms are present
Synthetic cannabinoids	Spice K_2	Symptoms like cannabis, plus: Hallucinations Delirium Psychosis Agitation Seizures Coma Respiratory depression	Supportive
Opioids			
Opiates • Extracted from plants (i.e., organic)	Heroin Opium Morphine Codeine	Hypoventilation Respiratory depression Miosis CNS depression	Naloxone
Opioids • Synthetic (i.e., made in a laboratory)	Hydrocodone Hydromorphone Oxycodone Methadone Fentanyl Carfentanyl		Naloxone May require larger and/or repeat doses for some synthetic opioids Some synthetic opioids do not respond to naloxone.

(continued)

TABLE 16.3.6 Drugs of Abuse (*continued*)

Class	Examples	Symptoms	Treatment
Sympathomimetics	Amphetamines Cocaine MDMA (aka ecstasy)	Tachycardia Hypertension Tachypnea Hyperthermia Diaphoresis Mydriasis SS may occur with MDMA toxicity	Supportive care Benzodiazepines for agitation Treatment of SS if present
Hallucinogens	LSD Psilocybin Ayahuasca/ dimethyltryptamine	Euphoria Synesthesia Visual and/or auditory hallucinations Tachycardia Hypertension Hyperthermia (rare) SS may occur with LSD intoxication	Supportive care Treatment of SS if present
NMDA antagonists	PCP Ketamine	Euphoria Hallucinations Hypertension Tachycardia Bizarre behavior (PCP) Psychomotor agitation Coma Laryngospasm (ketamine)	Supportive care Sedation when needed
Sedative Hypnotics			
Gamma hydroxybutyrate (GHB)		Bradycardia Hypotension Bradypnea or apnea Hypothermia CNS depression Coma Agitation Amnesia Myoclonus Seizures	Supportive care
Benzodiazepines	Alprazolam Diazepam Lorazepam Midazolam	Sedation Respiratory depression Ataxia (common in children)	Supportive care Flumazenil
Barbiturates	Butalbital Methohexital Pentobarbital Phenobarbital Primidone Thiopental	Sedation Coma Respiratory depression Hypotension Hypothermia Skin bullae	Supportive care MDAC Urinary alkalinization Hemodialysis
Imidazolines	Xylazine Tizanidine	Sedation Miosis Respiratory depression Hypotension Bradycardia Hypothermia	Supportive care

CNS, central nervous system; ECG, electrocardiogram; LSD, lysergic acid diethylamide; MDAC, multidose-activated charcoal; MDMA, 3,4-methylenedioxymethamphetamine; NMDA, *N*-methyl-D-aspartate; PCP, phencyclidine; SS, serotonin syndrome; THC: tetrahydrocannabinol.

Environmental Exposures

- Cyanide
  - Cyanide is a rapidly acting toxin that forms during combustion, is used for industrial purposes, metabolic product of amygdalin that is found in the pits and seeds of Rosaceae fruit (e.g., apricot, apple, peach, pear, plum, and bitter almonds), or can be ingested as a cyanide salt.
  - Mechanism and toxicity
    - Cyanide inhibits cytochrome oxidase to disrupt oxidative phosphorylation.
    - Anaerobic metabolism results in the formation of lactate and leads to metabolic acidosis.
    - Hydrogen cyanide (HCN) gas toxicity occurs within seconds.
    - Cyanide salt toxicity occurs within minutes.

- Cyanide toxicity from amygdalin ingestion requires consumption of large quantities and occurs within hours.
- Clinical features
  - Neurologic: headache, confusion, seizures, coma
  - GI: symptoms occur early; nausea, vomiting
  - Cardiovascular: hypertension, then arrhythmias and hemodynamic collapse
  - Respiratory: tachypnea, then pulmonary edema and respiratory failure
  - Odor: bitter almonds
- Diagnosis
  - Suspect in patients with rapid-onset coma, shock, and high AG metabolic acidosis
  - Laboratory evaluation
    - BMP, ABG, and lactate to assess for high AG metabolic acidosis
    - Venous blood gas (VBG) will show elevated oxygen saturation and will likely appear bright red like arterial blood due to reduced tissue extraction of oxygen.
    - Blood cyanide concentrations can be measured but will unlikely result in a clinically useful time frame.
- Treatment
  - Supportive care
    - Remove from exposure (if applicable).
  - Decontamination
    - Remove clothing and decontaminate skin (if applicable).
  - Antidote
    - Hydroxocobalamin
      - Reacts with cyanide to form cyanocobalamin (vitamin B_{12}), which is excreted in the urine
      - Preferred agent in all patients
      - Empiric treatment in patients with smoke exposure
    - Sodium nitrite and sodium thiosulfate
      - Contraindicated in patients with carbon monoxide toxicity and in pregnancy
      - Sodium nitrite: induces methemoglobinemia, which binds cyanide to form cyanmethemoglobin
      - Sodium thiosulfate: sulfur donor that complexes with cyanmethemoglobin to form thiocyanate, which is renally excreted
    - Cyanide antidote kit (discontinued in the United States)
      - Contraindicated in patients with carbon monoxide toxicity and in pregnancy
      - Amyl nitrates: inhaled nitrate induces methemoglobinemia.
      - Sodium nitrite: administered IV, once IV access established to induce methemoglobinemia
      - Sodium thiosulfate
  - HD
    - HD may be required to remove thiocyanate from patients with renal failure.

- Carbon monoxide (CO)
  - CO is a colorless, odorless gas produced by incomplete combustion of fuels and organic materials.
  - Sources of exposure include smoke inhalation from fires, vehicle exhaust, improperly vented gas stoves, and improperly functioning furnaces.
  - Mechanism and toxicity
    - CO binds hemoglobin with a higher affinity than oxygen to form carboxyhemoglobin (COHb), which impairs oxygen delivery (shifts oxyhemoglobin dissociation curve left) and causes cellular hypoxia.
    - Extravascular CO can bind cytochromes and NADPH reductase, causing impaired oxidative phosphorylation.
    - CO precipitates inflammatory cascade that causes cellular injury.
    - CO and cyanide poisoning can occur simultaneously following smoke inhalation.
    - Occurs from intentional and unintentional poisoning
  - Clinical features
    - Neurologic
      - Headache, dizziness, weakness, fatigue, confusion
      - Seizures, syncope, coma
      - Delayed sequelae: memory loss, personality changes, chorea
    - Cardiovascular: tachycardia, chest pain, myocardial ischemia, cardiac arrest
    - Respiratory: tachypnea, dyspnea, cough
    - GI: nausea, vomiting
    - Metabolic: lactic acidosis
    - Renal: rhabdomyolysis
  - Diagnosis
    - Suspect in patients with headache, nausea, and vomiting who are victims of fire or in cold climates, especially when multiple patients present with the same symptoms at the same time (i.e., a family)
    - Laboratory evaluation
      - COHb levels
        - COHb levels are elevated in smokers (up to 10%).
        - Inaccurate measurement occurs after hydroxocobalamin administration.
      - ABG
        - Pao_2 level may be normal as O_2 level reflects amount of dissolved oxygen, which is unaffected by CO poisoning.
        - Hemoglobin-bound O_2 will be reduced.
      - BMP and lactate
  - Treatment
    - Supportive care
      - Remove the patient from CO source.
      - Administer 100% oxygen via high-flow oxygen, or endotracheal intubation if required.
    - Antidote
      - Hyperbaric oxygen
        - Reduces CO half-life
        - Indications
          - COHb >25%
          - COHb >15% in pregnancy or evidence of fetal distress
          - LOC
          - Severe metabolic acidosis
          - End-organ dysfunction: coma, seizure, ECG changes and/or elevated troponin, respiratory failure, neurologic deficit
          - Persistent neurologic symptoms

- Methemoglobinemia
  - Mechanism and toxicity
    - Methemoglobin is formed when ferrous iron (Fe^{2+}) is oxidized to ferric iron (Fe^{3+}) in hemoglobin.

Ferric iron does not bind oxygen and also causes the remaining ferrous iron of hemoglobin to have increased affinity for oxygen. This results in a left shift of the oxyhemoglobin dissociation curve.
- Reduced oxygen delivery is a result of reduced oxygen binding by ferric iron and the increased affinity of remaining ferrous iron.
- Acquired methemoglobinemia can occur after exposure to nitrates and nitrites, sulfonamides, dapsone, phenazopyridine, local and topical anesthetics including benzocaine and lidocaine, and rasburicase, among other exposures.
- Congenital methemoglobinemia can occur as well.
- Patients with G6PD deficiency are predisposed to developing methemoglobinemia after exposure to suspect medications.

- Clinical features
  - Severity of symptoms correlates with methemoglobin level.
  - Neurologic: headache, lightheadedness, fatigue, lethargy, coma, seizure
  - Respiratory: tachypnea, dyspnea, hypoxia
  - Skin: cyanosis, pale, gray, or blue colored skin, lips, nailbeds
- Diagnosis
  - Suspect in a patient with cyanosis and/or hypoxia that does not resolve with supplemental oxygen
  - Laboratory evaluation
    - ABG
      - Appearance: chocolate brown color
      - Normal Pao_2
      - Normal Sao_2 (falsely elevated)
      - Elevated methemoglobin level (co-oximetry)
    - Pulse oximetry
      - Spo_2 will be ~85%, will not improve with supplemental oxygen.
    - Co-oximetry
      - Noninvasive device able to measure methemoglobin by its absorbance spectrum at 630 nm
- Treatment
  - Supportive care
    - Discontinue precipitating agents or remove the patient from exposure.
  - Antidote
    - Methylene blue: facilitates reduction of Fe^{3+} to Fe^{2+}
      - Indications: symptomatic patients
      - Contraindications: patients with G6PD deficiency
    - Ascorbic acid may be helpful in patients with contraindication to methylene blue (i.e., G6PD deficiency).

Toxic Alcohols

- Ethanol
  - Most common intoxication in the emergency department (ED). Can be found in cold medications, household cleaners, vanilla extract, aftershave, and mouthwash in addition to common forms
  - Mechanism
    - Ethanol is converted to acetaldehyde via ADH, which is converted to acetic acid via acetaldehyde dehydrogenase (Figure 16.3.5).

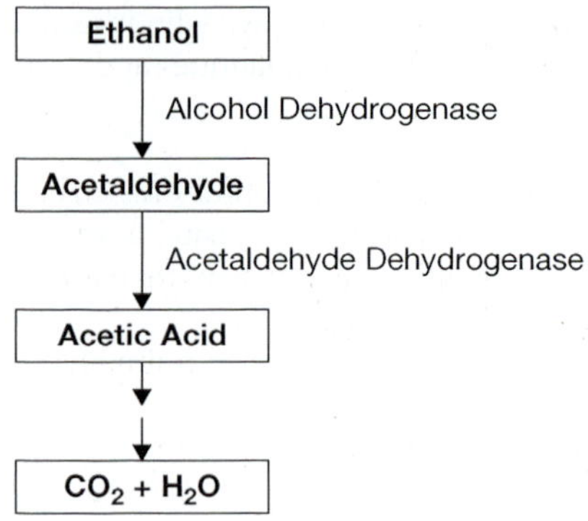

FIGURE 16.3.5 **Ethanol metabolism.**

    - Peak concentration: 1 hour
    - Elimination: hepatic by zero-order kinetics
  - Clinical features
    - Increased sociability may occur at low doses.
    - Slurred speech, nystagmus, ataxia, CNS and respiratory depression, and coma may occur at higher doses.
    - Patients with alcohol use disorder may be malnourished and have hypoglycemia, electrolyte abnormalities, depletion of folate, vitamin B_{12}, and thiamine.
  - Diagnosis
    - History and physical examination consistent with alcohol intoxication
    - Serum ethanol concentration
  - Treatment
    - Supportive care
    - Decontamination
      - Due to rapid absorption, GI decontamination has no role.
- Methanol
  - Found in windshield washing fluid, paint removers, solid cooking fuel, and used as an ethanol substitute as moonshine
  - Methanol produced in alcohol distillation process
  - Mechanism
    - Methanol is metabolized into the toxic metabolite, formaldehyde and formic acid (Figure 16.3.6).
    - Almost completely absorbed
    - Peak concentration: 1 hour
    - Elimination: hepatic by zero-order kinetics
  - Clinical features
    - Stage 1 (0-6 hours): mimics ethanol intoxication
      - Dizzy, ataxic, confused
      - Nausea, vomiting, abdominal pain

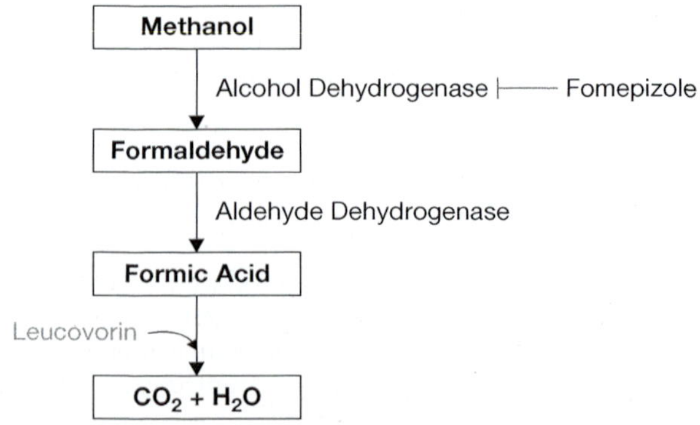

FIGURE 16.3.6 **Methanol metabolism.**

- Stage 2 (6-30 hours): latent phase may occur.
  - Inebriation resolves.
  - Can be asymptomatic
- Stage 3 (6-72 hours)
  - Blurred vision, central scotoma, hyperemic optic discs, blindness
  - Seizure, coma, cerebral edema, herniation
  - Cardiorespiratory failure
- Toxicity
  - Formic acid causes direct cellular injury to the retina and basal ganglia.
  - Serious toxicity at low volumes
  - Lethal dose: 1 g/kg
- Diagnosis
  - History and physical examination consistent with toxic alcohol ingestion
  - High osmolar gap
  - High AG metabolic acidosis
  - Visual changes
  - Serum methanol, ethanol, ethylene glycol, and isopropyl concentrations should be obtained. Although methanol, ethylene glycol, and isopropyl alcohol concentrations may not result quickly. Treatment should not wait until lab results are obtained.
- Treatment
  - Supportive care
    - Folic acid or leucovorin can be given to help facilitate metabolism of formic acid to carbon dioxide and water.
  - Decontamination
    - Due to rapid absorption, GI decontamination has no role.
  - Antidote
    - Fomepizole: inhibits ADH
  - HD
    - Indications
      - Serum methanol concentration ≥50 mg/dL
      - Severe acidosis
      - Evidence of end-organ damage (e.g., blindness)

- Ethylene glycol
  - Found in antifreeze, household cleaning products
  - May be consumed as an ethanol substitute or to inflict self-harm
  - Mechanism
    - Ethylene glycol is converted into the toxic metabolites, glycolic acid, oxalic acid, which can precipitate in the kidneys, causing renal failure (Figure 16.3.7).
    - Elimination: hepatic by first-order kinetics
  - Clinical features and toxicity
    - Stage 1 (30 minutes-12 hours)
      - Nausea, vomiting, abdominal pain
      - Ataxia, nystagmus
      - CNS depression, coma, seizure
    - Stage 2 (12-14 hours)
      - Myocardial dysfunction, shock
      - Tachypnea, ARDS
    - Stage 3 (24-72 hours)
      - Renal failure caused by glycolate-induced damage and tubule obstruction by oxalic acid
    - Stage 4
      - Late neurologic sequelae
  - Toxicity
    - Oxalic acid causes direct cellular injury to renal tubules.
    - Serious toxicity at low volumes
    - Lethal dose: 1 g/kg
  - Diagnosis
    - History and physical examination consistent with toxic alcohol ingestion
    - High osmolar gap
    - High AG metabolic acidosis
    - Elevated lactate
      - May represent true lactate elevation or may be falsely elevated due to inability to differentiate between lactate and glycolic acid or glyoxylic acid
      - Urinalysis (UA) may show oxalic acid crystals.
    - Acute renal failure
  - Treatment
    - Supportive care
      - Thiamine and pyridoxine may help facilitate conversion of oxalic acid to nontoxic metabolites.
    - Decontamination
      - Due to rapid absorption, GI decontamination has no role.

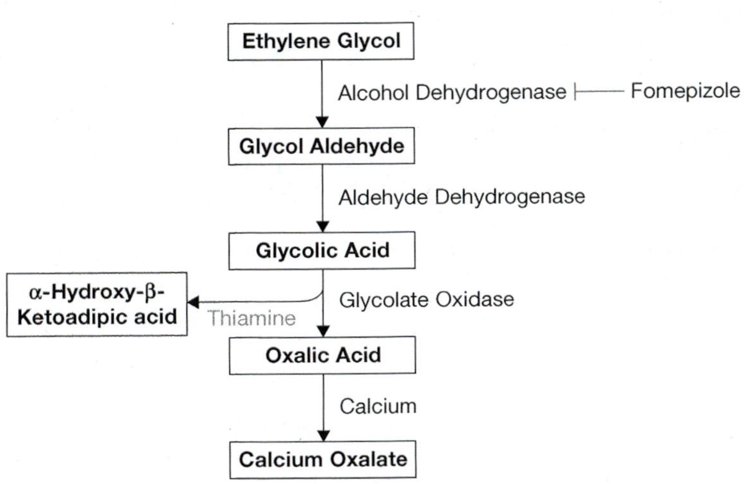

FIGURE 16.3.7 **Ethylene glycol metabolism.**

- Antidote
  - Fomepizole inhibits conversion of ethylene glycol to oxalic acid.
  - Ethanol can also be used as a competitive ADH inhibitor.
- HD
  - Indications
    - Serum ethylene glycol concentration >50 mg/dL
    - Severe acidosis
    - Evidence of end-organ damage (e.g., renal failure)

- Isopropyl alcohol
  - Sedative-hypnotic agent results in clinical intoxication similar to ethanol.
  - Found in disinfectants, antifreeze, hand sanitizers, solvents, and as a 70% solution in rubbing alcohol
  - Mechanism
    - Metabolized by ADH to acetone
    - Acetone is a ketone, which cannot be metabolized to an organic acid like methanol and ethylene glycol.
    - Peak concentration: 1 hour after ingestion
  - Toxicity and clinical features
    - Toxicity can occur after oral ingestion or via dermal exposure, especially in infants.
    - Symptoms include disinhibition, sedation, stupor, coma, nausea, vomiting, and abdominal pain.
    - May appreciate a fruity odor from the intoxicated patient
    - Massive ingestion: hematemesis, pulmonary edema, hemorrhage, tracheobronchitis, shock
  - Diagnosis
    - History and physical examination consistent with alcohol intoxication
    - High osmolar gap
    - No metabolic acidosis
    - "Ketosis without acidosis"
  - Treatment
    - Supportive care
    - Decontamination
      - Due to rapid absorption, GI decontamination has no role.
    - Antidote
      - No indication for fomepizole
    - HD should be considered after massive ingestion.
- Propylene glycol
  - Used as a diluent for commonly used medications, including lorazepam, diazepam, phenytoin, and phenobarbital. Also used in cosmetics and as a solvent
  - Mechanism
    - Propylene glycol is converted to lactaldehyde by ADH and to lactic acid by aldehyde dehydrogenase (Figure 16.3.8).
  - Toxicity and clinical features
    - Propylene glycol toxicity is dose and rate dependent.
    - Can cause intoxication similar to ethanol
    - Massive ingestions
      - Lactic acidosis, hypoglycemia, seizures, and coma
      - Cardiovascular: arrhythmias, hypotension, and shock
      - Renal: renal failure
  - Diagnosis
    - History and physical examination
    - Laboratory evaluation
      - Complete blood count (CBC), BMP, lactate, ABG, ECG

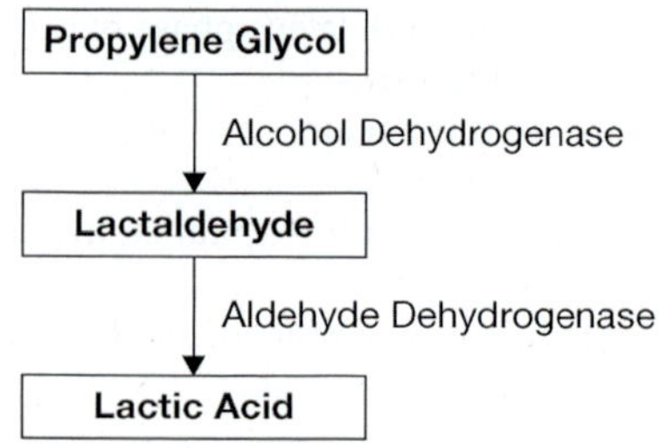

FIGURE 16.3.8 Propylene glycol metabolism.

  - Treatment
    - Supportive care
      - Stop the offending medication.
    - HD recommended
- Organophosphates and carbamates
  - Examples
    - Nerve gas: sarin, VX
    - Pesticides: parathion, chlorpyrifos, phosalone, diazinon
    - Medications: neostigmine, pyridostigmine, edrophonium, donepezil
  - Mechanism
    - Organophosphates bind to and inhibit AChE, leading to increased synaptic ACh and thus increased muscarinic and nicotinic receptor agonism.
    - AChE-organophosphorus compounds can undergo a conformation change (i.e., aging), which results in irreversible resistance to reactivation.
  - Clinical features
    - Cholinergic toxicity (Table 16.3.1)
      - Muscarinic effects mnemonic: SLUDGE and DUMBBELLSS
      - Nicotinic symptoms: muscle weakness, fasciculation, paralysis
    - Delirium, seizures, coma
  - Diagnosis
    - History and physical examination suggestive of exposure
  - Treatment
    - Supportive care
      - Close airway monitoring due to secretion production, depressed mental status, and nicotinic effects (i.e., weakness and paralysis)
    - Decontamination
      - Surface decontamination should occur immediately to prevent contamination of first responders and health care personnel.
    - Antidote
      - Atropine: anticholinergic used for patients with hemodynamically significant bradycardia and with excessive secretion burden
        - End point of therapy: drying of secretions
      - Pralidoxime (2-PAM): reactivates cholinesterase by displacing enzyme (i.e., cholinesterase inhibitor) from its receptor site
- Scombroid food poisoning
  - Associated with consuming improperly handled dark-meat fish including tuna, mahi-mahi, mackerel, sardine, marlin, and skipjack, among others. Can also occur after consuming contaminated Swiss cheese

- Toxicology
  - Scombroid poisoning occurs as a result of improperly stored fish at temperatures >4 °C/40 °F. These temperatures facilitate bacterial overgrowth that produce histidine decarboxylase, thus converting histidine to histamine and other biogenic amines.
  - High levels of histamine and other amines are heat and freeze stable.
- Clinical features
  - Signs and symptoms usually begin with an hour and are consistent with histamine poisoning.
  - Patients may report a peppery or metallic taste to the fish.
  - Neurologic: headache, lightheadedness, burry vision
  - GI: nausea, vomiting, diarrhea, abdominal cramping
  - Cardiovascular: tachycardia, palpitations; cardiac arrhythmias and shock are rare.
  - Respiratory: bronchospasm
  - Skin: cutaneous flushing, urticarial rash
- Diagnosis
  - History and physical examination
    - Rapid symptom onset after eating dark-meat fish or cheese
    - Flushing and urticarial rash with GI symptoms
    - Symptomatic improvement with antihistamine use
- Treatment
  - Supportive care
    - IV fluids and antiemetics as needed
  - Antidote: antihistamines directly treat the etiology of illness.

- Ciguatera
  - Foodborne illness caused by consuming reef fish contaminated by a heat-stable toxin produced by the dinoflagellate *Gambierdiscus toxicus*
  - Associated with eating barracuda, grouper, amberjack, moray eel, and red snapper, among others
  - Toxicology
    - Ciguatera fish poisoning is caused by multiple toxins, the most well known is ciguatoxin.
    - Ciguatoxin is a heat-stable, lipid-soluble, acid-resistant neurotoxin that causes voltage-dependent sodium channels to open, resulting in membrane depolarization.
  - Clinical features
    - Neurologic
      - Symptoms usually begin 3 to 72 hours after consumption.
      - Dysesthesia (hot-cold reversal), perioral paresthesia, pruritis, metallic taste in mouth, sensation of loose teeth, ataxia, and coma
    - Cardiovascular
      - Symptoms occur within hours.
      - Bradycardia, conduction delay, and hypotension
    - GI
      - Symptoms usually begin 3 to 6 hours after consumption.
      - Nausea, vomiting, diarrhea, and abdominal pain
  - Diagnosis
    - History and physical examination
    - Confirmation of ciguatoxin in the consumed fish, if possible
    - Ciguatera poisoning is a reportable condition in many states within the United States. However, all cases of ciguatera poisoning should be reported to local health authorities to identify potential outbreaks.
  - Treatment
    - Supportive care
      - Antiemetics and IV fluids as needed
      - Atropine is effective for symptomatic bradycardia.
      - Antihistamines for pruritis
      - Mannitol may be beneficial for neurologic effects.

Industrial Toxins

- Lead
  - Heavy metal used in manufacturing processes. Adult toxicity is primarily from occupational exposure. Pediatric toxicity is commonly from ingestion of lead-containing materials (e.g., paint, toys, water).
  - Mechanism
    - Lead inhibits many biologic processes including heme synthesis and many cellular enzymes.
    - Absorption: respiratory and GI tract, primarily
    - Half-life: 30 days
      - >10 years in patients with chronic exposure as lead is stored in bones
    - Elimination: renal
  - Clinical features
    - Some patients may be asymptomatic.
    - Developmental impacts: decreased learning and memory, impaired speech and hearing functions, lower IQ, early signs of attention-deficit/hyperactivity disorder (ADHD)
    - Neurologic: headache, difficulty concentrating, fatigue, irritability, lethargy, tremor, depression, short-term memory deficits. At high blood lead levels (BLLs), patients may develop encephalopathy and seizures.
    - GI: nausea, vomiting, abdominal pain and cramping, constipation, anorexia
    - Hematologic: anemia
    - Musculoskeletal: arthralgias, myalgias
    - Cutaneous: lead line on the gingival tissue
  - Lab evaluation
    - CBC with differential, BLL, erythrocyte protoporphyrin, BMP, liver panel, UA
  - Treatment
    - Chelation therapy should be guided under the supervision of a topic expert (i.e., clinical toxicologist).
    - Children
      - Asymptomatic children with BLL 45 to 69 μg/dL
      - Symptomatic children or BLL ≥70 μg/dL
        - Hospitalize, report case per local and national laws, and consult with toxicologist.
        - Asymptomatic children: succimer (2,3-dimercaptosuccinic acid, DMSA)
        - Symptomatic children: first, administer British anti-Lewisite (BAL), then administer IV $CaNa_2$-EDTA 48 hours later
    - Adults
      - Symptomatic patients with BLL >50 μg/dL
      - Most patients if BLL >80 μg/dL
      - All patients if BLL >100 μg/dL
- Mercury
  - Found in commercial products, dental fillings, and used during industrial processes, including electroplating

and mining. Historically used in thermometers. High mercury levels found in many fish
- Mercury toxicity occurs after exposure to the elemental form and to organic and inorganic mercury.
- Mechanism
  - Reacts with sulfhydryl groups to cause inhibition of multiple cellular enzymes
  - Elemental mercury
    - A volatile liquid at room temperature that readily forms a vapor. Exposure is primarily inhalational.
    - GI absorption is poor.
    - Elimination: small amount exhaled, primarily eliminated in feces
  - Inorganic mercury
    - Found as a mercury salt in various oxidation states
    - Exposure is primarily via ingestion or via dermal or mucosal absorption.
  - Organic mercury
    - Found as lipophilic organomercuric compounds, such as dimethylmercury and thimerosal
    - Found in high concentrations in many fish and in vaccines
- Clinical features—elemental mercury
  - Acute
    - Excessive salivation, gum inflammation
    - Cough, dyspnea, chest pain, pneumonitis, respiratory distress
    - Nausea, vomiting, diarrhea
    - Conjunctivitis and dermatitis
  - Chronic
    - Erethismus mercurialis, a constellation of symptoms including tremor, excitability, irritability, fearfulness, insomnia, memory loss, fatigue, weakness
    - Acrodynia, also known as "pink disease," is characterized by rash, edema, and desquamation of palms and soles.
    - Nausea, anorexia
    - Diaphoresis
    - Renal failure
- Clinical features—inorganic mercury
  - Acute
    - Metallic taste
    - Renal failure
    - Hemorrhagic gastroenteritis, massive volume loss leads to shock.
  - Chronic
    - Gingivitis, stomatitis
    - Irritability
    - Nephrotic syndrome
    - Acrodynia
- Clinical features—organic mercury
  - Acute
    - Nausea, vomiting, diarrhea
  - Chronic
    - Primarily neurologic toxicity, including paresthesias, ataxia, dysarthria, deafness
    - Acrodynia
- Toxicity
  - Elemental mercury: primary site of deposition is CNS.
  - Inorganic mercury: primary sites of deposition are the kidneys.
  - Organic mercury: primary sites of deposition are the CNS, kidneys, liver, and hair.
- Diagnosis
  - History and physical examination consistent with mercury exposure
  - May have work history including mining, smelting, electroplating, or work with mercury containing light bulbs or other mercury-containing products
  - Serum and urine mercury concentration
- Treatment
  - Supportive care
  - Antidote
    - Chelation with BAL/dimercaprol, or DMSA/succimer
    - Penicillamine is rarely used.

- Arsenic
  - Used in pesticides, wood preservatives, metal alloys, and in glass manufacturing
  - Can contaminate drinking water from soil runoff and mining
  - Also used in gas form, arsine, in semiconductor manufacturing, and during ore refining
  - Mechanism
    - Reacts with hydrogen, oxygen, chlorine, carbon, and sulfur and inhibits cellular oxidative phosphorylation
    - Good GI and dermal absorption
    - Elimination: renal
  - Toxicity
    - Acute
      - Neurologic: confusion, seizures, coma
      - GI: nausea, vomiting, diarrhea
    - Chronic
      - Can develop over months to years
      - Neurologic: peripheral neuropathy, headache, ataxia
      - Skin: hyperpigmentation, hyperkeratosis, transverse white lines on nails (i.e., mees lines)
      - Cancer: lung, bladder, skin, kidney, liver, prostate
    - Arsine gas
      - Primary toxicity occurs via inhalation.
      - Respiratory: pulmonary edema
      - GI: nausea, vomiting, abdominal pain
      - Hematologic: acute intravascular hemolysis
  - Diagnosis
    - History and physical examination consistent with exposure
    - Chronic exposure may result in insidious symptom onset. Consider in patients with occupational exposures.
    - 24-hour urine arsenic levels
  - Treatment
    - Supportive care
    - Antidote
      - Chelation with BAL or DMSA
- Hydrogen fluoride
  - Highly corrosive inorganic acid found in rust removers, automotive wheel cleaners, and is used in semiconductor production, among other uses
  - Mechanism
    - Directly caustic to tissues
    - Complexes with calcium and magnesium, leading to hypocalcemia and hypomagnesemia, respectively

- Toxicity
  - Toxicity can occur via dermal exposure or through ingestion.
  - Timing of symptom onset directly correlated with concentration.
- Clinical features
  - Hypocalcemia
    - Tetany, weakness, Chvostek sign
    - Dysrhythmias
  - Hypomagnesemia
    - Weakness, dysrhythmias
  - Hyperkalemia
    - ECG abnormalities, arrhythmias
  - Burns
    - Blistering with surrounding erythema, pain may continue due to extension into deep tissue.
- Diagnosis
  - History and physical examination consistent with ingestion or exposure
  - ECG findings suggestive of hypocalcemia
  - Serum calcium and ionized calcium
- Treatment
  - Supportive care
    - Calcium and magnesium supplementation
  - Decontamination
    - Copious irrigation with water to limit dermal exposure
  - Antidote
    - Calcium chloride or calcium gluconate
    - Calcium complexes with and neutralizes fluoride ions and can be administered as a topical agent for burns and IV for systemic toxicity.

Household Chemicals

- Hydrocarbons
  - Hydrocarbons are commonly found in household products, solvents, and used as fuels. These include butane, octane, benzene, toluene, naphthalene, and chloroform, among others.
  - Inhalants can be misused (i.e., huffing) for their euphoric effects.
  - Mechanism
    - Route of ingestion influences the toxicity.
  - Clinical features and toxicity
    - Neurologic
      - CNS depression related to direct neuronal injury and due to hypoxemia from pulmonary toxicity
      - Headache, ataxia, agitation
      - Chronic toxicity can result in cerebellar dysfunction, peripheral neuropathies, and leukoencephalopathy.
    - Respiratory: inhalational exposures can result in chemical pneumonitis and ARDS.
    - GI: nausea and vomiting
    - Cardiovascular: myocardial sensitization to catecholamines leads to arrhythmias.
  - Diagnosis
    - History and physical examination
    - Chest x-ray in patients with suspected inhalation injury
  - Treatment
    - Supportive care
- Caustics
  - Many household products are corrosive and may cause burns and tissue necrosis. These include bleaches, oven cleaners, degreasers, and toilet bowl cleaners.
  - Mechanism
    - Acids
      - Coagulative necrosis
    - Bases
      - Liquefactive necrosis
      - Deep tissue injury may occur slowly.
  - Clinical features and toxicity
    - Toxicity depends on agent and route of exposure.
    - Ingestion: chest and abdominal pain, vomiting, dysphagia, dysphonia, perforation
      - Scarring and strictures may develop after recovery.
    - Aspiration: airway burns, upper airway edema, stridor, airway obstruction
    - Skin: pain, burn
    - Eyes: pain, hyperemia, chemosis, vision changes, globe rupture
  - Diagnosis
    - History and physical examination consistent with exposure to caustic agent
  - Treatment
    - Supportive care
      - Early intubation if airway is involved
      - Urgent endoscopy may help for assessing severity.
      - Surgical consultation for GI perforation
    - Decontamination
      - Large-volume irrigation of skin for dermal exposures
- Electrical injuries
  - Injury patters differ depending on if victim is exposed to direct current (DC) or alternating current (AC).
  - Lightning delivers high-voltage DC, whereas electrical outlets deliver alternating current.
  - Mechanism
    - Direct electrical injury can cause ventricular arrhythmias.
    - Thermal injury
      - Tissue damage occurs as electrical energy is converted to thermal energy.
      - Higher resistance tissues (e.g., bones, skin, fat) heat up and may coagulate.
    - Electroporation
      - Electrical current disrupts cell membranes, causing cell death.
    - Mechanical trauma
      - Lightning strikes (i.e., high-voltage DC) can throw a victim's body and increase the risk of trauma. Lightning may also cause blast trauma or damage surrounding objects to expose the victim to blunt or penetrating trauma.
    - Mechanisms specific to lightning strikes
      - Direct: lightning strikes the victim.
      - Contact strike: lightning strikes nearby object that victim is touching.
      - Side-flash: electrical arc burn occurs when a nearby object is struck and the electrical current jumps through air to strike the victim.
      - Ground strike: lightning strikes the ground and travels to the victim via ground.

- Clinical features
  - Neurologic
    - DC: keraunoparalysis and autonomic dysfunction, tympanic membrane (TM) rupture, tinnitus, hearing loss, cataracts, vision loss
  - Cardiovascular
    - AC: ventricular arrhtyhmias
    - DC: asystole, myocardial damage
  - Dermal
    - AC: extensive tissue damage
    - DC: minor superficial burns, Lichtenburg figure (pathognomonic for lighting injury, appears as a superficial ferning pattern).
  - Renal
    - AKI, rhabdomyolysis
  - Musculoskeletal
    - Prolonged exposure to alternating current can stimulate muscle contraction and cause tetany.
    - Deep tissue injury can lead to edema, necrosis, and compartment syndrome.
- Diagnosis
  - History and physical examination
  - Obtain ECG to evaluate for conduction abnormalities.
- Treatment
  - Supportive care
    - Lightning strike victims in cardiac arrest should receive immediate intervention.
  - Special populations
    - Pregnancy: fetal mortality is high after high-voltage injury. Pregnant women should undergo fetal monitoring.
    - Pediatric: oral burns are common in young children who chew on power cords. Children with significant oral injuries should be admitted for closer monitoring.

Dysbarism

- Decompression sickness
  - Mechanism
    - Dissolved nitrogen saturates tissues under pressure as a diver descends. Upon ascent, nitrogen gas may precipitate out of solution to form bubbles. The location of these bubbles gives rise to the specific symptoms.
  - Risk factors
    - Increasing dive depth
    - Rapidity of ascent
    - Multiple dives during a short duration (i.e., cumulative dive duration and depth)
    - Air travel (i.e., decreased ambient pressure) within 24 hours following dive
    - Right-to-left shunt
    - Obesity
  - Clinical features
    - Onset is usually within 6 hours.
    - The bends: arthralgias and myalgias
    - The chokes: dyspnea, dry cough, chest pain
    - The staggers: vertigo, tinnitus, nausea
    - Skin bends: pruritis, burning
    - Neurologic: paresthesias, paralysis
    - Skin: purpura marmorata
  - Diagnosis
    - History and physical examination
    - Evaluate dive logs for cumulative duration and number of dives, depth, and decompression stops.
  - Treatment
    - Supportive care
      - Provide 100% oxygen and lay the patient flat.
      - Hydration (IV or PO)
    - Antidote
      - Hyperbaric oxygen therapy
- Arterial gas embolism
  - Severe form of decompression illness in which precipitated bubbles nucleate and embolize
  - Clinical features
    - Presents within 10 to 20 minutes of ascent
    - Cerebral embolism: stroke
    - Coronary artery embolism: myocardial infarction
    - Pulmonary embolism: dyspnea, hemoptysis, chest pain
  - Diagnosis
    - Suspect in any diver who surfaces unconsciousness or loses consciousness very soon after surfacing
  - Treatment
    - Supportive care
      - Provide 100% oxygen and lay the patient flat.
      - Hydration (IV or PO)
    - Antidote
      - Hyperbaric oxygen therapy
- Nitrogen narcosis
  - Results from breathing air under pressure at depths, typically, >30 m
  - Clinical features
    - Similar to alcohol intoxication
    - Symptoms worsen at increasing depths and include
      - Euphoria, poor judgment, slowed reaction time
      - Hallucinations and syncope
  - Treatment
    - Ascend to surface

Envenomation

- Viperidae family
  - Also known as pit vipers, the Viperidae family includes rattlesnakes (Crotalidae), copperheads (*Agkistrodon contortrix*), and cottonmouths (aka water moccasin, *Agkistrodon piscivorus*).
  - Majority of snake envenomations in the United States
  - Toxicity
    - Venom causes local tissue damage and systemic toxicity.
  - Clinical features
    - Dependent upon species
    - Local tissue
      - Pain, swelling, ecchymoses, and erythema
      - Bullae
    - Neurologic
      - Perioral paresthesia, dysarthria, dysphagia, myokymia, weakness, paralysis
    - GI
      - Nausea, vomiting, diarrhea
    - Cardiovascular
      - Tachycardia, hypotension

            - Renal
                - Rhabdomyolysis
            - Hematologic
                - Coagulopathy: thrombocytopenia, prolonged prothrombin time, and hypofibrinogenemia
        - Diagnosis
            - History and physical examination may or may not include bite marks.
            - Obtain CBC, PT/INR, PTT, and fibrinogen.
            - BMP and UA
        - Treatment
            - Supportive care
                - Immobilize extremity, minimize activity.
                - Do not use a tourniquet.
            - Antidote
                - Polyvalent Crotalinae ovine immune Fab (CroFab/FabAV)
- Elapidae family
    - Coral snakes are found in the United States, while cobras, kraits, and mambas are found outside the United States.
    - Toxicity
        - Coral snake venom irreversibly binds ACh receptors.
    - Clinical features
        - Local tissue damage
            - Pain and swelling
        - Neurologic
            - Weakness, paresthesias, paralysis
            - Diplopia, slurred speech, dysphagia
        - Respiratory paralysis
        - Hematologic
            - Coagulopathy not likely following North American coral snake bite
    - Treatment
        - Supportive care
            - Evaluate for muscle weakness or paralysis, intubate if needed.
            - Neostigmine unlikely to be beneficial for eastern or Texas coral snakebite. May be reasonable to trial for coral snakebites outside the United States
        - Antidote
            - Antivenom
- Black widow spider
    - *Latrodectus* spp is found in woodpiles, barns, outhouses, and sheds in the United States, Southern Canada, and some species are found globally.
    - Toxicity
        - Neurotoxin results in release of ACh and norepinephrine and causes muscle cramping and systemic effects.
    - Clinical features
        - Bite site: target lesion with pain and erythema
        - Cardiovascular: tachycardia, hypertension
        - GI: nausea, vomiting
        - Musculoskeletal: abdominal, back, leg pain and cramping
        - Children may present with severe symptoms, including seizures, and cardiac and respiratory failure.
    - Diagnosis
        - History and physical examination consistent with black widow bite in endemic regions
        - Consider in patients with a spider bite and abdominal pain or cramping.
    - Treatment
        - Supportive care
            - Opioid analgesia
            - Benzodiazepines for muscle spasms
        - Antidote
            - Black widow spider antivenom, reserved for severe symptoms and high-risk patients
- Brown recluse spider
    - *Loxosceles reclusa* is found in wood piles, under rocks, and in attics in the United States. *Loxosceles* sp are found globally in South America, South Africa, and Australia.
    - Toxicity
        - *Loxosceles* venom contains cytotoxic properties that cause local tissue damage (i.e., necrotic wound) and may cause systemic toxicity.
    - Clinical features
        - Bite site
            - Initially, painless. Small puncture marks with surrounding erythema.
            - Pain develops over 8 hours.
            - Bullae progress to necrosis over several days.
        - Systemic symptoms
            - Constitutional: fevers, chills
            - GI: nausea, vomiting
            - Renal: rhabdomyolysis
            - Hematologic: hemolytic anemia or disseminated intravascular coagulation (DIC)
    - Diagnosis
        - History and physical examination
        - Consider in patients with a spider bite and local necrotic wound.
        - Evaluate for systemic toxicity: CBC, BMP, UA, PT/INR, PTT, fibrinogen.
    - Treatment
        - Supportive care
            - Local wound care
            - Delayed debridement
        - Antidote
            - Antivenom is NOT available in the United States.

Recommended Reading

Alapat PM, Zimmerman JL. Toxicology in the critical care unit. *Chest*. 2008;133(4):1006-1013. doi:10.1378/chest.07-1840

Benson BE, Hoppu K, Troutman WG, et al. Position paper update: gastric lavage for gastrointestinal decontamination. *Clin Toxicol (Phila)*. 2013;51(3):140-146. doi:10.3109/15563650.2013.770154

Brooks DE, Levine M, O'Connor AD, French RNE, Curry SC. Toxicology in the ICU: Part 2: specific toxins. *Chest*. 2011;140(4):1072-1085. doi:10.1378/chest.10-2726

Calello DP, Liu KD, Wiegand TJ, et al. Extracorporeal treatment for metformin poisoning: systematic review and recommendations from the Extracorporeal Treatments in Poisoning Workgroup. *Crit Care Med*. 2015;43(8):1716-1730. doi:10.1097/CCM.0000000000001002

Cao D, Arens AM, Chow SL, et al. Part 10: Adult and pediatric special circumstances of resuscitation: 2025 American Heart Association Guidelines for cardiopulmonary resuscitation and emergency cardiovascular care. *Circulation*. 2025;152(16_suppl_2):S578-S672. doi:10.1161/CIR.0000000000001380

Caravati EM, Mégarbane B. Update of position papers on gastrointestinal decontamination for acute overdose. *Clin Toxicol (Phila)*. 2013;51(3):127. doi:10.3109/15563650.2013.772625

Dart RC, Mullins ME, Matoushek T, et al. Management of acetaminophen poisoning in the US and Canada: a consensus statement. *JAMA Netw Open*. 2023;6(8):e2327739. doi:10.1001/jamanetworkopen.2023.27739

Decker BS, Goldfarb DS, Dargan PI, et al. Extracorporeal treatment for lithium poisoning: systematic review and recommendations from the EXTRIP workgroup. *Clin J Am Soc Nephrol*. 2015;10(5):875-887. doi:10.2215/CJN.10021014

Fontana RJ, Liou I, Reuben A, et al. AASLD practice guidance on drug, herbal, and dietary supplement-induced liver injury. *Hepatology*. 2023; 77(3):1036-1065. doi:10.1002/hep.32689

Ghannoum M, Gosselin S, Hoffman RS, et al. Extracorporeal treatment for ethylene glycol poisoning: systematic review and recommendations from the EXTRIP workgroup. *Crit Care*. 2023;27(1):56. doi:10.1186/s13054-022-04227-2

Ghannoum M, Wiegand TJ, Liu KD, et al. Extracorporeal treatment for theophylline poisoning: systematic review and recommendations from the EXTRIP workgroup. *Clin Toxicol (Phila)*. 2015;53(4):215-229. doi:10.3109/15563650.2015.1014907

Ghannoum M, Yates C, Galvao TF, et al. Extracorporeal treatment for carbamazepine poisoning: systematic review and recommendations from the EXTRIP workgroup. *Clin Toxicol (Phila)*. 2014;52(10):993-1004. doi:10.3109/15563650.2014.973572

Hall AH, Rumack BH. Clinical toxicology of cyanide. *Ann Emerg Med*. 1986;15(9):1067-1074. doi:10.1016/s0196-0644(86)80131-7

Holstege CP, Borek HA. Toxidromes. *Crit Care Clin*. 2012;28(4):479-498. doi:10.1016/j.ccc.2012.07.008

Juurlink DN, Gosselin S, Kielstein JT, et al. Extracorporeal treatment for salicylate poisoning: systematic review and recommendations from the EXTRIP workgroup. *Ann Emerg Med*. 2015;66(2):165-181. doi:10.1016/j.annemergmed.2015.03.031

Kraut JA, Kurtz I. Toxic alcohol ingestions: clinical features, diagnosis, and management. *Clin J Am Soc Nephrol*. 2008;3(1):208-225. doi:10.2215/CJN.03220807

Kraut JA, Mullins ME. Toxic alcohols. *N Engl J Med*. 2018;378(3):270-280. doi:10.1056/NEJMra1615295

Lavonas EJ, Akpunonu PD, Arens AM, et al. 2023 American Heart Association focused update on the management of patients with cardiac arrest or life-threatening toxicity due to poisoning: an update to the American Heart Association Guidelines for Cardiopulmonary Resuscitation and Emergency Cardiovascular Care. *Circulation*. 2023;148(16):e149-e184. doi:10.1161/CIR.0000000000001161

Levine M, Brooks DE, Truitt CA, Wolk BJ, Boyer EW, Ruha AM. Toxicology in the ICU: Part 1: general overview and approach to treatment. *Chest*. 2011;140(3):795-806. doi:10.1378/chest.10-2548

Levine M, Ruha AM, Graeme K, Brooks DE, Canning J, Curry SC. Toxicology in the ICU: part 3: natural toxins. *Chest*. 2011;140(5):1357-1370. doi:10.1378/chest.11-0295

Mactier R, Laliberté M, Mardini J, et al. Extracorporeal treatment for barbiturate poisoning: recommendations from the EXTRIP workgroup. *Am J Kidney Dis*. 2014;64(3):347-358. doi:10.1053/j.ajkd.2014.04.031

Malhi GS, Tanious M, Das P, Coulston CM, Berk M. Potential mechanisms of action of lithium in bipolar disorder: current understanding. *CNS Drugs*. 2013;27(2):135-153. doi:10.1007/s40263-013-0039-0

Mehta AN, Emmett JB, Emmett M. GOLD MARK: an anion gap mnemonic for the 21st century. *Lancet*. 2008;372(9642):892. doi:10.1016/S0140-6736(08)61398-7

Mowry JB, Burdmann EA, Anseeuw K, et al. Extracorporeal treatment for digoxin poisoning: systematic review and recommendations from the EXTRIP workgroup. *Clin Toxicol (Phila)*. 2016;54(2):103-114. doi:10.3109/15563650.2015.1118488

Mowry JB, Shepherd G, Hoffman RS, et al. Extracorporeal treatments for isoniazid poisoning: systematic review and recommendations from the EXTRIP workgroup. *Pharmacotherapy*. 2021;41(5):463-478. doi:10.1002/phar.2519

Ornillo C, Harbord N. Fundaments of toxicology-approach to the poisoned patient. *Adv Chronic Kidney Dis*. 2020;27(1):5-10. doi:10.1053/j.ackd.2019.12.001

Purssell RA, Pudek M, Brubacher J, Abu-Laban RB. Derivation and validation of a formula to calculate the contribution of ethanol to the osmolal gap. *Ann Emerg Med*. 2001;38(6):653-659. doi:10.1067/mem.2001.119455

Reisinger A, Rabensteiner J, Hackl G. Diagnosis of acute intoxications in critically ill patients: focus on biomarkers—part 1: epidemiology, methodology and general overview. *Biomarkers*. 2020;25(1):9-19. doi:10.1080/1354750X.2019.1694994

Reisinger A, Rabensteiner J, Hackl G. Diagnosis of acute intoxications in critically ill patients: focus on biomarkers—part 2: markers for specific intoxications. *Biomarkers*. 2020;25(2):112-125. doi:10.1080/1354750X.2020.1725787

Riederer AM, Campleman SL, Carlson RG, et al. Acute poisonings from synthetic cannabinoids—50 U.S. Toxicology Investigators Consortium Registry Sites, 2010-2015. *MMWR Morb Mortal Wkly Rep*. 2016; 65(27):692-695. doi:10.15585/mmwr.mm6527a2

Roberts DM, Yates C, Megarbane B, et al. Recommendations for the role of extracorporeal treatments in the management of acute methanol poisoning: a systematic review and consensus statement. *Crit Care Med*. 2015;43(2):461-472. doi:10.1097/CCM.0000000000000708

Ross JA, Borek HA, Holstege CP, King JD. Toxic alcohol poisoning. *Emerg Med Clin North Am*. 2022;40(2):327-341. doi:10.1016/j.emc.2022.01.012

Rumack BH, Peterson RC, Koch GG, Amara IA. Acetaminophen overdose: 662 cases with evaluation of oral acetylcysteine treatment. *Arch Intern Med*. 1981;141(3 spec no):380-385. doi:10.1001/archinte.141.3.380

Santos CF, Gomes R. Syndrome of irreversible lithium-effectuated neurotoxicity (SILENT): a review. *Eur Psychiatry*. 2022;65(suppl 1):S717. doi:10.1192/j.eurpsy.2022.1850

Shepherd G, Velez LI. Role of hydroxocobalamin in acute cyanide poisoning. *Ann Pharmacother*. 2008;42(5):661-669. doi:10.1345/aph.1K559

Shingina A, Mukhtar N, Wakim-Fleming J, et al. Acute liver failure guidelines. *Am J Gastroenterol*. 2023;118(7):1128-1153. doi:10.14309/ajg.0000000000002340

Simpson MD, Cole JB. Developments in the epidemiology of calcium channel blocker poisoning and implications for management. *Curr Opin Crit Care*. 2024;30(6):603-610. doi:10.1097/MCC.0000000000001218

United States Environmental Protection Agency Office of Pesticide Programs. Chapter 5 Organophosphate Insecticides. 2013:43-55.

Weaver LK. Carbon monoxide poisoning. In: Richard E. Moon M, eds. *Hyperbaric Medicine Indications Manual*. 14th ed. Best Publishing Company; 2019:81-104.

Wightman RS, Nelson LS. Acetaminophen. In: Tintinalli JE, Yealy DM, Meckler GD, Stapczynski J, Cline DM, Thomas SH., eds. *Tintinalli's Emergency Medicine: A Comprehensive Study Guide*. 9th ed. McGraw-Hill Education; 2020.

SECTION 17

Transfusion Therapy

Section Editor: Marvin G. Chang

17.1

Transfusion Medicine

Patricia A. R. Brunker

Transfusion Therapy

- An integral part of the critical care practice is the administration of blood and blood component therapies. Intensivists must be knowledgeable about the indications, benefits, risks, and adverse effects associated with the use of various blood components.
- Transfusion support is usually required in case of decreased production, increased utilization, destruction, and loss or dysfunction of red cells, platelets (PLTs), or coagulation factors.

Available Blood Products

- Whole blood (WB) and low-titer O whole blood (LTOWB)
  - *General information*
    - WB is derived by phlebotomy of 450 to 500 mL of peripheral blood from eligible allogeneic donors. 14 mL of anticoagulant are present for each 100 mL of blood. If a PLT-sparing leukocyte reduction (LR) filter was used in collection, it contains ~5.5 $\times 10^{10}$ PLTs (see whole blood-derived platelets [WBD-PLTs] below).
    - Although occasionally used in pediatrics for ABO-identical recipients, WB is most commonly encountered in trauma resuscitation or emergent massive transfusion settings as LTOWB.
    - LTOWB is stored at 1 to 6 °C and has a variable outdated according to the anticoagulant. To be used in ABO-untyped individuals, the anti-A and anti-B isohemagglutinin titers of the product must be known prior to labeling to minimize passive hemolysis in non-O recipients. There is no standard titer threshold, although most LTOWB in the United States use a 1:200 limit. Typically, a maximum "out-of-group" plasma limit is set by hospitals and is around 600 mL of incompatible plasma or around 4 units of WB.
    - Since donor plasma is part of LTOWB, donors are males or never pregnant females to mitigate the risk of transfusion-related acute lung injury (TRALI; see later).
  - *Indications*
    - Like the familiar component (packed red blood cells [pRBCs]), WB is indicated in patients with symptomatic anemia to restore oxygen-carrying capacity.
    - In emergency settings or situations such as massive transfusion, when multiple blood components may be simultaneously indicated, LTOWB can be used.
      - Use has increased in military settings due to ease of administration (ie, infusing one bag with three blood components), but data in civilian trauma, including field administration by first responders, are mixed.
  - *Special considerations*
    - Leukocyte-reduced WB (LR-WB) can be manufactured using PLT-sparing LR filters, although some in vitro data suggest decreased hemostatic potential when compared to non–LR-WB.
    - Due partly to storage in refrigerated conditions, PLT function in WB is controversial, and most hospitals do not transfuse WB that is >15 days old but instead opt to manufacture pRBCs from residual inventory.
    - Send two specimens for ABO and Rh typing (as well as antibody screen determination) as promptly as possible to permit transitioning to type-specific component therapy after an initial WB resuscitation.
    - If available, RhD-negative LTOWB is preferred for children or women of childbearing age for whom RhD status is unknown; however, DO NOT DELAY administration of LTOWB that is RhD positive in emergent situations.
- RBCs
  - *General information*
    - pRBCs are obtained by centrifugation or apheresis (a centrifugal process where double-volume donations can be collected) methods from WB donations.
    - pRBCs are anticoagulated with citrate and are generally mixed with a preservative solution that increases the storage period to up to 42 days at 1 to 6 °C, depending on the preservative.

- One unit of compatible RBCs, which contains ~250 to 300 mL of volume with a hematocrit of 55% to 65%, will increase the hemoglobin (Hgb) level by ~1 g/dL or hematocrit by 3% in an average-sized, nonbleeding or hemolyzing adult.
- Donor RBCs must be ABO compatible (Table 17.1.1).

Indications

- RBCs are indicated in patients with symptomatic anemia to restore oxygen-carrying capacity.
- Hypovolemia of any cause without a significant reduction in cell mass should be managed with crystalloid/colloid solutions.
  - In the setting of massive bleeding (>1-2 L/h), RBCs should be considered a replacement solution.
- While the optimal threshold for transfusion is not established, the use of Hgb levels alone is discouraged.
  - The decision to transfuse or not should be based on the clinical situation (volume status, shock or hypoperfusion, duration and severity of anemia, and cardiopulmonary status).
- In hemodynamically stable patients without coronary artery disease (CAD), a lower Hgb trigger for transfusion (transfuse if Hgb <7) has proved to be as effective as a higher Hgb trigger (Hgb <10). Patients with CAD benefit from an Hgb trigger of 8.0 g/dL in most circumstances.

Special considerations

- LR-RBCs are generally prepared by prestorage filtration in the blood bank but can also be accomplished at the bedside.
- LR-RBCs are primarily indicated in the following situations:
  - Prevention of cytomegalovirus (CMV) in organ transplant recipients
  - Prevention of human leukocyte antigen (HLA) immunization (causing refractoriness to PLT transfusion)
  - Prevention of nonhemolytic febrile transfusion reaction
- Washed red cells are useful in preventing severe allergic transfusion reactions mediated by recipient antibodies (immunoglobulin E [IgE]) to donor soluble proteins.
  - The isotonic saline washing process virtually removes all the donor's plasma proteins.
  - Washing causes mechanical hemolysis and decreases RBC yield in the transfused product.
  - Washing blood products can introduce bacteria into the product.

TABLE 17.1.1 RBC and Plasma Compatibility

Recipient	RBC Donor	Fresh Frozen Plasma Donor
AB	AB, A, B, or O	AB
A	A or O	A or AB
B	B or O	B or AB
O	O	AB, A, B, or O
RhD+	RhD+ or RhD−	RhD+ or RhD−
RhD−	RhD−	RhD+ or RhD−

RBC, red blood cell.

  - Washed cells must be transfused within 24 hours if kept at 1 to 6 °C.
- Frozen red cells are cryoprotected with glycerol and can be stored for >10 years with good viability.
  - Once thawed and deglycerolized, they must be transfused within 24 hours.
  - This can be useful in military settings and for rare phenotypes but requires lead time in the laboratory.
- Although some retrospective studies suggest that transfusing blood stored for a prolonged period of time (>14 days of storage) may be associated with increased morbidity, no prospective data have confirmed such results, including randomized trials.

- PLTs

General information

- Designated as WBD-PLTs or single donor platelets (SDPs), according to the collection method
  - WBD-PLTs (50 mL) are prepared by centrifugation of individual WB units.
    - Typically, six WB-PLTs are pooled prior to transfusion to an adult recipient.
  - SDPs are collected from one single donor using various apheresis devices. SDPs can be collected in a platelet additive solution (PAS) that reduces the plasma content of the unit by about 60% to 70%. PAS may be helpful for patients with repeated allergic transfusion reactions or for giving O PLTs to non-O patients by diluting allergens and isohemagglutinins, respectively.
  - Both preparations are stored at room temperature (20-24 °C) and are licensed for a maximum of 5 days of storage. Alternative testing strategies allow for an extension of up to 7 days of storage.
  - They contain an appreciable volume of plasma. Although optimally released according to ABO compatibility with donor plasma, most adults can tolerate PLTs of any ABO type, and they are issued in a "first-in, first-out" manner.
  - Methods to pathogen reduce PLTs (as well as plasma and cryoprecipitate) are licensed in the United States and European Union (EU) using psoralens and ultraviolet (UV) light. Pathogen reduction allows for 5 days of storage without bacterial sampling, destroys lymphocytes better than irradiation, and renders a product "CMV-safe."
- ~30,000 to 60,000/mm^3 increase in the recipient's PLT count is expected for each SDP or pool of six WBD-PLTs administered.
- Apheresis PLTs and pooled WBD-PLTs have the same hemostatic efficacy.
- The efficacy and role of cold-stored PLTs for hemostasis (rather than prophylaxis) is controversial. Particularly since WB contains PLTs that have been stored in the cold and PLTs stored at room temperature have a short shelf-life, this is an active area of research.

Indications

- PLTs should be administered to correct a decrease in PLT count (thrombocytopenia) or function (thrombocytopathy).
- Given normal PLT function, the target count depends upon the indication for PLT transfusion (prophylactic or therapeutic).

- PLTs are typically maintained at >50,000/mm^3 for the therapeutic management of active bleeding, thrombocytopenia, and disorders of PLT function.
- PLTs are often maintained at >100,000mm^3 for central nervous system or multisystem trauma.
- For prophylactic purposes and to prevent spontaneous hemorrhage, PLTs should be transfused with PLTs of <10,000/mL.

Special considerations

- In the setting of heparin-induced thrombocytopenia, thrombotic thrombocytopenic purpura, and hemolytic-uremic syndrome, PLT transfusion should generally be *avoided* unless in the case of life-threatening bleeding where the benefits may outweigh the risks.
- ABO matching is not strictly necessary, but it is preferred with neonates and small volume pediatric patients who can develop hemolysis from passive transfer of isohemagglutinins (ie, anti-A, anti-B, or anti-A,B) from the donor plasma.
- PLT-related transfusion management decisions should always take into consideration the presence of circulating antiplatelet medications (aspirin [ASA], clopidogrel, GP IIb/IIIa antagonists, etc), herbal compounds (garlic, Danshen, etc), alloantibodies, and disorders with known effects on PLT functions like uremia, hypersplenism, disseminated intravascular coagulopathy (DIC), and sepsis.
- For surgery-related PLT management, see Table 17.1.2.

- Plasma products

Fresh frozen plasma (FFP)

- General information
  - Plasma is the remaining part of the WB after removal of PLTs and cellular elements, containing the clotting factors.
  - Serum refers to plasma from which the clotting factors have been removed and is not a transfusable blood product.

TABLE 17.1.2 Surgery-Related Platelet (PLT) Transfusion Management

Surgery	PLT Threshold for Transfusion
Procedure with expected insignificant blood loss/vaginal delivery	<10,000/mm^3
Surgical/OB patients with microvascular bleeding	<50,000/mm^3
Cardiothoracic surgery	No prophylaxis needed. Transfuse if microvascular bleeding with normal coagulation and PLTs <100,000/mm^3.
Neuro or ophthalmic surgery	>100,000/mm^3
Central line placement (CVP), paracentesis/thoracentesis, respiratory tract/gastrointestinal (GI) biopsies, lumbar puncture, sinus aspiration, dental extractions	>20,000/mm^3
Spinal/epidural anesthesia	No evidence-based data
Fiberoptic bronchoscopy/GI endoscopy without biopsy	>20,000/mm^3

  - The product is generally frozen within 8 hours of phlebotomy to prevent inactivation of factors V and VIII, which are temperature sensitive.
    - At a temperature <−18 °C, FFP can be stored for up to 1 year.
  - Before transfusion, the product must be thawed in a water bath at 37 °C for ~30 minutes. It is typically transfused within 24 hours.
  - If not, then thawed plasma can be stored for an additional 4 days at 1 to 6 °C with excellent hemostatic effect.
    - Factors V and VIII fall to 80% and 60% of normal in this case, respectively.
- Indications
  - Use FFP for the treatment of microvascular bleeding due to congenital or acquired coagulopathies resulting in prolongation of either the partial thromboplastin time (PTT) or prothrombin time (PT) >1.5 times normal.
- Special considerations
  - In general, sufficient hemostasis can be achieved when the activity of coagulation factors is at least 25% to 30% of normal and the level of fibrinogen is at least 75 to 100 mg/dL.
  - Therefore, for an average adult, a dose of ~10 to 15 mL/kg (3-5 units) FFP.
    - Donor plasma must be either ABO identical or ABO compatible with the recipient (Table 17.1.1).
  - Volume loading should be considered.
  - FFP should not be transfused prophylactically as a volume expander or as a source of nutrition.

Cryoprecipitate

- General information
  - Cryoprecipitate antihemophilic factor is prepared from a unit of FFP by thawing it at 4 °C (1-10 °C) and collecting (through centrifugation) the cold-insoluble precipitate that remains.
  - It can be stored at −18 °C for up to 1 year.
  - Cryoprecipitate contains concentrated levels of fibrinogen (150-250 mg), factor VIII:C (80-150 IU), factor VIII:vWF (von Willebrand factor), and factor XIII and fibronectin in 5 to 15 mL of plasma.
  - For fibrinogen replacement, 1 unit per 10 kg body weight increases plasma fibrinogen by ~50 to 70 mg in the absence of massive consumption/hemorrhage (minimum hemostatic level of fibrinogen is 70-100 mg/dL).
  - Usually available as prepooled bags from five donors
- Indications
  - Cryoprecipitate is used primarily to augment fibrinogen in the case of depleted levels because of massive hemorrhage or DIC.
  - It can be used prophylactically in nonbleeding perioperative or peripartum patients with congenital fibrinogen deficiencies or von Willebrand disease (vWD) (unresponsive to desmopressin).
  - Reversal of tissue plasminogen activator

Coagulation factors

- Plasma derivatives

- *Fibrinogen concentrates (RiaSTAP)*
  - Indicated for bleeding in congenital fibrinogen deficiency
- *Thrombin (Evithrom)*
- Topical product applicable to tissue when minor bleeding control is ineffective through standard procedures
- *Prothrombin complex concentrates (PCCs)*
  - "4-factor PCCs" (K-Centra, Octaplex, Beriplex) are concentrates of purified prothrombin proteins (factors II, VII, IX, and X).
    - The products also contain proteins C and S.
    - K-Centra is approved in the United States and is used for warfarin reversal.
  - Factor IX concentrates (Profiline, Bebulin, and Konyne) are available in the United States and contain three factors (II, IX, and X).
    - They are licensed for use in the treatment of factor IX deficiency (hemophilia B).
  - Activated PCCs (FEIBA) are also available in the United States.
    - They can be used to bypass the intrinsic pathway of the coagulation process and be used to treat patients with factor VIII or factor IX inhibitors.
    - Activated PCCs have a high potential for thrombotic side effects.

- Recombinant DNA produced coagulation factors.
  - *Factors VIII and IX*
    - Their production has been the most important in the evolution of the treatment of hemophilia. These factors are produced by cloning the genes for factors VIII (hemophilia A) and IX (hemophilia B).
  - *Factor VIIa (Novo-Seven)*
    - Provides rapid control of bleeding in patients with hemophilia A and B with inhibitors. Factor VIIa is also an effective treatment for congenital factor VII deficiency.
  - *Others*
    - Factor IX (BeneFIX): provides rapid control of bleeding in patients with hemophilia B. Used for perioperative management and prophylaxis
    - vWF (Vonvendi): for bleeding control, perioperative management, and prophylaxis, particularly for type 3 vWD

Compatibility Testing

- Pretransfusion compatibility testing is performed to prevent transfusion of incompatible blood that may result in a hemolytic transfusion reaction. Type & screen and crossmatch are crucial pretransfusion tests.
- Type
  - ABO group is determined by typing patient's RBCs using anti-A and anti-B reagents (forward type) or by testing the patient's serum against A and B reagent cells (reverse type).
  - In addition, patient's RBCs are tested with anti-D for the presence (RhD positive or "Rh positive") or absence (RhD negative) of the RhD antigen (a.k.a. "D antigen").
  - Many RhD variants exist, resulting in Rh types beyond simply "positive" or "negative."
- Screen
  - Screening involves incubating the patient's serum with two or three selected reagent red cell panels containing all of the critical non-ABO antigens.
  - The screen is considered positive if an antibody is detected in the patient's serum.
  - Antibodies causing a positive screen may be autoantibodies or alloantibodies. Interference may also occur from medication, including daratumumab (anti-CD38).
- Crossmatch
  - *Serologic*
    - Patient's serum is incubated with an aliquot of red cells from a specific donor.
    - Immediate spin—most useful for antibodies against ABO system antigens
      - Short incubation time (seconds) at room temperature
    - Anti-human globulin technique (indirect Coombs test)
      - Needs long incubation time (15-30 minutes) at 37 °C and is indicated for clinically significant non-ABO red cell antigens
  - *Electronic/computer*
    - For patients with no clinically significant antibodies and no history of a clinically significant antibody, an electronic or "computer" crossmatch may be performed instead of a serologic crossmatch, and it is based on validated computer algorithms.

Risks of Transfusion

- Immunologic complications
  - *Immediate*
    - Hemolytic transfusion reaction
      - It results from the destruction of donor RBCs by preformed recipient antibodies.
      - ABO incompatibility can result in fatal reactions with as little of 5 mL.
      - There is great variation in the clinical effects of an ABO-incompatible mistransfusion, ranging from no reaction to death.
      - Notify the blood bank IMMEDIATELY if a hemolytic reaction is suspected.
    - Allergic reactions
      - They usually occur as urticarial, wheezing, or angioedematous reactions.
      - There is no way to predict the occurrence of allergic reactions.
      - They usually respond to antihistamines, corticosteroids, and epinephrine.
      - Premedication is not indicated for most patients.
    - Anaphylactoid reactions
      - Characterized by autonomic dysregulation, dyspnea, pulmonary/laryngeal edema, and broncho/laryngospasm
      - They may occur in absolutely IgA-deficient patients with anti-IgA antibodies.
    - TRALI
      - Acutely increased permeability of pulmonary circulation leading to massive fluid and protein leakage into the alveoli and interstitium
      - It usually occurs within 6 hours of transfusion.

- TRALI results when the donor has antibodies against recipient's HLA.
- Antibodies against neutrophil antigen HNA-3a are also particularly dangerous.
- These antibodies bind to the recipient lungs and damage the endothelial-alveolar interface by activating the complement system.
- Donor antibodies to HLA (the cause of TRALI) are essentially restricted to multiparous female donors, who become HLA sensitized during their pregnancies.
  - Therefore, screening for the presence of HLA antibodies or exclusion of females with a history of pregnancy has significantly reduced the risk for TRALI.
- Therapy is supportive.

- Immune-mediated PLT destruction
  - It occurs in the recipient as a result of alloantibodies to HLA or PLT-specific antigens on transfused PLTs.
  - It causes PLT refractoriness: (ie, lack of the expected rise in PLT count posttransfusion). However, the cause of PLT refractoriness in post patients is nonimmune (ie, splenomegaly, sepsis, or other consumption).
- Febrile nonhemolytic reaction
  - It is defined as a temperature elevation by ≥1 °C during or up to 8 hours after a transfusion without another cause.
  - It may be the result of antibodies against white cells or the action of cytokines, either transfused or generated by the recipient.
  - It may accompany about 1% of transfusions.

Delayed

- Delayed hemolytic reaction
  - They occur more frequently than acute ones but are often mild.
  - Hemolysis is gradual (often 7-15 days posttransfusion), and jaundice, hemoglobinuria, and falling Hgb concentrations can gradually develop due to hemolysis of donor RBCs.
  - An anamnestic immune response to previous alloimmunization is often the cause.
- Alloimmunization
  - It can be toward antigen of red or white cells, PLTs, or plasma proteins and may occur unpredictably after transfusion.
  - If a component expressing the antigen to which the recipient has been previously immunized, hemolysis can be triggered.
  - Antibodies can decrease below the level of detection of routine screening tests so giving a FULL transfusion history to the blood bank is essential to respect all prior alloantibodies.
- Posttransfusion purpura (PTP)
  - PTP is a rare syndrome characterized by dramatic, sudden, and self-limiting thrombocytopenia 7 to 10 days after a blood transfusion in a patient previously sensitized (transfusion or pregnancy).
  - The reaction may be directed to a PLT antigen the patient lacks, and both the autologous and allogeneic PLTs are destroyed.
  - In a bleeding patient, high-dose intravenous immunoglobulin should be administered.
- Transfusion-associated graft-versus-host disease (TA-GVHD)
  - TA-GVHD is a rare but extremely dangerous complication with a 90% to 100% mortality rate.
  - It occurs when donor T lymphocytes react against recipient's tissues, particularly causing severe bone marrow suppression.
  - Development of TA-GVHD is possible even after a small number of T lymphocytes are transfused, if the recipient is unable to mount an immune response against transfused donor T lymphocytes (eg, in immunocompromised patients).
  - Irradiation of the product is the only approved preventive strategy at present for RBC components. PLTs can also undergo irradiation. Products that have ever been frozen without a cryoprotectant (eg, plasma or cryoprecipitate) do not require irradiation since leukocytes are extremely unlikely to survive the freezing and thawing processes.
  - Psoralen treatment during the pathogen reduction process is an additional approved method to mitigate TA-GVHD for PLT products in the United States.
  - Transfusions from family-related directed donors greatly increase the risk of TA-GVHD and MUST be irradiated.

Nonimmunologic complications

Infectious diseases

- Safety measures, such as improved screening tests, have dramatically reduced the risk of acquiring a viral infection from a blood transfusion. Recent estimates are as follows:
  - 1 in 200,000 to 1 in 360,000 for hepatitis B
  - 1 in 1 million to 1 in 2 million for hepatitis C
  - 1 in 1.5 million to 1 in 2 million for HIV
  - 1 in 2 million for human T-cell lymphoma/leukemia virus
- CMV may unpredictably be present in donor's white cells (up to 70% of donors).
  - It may be a concern in low-birth weight preterm infants of CMV-negative mothers and in immunocompromised patients.
  - LR, pathogen reduction, and CMV antibody screening of the component can reduce the risk in these subjects.
- Collections from states with endemic babesiosis are screened for antibodies to *Babesia* spp.
- There are no routinely available tests for the many other potentially transmissible infectious agents.
  - These agents include parvovirus, *Leishmania*, plasmodia, rickettsia, *Borrelia*, *Brucella*, prions, and certain Trypanosomes.

Bacterial contamination

- Bacterial contamination is rare but can cause acute, severe effects.
- Onset of high fever, severe chills, hypotension, or circulatory collapse during or immediately after transfusion should raise suspicion.
- PLTs stored at room temperature, products whose bag is opened by manipulation (eg, washing or

pooling without using a sterile dock) are at higher risk for bacterial contamination.
    - Pathogen reduction has reduced septic transfusion reactions in PLT products due to many bacteria, but rare cases, including organisms that cause biofilms, have been reported.
- *Transfusion-associated circulatory overload (TACO)*
    - It can occur after transfusion of excessive volume at a rapid rate and leads to pulmonary edema.
    - Patients with underlying heart failure, arrhythmias, renal failure, and pulmonary disease are at particular risk.
    - TACO is the leading cause of transfusion-associated mortality in the United States (32% of reported fatalities from 2017 to 2021).
- *Hypothermia*
    - Rapid infusion of large volumes of cold blood can depress body temperature.
    - Shock, surgery, and anesthesia increase the risk of hypothermia.
    - Blood warming devices should be considered in these situations.
- *Metabolic complications*
    - Citrate toxicity
        - Citrate toxicity results from a reduction of ionized calcium due to the presence of high citrate concentrations.
        - Patients with severe liver disease metabolize citrate slowly, and this leads to increased risk of rapid-onset hypocalcemia.
    - Other metabolic complications
        - Acidosis, alkalosis, and hyper-hypokalemia can accompany rapid/large volume transfusions.

SUGGESTED READINGS

American Association of Blood Banks; Standards Program Committee. *Standards for Blood Banks and Transfusion Services*. 34th ed. Association for the Advancement of Blood & Biotherapies; 2024.

American Society of Anesthesiologists Task Force on Perioperative Blood Management. Practice Guidelines for Perioperative Blood Management: An Updated Report by the American Society of Anesthesiologists Task Force on Perioperative Blood Management. *Anesthesiology*. 2015; 122(2),241-275.

Arynov A, Kaidarova D, Kabon B. Alternative blood transfusion triggers: a narrative review. 2024;24(1):71.

Bilgin YM, van de Watering LM, Eijsman L, et al. Double-blind, randomized controlled trial on the effect of leukocyte-depleted erythrocyte transfusions in cardiac valve surgery. *Circulation*. 2004;109:2755-2760.

British Committee for Standards in Haematology, Blood Transfusion Task Force. Guidelines for the use of platelet transfusions. *Br J Haematol*. 2003; 122:10-23.

Bulle EB, Klanderman RB, Pendergrast J, Cserti-Gazdewich C, Callum J, Vlaar AP. The recipe for TACO: a narrative review on the pathophysiology and potential mitigation strategies of transfusion-associated circulatory overload. *Blood Rev*. 2022;52:100891.

Carson JL, Stanworth SJ, Guyatt G, et al. Red blood cell transfusion: 2023 AABB international guidelines. *JAMA*. 2023;330(19):1892-1902.

Cohn CS, Shaz BH. Blood and its components. *JAMA*. 2023;330(19): 1903-1904.

De Rie MA, van der Plas-van Dalen CM, Engelfriet CP, von dem Borne AE. The serology of febrile transfusion reactions. *Vox Sang*. 1985;49:126-134.

Despotis GJ, Santoro SA, Spitznagel E, et al. On-site prothrombin time, activated partial thromboplastin time, and platelet count: a comparison between whole blood and laboratory assays with coagulation factor analysis in patients presenting for cardiac surgery. *Anesthesiology*. 1994; 80:338-351.

Dzik W, Rao A. Why do physicians request fresh frozen plasma? *Transfusion*. 2004;44(9):1393-1394.

Gajic O, Dzik WH, Toy P. Fresh frozen plasma and platelet transfusion for nonbleeding patients in the intensive care unit: benefit or harm? *Crit Care Med*. 2006;34:S170-S173.

Go AS, Leong TK, Sung SH, et al. Thromboembolism after treatment with 4-factor prothrombin complex concentrate or plasma for warfarin-related bleeding. *J Thromb Thrombolysis*. 2022;54(3):470-479.

Godbey EA. Whole blood transfusion: past, present, and future. *Clin Lab Med*. 2021;41(4):659-667.

Guinn NR, Resar LM, Frank SM. Perioperative management of patients for whom transfusion is not an option. *Anesthesiology*. 2021;134(6):939-948.

Hillyer CD, Emmens RK, Zago-Novaretti M, Berkman EM. Methods for the reduction of transfusion-transmitted cytomegalovirus infection: filtration versus the use of seronegative donor units. *Transfusion*. 1994; 34:929-934.

Juffermans NP, Aubron C, Duranteau J, et al. Transfusion in the mechanically ventilated patient. *Intensive Care Med*. 2020;46:2450-2457.

Kaufman RM, Djulbegovic B, Gernsheimer T, et al. Platelet transfusion: a clinical practice guideline from the AABB. *Ann Intern Med*. 2015;162(3): 205-213.

Klein H. Pathogen inactivation technology: cleansing the blood supply. *J Intern Med*. 2005;257:224-261.

Knopfelmacher AM. Transfusion reactions. *Oncologic Crit Care*. 2020;2: 1177-1190.

Koch CG, Li L, Sessler DI, et al. Duration of red-cell storage and complications after cardiac surgery. *N Engl J Med*. 2008;358:1229-1239.

Kochhar M, Neunert C. Immune thrombocytopenia: a review of upfront treatment strategies. *Blood Rev*. 2021;49:100822.

Kracalik I, Kent AG, Villa CH, et al. Posttransfusion sepsis attributable to bacterial contamination in platelet collection set manufacturing facility, United States. *Emerg Infect Dis*. 2023;29(10):1979.

Lehr AR, Hébert P, Fergusson D, Sabri E, Lacroix J. Association between length of storage of transfused packed RBC units and outcome of surgical critically ill adults: a subgroup analysis of the age of blood evaluation randomized trial. *Crit Care Med*. 2023;51(3):e73-e80.

Leslie SD, Toy PT. Laboratory hemostatic abnormalities in massively transfused patients given red blood cells and crystalloid. *Am J Clin Pathol*. 1991;96:770-773.

Napolitano LM, Kurek S, Luchette FA, et al. Clinical practice guideline: red blood cell transfusion in adult trauma and critical care. *Crit Care Med*. 2009;37:3124-3157.

O'Shaughnessy DF, Atterbury C, Bolton Maggs P, et al. Guidelines for the use of fresh-frozen plasma, cryoprecipitate and cryosupernatant. *Br J Haematol*. 2004;126:11-28.

Popovsky MA. Quality of blood components filtered before storage and at the beside: implications for transfusion practice. *Transfusion*. 1996;36: 470-474.

Raasveld SJ, De Bruin S, Reuland MC, et al. Red blood cell transfusion in the intensive care unit. *JAMA*. 2023;330(19):1852-1861.

Remy KE, Yazer MH, Saini A, et al. Effects of platelet-sparing leukocyte reduction and agitation methods on in vitro measures of hemostatic function in cold-stored whole blood. *J Trauma Acute Care Surg*. 2018; 84(6S):S104-S114.

Riess HB, Meier-Hellmann A, Motsch J, Elias M, Kursten FW, Dempfle CE. Prothrombin complex concentrate (Octaplex) in patients requiring immediate reversal of oral anticoagulation. *Thromb Res*. 2007;121:9-16.

Roback JD, Caldwell S, Carson J, et al. Evidence-based practice guidelines for plasma transfusion. *Transfusion*. 2010;50:1227-1239.

Sanders MR, Graeber JE. Posttransfusion graft-versus-host disease in infancy. *J Pediatr*. 1990;117:159-163.

Shah A, Oczkowski S, Aubron C, et al. Transfusion in critical care: past, present and future. *Transfus Med*. 2020;30(6):418-432.

Shander A, Hardy JF, Ozawa S, et al. A global definition of patient blood management. *Anesth Analg*. 2022;135(3):476-488.

Siegal DM, Belley-Côté EP, Lee SF, et al. Small-volume blood collection tubes to reduce transfusions in intensive care: the STRATUS randomized clinical trial. *JAMA*. 2023;330(19):1872-1881.

Slichter SJ, Davis K, Enright H, et al. Factors affecting posttransfusion platelet increments, platelet refractoriness, and platelet transfusion intervals in thrombocytopenic patients. *Blood*. 2005;105:4106-4114.

Van de Watering LM, Hermans J, Houbiers JG, et al. Beneficial effects of leukocyte depletion of transfused blood on postoperative complications in patients undergoing cardiac surgery: a randomized clinical trial. *Circulation*. 1998;97:562-568.

van der Horst RA, Rijnhout TW, Noorman F, et al. Whole blood transfusion in the treatment of acute hemorrhage, a systematic review and meta-analysis. *J Trauma Acute Care Surg*. 2023;95(2):256-266.

van der Meer PF, Klei TR, de Korte D. Quality of platelets in stored whole blood. *Transfus Med Rev*. 2020;34(4):234-241.

van Wonderen SF, Klanderman RB, Vlaar AP. Understanding transfusion-related acute lung injury (TRALI) and its complex pathophysiology. *Blood Transfus*. 2022;20(6):443.

Viel KR, Ameri A, Abshire TC, et al. Inhibitors of factor VIII in black patients with hemophilia. *N Engl J Med*. 2009;360:1618-1627.

Wiesen AR, Hospenthal DR, Byrd JC, Glass KL, Howard RS, Diehl LF. Equilibration of hemoglobin concentration after transfusion in medical inpatients not actively bleeding. *Ann Intern Med*. 1994;121:278-230.

SECTION 18

Transplants

Section Editor: Casey M. Luckhurst

18.1

Transplants: Lung, Heart, Liver, and Other Organs

Richard Teo and Leigh Anne Dageforde

Lung Transplantation

Common Causes to Remember (Table 18.1.1)

Epidemiology

- 2,743 lung transplants were performed in the United States in 2022.
- Most common indication in adults was restrictive lung disease (74%), followed by obstructive lung disease (18%).

Physiologic Considerations

- Bronchial artery circulation not restored, may affect lung parenchyma perfusion and bronchial anastomotic healing.
- Impaired lymphatic drainage increases fluid, immune cells, and inflammatory cytokines, which may increase the risk for primary graft dysfunction.
- Lung denervation leads to abnormalities of brain-lung cross talk (hypoxic vasoconstriction, cough reflex, Hering-Breuer reflex).

Potential Complications

- Primary graft dysfunction
  - A particular form of acute respiratory distress syndrome (ARDS) from ischemia-reperfusion injury
  - Occurs in 20% to 30% of recipients
  - Donor risk factors for primary graft dysfunction: donor age, comorbidities, tobacco use, donation after circulatory determination of death (DCD) status, ischemic time, undersized grafts
  - Recipient risk factors for primary graft dysfunction: recipient age, comorbidities, pulmonary diagnosis (idiopathic pulmonary fibrosis [IPF], sarcoidosis, pulmonary hypertension [PHTN]), need for mechanical ventilation or extracorporeal membrane oxygenation (ECMO) as a bridge to transplant, intraoperative transfusions, cardiopulmonary bypass, oxygen fracture at reperfusion
  - Graded 0 to 3 by the International Society of Heath and Lung Transplantation guidelines based on ratio of P:F ratio and infiltrates on chest x-ray (CXR)
  - Severe forms associated with short-term mortality and morbidity, chronic lung allograft dysfunction, and overall mortality
- Respiratory failure: donor or ventilator-associated pneumonia, acute rejection, bronchial anastomotic dehiscence, cardiogenic pulmonary edema, pulmonary vein stenosis, pulmonary embolism, hemothorax, lung or lobar torsion, phrenic nerve injury
- Shock: hemorrhagic, septic, cardiogenic (right or left ventricular failure), obstructive (tamponade, pulmonary embolism)
- Infection: pneumonia most common bacterial infection, *Pseudomonas* the most common cause; cytomegalovirus (CMV) most common viral infection, prophylaxis and surveillance commonly practiced
- Rejection: acute rejection in 50% of patients within 1 year posttransplant. Bronchoscopy commonly used to rule out infection and obtain transbronchial biopsies to confirm diagnosis
- Others: arrhythmias, pericarditis, gastroesophageal reflux, aspiration, immunosuppression side effects, central nervous system (CNS) complications, intensive care unit (ICU) myopathy

TABLE 18.1.1 Indications for Lung Transplantation and Postoperative Considerations

Indications	Postoperative Considerations
• Chronic obstructive pulmonary disease (COPD) • Idiopathic pulmonary fibrosis (IPF) • Cystic fibrosis (CF) • Alpha-1 antitrypsin deficiency • Pulmonary hypertension (PHTN)/Eisenmenger syndrome	• Ischemia-reperfusion injury • Primary graft dysfunction • Anastomotic dehiscence • Infection • Acute rejection • Adverse effects of immunosuppression

Postoperative Management

- Mechanical ventilation
  - Minimize ventilator-associated lung injury with protective settings, early weaning, and extubation
  - Initial ventilator settings: tidal volume (TV) 6 mL/kg predicted body weight (donor), inspiratory plateau pressure <30 cm H_2O, Spo_2 >90%, pH >2.5
  - Positive end-expiratory pressure (PEEP) adjusted according to the ARDS Network table, avoid PEEP >12 cm H_2O.
  - If P:F ratio <150, consider neuromuscular blockade and inhaled NO.
  - If P:F ratio <100, consider ECMO.
- Hemodynamics
  - Careful fluid management to avoid lung reperfusion injury
  - Requires accurate monitoring of cardiac preload, systemic and pulmonary arterial pressure and vascular resistance, cardiac output, and mixed venous oxygen saturation
  - Goal is to maintain adequate perfusion with the lowest possible cardiac output to reduce the risk of exacerbating lung edema induced by reperfusion injury.
  - Atrial fibrillation with an incidence of 20% to 39%

Outcomes

- Survival of lung transplantation recipients is currently 60% at 5 years (lower than in other solid organ transplants).
- Most limiting factor to long-term survival is the occurrence of obliterative bronchiolitis and its clinical correlate, bronchiolitis obliterans syndrome, which portends chronic rejection.

Heart Transplantation

Indications and Considerations to Remember (Table 18.1.2)

Epidemiology

- 3,668 heart transplants were performed in the United States in 2022.
- 74% of waitlisted patients rely on some form of life support (left ventricular assist device [LVAD], right ventricular assist device [RVAD], inotropes, intra-aortic balloon pump [IABP], ECMO, mechanical ventilator).
- Most common indication in adults cardiomyopathy (64%), followed by coronary artery disease (CAD) (26%)

TABLE 18.1.2 Indications for Heart Transplantation and Postoperative Considerations

Indications	Postoperative Considerations
• Ischemic cardiomyopathy • Congenital heart disease • Valvular disease • Autoimmune/metabolic disease • Pregnancy • Alcohol • Viral	• Denervation • Right ventricular (RV) dysfunction • Ischemia-reperfusion injury • Renal dysfunction/fluid overload • Technical/surgical complications

Physiologic Considerations

- Denervated heart dependent on circulating catecholamines
- Reinnervation generally occurs 1 year posttransplant.
- Various medications are ineffective in the denervated heart.
  - Digoxin has little effect on conduction and cannot be used for rate control in donor hearts developing atrial fibrillation (diltiazem, with a direct effect on the atrioventricular [AV] node, is preferred).
  - Atropine's parasympatholytic effect is negated; beta-adrenergic agonists, such as isoproterenol and epinephrine, are preferred.
  - Reflex tachycardia from nifedipine and hydralazine is absent.

Potential Complications

- Primary graft dysfunction
  - Diagnosis to be made within 24 hours post-op, classified into left ventricle or right ventricle.
  - Risk factors include donor and recipient characteristics, as well as operative factors.
  - May require mechanical circulatory support such as IABP, ECMO, or temporary ventricular assist device (VAD)
  - Associated with increased 30-day and 1-year mortality
- Refractory vasoplegic syndrome
  - No standard definition, generally hypotension within 24 hours post-op with cardiac index >2.2 L/kg/m^2 and systemic vascular resistance (SVR) <800 dyne·s/cm^5
  - Pathophysiology poorly understood
- Right heart failure or PHTN
  - Incidence around 6% for severe right heart failure after transplant
  - Pretransplant PHTN is a risk factor.
  - 45% of primary graft dysfunction with isolated right ventricular dysfunction, percutaneous right ventricular support useful
- Arrhythmias
  - Loss of parasympathetic innervation leads to higher resting heart rate (90-100) and decreased heart rate variability.
  - Afib, Aflutter, and supraventricular tachycardia (SVT) most common

TABLE 18.1.3 Indications for Heart Transplantation and Postoperative Considerations

Indications	Postoperative Considerations
• Alcohol-associated liver disease • Metabolic dysfunction–associated steatohepatitis • Hepatocellular carcinoma • Cholestatic liver disease • Hepatitis C • Hepatitis B • Autoimmune hepatitis • Other malignancy (cholangiocarcinoma, neuroendocrine tumor, colorectal liver metastasis) • Cryptogenic • Fulminant liver failure	• Bleeding • Primary graft nonfunction • Early allograft dysfunction • Hepatic artery/portal venous thrombosis • Biliary leaks/strictures • Small for size syndrome • Infectious • Effects of immunosuppressants

- Ventricular arrhythmias and sudden cardiac death account for 10% of post-heart transplant deaths.
- Sinus node dysfunction and AV block requiring pacemaker implantation are required in 2% to 15%.

Postoperative Management

- Hemodynamics
  - Inotropic support commonly required to support the newly implanted heart.
  - Preload, afterload, and contractility need to be optimized.
  - Low cardiac output and postoperative bleeding must be ruled out for cardiac tamponade.
  - Tricuspid regurgitation is the most common valvular abnormality (19%-84%).
- Rejection
  - Requires endomyocardial biopsies to monitor, diagnose, and classify
  - Majority of cases are subclinical; only 5% to 10% of cases produce significant hemodynamic compromise.
  - Rarely, can manifest as arrhythmias, orthopnea, fever, or dyspnea

Outcomes

- 1-year mortality is 20%, 5-year mortality is 30%.
- Posttransplant CAD
  - Major cause of late mortality
  - 50% incidence within 5 years after transplantation
  - Believed to be due to the recipient's predisposing diagnoses, donor age, rejection, and ischemia-reperfusion injury
  - Intravascular ultrasound is the diagnostic modality of choice due to low sensitivity of coronary angiography.

Liver Transplantation

Indications and Considerations to Remember (Table 18.1.3)

Epidemiology

- 9,527 liver transplants were performed in the United States in 2022.
- 94% were from deceased donors and 6% from living donors.
- Alcohol-associated liver disease is the most common indication for transplant (39%), followed by metabolic-associated steatohepatitis (MASH) (19%).

Key Pathophysiology

- End-stage liver disease affects every organ system.
- Transplantation results in the reversal of the majority of these perturbations.
- Some of which are noticeable within hours of transplantation, and some take months.
  - Neurologic: hepatic encephalopathy
  - Cardiovascular: generally a vasodilatory state; however, high incidence of cirrhotic cardiomyopathy. Alcohol-related cardiomyopathy may coexist.
  - Pulmonary: hepatopulmonary syndrome secondary to arteriovenous malformations (AVMs), portopulmonary hypertension secondary to vasoconstriction and vascular remodeling of pulmonary arteries, hepatic hydrothorax, abdominal ascites
  - Renal: hepatorenal syndrome types 1 and 2 carry increased mortality.
  - Heme: coagulopathy with thrombocytopenia and elevated international normalized ratio (INR)
    - Patients may be prothrombotic despite laboratory values.
    - Higher rates of portal vein thrombosis than the general population
    - Thromboelastography may be useful in determining targets to correct coagulopathy.
  - Immune disease (ID): immunocompromise, increased bacterial translocation from the gut
- Preoperative management and optimization of the effects of end-stage liver disease may correlate with improved outcomes.
- The effects of acute liver failure on organ systems differ slightly from chronic, cirrhotic liver disease, where acute liver failure has a high risk of cerebral edema from hyperammonemia, hypoglycemia, significant metabolic acidosis, renal failure, and hemodynamic instability.

Potential Complications

- Hepatic artery thrombosis
  - Occurs in about 5% of adult liver transplants
  - Leads to biliary complications, decreased patient, and allograft survival
  - Median arcuate ligament syndrome can decrease arterial inflow and predispose to hepatic artery thrombosis.
  - Graft salvage rates low (10%-40%), retransplantation often necessary
- Portal vein thrombosis
  - Most present with transaminitis, but can also present with ascites and gastrointestinal (GI) bleeding
  - Risk factors include preexisting portal vein thrombosis, use of venous conduits, prior shunt surgery, and small portal vein size.
- Early allograft dysfunction (EAD): bilirubin ≥10 mg/dL on day 7, INR ≥1.6 on day 7, and alanine transaminase (ALT) or aspartate transaminase (AST) >2,000 IU/L within the first 7 days
- Primary nonfunction: devastating irreversible extreme of EAD, extent of injury not compatible with survival, urgent retransplantation required for rescue
- Ischemic cholangiopathy: diffuse biliary strictures secondary to prolonged warm ischemia time, typically in DCD grafts
- Small for size syndrome: insufficient liver mass to support the metabolic demand of the patient, seen in living donor liver transplant and partial grafts
- Rejection: often treated empirically with steroids in the early post-op period, especially if tacrolimus levels not therapeutic, biopsy required to differentiate from other causes of liver injury that is, biliary obstruction/drug-induced liver injury

Postoperative Management

- Bleeding
  - Some patients require transfusion of packed red blood cells (PRBCs) after transplant. Many transplant teams will tolerate up to 6 to 8 units of PRBC transfusion before returning to the operating room for a washout.

    - Waiting close to 24 hours prior to a takeback for a washout gives the liver time to function.
    - The drains often sufficiently manage the blood, and hematomas are not always found in the operating room. Isolated sources of bleeding are also not often identified.
- Assessment of graft function
- Clearance of lactate, correction of coagulopathy commonly used. Some transplant teams will request that coagulopathy not be corrected with fresh frozen plasma (FFP) or cryoprecipitate so the trend can be followed.
- Degree of transaminase elevation in general reflective of the extent of ischemic reperfusion injury
- Bilirubin peaks after transaminases.
- Doppler ultrasound used to assess the patency of hepatic vasculature
- Acute kidney injury
    - Some patients may have ongoing renal replacement therapy needs after transplant, either from ongoing hepatorenal syndrome or due to the effects of blood loss and hemodynamic changes perioperatively.
    - Patients who progress to end-stage renal disease (ESRD) after liver transplant do become candidates for an expedited "safety net" kidney transplant.

Outcomes

- 1-year mortality is 7%, 5-year mortality is 20%.

Other Organs

Kidney Transplantation

- Treatment of choice for ESRD
- Improved outcomes compared to dialysis for patients in ever-increasing age groups and with increased cardiovascular disease
- High incidence of CAD in patients with ESRD (35%-50%), even higher in those with diabetes (50%-85%)
- Most common perioperative complication seen in the ICU is related to CAD, with incidence as high as 6.1%. Management is same as with other patients. Discussion with transplant surgical team surrounding antiplatelet and anticoagulation therapy in regard to bleeding risk is needed.
- Older patients are at higher risk of complications from infection and immunosuppression.
- Delayed graft function requiring dialysis is common in up to 30% to 50% of kidney transplant recipients. Dialysis requirements can be continued for up to 6 months, and recipients can still go on to have a functional kidney. Just because a recipient is on dialysis does not mean the kidney has failed.

Pancreas Transplantation

- Performed as simultaneous pancreas-kidney transplant, pancreas transplant alone, or pancreas after kidney transplant
- Volume decreasing in the United States due to the improvement in insulin delivery systems, continuous glucose monitoring technologies, and more stringent donor and recipient selection
- Potential complications: venous thrombosis (10%-35%), enteric anastomotic leak, graft pancreatitis, intra-abdominal sepsis, mycotic aneurysm

Miscellaneous

- Many other organ transplants, including intestinal transplant, multivisceral transplant (combinations of liver, small intestine, pancreas, stomach), and vascularized composite allograft (hand, penile, uterine, face), transplant may present to the ICU.
    - Care of patients guided by principles of surgical complications and immunosuppression
- Neurologic dysfunction posttransplantation is common, and etiologies include stroke, seizures related to calcineurin inhibitors, opportunistic infections, myopathy related to steroids, and encephalopathy
- Immunosuppressive agents have significant side effects in addition to immunosuppression, including renal failure or acute kidney injury, altered glucose metabolism, neurologic complications, drug-drug interactions, and anaphylactoid reactions
- Immunosuppression regimens vary by center, in general:
    - Induction with basiliximab, thymoglobulin, alemtuzumab, and/or corticosteroids, or none
    - Maintenance with triple-drug combination of a calcineurin inhibitor (tacrolimus or cyclosporine), a cell cycle inhibitor (mycophenolate or azathioprine), and corticosteroids. Some centers may use mTOR inhibitors (everolimus or sirolimus) that do impair wound healing and should be considered with subsequent operations.
- Especially for the first 6 months to a year after transplant, transplant patients are at increased risk for opportunistic infections, including Pneumocystis pneumonia (PCP) and CMV, and may be on sulfamethoxazole/trimethoprim or atovaquone (PCP prophylaxis) and famciclovir or valacyclovir (CMV prophylaxis). These medications should be continued in the ICU.
- Donor-derived infections should be on the differential when pursuing an infectious workup.
- Novel perfusion technologies (normothermic/hypothermic machine perfusion, normothermic regional perfusion, ex vivo lung perfusion) are increasingly utilized in the resuscitation, preservation, and assessment of allografts; expanding the donor pool—in particular with DCDs and marginal allografts.

SUGGESTED READINGS

Adegunsoye A, Strek ME, Garrity E, et al. Comprehensive care of the lung transplant patient. *Chest*. 2017;152(1):150-164.

Aref A, Zayan T, Pararajasingam R, Sharma A, Halawa A. Pancreatic transplantation: brief review of the current evidence. *World J Transplant*. 2019; 9(4):81-93.

Bittar J, Arenas P, Chiurchiu C, et al. Renal transplantation in high cardiovascular risk patients. *Transplant Rev*. 2009;23:224-234.

Diamond JM, Arcasoy S, Kennedy CC, et al. Report of the International Society for Heart and Lung Transplantation Working Group on primary lung graft dysfunction, part II: epidemiology, risk factors, and outcomes-A 2016 Consensus Group statement of the International Society for Heart and Lung Transplantation. *J Heart Lung Transplant*. 2017;36:1104-1113.

Di Nardo M, Tikkanen J, Husain S, et al. Postoperative management of lung transplant recipients in the intensive care unit. *Anesthesiology*. 2022;136:482-499.

Kramer DJ, Siegal EM, Frogge SJ, Chadha MS. Perioperative management of the liver transplant recipient. *Crit Care Clin*. 2019;35(1):95-105.

Nesseler N, Mansour A, Cholley B, et al. Perioperative management of heart transplantation: a clinical review. *Anesthesiology*. 2023;139:493-510.

Olthoff KM, Kulik L, Samstein B, et al. Validation of a current definition of early allograft dysfunction in liver transplant recipients and analysis of risk factors. *Liver Transpl*. 2010;16(8):943-949.

Velleca A, Shullo MA, Dhital K, et al. The International Society for Heart and Lung Transplantation (ISHLT) guidelines for the care of heart transplant recipients. *J Heart Lung Transplant*. 2023;42(5):e1-e141.

18.2

Organ Donation

Alban Longchamp

Organ Procurement and Allocation

- In the United States, Organ Procurement Organizations (OPOs) are federally designated entities responsible for identifying potential organ donors, obtaining authorization for donation, determining donor medical suitability, and coordinating the recovery and allocation of donated organs.
- Each OPO serves a defined geographic area and acts as the local operational arm of the national system overseen by the Organ Procurement and Transplantation Network (OPTN).
- The OPTN maintains a computerized national waitlist of transplant candidates and sets policies to promote the equitable allocation of organs.
- Its overarching mission is to maximize the recovery and efficient, fair distribution of a scarce resource: donated deceased donor organs. OPOs are members of the OPTN and are regulated by both the OPTN (under the authority of the United Network for Organ Sharing, or UNOS) and the Centers for Medicare & Medicaid Services (CMS).
- OPOs work in close partnership with donor hospitals, transplant centers, and transplant surgeons to facilitate organ recovery and transplantation.
- Similar organ procurement systems exist globally in countries where deceased donor transplantation is prevalent.
- While the institutional frameworks may vary, ranging from centralized national agencies to regionally coordinated networks, all share a focus on regulated organ stewardship and ethical distribution practices. In all cases, donation activities function under the oversight of national authorities and are anchored by a legal framework that authorizes organ donation, defines institutional responsibilities, sets allocation criteria, and outlines a sustainable financing model.

Deceased Donor Management

- Organ transplantation is the best therapy for patients with end-stage failure.
- Over the past few decades, advances in surgical techniques, critical care, and immunosuppression have dramatically improved outcomes after transplantation, leading to a significant expansion in both indications and patient eligibility.
- This increased utility, however, has not been matched by a proportional increase in the availability of donor organs. As a result, the gap between the number of patients waiting for organs and those receiving transplants continues to increase.
- Organ donation can occur either from living donors or from deceased donors.
  - Deceased organ donation requires that the process of death occurs in a manner compatible with organ preservation, most often within an intensive care unit (ICU).
  - Deceased donors are classified based on the method of death determination: either donation after brain death (DBD) or donation after circulatory determination of death (DCD).
    - In DBD, death is diagnosed based on the irreversible cessation of all brain activity.
    - In DCD, donation occurs after cessation of circulatory and respiratory function.
  - These two pathways differ in both ethical and physiologic considerations, and they require distinct approaches to donor management.

Shifting Landscape of Deceased Donation

- Historically, DBD donors comprised the vast majority of deceased organ donors. However, over the past decade, DCD has become increasingly prevalent.
- In the United States, DCD now accounts for approximately 40% to 50% of all deceased donors, representing a dramatic increase in adoption across transplant centers.
- This rise has been facilitated by improved protocols for DCD organ recovery, advances in organ preservation technologies (eg, normothermic regional perfusion, ex vivo machine perfusion), and growing public and institutional support for donation under circulatory criteria.
- Despite the increase in DCD activity, DBD donors continue to yield a higher number of transplantable organs per donor. This is due to the absence of warm ischemic injury and the more controlled physiologic environment associated with brain death.
- Nonetheless, DCD remains an essential and growing component of the donor pool, particularly for kidney and liver transplantation, and increasingly for heart and lung transplantation.

Critical Care Management of the Deceased Donor

- The success of deceased organ donation and the quality of transplanted organs depend heavily on meticulous donor management.
- The process begins in the ICU with the recognition of a catastrophic brain injury or terminal illness and often continues beyond the formal declaration of death.
- Effective donor management requires close coordination between the ICU team, transplant coordinators, and the local OPO.
- Timely identification of a potential donor and early engagement with families are crucial steps in facilitating successful organ donation.
- Discussions regarding the patient's wishes, advance directives, or registration in a donor registry should be initiated early.
- In the absence of documented consent, discussions with next-of-kin should be handled with compassion, ideally by staff trained in donor family communication.

Post-Death Physiologic Management

- Following the declaration of death, either by neurologic or circulatory criteria, a cascade of physiologic changes occurs that can jeopardize organ viability. These include:
  - Hemodynamic instability (eg, hypotension, vasoplegia)
  - Hormonal dysregulation (eg, adrenal insufficiency, thyroid hormone depletion)
  - Systemic inflammatory response
  - Electrolyte abnormalities
  - Coagulopathy
- If not managed proactively, these changes can result in the loss of transplantable organs.
  - Up to 25% of brain-dead donors may experience hemodynamic collapse prior to procurement, leading to a missed opportunity for transplantation.
  - Donor management is increasingly supported by dedicated donor management teams, often composed of critical care physicians in collaboration with OPO staff.
- To mitigate these risks, standardized donor management protocols include:
  - Hemodynamic optimization: maintenance of adequate perfusion pressure using fluids and vasopressors
  - Hormonal replacement therapy: administration of corticosteroids, thyroid hormones, insulin, and vasopressin to stabilize cardiovascular function and improve organ perfusion
  - Ventilatory strategies: lung-protective ventilation to minimize atelectasis and barotrauma, particularly important for lung donation
  - Metabolic and electrolyte management: timely correction of sodium, potassium, calcium, and acid-base abnormalities
  - Temperature control: normothermia to prevent coagulopathy and metabolic dysfunction
- DCD donors present unique logistical and physiologic challenges.
  - In these cases, organ recovery occurs after a period of warm ischemia following withdrawal of life-sustaining therapies.
  - The interval between circulatory arrest and organ perfusion initiation must be minimized to reduce ischemic injury.
  - With appropriate donor selection, timing, and organ preservation strategies (see later), outcomes from DCD organs can be comparable to those from DBD donors.
  - The increased use of DCD, especially in high-volume centers, has been critical to expanding the donor pool.

Outcomes and Future Directions

- Recent data from the United States show that in 2023, there were over 16,000 deceased donors, resulting in >40,000 transplanted organs.
- The average number of organs transplanted per donor remains around 3, although efforts to increase utilization per donor continue.
- Innovations such as machine perfusion, biomarker-guided donor assessment, and real-time organ viability testing are poised to further improve donor management and expand the boundaries of transplantable organs.
- The management of deceased organ donors is a complex but critical component of the transplantation process.
- Timely identification, sensitive communication with families, and standardized critical care protocols are essential to optimize organ recovery and recipient outcomes.

Organ Procurement After Brain Death

Cardiovascular Effects of Brain Death

- The rapid rise in intracranial pressure during brain death leads to ischemic injury from the cerebrum to the spinal cord, culminating in medullary herniation and vagal ischemia.
- This triggers a catecholamine storm: initial hypertension and tachycardia driven by sympathetic overactivity and peripheral vasoconstriction
  - This surge paradoxically increases coronary flow but impairs myocardial perfusion, leading to global ischemia, subendocardial necrosis, hemorrhage, and mononuclear infiltration.
    - The severity of myocardial injury tends to correlate with the magnitude of the intracranial insult and catecholamine release.
  - Following the hypertensive phase, systemic vascular resistance declines (often due to spinal ischemia), resulting in hypotension from vasodilation, hypovolemia, and impaired autoregulation.
  - These changes produce widespread hypoperfusion and endothelial dysfunction if not promptly addressed.
  - Effective donor hemodynamic management (including fluid resuscitation, vasoactive support, and hormonal therapy) is essential to preserve organ quality prior to procurement.

Endocrine Dysregulation After Brain Death

Brain death induces an endocrine crisis: an acute catecholamine surge is followed by posterior pituitary failure and anterior pituitary dysfunction of variable severity.

- Posterior pituitary failure: up to 80% of donors develop diabetes insipidus, leading to polyuria, hypernatremia, hypovolemia, and further cardiovascular instability. Synthetic vasopressin or desmopressin (DDAVP) is thus essential.
- Thyroid axis: most donors exhibit a "sick euthyroid syndrome," with decreased T_3 (60%-80%), variable T_4, and normal thyroid-stimulating hormone (TSH) rather than true hypothyroidism. Routine T_3/T_4 supplementation is controversial and generally reserved for unstable donors or those with poor cardiac function.
- Adrenal function: though cortisol levels often remain normal, up to 76% of donors do not respond to adrenocorticotropic hormone (ACTH) stimulation, suggesting subclinical adrenal insufficiency. Corticosteroid therapy is frequently used to modulate inflammation and reduce vasopressor dependence.
- Early inflammatory cascades are characterized by elevated cytokines (tumor necrosis factor alpha [TNF-α], interleukin-6 [IL-6]), chemokines, and adhesion molecules (intercellular adhesion molecule 1 [ICAM-1], vascular cell adhesion molecule 1 [VCAM-1]), promoting immune cell infiltration, enhancing immunogenicity, which predisposes to acute rejection and graft dysfunction.

Organ Procurement After Circulatory Death

Definition and Classification

- DCD refers to organ donation when death is declared based on irreversible loss of cardiopulmonary function, typically after withdrawal of life-sustaining therapy in patients who do not meet neurologic death criteria.
- DCD is classified under the Maastricht criteria as follows:
  - Category I: dead on arrival at the hospital
  - Category II: death following unsuccessful resuscitation
  - Category III (controlled DCD): death following planned withdrawal of life support
  - Category IV: cardiac arrest in a patient previously declared brain dead
- Controlled and uncontrolled DCD are differentiated by the setting and process of death.
  - In uncontrolled settings (categories I/II), patients typically arrest outside the ICU, and selected centers may use extracorporeal support (eg, extracorporeal membrane oxygenation [ECMO] or regional perfusion) under protocolized pathways.
  - In controlled DCD (category III), death occurs after withdrawal of support in an ICU or operating room, followed by rapid declaration of death and expedited procurement.

Technical and Ethical Protocols

- In controlled DCD, decisions to withdraw care are made independently of the transplant team.
- Premortem procedures, including vascular access placement or heparin administration, are permitted with explicit consent from the next-of-kin.
- After death is declared, typically following a 2- to 5-minute observation period, organ recovery begins with urgent perfusion and cooling to minimize warm ischemic injury.
- Functional warm ischemia time (fWIT), from physiologic deterioration to organ perfusion, is a major determinant of organ viability.
- For abdominal organs, prolonged fWIT has been shown to negatively impacts graft function.
- Technologies such as normothermic regional perfusion (NRP) and ex vivo perfusion are increasingly used to mitigate ischemic injury and improve transplant outcomes.

Outcomes and Organ-Specific Findings

- DCD kidneys are now widely accepted and commonly used.
  - A large registry study (2010-2021) found that long-term outcomes of DCD kidneys are comparable to DBD kidneys, especially when the Kidney Donor Risk Profile Index (KDPI) is low.
  - Delayed graft function is more frequent in DCD recipients, but graft survival at 10 years remains similar to that from DBD donors.
- DCD liver transplantation has historically been associated with higher rates of biliary complications and graft loss.
  - However, the utilization of ex vivo normothermic machine perfusion (NMP) demonstrated that this technology was able to reduce posttransplant early allograft dysfunction and ischemic biliary complications.
  - The utilization of NMP has resulted in increased use of DCD livers, with contemporary outcome similar comparable to those of DBD livers.
  - A recent meta-analysis of comparing DCD and DBD suggested significant long-term survival advantage of DCD lung transplant despite an initial small increased mortality risk in the short-term.
- In multiple studies conducted in recent years, survival outcomes assessed up to 5 years after transplant in DCD heart recipients have been similar to those with DBD heart.
  - Similarly to the liver, the utilization of NMP resulted in high rate of DCD heart utilization for transplantation with excellent patient and graft survival outcomes compared to DBD donor hearts, supporting the use of DCD/NMP to expand the donor pool.
- DCD donation has become an essential component of modern organ transplantation.
  - With proper donor selection, technical execution, and postmortem management, organs recovered from DCD donors can offer outcomes equivalent to those from brain-dead donors.
  - The expansion of machine perfusion technologies and standardized procurement protocols continues to improve the safety, feasibility, and results of DCD organ transplantation across all major solid organs.

SUGGESTED READINGS

Au AK, Bell MJ. Severe postoperative hyponatremia after pediatric intracranial tumor surgery—is this preventable? *Pediatr Crit Care Med.* 2014;15:497-498.

Centers for Medicare & Medicaid Services. *Organ Procurement Organizations (OPOs).* https://www.cms.gov/medicare/health-safety-standards/conditions-coverage-participation/organ-procurement-organizations-opo

Domínguez-Gil B, Delmonico FL, Shaheen FA, et al. The critical pathway for deceased donation: reportable uniformity in the approach to deceased donation. *Transpl Int.* 2011;24:373-378.

Israni AK, Zaun DA, Martinez A, et al. OPTN/SRTR 2023 annual data report: deceased organ donation. *Am J Transplant*. 2025;25:S490-S517.

Kharawala A, Nagraj S, Seo J, et al. Donation after circulatory death heart transplant: current state and future directions. *Circ Heart Fail*. 2024;17:e011678.

Markmann JF, Abouljoud MS, Ghobrial RM, et al. Impact of portable normothermic blood-based machine perfusion on outcomes of liver transplant: the OCS liver PROTECT randomized clinical trial. *JAMA Surg*. 2022; 157:189-198.

Meyfroidt G, Gunst J, Martin-Loeches I, et al. Management of the brain-dead donor in the ICU: general and specific therapy to improve transplantable organ quality. *Intensive Care Med*. 2019;45:343-353.

Nasralla D, Coussios CC, Mergental H, et al. A randomized trial of normothermic preservation in liver transplantation. *Nature*. 2018;557:50-56.

Organ Procurement and Transplantation Network. https://optn.transplant.hrsa.gov/

Schroder JN, Patel CB, DeVore AD, et al. Transplantation outcomes with donor hearts after circulatory death. *N Engl J Med*. 2023;388:2121-2131.

Wojda TR, Stawicki SP, Yandle KP, et al. Keys to successful organ procurement: an experience-based review of clinical practices at a high-performing health-care organization. *Int J Crit Illn Inj Sci*. 2017;7:91-100.

SECTION 19

Trauma Management

Section Editor: Casey M. Luckhurst

19.1

Fluid Resuscitation/ Transfusion Guidelines

Matthew Elson and Jonathan Parks

Definitions

- The primary focus in the management of shock is to identify the origin and treat accordingly.
- This chapter focuses on fluid resuscitation and transfusion in trauma, which is primarily related to hypovolemic, specifically hemorrhagic, and shock, though can be translated to the treatment of other causes of hemorrhagic shock, including intraoperative, postoperative, and gastrointestinal bleeding.
- The primary effort should focus on hemorrhage control.
- Time to definitive hemorrhage control has the single greatest effect on mortality.

Epidemiology of Shock in Trauma

- ~5% of patients with trauma present to the emergency department in severe shock.
- The most common etiology of shock in the injured patient is hemorrhage, which should be assumed until proven otherwise.
- Shock accounts for 20% to 40% of all mortality in trauma.
- Other causes of shock include neurogenic, cardiogenic, obstructive, distributive, and other forms of hypovolemia.

Diagnosis of Shock and Resuscitation Monitoring

- Shock is the state of inadequate tissue perfusion due to the imbalance of oxygen delivery (supply) and tissue requirements (demand).
- Hemorrhagic shock can be divided into different classes depending on the volume of blood/percent of total blood volume lost.
    - Notably, tachycardia, hypotension, and altered mental status are not present until a significant blood volume has been lost; thus, a high index of suspicion must be held for all presenting patients.
    - Narrowed pulse pressure may be the first subtle indication of impending severe shock.
- Various scoring systems have been developed to help predict patients who will require massive transfusion of blood products, such as the Assessment of Blood Consumption score, which incorporates a patient's heart rate, blood pressure, FAST examination, and mechanism.
- The use of pulmonary artery catheters has fallen out of favor in patients with trauma and is primarily reserved for patients in an undifferentiated shock or in a mixed shock where a cardiogenic component is suspected.
- Normalization of markers of resuscitation, such as arterial pH, bicarbonate, base deficit, and lactate, can be used as end points; however, a patient's overall clinical picture must be taken into account.
- Viscoelastic testing using thromboelastography/rotational thromboelastometry (TEG/ROTEM) can provide more specific goal-directed resuscitation using component therapy; however, this takes time to result and is often not available at initial presentation.

Damage Control Resuscitation

- Overall aim is to prevent the "lethal triad of trauma" (hypothermia, acidosis, and coagulopathy), which can quickly become irreversible.
- Again, early recognition is key, with a focus on rapid transport of patients to a trauma facility and definitive hemorrhage control.
- Permissive hypotension
    - Refers to the concept of limiting fluid resuscitation to the minimum required to maintain adequate organ perfusion (particularly the heart and brain) until the underlying cause has been addressed
    - Resuscitation is targeted to avoid complete hemodynamic collapse, rather than to normalize blood pressure.

TABLE 19.1.1 Composition of Saline Solutions

Solution	Sodium (mEq/L)	Potassium (mEq/L)	Chloride (mEq/L)	Osmolarity	Other
Lactated Ringer	130	4	109	273	Lactate = 28 Calcium = 3
Hypertonic saline (3% NaCl)	513		513	1,026	
Normal saline (0.9% NaCl)	154		154	308	

- Typically, a systolic blood pressure of 80 to 90 mm Hg is targeted as long as the patient is mentating appropriately.
- Shown to improve mortality, decrease further blood loss, and decrease transfusion requirements
- Temporary hemorrhage control with adjuncts such as pelvic binders, tourniquets, traction splints, and compression dressings, until definitive hemorrhage control is obtained.
- Minimization of crystalloids to prevent further dilutional coagulopathy
- Utilization of balanced blood product (whole blood vs component therapy) as the primary resuscitation fluid
  - Massive transfusion protocols can deliver large volumes of predetermined ratios of blood product at defined time intervals.
- Goal-directed correction of coagulopathy using viscoelastic testing, as available
- The use of adjuncts, such as tranexamic acid (TXA), can help treat hyperfibrinolysis when present on viscoelastic testing, and empiric use may help prevent further hemorrhage, but use must be cautioned in patients with traumatic brain injury.

Fluid Choices (See Tables 19.1.1 and 19.1.2)

- Crystalloids
  - Though still recommended as the initial resuscitation fluid by Advanced Trauma Life Support, blood products should be used preferentially when available for the reasons mentioned earlier.
  - Lactated Ringer is preferred to normal saline due to lower risk of hyperchloremic metabolic acidosis.
- Hypertonic saline
  - There is no compelling evidence to support the routine use of hypertonic saline for resuscitation.
  - Excluding this, 3% and 23.4% NaCl are effective measures to control intracranial pressure in patients with traumatic brain injury.
- Colloids
  - The protein content allows colloids to remain intravascular and generate an oncotic pressure that shifts fluid from the intracellular to the intravascular space.
  - May improve microvascular perfusion, but are much more expensive than crystalloids, and have been implicated in a variety of damaging immunologic effects
  - Synthetic colloids have also been associated with coagulopathy in high doses.
  - Dextran has been implicated in lethal cases of anaphylaxis, pulmonary edema, and platelet dysfunction, as well as renal damage.
  - Multiple trials have demonstrated no difference in outcomes of critically ill patients comparing crystalloid versus colloid resuscitation.
- Blood products
  - Should be used as the primary resuscitation fluid in hemorrhaging patients, when available
  - Can reestablish the coagulation system in the bleeding patient
  - Drawbacks include cost, the risk of transfusion reactions, and transmission of blood-borne pathogens.
  - Rapid availability is usually achieved through the use of low-titer, type O blood until type-specific and cross-matched units are available.
  - The transfusion of plasma, platelets, and red blood cells in a 1:1:1 ratio has been shown to have improved outcomes, including hemostasis rates and survival.
  - The early use of plasma, particularly in the prehospital setting, has also been shown to have improved mortality.
  - Whole blood use in the civilian setting is relatively new; however, research in the combat setting has shown improved outcomes, including survival, compared to traditional component therapy.

TABLE 19.1.2 Composition of Colloid Solutions

Solution	Sodium (mEq/L)	Potassium (mEq/L)	Chloride (mEq/L)	Osmolarity	Other
Albumin 5%	145-154		154	~300	Albumin = 50 g/L
Hextend	145-154	3	124	~307	Hydroxyethyl starch = 60 g/L Lactate = 28 mEq/L Calcium = 5 mEq/L Magnesium = 0.9 mEq/L Dextrose = 0.99 g/L

SUGGESTED READINGS

Cannon JW, Khan MA, Raja AS, et al. Damage control resuscitation in patients with severe traumatic hemorrhage: a practice management guideline from the Eastern Association for the Surgery of Trauma. *J Trauma Acute Care Surg*. 2017;82(3):605-617.

Cotton BA, Dossett LA, Haut ER, et al. Multicenter validation of a simplified score to predict massive transfusion in trauma. *J Trauma*. 2010;69(suppl 1): S33-S39.

CRASH-3 Trial Collaborators. Effects of tranexamic acid on death, disability, vascular occlusive events and other morbidities in patients with acute traumatic brain injury (CRASH-3): a randomised, placebo-controlled trial. *Lancet*. 2019;394(10210):1713-1723.

Holcomb JB, Tilley BC, Baraniuk S, et al. Transfusion of plasma, platelets, and red blood cells in a 1:1:1 vs a 1:1:2 ratio and mortality in patients with severe trauma: the PROPPR randomized clinical trial. *JAMA*. 2015; 313(5):471-482.

Shakur H, Roberts I, Bautista R, et al. Effects of tranexamic acid on death, vascular occlusive events, and blood transfusion in trauma patients with significant haemorrhage (CRASH-2): a randomised, placebo-controlled trial. *Lancet*. 2010;376(9734):23-32.

Sperry JL, Guyette FX, Brown JB, et al. Prehospital plasma during air medical transport in trauma patients at risk for hemorrhagic shock. *N Engl J Med*. 2018;379(4):315-326.

Stewart BT, Maier RV. Management of shock. In: Mattox KL, Moore EE, Feliciano DV, ed. *Trauma*. 9th ed. McGraw-Hill; 2020.

Tran A, Yates J, Lau A, et al. Permissive hypotension versus conventional resuscitation strategies in adult trauma patients with hemorrhagic shock: a systematic review and meta-analysis of randomized controlled trials. *J Trauma Acute Care Surg*. 2018;84(5):802-808.

19.2

Basic Management

John Luckoski and Michael P. DeWane

Epidemiology (in the United States)

- Trauma is the leading cause of death between the ages 1 and 44.
  - It is the fifth overall leading cause of death in the United States.
- Blunt trauma is more common than penetrating trauma.
  - Motor vehicle crashes are the leading cause of death for persons aged 5 to 34 years, >30,000 deaths annually.
- Penetrating abdominal trauma affects 35% of patients in urban trauma centers and up to 12% of nonurban centers.
  - ~90% of patients with penetrating trauma are male.

Differential Diagnosis of Hypotension in the Patient With Trauma

- Hypovolemic shock
  - Hemorrhage is the most common etiology and must be ruled out first. Possible locations of hemorrhage include:
    - Thorax, abdomen, pelvis/retroperitoneum, extremities, external (scene of the trauma)
      - Closed intracranial hemorrhage cannot cause hemorrhagic shock.
  - For most extremity hemorrhage, direct manual compression or suture ligation is sufficient.
  - Failing this, proximal tourniquet control is recommended until operative repair is achieved.
  - In patients with an identified open-book pelvic fracture, a pelvic binder may be used to assist as a bridge to definitive hemorrhagic control.
    - Definitive control may include angioembolization or operative external fixation.
      - Operative preperitoneal pelvic packing may be utilized as an additional bridge to definitive treatment.
  - Obstructive shock—tension pneumothorax and cardiac tamponade
    - Similar "tension physiology": hypotension, tachycardia, distended neck veins
  - Tension pneumothorax results in mediastinal shift, which causes compression of cardiac venous return.
    - Tension physiology is a dynamic process and worsens as mediastinal shifts increase.
    - Clinical diagnosis treated with finger or needle decompression followed by formal chest tube placement
    - Adults: fourth or fifth intercostal space in the middle axillary line
    - Children: second intercostal space in the midclavicular line
  - Cardiac tamponade limits diastolic filling and subsequent cardiac output. Most commonly caused by penetrating thoracic trauma
    - Cardiac focused assessment with sonography for trauma (FAST) examination is the gold standard diagnostic imaging modality.
    - Unstable patients with cardiac tamponade require immediate emergency department (ED) resuscitative thoracotomy to relieve the tamponade.
    - Patients with traumatic pericardial effusion with stable vital signs may be transported to the operating room for pericardial window and further definitive operative treatment.
- Neurogenic shock
  - Spinal cord injury above the T1 level results in sympathectomy and loss of vasomotor tone. In the patient who is euvolemic, hypotension is treated with vasopressors.
    - Clinically presents as hypotension without tachycardia nor peripheral vasoconstriction

- Cardiogenic shock
  - In patients with trauma with preexisting cardiac disease or those suffering blunt cardiac injury, hypotension may result from cardiac failure. Treatment is supportive.
    - Blunt thoracic trauma should be evaluated with electrocardiogram (ECG) monitoring to evaluate for dysrhythmias.

Management and Treatment

- Airway
  - Indications for posttraumatic intubation: inability to protect airway (Glasgow Coma Scale [GCS] <8), extensive facial trauma, hypoxia/hypoventilation, impending airway compromise, combativeness (to facilitate comprehensive evaluation)
  - Rapid-sequence induction should be performed in all patients with trauma requiring intubation.
  - Cervical spine (C-spine) immobilization is a critical aspect of airway management.
    - Cervical immobilization is not mandatory in penetrating trauma.
  - For blunt mechanism injury, the cervical collar may be removed for intubation with in line stabilization provided.
- Breathing
  - Asymmetric breath sounds may result from a large pneumothorax and/or hemothorax.
  - Chest x-ray (CXR) and thoracic ultrasound may be used as adjuncts to the physical examination.
    - On a supine chest film, secondary signs of pneumothorax may be the only signs present: rib fractures, subcutaneous emphysema, or a unilateral deep sulcus sign.
  - In an unstable patient with asymmetrical breath sounds, needle decompression or finger thoracostomy should be performed prior to intubation as positive pressure ventilation can exacerbate a tension pneumothorax.
    - In a stable patient requiring positive pressure ventilation, chest tube placement is not always mandatory in the presence of a pneumothorax. Close monitoring is warranted.
- Circulation
  - In unstable patients, the ideal intravenous (IV) catheters for resuscitation are short and wide: large-bore (14-18 g) peripheral access (at least two) or central introducer (subclavian or femoral) access is preferred.
    - Intraosseous (IO) access is recommended if IV access proves difficult.
  - Once tension physiology is excluded as a cause of shock, hypotension in patients with trauma should be considered secondary to blood loss.
  - Clinical signs of shock included mental status, pallor, and tachycardia, though no single sign is perfectly sensitive nor specific.
  - Whole blood and blood products (over crystalloid) should be first line in the resuscitation of a patient with trauma.
    - Excessive crystalloid resuscitation is strongly discouraged; resuscitation >1.5 L increases mortality odds ratio.
  - A *massive transfusion protocol* should be utilized in a patient requiring >4 units of blood product within 1 hour, or 10 units within the first 24 hours of presentation.
    - Fresh frozen plasma (FFP) should be transfused empirically.
    - Massive transfusion should be performed in a 1:1:1 manner with packed red blood cell (pRBC), FFP, and platelets, respectively.
    - Growing body of evidence supports whole blood as an initial resuscitation product; however, limited by institution.
- Hypotensive resuscitation—in patients with significant vascular injury requiring operative repair, a strategy of tolerating hypotension improved survival outcomes.
  - Currently, military guidelines recommend withholding fluids in a patient with a normal mental status and palpable radial pulse.
  - This strategy should not be exercised if there is suspicion of traumatic brain injury (TBI).
- C-spine evaluation
  - The National Emergency X-radiography Utilization Study (NEXUS) criteria for clinical removal of a cervical collar include the absence of posterior midline C-spine tenderness, absence of focal neurologic deficit, normal level of alertness, absence of intoxication, and absence of painful distracting injury.
  - Patients who do not meet the abovementioned clinical decision rules require radiographic evaluation: computed tomography (CT) is recommended as plain films are not sufficiently sensitive to detect clinically significant fractures.
    - Negative high-quality C-spine CT result alone is often sufficient for C-spine clearance, even in obtunded patients; however, no consensus guidelines have been reached.
    - Long-term C-collar use carries the risk of pressure ulcers and difficulties with airway and central line management.
    - Magnetic resonance imaging (MRI) is the gold standard imaging modality to evaluate spinal cord and ligamentous injury if there is concern for neurologic injury.
  - Blunt cerebrovascular injury (BCVI)
    - Rare but potentially devastating cause of stroke, Horner syndrome, and possible hemorrhage
      - Grade I to V Denver Criteria (Table 19.2.1)

TABLE 19.2.1 Denver Criteria for BCVI

Grade	Scale
I	Irregularity of the vessel wall or dissection/intramural hematoma with <25% luminal stenosis
II	Intraluminal thrombus or raised intimal flap, or dissection/intramural hematoma with ≥25% luminal stenosis
III	Pseudoaneurysms
IV	Vessel occlusion
V	Vessel transection

BCVI, blunt cerebrovascular injury.

From Grabowski G, Robertson RN, Barton BM, Cairns MA, Webb SW. Blunt cerebrovascular injury in cervical spine fractures: are more-liberal screening criteria warranted? *Global Spine J*. 2016;6(7):679-685, Table 1.

- Risk factors include LeFort fractures II+III, severe TBI w/GCS <6, upper rib fractures, hanging injuries, and basilar skull fractures.
- Screen for BCVI with computed tomographic angiogram (CTA) neck in high-risk patients, treatment varies with the grade of injury.

- Penetrating injuries
  - Neck
  - Sharp/puncture injuries to the neck deep to the platysma are considered penetrating.
  - Patients with clinical evidence of vascular, neurologic, or aerodigestive injury require formal operative exploration.
    - Signs include air bubbling from a wound, "hard" signs of vascular injury, including expanding hematoma, pulsatile blood flow, and palpable thrill.
  - In the absence of obvious injury, diagnostic workup should include CTA, with or without esophagram, esophagoscopy, and bronchoscopy.
  - Chest
  - Barring cardiac or great vessel injury, the majority of penetrating thoracic injuries may be managed by tube thoracostomy alone.
    - A chest tube should be placed empirically prior to imaging if evidence of respiratory compromise or tension physiology exists in a known penetrating injury.
  - Indications for thoracotomy include >1,500 mL initial chest tube output, 150 to 200 mL/h for 2 to 4 hours, massive air leak, and hemodynamic instability.
  - Abdomen
    - Anterior abdominal stab wounds—must penetrate deep to the anterior rectus sheath to be considered penetrating—are indications for exploratory laparotomy.
    - Clinically concerning signs include hemodynamic instability, peritonitis, and evisceration.
    - Alert and oriented patients with normal vital signs without peritonitis can be admitted for 24 hours of observational nonoperative management; however, this is an institution-dependent and resource-limited clinical decision.
    - Gunshot wounds to the abdomen should be explored operatively.
  - Thoracoabdominal
    - For left-sided injuries, diagnostic laparoscopy should be performed to evaluate for diaphragmatic injury. Left-sided diaphragm injury requires formal repair.
  - Extremities
    - "Hard" signs of vascular injury, which require immediate operative exploration, include pulsatile hemorrhage, expanding hematoma, thrill or bruit, and distal ischemia/absent distal pulse.
    - "Soft" signs that require CTA include small hematoma, moderate hemorrhage, proximity to major vascular structures, and associated nerve injury.
- Blunt injuries
  - Imaging
    - In blunt injury, CXR and pelvic x-ray should be obtained in the resuscitation bay to evaluate for hemothorax and pelvic fractures as possible sources of bleeding as a target for immediate intervention.
    - FAST is a useful tool to evaluate for the presence of hemoperitoneum, pericardial tamponade, and pneumothorax/hemothorax.
      - The four traditional views are pericardial view, hepatorenal recess (Morison pouch), splenorenal recess, and bladder view.
      - Extended FAST (eFAST) includes thoracic ultrasound and has been reported to be more sensitive than CXR in the detection of pneumothorax.
      - Limitations of the FAST: operator dependent, cannot assess retroperitoneum, cannot assess for hollow organ injury, inaccurate in the assessment of penetrating injury
    - Unstable patients should not be transported to CT scan.
    - Diagnostic peritoneal lavage (DPL) is a mostly historical procedure, as it has been replaced by FAST in the evaluation of a patient with unstable blunt trauma to rule out intra-abdominal hemorrhage.
  - Stable patients
    - CT "pan scan" of head, neck, chest, abdomen, and pelvis should be performed liberally to assess for occult injury in stable high-energy blunt mechanism patients. Physical examination, plain films, and FAST are not sufficiently sensitive to detect clinically significant injuries. CTA should be utilized if there is suspicion of arterial injury.
    - In a hemodynamically stable patient, solid organ injury with active "blush" on CTA scan may be managed with angioembolization.
    - Free air, peritonitis, diaphragm rupture, and declining clinical status are indications for operative management.
  - Unstable patients
    - An unstable patient with a positive FAST should undergo exploratory laparotomy.
    - With a negative FAST scan and open-book pelvic fracture, a pelvic binder should be placed and strong consideration should be given for pelvic angioembolization.
    - If a significant delay is anticipated, the patient should be taken to the operating room for emergency pelvic external fixation and preperitoneal pelvic packing.
- ED resuscitative thoracotomy
  - This extreme measure should be performed only as a temporizing measure and should not be performed if a surgeon and operating room are not immediately available.
  - Indications
    - Penetrating trauma—prehospital cardiopulmonary resuscitation (CPR) for <15 minutes or loss of vital signs in the ED
    - Blunt trauma—loss of vital signs in the ED with a potentially correctable source of bleeding

SUGGESTED READINGS

American College of Surgeons. *Advanced Trauma Life Support®: Student Course Manual*. 10th ed. American College of Surgeons; 2018.

Bickell WH, Wall MJ, Pepe, PE, et al. Immediate versus delayed fluid resuscitation for hypotensive patients with penetrating torso injuries. *N Engl J Med*. 1994;331(17):1105-1109.

Biffl WLK, Krista L, Cothren CC, et al. Management of patients with anterior abdominal stab wounds: a western trauma association multicenter trial. *J Trauma*. 2009;66:1294-1301.

Blaivas M, Lyon M, Duggal S. A prospective comparison of supine chest radiography and bedside ultrasound for the diagnosis of traumatic pneumothorax. *Acad Emerg Med*. 2005;12(9):844-849.

Bracken MBS, Jo M, Holford TR, et al. Administration of methylprednisolone for 24 or 48 hours or tirilazad mesylate for 48 hours in the treatment of acute spinal cord injury: results of the Third National Acute Spinal Cord Injury Randomized Controlled Trial. *JAMA*. 1997;277(20):1597-1604.

Hoffman JR, Mower WR, Wolfson AB, Todd KH, Zucker MI; National Emergency X-Radiography Utilization Study Group. Validity of a set of clinical criteria to rule out injury to the cervical spine in patients with blunt trauma. *N Engl J Med*. 2000;343(2):94-99.

Kragh JF, Walters TJ, Baer DG, et al. Survival with emergency tourniquet use to stop bleeding in major limb trauma. *Ann Surg*. 2009;249:1-7.

Lotfollahzadeh S, Burns B. Penetrating abdominal trauma.]. In: *StatPearls* [Internet]. StatPearls Publishing; Updated June 3, 2023. https://www.ncbi.nlm.nih.gov/books/NBK459123/

Stiell IG, Wells GA, Vandemheen KL, et al. The Canadian C-spine rule for radiography in alert and stable trauma patients. *JAMA*. 2001;286(15): 1841-1848.

19.3

FAST: Focused Assessment With Sonography

John Luckoski and Michael P. DeWane

Definitions

- FAST uses four ultrasound views to assess for fluid in the abdomen and pericardium.
- Extended FAST (eFAST) can additionally evaluate for hemothorax/pneumothorax.
- The skills can be acquired with short, structured training and at least 25 to 50 examinations.
- In the hands of the experienced operator, FAST can be completed in 2 to 3 minutes.
- FAST can provide information on:
  - Intraperitoneal fluid in blunt abdominal trauma, with a sensitivity of 80% to 90% and a specificity approaching that of diagnostic peritoneal lavage (DPL) and computed tomography (CT)
  - Pericardial fluid, with a sensitivity of 100% sensitivity and 97% specificity
- The abdominal portion of the FAST examination is most useful in the patient with unstable blunt trauma, while pericardial tamponade is most commonly seen in penetrating trauma.
  - FAST examination should not delay rapid transport to a CT scan if appropriate sonographic windows are not readily achieved.
  - If hemoperitoneum or pericardial tamponade is seen on FAST in an unstable patient, the patient should proceed directly to the operating room for definitive management.

Advantages

- Can be performed simultaneously with other management and as part of initial resuscitation efforts
- Can obviate the need for urgent CT and the transport of the patient out of the resuscitation area
- Rapid—complete FAST can be performed in under 3 minutes in trained hands; may improve surgical triage and time to definitive operative management for patients with hemoperitoneum
- Skills can be acquired with 10 to 16 hours of didactic training and 25 to 50 completed scans.
  - Maximal operator sensitivity occurs in the 50 to 200 scan experience range.

Limitations

- Poor sensitivity to assess for retroperitoneal bleeding or solid organ injury
- Operator dependent and requires sufficient experience for improved negative predictive value
- Can be technically difficult in the patient who is obese and where subcutaneous emphysema may obscure images

FAST Technique

- Aims to answer two questions:
  - Is there fluid in the abdomen?
  - Is there fluid in the pericardium?
- The standard FAST examination requires interrogation of four areas (Table 19.3.1); isolated abdominal or cardiac

TABLE 19.3.1 Four Areas of the Fast Scan

View	Probe Position	Viscera Assessed	Site of Fluid	Notes
1. Subxiphoid[a] (Figure 19.3.1A)	Nearly flat beneath xiphisternum	Pericardial sac, ventricle walls	Within pericardium	Uses liver as "echogenic" window
2. Hepatorenal (Figure 19.3.1B)	R side MAL 9–10th rib	Liver, right kidney	Morrison pouch/right paracolic gutter	Most likely area for fluid accumulation in abdomen
3. Splenorenal	L side PAL 8–9th rib	Spleen, left kidney	Splenorenal space/left paracolic gutter	Investigate subdiaphragmatic space above the spleen
4. Latitudinal and longitudinal pelvic views (Figure 19.3.1C)	Just superior to pubic symphysis-angled inferiorly	Bladder, rectum, prostate	Pouch of Douglas (F) Rectovesical pouch (M)	Sensitive for small volumes of fluid

All can be acquired with 2-5 MHz curvilinear abdominal probe.
F, female; M, male; MAL, midaxillary line; PAL, posterior axillary line.
[a]Cardiac probe preferred (not essential) for cardiac view.

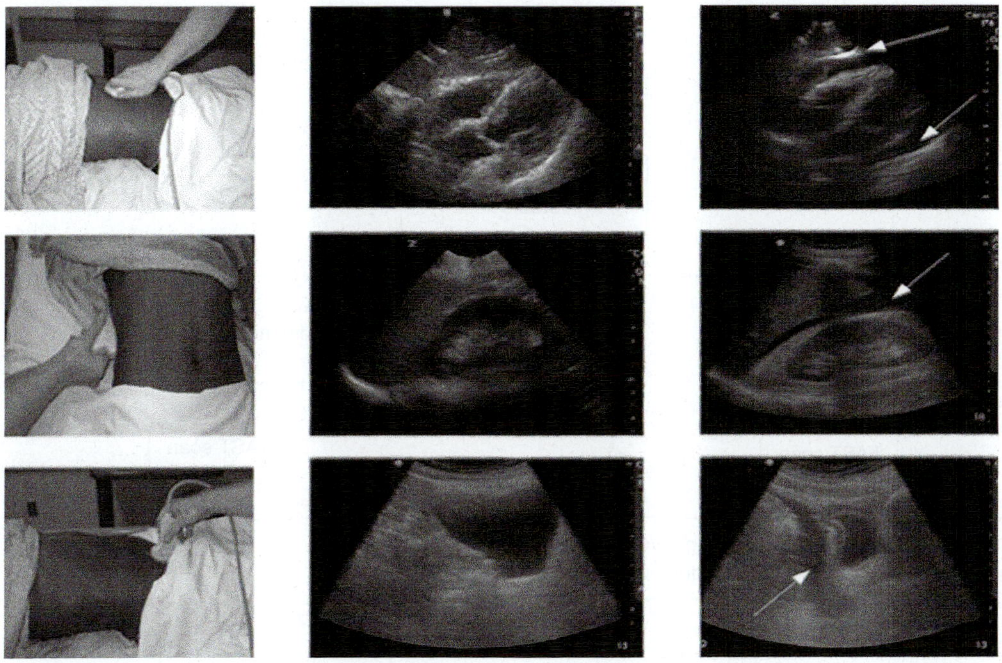

FIGURE 19.3.1 **A.** Subxiphoid. Upper arrow denotes pericardium, and lower arrow is fluid. **B.** Hepatorenal. Arrow denotes fluid in Morrison pouch. **C.** Pelvic: Longitudinal view. Arrow denotes pelvic fluid. B, bladder; L, liver; K, kidney.

ultrasound may be indicated clinically, but this is not a complete "FAST" by consensus definition.

- When assessing Morrison pouch (hepatorenal recess) and the splenorenal recess, the inferior pole of the kidney must be visualized for the examination to be declared negative; small pockets of fluid may accumulate here and, if not imaged, can yield a false-negative scan.
- A parasternal long view of the heart may be substituted if a subxiphoid is technically difficult.
- *Abdominal views* (Figure 19.3.1)
  - The most common sources of bleeding identifiable on ultrasound in blunt traumatic hemoperitoneum are the liver and the spleen. These usually present as fluid in the hepatorenal or splenorenal recesses on FAST.
    - Ultrasound was positive when an average of 617 mL (standard deviation [SD] 173 mL) of fluid had been infused.
    - Ultrasound was positive in 97% of cases when >1 L of fluid infused versus 10% when <400 mL infused.
    - Amount of fluid required for a positive scan did not vary with height, weight, age, or gender.
  - Quoted sensitivities and specificities of ultrasound vary widely depending on the end point being measured. Studies have shown that FAST performed by surgeons and emergency medicine (EM) physicians detects hemoperitoneum, with 80% to 86% sensitivity and 97% to 99% specificity; false-negatives tend to have lower volumes of fluid (ie, <500 mL).
- *Pericardium*
  - Ultrasound sensitivity for hemopericardium approaches 100% sensitivity and 97% specificity.
  - Prompt use of ultrasound in penetrating cardiac injury can improve surgical triage and direct aggressive resuscitation, potentially improving patients' survival and neurologic outcomes.
  - While traumatic pericardial effusion is uncommon in blunt trauma, it is easily excluded with the highly sensitive cardiac view.
- *Algorithms* (Figures 19.3.2 and 19.3.3)
  - In patients who are unstable or hypotensive, the role of FAST is generally clear.
    - Positive FAST: indicates intra-abdominal source of bleeding and the need for laparotomy
    - Negative FAST: has a high negative predictive value for intra-abdominal injury as the source of hypotension; strongly suggests that intra-abdominal bleeding is not the source of shock
      - Patients with unstable trauma with a negative FAST should be adequately resuscitated to determine the source of their shock and next clinical steps.

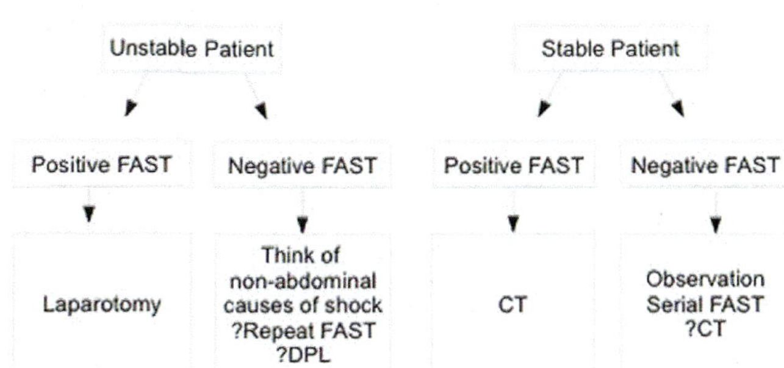

FIGURE 19.3.2 **Suggested clinical FAST algorithm for a patient with trauma.** CT, computed tomography; DPL, diagnostic peritoneal lavage. Adapted from Noble V, Nelson B. Focused assessment with sonography in trauma. In: *Manual of Emergency and Critical Care Ultrasound.* 2nd ed. Cambridge University Press; 2011:23-49.

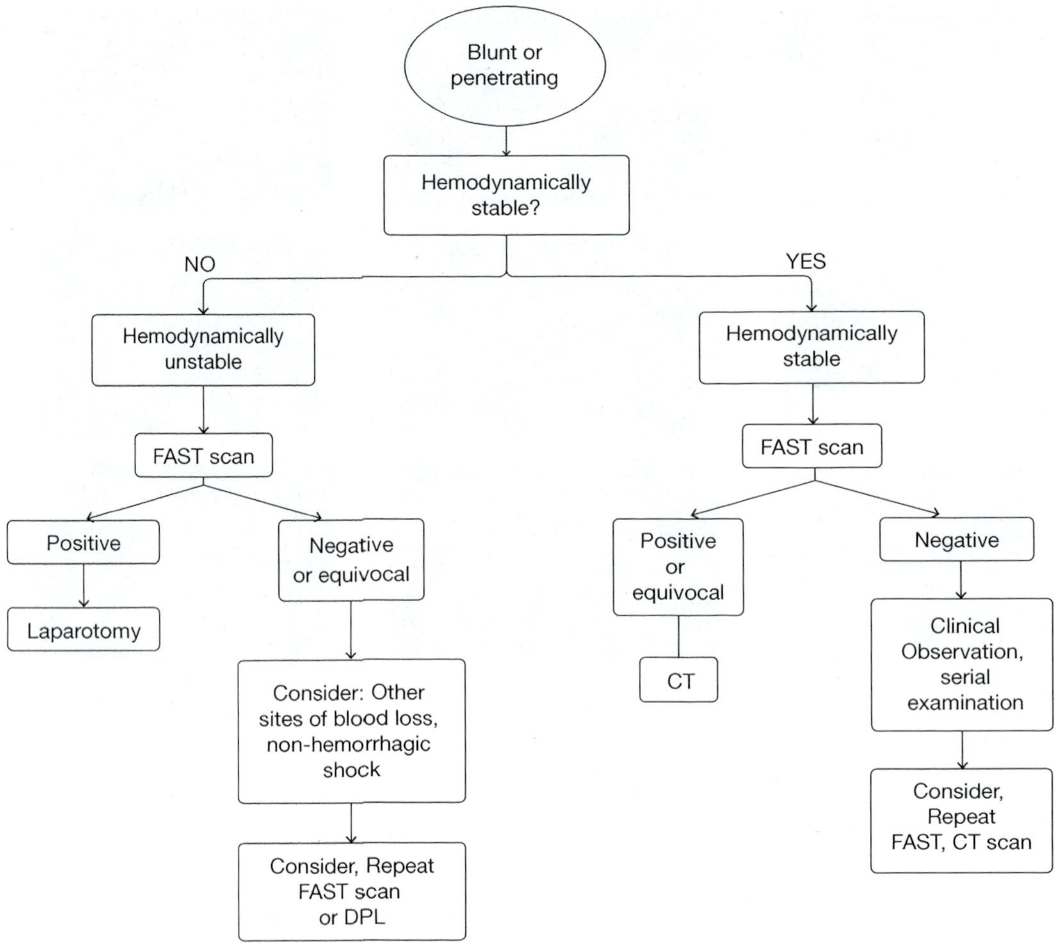

FIGURE 19.3.3 Management of blunt or penetrating trauma. CT, computed tomography; DPL, diagnostic peritoneal lavage.

- A positive FAST in a stable patient can be monitored and managed nonoperatively (correction of coagulopathy and possible infrared [IR] angioembolization).

- With stable or normotensive patients, the role is less clear.
  - Positive FAST: may indicate potential for deterioration and higher likelihood of need for laparotomy, warranting observation with serial ultrasound examination, or computed tomographic angiography (CTA)
  - Negative FAST: less likely to develop significant intra-abdominal hemorrhage. May require evaluation for other injuries

SUGGESTED READINGS

Branney SW, Wolfe RE, Moore EE, et al. Quantitative sensitivity of ultrasound in detecting free intraperitoneal fluid. *J Trauma.* 1995;39(2):375-380.

Korner M, Krotz MM, Degenhart C, Klaus-Jurgen P, Reiser M, Linsenmaier U. Current role of emergency ultrasound in patients with major trauma. *Radiographics.* 2008;28:225-244.

Mckenny K, McKenny M, Cohn S, et al. Hemoperitoneum score helps determine need for therapeutic laparotomy. *J Trauma.* 2001;50:650-656.

Melniker L, Leibner E, McKenny M, Lopez P, Briggs W, Mancuso C. Randomised controlled clinical trial of point-of-care, limited ultrasonography for trauma in the emergency dept: the first sonography outcomes assessment program trial. *Ann Emerg Med.* 2006;48(3):227-235.

Moylan M, Newgard CD, Ma OJ, Sabbaj A, Rogers T, Douglas R. Association between a positive ED FAST and therapeutic laparotomy in normotensive blunt trauma patients. *J Emerg Med.* 2007;33(3):265-271.

Noble V, Nelson B. Focused assessment with sonography in trauma. In: *Manual of Emergency and Critical Care Ultrasound.* 2nd ed. Cambridge University Press; 2011:23-49.

Rozycki G, Ballard R, Feliciano D, Schmidt J, Pennington S. Surgeon-performed ultrasound for the assessment of truncal injuries: lessons learned from 1540 patients. *Ann Surg.* 1998;228(4):557-567.

Scalea TM, Rodriguez A, Chiu WC, et al. Focused assessment with sonography for trauma (FAST): results from an International Consensus Conference. *J Trauma.* 1999;46(3):466-472.

Thomas B, Falcone RE, Vasquez D, et al. Ultrasound evaluation of blunt abdominal trauma: program implementation, initial experience, and learning curve. *J Trauma.* 1997;42(3):384-388.

19.4

Complications

Moustafa Abdalla, Lydia Maurer, and Jason Brocker

Neurologic

- Cerebrospinal fluid (CSF) fistula
  - Traumatic CSF leakage (rhinorrhea, otorrhea, or direct leakage from the wound) complicates 2% to 4% of all head traumas, and 12% to 30% of all basilar skull fractures.
  - Beta-2 transferrin assay of the fluid is highly specific for confirming CSF leakage.
  - The majority resolve spontaneously within a few days with conservative measures, including bed rest, head elevation, and avoidance of activities that increase intracranial pressure.
  - Persistent drainage may require placement of a lumbar drain or surgical repair.
  - The overall risk of meningitis in patients with persistent CSF rhinorrhea is 10% to 20%.
  - Prolonged prophylactic antibiotics do not reduce this risk and are associated with the selection of resistant microorganisms.
- Hypopituitarism
  - Common after moderate-to-severe traumatic brain injury, affecting 20% to 40% of patients
  - Growth hormone deficiency is the most frequently observed deficiency in these patients.
  - Early testing for pituitary dysfunction is not recommended; however, if there is clinical suspicion of cortisol insufficiency (eg, secondary to anterior pituitary dysfunction) with unexplained hypotension or hypoglycemia or cranial diabetes insipidus (DI) (posterior pituitary dysfunction) with sudden large urine losses and unexpected hypernatremia, patients should be tested and managed clinically.
  - Patients admitted for >48 hours for the management of traumatic brain injury should undergo screening for pituitary dysfunction at 3 to 6 months (British Neurotrauma Group guidance 2017).
- DI
  - Incidence after severe head injury varies markedly, with estimates ranging from 2.6% to 51%, highlighting the difficulty of making a definitive diagnosis with confounding factors (eg, aggressive resuscitation).
  - Although cranial DI usually resolves spontaneously, it is a predictor of mortality and of other long-term pituitary deficits.
  - Clinically manifests as hypotonic polyuria and hypernatremia; evaluate serum creatinine, serum electrolytes, plasma glucose, and paired plasma-urine osmolality as part of the workup.
  - Treatment of new-onset DI involves administering desmopressin (DDAVP) to control diuresis, managing fluid balance with intravenous (IV) hypotonic fluids to prevent dehydration and correct hypernatremia, and closely monitoring urine output, serum sodium levels, and overall fluid status to adjust treatment as needed.
  - It is important to note that *hypernatremia* may be a *protective mechanism* in patients with elevated intracranial pressures.
- Syndrome of inappropriate antidiuretic hormone secretion (SIADH)
  - Incidence after severe head injury is about 15%; be sure to exclude renal, adrenal, and/or thyroid dysfunction as contributing factors.
  - Presents as hyponatremia and concentrated urine (usually UOsm >300 mOsm) due to excessive water retention in the context of *euvolemia* or *hypervolemia*; usually resolves spontaneously
  - Treatment is fluid restriction and/or hypertonic saline if symptomatic; demeclocycline may be used in refractory cases.
- Cerebral salt wasting syndrome (CSWS)
  - Key diagnostic features include polyuria with high urine sodium concentration and *hypo*natremia (typically <135 mmol/L).
  - Unlike SIADH, CSWS results in *hypovolemia* due to excessive intravascular fluid loss.
  - Treatment is aggressive hydration and sodium repletion; careful monitoring is essential to avoid over-(or under-) correction and the speed of this correction.
  - May require mineralocorticoid therapy (fludrocortisone) or DDAVP (ADH analog)
- Posttraumatic seizures
  - The prevalence of posttraumatic seizures is severity dependent—mild traumatic brain injury (TBI) (1%-2%), moderate TBI (4%-7%), and severe TBI (10%-20%), with more than half being nonconvulsive—most commonly associated with penetrating injuries, followed by subdural hematomas (SDHs) and intraparenchymal contusions.
  - Early (<7 days)—routine seizure prophylaxis (phenytoin or levetiracetam) is recommended for the first week postinjury.
  - Late (>7 days)—is associated with worse outcomes; seizure prophylaxis beyond 7 days does not decrease the incidence of late posttraumatic epilepsy.
- Paroxysmal sympathetic hyperactivity (PSH; "sympathetic storming")
  - Occurs in up to 33% of patients with severe TBI
  - Characterized by fever, diaphoresis, tachycardia, tachypnea, hypertension, and pupillary dilation; episodes are usually unprovoked (multiple episodes per day and usually >30 minutes) and commonly occur during weaning of sedatives and narcotics.
  - "PSH Assessment Measure" (PSH-AM) is a tool used to standardize the diagnosis and severity assessment, considering both clinical features and the frequency of episodes.
  - Treatment is symptom directed and may include baclofen, narcotics, benzodiazepines, propranolol, clonidine, and dantrolene.

Vascular

- Blunt cerebrovascular injury (BCVI)—rare entity (0.1%-2.7%); high incidence of neurologic morbidity (40%) and mortality
- Diagnosis, in both children and adults, should be considered with any hard signs of vascular injury, or if asymptomatic, if the following risk factors are present: Glasgow Coma Scale (GCS) <8, petrous bone fracture, diffuse axonal injury, cervical spine fractures (particularly with C1-C3 fractures or fractures through the foramen transversarium), cervical spine fractures with rotation or subluxation, and Le Fort II and III facial fractures (EAST BCVI guidelines 2012).
- Screening modality is either computed tomographic angiography or traditional angiography; duplex ultrasound (US) is not adequate for screening.
- In the absence of contraindications, low-grade injuries (grade I: intimal irregularity with <25% narrowing, dissection; or grade II: intramural hematoma with >25% narrowing) should be treated with aspirin or heparin.
- For high-grade injuries (grade III: pseudoaneurysms, grade IV: occlusion, grade V: transection with extravasation), consult neurosurgery and/or interventional radiology to determine the most appropriate treatment, which may include anticoagulation, endovascular stenting, or open intervention, depending on the institution.

Chest

- Retained hemothorax despite tube thoracostomy placement—use of fibrinolytic agents (eg, tissue plasminogen activator [tPA] combined with DNase) and early thoracoscopy (<7 days postinjury) is associated with decreased complications and shorter hospital stays.
- Pulmonary contusion—morbidity correlates with excessive fluid resuscitation, which exacerbates pulmonary edema and worsens lung injury; there are higher rates of respiratory complications (including pneumonia and acute respiratory distress syndrome [ARDS]) in patients with severe contusions.
- Pulmonary embolism—all patients with trauma should be considered high risk for thromboembolic complications; in the absence of contraindications, chemoprophylaxis with enoxaparin should be administered within 24 hours (AAST [American Association for the Surgery of Trauma] Critical Care Committee Clinical Consensus Document 2021).

Abdomen

- Liver—complications after high-grade liver injury with or without angioembolization are frequent (70%) and include biliary leak, intra-abdominal hypertension, inflammatory peritonitis, hepatic necrosis and abscess formation, gallbladder infarction, and compressive subcapsular hematoma.
  - Success of nonoperative management (NOM) depends on the grade of (blunt) liver injury (Brillantino et al 2019):
    - Grade I and II injuries: overwhelmingly managed nonoperatively, with success rates approaching 90% to 95%
    - Grade III injuries: Success rates for NOM are around 70% to 85%.
    - Grade IV and V injuries: these are more likely to require surgical intervention, with success rates for NOM around 50% to 70%.
  - Hemobilia—classic Quincke triad: abdominal pain, jaundice, gastrointestinal bleeding
    - May present as delayed hematemesis
    - Treated with angioembolization
  - Abscess—most frequent infectious complication after liver injury; most commonly treated by antibiosis and percutaneous drainage
- Hepatic necrosis—has been reported in as high as 41% of patients undergoing angioembolization for blunt liver injury. Early formal operative lobectomy should be considered in cases of extensive necrosis or failure of less invasive measures.
- Biloma/bile leak—managed with drainage with or without endoscopic retrograde cholangiopancreatography (ERCP) stent/sphincterotomy
- Spleen
  - Similar to traumatic blunt liver injury, failure of NOM occurs in almost 40% of high-grade (4 and 5) splenic injuries.
  - Angioembolization may increase the nonoperative salvage rate for patients with splenic injuries; consider angioembolization for >grade III injuries, presence of a contrast extravasation, moderate hemoperitoneum, or clinical evidence of ongoing splenic bleeding (EAST 2019).
  - Complications of splenic angioembolization include postembolization syndrome (fever, pain, elevated white blood cell [WBC]), splenic infarction, rebleeding, abscess formation, and, rarely, delayed splenic rupture. Proximal embolization has a higher risk of splenic infarction, while distal embolization is more associated with abscess formation.
  - Splenectomy remains the standard of care for the unstable patient with high-grade splenic injury.
  - Delayed splenic rupture
    - Incidence of delayed splenic rupture ranges from 0.5% to 6% among patients with blunt splenic injuries.
    - Can occur secondary to pseudoaneurysms; other factors include subcapsular hematomas, pseudocyst formations, delayed splenic infarctions, and incomplete healing.
    - It typically occurs within the first week postinjury, although cases have been reported up to 14 days postinjury, with rare instances occurring beyond this period.
  - Overwhelming postsplenectomy sepsis
    - Rare in adults; rare in posttraumatic splenectomy
    - Postsplenectomy vaccines should be initiated before discharge from the hospital, with planned follow-up vaccinations at trauma clinic, primary care physician (PCP), or emergency department (ED)/urgent care.
  - Splenic infarction
    - Secondary to angioembolization; may result in splenic abscess and may ultimately require splenectomy

- Kidney
  - High-grade injuries managed nonoperatively have a complication rate between 11% and 20%; the vast majority of these complications may be managed percutaneously.
  - Abscess—accounts for 50% of complications
  - Urinoma—consider dedicated cross-sectional imaging (with both a noncontrast phase, arterial IV contrast phase, and a delayed phase); aspiration and/or a rising serum creatinine may also help with diagnosis.
  - Ureteral stricture
  - Pseudoaneurysm
  - Delayed renovascular hypertension, likely secondary to vascular injury and scarring with stenosis and reduced renal blood resulting in activation of the renin-angiotensin cascade

Pelvis

- Rebleeding—after angioembolization, this may occur in up to 18%.
- Gluteal necrosis—infrequent but highly morbid complication after bilateral internal iliac artery embolization
- Neurologic complications—10% to 15% incidence; treatment involves fracture stabilization and aggressive physical therapy for muscle strengthening and prevention of contractures.
- Genitourinary tract injury—incidence among all patients with trauma with pelvic fractures is 5%; includes bladder injury (ranging from contusions to partial or complete ruptures) and urethral injuries (more common in men).
  - Diagnostic imaging modalities include CT cystogram (for suspected bladder injury) or retrograde urethrography (for suspected urethral injuries).
  - Minor urinary tract injuries may be managed conservatively with catheterization to decompress the bladder and allow healing.
- Avascular necrosis of the femoral head—mostly associated with posterior fracture dislocations (10% incidence). Prompt reduction within 6 hours of the dislocation significantly improves blood flow, reducing the likelihood of permanent damage.

Extremities

- Fat embolism syndrome
  - Reported incidence in up to 10% of patients with long bone and pelvic fractures
  - Classic triad: confusion/neurologic impairment, dyspnea, upper torso petechiae
  - Gurd criteria: major criteria (respiratory symptoms, cerebral signs, petechial rash) and minor criteria (tachycardia, fever, retinal changes, renal dysfunction, thrombocytopenia, anemia, elevated erythrocyte sedimentation rate [ESR]) can help in diagnosis.
  - Treatment is primarily supportive; mortality rate ~10%.
  - Early operative fracture fixation is associated with decreased incidence.
- Compartment syndrome
  - Can occur in any extremity and also in the gluteal compartments; high level of suspicion and vigilance is required.
  - Can occur in the *absence* of fractures (eg, patients found down, massive fluid resuscitation); it is, however, more common in certain types of fractures (particularly tibial fractures), where incidence can be as high as 10% to 30%, as well as with crush injuries and high-energy mechanisms.
  - Pain (out of proportion) and paresthesias are the earliest symptoms; pallor and pulselessness are late findings.
  - Compartment pressures >30 mm Hg or a delta pressure (diastolic blood pressure minus compartment pressure) <30 mm Hg are indicative of compartment syndrome.
  - Diagnosis is primarily clinical; measuring compartment pressures is neither necessary nor indicated for operative decompression.

Acknowledgments

We gratefully acknowledge the contributions of previous edition author(s), Dante Yeh, as portions of those chapters have been retained in this revision.

SUGGESTED READINGS

Anand RJ, Ferrada PA, Darwin PE, Bochicchio GV, Scalea TM. Endoscopic retrograde cholangiopancreatography is an effective treatment for bile leak after severe liver trauma. *J Trauma*. 2011;71(2):480-485.

Bjurlin MA, Fantus RJ, Mellett MM, Goble SM, Hollowell CM. Genitourinary injuries in pelvic fracture morbidity and mortality using the National Trauma Data Bank. *J Trauma*. 2009;67(3):1033-1039.

Brillantino A, Iacobellis F, Festa P, et al. Non-operative management of blunt liver trauma: safety, efficacy and complications of a standardized treatment protocol. *Bull Emerg Trauma*. 2019;7(1):49-54.

Bromberg WJ, Collier BC, Diebel LN, et al. Blunt cerebrovascular injury practice management guidelines: the Eastern Association for the Surgery of Trauma. *J Trauma*. 2012;73(5 suppl 4):S326-S332.

Bukur M, Inaba K, Barmparas G, et al. Routine follow-up imaging of kidney injuries may not be justified. *J Trauma*. 2011;70(5):1229-1233.

Dabbs DN, Stein DM, Philosophe B, Scalea TM. Treatment of major hepatic necrosis: lobectomy versus serial debridement. *J Trauma*. 2010;69(3):562-567.

Daudia A, Biswas D, Jones NS. Risk of meningitis with cerebrospinal fluid rhinorrhea. *Ann Otol Rhinol Laryngol*. 2007;116(12):902-905.

Friedman JA, Ebersold MJ, Quast LM. Post-traumatic cerebrospinal fluid leakage. *World J Surg*. 2001;25(8):1062-1066.

Kim DY, Biffl W, Bokhari F, et al. Evaluation and management of blunt cerebrovascular injury: a practice management guideline from the Eastern Association for the Surgery of Trauma. *J Trauma Acute Care Surg*. 2020;88(6):875-887.

Kozar RA, Crandall M, Shanmuganathan K, et al. Management of adult blunt splenic trauma: a practice management guideline from the Eastern Association for the Surgery of Trauma. *J Trauma Acute Care Surg*. 2020;89(6):1146-1158.

Letoublon C, Morra I, Chen Y, Monnin V, Voirin D, Arvieux C. Hepatic arterial embolization in the management of blunt hepatic trauma: indications and complications. *J Trauma*. 2011;70(5):1032-1036.

Meyfroidt G, Baguley IJ, Menon DK. Paroxysmal sympathetic hyperactivity: the storm after acute brain injury. *Lancet Neurol*. 2017;16(9):721-729.

Rahman NM, Maskell NA, Davies CWH, Hedley EL, Nunn AJ, Gleeson FV. The use of intrapleural tPA and DNase in pleural infection. *N Engl J Med*. 2011;365(6):518-526.

Rappold JF, Sheppard FR, Carmichael SP II, et al. Venous thromboembolism prophylaxis in the trauma intensive care unit: an American Association for the Surgery of Trauma Critical Care Committee Clinical Consensus Document. *Trauma Surg Acute Care Open*. 2021;6(1):e000643.

Schnuriger B, Inaba K, Konstantinidis A, Lustenberger T, Chan LS, Demetriades D. Outcomes of proximal versus distal splenic artery embolization after trauma: a systematic review and meta-analysis. *J Trauma*. 2011;70(1):252-260.

Smith JW, Franklin GA, Harbrecht BG, Richardson JD. Early VATS for blunt chest trauma: a management technique underutilized by acute care surgeons. *J Trauma*. 2011;71(1):102-107.

Stassen NA, Bhullar I, Cheng JD, et al. Selective nonoperative management of blunt splenic injury: an Eastern Association for the Surgery of Trauma practice management guideline. *J Trauma Acute Care Surg*. 2019;88(3):457-467.

Tan CL, Alavi SA, Baldeweg SE, et al. The screening and management of pituitary dysfunction following traumatic brain injury in adults: British Neurotrauma Group guidance. *J Neurol Neurosurg Psychiatry*. 2017; 88(11):971-981.

Velmahos GC, Toutouzas KG, Radin R, et al. High success with nonoperative management of blunt hepatic trauma: the liver is a sturdy organ. *Arch Surg*. 2003;138(5):475-480; discussion 480-481.

Velmahos GC, Zacharias N, Emhoff TA, et al. Management of the most severely injured spleen: a multicenter study of the Research Consortium of New England Centers for Trauma (ReCONECT). *Arch Surg*. 2010; 145(5):456-460.

Vespa PM, Nuwer MR, Nenov V, et al. Increased incidence and impact of nonconvulsive and convulsive seizures after traumatic brain injury as detected by continuous electroencephalographic monitoring. *J Neurosurg*. 1999;91(5):750-760.

Williams B, Carnes A, Lowry J. Beta-2 transferrin in the identification of cerebrospinal fluid. *Clin Chem Lab Med*. 2013;51(8):1633-1637.

Zarzaur BL, Vashi S, Magnotti LJ, Croce MA, Fabian TC. The real risk of splenectomy after discharge home following nonoperative management of blunt splenic injury. *J Trauma*. 2009;66(6):1531-1536; discussion 1536-1538.

SECTION 20

Pediatric Emergencies

Section Editor: Edward A. Bittner

20.1

Airway and Pulmonary Emergencies

Lakshmi Nemani and Christoph G.S. Nabzdyk

Respiratory distress is a frequent cause of pediatric emergency department visits, and cardiac arrest in children most commonly occurs due to respiratory failure. Conditions of the upper airway (croup, epiglottitis, bacterial tracheitis, retropharyngeal/peritonsillar abscess, foreign body obstruction) and lower airway (bronchiolitis, asthma, pneumonia) can cause respiratory emergencies in the pediatric population. When these conditions progress to respiratory failure, intubation and mechanical ventilation versus noninvasive ventilation (NIV) strategies may be required. When managing the pediatric airway, it is important to note several key factors that distinguish infants' and children's airway anatomy and physiology from that of adults.

The Pediatric Airway: Anatomy and Physiology

Anatomy

- Large occiput necessitating alignment of the external auditory meatus with the sternal notch
- Superior/anterior glottic opening
- Large, "floppy" epiglottis requiring lifting with a straight blade to expose the airway

Physiology

- Smaller lung volumes making patients vulnerable to barotrauma during mask ventilation
- Higher metabolic rate (VO_2) and lower functional residual capacity (FRC) (high VO_2:FRC ratio) leading to rapid desaturation and significantly shorter safe apneic times compared with adults

Upper Airway Emergencies

Croup (Laryngotracheobronchitis)

- Definition: viral infection (usually parainfluenza) causing subglottic edema
- Epidemiology: peak incidence among children aged 6 months to 3 years
- Presentation: nontoxic appearing, upper respiratory infection (URI) followed by a barky cough, hoarseness, inspiratory stridor, and respiratory distress
- Imaging: "steeple" sign, or subglottic narrowing on posterior-anterior x-ray
- Management: one dose of 0.6 mg/kg of oral dexamethasone if able, otherwise parenteral; nebulized racemic epinephrine if stridor at rest; heliox does not provide added benefit compared with standard treatment and should be avoided in children requiring supplemental oxygen.
- Special considerations: altered mental status, somnolence, and poor air movement suggest severe croup and impending respiratory failure. Intubation should be pursued in a controlled setting with several smaller sized endotracheal tubes (ETT) available in anticipation of a swollen airway.

Epiglottitis (Supraglottitis)

- Definition: bacterial infection leading to swollen epiglottis with risk for airway obstruction
- Epidemiology: historically most common in 2- to 6-year-olds, but currently more often diagnosed in older children. Fewer cases are attributable to *Haemophilus influenzae* type B (HIB) after the vaccine was introduced in 1985, but nontypable *H. influenzae* remains the most common cause. Other pathogens include *Streptococcus pneumoniae*, *Staphylococcus aureus*, and group A *Streptococcus*.
- Presentation: toxic appearing, abrupt onset, stridor, tripoding, fever, muffled voice, dysphagia, sore throat, NO cough
- Imaging: "thumbprint" sign, or thickened epiglottic folds, on lateral x-ray
- Management: keep child calm preferably in caregiver's arms, intubation in the operating room with anesthesia and surgery present, broad-spectrum intravenous (IV)

antibiotics. Steroids are frequently given, but there is no compelling evidence to suggest their efficacy.
- Special considerations: symptoms progress quickly; drooling may be a sign of impending airway compromise.

Bacterial Tracheitis

- Definition: bacterial superinfection of the trachea and bronchi, causing edema, pseudomembrane formation, and possible complete airway obstruction
- Epidemiology: usually affects children around 3 years old in the fall and winter months. Usually polymicrobial
- Presentation: toxic appearing, fever, preceding URI, stridor, tachypnea, respiratory distress, purulent debris in trachea, sometimes wheezing, progresses to respiratory failure over days (less abrupt than epiglottitis)
- Imaging: subglottic and tracheal narrowing on lateral x-ray, irregular tracheal contour
- Management: if impending respiratory failure, pursue intubation with a small ETT (1 mm smaller than calculated for age), given airway edema; broad-spectrum IV antibiotics
- Special considerations: historically mortality rate was as high as 40% but is more recently quoted between 3% and 20%. Monitor for toxic shock syndrome, given *S. aureus* and *Streptococcus pneumoniae* are two common pathogens. Frequent ETT suctioning and/or bronchoscopy to remove debris from the trachea may be needed.

Retropharyngeal Pharyngeal Abscess

- Definition: abscess forming bacterial infection filling the retropharyngeal space between the posterior wall of esophagus (retropharyngeal fascia) and the anterior border of cervical vertebrae (prevertebral fascia)
- Epidemiology: children younger than 5 years of age, uncommon in older population because retropharyngeal lymph nodes regress in adolescence. Common pathogens include: group A beta-hemolytic *Streptococcus* and *S. aureus* (including methicillin-resistant *S. aureus*)
- Presentation: toxic appearing, fever, sore throat, stridor, drooling, nuchal rigidity and torticollis, respiratory distress. Onset less abrupt onset than epiglottitis
- Imaging: lateral neck x-ray with neck extension during inspiration shows widened prevertebral space (cutoff >7 mm at C2, >14 mm at C6)
- Management: broad-spectrum IV antibiotics, intubation or surgical airway if concerned for impending respiratory failure/airway obstruction, pediatric otolaryngology consultation for surgical management depending on the size of abscess and response to antibiotics
- Special considerations: computed tomography (CT) scan indicated for surgical planning; retropharyngeal pharyngeal abscess (RPA) can cause several severe complications including mediastinitis and carotid artery aneurysm/rupture.

Peritonsillar Abscess

- Definition: purulent material in the peritonsillar fossa
- Epidemiology: usually occurs in adolescents; often polymicrobial
- Presentation: fever, sore throat, voice changes, drooling, trismus, uvula deviation away from asymmetric swelling on the affected side
- Imaging: ultrasound, CT scan to confirm abscess/fluid collection when unresponsive to treatment or unsure of diagnosis
- Management: broad-spectrum IV antibiotics, needle aspiration versus incision and drainage (I&D), supportive care with fluids and analgesia. Does not require inpatient admission if patient is tolerating fluids and medications by mouth
- Special considerations: injury to the internal carotid artery is a potential complication during needle aspiration and I&D.

Foreign Body Aspiration

- Epidemiology: usually children up to 5 years old
- Presentation: nontoxic appearing, sudden onset, stridor, can also present similarly to a lower airway process with coughing, unilateral wheezing, and decreased breath sounds

  Imaging: radiopaque foreign bodies, air trapping, atelectasis, or unilateral differences in aeration may be seen on inspiratory and expiratory chest x-rays; nasal fiberoptic scope can be used for direct visualization of objects in the hypopharynx.
- Management: avoid causing agitation as this can worsen airway resistance; if the child can cough and talk, allow them to remain in a position of comfort and provide supplemental oxygen; if the object is visible, forceps may be used to attempt retrieval; otherwise, laryngoscopy or bronchoscopy may be needed to remove the foreign body.
- Special considerations: for complete airway obstruction trial back blows/chest thrusts (for children <1 year or above) or abdominal thrusts (only for children >1 year old). Further complications from foreign body aspiration may include airway perforation, infection, and mediastinitis.

Lower Airway Emergencies

Bronchiolitis

- Definition: viral infection leading to inflammation and obstruction of the small airways
- Epidemiology: usually caused by respiratory syncytial virus in winter and early spring and affects mostly children under 2 years of age
- Presentation: URI symptoms with upper airway secretions for several days followed by lower airway symptoms (cough, tachypnea, retractions, wheezing, rales), inflammation, mucous, and debris
- Management: supportive care with hydration, pulmonary toilet. Saline nebulizers may reduce respiratory illness severity score and hospitalization risk. Bronchodilators and steroids have not proven effective in routine management.
- Special considerations: consider admission for patients <6 weeks old, requiring supplemental oxygen, IV fluids, or those with underlying lung disease.

Asthma

- Definition: inflammation of the airway with hyperreactivity leading to bronchospasm and airway obstruction
- Epidemiology: most common in school-aged children and adolescents 5 to 17 years old. Exacerbations can be triggered by viral upper respiratory infections, weather changes, or known environmental allergens.

- Presentation: wheezing, tachypnea, cough, and increased work of breathing/use of accessory muscles progressing to bradypnea, absent breath sounds, and hypoxia
- Management: B_2 agonists such as albuterol (metered-dose inhaler > nebulizer), anticholinergic bronchodilator such as ipratropium, systemic corticosteroids such as dexamethasone; IV magnesium and subcutaneous/intramuscular epinephrine for refractory cases; evidence on the efficacy of heliox is mixed.
- Special considerations: altered mental status, lack of breath sounds, hypoxia, and pulsus paradoxus are signs of critical airflow obstruction and should trigger consideration of intubation.

Pneumonia

- Definition: lower respiratory infection
- Epidemiology: pneumonia is a leading cause of pediatric mortality globally and a leading cause of emergency department presentation in the United States. Most likely etiologies of pneumonia vary by age group: maternally transmitted organisms in neonates, Chlamydophila trachomatis in early infants aged 2 to 12 weeks, bacterial pneumonias in infants aged 3 to 4 months, viruses in children under 2 years, and pneumococcal and atypical organisms in children aged 2 to 5 years. In children aged 5 to 13 years, *S. pneumoniae* is the most common pathogen causing pneumonia, but *Mycoplasma pneumoniae* is common as well.
- Presentation: presentation is nonspecific and may vary depending on the patient's age and etiology of the illness. Symptoms may include fever, cough, and respiratory distress with rhonchi or decreased breath sounds heard on chest auscultation.
- Imaging: while a lobar infiltrate may be seen on chest x-ray, imaging findings may be nonspecific in viral and atypical pneumonias.
- Management: supportive care and antibiotics targeted toward the causative organism
- Special considerations: dehydration, hypoxemia, and signs of hemodynamic instability warrant admission.

Ventilation Strategies

- NIV strategies, such as continuous positive airway pressure (CPAP) and bilevel positive airway pressure (BIPAP), are an option for supporting children with hypoxic and/or hypercapnic respiratory failure. NIV is contraindicated in patients with airway obstruction, diminished consciousness, apnea, inability to manage secretions, absent airway reflexes, active nausea/vomiting, and severe hemodynamic instability. Complications such as barotrauma and volutrauma are possible with NIV if device pressure and flow are not carefully monitored.
- High-flow nasal cannula (HFNC), in contrast to NIV, is indicated for only hypoxemic respiratory failure as it does not effectively increase alveolar ventilation. Apnea, airway obstruction, and hypercarbic respiratory failure are contraindications to HFNC. Barotrauma remains a possible complication, especially if the flow rate is inappropriately high for the patient's weight, but was also reported at lower flow rates.
- The upper airway emergencies described earlier may progress to respiratory failure and airway closure, requiring securing of the airway with an ETT. While not an appropriate substitute for definitive airway management, HFNC can additionally be used to passively oxygenate children and prolong safe apnea times peri-intubation, and CPAP/BIPAP can be used to preoxygenate prior to intubation.

SUGGESTED READINGS

Akhavan M. Beyond pharyngitis: retropharyngeal abscess, peritonsillar abscess, epiglottitis, bacterial tracheitis, and postoperative tonsillectomy. *Emerg Med Clin N Am*. 2021;39:661-675.

Choi J, Lee GL. Common pediatric respiratory emergencies. *Emerg Med Clin N Am*. 2012;30:529-563.

Dalziel SR, Haskell L, O'Brien S, et al. Bronchiolitis. *Lancet*. 2022;400:392-406.

Ebeledike C, Ahmad T. Pediatric pneumonia. In: *StatPearls* [Internet]. StatPearls Publishing; 2024.

Guerra AM, Waseem M. Epiglottitis. In: *StatPearls* [Internet]. StatPearls Publishing; 2024.

Hegde S, Prodhan P. Serious air leak syndrome complicating high-flow nasal cannula therapy: a report of 3 cases. *Pediatrics*. 2013;131(3):e939-e944.

House SA, Gadomski AM, Ralston SL. Evaluating the placebo status of nebulized normal saline in patients with acute viral bronchiolitis: a systematic review and meta-analysis. *JAMA Pediatr*. 2020;174(3):250-259.

Lim CA, Whitney R, Rose JM. Airway foreign bodies. In: Rose E ed. *Pediatric Emergencies: A Practical, Clinical Guide*. Oxford University Press; 2021:37-50.

Miller KA, Nagler J. Emergent airway management in pediatrics. In: Rose E ed. *Pediatric Emergencies: A Practical, Clinical Guide*. Oxford University Press; 2021:37-50.

Rahim N, Uraizee A, Rao A, Finkel L. Pediatric respiratory emergencies—recognition, approach, and management. *Pediatr Ann*. 2023;52(4):e146-e152.

Sequera-Ramos L, Garcia-Marcinkiewicz A, Riva T, Fuchs A. Noninvasive ventilation in children: a review for the pediatric anesthesiologist. *Pediatr Anesth*. 2022;32:262-272.

Sharma GD, Conrad C. Croup, epiglottitis, and bacterial tracheitis. In: American Academy of Pediatrics Section on Pediatric Pulmonology; Light MJ, Blaisdell CJ, Homnick DN, ed. *Pediatric Pulmonology*. American Academy of Pediatrics; 2011:347-363.

20.2

Surgical Emergencies

Michael Flaherty

Surgical Emergencies

Omphalocele

- Abdominal contents herniate *through* the umbilicus (usually bowel, possibly liver).
- Supraumbilical portions outside the abdominal wall covered by the peritoneum and amniotic sac
- Caused by a defect in the folding of the embryonic disc
- Associated with gastrointestinal (GI) and cardiac defects
- Treatment
  - Naso/orogastric tube to intermittent suction
  - Do not attempt to reduce.
  - Wrap sac with sterile, saline-soaked gauze and dressing to preserve heat and minimize fluid losses.
  - If sac ruptured, cover with saline gauze and rapid surgical intervention needed.
  - Plastic wrap to support sac on the abdomen to support the abdominal contents
  - Broad-spectrum antibiotics
  - Surgical repair primarily or in stages depending on size

Gastroschisis

- Herniation of intestine through the abdominal wall *lateral* to the umbilicus (usually bowel, possibly gonads)
- Compared to omphalocele:
  - No covering sac
  - Smaller
  - Fewer associated abnormalities
    - Can be associated with atresia of the small bowel
- Treatment
  - Surgical emergency
  - Wrap the bowel with sterile saline dressings covered with plastic wrap.
  - Nasogastric tube to suction
  - Wrap infant to reduce heat loss.
  - Broad-spectrum antibiotics
  - Surgical repair almost always done in stages.

Congenital Diaphragmatic Hernia

- Herniation of abdominal contents into the thoracic cavity
  - 85% left sided
  - Scaphoid abdomen, bowel sounds in the chest, respiratory distress
- Pulmonary hypoplasia and pulmonary hypertension are the most serious sequelae.
- Management
  - Intubation and mechanical ventilation required, often need high-frequency oscillatory ventilation or extracorporeal membrane oxygenation (ECMO)
  - Selective use of surfactant
  - Medical management of pulmonary hypertension
  - Operative repair with balanced chest drainage required or will have high transalveolar pressure gradients.

Tracheoesophageal Fistula

- Four types: most common is esophageal atresia with distal tracheoesophageal fistula.
- Associated with both cardiac and GI abnormalities
- VACTERL syndrome: vertebral, anal, cardiac, tracheal, esophageal, renal, and limb defects
- Treatment: prone positioning with the head of bed up 60 degrees, NPO, and surgical repair

Necrotizing Enterocolitis

- Inflammation and ischemia of the lower GI tract
- Most often in preterm infants, but can be seen in term infants
- Possible etiologies: hypoxemia, hypotension, infection/systemic inflammatory response syndrome (SIRS)
- Signs: abdominal distension, feeding intolerance, lethargy, bloody stool (gross or occult), pneumatosis intestinalis (intramural gas), or portal venous gas on plain radiographs
- Management: NPO, gastric decompression, antibiotics, pediatric surgery consultation
- Most resolve medically, resection of the intestine if pneumoperitoneum, no improvement with medical management

Malrotation With Volvulus

- Posterior fixation of the intestinal mesentery due to malrotation in utero predisposes to intestine twisting on itself, causing ischemia
- Most commonly seen in children less than 1 month of age, later diagnosis possible
- Signs: bilious vomiting, ill appearing, upper GI with small bowel follow-through shows C-loop of duodenum and small bowel to the right of the spine

Pyloric Stenosis

- Gastric outlet obstruction due to hypertrophy of pylorus
- Manifests between 2 and 8 weeks of life
- Males more than females
- Signs: nonbilious projectile vomiting, hungry infant, dehydration with hypokalemic, hypochloremic metabolic alkalosis
- Management: ultrasound to confirm diagnosis, gastric decompression, pediatric surgery consultation, operative repair once metabolic derangements corrected

Meckel Diverticulum

- Remnant of the omphalomesenteric duct that usually contains gastric or pancreatic tissue
- Rule of 2s: 2% of the population, 2% get complications, most often symptomatic around age 2, 2 in long, 2 ft from the ileocecal valve, 1/2 contain gastric mucosa
- Painless rectal bleeding
- Diagnoses with “Meckel scan” (technetium-99m pertechnetate)

Intussusception

- Telescoping of one part of bowel into another causing bowel ischemia
- Majority are ileocolic.
- Profound lethargy can be the only presenting sign.
- Intermittent pain, often raising knees to chest
- Rectal bleeding common, but classic "currant jelly" bleed rarely seen
- Abdominal x-ray (AXR) may show paucity of gas in the right lower quadrant +/− air fluid levels.
- Ultrasound is usually the first diagnostic test of choice.
- Air enema can be used for diagnosis and is the method of choice to reduce.
- Surgery if air enema fails or intussusception recurs
- Consider lead point (Meckel, polyp, lymphoma) as cause, especially in children older than 5 years, who are less likely to have spontaneous intussusception.

Biliary Atresia

- Most common reason for pediatric liver transplantation
- Presents with prolonged and obstructive jaundice (direct/conjugated hyperbilirubinemia), alcoholic stools, dark urine, hepatomegaly
- Affects both intrahepatic and extrahepatic ducts
  - Type I: common bile duct and proximal cystic biliary duct
  - Type II: common hepatic duct
  - Type III: (most common) affects the entire extrahepatic biliary tree
- Progresses to cirrhosis, portal hypertension, and fulminant liver failure if not treated
- Kasai procedure (hepatoportoenterostomy) is the initial surgical treatment.
  - Most successful if performed prior up to the age of 8 weeks
  - Successful in over half of patients in clearing jaundice, and they will subsequently have an 80% chance of reaching adolescence without the need for transplantation.
- Medical management consists of antibiotics, ursodeoxycholic acid to improve the flow of bile and nutritional support/fat-soluble vitamin supplementation.
- 10-year survival after liver transplant is >80%.

SUGGESTED READINGS

Advanced Trauma Life Support for Doctors. *ATLS Student Course Manual*. 10th ed. Committee on Trauma of American College of Surgeons; 2018.

D'Agostino J. Pediatric airway nightmares. *Emerg Med Clin N Am*. 2010; 28(1):119-126.

Eicher DJ, Wagner CL, Katikaneni LP, et al. Moderate hypothermia in neonatal encephalopathy: safety outcomes. *Pediatr Neurol*. 2005;32(1): 18-24.

Harper MB, Fleisher, GR. Infectious disease emergencies. In: Fleisher GR, Ludwig S, eds. *Textbook of Pediatric Emergency Medicine*. 6th ed. Lippincott, Williams & Wilkins; 2010:303-322.

Hopkins A, Lahiri T, Salerno R, Heath B. Changing epidemiology of life-threatening upper airway infections: the reemergence of bacterial tracheitis. *Pediatrics*. 2006;118(4):1418-1421.

Neu, J, Walker, WA. Necrotizing enterocolitis. *N Engl J Med*. 2011;364(3): 255-264.

Pickering LJ, ed. *Red Book: 2024 Report of the Committee on Infectious Diseases*. 33rd ed. American Academy of Pediatrics; 2024.

Shargorodsky J, Whittemore KR, Lee GS. Bacterial tracheitis: a therapeutic approach. *Laryngoscope*. 2010;120(12):2498-2501.

Skarsgard ED. Management of gastroschisis. *Curr Opin Pediatr*. 2016; 28(3):363-369.

20.3

Cardiovascular Emergencies

Michael Salt and Lisa Bartucca

Cardiovascular Emergencies

- Age-related presentation of various congenital cardiac anomalies
  - 0 to 4 weeks: ductal-dependent lesions as the ductus arteriosus closes
    - Hypoplastic left heart syndrome
    - Aortic stenosis, interrupted aortic arch, coarctation of the aorta
    - Transposition of the great arteries
    - Tetralogy of Fallot
    - Truncus arteriosus
    - Total anomalous venous return
    - Tricuspid atresia
    - Pulmonary atresia
  - 6 weeks to 3 months: lesion causing significant left-to-right shunt as pulmonary vascular resistance falls
    - Anomalous left coronary artery from the pulmonary artery (ALCAPA)
      - Often irritable and difficult to console due to angina
    - Large ventricular septal defect
- Cardiogenic shock
  - Four etiologies
    - Congenital heart disease with poor cardiac output (hypoplastic left heart syndrome, coarctation of the aorta)
    - Cardiac muscle disorders (primary neuromuscular disorders, myocarditis)
    - Dysrhythmias (supraventricular tachycardia [SVT], complete atrioventricular [AV] block)
    - Metabolic disorders (hypoglycemia, adrenal insufficiency, rare inborn errors of metabolism)
    - Noncardiac conditions leading to cardiogenic shock: bilateral pneumothoraces, cardiac tamponade
  - Typical appearance of cardiogenic shock: poor feeding, mottled, cold, lethargic, poor urine output, hypotensive, tachycardic or bradycardic, enlarged liver, prolonged capillary refill, rales, elevated central venous pressure (CVP) >10, acidosis, hypoglycemia

  - Initial management: support airway, obtain access; if etiology of shock unclear, administer small bolus (no >10 mL/kg normal saline [NS]) and then reevaluate for the development of rales, enlarged liver, and gallop.
  - Pharmacologic agents
    - Choice of agent and dosing should be tailored to the individual patient, consider:
      - Dopamine, dobutamine, or epinephrine for inotropic support
      - Milrinone for afterload reduction
      - Prostaglandins (PGE1) for any neonate presenting with suspected cardiogenic shock until a ductal-dependent lesion has been ruled out by ECHO
      - Norepinephrine if concern for septic shock
      - May cause apnea, so be prepared to intubate
      - May cause hypotension, so be prepared to start a vasopressor
      - May cause fever
    - Inhaled nitric oxide for lesions associated with right ventricular failure, such as, persistent pulmonary hypertension
- Life-threatening arrhythmias
  - SVT
    - May be associated with Wolff-Parkinson-White syndrome
    - Children may present with nonspecific history of poor feeding, inconsolable crying, fussy behavior, rales, enlarged liver, and large heart with pulmonary edema on chest radiograph.
    - SVT versus sinus tachycardia
      - SVT: >220 bpm in infants, >180 in children, abrupt onset, absent p waves, no variability
      - ST: <220 in infants, <180 in children, gradual onset, p waves present, +variability, usually responds to fever control and volume
    - Treatment
      - Stable SVT (signs of good end-organ perfusion)
        - Vagal maneuvers (ice to face, have child blow bubbles, bear down, knee to chest)
        - Adenosine (very short half-life, so must administer quickly with rapid flush through a peripheral intravenous line [PIV] placed as close to the heart as possible before drug is hydrolyzed)
      - Unstable SVT
        - Synchronized cardioversion at 0.5 to 1 J/kg with defibrillator ready in case of fatal arrhythmia; have electrocardiogram (ECG) running to capture transient normal sinus rhythm (NSR) in the event that patient reverts into SVT

SUGGESTED READINGS

Advanced Trauma Life Support for Doctors. *ATLS Student Course Manual*. 10th ed. American College of Surgeons; 2018.

American Heart Association. *Pediatric Advanced Life Support Provider Manual*. American Academy of Pediatrics; 2020.

Maconochie IK, Aickin R, Hazinski MF, et al; on behalf of the Pediatric Life Support Collaborators. Pediatric life support: 2020 International Consensus on Cardiopulmonary Resuscitation and Emergency Cardiovascular Care Science with Treatment Recommendations. *Circulation*. 2020;142(suppl 1):S140-S184.

Topjian AA, Raymond TT, Atkins D, et al; on behalf of the Pediatric Basic and Advanced Life Support Collaborators. Part 4: pediatric basic and advanced life support: 2020 American Heart Association guidelines for cardiopulmonary resuscitation and emergency cardiovascular care. *Circulation*. 2020;142(suppl 2):S469-S523.

Van Diepen S, Katz JN, Albert NM, et al. Contemporary management of cardiogenic shock: a scientific statement from the American Heart Association. *Circulation*. 2017;136:e232-e268.

SECTION 21

Advanced Cardiac Life Support (ACLS) and Advanced Trauma Life Support (ATLS)

Section Editor: Edward A. Bittner

21.1

Advanced Cardiovascular Life Support and Advanced Trauma Life Support Guidelines

Sophia Bechek and Jean Kwo

Advanced Cardiovascular Life Support and Advanced Trauma Life Support Guidelines

Key Points

- Survival from cardiac arrest depends on rapid recognition, performance of high-quality cardiopulmonary resuscitation (CPR), early defibrillation of malignant shockable rhythms and treatment of underlying causes.
- High-quality CPR includes adequate compression depth (at least 2 in [5 cm]) and rate (100-120/min) allowing chest recoil with minimal interruptions in compressions.
- Epinephrine along with high-quality CPR improves survival.
- Consider extracorporeal cardiopulmonary resuscitation (ECPR) for cardiac arrest refractory to ACLS in select patients in experienced extracorporeal membrane oxygenation centers.
- Recognize changes in the trauma patient's status by repeating primary and secondary surveys frequently.
- Initial resuscitation with 1 L crystalloid. If patient requires more resuscitation, move to blood products.
- Use a tourniquet to control severe extremity bleeding.
- Have a low threshold to transfer the patient if their needs exceed your facilities capabilities.
- Early and successful treatment during advanced cardiovascular life support and advanced trauma life support (ACLS/ATLS) protocols starts with effective communication and leadership by a team leader.

Common Themes to Remember

ACLS	ATLS
• High-quality CPR (100-120/min; >2 in) • Minimize interruptions in chest compressions. • Compressions, airway, breathing (CAB)	• Primary ABCDE/Secondary ABCDE • Airway maintenance with restriction of cervical spine motion • Breathing and "normal" ventilation (avoid hypoventilation)
• In cardiac arrest, epinephrine 1 mg every 3-5 min	• Circulation with hemorrhage control • Disability: neurologic status • Exposure/Environmental control: completely undress the patient, but prevent hypothermia

ACLS, advanced cardiovascular life support; ATLS, advanced trauma life support; CPR, cardiopulmonary resuscitation; ABCDE, airway, breathing, circulation, disability,exposure.

Epidemiology

- Leading cause of death overall is diseases of the heart—over 700,000 annually.
- Leading cause of death from ages 1 to 44 years is accidents (unintentional injuries)—over 220,000 annually.

- Trauma is a leading cause of mortality globally and affects low- and middle-income countries disproportionately.

Key Pathophysiology

- ACLS: 5 Hs and 5 Ts (discussed in detail below)
- ATLS: Identify life-threatening injuries and treat.

Advanced Cardiovascular Life Support Guidelines

- Most recent guidelines published in 2020 with a focused update in 2023. Key changes from earlier versions:
  - Affirmation that epinephrine significantly increases return to spontaneous circulation (ROSC) and improves survival, particularly in patients with nonshockable rhythms
  - Vasopressin alone or vasopressin (20 IU) and methylprednisolone (40 mg) after first dose of epinephrine can be considered in patients with cardiac arrest.
  - Amiodarone OR lidocaine can be used for ventricular fibrillation/pulseless ventricular tachycardia if defibrillation fails to achieve ROSC.
  - Routine administration of calcium, magnesium, and sodium bicarbonate in cardiac arrest is not recommended.
  - Atropine IV dose for hemodynamically significant bradycardia is 1 mg (increased from 0.5 mg).
  - Continuous arterial blood pressure and end-tidal CO_2 monitoring can be used to assess CPR quality.
  - Intravenous (IV) access is preferred to intraosseous (IO) for medication administration during ALCS, though the latter is acceptable if IV access is unavailable.
  - Emergent coronary angiography is not routinely recommended in patients after cardiac arrest unless they exhibit signs of significant myocardial ischemia (eg, ST-segment elevation, shock, electrical instability).
  - Postarrest temperature goal of 32 to 37.5 °C (updated from 32 to 36 °C) for patients who do not follow commands after ROSC
  - Trial of antiepileptic medication may be reasonable in survivors of cardiac arrest with concerning electroencephalogram (EEG) patterns.
  - Use of ECPR for cardiac arrest refractory to ACLS is reasonable in select patients in experienced extracorporeal membrane oxygenation centers.
- Management of cardiac arrest: ventricular fibrillation (VF), pulseless ventricular tachycardia (VT), pulseless electrical activity (PEA), and asystole
  - Shout for help/activate emergency response.
  - Start high-quality CPR. "Push hard and fast" (depth 2 in, rate100-120/min for rate) and allow complete chest recoil.
  - Every second without CPR means a lack of cardiac and cerebral perfusion.
  - Look for reversible causes: the 5 Hs and 5 Ts (see Table 21.1.1 and Figure 21.1.1.)
  - VF (disorganized electrical activity) or pulseless VT (organized electric activity of the ventricular myocardium)
    - Defibrillation for VF/pulseless VT is the only therapy proven to increase survival to hospital discharge and should be delivered as soon as possible.

TABLE 21.1.1 The Five Hs and Ts

Hs	Ts
Hypoxia	Toxins
Hypovolemia	Tamponade
Hydrogen ion (acidosis)	Tension pneumothorax
Hypo-/hyperkalemia	Thrombosis—pulmonary
Hypothermia	Thrombosis—cardiac

    - Biphasic defibrillation: Use initial energy dose of 120 to 200 J.
    - Monophasic defibrillation: Use initial energy dose of 360 J.
    - After initial shock, resume CPR immediately for 2 minutes before the next rhythm check.
    - If VF or pulseless VT persists after at least one shock and a cycle of CPR, epinephrine 1 mg should be given every 3 to 5 minutes.
    - Amiodarone or lidocaine (see Table 21.1.2) may be given if VF/VT is refractory to above treatments.
  - Asystole/PEA
    - Identification of a nonshockable rhythm should lead to immediate implementation of CPR for 2 minutes.
    - Epinephrine should be given every 3 to 5 minutes.
    - Look for reversible causes: 5 Hs and 5 Ts (see Table 21.1.1)
  - Special considerations for the pregnant patient in cardiac arrest
    - Maintain continuous manual left uterine displacement to minimize aortocaval compression by gravid uterus.
    - Maternal arrest team consisting of obstetric, neonatal, anesthesia, intensive care, and cardiac arrest services
    - Consider causes of arrest (see Table 21.1.3).
    - Airway management by the most experienced provider
    - Prioritize oxygenation as pregnant patients are more prone to hypoxia.
    - IV access should be above the diaphragm.
    - If receiving magnesium IV, stop and give calcium chloride or gluconate.
    - Perform perimortem cesarean delivery if no ROSC within 5 minutes.
    - Fetal monitoring should *not* be performed given potential interference and distraction from resuscitation.
    - Targeted temperature management for patients are comatose after arrest, with continuous monitoring for fetal bradycardia.
  - Return of spontaneous circulation
    - Sustained return of pulse and blood pressure
    - Sustained increase in end-tidal CO_2
    - If intra-arterial monitoring available, sustained arterial pressure waves
    - Sustained plethysmography tracings on pulse oximetry
  - Post arrest care
    - Manage airway and respiration.
      - Place endotracheal tube if not already placed.
      - Ensure adequate oxygenation (O_2 saturation 92%-98%) and ventilation (normocapnia).
        - Consider lung protective ventilation.

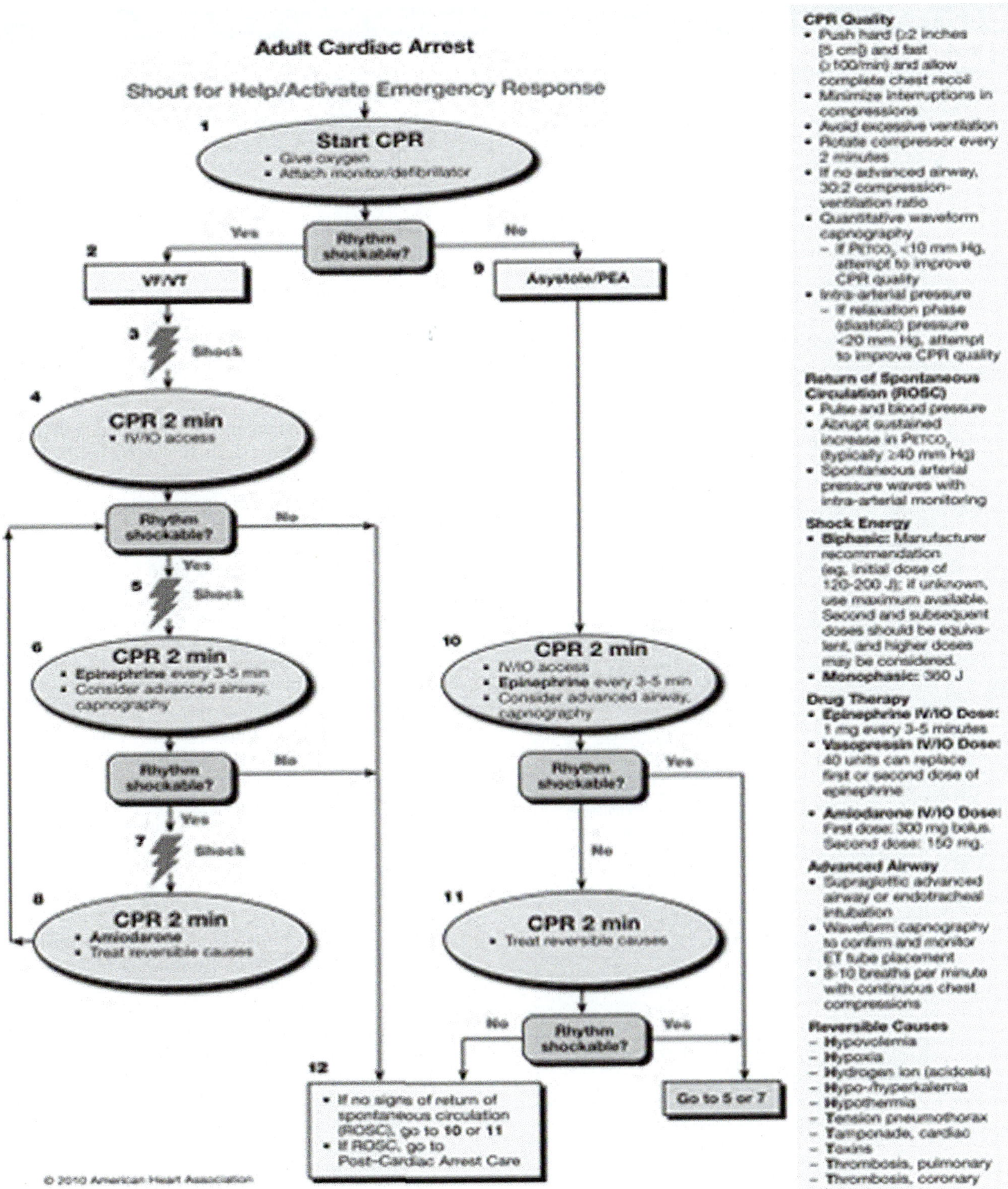

FIGURE 21.1.1 Adult cardiac arrest algorithm. CPR, cardiopulmonary resuscitation; IV/IO, intravenous/intraosseous; PEA, pulseless electrical activity; ROSC, return of spontaneous circulation; VF/VT, ventricular tachycardia/ ventricular fibrillation. (© American Heart Association.)

TABLE 21.1.2 ACLS Pharmacology

Drug Name	Dose	Note
Epinephrine	1 mg	No evidence for use of higher doses
Vasopressin	20 IU	Can be considered after first dose of epinephrine in patients with cardiac arrest
Amiodarone	300 mg first dose 150 mg second dose	VF/pulseless VT if defibrillation fails to achieve ROSC
Amiodarone	150 mg over 10 min Maintenance infusion: 1 mg/min × 6 h	For stable wide-complex tachycardia with pulse
Lidocaine	1-1.5 mg/kg first dose 0.5-0.75 mg/kg second dose	VF/pulseless VT if defibrillation fails to achieve ROSC
Magnesium sulfate	1-2 g in 50-100 mL D5W or NS over 5-60 min	For polymorphic VT associated with a long QT interval (torsades de pointes)
Atropine	1 mg every 3-5 min, max dose 3 mg	For symptomatic bradycardia
Dopamine	5-20 μg/kg/min	For symptomatic bradycardia unresponsive to atropine Titrate dose to HR response.
Epinephrine	2-10 μg/min	For symptomatic bradycardia unresponsive to atropine Titrate dose to HR response.
Adenosine	Initial dose: 6 mg IV followed by 20 mL flush Second dose: 12 mg IV followed by 20 mL flush	For hemodynamically stable patients with regular, monomorphic tachycardia
Procainamide	20-50 mg/min until arrhythmia controlled, QRS increase >50% or max dose of 17 mg/kg given Maintenance infusion: 1-4 mg/min	Avoid in patients with prolonged QT or CHF.
Sotalol	100 mg (1.5 mg/kg over 5 min)	Avoid if QT prolonged.

CHF, congestive heart failure; D5W, dextrose 5% in water; HR, heart rate; NS, normal saline; ROSC, return of spontaneous circulation; VF ventricular fibrillation; VT ventricular tachycardia.

TABLE 21.1.3 Potential Causes of Cardiac Arrest in the Pregnant Patient

Anesthetic complications and drugs
Hemorrhage
Cardiovascular
Embolic
Fever
Hypertension
Other causes of cardiac arrest—see Table 21.1.1

TABLE 21.1.4 Potential Causes of Bradycardia

Hypoxia
Electrolyte abnormality
Myocardial ischemia/infarction
Drugs/Toxins (eg, calcium channel blockers, β-blockers, digoxin, cholinergic agents)

- Ensure adequate circulation.
  - Systolic blood pressure >90 mm Hg, mean arterial pressure >65 mm Hg
    - Administer crystalloid as needed.
    - Administer vasopressor or inotropic agent as needed.
- Evaluation for emergent cardiac intervention and targeted temperature management should occur concurrently.
  - Emergent cardiac intervention for:
    - ST-elevation myocardial infarction (STEMI)
    - Cardiogenic shock (including need for mechanical circulatory support)
- Targeted temperature management for patients who are comatose after arrest
  - Obtain CT scan of brain.
  - Target temperature 32 to 36 °C for 24 hours
  - Use cooling device with feedback loop.
  - Continuously measure core temperature.
  - Continuous or intermittent EEG monitoring
- Continue to evaluate and treat reversible etiologies.

○ Treatment of symptomatic bradycardia and tachycardia

- Adult bradycardia (Heart rate <50/min with a pulse)
  - Maintain airway and oxygenation; obtain IV access; 12-lead electrocardiogram (ECG).
  - Consider and treat possible causes (see Table 21.1.4 and Figure 21.1.2).
  - If bradycardia is associated with symptoms (hypotension, altered mental status, chest pain, heart failure)
  - Give atropine every 3 to 5 minutes (see Table 21.1.2).
  - Use atropine cautiously in the presence of acute coronary ischemia or myocardial infarction (MI) as it can cause tachycardia.
  - Atropine may be ineffective in patients who have undergone cardiac transplantation.
  - Transcutaneous pacing may be indicated if atropine is ineffective or when IV/IO access is not available.
  - IV infusions of adrenergic agonists (eg, epinephrine, dopamine, see Table 21.1.2) can be used in conjunction with or as an alternative to transcutaneous pacing.
  - Obtain cardiology consult when appropriate.
  - Consider transvenous pacing.
- Adult tachycardia (HR ≥150/min with a pulse, see Table 21.1.5)
  - Maintain airway and oxygenation; obtain IV access.
  - If unstable: acutely altered mental status, chest pain, acute heart failure, hypotension
    - Perform immediate synchronized cardioversion (use device's recommended energy level).
    - Consider adenosine for unstable regular narrow-complex tachycardia.

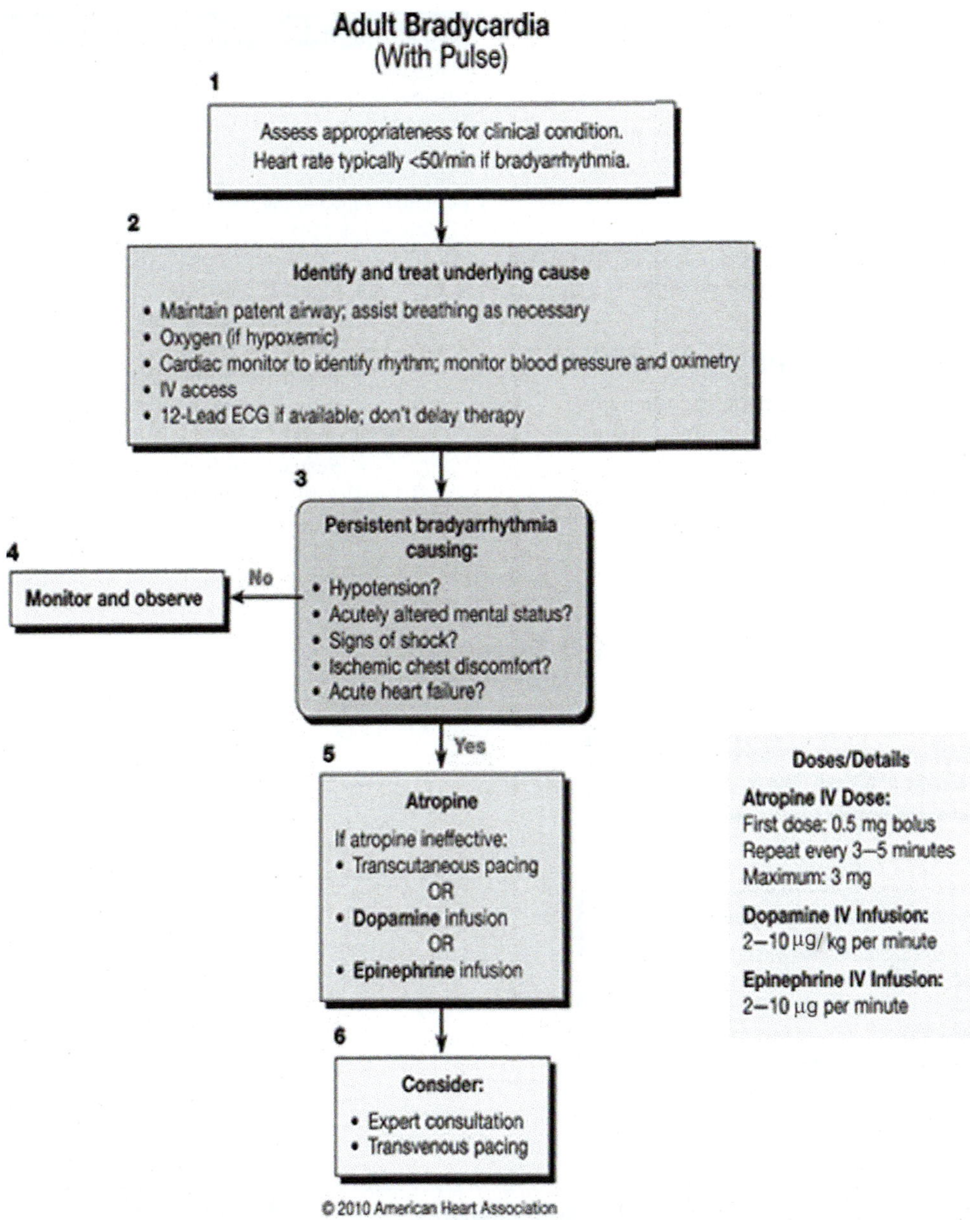

FIGURE 21.1.2 Adult bradycardia (with pulse) algorithm. ECG, electrocardiogram; IV, intravenous. (© American Heart Association.)

TABLE 21.1.5 Tachyarrhythmias

Wide-complex tachycardia HR >150, QRS duration >120 ms	Aberrant conduction of SVT Preexcited tachycardias (Wolff-Parkinson-White) Ventricular tachycardia Rapid ventricularly paced rhythm in patient with pacemaker
Narrow-complex tachycardia (QRS duration <120 ms)	Sinus tachycardia Atrial fibrillation Atrial flutter AV nodal reentry Accessory pathway tachycardia Multifocal atrial tachycardia Junctional tachycardia

AV, atrioventricular, HR, heart rate; SVT, supraventricular tachycardia.

- Defibrillation for unstable irregular, wide-complex tachycardia
- If stable, obtain 12-lead electrocardiogram (EKG) diagnose the arrhythmia (with expert consultation as required)
- Determine if rhythm is (1) narrow-complex or wide-complex, (2) regular or irregular.
- Narrow QRS-complex (Supraventricular Tachycardia [SVT]) tachycardias (QRS <0.12)
  - Vagal maneuvers
  - Adenosine for patients with regular, monomorphic tachycardia to aid rhythm diagnosis. (It will terminate tachycardias caused by atrioventricular (AV) reentry and will slow ventricular response to atrial arrhythmias.)
  - Beta-blocker or calcium channel blocker

- Use calcium channel blockers with caution as they can accelerate preexcited atrial arrhythmias.
- Wide QRS-complex tachycardias (QRS ≥0.12 second)
  - Adenosine if regular and monomorphic (SVT with aberrancy)—see Table 21.1.2.
  - Antiarrhythmic infusion (see Table 21.1.2 and Figure 21.1.3)
  - Magnesium for polymorphic VT associated with a long QT interval (torsades de pointes)

Advance Trauma Life Support Guidelines

- Timing is essential: ATLS is a systematic approach for assessment and treatment of critically injured patients (see Table 21.1.6).
  - Preparation
    - Prehospital
      - Maintain airway.
      - Immobilize patient.
      - Control bleeding.
      - Minimize scene time: transport immediately to closest facility.
      - Report information needed to hospital so trauma team members can be mobilized.
    - Hospital
      - Resuscitation area available
      - Airway equipment working and easily accessible
      - Warmed IV crystalloid solutions available
      - Additional medical assistance available if needed
      - Laboratory/radiology services available

TABLE 21.1.6 Components of ACLS Initial Assessment
Preparation
Triage
Primary survey (ABCDEs)
Consider need for patient transfer.
Secondary survey
Continued monitoring/reevaluation after resuscitation
Definitive care

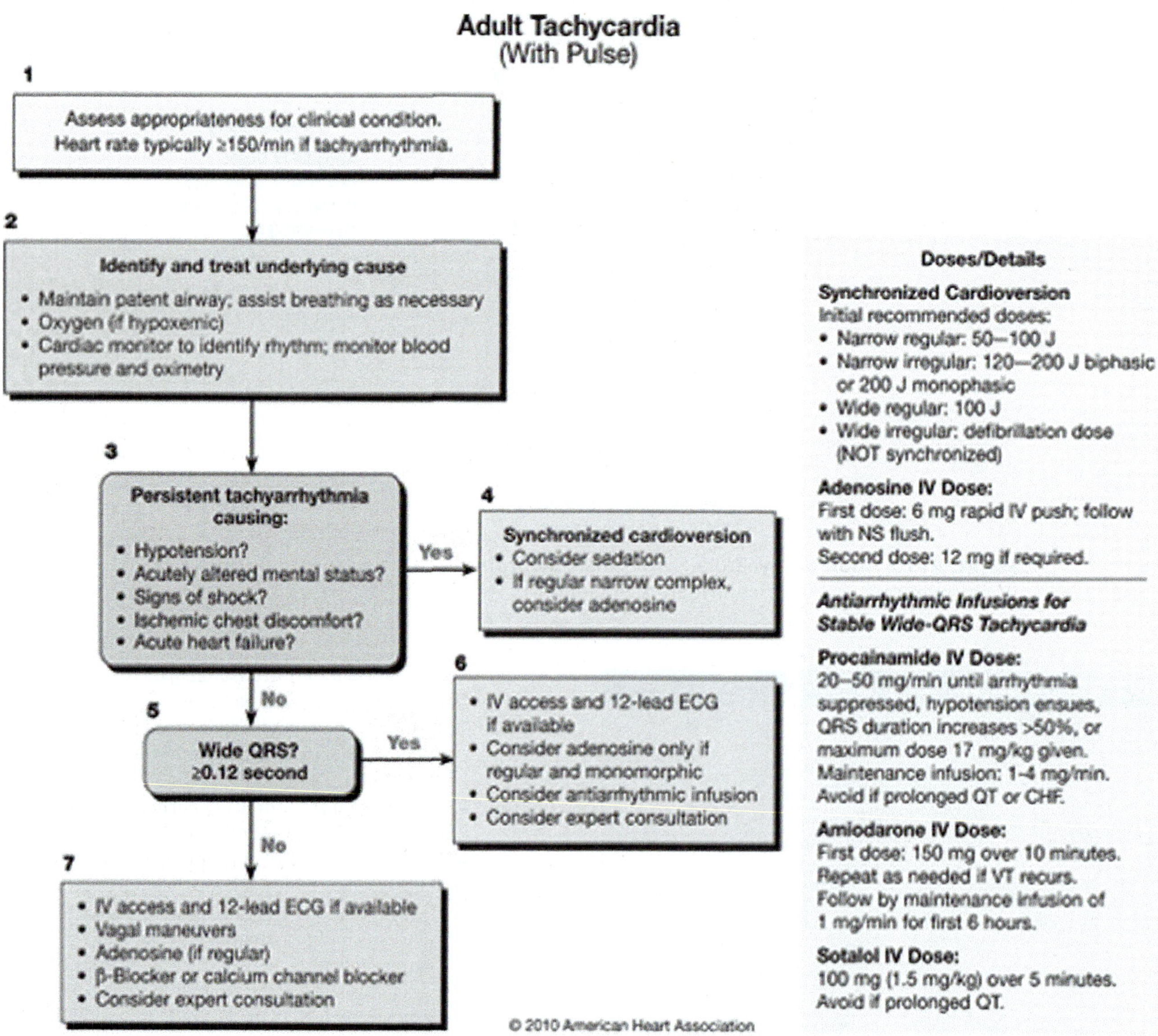

FIGURE 21.1.3 Adult tachycardia (with pulse) algorithm. ECG, electrocardiogram; IV, intravenous. (© American Heart Association.)

- Triage
  - Sorting of patients based on severity of injuries and resources available
- Primary survey
  - Rapid identification of life-threatening conditions with simultaneous resuscitation using ABCDEs
  - Should be repeated whenever a patient's status changes
    - Airway—Unlike ACLS, airway evaluation is paramount to avoid compromised oxygen delivery to brain and other vital structures.
      - Assess airway patency and if needed, maintain patency with:
        - Jaw thrust, chin lift in conjunction with keeping spine stabilized.
        - Nasal or oral away (caution in head/facial injuries).
      - Consider definitive airway (tube within trachea with cuff inflated below vocal cords) if:
        - Altered level of consciousness (Glasgow Coma Scale [GCS] ≤8 requires prompt intubation).
        - Maxillofacial trauma.
        - Neck injuries (both penetrating and blunt).
        - Laryngeal trauma.
      - Drug assisted intubation (administration of induction agents, sedatives, neuromuscular blocking agents) for patients with intact gag reflex.
      - Consider supraglottic devices (eg, LMA) for patients who fail initial intubation attempt.
      - Videolaryngoscopy may be beneficial.
      - Assume presence of spinal injury. Avoid excessive movement of cervical spine.
    - Breathing
      - Assess adequacy of ventilation.
        - Look for tachypnea, increased work of breathing.
        - Obtain arterial or venous blood gas.
        - Examination: Look for adequate, symmetric chest rise, auscultate for equal, bilateral lung sounds.
        - Use pulse oximetry, capnography to assess adequacy of oxygenation and ventilation.
      - Decompress hemothorax/pneumothorax.
      - Definitive airway if inadequate ventilation
      - Watch for complications of positive pressure ventilation (barotrauma, tension pneumothorax).
    - Circulation
      - Shock = inadequate tissue perfusion
      - Most common cause of shock is hemorrhage.
      - Four classes of hemorrhagic shock based on:
        - Percent of blood volume lost.
        - Heart rate.
        - Pulse pressure.
        - Respiratory rate.
        - Urine output.
        - Glasgow coma scale.
        - Base deficit.
        - Need for blood products.
      - Stop the bleeding (consider external and internal sources of bleeding).
        - Use tourniquet for extremity bleeding.
      - Initial resuscitation: up to 1 L warmed crystalloid
      - Subsequent resuscitation with blood products (whole blood, packed red blood cells [pRBCs], plasma, platelets)
      - Massive transfusion defined as >10 units of pRBCs over 24 hours or more than 4 units of pRBCs in 1 hour
      - Watch for coagulopathy.
        - Viscoelastic testing may be useful.
        - Consider reversal agents for patients on anticoagulants or antiplatelet medications.
        - Give tranexamic acid (TXA) within 3 hours.
        - Keep patient warm.
      - Always keep in mind other causes of shock:
        - Cardiogenic
        - Obstructive (cardiac tamponade, tension pneumothorax)
        - Neurogenic
        - Sepsis
    - Disability—neurologic exam
      - Determine GCS.
      - Examine and document pupils for size, reaction, and equality.
      - Decreased level of consciousness can be sign of decreased cerebral perfusion.
    - Exposure—complete examination
      - Complete exposure of patient to examine for additional injuries but prevent hypothermia
  - Secondary survey
    - Done after resuscitation and stabilization of patient
    - Obtain patient history including allergies, current medications, past illnesses/pregnancy, last meal, events/environment related to injury.
    - Injuries differ depending on injury mechanism:
      - Blunt
      - Penetrating
      - Thermal
      - Hazardous environment: exposure to chemicals, toxins, radiation
    - Physical examination
      - Head and maxillofacial
      - Cervical spine and neck
      - Chest
      - Abdomen and pelvis
      - Perineum/rectum/vagina
      - Musculoskeletal
      - Neurologic
      - Adjuncts to secondary survey
        - Diagnostic tests to identify injuries (eg, x-rays, CT scans, angiograms, bronchoscopy)
    - Trauma patients need constant reevaluation and a high index of suspicion for missed, life-threatening injuries.
    - Consider need for transfer to higher level of care.

SUGGESTED READINGS

American Heart Association. *Highlights of the 2020 American Heart Association: Guidelines for CPR and ECC*. Accessed June 3, 2024. https://cpr.heart.org/-/media/cpr-files/cpr-guidelines-files/highlights/hghlghts_2020_ecc_guidelines_english.pdf

Apfelbaum JL, Hagberg CA, Connis RT, et al. 2022 American Society of Anesthesiologists Practice guidelines for management of the difficult airway. *Anesthesiology*. 2022;136:31-81.

CRASH-2 trial collaborators, Shakur H, Roberts I, Bautista R, et al. Effects of tranexamic acid on death, vascular occlusive events, and blood transfusion in trauma patients with significant haemorrhage (CRASH-2): a randomised, placebo-controlled trial. *Lancet*. 2010;376:23-32.

Gottlieb M, Alerhand S. Managing cardiac arrest using ultrasound. *Ann Emerg Med*. 2023;81:532-542.

Holcomb JB, Tilley BC, Baraniuk S. Transfusion of plasma, platelets, and red blood cells in a 1:1:1 vs a 1:1:2 ratio and mortality in patients with severe trauma: the PROPPR randomized clinical trial. *JAMA*. 2015;313:471-482.

Low CJW, Ramanathan K, Ling RR, et al. Extracorporeal cardiopulmonary resuscitation versus conventional cardiopulmonary resuscitation in adults with cardiac arrest: a comparative meta-analysis and trial sequential analysis. *Lancet Respir Med*. 2023;11:883-893.

Mutschler A, Nienaber U, Brockamp T, et al. A critical reappraisal of the ATLS classification of hypovolaemic shock: does it really reflect clinical reality? *Resuscitation*. 2013;84:309-313.

Panchal AP, Bartos JA, Cabanas JG, et al. Part 3: adult advanced cardiovascular life support: 2020 American Heart Association guidelines for cardiopulmonary resuscitation and emergency cardiovascular care. *Circulation*. 2020;142(suppl 2):S366-S468.

Perkins GD, Ji C, Deakin CD, et al. A randomized trial of epinephrine in out-of-hospital cardiac arrest. *N Engl J Med*. 2018;379:711-721.

Perman SM, Elmer J, Maciel CB, et al. 2023 American Heart Association focused update on adult advanced cardiovascular life support: an update to the American Heart Association guidelines for cardiopulmonary resuscitation and emergency cardiovascular care. *Circulation*. 2023;149:e254-e273.

Rossaint R, Afshari A, Bouillon B, et al. The European guideline on management of major bleeding and coagulopathy following trauma: sixth edition. *Crit Care*. 2023;27:80.

Sayve AC, Neal MD, Leeper CM. Viscoelastic monitoring in trauma resuscitation. *Transfusion*. 2020;60:33-51.

Stewart RM, Rotondo MF, Henry SM, et al. for American College of Surgeons, Committee on Trauma. Initial assessment and management in: Advanced Trauma Life Support Program; ATLS 10th edition, 2018. pp 2-21.

SECTION 22

Point-of-Care Ultrasound in the ICU

Section Editor: Marvin G. Chang

22.1

Point-of-Care Ultrasound in the ICU

Tenzing T. Lama and Marvin G. Chang

Key Points

- Point-of-care ultrasound (POCUS) is a bedside imaging technique that is noninvasive, free of radiation, and cost-effective, allowing for real-time clinical assessments and decision-making.
- POCUS may reduce reliance on traditional imaging modalities, minimizing delays in diagnosis and intervention, particularly in critically ill patients.
- Facilitates multiorgan assessments, procedural guidance, evaluation of hemodynamics and volume status, and guides therapeutic treatments
- Serial evaluations allow monitoring of patients' conditions over time and optimization of patient care.

Main Variables that Determine Ultrasound Image Quality

- Frequency
  - Largely determined by transducer selection
  - High-frequency transducers provide excellent resolution but limit the depth at which structures can be viewed.
    - For structures close to the body surface → high-frequency transducer
    - For deep structures → low-frequency transducer
- Depth
  - Increasing depth allows the user to view more structures.
  - Increased depth causes a reduction in resolution.
  - Optimized depth ensures the area of interest occupies the central portion of the image, balancing resolution and visibility.
- Gain
  - Increasing gain increases the intensity, or brightness, of the image.
  - Under-gained images are too dark to interpret.
  - Over-gained images are too bright to interpret.

Ways to Manipulate the Ultrasound Transducer

- *Slide*
  - Move to a different location on the body to find a better acoustic window.
- *Tilt*
  - Move the "tail" of the probe cephalad or caudad while keeping the probe in the same location.
- *Rotate*

To achieve optimal imaging, the user must alter *only* the location *or* the tilt *or* the rotation about an axis at one time.

Focused Transthoracic Echocardiography

- Focused transthoracic echocardiography (TTE) is a limited bedside ultrasound technique that employs a qualitative and semi-quantitative approach, using standardized views and a systematic method to address specific clinical questions, facilitating rapid decision-making and real-time management in acute settings.
- Unlike advanced echocardiography (beyond the scope of this chapter), which requires comprehensive training and certification (eg, through the National Board of Echocardiography's Examination of Special Competence in Critical Care Echocardiography), focused TTE is designed for goal-directed, qualitative assessments rather than detailed, quantitative analyses of cardiac structure and function, as discussed in this chapter.

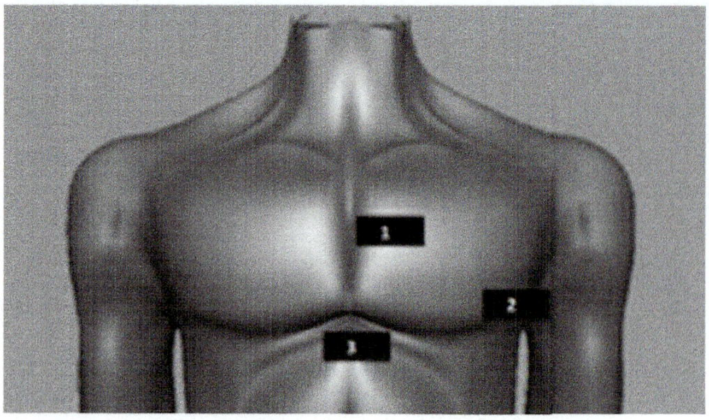

FIGURE 22.1.1 Focused TTE utilizes standardized anatomic "windows" to view the heart. Positions 1–3 correspond to the parasternal, apical, and subcostal windows, respectively. (Reprinted with permission from authors, Ferrada P, Murthi S, Anand RJ, et al. Transthoracic focused rapid echocardiographic examination: real-time evaluation of fluid status in critically ill trauma patients. *J Trauma.* 2011;70(1):56-62.)

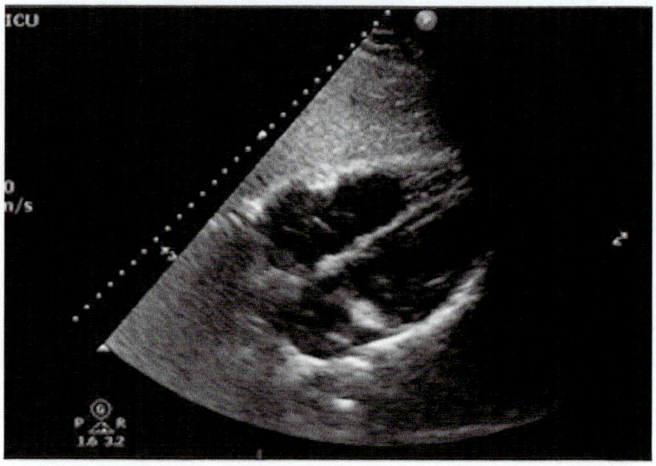

FIGURE 22.1.2 Normal subcostal four-chamber view during focused echocardiography. This window is considered the most reliable for diagnosing a significant pericardial effusion and cardiac tamponade, and is the primary window used to guide a bedside pericardiocentesis.

- Focused TTE utilizes standardized anatomic "windows" to view the heart (Figure 22.1.1):
  1. Parasternal
  2. Apical
  3. Subcostal
     - A phased array transducer is ideal for TTE because its small footprint allows it to navigate narrow intercostal spaces between ribs that impede ultrasound waves. Its design enables electronic steering of the ultrasound beam, creating a sector-shaped field of view essential for performing a comprehensive cardiac assessment.

Goals of Focused Transthoracic Echocardiography

Answer specific clinical questions in a systematic approach:

- Left ventricle
  - Size/dilation
  - Left ventricular outflow tract evaluation for obstruction during systole
  - Systolic function
    - Hyperdynamic, normal, depressed, or severely depressed
    - Global or regional wall motion abnormalities
- Right ventricle
  - Size/dilation
  - Systolic function
    - Normal or depressed
- Pericardial effusion: present or absent
  - The subcostal view is the best initial view for assessing pericardial effusion due to its ability to provide a clear, unobstructed image of the pericardial space; confirmation in other echocardiographic views is recommended to rule out artifacts and ensure diagnostic accuracy.
  - Evidence of tamponade: right atrial systolic and ventricular diastolic collapse, plethoric inferior vena cava (IVC)
- Valves
  - Gross appearance on 2D imaging
  - Color Doppler for regurgitation and stenosis
- Inferior vena cava
  - Underfilled, normal, or plethoric
- Pleural effusion: present or absent

Normal subcostal four-chamber view during focused echocardiography (Figure 22.1.2)

Detection of Severe Hypovolemia

- Hyperdynamic left ventricle
  - Near or complete effacement of the small left ventricular cavity
  - Can also be observed in vasodilatory states such as sepsis and during anesthesia; findings should be interpreted in the clinical context and not in isolation
  - Ejection fraction approaches 100%.
- IVC evaluation in the setting of shock
  - Static IVC measurements correlate more strongly with central venous pressure (CVP) than fluid responsiveness. Of note, dynamic measurements (eg, left ventricular outflow tract velocity-time integral [LVOT VTI]) provide a more accurate assessment of fluid responsiveness but require advanced echocardiography skills.
  - A large IVC (>2.1 cm) with minimal respiratory variation may, in the appropriate clinical context, suggest the patient is unlikely to be fluid responsive. Potential confounders include significant tricuspid regurgitation, pulmonary hypertension, right ventricular (RV) failure, and pericardial effusion.
  - A small IVC (<2.1 cm) with marked respiratory variation may suggest that the patient will likely be fluid responsive in the appropriate clinical context.

Basics of Lung Ultrasonography

Lung ultrasound involves the interpretation of stereotypical patterns of artifacts.

- A-lines
  - Normal aerated lung causes horizontal reverberation artifacts, representing reflection from the air-pleura interface.

    - Prominent A-lines may also be observed in conditions with increased lung aeration, such as chronic obstructive pulmonary disease (COPD) exacerbations, pneumothorax, or pulmonary hyperinflation.
- B-lines
    - B-lines are bright vertical lines that extend from the most superficial aspect of the display to the edge of the display and move back and forth as breathing occurs and erase A-lines.
    - Number of B-lines correlates with the severity of interstitial or alveolar fluid accumulation.
    - Three or more B-lines, or confluent B-lines, in a single interspace are considered abnormal.
    - While commonly associated with interstitial edema (ie, cardiogenic pulmonary edema), B-lines may also appear in any disease process that causes an alveolar-interstitial syndrome like pneumonia, acute respiratory distress syndrome (ARDS), pulmonary fibrosis, diffuse alveolar hemorrhage, or pulmonary contusion.

Evaluation for Pneumothorax

"Lung sliding" effectively rules out pneumothorax at the site of the ultrasound transducer.

- Perform the scan in the sagittal plane using a high-frequency linear transducer, which provides high-resolution imaging of superficial structures, particularly the pleural line.
    - Identify rib shadows with a bright pleural line in between the ribs (commonly referred to as the "bat sign").
    - In the absence of pneumothorax, the apposition of the visceral pleura against the parietal pleura creates a characteristic pleural pattern known as "lung sliding," observed as shimmering or to-and-fro movement of the pleural line that is synchronized with the patient's respiratory cycle.
    - Positioning dependence of absent lung sliding in pneumothorax:
        - In supine patients, the absence of lung sliding due to pneumothorax is most likely observed in the anterior chest, typically around the second and third intercostal space along the midclavicular line, as air accumulates in the least dependent areas.
        - In an upright patient, it is most likely seen in the apical regions, as air rises to the highest point within the pleural space.
    - M-mode imaging, which records motion over time along a single ultrasound line, can assist in pneumothorax evaluation.
        - In a normal lung, the "sandy beach" or "seashore" sign is observed, reflecting dynamic lung sliding below the pleural line.
        - In pneumothorax, the "barcode" or "stratosphere" sign appears due to the absence of lung sliding, with the pleural line remaining static because air in the pleural space prevents ultrasound waves from being transmitted beyond the parietal pleura.
    - Scan multiple locations on the right and left chest systematically to rule out pneumothorax.
    - A variety of lung and pleural pathologies can also cause a lack of lung sliding and is not specific for pneumothorax.
        - Conditions causing absent lung sliding include pneumothorax, ARDS, atelectasis, pleural disease, apnea, mucus plugging, and mainstem intubation.
        - The identification of a lung point, representing the transition between lung sliding and absent lung sliding, is a highly specific ultrasound finding for pneumothorax.
        - Certain findings, such as B-lines, lung pulse (a subtle rhythmic movement of the pleural line synchronized with cardiac activity), subpleural consolidations, or the absence of a lung point, can help rule out pneumothorax at the site of the ultrasound probe and suggest alternative causes for the absence of lung sliding.

Pleural Effusion

- A low-frequency curvilinear or phased array transducer is preferred as it provides sufficient depth penetration to visualize deeper structures, including pleural fluid and adjacent lung tissue.
- Free fluid appears anechoic (black) on the ultrasound display.
    - Simple pleural effusion: anechoic (black) appearance on ultrasound, indicating clear fluid
    - Complex pleural effusion: presence of heterogeneous contents (ie, internal echoes), septations, or loculations that may suggest conditions such as infection, hemorrhage, or malignancy.
- Large pleural fluid collections collapse the adjacent lung.
    - Airless, atelectatic lung can be seen moving within the pleural fluid.
        - Appears gray and grainy, similar to liver tissue or "hepatization"
        - Static air bronchograms are hyperechoic (bright) linear or punctate structures within consolidated lung tissue that remain stationary during respiration, often indicating conditions like atelectasis, where air is trapped in the bronchi due to obstruction.
        - Dynamic air bronchograms, in contrast, exhibit movement synchronous with the respiratory cycle, suggesting the presence of patent airways within consolidated lung regions commonly associated with pneumonia.
    - Ultrasound can help determine whether thoracentesis or thoracostomy tube placement would be possible and can be used for procedural guidance.

Focused Assessment With Sonography for TraumaExam

- To evaluate for free fluid (blood) and cardiac activity in trauma patients, particularly those suffering from shock
- Positive (free fluid present) or negative (free fluid not present) result of the focused assessment with sonography for trauma (FAST) exam aids in decision-making regarding the need for immediate surgery versus ongoing workup.
- A curvilinear or phased array transducer is typically used given that these transducers operate at low frequencies, balancing the need for adequate tissue penetration and image resolution.
- FAST exam examines four areas:
    - Right upper quadrant: for blood between the diaphragm and liver, between liver and kidney, or around the kidney
    - Left upper quadrant: for blood between diaphragm and spleen, between spleen and kidney, or around the kidney

- Heart and pericardial space: for evidence of cardiac activity and pericardial fluid
- Pelvis: for free fluid around the bladder

- Sensitivity of the FAST exam depends on the location of the free fluid, the position of the patient, and the quality of imaging and interpretation.
  - In general, the FAST exam is capable of detecting free fluid greater than 250 mL.

Vascular Access

- High-frequency transducer typically utilized given excellent resolution of vessels at relatively shallow depths.
- Imaging of the internal jugular vein commonly performed in short axis (in cross-section)
  - Shows relationship between the internal jugular vein and the carotid artery
  - Reduces the risk of carotid artery puncture and reduces the number of attempts
- Similar technique can be applied to the femoral vein.
- A short or long axis view of the subclavian/axillary vein can also be used.
- Facilitation of placement of arterial catheters in both superficial (eg, radial) and deep (eg, femoral, axillary, brachial) vessels
- Facilitation of placement of peripheral intravenous lines

Deep Venous Thrombosis

- Most lower extremity deep venous thromboses (DVTs) are located at the branch points of the venous system (ie, junction of the common femoral vein with the greater saphenous vein, popliteal vein).
- Typically performed with a high-frequency transducer for imaging of superficial veins, and a lower frequency transducer as necessary for visualization of deeper veins, particularly in obese patients
  - Apply gentle pressure along the vein to assess compressibility in a systematic fashion; 5 to 10 cm of vein should be assessed in both the femoral and popliteal regions to ensure a thorough evaluation.
  - If common femoral vein and popliteal veins are fully compressible and no thrombus is visualized, the patient is unlikely to have a clinically significant DVT.
  - Lack of full compressibility is the primary diagnostic sign of DVT.

Training in POCUS

- Acquire hands-on skills by training under the guidance of an experienced POCUS practitioner or simulator.
- Attend local, regional, and national courses in critical care ultrasound.
- Read textbooks and peer-reviewed manuscripts.
- Question and answer resources.
- Utilize online resources.
  - Full curricula in critical care ultrasound are available through professional organizations and training programs.
  - Sites with example images and cine loops
- Feedback on acquired images by experienced POCUS practitioners
- Engage in continuing medical education to ensure updated on advancements, skills, and interpretation of images.
- Maintain proficiency through regular practice, periodic assessments, image review, and integrating ultrasound into routine clinical decision-making.

Acknowledgments

We gratefully acknowledge the contributions of previous edition author, Daniel W. Johnson, as portions of those chapters have been retained in this revision.

SUGGESTED READINGS

Beshara M, Bittner EA, Goffi A, Berra L, Chang MG. Nuts and bolts of lung ultrasound: utility, scanning techniques, protocols, and findings in common pathologies. *Crit Care*. 2024;28(1):328.

Bhattacharjee S, Maitra S, Baidya DK. Comparison between ultrasound guided technique and digital palpation technique for radial artery cannulation in adult patients: an updated meta-analysis of randomized controlled trials. *J Clin Anesth*. 2018;47:54-59.

Buda N, Mendrala K, Skoczyński S, et al. Basics of point-of-care lung ultrasonography. *N Engl J Med*. 2023;389(21):e44.

Chang MG, Sonny A, Tainter CR, et al, eds. *Critical Care Echocardiography Review: 1200+ Questions and Answers*. Lippincott Williams & Wilkins; 2021.

Díaz-Gómez JL, Mayo PH, Koenig SJ. Point-of-care ultrasonography. *N Engl J Med*. 2021;385:1593-1602.

Frankel HL, Kirkpatrick AW, Elbarbary M, et al. Guidelines for the appropriate use of bedside general and cardiac ultrasonography in the evaluation of critically ill patients—part I: general ultrasonography. *Crit Care Med*. 2015;43:2479-2502.

Gibson LE, White-Dzuro GA, Lindsay PJ, Berg SM, Bittner EA, Chang MG. Ensuring competency in focused cardiac ultrasound: a systematic review of training programs. *J Intensive Care*. 2020;8(1):93.

Mojoli F, Bouhemad B, Mongodi S, Lichtenstein D. Lung ultrasound for critically ill patients. *Am J Respir Crit Care Med*. 2019;199:701-714.

Narula J, Chandrashekhar Y, Braunwald E. Time to add a fifth pillar to bedside physical examination: inspection, palpation, percussion, auscultation, and insonation. *JAMA Cardiol*. 2018;3:346-350.

Orso D, Paoli I, Piani T, Cilenti FL, Cristiani L, Guglielmo N. Accuracy of ultrasonographic measurements of inferior vena cava to determine fluid responsiveness: a systematic review and meta-analysis. *J Intensive Care Med*. 2020;35:354-363.

Singh J, Matern LH, Bittner EA, Chang MG. Characteristics of simulation-based point-of-care ultrasound education: a systematic review of MedEdPORTAL curricula. *Cureus*. 2022;14(2):e22249.

Vieillard-Baron A, Evrard B, Repessé X, et al. Limited value of end-expiratory inferior vena cava diameter to predict fluid responsiveness impact of intra-abdominal pressure. *Intensive Care Med*. 2018;44:197-203.

SECTION 23

Burns and Thermal Injuries

Section Editor: Edward A. Bittner

23.1

Burns and Thermal Injuries

Stefano Spina and Sean A. Hickey

Definitions

- Burn: a burn is defined as a traumatic injury involving the skin and subcutaneous tissues primarily caused by heat, electricity, chemicals, friction, or radiation and is classified according to burn depth and the percentage of the total body surface area (TBSA) involved.
- Burn depth: burns are categorized into four main types based on their depth: first degree (superficial), second degree (superficial and deep partial thickness), and third degree (full thickness) (Table 23.1.1).
  - Burn depth depends on four main factors: the temperature of the offending agent, the duration of contact, the thickness of the affected skin and dermis, and the blood supply to the area of injury.
  - Clinical determination of burn depth is best performed 48 to 72 hours postinjury.
  - First-degree burns affect the epidermis and do not cause blistering or open wounds.
    - Skin is erythematous and painful to touch.
  - Second-degree burns (partial thickness) extend through the epidermis and into the dermis.
    - Superficial partial-thickness burns involve injury to the papillary dermis and are characterized by erythema and blistering.
    - Deep partial-thickness burns involve injury to the reticular dermis and are characterized by decreased capillary refill, often appearing dry with a white or waxy appearance.
  - Third-degree (full-thickness) burns destroy the entire epidermis and dermis, including dermal appendages, resulting in a white, brown, or black charred appearance with visible coagulated vessels.
    - The dry, leathery tissue formed is known as eschar.
    - Unless they are very small (<5 cm), full-thickness burns require excision and skin grafting.
- Burn size: TBSA of a burn wound is the percentage of the total surface area of the skin that has been affected by partial- or full-thickness burns.
  - The "Rule of Nines" divides the body into sections, each representing ~9% (or multiples of 9%) of the TBSA (Figure 23.1.1).
    - Head and neck: 9% of TBSA
    - Each upper extremity: 9% of TBSA

TABLE 23.1.1 Burn Depth Classification: Layers Involved, Clinical Features, and Treatment Approaches

	Burn Depth			
	Superficial (First Degree)	**Partial Thickness (Superficial Second Degree)**	**Partial Thickness (Deep Second Degree)**	**Full Thickness (Third Degree)**
Layers Involved	Epidermis	Papillary dermis	Reticular dermis	Subcutaneous tissue
Visual Characteristics	Red, dry, intact skin	Red, blistered, blanches with pressure	Pale, mottled, delayed to no blanching	Tough, leathery
Sensation/Pain	Very painful	Very painful	Diminished pain with deep pressure only	Painless
Healing and Treatment	Aloe, moisturizer salves for comfort	Local wound care/topical antimicrobial ointments and dressings	Local wound care/topical antimicrobial ointments and dressings vs excision and autografting	Excision and grafting

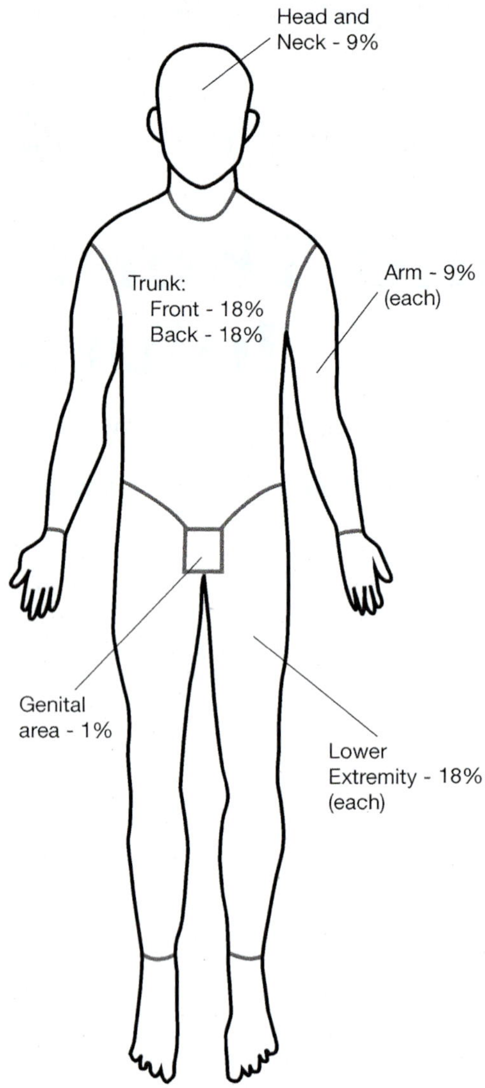

FIGURE 23.1.1 Rule of nines, which divides the body into sections, each representing ~9% (or multiples of 9%) of the total body surface area.

- Each lower extremity: 18% of TBSA (9% for the front, 9% for the back)
- Anterior trunk: 18% of TBSA
- Posterior trunk: 18% of TBSA
- Perineum: 1% of TBSA
- First-degree burns are not included in TBSA calculations.
- The "Rule of Nines" is not valid in children due to relatively larger heads and smaller limbs when compared to adults.

- Palmar method: The size of the patient's palm (including fingers) represents ~1% of their TBSA.
  - Useful for estimating scattered burns in children and adults
  - Less accurate for larger burns
- Lund and Browder chart: provides a more accurate and detailed assessment of TBSA, especially in children, by accounting for the varying proportions of body segments across different ages (Figure 23.1.2)
  - Can delay initial burn size estimation in emergency situations where rapid assessment is critical
- New tools based on computer-assisted programs to improve burn size estimation are also under investigation.

Epidemiology

- Nearly 11 million people worldwide require medical attention for burn injuries annually.
  - ~180,000 people die from burns each year, predominantly in low- and middle-income countries.
  - House fires account for 5.8 deaths per 100,000 individuals.
  - Globally, burn injury is the fourth most common cause of civilian traumatic injury.
- In the United States, burn injuries resulted in 398,000 emergency department visits and 60,000 hospital admissions.
  - ~3,200 deaths annually
  - House fires account for 1.2 deaths per 100,000 individuals.
    - Smoke inhalation injury is responsible for 75% of burn-related deaths at the scene.
    - In the United States, more than two-thirds of all burns occur in residential settings, with scald injuries being the most common type among young children.
    - Children under 5 years of age account for 25% of all burn injuries.
    - Risk factors for burn injury include:
  - Children under 5 and adults over 65 years of age
  - Male gender
  - Low socioeconomic status
  - Disability
  - Homelessness
  - Psychiatric disorders
  - Tobacco use disorder and active drug or alcohol abuse
    - Risk prediction of mortality can be estimated through the revised Baux score, which combines patient age, % TBSA, and presence of inhalation injury.

Pathophysiology

- Initial injury and local response
  - Deep thermal burns cause immediate coagulation of cellular proteins and necrosis of the affected tissues.
  - Inflammatory response
    - Cytokine release: tumor necrosis factor alpha (TNF-α), interleukin-1 (IL-1), IL-6, and other mediators
    - Vasodilation and increased permeability: histamine, prostaglandins, and bradykinin
      - Increased capillary permeability leads to fluid leakage into the interstitial space.
        - Contributes to hypovolemia, systemic edema, and increased pressure within subcutaneous tissues
      - Pain and sensory changes: activation of nociceptors and release of pain mediators
- Systemic response
  - Burns covering >20% TBSA are likely to trigger a systemic inflammatory response, leading to systemic effects such as hypovolemia, shock, hypermetabolism, and alterations in endocrine function and immune response.

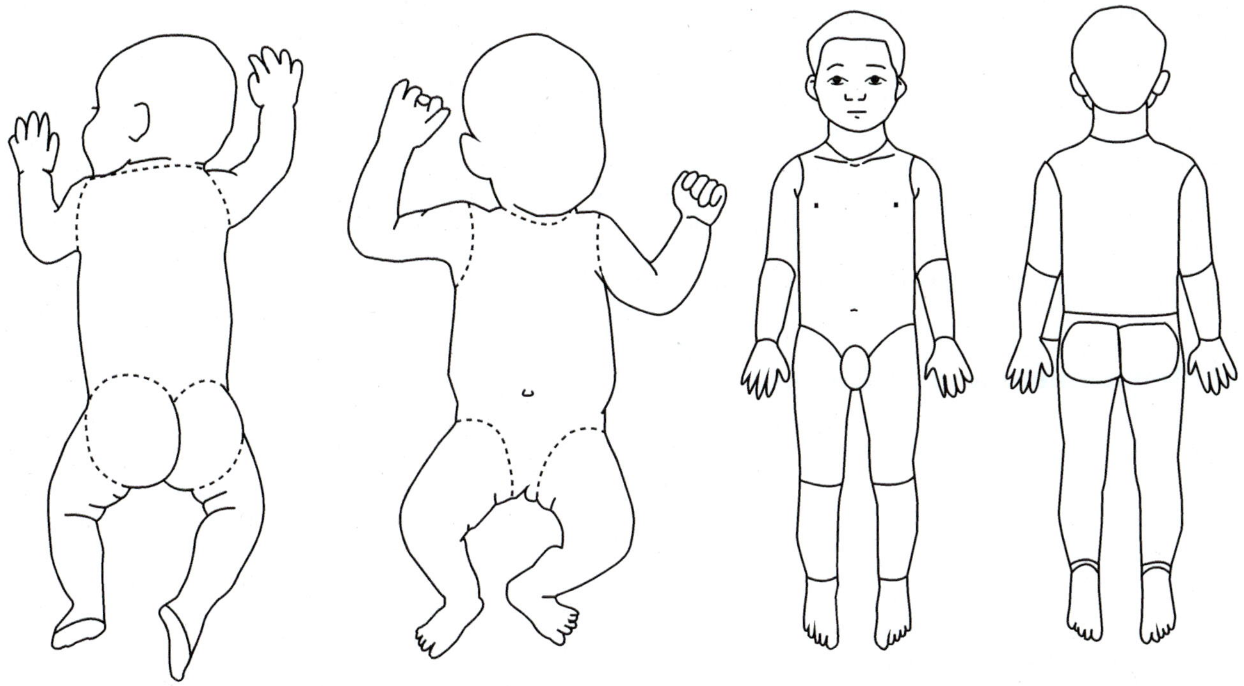

Area	Birth - 1 yr.	1-4 yrs.	5-9 yrs.	10-14 yrs.	15 yrs.	Adult	2°**	3°**
Head	19	17	13	11	9	7		
Neck	2	2	2	2	2	2		
Anterior Trunk	13	13	13	13	13	13		
Posterior Trunk	13	13	13	13	13	13		
RIGHT Buttock	2.5	2.5	2.5	2.5	2.5	2.5		
LEFT Buttock	2.5	2.5	2.5	2.5	2.5	2.5		
Genitalia	1	1	1	1	1	1		
RIGHT Upper Arm	4	4	4	4	4	4		
LEFT Upper Arm	4	4	4	4	4	4		
RIGHT Lower Arm	3	3	3	3	3	3		
LEFT Lower Arm	3	3	3	3	3	3		
RIGHT Hand	2.5	2.5	2.5	2.5	2.5	2.5		
LEFT Hand	2.5	2.5	2.5	2.5	2.5	2.5		
RIGHT Hand	5.5	6.5	8	8.5	9	9.5		
LEFT Thigh	5.5	6.5	8	8.5	9	9.5		
RIGHT Lower Leg	5	5	5.5	6	6.5	7		
LEFT Lower Leg	5	5	5.5	6	6.5	7		
RIGHT Foot	3.5	3.5	3.5	3.5	3.5	3.5		
LEFT Foot	3.5	3.5	3.5	3.5	3.5	3.5		

Total 2° ________

Total 3° ________

Total ________

**Only 2° and 3° burns are included in the total TBSA burn percent.

FIGURE 23.1.2 Pediatric Lund-Browder chart, which provides a more accurate and detailed assessment of total body surface area (TBSA) in children by accounting for the varying proportions of body segments across different ages.

- *Ebb phase*: first 72 to 96 hours after injury, with hypometabolism, decreased tissue perfusion, low cardiac output, and low intravascular volume
- *Flow phase*: can persist for several weeks/months after injury, with increased catecholamines, glucocorticoids, and glucagon levels leading to increased catabolism, immune dysregulation, and potential multiorgan failure

- Burn shock: characterized by a combination of hypovolemic and distributive shock, resulting from extensive fluid loss and systemic inflammatory response
  - Distributive shock component
    - Systemic inflammatory response causes widespread vasodilation.
    - Capillary leak: increased capillary permeability leads to the leakage of intravascular fluid and proteins into the interstitial spaces.
  - Hypovolemic shock component
    - Evaporation: significant fluid loss occurs through evaporative losses directly from the exposed burn surfaces
    - Exudation: intravascular fluid and proteins leak into the interstitial spaces due to increased capillary permeability.
  - Despite ongoing fluid loss, the vasodilatory effects of inflammatory mediators lead to decreased systemic vascular resistance, decreased cardiac output, worsening tachycardia, and hypotension.

- Hypermetabolic response: caused by increased levels of circulating catecholamines, glucocorticoids, and glucagon
  - Metabolism can increase to twice the normal rate.
  - Increased protein catabolism with negative nitrogen balance contributes to muscle wasting and weight loss.
  - Glucose intolerance and insulin resistance
- Large TBSA burns cause significant immunosuppression and disruption of both the innate and adaptive immune responses, resulting in a higher incidence of bacterial, viral, and fungal infections.

Initial Management and Treatment

- Major burns should be considered traumatic injuries and managed according to the Advanced Trauma Life Support (ATLS) protocols.
  - ABCDE:
    - A. Airway assessment
      - The establishment of an airway is the priority. Consider cervical and full spine immobilization when associated trauma is suspected.
      - Indications for tracheal intubation
        - Impaired mental status (concomitant head trauma; impairment due to substance use; underlying medical conditions)
        - Respiratory distress in the setting of inhalation injury
        - Patients with deep burns to the head and neck
        - Large TBSA burns that require a large volume of resuscitation leading significant interstitial/airway edema
    - B. Breathing and ventilation assessment
      - Full-thickness burns of the trunk demonstrate a low compliance and may affect ventilation dynamics.
        - Early escharotomy is warranted to facilitate proper ventilation when circumferential truncal burns are present.
      - Impaired gas exchange might result from carbon monoxide and/or cyanide toxicity.
        - Carbon monoxide toxicity: initial treatment is 100% inhaled oxygen.
        - Cyanide toxicity: consider intravenous (IV) hydroxocobalamin administration.
    - C. Circulation with hemorrhage control
      - Do not expect *immediate* hemodynamic instability after a major burn. However, hemodynamic changes are present in the first 24 to 48 hours.
      - Reliable IV access must be established as soon as possible, either in the form of two large-bore peripheral lines (14-16 gauge) or a central venous catheter.
        - If necessary, access can be placed through burned skin.
      - Arterial catheterization is also recommended for larger sized burns and in patients with significant comorbidities and cardiac or respiratory concerns.
    - D. Disability (neurologic evaluation)
      - Brief neurologic examination, including Glasgow Coma Scale (GCS), pupil size and reactivity, and motor function
    - E. Exposure and environmental control
      - Completely undress the patient while preventing hypothermia.
        - Use warm blankets, warm IV fluids, and ambient temperature control.
    - Complete a secondary survey to identify all injuries.
- Large volume fluid resuscitation
  - An indwelling Foley catheter should be placed in all burns >20% TBSA in adults and considered for pediatric burns of >15% TBSA.
  - Modified Parkland formula (2-4 mL × %TBSA × actual body weight [kg]) is used to calculate the initial fluid requirement for burns >20% TBSA in adults. Of note, burn size >15% TBSA is commonly used for initiation of Parkland resuscitation in pediatric patients aged 12 years or younger.
    - Half of the calculated volume is given as an hourly infusion rate over the first 8 hours from the initial time of injury; the second half is infused over the next 16 hours.
    - Lactated Ringer (LR) solution is the crystalloid of choice for most patients.
      - LR decreases the potential for metabolic acidosis with respect to normal saline infusion.
    - Pediatric patients should receive LR with 5% dextrose at a maintenance rate, which should be deducted from their total Parkland formula resuscitation volume.
    - Time delays and any fluids administered during transport to the treatment center must also be accounted for in the resuscitation plan.
    - Example: A 70-kg adult with 50% TBSA second- and third-degree burns presents 2 hours after injury. The patient received 2 L (2,000 mL) of LR en route.
      - Calculation (Parkland Formula):
        - 4 mL LR × 70 kg × 50% TBSA = 14,000 mL LR in first 24 hours
          - First 8 Hours:
            - Total required in first 8 hours: 7,000 mL LR
            - Fluid already given: 2,000 mL LR
            - Remaining fluid: 7,000 − 2,000 = 5,000 mL LR
            - Time left: 6 hours
            - Infusion rate: 5,000 ÷ 6 = ~830 mL/h LR
          - Next 16 Hours:
            - Total required: 7,000 mL LR
            - Infusion rate: 7,000 ÷ 16 = ~440 mL/h LR
    - Crystalloid bolus infusion should be avoided, except in cases of hemodynamic instability.
      - Patients who are hypotensive should receive a fluid bolus and a one-third increase in fluid infusion.
    - Overly aggressive resuscitation can have deleterious effects, leading to exacerbating pulmonary edema, heart failure, renal failure, abdominal compartment syndrome, and ocular compartment syndrome.
    - Administration of a 5% albumin infusion may be used as an adjunct to the calculated LR infusion to decrease overall resuscitation volume requirements.
    - Special considerations
      - Inhalation injury
        - Additional fluid requirements due to increased capillary permeability

- Electrical injury
  - Potential for deeper tissue damage and myoglobinuria, requiring higher fluid volumes
- Pediatric patients
  - Adjustment in fluid volumes due to different body surface area to weight ratios
- If the patient is not resuscitating appropriately, consideration should be given to instituting advanced hemodynamic monitoring.
- Once resuscitation is complete, usually after 24 hours, the crystalloid rate can be slowly decreased by 10% per hour while monitoring end point resuscitation parameters.
- Resuscitation parameters: successful fluid resuscitation should be guided by the normalization of vital signs/hemodynamic and laboratory parameters:
  - A goal urine output of 0.5 to 1 mL/kg/h in adults and 1 to 1.5 mL/kg/h in children
    - Indicates adequate renal perfusion and overall fluid balance
  - Base deficit/excess
  - Serum lactate
  - Serum bicarbonate
  - Venous oxygen saturation
  - Thermodilution-derived variables
  - Stroke volume or pulse pressure variation
- Other therapies with unclear benefit in large TBSA burns
  - High-dose vitamin C (66 mg/kg/h for 24 hours) might have some benefits, given its antioxidant and reactive oxygen species scavenging effects. However, concerns about renal injury have been reported.
  - Plasma exchange and hemofiltration

- Initial wound management
  - Goals: prevent infection, manage pain, prevent wound desiccation by providing a moist wound environment, and prepare for definitive wound closure.
  - Most used topical antimicrobial agents
    - Bacitracin/polymyxin B
      - Soothing on application
      - Limited effectiveness in controlling localized burn wound infections
      - Prolonged use is associated with hypersensitivity reactions.
    - Silver sulfadiazine
      - Painless to apply with broad-spectrum activity against Gram-positive and Gram-negative organisms
      - Does not penetrate eschar and may retard wound healing
      - May cause self-limiting neutropenia
    - Mafenide acetate
      - Broad-spectrum activity against Gram-positive and Gram-negative organisms and can penetrate eschar
      - Painful on application
      - When used in large quantities, it is associated with metabolic acidosis due to carbonic anhydrase inhibition.
    - Silver nitrate
      - Painless to apply with broad-spectrum activity against Gram-positive and Gram-negative organisms
      - Can cause methemoglobinemia and electrolyte disturbances (hyponatremia and hypochloremia)
    - Sodium hypochlorite and hypochlorous acid
      - Broad-spectrum antimicrobial coverage
      - Sodium hypochlorite can cause skin irritation at high concentrations.
  - Superficial and deep partial-thickness burns are most commonly treated with daily application of a topical antimicrobial ointment/cream (eg, bacitracin, mupirocin, Sulfamylon cream, silver sulfadiazine) and securing the dressing with a dry gauze wrap.
    - Additional wound care options are application of a dry gauze sterile dressing over top of the burn injury and soaking the dressing/wound with solutions containing: mafenide acetate (if available), silver nitrate, sodium hypochlorite, or hypochlorous acid.
    - Superficial partial-thickness burns usually heal within 1 to 2 weeks.
    - Deep partial-thickness burns may need excisional debridement and autografting if not expected to heal within 3 weeks.
  - Third-degree burn wounds are treated initially with daily topical antimicrobial agents.
    - If the burn injury >3 to 5 cm in diameter, early excision and autografting are recommended to obtain durable wound closure.
  - There is no role for the prophylactic use of systemic antibiotics for burn wounds.

Surgical Excision of Burn Wounds and Wound Closure

- Debridement of deep partial-thickness and third-degree burn wounds
  - Timing
    - Early excision/debridement: recommended within the first 48 to 72 hours
      - Benefits: reduced risk of infection, decreased inflammatory response, and improved survival rates for large TBSA burn wounds
  - Debridement techniques
    - Tangential excision: sequential removal of thin layers of eschar until viable tissue (punctate bleeding) is reached
      - Advantages: preserves the maximum amount of viable tissue and improves cosmetic outcome with respect to fascial excision
      - Disadvantages: requires surgical expertise and is associated with increased operative blood loss with respect to fascial excision
    - Fascial excision: removal of the burn wound and subcutaneous tissue down to the level of fascia
      - Advantages: a faster and simpler surgical technique with reduced blood loss with respect to tangential excision
      - Disadvantages: poor cosmetic outcomes due to loss of subcutaneous tissue and body contour
    - Enzymatic excision: Anacaulase-bcdb is an enzymatic debriding agent derived from bromelain (pineapple stem extract) that removes eschar in deep partial-thickness and full-thickness burns while preserving viable dermis (NEXOBRID).

          - Advantages: preserves viable dermis, potentially reducing the need for grafting
          - Disadvantages: requires careful application technique to ensure full eschar removal
- Wound closure techniques
    - Wound closure is essential to prevent infection, reduce fluid loss, and improve healing.
    - Options include autografts, allografts, xenografts, cultured cells, autologous cell suspensions, and tissue matrices.
        - Autograft (gold standard)
            - Harvesting: dermatome is used to harvest skin at a depth of 0.008 to 0.015 in.
            - Meshing: allows fluid drainage and expansion
            - Healing: donor sites become superficial wounds that heal in 2 weeks, and the site can be reharvested.
            - Complications: graft failure from inadequate excision, infection, hematomas or seromas
        - Allograft (cadaver skin—temporary coverage)
            - Used when donor sites are limited, allowing time for healing and reharvesting
            - Not permanent: rejected within several weeks
            - Risk: potential disease transmission, though rare
        - Xenograft (porcine or fish skin—temporary coverage)
            - Similar use as allograft
        - Cultured epithelial autografts (carcinoembryonic antigen [CEA], grown from patient's cells)
            - Used for large TBSA burns with minimal donor sites
            - Limitations: fragile, high failure rates, slow to prepare, high cost
        - Autologous cell suspension therapy
            - Uses a small skin biopsy to create a spray-on suspension of keratinocytes, fibroblasts, and melanocytes
            - Advantages: expands coverage, reduces need for meshing, improves pigmentation
            - Limitations: less effective on deep wounds, requires viable dermis for success
        - Tissue matrices (dermal substitutes)
            - Used in deep burns lacking dermis to prepare for later grafting
            - Pros: promotes vascularization and dermal regeneration
            - Cons: requires a two-stage procedure, costly, risk of infection

Nonthermal Burn Injuries and Their Management

- Electrical burns
    - Account for 3% to 4% of burn center admissions
    - Classified by voltage exposure
        - Low voltage (<1,000 V)—common in household injuries where appliances require 120 or 240 V
            - Tissue injury is at the site of contact.
        - High voltage (>1,000 V)—common in industrial settings
            - Associated with extensive deep tissue damage, myonecrosis, rhabdomyolysis, compartment syndrome, arrhythmias, and cardiac arrest
            - Myoglobinuria from muscle breakdown may lead to acute kidney injury.
            - Tetanic contractions may cause fractures/dislocations.
            - Associated with flame burns from ignited clothing
    - Pathophysiology of electrical burns
        - Muscle and nerve tissue have low resistance, allowing current to pass through and cause deep injuries.
        - Tissue damage occurs internally and may be more extensive than skin involvement.
    - Initial management of high-voltage electrical injury
        - Primary survey (ABCs) and trauma evaluation due to potential associated injuries
        - Telemetry and serial cardiac enzymes are indicated for patients with:
            - Cardiac arrest at the scene
            - Abnormal electrocardiogram (ECG) on initial evaluation
        - Serial ECGs are not indicated if the initial ECG is normal.
        - Crystalloid hydration is standard; bicarbonate/mannitol use remains controversial.
            - Higher volume needs than thermal burns due to deep tissue injury
        - Serial neurovascular examinations to detect evolving compartment syndrome
            - Fasciotomy/escharotomy if:
                - Severe limb swelling with impending ischemia
                - Tissue pressure exceeds 30 cm H_2O.
    - Long-term complications
        - Delayed neurologic deficits (peripheral neuropathy, neurocognitive dysfunction)
        - Cataract formation months to years postinjury
- Chemical burns
    - Definition: chemical burns result from contact with household cleaners, industrial products, or laboratory chemicals.
    - Severity of injury is determined by the chemical's type, concentration, volume, and duration of exposure.
    - Obtain poison control guidance if the chemical composition is unknown.
    - Assess for inhalation injury and systemic toxicity.
    - Acid burns
        - Common agents: sulfuric acid, nitric acid, hydrochloric acid, phosphoric acid, hydrofluoric acid (HFA)
        - Pathophysiology
            - Acids donate protons (H^+ ions), leading to protein denaturation by hydrolysis of cellular structures, which disrupts cell integrity.
                - Leads to coagulation necrosis with the formation of a thick eschar, which limits further chemical penetration, making acid burns typically less deep than alkali burns.
    - Alkali burns
        - Common agents: ammonia, bleach, lye, sodium hydroxide, potassium hydroxide, cement
        - Pathophysiology
            - Hydroxide (–OH) moiety acts as a proton acceptor, causing liquefactive (colliquative) necrosis, leading to deep tissue penetration, fat saponification, and progressive protein denaturation.
            - Fat saponification occurs due to the reaction of hydroxide ions with lipids, breaking down cell membranes.

- Irreversible protein denaturation contributes to extensive, progressive tissue damage, often appearing worse over time.
- Initial care and management of chemical burns
  - Remove contaminated clothing, jewelry, and shoes
  - Brush off dry chemical powders before irrigation
  - Copious tap water irrigation for at least 30 minutes unless contraindicated
    - Alkaline burns require prolonged irrigation due to poor water solubility.
  - Assess completeness of irrigation:
    - Soapy feel on gloved fingers suggests residual alkali.
    - Litmus paper can confirm neutralization.
  - Contraindications to immediate water irrigation
    - Dry lime (calcium oxide)—reacts with water to form heat
    - Phenols—poorly soluble in water, use polyethylene glycol (PEG) or isopropyl alcohol for decontamination
    - Elemental metals (sodium, lithium, cesium, potassium, magnesium)—contact with water triggers an exothermic reaction; use mineral oil for decontamination.
  - No role for neutralization of acids or alkalis (exothermic reactions may worsen burns)
  - Unique toxicity of hydrofluoric acid burns
    - Weak acid with highly toxic effects due to fluoride ion penetration
    - Fluoride ions rapidly bind calcium and magnesium, leading to:
      - Extensive tissue destruction (liquefactive necrosis)
      - Severe electrolyte imbalances
        - Hypocalcemia, hypomagnesemia, and hyperkalemia
    - **Management**
      - Immediate irrigation
      - Topical and/or intradermal calcium gluconate to affected tissues
      - Intra-arterial calcium gluconate infusion (for large or severe burns)
      - Monitor serum calcium, magnesium, and potassium levels.

Special Considerations

- Inhalation injury
  - Occurs in fire and smoke exposure in enclosed spaces
  - Affects one-third of patients with flame burn, increasing morbidity and mortality
  - It can impact the upper airway, tracheobronchial tree, and lung parenchyma and cause systemic toxicity.
  - 50% develop pneumonia; 20% develop acute respiratory distress syndrome (ARDS).
  - Signs and symptoms
    - Facial burns, singed nasal hairs, carbonaceous sputum, cough, tachypnea
    - Hoarseness, stridor, hypoxia, bronchospasm
    - Upper airway edema can rapidly progress, necessitating early endotracheal intubation.
    - Bronchoscopy confirms diagnosis (edema, erythema, mucosal sloughing, subglottic soot).
  - Pathophysiology
    - Rarely from direct thermal injury
    - Primarily caused by toxic smoke byproducts, leading to chemical pneumonitis
      - Exception: high-pressure steam inhalation can injure the lower airway.
  - Treatment
    - Supportive care: head elevation (30 degree), aerosolized bronchodilators, airway clearance (*N*-acetylcysteine, heparin, chest physiotherapy)
    - No role for steroids or prophylactic antibiotics
- Carbon monoxide (CO) toxicity
  - High affinity for hemoglobin (>200× oxygen affinity)
  - Pulse oximetry is unreliable; confirm with arterial blood gas
  - Treatment
    - 100% oxygen (reduces CO half-life from ~4 hours to ~30-90 minutes)
    - Hyperbaric oxygen therapy (HBO) is controversial.
      - Critically ill patients may not tolerate HBO therapy.
- Cyanide toxicity
  - Present in ~30% of CO toxicity cases
  - Cyanide binds cytochrome oxidase, halting cellular respiration and leading to lactic acidosis.
  - Difficult to diagnose in the first 24 hours; suspect in cases with elevated lactate (>10 mmol/L)
  - Treatment

Hydroxocobalamin (vitamin B_{12} analog) binds cyanide to form cyanocobalamin, excreted in urine.

Referral Criteria

- American Burn Association (ABA) referral criteria (Table 23.1.2):
  - Extent of burn injury
    - Partial-thickness burns
      - Burns >10% TBSA
    - Full-thickness burns
      - Burns of any size requiring specialized care
  - Location of burn injury
    - Critical areas: burns involving the face, hands, genitalia, perineum, or burns overlying major joints
  - Type of burn injury
    - Electrical burns including lightning injury
    - Chemical burns of any type
    - Inhalation injury with evidence of respiratory tract burn or significant exposure to smoke and/or noxious gases
  - Patients with complex preexisting medical, or complex social/psychiatric, conditions
  - Burn injury in a patient with concomitant non–burn-related trauma

Survival Following Burn Injury

- Advancements in burn care and multidisciplinary management have significantly improved survival rates.
- Children and adults with burns covering up to 70% TBSA now have a <10% mortality rate due to modern treatment protocols.

TABLE 23.1.2 ABA Referral Criteria

Category	Immediate Transfer Consideration	Consultation Recommended
Thermal Burns	• Partial-thickness burns ≥10% TBSA • Deep burns on face, hands, feet, genitalia, perineum, joints • Burns with comorbidities or trauma • Circumferential burns • Uncontrolled pain	• Partial-thickness burns <10% TBSA • Any potentially deep burns of any size
Inhalation Injury	All patients with suspected inhalation injury	Patients with signs of potential inhalation, such as facial, ash burns, singed facial hairs, or smoke exposure
Pediatrics (≤14 y, <30 kg)	Consider transfer for pain, dressing changes, rehab, caregiver needs, or suspected abuse.	
Chemical Burns	All chemical injuries	
Electrical Burns	• High voltage (≥1,000 V) • Lightning injuries	Low voltage (<1,000 V): Consider follow-up for delayed symptoms/vision issues.

ABA: American Burn Association; TBSA: total body surface area.

- Mortality rates have decreased dramatically over the past 30 years, largely due to:
  - Improved prevention efforts (fire safety regulations, public awareness)
  - Early excision and grafting, reducing infection risk and improving wound healing
  - Advancements in intensive care, including fluid resuscitation, infection control, and ventilatory support

Long-Term Rehabilitation and Quality of Life

- Burn survivors face increased risks of:
  - Trauma-related complications (eg, chronic wounds, neuropathy)
  - Mental health challenges, including posttraumatic stress disorder (PTSD), depression, and anxiety
  - Reduced quality of life and difficulties returning to work
- Comprehensive postburn care includes:
  - Physical rehabilitation (occupational and physical therapy)
  - Psychosocial support (counseling, peer support groups)
  - Ongoing medical follow-up for scar management and reconstructive needs

SUGGESTED READINGS

Bittner EA, Shank E, Woodson L, Martyn JA. Acute and perioperative care of the burn-injured patient. *Anesthesiology*. 2015;122(2):448-464.

Cartotto R, Burmeister DM, Kubasiak JC. Burn shock and resuscitation: review and state of the science. *J Burn Care Res*. 2022:irac025.

Cartotto R, Johnson LS, Savetamal A, et al. American Burn Association clinical practice guidelines on burn shock resuscitation. *J Burn Care Res*. 2024;45(3):565-589.

Herndon DN. *Total Burn Care*. 5th ed. Elsevier; 2017.

Sheridan RL. *Burns: A Practical Approach to Immediate Treatment and Long-Term Care*. 1st ed. Thieme; 2011.

SECTION 24

Disaster Management, Exposures, and Other Environmental Injuries

Section Editor: Edward A. Bittner

24.1 Mass Casualty, Triage, and Epidemic/Pandemic Response

Karim Fikry

Mass Casualty Incidents

Definition and Characteristics

A mass casualty incident (MCI) is an event that overwhelms the local health care system, with the number of casualties exceeding the available resources. MCIs can result from natural disasters, accidents, terrorist attacks, or industrial accidents. The key characteristics of MCIs include:

- **Sudden onset:** MCIs often occur without warning, requiring immediate and decisive action.
- **Resource limitations:** the number of injured or affected individuals surpasses the available medical resources, including personnel, equipment, and facilities.
- **Need for rapid triage:** efficient triage systems are essential to prioritize patients based on the severity of their conditions.

Phases of Mass Casualty Incident Response

- **Preincident planning and preparedness**
  - Developing MCI protocols and disaster plans
  - Training health care personnel in disaster response
  - Conducting drills and simulations to ensure readiness
- **Incident response**
  - Rapid assessment of the scene and initial triage
  - Establishing command and communication structures
  - Coordinating with local, regional, and national emergency services
- **Postincident recovery**
  - Continuation of medical care for survivors
  - Mental health support for patients and health care providers
  - Evaluating and revising response plans based on lessons learned

Triage in Critical Care

Principles of Triage

Triage is the process of sorting patients based on the urgency of their medical needs. The primary goal is to maximize the number of survivors by ensuring that limited resources are used where they can have the most significant impact. The principles of triage include:

- **Immediate (red):** patients requiring immediate lifesaving interventions
- **Delayed (yellow):** patients who need significant medical intervention but can tolerate a delay
- **Minimal (green):** patients with minor injuries who can wait or are capable of self-care
- **Expectant (black):** patients with severe injuries unlikely to survive, given the resource constraints

Triage Systems

Several triage systems are utilized in critical care settings, including:

- **Simple Triage and Rapid Treatment**
  - Utilizes a quick assessment based on respiratory rate, perfusion, and mental status
  - Effective for use in prehospital and mass casualty settings

- **Sort, Assess, Lifesaving interventions, treatment/transport**
  - A more comprehensive system that includes reassessment and lifesaving interventions
  - **Emergency Severity Index**
  - A five-level triage system used primarily in emergency departments
  - Considers both the severity of the condition and the resources required

Triage Steps in Mass Casualty Incidents

- **Initial triage**
  - Conducted at the scene of the incident by first responders
  - Patients are rapidly assessed and tagged with colored labels indicating their triage category.
  - The primary goal is to identify those who need immediate care and those who can wait.
- **Secondary triage**
  - Performed once patients are transported to a medical facility or a more controlled environment
  - More thorough assessment and recategorization based on updated clinical information
  - Helps ensure that patients receive the appropriate level of care based on their evolving conditions

Key Considerations

- **Speed and efficiency**
  - Triage must be performed quickly and efficiently to manage large numbers of casualties.
  - The use of simple, easy-to-remember criteria is essential for rapid decision-making.
- **Resource allocation**
  - Triage aims to make the best use of limited resources, ensuring that they are directed where they can save the most lives.
  - Decisions often involve difficult ethical considerations, especially when resources are extremely scarce.
- **Flexibility**
  - Triage categories are not fixed and can change as patients' conditions evolve.
  - Continuous reassessment is crucial to ensure patients receive appropriate care as their needs change.
- **Communication**
  - Effective communication among first responders, medical personnel, and incident command is vital for successful triage operations.
  - Clear and consistent use of triage tags and documentation helps maintain an organized response.

Epidemic and Pandemic Response

Preparedness and Planning

Effective response to epidemics and pandemics requires comprehensive planning and preparedness, including:

- **Surveillance and early detection**
  - Implementing robust surveillance systems to detect outbreaks early
  - Utilizing data analytics and modeling to predict spread and impact
- **Capacity building**
  - Expanding health care infrastructure to handle surges in patient volume
  - Training health care workers in infection control and outbreak management
- **Stockpiling resources**
  - Maintaining reserves of essential supplies, such as personal protective equipment (PPE), medications, and ventilators

Response Strategies

- **Infection control measures**
  - Implementing quarantine and isolation protocols
  - Ensuring adherence to hygiene and sanitation practices
- **Health care system adaptations**
  - Repurposing facilities and redistributing resources to areas of greatest need
  - Utilizing telemedicine and remote monitoring to reduce the burden on health care facilities
- **Vaccination and treatment**
  - Accelerating the development and distribution of vaccines
  - Ensuring equitable access to treatments and therapeutics

Ethical Considerations

- **Resource allocation**
  - Making difficult decisions about the allocation of scarce resources
  - Balancing individual patient needs with public health priorities
- **Equity and access**
  - Ensuring that vulnerable populations receive appropriate care and support
  - Addressing disparities in health care access and outcomes

Conclusion

Critical care medicine is integral to the effective management of MCIs, triage situations, and epidemic/pandemic responses. By adhering to established principles and continually refining strategies based on experience and research, health care providers can save lives and mitigate the impact of these challenging scenarios. Preparedness, adaptability, and ethical decision-making are key components of successful critical care in times of crisis.

Specialized Areas Responses

Management of Biologic, Chemical, and Nuclear Exposure

Managing exposures to biologic, chemical, and nuclear agents requires a comprehensive approach involving immediate- and long-term medical care, decontamination, and public health interventions. An overview of the management strategies for each type of exposure is explained here.

Biologic Exposure

Types of Biologic Agents

Biologic agents include bacteria, viruses, fungi, and toxins that can cause disease. Examples include anthrax, smallpox, plague, and botulinum toxin.

Management Strategies

- Detection and diagnosis
    - Rapid identification of the biologic agent through clinical signs, symptoms, and laboratory tests
    - Use of surveillance systems to detect outbreaks and track the spread of disease
- Isolation and quarantine
    - Isolation of infected individuals to prevent the spread of the disease
    - Quarantine of exposed individuals who are not yet symptomatic
- Medical treatment
    - Administration of appropriate antibiotics, antivirals, or antitoxins based on the specific agent
    - Supportive care to manage symptoms and complications, such as respiratory support for severe infections
- Vaccination
    - Use of vaccines for prevention and postexposure prophylaxis if available
    - Mass vaccination campaigns in the event of a large-scale outbreak
- Infection control measures
    - Implementation of strict hygiene and sanitation practices
    - Use PPE by health care workers and first responders
- Public health interventions
    - Public education on the signs and symptoms of infection and prevention measures
    - Coordination with local, state, and federal health agencies for a coordinated response

Chemical Exposure

Types of Chemical Agents

Chemical agents include toxic industrial chemicals and chemical warfare agents such as nerve agents (sarin, VX), blister agents (mustard gas), and choking agents (chlorine).

Management Strategies

- Detection and diagnosis
    - Rapid identification of the chemical agent through clinical signs, symptoms, and environmental detection methods
    - Use of poison control centers for guidance on diagnosis and treatment
- Decontamination
    - Immediate removal of contaminated clothing and thorough washing of exposed skin with soap and water
    - Use of specialized decontamination units for MCIs
- Medical treatment
    - Administration of specific antidotes, such as atropine and pralidoxime, for nerve agent exposure
    - Supportive care for respiratory distress, seizures, and other symptoms
- Protective measures
    - Use of PPE by health care workers and first responders to prevent secondary contamination
    - Establishment of hot, warm, and cold zones to manage the scene and prevent the spread of contamination
- Public health interventions
    - Evacuation and shelter-in-place orders for affected populations
    - Public education on recognition of chemical exposure and self-protection measures

Nuclear Exposure

Types of Nuclear Agents

Nuclear incidents involve exposure to radioactive materials from nuclear power plant accidents, radiologic dispersal devices (dirty bombs), or nuclear weapons.

Management Strategies

- Detection and diagnosis
    - Use of radiation detection devices to assess exposure levels
    - Clinical evaluation for signs of acute radiation syndrome (ARS), including nausea, vomiting, and decreased blood cell counts
- Decontamination
    - Removal of contaminated clothing and thorough washing of exposed skin
    - Use of decontamination showers and facilities for mass decontamination
- Medical treatment
    - Administration of potassium iodide (KI) to block radioactive iodine uptake by the thyroid
    - Use of colony-stimulating factors to support bone marrow recovery in ARS
    - Supportive care for burns, trauma, and other injuries
- Protective measures
    - Use of PPE by health care workers and first responders to prevent internal and external contamination
    - Establishment of exclusion zones to limit access to contaminated areas
- Public health interventions
    - Evacuation and sheltering of affected populations based on radiation plume modeling and exposure levels
    - Public education on measures to reduce radiation exposure, such as staying indoors and using shielding materials

SUGGESTED READINGS

Blumenstock J, Bakker G, Jarris PE. Measuring preparedness: the National Health Security Preparedness Index. *J Public Health Manag Pract*. 2014;20(3):361-363.

Centers for Disease Control and Prevention (CDC). *Interim Prepandemic Planning Guidance: Community Strategy for Pandemic Influenza Mitigation in the United States—Early, Targeted, Layered Use of Nonpharmaceutical Interventions*. CDC; 2007. http://www.flu.gov/planning-preparedness/community/community_mitigation.pdf

Centers for Disease Control and Prevention (CDC). *Interim Operational Considerations for Implementing the Shielding Approach to Prevent COVID-19 Infections in Humanitarian Settings*. 2020. https://stacks.cdc.gov/view/cdc/117081

Fink BN, Rega PP, Sexton ME, Wishner C. START vs. SALT triage: which is preferred by the 21st century health care student? *Prehosp Disaster Med*. 2018;33:381.

Hick JL, Barbera JA, Kelen GD. Refining surge capacity: conventional, contingency, and crisis capacity. *Disaster Med Public Health Prep*. 2009;3(1):S59-S67.

Hick JL, Einav S, Hanfling D, et al; Task Force for Mass Critical Care; Task Force for Mass Critical Care. Surge capacity principles: care of the critically ill and injured during pandemics and disasters: CHEST consensus statement. *Chest*. 2014;146(4 suppl):e1S-e16S.

Pole T, Marcozzi D, Hunt RC. Interrupting my shift: disaster preparedness and response. *Ann Emerg Med*. 2013;63:584-588.

Rawlings A, Brandt L, Ferreres A, Asbun H, Shadduck P. Ethical considerations for allocation of scarce resources and alterations in surgical care during a pandemic. *Surg Endosc*. 2021;35(5):2217-2222.

Rubinson L. Nuzzo JB, Talmor DS, et al. Augmentation of hospital critical care capacity after bioterrorist attacks or epidemics: recommendations of the Working Group on Emergency Mass Critical Care. *Crit Care Med*. 2005;36(1):S275-S280.

Sax DR, Warton EM, Mark DG, et al; Kaiser Permanente CREST (Clinical Research on Emergency Services & Treatments) Network. Evaluation of the Emergency Severity Index in US emergency departments for the rate of mistriage. *JAMA Netw Open*. 2023;6(3):e233404.

Usoro A, Mehmood A, Rapaport S, et al. A scoping review of the essential components of emergency medical response systems for mass casualty incidents. *Disaster Med Public Health Prep*. 2023;17:e274.

World Health Organization. *WHO Global Influenza Preparedness Plan: The Role of WHO and Recommendations for National Measures Before and During Pandemics*. World Health Organization; 2005. http://www.who.int/csr/resources/publications/influenza/WHO_CDS_CSR_GIP_2005_5.pdf

World Health Organization. Pandemic influenza preparedness and response: a WHO guidance document. 2010. https://iris.who.int/handle/10665/44123

World Health Organization. Vaccination in acute humanitarian emergencies: a framework for decision making. 2017. https://www.who.int/publications/i/item/WHO-IVB-17.03

World Health Organization. Enhancing preparedness for an equitable response to pandemic influenza and other respiratory viral diseases. 2024. https://www.emro.who.int/pip-framework/index.html

24.2

Chemical, Biological, Radiological, and Nuclear Exposures

Sandra Carvajal-Raga and Anahat Dhillon

Definition

- Chemical, Biological, Radiological, and Nuclear (CBRN) exposure poses unique challenges for health care providers due to the diverse nature of the agents involved and their profound effects on human health.
- Early detection and triage, rapid decontamination, and immediate control over the radius of exposure are critical elements in the management of nuclear, radiologic, chemical, and/or biologic exposures.
- Protection of first responders, health care personnel, and the public is as important as caring for exposed individuals in order to minimize the overall impact of nuclear, radiologic, chemical, and/or biologic exposures.

Common Causes to Remember

CBRN agents pose a serious risk to human health and safety, with the potential for mass casualties in both military and civilian settings. These are some modern-day examples of CBRN exposures:

- Chemical: Syrian Chemical Attacks with sarin and chlorine gas 2017 to 2018
- Biologic: Ebola outbreaks in West Africa 2014 to 2016 and resurgence in Guinea in 2021
- Radiologic: Fukushima Nuclear Power Plant disaster in 2011, causing ongoing radiation exposure when contaminated water was released in 2021
- Nuclear: wildfires in the Chernobyl exclusion zone in 2020 re-released radioactive particles, underlining persistent risks from historical nuclear incidents

Epidemiology

- The Global Incident Map (http://www.globalincidentmap.com) displays the enormity of the current global threat of terrorism.
- High-explosive events remain the most common type of terrorist activity and are, therefore, easy to detect; a higher index of suspicion is required to identify CBRN attacks.
- Chemical exposures
  - In 2020, there were 2,079 cases of organophosphate poisoning and no fatalities, usually these events, were from occupational exposure or accidental ingestion; Organophosphate poisoning remains a global concern, particularly in low- and middle-income countries, but the United States has seen fewer cases due to stricter regulations and improved safety measures. The World Health Organization (WHO) estimates that around 200,000 deaths occur annually due to pesticide poisoning, with organophosphates being a major contributor.
  - The most common cause of cyanide poisoning in the United States is related to household fires; up to 35% to 40% of fire-related deaths involve cyanide toxicity in addition to carbon monoxide exposure.
  - Since 2010, there have been several instances of chemical weapons use in the Middle East, particularly in Syria, leading to significant casualties. The Syrian Civil War has been the focal point of most chemical attacks, with multiple confirmed incidents involving chemical agents like sarin, chlorine, and mustard gas. Estimates vary, but chemical attacks in Syria alone are believed to have caused over 1,500 to 2,000 deaths since 2010, with thousands more injured. Survivors of chemical attacks often suffer from long-term respiratory issues, neurologic damage, and psychological trauma.
- Biologic exposures
  - Since 2015, several biologic exposure events have occurred, ranging from naturally occurring pandemics to deliberate use of biologic agents in bioterrorism.

These exposures have underscored the vulnerability of global public health systems to both natural and man-made biologic threats.
  - The 2014-2016 West Africa outbreak was the largest Ebola epidemic to date, with more than 28,000 cases and 11,000 deaths across Guinea, Liberia, and Sierra Leone.
  - The Zika virus epidemic spread rapidly through South and Central America, with over 500,000 suspected cases reported. Zika infection during pregnancy was linked to severe birth defects, including microcephaly. The outbreak raised awareness of the global threat posed by mosquito-borne viruses.
  - While naturally occurring anthrax outbreaks have been rare, concerns about the use of anthrax as a biologic weapon have persisted. Deliberate releases of anthrax spores through contaminated mail (such as the 2001 anthrax attacks) have resulted in heightened biosecurity measures.
  - As of 2024, COVID-19 has resulted in over 780 million confirmed cases and nearly 7 million deaths worldwide. The virus primarily spreads through respiratory droplets, but it can also transmit via aerosols in enclosed spaces. The pandemic has caused immense strain on health care systems globally, leading to high morbidity and mortality rates, particularly among older populations and individuals with comorbidities.
- Nuclear and radiologic exposures
  - Two major databases track radiation accidents: Oak Ridge Institute for Science and Education (ORIS) in the United States and Institut de Radioprotection et de Sûreté Nucléaire (IRSN) in Europe.
  - Since 2000, there has been a reduction in radiation accident exposure; most reported cases are related to occupational exposures rather than large-scale radiation accidents.
  - On March 11, 2011, a magnitude 9.0 earthquake and subsequent tsunami triggered the meltdown at Fukushima Daiichi Nuclear Power Plant in Japan, resulting in the release of radioactive materials. Despite initial fears, comprehensive epidemiologic studies, including those from the WHO and United Nations Scientific Committee on the Effects of Atomic Radiation (UNSCEAR), have shown no significant increase in overall cancer rates attributable to the radiation exposure, though increased thyroid cancer screening has led to the detection of more cases.
  - A study of nuclear industry workers published by the International Agency for Research on Cancer (IARC) in 2015 found a small but statistically significant increase in cancer risk, particularly for leukemia, among long-term workers exposed to low doses of ionizing radiation.

Key Pathophysiology

- Chemical exposures
  - Most likely to occur within enclosed spaces (eg, shopping malls) since the effects of chemicals dissipate rapidly when victims are removed from the area of exposure
  - Easily detectable in the sense that symptoms are rapid in onset and multiple people in close proximity will have similar presentations
  - Each major category has specific mechanisms of action:
    - Asphyxiants (suffocation agents): interfere with the availability of oxygen for cellular respiration (eg, hydrogen cyanide, arsine)
    - Cholinesterase inhibitors (nerve gases): inhibit acetylcholinesterase activity (eg, sarin, VX)
    - Pulmonary irritants (choking agents): act directly by damaging the upper airway and pulmonary tissue (eg, chlorine, ammonia)
    - Vesicants (blistering agents): cause direct chemical burns in epithelial tissue; interfere with DNA synthesis and cell division (eg, sulfur mustard, Lewisite)
  - Handheld chemical detectors exist; they are more accurate than handheld biologic detectors, but less reliable than radiation detectors.
- Biologic exposures
  - Terrorists use of biologic weapons would likely be through aerosol dissemination, given the significantly higher likelihood of mass casualties.
  - The U.S. Centers for Disease Control and Prevention have identified a number of pathogens that could be used in biologic terrorism and ranked them:
    - Category A: can be grown easily in large quantities, are particularly well suited to airborne dissemination, and are resistant to destruction (eg, anthrax, smallpox)
    - Category B: moderately easy to spread, may require enhanced diagnostic or surveillance techniques to monitor, and generally less destructive than category A (eg, ricin, brucellosis)
    - Category C: include pathogens that could be engineered for mass dissemination because of ease of availability and have significant potential for morbidity and/or mortality (eg, hantavirus, multidrug-resistant tuberculosis)
  - The US anthrax letter incidents in 2001 presented a novel method of biologic terrorism, which is less effective than high-volume aerosolized delivery, but is significantly more covert.
  - Nuclear and radiologic exposures
  - Nuclear explosions are obvious and considered "overt" events; release of radionuclear material into the food/water supply or into ventilation systems is considered a "covert" event.
  - Mixed "overt" and "covert" events include the use of radiologic dispersion devices ("dirty bombs"), where the explosion would be rapidly detected, but the presence of radiation would only be apparent if detectors are used by first responders.
  - Most commonly used predictor of acute symptoms is the whole-body absorbed dose of gamma radiation (Gy = Gray units).
  - Radiation sickness is caused by exposure to radiation doses >0.1 Gy over a short period of time (eg, >0.1 Gy/h).

Differential Diagnosis

- Chemical exposures
  - Four basic clinical syndromes may occur after exposure to chemical agents:
    - Asphyxiants: cellular hypoxia leads to marked central nervous system, cardiovascular, and respiratory derangements; cyanide is often described as having

a bitter almond smell, while arsine is described as having a garlic smell.
    - Cholinesterase inhibitors: cause miosis, secretions, fasciculations, rhinorrhea, wheezing, and seizures
    - Pulmonary irritants: present with cough, chest tightness, wheezing, and noncardiogenic pulmonary edema; phosgene is colorless and smells like freshly mowed hay, chlorine is greenish yellow and has a pungent smell, ammonia is colorless with a characteristic smell associated with conventional household cleaners
    - Vesicants: result in extremely painful eye injuries, vesicular skin lesions, respiratory distress, damage to the epithelial lining of the gastrointestinal tract, and leukopenia
  - Each major category of chemical agents is associated with very distinct signs and symptoms, which may be helpful in early recognition and management by early responders.
- Biologic exposures
  - Clinical manifestations of most biologic agents involve nonspecific influenza-like symptoms; therefore, clinicians must have a high suspicion for terrorism-related release of biologic agents for timely detection.
  - Appropriate collection of clinical specimens within the first 24 hours is crucial for timely detection; nasal swab and sputum are usually sent for culture and polymerase chain reaction testing; fluorescein antibody testing is sometimes helpful to detect tularemia.
  - Serum is needed for toxin assays when botulism is suspected.
  - The route of exposure may determine observed signs and symptoms; for example, inhaled ricin is associated with respiratory distress, fever, cough, and pulmonary edema within 8 hours of exposure versus ingestion that is associated with vomiting, bloody diarrhea, and dehydration within 6 hours of exposure.
  - Nuclear and radiologic exposures
  - Burn-like wounds without a history consistent with a thermal injury should prompt clinicians to inquire about the possibility of radiation exposure.
  - Acute radiation syndrome (ARS) is divided into three main presentations:
    - Hematopoietic: aplastic anemia can be seen with exposure doses around 0.25 Gy but is more pronounced at doses >1 Gy; typically manifests as infections (from a sudden drop in white blood cell [WBC]), bleeding (from a sudden drop in platelets), and anemia (from a combination of bleeding and a sudden drop in red blood cell [RBC] production).
    - Gastrointestinal: nausea, vomiting, loss of appetite, and abdominal pain are usually seen within 2 hours with exposure doses of 6 to 30 Gy; time to onset of nausea is often an indicator of the severity of whole-body exposure.
    - Neurologic: can be observed with exposure doses around 10 Gy but is significantly more pronounced at doses >30 Gy; dizziness, headache, and/or decreased level of consciousness occurring within minutes to a few hours are invariably fatal.
  - Unless radiation exposure is high, patients may not experience immediate symptoms; sometimes, a nonspecific prodrome (nausea, vomiting, headaches, fatigue, fever, and a short period of skin erythema) may precede ARS at radiation doses starting around 0.35 Gy.

Management and Treatment

- Managing CBRN exposures involves a multifaceted approach for both first responders and patients. Rapid decontamination, use of personal protective equipment (PPE), and specific antidotes or treatments are critical for mitigating the effects of CBRN agents.
- Chemical exposures
  - Initial management includes moving affected persons out of enclosed spaces and to dedicated decontamination sites.
  - Decontamination starts with removal of all clothing followed by washing with soap and water for at least 15 minutes.
  - Eyes should be flushed with water for at least 10 minutes; mouth and nose should also be thoroughly flushed to eliminate residue.
  - Full-body protection, including a self-contained breathing apparatus (SCBA), is necessary.
  - Asphyxiants
    - 100% oxygen should be instituted as soon as possible.
    - Cyanide poisoning may require the administration of intravenous (IV) sodium nitrite (300 mg over 5-15 minutes), followed by sodium thiosulfate (12.5 g slow push); not recommended in the setting of significant hypoxia or concurrent carbon monoxide poisoning as nitrite-induced methemoglobinemia may cause further injury; in such cases, thiosulfate only or hydroxocobalamin should be considered.
    - No specific antidotes exist for arsine; therapy is mostly supportive and directed at the end-organ ramifications of its characteristic hemolysis syndrome (eg, renal failure).
  - Cholinesterase inhibitors
    - Topical application of reactive skin decontamination lotion (RSDL) acts within seconds to neutralize any chemicals present on the skin.
    - Initial atropine dose (2-4 mg IV) should be administered and redosed every 5 to 10 minutes until muscarinic symptoms disappear.
    - Pralidoxime (1-2 g) should be administered as soon as possible.
    - Other supportive measures (eg, airway patency, management of shock, seizure therapy) should continue as needed.
  - Pulmonary irritants
    - Bronchospasm is treated with bronchodilators and corticosteroids.
    - Mechanical ventilation and more focused therapy may be required in cases of acute respiratory distress syndrome (ARDS).
    - Eyes should be treated with a mydriatic and a topical antibiotic.
  - Vesicants
    - No specific drug is available to counteract the effects of mustard gas on the skin, eyes, and lungs; treatment is mainly supportive.

    - Immediate topical application of RSDL may assist with effective decontamination of sulfur mustard exposure.
    - The topical antidote dimercaprol is effective against Lewisite if applied immediately to the skin and eyes.
- Biologic exposures
  - Initial management includes moving affected persons into quarantined decontamination sites.
  - Decontamination starts with the removal of all clothing, followed by copious washing with soap and water.
  - Exposed surfaces, artifacts, and clothing may be decontaminated with a 0.5% sodium hypochlorite solution; it should not be used on human skin.
  - No proven commercially available antidotes exist; therapy is predominantly supportive; gastric lavage and activated charcoal may be considered in cases where pathogens may have been ingested.
  - Antitoxins to ricin, anthrax, and botulinum do exist; a monoclonal antibody against inhalational anthrax was recently approved by the U.S. Food and Drug Administration but is only maintained in the U.S. Office of Health Preparedness and Response's Strategic National Stockpile.
  - Ciprofloxacin and doxycycline may be used for chemoprophylaxis against anthrax, tularemia, and the plague.
  - Trimethoprim-sulfamethoxazole may have a role in chemoprophylaxis for glanders and melioidosis.
  - Combination therapy with doxycycline and rifampin for 21 days is the preferred chemoprophylaxis regimen for brucellosis.
  - Nuclear and radiologic exposures
  - Immediate management involves:
    - Minimizing the time of radiation exposure
    - Increasing the distance from the radiation source
    - Shielding from radiation
    - Minimizing incorporation into the body by use of PPE (eg, use of gas/dust mask)
  - Once immediate measures have been instituted, clinicians should:
    - Confirm the history and evidence of exposure
    - Process biologic samples such as complete blood counts (an absolute lymphocyte count decrease in 6-48 hours predicts toxicity; in severe cases, patients may require bone marrow transplantation)
    - Swab all body orifices; if internal radiation contamination is suspected, providers should also collect urine, feces, and gastric secretions.
    - Specific antidotes (eg, potassium iodide to protect the thyroid) should be considered.
  - Emesis predicts toxicity (immediate and up to 2 hours postexposure indicates a significant radiation dose).
  - Treatment is generally supportive; antibiotics, blood products, colony-stimulating factors, and stem cell transplant when clinically indicated.

Outcomes

- Chemical exposures
  - Asphyxiants
    - While intranasal sodium nitrite is beneficial in situations where IV access may be delayed, switching to parenteral dosing as soon as possible improves cyanide clearance.
    - Dicobalt edetate is approved in Europe and Australia as a chelating agent for cyanide toxicity; though effective, the known potential side effects warrant significant caution before considering its use.
    - High-dose hydroxocobalamin is used for cyanide toxicity since it is effective and has a much lower side-effect profile than dicobalt edetate or sodium nitrate (ie, does not result in methemoglobinemia).
    - Diuresis is recommended to prevent heme-pigment nephropathy following hemolysis syndrome from arsine toxicity; dialysis is not effective in removing arsine.
  - Cholinesterase inhibitors
    - RSDL has been used by the US Armed Forces to demonstrate effectiveness.
    - Hallmark of therapy is the administration of atropine and pralidoxime as soon as possible.
    - Atropine doses >200 mg in the first 24 hours have been reported.
    - In refractory cases of toxicity following bolus doses of pralidoxime, continuous infusions at 8 mg/kg/h have been used.
    - Organophosphates are particularly lipid soluble and remain in the body for several weeks, potentially continuing to cause symptoms; atropine and pralidoxime should be continue to be administered until there are no more symptoms.
    - Intramuscular administration of both atropine and pralidoxime is effective and is particularly helpful when IV access is delayed or a prolonged duration of therapy is indicated.
  - Pulmonary irritants
    - Symptoms are usually delayed and typically related to the concentration of the irritant; high pulmonary concentrations can result in fatality within 10 minutes.
    - Signs of acute lung injury within 4 hours of exposure are associated with a low likelihood of survival.
    - Toxic ammonia exposure is remarkable for deep burns and blisters that look like frostbite as well as opaque corneas and cataracts.
  - Vesicants
    - In general, vesicants are designed to incapacitate victims; mortality rate is usually ~4% and typically related to secondary complications.
    - Early respiratory symptoms include sore throat, cough, and hoarseness, followed by shortness of breath in ~12 hours postexposure; bacterial pneumonia may be appreciated 3 to 4 days after exposure.
    - Early skin symptoms of mustard gas exposure include redness followed by pain and itching; blisters appear 16 hours postexposure, reaching a maximum by the third postexposure day.
    - Corneal symptoms, eye pain, and eyelid swelling occur ~12 hours post mustard gas exposure; blindness is uncommon, though corneal damage can be chronic and progressive.
    - Skin and eye symptoms begin immediately with Lewisite exposure.

- Biologic exposures
  - Regular soap and water are as effective in the removal of spores (eg, anthrax) as antimicrobial soap or 2% chlorhexidine gluconate; ethyl alcohol waterless rub is not active against these spores.
  - The value of mass vaccination after a biologic event is unclear; under special circumstances, vaccines against anthrax, botulinum, cholera, Q fever, and viral encephalitides/hemorrhagic fevers may be obtained from the U.S. Centers for Disease Control and Prevention.
- Nuclear and radiologic exposures
  - While there is a direct relationship between the degree of neutropenia after exposure to radiation and the risk of infections, there are no controlled studies of therapeutic interventions in humans.
  - Current recommendations for antimicrobial therapy following radiation poisoning are based on case reports and animal research, which support the use of broad-spectrum Gram-positive and Gram-negative coverage while avoiding the use of agents that target strict anaerobic components of the gut flora (eg, metronidazole).
  - Despite timely supportive therapy, mortality rate increases significantly with escalating exposure doses:
    - 1 to 2 Gy: 0% to 5% within 6 to 8 weeks
    - 2 to 6 Gy: 5% to 50% within 4 to 6 weeks
    - 6 to 8 Gy: 50% to 100% within 2 to 4 weeks
    - 8 to 30 Gy: 100% within 2 days to 2 weeks
    - >30 Gy: 100% within 1 to 2 days

SUGGESTED READINGS

Bozeman WP, Dilbero D, Schauben JL. Biologic and chemical weapons of mass destruction. *Emerg Med Clin North Am.* 2002;20(4):975.

Chalela JA, Burnett T. Chemical terrorism for the intensivist. *Mil Med.* 2012;177(5):495-500.

Christian MD. Biowarfare and bioterrorism. *Crit Care Clin.* 2013;29(3):717-756.

Coleman CN, Stone HB, Moulder JE, et al. Medical management of acute radiation syndrome: recommendations of the Strategic National Stockpile Radiation Working Group. *Ann Intern Med.* 2011;154(9):573-578.

D'Errico R, Volpe A, D'Errico L. Chemical warfare agents: toxicity at low levels and their pre-exposure management. *J Occup Environ Hyg.* 2013;10(1):1-7.

Fowler RA, Fletcher T, Fischer WA II, et al. Caring for critically ill patients with Ebola virus disease. *Perspect Infect Dis.* 2014;384(9959):498-503.

Goans RE, Waselenko JK. Medical management of radiological casualties: current concepts. *BJR Suppl.* 2012;35:93-100.

Greenfield RA, Brown BR, Hutchins JB, et al. Microbiological, biological, and chemical weapons of warfare and terrorism. *Am J Med Sci.* 2002;323(6):326.

Hendrickson RG, Hedges JR. Introduction—what critical care practitioners should know about terrorism agents. *Crit Care Clin.* 2005;21(4):641-652.

Khan AS, Levitt AM, Sage MJ. Biological and chemical terrorism: strategic plan for preparedness and response. *Emerg Infect Dis.* 2010;6(6):579-590.

McDonnel G, Russell AD. Antiseptics and disinfectants: activity, action, and resistance. *Clin Microbiol Rev.* 2015;28(1):147-176.

Mettler FA Jr, Voelz GL. Major radiation exposure-what to expect and how to respond. *N Engl J Med.* 2002;346(20):1554.

Thompson J, Rehn M, Lossius HM, Lockey D. Risks to emergency medical responders at terrorist incidents: a narrative review of the medical literature. *Crit Care.* 2014;18(5):521.

Titus E, Lemmer G, Slagley J, Eninger R. A review of CBRN topics related to military and civilian patient exposure and decontamination. *Am J Disaster Med.* 2019;14(2):137-149.

Waselenko JK, MacVittie TJ, Blakely WF, et al. Medical management of the acute radiation syndrome: recommendations of the Strategic National Stockpile Radiation Working Group. *Ann Intern Med.* 2004;140(12):1037.

White SM. Chemical and biological weapons: implications for anaesthesia and intensive care. *Br J Anaesth.* 2002;89(2):3.

24.3

Drowning

Timothy G. Gaulton

Definition

- World Health Organization definition: "Drowning is the process of experiencing respiratory impairment from submersion/immersion in liquid."
  - Immersion—upper airway above water
  - Submersion—upper airway below water
  - Fatal drowning—death
  - Nonfatal drowning—morbidity or no morbidity
  - Rescue—intervention that prevents progression to respiratory impairment

Epidemiology

- Drowning is one of the leading causes of death from unintentional injury worldwide, accounting for nearly 300,000 reported deaths.
  - Drowning rates are >3 times higher in low- and middle-income countries than in high-income countries.
  - In the United States, drowning death rates have increased since 2020.
- Nonfatal drowning cases resulting in hospital care are over twice as common as fatal cases.
- Over 90% of drowning cases are preventable.

Risk Factors

- Males have twice the drowning death rate than females due to increased exposure to water and riskier behaviors (eg, swimming alone, alcohol use).
- Children (<14 years) have an elevated risk due to a lack of swimming skills and an underdeveloped ability to assess risk.
  - The risk increases without adult supervision.

- Other individual risk factors include alcohol use, epilepsy, and concomitant trauma.
- Systemic risk factors include poverty and inequality, rural residency, and water exposure.

Key Pathophysiology

Submersion

- Begins with breath holding
  - First phase (easy-going) with the absence of respiratory muscle activity
  - Second phase (struggle) with inspiratory muscle contractions
- Length of breath-hold depends on:
  - Metabolic rate, carbon dioxide and oxygen storage capacity, tolerance of unpleasant sensations, water temperature, prior hyperventilation
  - The diving response may preserve oxygen consumption during apnea.
    - Results in bradycardia, peripheral vasoconstriction, and hypertension
    - Less active in adults than in kids
    - Large interindividual differences
- Aspiration of water
  - Activation of upper airway reflexes
    - Coughing occurs.
    - Stimulation of the laryngeal mucosa may result in laryngeal closure (laryngospasm) that prevents water from entering the lungs.
    - Forced ventilatory movement against a closed glottis can cause mechanical lung injury.
    - Hypoxemia will terminate laryngospasm.
  - Impairs and washes out surfactant
  - Disrupts the alveolar-capillary membrane integrity
  - This leads to alveolar edema and acute respiratory distress syndrome (ARDS).
    - Can occur with aspiration of 1 mL/kg of water
    - Injury is similar with fresh or salt water.
- Cardiac arrhythmias
  - Increased in cold water due to vagal stimulation
  - May occur with cessation of breath-hold

Immersion

- Most drowning events occur at temperatures below thermoneutral (35 °C ± 0.5).
- Cold-water immersion (<~25 °C)
  - Results in hyperventilation, increased cardiac output, and peripheral vasoconstriction via cutaneous cold receptors
  - The inability to breath-hold increases the probability of aspiration.
  - Progressive hypothermia results in coma, ventricular arrhythmias, and death.
- Hold-water immersion (>38 °C)
  - Limited evaporation of sweat above water
  - Decreased peripheral vascular resistance contributes to orthostatic hypotension and syncope with standing.

Management and Treatment

Prehospital Resuscitation

- In 2024, the American Heart Association released updated guidelines on resuscitation following drowning.
- While prevention is critical, once the drowning process begins, rescuers should follow the Drowning Chain of Survival:
  - Recognize distress and send for help.
  - Provide flotation to prevent submersion.
    - Untrained rescuers must avoid dangerous rescue responses that would make them another victim.
  - Remove the victim from water when safe to do so and in the most feasible position so as not to delay resuscitation.
  - Provide care as needed using Basic Life Support (BLS) and Advanced Life Support (ALS).
    - However, most cases do not require cardiopulmonary resuscitation (CPR) (<0.5% of all rescues).
- BLS
  - For trained rescuers, in-water rescue breathing to an unresponsive individual may result in improved survival but only if safety is not compromised.
  - Once out of the water, presume cardiac arrest if no signs of normal breathing and consciousness.
  - Initiate rescue breathing followed by chest compressions in the supine position without an initial pulse check to prevent delay.
    - Rescue breaths are important as cardiac arrest from drowning is often due to hypoxemia.
    - Compression-only CPR may reduce survival.
    - Provide rescue breaths by first means available (eg, mouth-to-mouth, bag-mask ventilation) in a ratio of 2 breaths to 30 compressions.
  - Placement of automatic external defibrillators should occur after CPR with rescue breaths is initiated.
    - Initial shockable rhythms account for a minority of cardiac arrests following drowning.
  - Injuries to the cervical spine are infrequent in persons who are drowning; immobilization of the spine in the water is indicated only in cases in which head or neck injury is strongly suspected (eg, accidents involving diving, waterskiing, surfing).
  - If the person is unconscious but breathing, the recovery position (lateral decubitus) should be used.
  - Regurgitation of stomach contents may occur during resuscitation.
    - However, avoid efforts to expel water from the airway (using abdominal thrusts or placing the person head down) because they delay the initiation of ventilation and increase the risk of vomiting.
- ALS
  - Notify ALS teams as soon as possible.
  - Provide supplemental oxygen if available as hypoxemia is associated with worse outcomes.
  - In cases of cardiac arrest, placement of an advanced airway to deliver positive airway pressure should be initiated as soon as possible.
    - Supraglottic airways are an alternative to tracheal tubes, depending on the skill of the operator, but may increase aspiration.

- Although fluid may appear in the tracheal tube due to pulmonary edema, suctioning results in loss of airway pressure.
- Peripheral venous access is the preferred route for drug administration, while intraosseous access is an alternative route.
- Endotracheal administration of drugs is not recommended.
- If hypotension is not corrected by oxygenation, a rapid crystalloid infusion should be administered, regardless of whether salt water or fresh water has been aspirated.

Emergency Department Care

- Following stabilization of the airway, oxygenation, and circulation, check body temperature, given the high co-incidence of hypothermia.
- Place gastric tube as water is likely to have been swallowed.
- Metabolic acidosis occurs in most patients and is usually corrected by the patient's spontaneous effort to increase minute ventilation or by setting a higher minute ventilation on the mechanical ventilator.
  - Routine use of sodium bicarbonate is not recommended.
- History of events surrounding the drowning incident should include information on the rescue, resuscitation activities, and any current or previous illness.
  - Drowning can be precipitated by an injury or medical condition (eg, trauma, seizure, cardiac arrhythmia).
  - If the person remains unresponsive without an obvious cause, a toxicologic investigation and computed tomography of the head and neck should be considered.
- Patients with adequate arterial oxygenation without adjuvant therapy and with no other associated morbidity can be safely discharged.
- Patients whose clinical status deteriorates are admitted to an intermediate care unit for prolonged observation or intensive care unit (ICU) if intubation and mechanical ventilation are needed.

Intensive Care Unit Care

Respiratory System

- Drowning and subsequent resuscitation result in alveolar edema and the development of ARDS.
- Guidelines for ventilation in ARDS, including positive end-expiratory pressure (PEEP) titration, should be followed.
- Since a temporary and local insult causes the pulmonary injury, patients with pulmonary distress due to a drowning tend to recover much faster than patients with ARDS of other etiologies, and late pulmonary sequelae are uncommon.
- It is usually best not to initiate weaning from mechanical ventilation for at least 24 hours, even when gas exchange appears to be adequate, since the local pulmonary injury may not have resolved sufficiently.
- Data on prophylactic antibiotics, steroids, and diuretics are observational and may be initiated depending on clinical progression and available evidence.
- Aspiration of swimming pool water rarely results in pneumonia.
- Early-onset pneumonia can be due to the aspiration of polluted water, endogenous flora, or gastric contents.

Circulatory System

- In most persons rescued from drowning, blood pressure stabilizes after oxygenation, fluid resuscitation, and restoration of normal body temperature.
- Early cardiac dysfunction can occur secondary to stress cardiomyopathy and can be diagnosed with echocardiography.
- No evidence supports the use of a specific fluid therapy, diuretics, or water restriction in persons who have been rescued from drowning in salt water or fresh water.
- Extracorporeal membrane oxygenation may be considered in cases of refractory shock or pulmonary failure and allows for controlled rewarming.

Neurologic System

- Permanent neurologic damage is the most concerning outcome in persons who have been resuscitated after a drowning incident.
- Persons who are comatose or have neurologic deterioration should undergo intensive assessment and care.
- The goals are to achieve normal values for glucose, partial pressure of oxygen and carbon dioxide, and avoid any factors that increase brain metabolism.
- Target temperature management may be neuroprotective.
- Duration of submersion and risk of death or severe neurologic impairment after hospital discharge:
  - 0 to 5 minutes—10%
  - 6 to 10 minutes—56%
  - 11 to 25 minutes—88%
  - >25 minutes—99.9%

SUGGESTED READINGS

Bierens JJ, Lunetta P, Tipton M, et al. Physiology of drowning: a review. *Physiology (Bethesda)*. 2016;31(2):147-166.

Clemens T, Moreland B, Mack KA, et al. Vital signs: drowning death rates, self-reported swimming skill, swimming lesson participation, and recreational water exposure—United States, 2019-2023. *MMWR Morb Mortal Wkly Rep*. 2024;73(20):467-473.

Dezfulian C, McCallin TE, Bierens J, et al. 2024 American Heart Association and American Academy of Pediatrics Focused Update on special circumstances: resuscitation following drowning: an update to the American Heart Association Guidelines for Cardiopulmonary Resuscitation and Emergency Cardiovascular Care. *Circulation*. 2024;150(23):e501-e516.

Szpilman D, Morgan PJ. Management for the drowning patient. *Chest*. 2021;159(4):1473-1483.

Szpilman D, Soares M. In-water resuscitation—is it worthwhile? *Resuscitation*. 2004;63(1):25-31.

WHO Guidelines Approved by the Guidelines Review Committee. *WHO Guideline on the Prevention of Drowning Through Provision of Day-Care, and Basic Swimming and Water Safety Skills*. World Health Organization; 2021.

Yoshimura S, Kiguchi T, Nishioka N, et al. Association of pre-hospital tracheal intubation with outcomes after out-of-hospital cardiac arrest by drowning comparing to supraglottic airway device: a nationwide propensity score-matched cohort study. *Resuscitation*. 2024;197:110129.

24.4

Hanging and Strangulation Injuries

Mina Ghobrial, Brian W. Chin, Kylee Greider, and Ulrich H. Schmidt

Epidemiology

- Hanging is the second most common method of suicide in the United States.
- Strangulation is a common form of assault in domestic disputes, and women have a 4 to 11 times greater lifetime risk of being victimized.
- Strangulation injuries accounted for ~1.2% of emergency department visits for intimate partner violence between 2006 and 2014 (Patch et al 2021).
  - Lifetime prevalence of nonfatal intimate partner strangulation in the United States is ~10% (11 million women).
- For suicidal hanging/strangulation, drug/alcohol ingestion is present in up to 70% of cases (Penney et al 2002).

Terminology

Medical providers, first responders, and law enforcement use varying terms to describe forceful compression of the head and neck. Different forces and pressures can compress and damage neck structures. It is important to understand not only the varying mechanisms of hanging but also the warning signs for the areas involved.

Hanging

Long-Drop Hanging

- Judicial hanging is still used as a method of execution in parts of the world.
  - Knot is placed anteriorly (submental).
  - Drop distance is usually the same as the subject's height.
- Often results in high cervical fracture and spinal cord transection
- The goal of long-drop length is for a quick death from cervical fracture. Failure to achieve this often results in slower death from asphyxiation.
- Excessive drop lengths can result in decapitation.

Short-Drop Hanging

- Cervical spine injury is significantly less frequent for drop distances <1 m.
- Anterior placement of the knot poses a greater risk for high cervical spine injury.
  - Hyperextension of the neck is the classic mechanism associated with the "Hangman fracture."
    - Hangman fracture: bilateral fracture extending across the pars interarticularis of the second cervical vertebrae with associated traumatic subluxation of the second cervical vertebrae on the third cervical vertebrae.
  - Older age, possibly secondary to poor bone quality, is a risk factor.

Near-Hanging

- Full suspension of body weight by the neck never achieved

Strangulation

Ligature Strangulation

- Strangulation using a rope, chain, or other string-like object to apply compressive forces to the neck

Manual Strangulation

- Using two hands to encircle the neck to apply compressive forces to the neck

Postural Strangulation

- Unidirectional compression of the neck, usually against an object
- Commonly seen in martial arts and law enforcement as a method of submission

Evaluation

Signs, symptoms, and presentations of injuries within different areas of the head and neck

Cervical Spine Injury

- More common with longer drop heights (>1 m)
  - Nonjudicial long-drop hangings are exceedingly rare.

Nervous System Injury

- Spinal cord trauma from high C-spine injury can often result in spinal shock.
- Significant elevation in vagal tone from carotid sinus pressure may result in reflex bradycardia and cardiac arrest.
- Acute cerebral venous outflow tract obstruction from bilateral jugular compression can result in rapid loss of consciousness, cerebral edema, and parenchymal hemorrhage.
- Patients often have subarachnoid hemorrhages. May result from rupture/disruption of carotid or vertebral arteries.

Vascular Injury

- Jugular venous compression
  - ~2 kg of force required for obstruction.
  - Patients can suffer significant neurologic injury from resulting venous outflow obstruction, leading to cerebral edema, elevated intracranial pressure, and ultimately herniation.
- Arterial compression
  - ~3.5 kg required for obstruction.
  - Obstruction of arterial flow is the mechanism behind the rapid loss of consciousness.
- Direct traction on vessels can result in dissection.
  - Carotid arteries are often affected. One study demonstrated carotid artery damage in nearly half of the cases.

- Vertebral artery injury has also been previously described to occur in up to one-fourth of these patients (Saternus 1984).
- Vertebral artery dissection can occur and is suspected to be a mechanism of subarachnoid hemorrhage.

Respiratory Injury

- 15 kg of force required to obstruct the trachea.
- Children are at much higher risk of neck compression due to anatomically smaller larynx and less rigid tissues.
- Direct compression can result in fractures of the hyoid and breakage of the thyroid, cricoid, and tracheal ring cartilage.

Skin and Soft Tissue Injury

- Most commonly abrasions or skin tears overlying areas where pressure was applied
- Soft tissue injuries may extend deeper, particularly in hanging injuries where autopsies have demonstrated hematomas of the soft tissue of the neck and hemorrhage extending into the mediastinum.

Treatment/Management

Initial

- Remove any objects around the neck.
- Prioritize airway protection and maximize cerebral blood flow.
- Consider head of bed elevation for possible cerebral edema.
- Place in cervical collar.
  - Although spinal cord injury is rare, complications are devastating.
  - Of particular concern in anterior knots
  - Significant injury to ligaments can occur. Consider magnetic resonance imaging (MRI) for further evaluation.
- Previously, symptom-based decision tools were recommended for determining the need for computed tomography (CT). However, retrospective studies show symptoms such as loss of consciousness or headache have low positive predictive value for significant injury.
- CT studies of the head and neck, including angiography, aid in the evaluation of vascular injury and subarachnoid hemorrhage. MRI may be more sensitive but is not always readily available.
- Advanced imaging should be obtained if Glasgow Coma Scale (GCS) <15, there is a focal neurologic deficit, or if the patient has dysphagia or high suspicion for airway injury.
- Full-body examination is important to identify other injuries and may help the clinician identify patterns of abuse. This is especially important for children.
- If patient is asymptomatic, they can be discharged with strict return precautions.
- If patient presents with significant symptoms, observation is often warranted to monitor for delayed symptoms.

Delayed

- Acute respiratory distress syndrome (ARDS) can develop, although the mechanism is unclear.
  - Could result from increased intrathoracic pressure against an obstructed trachea
  - Possible neurogenic component behind the development of pulmonary edema
  - Treatment is supportive and can require intensive care unit (ICU) management.
- A significant number of hanging/near-hanging victims develop subarachnoid hemorrhage. Although the exact mechanism is not firmly established, vertebral artery injury/rupture might contribute to it.
- Cerebral infarction
  - Anoxic brain injury can lead to significant cerebral edema and persistent neurologic deficits.
  - Carotid dissection is a common traumatic complication that may lead to subsequent thrombus formation and embolic stroke.
- Patients may develop seizures as a sequelae of neurologic insults. Neurosurgery consultation may be warranted to provide recommendations on antiepileptics.

Prognosis

- Patients can have significant neurologic side effects from an event/injury, but the specific prognosis is variable and dependent on environmental factors/nature of the injury.
- Survival rates are highly variable, with studies citing ranges between 23% and 80%. This is perhaps reflective of different populations and methodologies.
- Poor prognostic factors include prolonged hanging time, with one Japanese study citing an average difference of 11.8 minutes between survivors and nonsurvivors (Matsuyama et al 2004).
- Other poor prognostic factors include:
  - Presence of cardiopulmonary arrest
  - Low GCS

Social/Environmental Considerations

- Careful assessment for continued suicidality to assess if the patient has additional psychiatric care needs
- Given the prevalence of strangulation in domestic disputes, it is prudent to ensure discharge to a safe environment. Nonfatal strangulation is one of the strongest predictors of future violence and homicide. Because of this, these cases are often looked at as attempted homicide.
- Forensic involvement may be necessary, especially in cases where law enforcement is involved.
- The American College of Emergency Physicians (ACEP) currently recommends that all emergency physicians and emergency departments assess all victims of intimate partner and sexual violence, child and older maltreatment, and neglect for strangulation injuries.
- Law enforcement has utilized forceful vascular restraint as an attempt to gain compliance without the use of deadly weapons. The aim of this type of restraint is to compress the venous system only. Fatal outcomes happened due to more significant pressure using the officer's knee.
- Neck compression is seen in competitive sports, such as martial arts and sport fighting. Terms such as "chokehold" are often used, but vascular compression is the correct nomenclature.
- Neck compression occurs in erotic sexual practices. It is important for clinicians to attempt to differentiate these behaviors from intimate partner violence.

Prevention

- Pediatric hanging: rare but can occur with items in the household, such as window blind cords. Appropriate safeguarding of the home and supervision are important.
- Pediatric strangulation
  - Majority of events are accidental and related to car windows, electrical cords, entrapment between large items of furniture, clothing/jewelry items with drawstrings or circumferential neck wraps (scarves/necklaces), and outdoor toys involving rope swings. Awareness and supervision are important.
  - Nonaccidental trauma and physical abuse are also important to consider. Pediatricians and emergency medicine providers should maintain a high index of suspicion for this in individuals presenting with trauma or evidence of maltreatment
- Adult hanging/strangulation
  - Specific precautions for inpatient psychiatric settings: remove or limit lanyards, circumferential garments, bedding, and doors that can serve as anchor points, and social work services to connect individuals with appropriate resources
  - Outpatient: suicide hotline, law enforcement intervention, recognition of at-risk behaviors by emergency medicine, primary care providers, and psychiatric providers; access to appropriate mental health services
  - Workplace safety practices to limit accidental hanging and strangulation trauma

Conclusion

- Hanging is the second most common method of suicide in the United States.
- Strangulation is a common form of intimate partner violence.
- Hanging can be further differentiated by the drop distance.
  - Long-drop hanging is considered a drop distance of at least the height of the individual.
  - Cervical spine injury, such as Hangman fracture and spinal cord transection, can occur in both long-drop and short-drop hanging, though more common in the former.
  - Near-hanging occurs when the full suspension of body weight body weight suspension by the neck is not achieved.
- Strangulation can occur by ligature, manually with hands, or through direct unidirectional compression of the neck (postural hanging).
- Patients who experience hanging or strangulation should be evaluated for cervical spine, neurologic, vascular, respiratory, and skin/soft tissue injury.
  - Depending on the clinical scenario, evaluation may include CT imaging with consideration for angiographic evaluation of vessels in the head and neck, MRI to further assess for spinal cord/ligamentous injury, and radiographic imaging to assess for pulmonary edema and tracheal injury.
- Initial management includes urgently addressing airway concerns, protecting the cervical spine, and evaluating for acute injuries. Ongoing evaluation for ARDS and subarachnoid hemorrhage should be performed in appropriate clinical scenarios.
- Preventing accidental and nonaccidental incidents of hanging and strangulation is critical. Implementing appropriate workplace, hospital, and home safeguards may prevent occurrences. Health care workers should evaluate for other risk factors associated with these mechanisms of injury, including psychiatric care needs.

SUGGESTED READINGS

Dunn RJ, Sukhija K, Lopez RA. Strangulation Injuries. *In: StatPearls*. StatPearls Publishing; 2023.

Ghodake D, Mohite S, Desai H. Histopathological study of carotid arteries in deaths due to hanging. *Medico-Legal Update*. 2014;14(1):123-126.

Gunnell D, Bennewith O, Hawton K, Simkin S, Kapur N. 2005. The epidemiology and prevention of suicide by hanging: a systematic review. *Int J Epidemiol*. 34(2):433-442.

Iserson KV. Strangulation: a review of ligature, manual, and postural neck compression injuries. *Ann Emerg Med*. 1984;13(3):179-185.

Le Blanc-Louvry I, Papin F, Vaz E, Proust B. Cervical arterial injury after strangulation—different types of arterial lesions. *J Forensic Sci*. 2013; 58(6):1640-1643.

Matsuyama T, Okuchi K, Seki T, Murao Y. Prognostic factors in hanging injuries. *Am J Emerg Med*. 2004;22(3):207-210.

Mills PD, King LA, Watts BV, Hemphill RR. Inpatient suicide on mental health units in Veterans Affairs (VA) hospitals: avoiding environmental hazards. *Gen Hosp Psychiatry*. 2013;35(5):528-536.

Nikolić S, Živković V. Cervical spine injuries in suicidal hanging without a long-drop—patterns and possible underlying mechanisms of injury: an autopsy study. *Forensic Sci Med Pathol*. 2014;10(2):193-197.

Patch M, Farag YMK, Anderson JC, Perrin N, Kelen G, Campbell J. United States ED visits by adult women for nonfatal intimate partner strangulation, 2006 to 2014: prevalence and associated characteristics. *J Emerg Nurs*. 2021;47(3):437-448.

Penney DJ, Stewart AHL, Parr MJA. Prognostic outcome indicators following hanging injuries. *Resuscitation*. 2002;54(1):27-29.

Rayes M, Mittal M, Rengachary SS, Mittal S. Hangman's fracture: a historical and biomechanical perspective. *J Neurosurg Spine*. 2011;14(2):198-208.

Saternus KS. Injury of the vertebral artery in suicidal hanging. *Forensic Sci Int*. 1984;25(4):265-275.

Sorenson SB, Joshi M, Sivitz E. A systematic review of the epidemiology of nonfatal strangulation, a human rights and health concern. *Am J Public Health*. 2014;104(11):e54-e61.

Stellpflug SJ, Weber W, Dietrich A, et al. Approach considerations for the management of strangulation in the emergency department. *JACEP Open*. 2022;3:e12711.

Todd NV. Priapism in acute spinal cord injury. *Spinal Cord*. 2011;49(9): 1033-1035.

Wallace SK, Cohen WA, Stern EJ, Reay DT. Judicial hanging: postmortem radiographic, CT, and MR imaging features with autopsy confirmation. *Radiology*. 1994;193(1):263-267.

24.5

Altitude Injury

Timothy G. Gaulton

Altitude injury is an acute condition that results from exposure to low oxygen levels at high altitudes.

Key Points

- The ascent to high altitude decreases barometric pressure and lowers the inspired partial pressure of atmospheric oxygen.
- The rapidity of ascent, altitude, and degree of physical exertion are key determinants of injury development and severity.
- Symptoms are often mild (eg, headache and fatigue) yet can be life-threatening and progress to respiratory distress and coma.
- Acclimatization is an adaptive, multisystem physiologic process that improves tolerance to high altitudes and can take days to weeks.
- Controlling the rate of ascent is the primary preventive measure for altitude injury.
- Preventive pharmacotherapies include acetazolamide and dexamethasone.

Epidemiology

- The incidence of altitude injury increases at >2,400 m (8,000 ft) of elevation.
- The incidence varies based on prior acclimatization and individual physiologic and genetic factors that impact oxygen-carrying capacity, alveolar ventilation, and the ventilatory and pulmonary artery responses to hypoxemia.
- Notable patient risk factors include a history of acute altitude illness, obesity, migraines, and younger age.

Key Pathophysiology

- The fractional concentration of oxygen, saturated vapor pressure of water, and barometric pressure determine the partial pressure of oxygen.
- Even at the highest terrestrial elevations, the fractional concentration of oxygen and vapor pressure remain constant.
- At the summit of Mount Everest, the average partial pressure of arterial oxygen in acclimatized climbers breathing ambient air is 24.6 mm Hg.
- Hypobaric hypoxemia triggers hemodynamic and neurohormonal responses that alter tissue perfusion and capillary integrity.
- Hypoxemia constricts the pulmonary vasculature, elevating pulmonary artery pressure and promoting the development of noncardiogenic protein-rich alveolar edema via capillary stress fracture.
- Hypoxemia dilates the cerebral vasculature, increasing cerebral volume and blood-brain barrier permeability.

Clinical Features

- Mild forms of disease—acute mountain sickness (AMS)
  - Symptoms include headache, fatigue, lightheadedness, nausea and vomiting, and disturbed sleep, which can occur within 6 to 12 hours, depending on the ascent rate.
  - Oxygen saturation via pulse oximeter does not correlate with AMS development.
- Severe forms of disease
  - High altitude cerebral edema (HACE)
    - Potential continuum with AMS
    - Progressive decline in neurologic function (irritability, confusion, impaired cognition) that can lead to coma
    - Initial symptoms are often mistaken for physical exhaustion.
    - Neuroimaging often reveals cerebral edema and microhemorrhage.
  - High altitude pulmonary edema (HAPE)
    - Dyspnea at rest, tachypnea, coughing, hemoptysis
    - Inspiratory crackles on auscultation
    - Lower oxygen saturation compared to the expected value at a given altitude

Treatment

- Mild symptoms
  - Symptomatic treatment (eg, analgesics, antiemetics)
  - Halting ascent
  - Limiting physical activity
  - Acetazolamide (oral): adults—250 mg every 12 hours; pediatrics—2.5 mg/kg every 12 hours (maximum: 250 mg per dose)
- Severe cases
  - Supplemental oxygen is a first-line treatment.
  - Descent is indicated at higher altitudes, if oxygen is unavailable, or with persistent severe symptoms.
  - Other treatment considerations include:
    - HAPE
      - Noninvasive positive airway pressure to improve gas exchange
      - Pharmacologic therapies to reduce pulmonary artery pressure (calcium channel blockers, phosphodiesterase-5 inhibitors) have limited established efficacy.
    - HACE
      - Dexamethasone (oral, intramuscular [IM], intravenous [IV]): adults—8 mg once then 4 mg every 6 hours; pediatrics—0.15 mg/kg every 6 hours (maximum: 4 mg per dose)
      - Hyperbaric therapy via a portable, manually inflated hyperbaric chamber may be lifesaving in the absence of supplemental oxygen.

Prevention

- Nonpharmacologic measures
  - Gradual ascent depending on the individual risk of developing acute altitude injury
- Pharmacologic measures
  - Acetazolamide (oral): adults—125 mg every 12 hours; pediatrics—1.25 mg/kg
    - Accelerates acclimatization to high altitude

- Dexamethasone (oral, IM, IV): adults—4 mg every 12 hours; pediatrics—not recommended for prophylaxis
  - Can be administered in cases where acetazolamide is contraindicated due to allergy.
  - Does not accelerate acclimatization to high altitude

SUGGESTED READINGS

Grocott MP, Martin DS, Levett DZ, McMorrow R, Windsor J, Montgomery HE; Caudwell Xtreme Everest Research Group. Arterial blood gases and oxygen content in climbers on Mount Everest. *N Engl J Med*. 2009; 360(2):140-149.

Hackett PH, Roach RC. High-altitude illness. *N Engl J Med*. 2001; 345(2):107-114.

Larson EB, Roach RC, Schoene RB, Hornbein TF. Acute mountain sickness and acetazolamide: clinical efficacy and effect on ventilation. *JAMA*. 1982;248(3):328-332.

Luks AM. Physiology in medicine: a physiologic approach to prevention and treatment of acute high-altitude illnesses. *J Appl Physiol (1985)*. 2015;118(5):509-519.

Luks AM, Beidleman BA, Freer L, et al. Wilderness Medical Society clinical practice guidelines for the prevention, diagnosis, and treatment of acute altitude illness: 2024 update. *Wilderness Environ Med*. 2024; 35(1_suppl):2S-19S.

Richalet JP, Larmignat P, Poitrine E, Letournel M, Canouï-Poitrine F. Physiological risk factors for severe high-altitude illness: a prospective cohort study. *Am J Respir Crit Care Med*. 2012;185(2):192-198.

Rock PB, Johnson TS, Larsen RF, Fulco CS, Trad LA, Cymerman A. Dexamethasone as prophylaxis for acute mountain sickness: effect of dose level. *Chest*. 1989;95(3):568-573.

Swenson ER, Maggiorini M, Mongovin S, et al. Pathogenesis of high-altitude pulmonary edema: inflammation is not an etiologic factor [published correction appears in *JAMA*. 2002;288(9):1064]. *JAMA*. 2002;287(17):2228-2235.

Wilkins MR, Ghofrani HA, Weissmann N, Aldashev A, Zhao L. Pathophysiology and treatment of high-altitude pulmonary vascular disease. *Circulation*. 2015;131(6):582-590.

SECTION 25

Intensive Care Unit Prophylaxis

Section Editor: Raghu R. Chivukula

25.1

Prophylaxes and Harm Reduction in the Intensive Care Unit

Emmett A. Kistler and Christopher M. Worsham

Overview

- Definitions
  - Medical error: failure of intent and/or execution that exposes a patient to possible harm
  - Adverse event: medical management that results in harm. Adverse events can be either preventable or unpreventable.
  - Harm: unintended injury that requires additional monitoring, treatment, hospitalization, or results in death. Harm can manifest in many ways, including physical, emotional, and financial injury.
- Adverse events in the intensive care unit (ICU)
  - Adverse events are common, affecting 10% to 20% of critically ill patients.
  - About half of adverse events are avoidable.
  - Adverse events have significant ramifications, including increased length of ICU stay, prolonged disability, and worsened mortality.
  - Adverse events also contribute to increased costs for payers and providers. The Centers for Medicare & Medicaid Services (CMS) does not reimburse for preventable events, such as catheter-associated urinary tract infections (CAUTIs).
- Rationale for prophylaxis in the ICU
  - Implementing efforts to reduce adverse events and harm supports higher quality of care and better patient outcomes.
  - Monitoring, reporting, and reducing certain preventable conditions are also required by regulatory bodies such as CMS.
  - Prophylaxes reduce the risk of adverse events, but rarely do they completely eliminate these risks, many of which are secondary to the underlying critical illness.
  - Evidence-based practices and guidelines inform prophylaxis and harm reduction strategies for venous thromboembolism, gastrointestinal (GI) bleeding, nosocomial infections, delirium, and post-intensive care syndrome (PICS).

Venous Thromboembolism

- Background
  - Venous thromboembolic events (VTEs) consist of deep vein thromboses and pulmonary emboli.
  - VTEs are common phenomena among critically ill patients.
  - Hospital-acquired VTEs are associated with worsened outcomes, including increased ICU length of stay and duration of mechanical ventilation.
  - The risk of VTE can be reduced with prophylaxis.
  - However, even with appropriate pharmacologic prophylaxis, VTE can still occur in up to one-fifth of critically ill patients.
  - There are different strategies for VTE prophylaxis, and even prophylactically dosed anticoagulation can have adverse effects.
  - Not all patients require VTE prophylaxis.
- Risk assessment
  - The decision to provide thromboprophylaxis hinges upon a patient's risk of VTE and risk of bleeding, both of which may change over the course of an ICU admission.
  - Risk factors for VTE include patient attributes (age, immobilization), chronic comorbidities (malignancy, prior VTE), acute conditions (infection, myocardial infarction), and features of the hospitalization (length of stay, surgical admission).
  - Evidence-based models guide prophylactic management strategy according to the number of risk factors present.

- Frequently utilized models include the Geneva score, the Padua score, and the International Medical Prevention Registry on Venous Thromboembolism (IMPROVE).
- A 2024 head-to-head comparison found that the Geneva score was the most sensitive, while IMPROVE was the most specific. However, the overall prognostic performance of all of the risk assessment models was suboptimal, indicating the need for more accurate models.

- Prophylaxis strategies
  - Pharmacologic
    - Low-molecular-weight heparins (LMWHs, eg, dalteparin, enoxaparin)
      - LMWH activates antithrombin III, which then binds to factor Xa and prevents activation of the final step of the common pathway.
      - LMWHs are given as subcutaneous injections. Frequency of dosing depends on which agent is used.
      - LMWHs are supported by systematic reviews and society guidelines as the pharmacologic thromboprophylaxis of choice.
      - Compared to unfractionated heparin (UFH), LMWHs offer superior VTE risk reduction without an associated increased risk of bleeding.
      - Severe renal insufficiency necessitates LMWH dose reduction or rotation to UFH.
    - UFH
      - UFH activates antithrombin III, preventing fibrin formation and inhibiting thrombin-induced activation of coagulation factors V and VIII.
      - UFH is also administered subcutaneously.
      - UFH is dosed 2 or 3 times daily. Thrice-daily dosing is associated with decreased risk of VTE but with increased risk of bleeding.
      - UFH dosing frequency should be determined based on the patient's individual risk of VTE and bleed. An elevated body mass index also favors administering UFH 3 times per day.
    - Other agents
      - There is insufficient evidence to support the use of direct-acting oral anticoagulants or vitamin K antagonists for VTE prophylaxis in hospitalized patients.
      - Therapeutically dosed pharmacologic anticoagulation for acute or chronic indications supplants the need for prophylactic anticoagulation.
    - Leeway periods
      - While patients recovering from surgical procedures such as orthopedic and trauma interventions are at higher risk for VTE, prophylactic anticoagulation should not be immediately initiated to limit perioperative bleeding and other sequelae.
      - These leeway times differ according to the surgery.
        - Most general surgical and orthopedic procedures: 24 hours
        - Transplant or trauma: 48 hours
        - Spinal surgery: 5 days
      - Best practice is to consult with the primary surgical team prior to initiating prophylactic anticoagulation directly after an operation.
    - Thromboprophylaxis monitoring
      - There is no consensus regarding the routine use of anti-factor Xa levels or partial thromboplastin time (PTT) testing to confirm appropriate levels of prophylactic anticoagulation.
      - Anti-Xa levels and PTT levels may offer value in patients with intensely hypercoagulable states, patients who develop VTE despite presumably prophylaxis, and patients who develop significant bleeding on prophylactically dosed LMWH or UFH.
  - Mechanical
    - Mechanical thromboprophylaxis entails external pressure applied to a patient's lower extremities to reduce blood stasis and formation of clot.
    - Examples include intermittent or sequential pneumatic compression devices and compression stockings.
    - Mechanical thromboprophylaxis likely reduces the risk of deep venous thrombosis (DVT) compared to no VTE prophylaxis.
    - Current evidence—which is limited—suggests that combining mechanical and pharmacologic prophylaxis does not offer an additive benefit.
    - Combined mechanical and pharmacologic prophylaxes are not endorsed by most guidelines, except in patients at high risk of VTE (eg, following orthopedic surgery, spinal cord injury).
    - In addition to these high-risk patients, the main indications for mechanical VTE prophylaxis are in patients with contraindications to chemical prophylaxis.
    - Mechanical thromboprophylaxis may contribute to skin breakdown, discomfort, and delirium, although the literature is mixed as to the significance of these concerns.
- Contraindications to VTE prophylaxis
  - Absolute contraindications
    - Major active bleed or recent bleed including, but not limited to:
      - Active GI bleed
      - Active postoperative bleed
      - Recent trauma
      - Intraocular surgery within the last 2 weeks
      - Intracranial hemorrhage within the last year
    - Increased risk of bleeding
      - Thrombocytopenia (platelet count $<50,000/m^3$)
      - Recent or upcoming epidural
    - Heparin-induced thrombocytopenia
    - Already receiving therapeutic anticoagulation
  - Relative contraindications
    - Coagulopathy
    - Severe liver failure with coagulopathy (eg, international normalized ratio [INR] >1.5)
    - Severe renal impairment
    - Hypertensive urgency/emergency
  - If there is clinical equipoise as to whether a clinical circumstance comprises a contraindication to prophylactic anticoagulation, consider discussing with the relevant consultant.

Stress Ulcer and Gastrointestinal Bleeding

- Background
  - Critical illness can provoke stress ulcers in the upper GI tract, which can, in turn, precipitate clinically significant bleeding.
  - Clinically significant bleeding is defined as bleeding associated with hemodynamic changes, a prominent drop in hemoglobin level, transfusion of at least two units of blood, evidence of bleeding on endoscopy, or need for surgery.
  - About 4% of critically ill patients develop clinically significant GI bleeds.
  - Not all ICU patients require prophylaxis against stress ulcers and GI bleeding. GI bleeding prophylaxis is likely overutilized.
  - Gastric acid–suppressing medications are generally well tolerated but may have some adverse effects, including increased risk of infections such as pneumonia as well as altered metabolism of other medications.
  - Patients receiving gastric acid–suppressing medications for alternative reasons, such as gastroesophageal reflux disease, should usually continue to receive these medications while critically ill, even if they do not otherwise meet criteria for stress ulcer and GI bleeding prophylaxis.
- Risks stratification for prophylaxis
  - Current guidelines divide ICU patients into tiers based on risk factors for GI bleeds synthesized by systematic reviews.
    - Stress ulcer and GI bleeding prophylaxis are recommended for patients at high and highest risk of GI bleeding (≥4% risk of bleeding).
    - Patients at moderate risk of GI bleeding (2%-4%) may be considered for prophylaxis on a case-by-case basis; the default recommendation is that routine prophylaxis is not needed.
    - Patients at low risk for GI bleeding should not routinely receive prophylaxis.
    - If an ICU patient receiving GI prophylaxis transitions to a lower risk tier, GI prophylaxis should usually be discontinued.
- Tiers and associated risk factors
  - Highest risk of GI bleed (incidence of 8%-10%)
    - Mechanical ventilation without enteral nutrition
    - Chronic liver disease
  - High risk of GI bleed (4%-8%)
    - Coagulopathy (INR >1.7 while not on anticoagulation, platelets <80,000 per microliter)
    - ≥2 factors from moderate-risk category
  - Moderate risk of GI bleed (2%-4%)
    - Mechanical ventilation with enteral nutrition
    - Acute kidney injury
    - Sepsis
    - Shock
  - Low risk of GI bleed (1%-2%)
    - Acute liver failure
    - Use of steroids, immunosuppression, or anticoagulation
    - Active malignancy
    - Male gender
    - Critically ill patients with no other risk factors
- Gastric acid suppressants
  - Gastric acid suppressants such as proton pump inhibitors (PPIs) and histamine-2 receptor antagonists (H2RAs) can reduce the risk of GI bleeding by up to 3% to 5%. The degree of risk reduction depends upon the baseline risk of GI bleeding.
  - PPIs
    - PPIs are the most utilized GI prophylaxis and are considered the agent of choice compared to H2RAs, although comparative data regarding efficacy and adverse effects are not robust.
    - PPIs are dosed once daily for GI prophylaxis.
    - Intravenous (IV) and enteral formulations are considered equally effective. The availability of enteral access, perceived effectiveness of gut absorption, and cost considerations (IV is usually more expensive) may influence the choice of one route over the other. The default choice should be the enteral formulation.
  - H2RAs
    - H2RAs are less commonly utilized; they may be favored in patients receiving other medications whose metabolism is impacted by PPIs.
    - H2RAs are dosed 2 to 3 times per day.
    - As with PPIs, IV and enteral formulations are considered equally effective.
  - Sucralfate
    - Sucralfate is not recommended as a GI prophylaxis.
    - Available evidence suggests that sucralfate is inferior to H2RA and PPIs.
    - Sucralfate can only be administered orally and is given 4 times per day.

Nosocomial Infections

- Background
  - Nosocomial infections, including device-related infections, occur disproportionately among ICU patients relative to other hospitalized patients and contribute to worsened outcomes including mortality.
  - While ICU patients carry inherently higher nonmodifiable risk for infection due to their acute illness, steps can be taken to reduce the modifiable risk of certain infections.
  - In 2022, the Centers for Disease Control and Prevention (CDC) estimated ~50,000 nosocomial infections occurred in ICUs across the United States.
  - Rates have generally been falling nationally thanks to increased adoption of preventive care.
- Catheter Associated Urinary Tract Infections (CAUTIs)
  - Background
    - CAUTI is a common nosocomial infection, as urinary catheters allow bacteria to enter the urinary tract, which can lead to urinary tract infections (UTIs).
    - Diagnosis is established by the presence of bacteriuria as well as signs and symptoms of a UTI in a patient with an indwelling urinary catheter.

- If CAUTI is suspected, urine culture should ideally be collected as a mid-stream sample after removal of prior catheter, or alternatively after a new catheter has been placed if a patient is unable to pass urine. Samples should be taken from the catheter port and not the drainage bag.
- Appropriate use of an indwelling urinary catheter includes:
  - Acute urinary retention or bladder outlet obstruction
  - Need for accurate hourly measurements of urinary output in critically ill patients
  - Perioperative use for certain surgeries
  - To assist in healing of open sacral or perineal wounds
  - Prolonged immobilization (eg, unstable spine)
  - Comfort at end-of-life care
- Incontinence alone is *not* an indication for an indwelling urinary catheter.

Risk assessment

- Any patient with an indwelling urinary catheter is at risk for CAUTI.
- The longer a urinary catheter is in place, the higher the risk of CAUTI.
- Other risk factors such as female sex, increased age, and diabetes have been identified.

Prophylactic strategies

- Daily assessment of whether a urinary catheter is no longer necessary and can be removed.
- Ensure that equipment necessary for appropriate use and sterile placement of indwelling catheters, including bladder scanners, are available and used.
- Nonindwelling urinary systems including urinals, straight catheters, and external urinary catheters should also be readily available and used as an alternative to indwelling catheters.
- Placement, maintenance, and removal practices to minimize infectious risk should be protocolized and performed by health care workers trained in this specific procedure.
- Urine-culturing practices for patients with or without indwelling catheters should be protocolized in coordination with hospital infection control and microbiology labs.

Catheter-related bloodstream infections (CRBSIs)

Background

- Any indwelling vascular catheter used in routine hospital care—central venous catheters (CVCs) in addition to peripheral venous catheters (PIVs), peripheral arterial catheters, peripherally inserted central venous catheters (PICCs), and midline catheters—provides a pathway for bacteria into the bloodstream.

Risk assessment

- CVCs are generally at the highest risk of bloodstream infection.
- Risk factors for CVC-associated bloodstream infections include:
  - Prolonged hospitalization prior to placement
  - Prolonged duration of catheterization
  - Multiple-lumen catheters
  - Multiple catheters
  - Neutropenia
  - Body mass index >40
  - Parenteral nutrition
  - Reduced nurse-to-patient ratio in the ICU
  - Poor catheter care
  - Heavy microbial colonization at the insertion site

Strategies to prevent infections from peripheral and midline catheters

- Upper extremity site is ideal.
- Use a midline catheter or PICC when the duration of IV therapy is expected to last >6 days.
- Prompt removal upon recognition of signs of phlebitis, infection, or malfunction

Strategies to prevent infections from CVCs

- Daily chlorhexidine baths can reduce risk in the ICU.
- Prior to and during insertion:
  - Ensure that CVC is necessary for care versus other vascular catheters with lower infection risk.
  - Use a structured process (eg, checklist) to ensure adherence to all infection control practices for sterile placement.
  - Use an all-inclusive catheter cart or kit to ensure quick and easy access to all necessary sterile supplies.
  - Site preference for nontunneled CVC is subclavian > jugular > femoral; site selection may be individualized based on patient and operator factors.
  - Use ultrasound guidance.
  - Use maximal sterile barrier precautions.
  - Use chlorhexidine for skin preparation.
- After insertion
  - Use chlorhexidine-containing dressings; change dressing if soiled, loose, or damp, or every week until removed.
  - Disinfect prior to accessing catheter.
  - Replace infusion sets (medications, tubing, and other connected parts) at regular intervals up to 7 days.
  - Ensure proper nurse:patient ratios.
  - ICU-based nurses reduce risk of infection compared float nurses.
  - Do *not* routinely replace catheters unless they were placed under nonsterile conditions, in which case they should be replaced within 48 hours.

Ventilator-associated pneumonia (VAP), ventilator-associated events (VAEs), and nonventilator hospital-acquired pneumonia (NV-HAP)

Background

- Lower respiratory infection is common in ICU patients for both ventilated and nonventilated patients.
- Despite their prevalence, obtaining a definitive diagnosis of ventilator-related infections can be difficult.
- The CDC National Healthcare Safety Network implemented a VAE surveillance system to standardize identification.
  - Ventilator-associated conditions (VACs) entail sustained worsening of respiratory status (increase in positive end-expiratory pressure ≥3 cm H_2O or increase in fraction of inspired oxygen by ≥0.2 for 2 days).
  - Infection-related ventilator-associated complications (IVACs) consist of VAC with abnormal temperature (<36 °C or >38 °C) and/or white blood cell counts (≤4,000 or ≥12,000 cells/mm^3).

            - Possible and probable VAPs are characterized by a sustained worsening of respiratory status requiring increased ventilatory support, presence of abnormal temperature or white blood cell count, and microbiology data confirming a pathologic organism.
        - The diagnostic and management implications of the abovementioned definition are not yet defined, but the surveillance system facilitates widespread, uniform collection, and analysis of data pertaining to VAEs.
        - Guideline-based prevention interventions outline steps taken to reduce outcomes like duration of mechanical ventilation, ICU or hospital length of stay, mortality, VAEs, antibiotic use, or costs.
    - Risk assessment
        - Patients receiving ventilatory support are at increased risk of pneumonia and VAE.
        - Patients with underlying lung disease and dysphagia are at even higher risk of adverse outcomes.
    - Prophylactic strategies for mechanically ventilated patients
        - Use a protocol to minimize sedation.
        - Sedation strategies should focus on using multiple drugs like propofol, dexmedetomidine, analgesics, and antipsychotics for the management of agitation and dyspnea rather than benzodiazepines.
        - Perform daily spontaneous breathing trials (SBTs) to assess whether the patient is ready to extubate.
        - Brush teeth daily but *without* chlorhexidine.
        - Elevate head of bed to 30 to 45 degrees.
        - Steps to take as early as reasonable
            - Exercise and mobilize.
            - Provide enteral, rather than IV, feeding.
        - Only change ventilator circuit if it is soiled or malfunctioning.
    - Prophylactic strategies for patients who are not mechanically ventilated
        - Avoid intubation (and reintubation) using high-flow nasal oxygen or noninvasive positive pressure if appropriate.
        - Monitor for and treat dysphagia.
        - Take steps to avoid nosocomial transmission of viral illnesses from other patients, family members, or clinicians.
        - Daily oral care.
- *Clostridioides difficile* infection (CDI)
    - Background
        - CDI is common in hospitalized patients and a significant source of morbidity and mortality.
        - Infection can arise after disruption to the normal fecal bacterial flora, most often from antibiotics, in a patient who is colonized or exposed to bacterial spores, such as from the hands of health care workers.
        - A nosocomial CDI is defined as CDI symptom onset on or after hospital day 4 with a positive nucleic acid amplification test or toxin test.
    - Risk assessment
        - Receipt of antibiotics is the primary risk factor due to the disruption they can cause to the normal fecal flora.
        - Other risk factors include advanced age, prolonged hospitalization, GI surgery, enteral feeding tubes, chemotherapy, inflammatory bowel disease, and solid organ transplant.
        - Use of PPIs may be a risk factor for CDI.
    - Prophylactic strategies
        - Outside of reducing exposure to antibiotics, evidence quality for other prophylactic measures against CDI is low.
        - Antibiotic stewardship programs can reduce exposure to antibiotics that place patients at risk for CDI.
        - Isolate and initiate contact precautions for patients with suspected CDI until ruled out.
        - Diagnostic stewardship programs and inpatient CDI protocols can help ensure patients are appropriately tested, results of diagnostic tests are appropriately interpreted, and results of positive tests acted upon in a timely manner.
            - Nucleic acid amplification tests are very sensitive tests for the presence of *C. difficile*, but they cannot determine the difference between colonization and infection.
            - Toxin tests are less sensitive but have higher predictive ability for detecting active infection.
            - Depending on available tests, multi-step testing algorithms can help improve diagnostic accuracy.
            - Diagnostic stewardship entails:
                - Deferring testing patients without diarrhea unless they have other signs of CDI (eg, ileus or toxic megacolon)
                - Holding laxatives to see if they are the cause of diarrhea before testing.
                - Deciding not to test for cure of CDI, only monitor symptoms.
        - Clean the environment and any contaminated equipment with appropriate cleansers.

Delirium

- Background
    - Delirium is an acute confusional state characterized by disturbances in attention, awareness, cognition, and orientation that can present in either hypoactive or hyperactive states.
    - Delirium is very common in the ICU, with incidence rates estimated from 20% to 84% depending on the severity of critical illness.
    - Delirium is associated with adverse outcomes during the acute hospitalization, mortality, as well as long-term adverse outcomes, such as cognitive dysfunction that is considered part of the PICS.
- Risk assessment
    - Any patient with acute critical illness is at increased risk for delirium, but the risk is higher in patients with more severe and longer duration of critical illness.
    - Other risk factors include older age, frailty, predisposing medications, and complex surgery.
- Prophylactic strategies
    - There are no strategies that have been definitively shown to reliably prevent delirium in the ICU, including prophylactic antipsychotic administration.
        - Antipsychotics can play a role in managing agitated delirium.
    - Avoid known precipitating factors such as medications (eg, benzodiazepines), uncontrolled pain, and unnecessarily prolonged duration of sedation or mechanical ventilation.

- Studies of low-risk, low-cost nonpharmacological interventions are lacking to be able to evaluate their effectiveness for ICU delirium. Many of these interventions simply represent human-centric care, and studies suggest benefits in the general hospital population. These may also benefit ICU patients in the short and long term.
  - Early mobilization
  - For awake patients, frequent reorientation, hearing and vision adaptations, adequate nutrition and hydration, and optimal sleep.
  - Extended family visitation at the bedside.
  - Daily interruption of sedation ("sedation vacations") has not been shown to reduce delirium but is important for daily evaluation of readiness to extubate.
- The "ABCDEF Bundle," a tool to help clinicians consider many aspects of high-quality ICU care, may be helpful in reducing ICU delirium by employing the abovementioned interventions and improving holistic care of the ICU patient:
  - Assess, prevent, and manage pain
  - Both spontaneous awakening trials (SAT) and SBTs daily
  - Choice of sedation and analgesia individualized
  - Delirium assessment, prevention, and management
  - Early mobility and exercise
  - Family engagement and empowerment at the bedside

Post-Intensive Care Syndrome

- Background
  - PICS is defined as new or worsening impairments in physical, cognitive, or mental health status after critical illness persisting beyond the acute care hospitalization. Adverse outcomes include:
    - Mental health conditions can include anxiety, posttraumatic stress disorder (PTSD), and depression.
      - PICS-F is the designation for mental health aspects of PICS affecting family members of critically ill patients who are at risk for the abovementioned mental health conditions as well as complicated grief.
    - Cognitive impairment conditions can include deficits in executive function, memory, attention, visuospatial processing, and mental processing speed.
    - Physical impairments related to pulmonary function, specific neuromuscular problems, or general functional capacity.
    - New research has shed additional light on other symptoms experienced by patients following critical illness, including chronic fatigue, chronic pain, and unemployment.
- Risk assessment
  - Any patient with acute critical illness is at risk for PICS.
  - Risk is higher in patients with critical illness that is more severe, requires more interventions, and of longer duration.
  - Preexisting physical impairments, lung disease, cognitive impairments, or psychiatric conditions also place patients at higher risk of PICS.
- Prophylactic strategies
  - Prevention of PICS and its component symptoms is a relatively new area of research, and as such, evidence for PICS prophylaxis among ICU patients is limited.
  - Interventions aimed at reducing the duration and severity of critical illness, avoiding complications, and promoting patient-centered care that have a variety of other known benefits may help reduce PICS.
  - The ABCDEF Bundle covers a variety of daily interventions that provide a variety of benefits and may reduce the risk of PICS.
  - Maintaining an ICU diary that allows patients to read details of their hospitalization that they cannot remember can reduce the risk of depression and anxiety symptoms of PICS for both patients and family members.
  - Facilitating proactive communication between ICU clinicians and family members, either through individuals or protocols, may reduce psychological distress that can lead to PICS-F for family members of dying patients.

Incorporating Prophylaxes and Risk Reduction Into Intensive Care Unit Routine Care

- Background
  - Measures to reduce the risk of VTE, GI bleeding, delirium, and infectious complications are valuable but may become an afterthought amidst high acuity clinical issues, an overabundance of data, and a multitude of competing tasks in the ICU.
  - Ensuring that the abovementioned strategies are integrated into day-to-day care requires intentional augmentations to workflow, electronic health records, and culture.
  - Prophylaxis and harm reduction strategies should not fall to one member of the ICU team but instead comprise an interdisciplinary responsibility facilitated by system-level interventions.
- Strategies to increase compliance
  - Rounding checklists: at the end of rounds review harm reduction measures for each patient.
  - Templated documentation: at the end of physician ICU note templates in electronic medical record systems, construct a mandatory field that serves as a checklist for VTE, GI bleed, infectious, and other prophylaxes.
  - Daily rounding: the ICU team member formulating the plan for the patient reviews a checklist each day regarding which prophylaxes and measures are present, which are being intentionally held, and what changes should be made.
  - Nursing-driven protocols: establish protocols for key aspects of care (eg, Foley catheter maintenance, VAP bundle implementation), which include step-by-step descriptions and contingencies. Supplement protocols with educational sessions.
  - Order sets: collaborate with pharmacy and other team members to build order sets that prompt users to consider the need for prophylaxes and easily access different options. Incorporate these orders into admission and transfer order sets to increase routine use.

    - Automation: develop algorithms to identify patients at high risk of certain issues (eg, IMPROVE score for VTE risk), which trigger best practice alerts prompting providers to order associated prophylaxes or document why it is being withheld.
- Key example: ICU Liberation Bundle
    - Background
        - The ICU Liberation or ABCDEF Bundle is an evidence-based, society-recommended collection of assessments and interventions intended to be reviewed daily for each ICU patient.
        - The ABCDEF Bundle has been found to improve a multitude of outcomes, including mortality, ICU readmission, delirium, and the use of physical restraints.
        - The ABCDEF Bundle utilizes objective evaluations such as the Critical Care Pain Observation Tool (CPOT), Richmond Agitation and Sedation Scale (RASS), and Confusion Assessment Method for the ICU (CAM-ICU) to inform management decisions.
        - The ABCDEF Bundle relies on input from nurses, physicians, respiratory therapists, pharmacists, the patient, and family members.
    - Contents
        - Assess, prevent, and manage pain
        - Both SATs and SBTs daily
        - Choice of sedation and analgesia individualized
        - Delirium assessment, prevention, and management
        - Early mobility and exercise
        - Family engagement and empowerment at the bedside
    - Implementation
        - Like any major quality and safety intervention, implementation of the ABCDEF Bundle requires a comprehensive approach supported by local and institutional leadership.
        - Understanding the current state of preventive practices (strengths and opportunities for improvement), staff knowledge, and local safety culture is a key first step.
        - This knowledge will inform communication strategies and implementation approaches.
        - Following implementation, routine data gathering and analysis is key to ensuring continued success and identifying subsequent modifications.
        - Toolkits are available online to guide implementation.

Take-Home Points

- ICU patients are at elevated risk for adverse events for a multitude of reasons. Some of these adverse events are preventable. The risk of some preventable adverse events can be modulated but typically not eliminated with specific management strategies.
- An ICU patient's risk of preventable adverse events may change over the course of their admission. Prophylaxis strategies should be adapted accordingly, including cessation of prophylaxis once it is no longer indicated.
- Incorporating interdisciplinary harm reduction strategies into everyday workflows, such as checklists at the end of daily rounds, can help ensure that the optimal prophylactic strategies are in place and that preventive measures such as removing unnecessary invasive lines removal are frequently revisited.

SUGGESTED READINGS

Agency for Healthcare Research and Quality. Chapter 4. Choose the Model to Assess VTE and Bleeding Risk. In: *Preventing Hospital-Associated Venous Thromboembolism: A Guide for Effective Quality Improvement*. Agency for Healthcare Research and Quality; 2016. Updated October 2022. Accessed July 6, 2024. https://www.ahrq.gov/patient-safety/settings/hospital/vtguide/guide4.html

Agency for Healthcare Research and Quality Patient Safety Network. *Patient Safety 101*. AHRQ PSNet; 2019. Accessed June 30, 2023. https://psnet.ahrq.gov/primer/patient-safety-101

Arabi YM, Al-Hameed F, Burns KEA, et al; Saudi Critical Care Trials Group. Adjunctive intermittent pneumatic compression for venous thromboprophylaxis. *N Engl J Med*. 2019; 380:1305-1315.

Barbar S, Noventa F, Rossetto V, et al. A risk assessment model for the identification of hospitalized medical patients at risk for venous thromboembolism: the Padua Prediction Score. *J Thromb Haemost*. 2010; 8(11):2450-2457.

Buetti N, Marschall J, Drees M, et al. Strategies to prevent central line-associated bloodstream infections in acute-care hospitals: 2022 Update. *Infect Control Hosp Epidemiol*. 2022;43(5):553-569.

Centers for Disease Control and Prevention. *Ventilator-Associated Event*. National Healthcare Safety Network; 2024. Accessed July 30, 2024. https://www.cdc.gov/nhsn/pdfs/pscmanual/10-vae_final.pdf

Darzi AJ, Repp AB, Spencer FA, et al. Risk-assessment models for VTE and bleeding in hospitalized medical patients: an overview of systematic reviews. *Blood Adv*. 2020;4(19):4929-4944.

Forster AJ, Kyeremanteng K, Hooper J, Shojania KG, van Walraven C. The impact of adverse events in the intensive care unit on hospital mortality and length of stay. *BMC Health Serv Res*. 2008;8:259

Fridkin SK, Welbel SF, Weinstein RA. Magnitude and prevention of nosocomial infections in the intensive care unit. *Infect Dis Clin North Am*. 1997;11(2):479-496.

Häfliger E, Kopp B, Darbellay Farhoumand P, et al. Risk assessment models for venous thromboembolism in medical inpatients. *JAMA Netw Open*. 2024;7(5):e249980.

Helms J, Middeldorp S, Spyropoulos AC. Thromboprophylaxis in critical care. *Intensive Care Med*. 2023;49:75-78.

Herling SF, Greve IE, Vasilevskis EE, et al. Interventions for preventing intensive care unit delirium in adults. *Cochrane Database Syst Rev*. 2018;11(11):CD009783.

Hirsh J, Anand SS, Halperin JL, Fuster V; American Heart Association. Guide to anticoagulant therapy: Heparin: a statement for healthcare professionals from the American Heart Association. *Circulation*. 2001; 103(24):2994-3018.

Hiser SL, Fatima A, Ali M, Needham DM. Post-intensive care syndrome (PICS): recent updates. *J Intensive Care*. 2023;11(1):23.

Hshieh TT, Yue J, Oh E, et al. Effectiveness of multicomponent nonpharmacological delirium interventions: a meta-analysis. *JAMA Intern Med*. 2015;175(4):512-520.

Institute of Medicine (US) Committee on Quality of Health Care in America. *To Err is Human: Building a Safer Health System*. Kohn LT, Corrigan JM, Donaldson MS, eds. National Academies Press (US); 2000.

Klompas M, Branson R, Cawcutt K, et al. Strategies to prevent ventilator-associated pneumonia, ventilator-associated events, and nonventilator hospital-acquired pneumonia in acute-care hospitals: 2022 update. *Infect Control Hosp Epidemiol*. 2022;43(6):687-713.

Kociolek LK, Gerding DN, Carrico R, et al. Strategies to prevent Clostridioides difficile infections in acute-care hospitals: 2022 update. *Infect Control Hosp Epidemiol*. 2023;44(4):527-549.

Lyman GH, Carrier M, Ay C, et al. American Society of Hematology 2021 guidelines for management of venous thromboembolism: prevention and treatment in patients with cancer. *Blood Adv*. 2021;5:927-974.

Makary MA, Daniel M. Medical error-the third leading cause of death in the US. *BMJ*. 2016;353:i2139.

Marra A, Ely EW, Pandharipande PP, Patel MB. The ABCDEF bundle in critical care. *Crit Care Clin*. 2017;33(2):225-243.

McIlroy PA, King RS, Garrouste-Orgeas M, Tabah A, Ramanan M. The effect of ICU diaries on psychological outcomes and quality of life of survivors of critical illness and their relatives: a systematic review and meta-analysis. *Crit Care Med*. 2019;47(2):273-279.

Molina FJ, Rivera PT, Cardona A, et al. Adverse events in critical care: search and active detection through the Trigger Tool. *World J Crit Care Med*. 2018;7(1):9-15.

Needham DM, Davidson J, Cohen H, et al. Improving long-term outcomes after discharge from intensive care unit: report from a stakeholders' conference. *Crit Care Med*. 2012;40(2):502-509.

O'Grady NP, Alexander M, Burns LA, et al. Guidelines for the prevention of intravascular catheter-related infections. *Clin Infect Dis*. 2011; 52(9):e162-e193.

Ouellette DR, Patel S, Girard TD, et al. Liberation from mechanical ventilation in critically ill adults: an official American College of Chest Physicians/American Thoracic Society clinical practice guideline: inspiratory pressure augmentation during spontaneous breathing trials, protocols minimizing sedation, and noninvasive ventilation immediately after extubation. *Chest*. 2017;151(1):166-180.

Pronovost P, Needham D, Berenholtz S, et al. An intervention to decrease catheter-related bloodstream infections in the ICU. *N Engl J Med*. 2006; 355(26):2725-2732.

Pun BT, Balas MC, Barnes-Daly MA, et al. Caring for critically ill patients with the ABCDEF Bundle: Results of the ICU Liberation Collaborative in Over 15,000 Adults. *Crit Care Med*. 2019;47(1):3-14.

Rhoads SL, Trikalinos TA, Levy MM, Amass T. Intensive care based interventions to reduce family member stress disorders: a systematic review of the literature. *J Crit Care Med (Targu Mures)*. 2022;8(3):145-155.

Rosa RG, Tonietto TF, da Silva DB, et al. Effectiveness and safety of an extended ICU visitation model for delirium prevention: a before and after study. *Crit Care Med*. 2017;45(10):1660-1667.

Rothschild JM, Landrigan CP, Cronin JW, et al. The Critical Care Safety Study: the incidence and nature of adverse events and serious medical errors in intensive care. *Crit Care Med*. 2005;33(8):1694-700.

Society of Critical Care Medicine. *ICU Liberation Bundle (A-F)*. Society of Critical Care Medicine. Accessed July 6, 2024. https://www.sccm.org/iculiberation/abcdef-bundles

Ye Z, Reintam Blaser A, Lytvyn L, et al. Gastrointestinal bleeding prophylaxis for critically ill patients: a clinical practice guideline. *BMJ*. 2020; 368:l6722.

SECTION 26

Procedures

Section Editor: Casey M. Luckhurst

26.1

Tracheostomy

Danny Wang and Nikhil Panda

Overview

- Tracheostomy was originally performed to relieve airway obstruction or provide access to the upper airway when oral endotracheal intubation was impossible.
- Now, tracheostomy is often performed electively to facilitate ventilatory weaning and prevent complications associated with prolonged intubation.
- Tracheostomy can be performed via an open surgical approach or percutaneously; here, we discuss primarily percutaneous tracheostomy, which is more frequently encountered in intensive care settings.

Indications

- Tracheostomy can be performed electively or emergently (see Table 26.1.1).

Contraindications

- Inability to tolerate short periods of apnea safely is the only *absolute contraindication* to percutaneous tracheostomy.
- Tracheostomy should not be attempted in patients requiring FiO_2 >50% or positive end-expiratory pressure (PEEP) >12 mm Hg.

TABLE 26.1.1 Indications for Tracheostomy

Elective
• Prolonged mechanical ventilation, including anticipated prolonged intubation (eg, neurologic injury)
• Impending upper airway obstruction (eg, tumor)
• Secretion management
Emergency
• Inability to intubate:
• Mechanical oral or laryngotracheal obstruction (eg, facial trauma, laryngeal edema)
• Difficult anatomy

- Tracheostomy should be deferred in patients with uncontrolled coagulopathy, cellulitis of the neck, or cervical spine instability.
- Patients with primary tracheal pathology (eg, airway tumors) may benefit from an open rather than percutaneous tracheostomy.
- Prior tracheostomy and/or neck surgery are not contraindications to tracheostomy.

Equipment

- Tracheostomy tubes can be:
  - Plastic (polyvinyl chloride or silicone) or metal (silver or stainless steel)
  - Uncuffed or cuffed
  - Nonfenestrated or fenestrated
- A cuff provides an airway seal, which allows for positive pressure ventilation, and reduces aspiration of secretions.
- Modern cuffs are typically air filled with low pressure and higher volume.
- Higher cuff pressures may cause tissue ischemia, tracheomalacia, and, eventually, tracheal stenosis; cuff pressures generally should not exceed 25 cm H_2O.
- Fenestrated tubes have an additional opening in the posterior portion above the cuff, which, in theory, permit upper airway airflow and facilitate speech. However, these fenestrations are prone to occlusion from secretions.
- Tracheostomy appliance specifications include the outer diameter, inner diameter, and length (angle or curved, standard or extra length, fixed length, or adjustable flange).
- Adjustment in horizontal or vertical length can be helpful in patients with excess soft tissue or longer trachea.
- Tubes can have a single or dual cannula:
  - Dual cannula tubes possess an inner cannula needed to connect to a ventilator.
  - Inner cannulae allow for frequent cleaning to prevent obstruction by secretions.
  - Disadvantages include a smaller internal diameter, which may increase the work of breathing and paradoxically trap secretions.
- Tracheostomy tubes can be changed after there is a mature tract from the skin to the airway, typically at least 7 days after the procedure.
- If a tracheostomy tube becomes dislodged before there is a mature tract, no immediate attempt should be made

to replace the tube, and the patient should first be orotracheally intubated to control the airway if there is ongoing respiratory distress.

Procedure

- Successful performance of bedside percutaneous tracheostomy is related to expertise of the operator and ancillary personnel.
- Requisite team members: operator and assistant, intensive care nurse, bronchoscopist, respiratory therapist
- Requisite equipment
  - Scalpel
  - Hemostat
  - Introducer needle (gauge compatible with guidewire)
  - Syringe
  - J-tip guidewire
  - Lubricating jelly
  - Introducer dilator
  - Guiding catheter
  - Percutaneous tracheostomy dilator
  - Tracheostomy loading dilator (compatible with tracheostomy)
  - Tracheostomy
  - Double swivel connector
  - Tracheostomy tube holder (tracheostomy tie)
  - Bronchoscope
  - Bronchoscopy tower (video monitor, video processor, light source, suction)
- Preprocedural preparation: preoxygenate with FIO_2 at 100%; analgesia with intravenous (IV) short-acting opioid (eg, fentanyl); sedation with IV short-acting agent (eg, propofol); paralysis with IV short-acting agent (eg, rocuronium).
- Positioning: supine with shoulders supported anteriorly to facilitate neck extension.
- Key anatomic landmarks to identify include thyroid cartilage, cricoid cartilage, and sternal notch.
- Tracheostomy procedure steps
  - Huddle with team and time-out.
  - Sterilely prep and drape the anterior neck allowing for ready access to the endotracheal tube.
  - Make a 2 to 3 cm midline, vertical incision below the cricoid cartilage.
  - Using a hemostat, bluntly dissect the pretracheal soft tissue down to the level of the tracheal rings.
  - (Optional) For patients on anticoagulation or predisposed to bleeding, placement, but not tying, of a removable purse-string suture may facilitate hemostasis after the procedure.
  - Advance bronchoscope through the endotracheal tube to survey the airway and align end of camera with the tip of the tube.
  - Deflate the tube cuff and slowly withdraw the endotracheal tube and the bronchoscope until the subglottic landmarks are identified.
  - Insert the introducer needle between the second and third tracheal rings with the bevel pointed downward and needle perpendicular to the trachea.
  - Pass the guidewire through the introducer needle until just beyond the carina.
  - Via Seldinger technique, exchange the introducer needle for the introducer dilator followed by the percutaneous tracheostomy dilator.
  - Pass the tracheostomy loaded with the appropriate size loading dilator and guiding catheter over the guidewire.
  - After the tube is placed, remove the loading dilator, guiding catheter, and guidewire.
  - Inflate the tracheostomy cuff and ventilate through the tracheostomy once proper placement is confirmed.
  - Secure tracheostomy and tie sutures if necessary.
- Direct bronchoscopic visualization during the procedure through the existing endotracheal tube is recommended to ensure proper placement and reduce the risk of inadvertent extubation.
- Initial tracheostomy placement should be confirmed by four methods when possible:
  - Bronchoscopic visualization of the carina through the tracheostomy
  - Bronchoscopic visualization of proper tracheostomy seating from above the tracheostomy
  - End-tidal CO_2
  - Chest wall rise

Complications

- The most severe complication during a tracheostomy procedure is failure to establish an airway, which may result in hypoxemic cardiac arrest, hypoxemic brain injury, or death.
- Minor bleeding along the tract of the tracheostomy can result in respiratory compromise.
- Massive hemorrhage due to a tracheoinnominate fistula (TIF) is a rare but devastating complication:
  - This presents as a sentinel bleed usually 1 to 2 weeks after tracheostomy.
  - Bronchoscopy or computed tomographic (CT) angiography of the head, neck, and chest may be useful in the diagnosis of TIF but has limited sensitivity.
- See Table 26.1.2 for a complete list of complications with tracheostomy.

Outcomes After Tracheostomy

- There are several potential benefits of subglottic ventilation (Table 26.1.3).

TABLE 26.1.2 Complications of Tracheostomy
• Failure to establish an airway
• Inadvertent decannulation
• Subcutaneous emphysema
• Pneumothorax
• Pneumomediastinum
• Aspiration
• Bleeding
• Infection
• Tracheal granulations
• Subglottic stenosis
• Tracheal stenosis
• Tracheoinnominate fistula
• Posterior tracheal wall perforation/esophageal injury

TABLE 26.1.3 Potential Benefits of Tracheostomy

- Decrease in ventilator dead space
- Decreased airway resistance
- Ease of suctioning
- Reduced orolabial and laryngeal trauma
- Increased patient comfort
- Reduced requirement for sedation
- Increased patient mobility
- Shorter duration of mechanical ventilation
- Ability to transfer spontaneously breathing patients to non-ICU settings
- Ease of tube replacement (once tract matures)
- Increased ability for the patient to communicate
- Variable capacity for oral intake of nutrition and medication

ICU, intensive care unit.

Troubleshooting Common Issues After Tracheostomy

- Cuff issues: cuff leak and elevated cuff pressures
  - Common causes of loss of tidal volume around the tracheostomy are underfilled cuff, damaged cuff, tracheomalacia, malpositioned orogastric/nasogastric tubes, or high ventilatory pressures.
  - Common causes of elevated cuff pressures include overfilled cuff or a malpositioned tracheostomy appliance with angulation or herniation of the cuff.
  - Initial management involves checking the cuff pressure and adjusting the ventilatory settings, followed by transoral bronchoscopy to directly visualize the position of the tracheostomy appliance and inflated balloon.
  - Tracheostomy exchange may be performed if a damaged cuff, malpositioning, or tracheal anomalies are suspected and initial maneuvers are unsuccessful in addressing the issue.
  - Special care should be taken whenever an airway exchange is performed.
  - Patients requiring increasing ventilatory settings despite initial optimization may require an upsizing or reintubation.
- Peristomal bleeding
  - Minor peristomal bleeding is most commonly seen immediately after the initial tracheostomy procedure; peristomal bleeding can present at a later time related to the formation of friable granulation tissue.
  - Initial evaluation should include workup of coagulopathy and holding anticoagulation if possible.
  - Hemostatic agents such as oxidized cellulose or topical silver nitrate may be used around the stoma.
  - Placement of a temporary purse-string suture around the tracheostomy stoma may be helpful in achieving hemostasis.
  - Generally, hemostatic agents and sutures should be removed within 48 to 72 hours to avoid infection or tissue necrosis.
  - Any peristomal bleeding that involves the lower airways should be evaluated promptly with bronchoscopy as this could lead to respiratory compromise.
- Peristomal infection
  - Tracheostomy stomas are inherently exposed to bacterial flora from the mouth and lower airways.
  - Peristomal infections typically present with cellulitis around the incision site with or without purulence.
  - Initial management should involve antibiotics, wound cleansing, and gentle debridement if necessary.
  - Prevention of peristomal infections with regular cleaning and routine pulmonary hygiene is critical.
  - Overly tightened tracheostomy ties can cause venous congestion and tissue necrosis leading to infection.

Other Considerations

- Timing of tracheostomy in endotracheally intubated patients
  - Early tracheostomy (<7 days after intubation) has been shown to reduce duration of mechanical ventilation, ventilator-associated pneumonia, and intensive care unit (ICU) length of stay.
  - The timing of tracheostomy should be individualized to each patient and must reflect their anticipated clinical status, readiness to wean from the ventilator, and possible benefits from tracheostomy.
  - Emergency tracheostomy can be an effective means for emergent airway access. However, this requires additional preparation and an experienced operator.
- Weaning and decannulation
  - As the need for ventilatory support and secretion clearance decreases, patients may have their tracheostomy tubes downsized to advance care.
  - A one-way valve, such as a Passy-Muir valve, permits laryngeal airflow during expiration and enable speech.
  - Specific weaning strategies are institution dependent: some consider it after the tracheostomy tube has been capped for 48 hours, whereas others consider it once a speaking-valve is tolerated.
  - It is important to *never* place a speaking-valve or cap a nonfenestrated tube with the cuff inflated, as this causes complete airway obstruction.
  - It is standard practice when decannulating a patient to simply remove the tracheostomy tube and allow the wound to heal by secondary intention.

SUGGESTED READINGS

Allan JS, Wright CD. Tracheoinnominate fistula: diagnosis and management. *Chest Surg Clin N Am*. 2003;13(2):331-341.

Chorath K, Hoang A, Rajasekaran K, Moreira A. Association of Early vs Late Tracheostomy Placement With Pneumonia and Ventilator Days in Critically Ill Patients: a meta-analysis. *JAMA Otolaryngol Head Neck Surg*. 2021;147(5):450-459.

Ciaglia P, Firsching R, Syniec C. Elective percutaneous dilatational tracheostomy: a new simple bedside procedure; preliminary report. *Chest*. 1985; 87(6):715-759.

Hashimoto DA, Axtell AL, Auchincloss HG. Percutaneous tracheostomy. *N Engl J Med*. 2020;383(20):e112.

Hess DR, Altobelli NP. Tracheostomy tubes. *Respir Care*. 2014;59(6):956-973.

Holevar M, Dunham JC, Brautigan R, et al. Practice management guidelines for timing of tracheostomy: the EAST Practice Management Guidelines Work Group. *J Trauma*. 2009;67(4):870-874.

McGrath BA, Bates L, Atkinson D, Moore JA; National Tracheostomy Safety Project. Multidisciplinary guidelines for the management of tracheostomy and laryngectomy airway emergencies. *Anaesthesia*. 2012;67(9): 1025-1041.

Mussa CC, Gomaa D, Rowley DD, Schmidt U, Ginier E, Strickland SL. AARC Clinical Practice Guideline: management of adult patients with tracheostomy in the acute care setting. *Respir Care*. 2021;66(1):156-169.

Siempos II, Ntaidou TK, Filippidis FT, Choi AMK. Effect of early versus late or no tracheostomy on mortality and pneumonia of critically ill patients receiving mechanical ventilation: a systematic review and meta-analysis. *Lancet Respir Med*. 2015;3(2):150-158.

Sugerman HJ, Wolfe L, Pasquale MD, et al. Multicenter, randomized, prospective trial of early tracheostomy. *J Trauma*. 1997;43(5):741-747.

Terragni PP, Antonelli M, Fumagalli R, et al. Early vs late tracheotomy for prevention of pneumonia in mechanically ventilated adult ICU patients: a randomized controlled trial. *JAMA*. 2010;303(15):1483-1489.

Young D, Harrison DA, Cuthbertson BH, Rowan K, TracMan C. Effect of early vs late tracheostomy placement on survival in patients receiving mechanical ventilation: the TracMan randomized trial. *JAMA*. 2013; 309(20):2121-2129.

Zouk AN, Batra H. Managing complications of percutaneous tracheostomy and gastrostomy. *J Thorac Dis*. 2021;13(8):5314-5330.

26.2

Cricothyroidotomy

Kristina Bermas

Cricothyroidotomy (Cricothyrotomy)

- An emergent procedure to surgically introduce a tube into the airway through an incision made in the skin and cricothyroid membrane (CTM)

Indications and Contraindications

- An emergent cricothyroidotomy is indicated in a "Cannot Intubate, Cannot Oxygenate" (CICO) scenario. These situations can occur in patients with:
  - Significant oral or maxillofacial trauma
  - Cervical spine trauma
  - Limited oral or nasal access (such as from bleeding, emesis, obstructing lesions, soft tissue swelling, trismus, or anatomic abnormalities)

  When time and situation allow, tracheostomy (see Section 27.1: ICU Transport) is usually preferred.
- Relative contraindications to cricothyroidotomy include:
  - Laryngotracheal disruption
  - Distortion of neck anatomy due to disease or injury
  - Preexisting laryngeal diseases, such as cancer, acute or chronic inflammation, or epiglottitis
  - Subglottic stenosis
  - Bleeding diathesis or history of coagulopathy
  - Insertion site infection
  - Children <12 years of age
- In a CICO scenario, there are no absolute contraindications to cricothyroidotomy.

Complications

- Studies show complication rates varying from 0% to 54% depending on clinical scenario, personnel training, and procedure location.
- Immediate complications include bleeding, tracheal injury, tracheal cartilage laceration, and creation of a false tract.
- Late complications include voice change, subglottic stenosis, and infection.
- Voice change is the most common complication, occurring in up to 50% of cases.
- Subglottic stenosis is the most frequently reported major complication after cricothyroidotomy.
- Complication rate is higher in the pediatric population. Pneumothorax is the most common complication in children (5%-7%).
- The mortality rate in children is up to 8.7%.

Anatomy

- The CTM measures 10 mm in height and 22 mm in width and is located in the anterior neck between the thyroid cartilage superiorly and the cricoid cartilage inferiorly.
- The cricothyroid space can be easily identified by palpating a slight dip or indentation in the skin immediately below the laryngeal prominence.
- The CTM can be difficult to palpate in children and in patients who are obese or pregnant.
- Studies have shown that ultrasound can help identify the CTM accurately, though more time-consuming.

Procedure

- There are several techniques currently used for cricothyrotomy. In general, there are open surgical techniques and a Seldinger technique.
- Figure 26.2.1 shows the pertinent landmarks and the first three steps in an open technique. The variation lies in the fourth step, where either a tracheal hook or a bougie is used.
  - *Standard technique*
    - Identify the CTM and make a vertical incision on the skin overlying it.
    - Bluntly dissect down to the CTM and incise it horizontally.
    - Use tracheal hook under the thyroid cartilage and the Trousseau dilator to enlarge CTM incision vertically.
    - Insert tube between the teeth of Trousseau dilator.
  - *Scalpel-Finger-Bougie technique*
    - Identify the CTM and make a vertical incision on the skin overlying it.
    - Bluntly dissect down to the CTM and incise it horizontally.
    - Insert finger into the trachea and guide the bougie in, directed caudally.
    - Pass a 6.0 cuffed endotracheal tube (ETT) over the bougie and into the trachea, then withdraw the bougie.
  - *Seldinger technique*
    - Catheter over needle is inserted into the trachea through the CTM while aspirating for air.

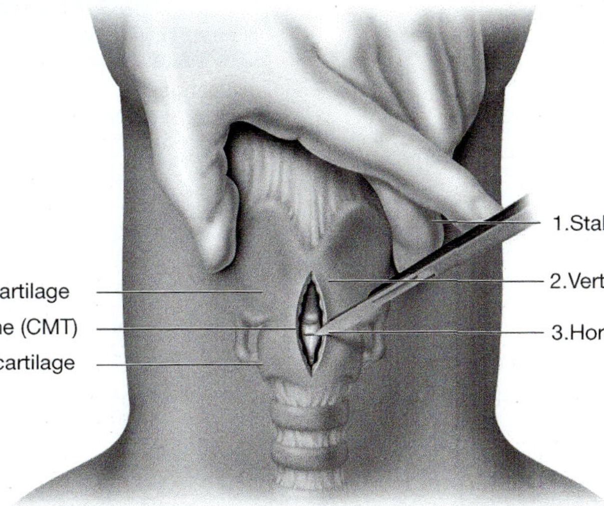

FIGURE 26.2.1 Pertinent landmarks and the first three steps of an open cricothyroidotomy. (From Bair AE, Caro DA. Surgical airway management. In: Brown CA III, Sakles JC, Mick NW, eds. *The Walls Manual of Emergency Airway Management*. 5th ed. Wolters Kluwer; 2018:209-231. Figure 19.6A.)

  - Needle is removed, leaving the catheter in the trachea.
  - Guidewire is introduced through the catheter, then the catheter is removed.
  - A small incision is made in the skin and CTM.
  - The combined tissue dilator-airway catheter unit is advanced over the wire, through the skin incision, and into the trachea.
  - The dilator and guidewire are removed together, leaving the airway catheter in the trachea.
- The Difficult Airway Society deems the scalpel cricothyroidotomy as the fastest and most reliable method, using a #10 scalpel, bougie, and 6.0 cuffed ETT.
- The Seldinger technique appears to lessen the incidence of bleeding and promote a more precise technique of insertion.
- ETT position should be confirmed by the usual methods (auscultation, end-tidal CO_2 monitoring, and chest x-ray).
- If using an ETT, avoid advancing it too far in order to avoid mainstem intubation.
- The tube can be secured using a suture or fabric tape. However, it has been shown that the suture technique was superior in stabilizing an ETT when compared to using a fabric tape tied around the patient's neck, regardless of the tying techniques.

Other Considerations

- There are several commercially available cricothyrotomy kits, but studies have not shown a significant difference in their success rates in comparison with each other.
- Commonly used ETT sizes are 5.0 to 6.0. Alternatively, tracheostomy tubes may be easier to handle.
- Emergent cricothyrotomy is largely a tactile procedure; the field can become bloody after initial incision, obscuring the view of any landmarks.
- Postprocedural care includes appropriate ventilator settings, sedation, and analgesia.
- Consultation with surgery or otolaryngology may be necessary with regard to decannulation or conversion to a formal tracheostomy.

SUGGESTED READINGS

Benumof JL. *Airway Management Elsevier Health Sciences*. MO. Principles and Practice; 1996.

Caparosa RJ, Zavatsky AR. Practical aspects of the cricothyroid space. *Laryngoscope*. 1957;67:577.

Frerk C, Mitchell VS, McNarry AF, et al. Difficult Airway Society 2015 guidelines for management of unanticipated difficult intubation in adults. *Br J Anaesth*. 2015;115(6):827-848.

George N, Consunji G, Storkersen J, et al. Comparison of emergency airway management techniques in the performance of emergent cricothyrotomy. *Int J Emerg Med*. 2022;15(1):24.

Glassenburg R, Vaisrub N, Albright G. The incidence of failed intubation in obstetrics: is there an irreducible minimum abstracted? *Anesthesiology*. 1990;73:A1061.

Groombridge CJ, Maini A, Mathew J, et al. Comparing methods to secure a tracheal tube placed via a surgical cricothyroidotomy: a randomised controlled study in cadavers. *Scand J Trauma Resusc Emerg Med*. 2021; 29(1):104.

Jackson IJB, Choudhry AK, Ryan DW, et al. Minitracheostomy: Seldinger—assessment of a new technique. *Anaesthesia*. 1991;46:475.

Kress TD, Balasubramanian S. Cricothyroidotomy. *Ann Emerg Med*. 1982; 11:197.

Lyons G. Failed intubation. *Anaesthesia*. 1985;40:759.

McKenna P, Desai NM, Tariq A, Morley EJ. Cricothyrotomy. In: *StatPearls* [Internet]. StatPearls Publishing; 2023.

Nakazawa H, Uzawa K, Tokumine J, Lefor AK, Motoyasu A, Yorozu T. Airway ultrasound for patients anticipated to have a difficult airway: perspective for personalized medicine. *World J Clin Cases*. 2023;11(9): 1951-1962.

Schaumann N, Lorenz V, Schellongowski P, et al. Evaluation of Seldinger technique emergency cricothyroidotomy versus standard surgical cricothyroidotomy in 200 cadavers. *Anesthesiology*. 2005;102(1):7.

Sise MJ, Shackford SR, Cruickshank JC, et al. Cricothyroidotomy for long-term tracheal access: a prospective analysis of morbidity and mortality in 76 patients. *Ann Surg*. 1984;200:13.

Tunstall ME. Failed intubation in the parturient. *Can J Anaesth*. 1989;36:611.

26.3

Bronchoscopy

Samantha E. Halpern and Nikhil Panda

Overview

- For certification, the American College of Chest Physicians recommends that the bronchoscopist complete the following number of bronchoscopies:
    - 100 bronchoscopies for initial certification
    - 25 bronchoscopies per year to maintain certification
- There are multiple types of bronchoscopy, including flexible, rigid, virtual/navigational, and robot assisted. We focus here on flexible bronchoscopy (Table 26.3.1).

Indications and Contraindications in the Intensive Care Unit

See Table 26.3.2 *for additional details.*

Complications

See Table 26.3.3 *for additional details.*

- Complication rate is low (~1%).
- Most complications are from biopsies, especially bleeding and pneumothorax.
- Self-limited fever is common after bronchoalveolar lavage (BAL, up to one-third of patients).

Equipment

- The flexible bronchoscope (typically) has the following parts:
    - 55 to 60 cm scope with 4 to 6 mm outer diameter and 2 to 3 mm working channel
    - Light source
    - Image transmission device (fiberoptic or charge-coupled device camera)
    - Working channel for instruments or lavage
    - Suction channel
    - Mechanical mechanism to flex and extend the distal end of the scope
- Other necessary equipment:
    - Sedating medications
    - Topical anesthetic (delivered via nebulizer, atomization device, or direct instillation in working channel)
    - Saline flushes
    - Suction
    - Equipment to endotracheally intubate if needed
    - Ventilator adaptor with silicone lubricant for patients with endotracheal or tracheostomy tube in place

TABLE 26.3.2 Common and Major Complications of Bronchoscopy

Indications	Relative Contraindications
• Evaluation of pulmonary infection	• Unstable cardiac disease
• Hemoptysis[a]	• Inability to cooperate
• Evaluation of airway pathology (burn, fistula, mass, mucus plug, trauma, foreign body)	• Unstable/immobile cervical spine
• Endotracheal tube management (intubation, confirmation, change)	• Hemodynamic instability
• Surveillance (ie, post-lung transplant)	• Asthma/chronic obstructive pulmonary disease exacerbation
	• Severe hypoxemia
	• Coagulopathy (especially for brushing, needle aspiration, and biopsy)
	• Severe pulmonary hypertension
	• Increased intracranial pressure
	• Pregnancy

ICU, intensive care unit.
[a]Massive hemoptysis may require rigid bronchoscopy for adequate control.

TABLE 26.3.1 Types of Bronchoscopy

Flexible Bronchoscopy	Rigid Bronchoscopy	Virtual/Navigational Bronchoscopy	Robot-Assisted Bronchoscopy
• Can be performed at bedside or in an operating or dedicated procedure room	• Typically requires an operating or dedicated procedure room	• Requires high-resolution CT mapping followed by bronchoscopy in an operating or dedicated procedure room	• Requires an operating or dedicated procedure room with robotic capabilities and trained personnel
• Typically requires sedation and topical anesthesia	• Typically requires general anesthesia	• Typically requires general anesthesia	• Typically requires general anesthesia
• Flexible and small-diameter device	• Rigid and large-diameter device	• Ultrathin flexible device	• Flexible and small-diameter device
• Only certain interventions and diagnostic studies can be done	• Wide range of procedures can be done	• Primarily used to obtain tissue from beyond segmental bronchi	• Primarily used to obtain tissue from beyond segmental bronchi

CT, computed tomography.

TABLE 26.3.3 Common and Major Complications of Bronchoscopy

Most Common Complications	Major Complications
• Fever	• Pneumothorax (0.1%)
• Transient hypotension from sedation	• Epistaxis/Bleeding (0.2%)[a]
• Bronchospasm	• Respiratory failure (<0.1%)
• Hypoxemia	• Death (<0.04%)
• Nausea and vomiting	
• Cardiac arrhythmias	
• Infection	
• Vasovagal syncope	
• Laryngospasm	
• Seizure	
• Bacteremia	
• Laryngeal edema	
• Laryngeal injury	

ICU, intensive care unit.
[a]Minor bleeding is common, affecting nearly 90% of patients.

- Cardiac and respiratory monitors
- Airway sampling and collection devices
- Bite block for oral approach

Anatomy

- Classification system: Jackson-Huber, including lobes and segments

Jackson-Huber Classification

- Right upper lobe (RUL)
  - Apical, posterior, anterior
- Right middle lobe (RML)
  - Lateral, medial
- Right lower lobe (RLL)
  - Superior/apical, medial basal, anterior basal, lateral basal, posterior basal
- Left upper lobe (LUL)
  - Superior division: apicoposterior, anterior
  - Lingular division: superior, inferior
- Left lower lobe (LLL)
  - Superior/apical, anteromedial basal, lateral basal, posterior basal
- Trachea begins at the cricoid cartilage; ~1/3 extrathoracic (above sternal notch) and dependent on cervical spinal pathology (eg, scoliosis, kyphosis).
  - Adult trachea is 10 to 13 cm in length, with an average inner diameter of 2.5 cm.
  - 18 to 24 incomplete cartilage rings
  - The membranous wall and longitudinal fibers of the trachealis muscle provide orientation.
- Main carina branches into the right and left main bronchus at the level of the sternal notch.
  - Left main bronchus is typically 10 to 15 degrees higher than right.
- Right bronchus is ~2 cm in length.
  - First branch is the RUL bronchus, visualizing three segmental bronchi.
  - Right bronchus then becomes the bronchus intermedius, ~2 to 2.5 cm in length.
  - The bronchus intermedius divides into the RML and RLL bronchi; the membranous wall leads the bronchoscopist to the RLL.
- Left bronchus is ~5 cm in length.
  - Divides into the LUL and LLL bronchi.
  - The LUL bronchus branches into the superior division and lingular division.
  - The LLL is identified by following the membranous wall.

Procedure

- Sedation and anesthesia
  - Telemetry and pulse oximetry monitoring with audible alarm for desaturation and bradycardia
  - Conscious sedation is typically recommended along with topical anesthesia.
  - Topical
    - Nebulize or atomize 1% or 2% lidocaine; awake patients can gargle lidocaine.
    - Spray above and below the vocal cords.
- Procedure
  - Preoxygenate the patient.
  - Enter through either nose, mouth, endotracheal tube, or tracheostomy tube.
    - Inner diameter ≥7.5 mm is required to pass a standard flexible bronchoscope through an endotracheal or tracheostomy tube.
  - Visualize and inspect the posterior pharynx and vocal cords.
  - Deliver additional direct topical anesthesia through the working channel.
  - Have the patient take a deep breath and pass the scope during inspiration.
  - Visualize and inspect the trachea, mainstem bronchi, and segmental bronchi.
- Basic diagnostic and therapeutic procedures
  - BAL: used to obtain cytologic material from distal airways and alveoli
    - Attach specimen trap to suction channel.
    - Wedge bronchoscope in the fourth or fifth order bronchi toward lesion of interest.
    - Instill 100 to 200 mL of sterile saline in serial 30 to 60 mL aliquots.
    - Suction saline back into specimen trap.
      - Typically less than half of the volume instilled returns
    - Samples needed for laboratory testing
      - For microbiology, obtain samples before or within 48 hours of antibiotic use.
      - 5 to 20 mL for cell count and differential, Gram stain, fungal, and cultures
      - 5 to 10 mL for flow cytometry and cell markers
      - 15 mL for cytology
    - Poor sample
      - Lack of alveolar macrophages
      - Epithelial cells >5%
  - Bronchial washing: used for microbiologic evaluation of central airways
    - Similar to BAL, but no need to wedge the bronchoscope
    - Instill 5 to 50 mL of sterile saline.
    - Quickly aspirate into specimen trap.

- Samples needed for laboratory testing
  - For microbiology, obtain samples before or within 48 hours of antibiotic use.
  - 5 to 15 mL for microbiologic testing
  - 10 mL for cytology
- Higher risk of oral flora contamination than BAL

- Brushing: used to obtain cytologic specimens from mucosal lesions
  - Advance bronchoscope near the lesion of interest.
  - Deploy the brush.
  - Briskly rub the lesion multiple times.
- Endobronchial biopsy: used to obtain tissue for pathologic examination
  - Wedge bronchoscope in the target airway.
  - Advance closed biopsy forceps into the target segment until gentle resistance is met.
  - Pull back 1 to 2 cm, then open forceps and readvance to point of resistance.
  - Close the forceps on the target lesion and retract. Perform several biopsies in succession.
  - Maintain bronchoscope in wedged position for at least 1 minute for hemostasis.

Other Considerations

- Advanced diagnostic and therapeutic procedures
  - Laser resection/tumor debulking
  - Photodynamic therapy
  - Electrocautery
  - Cryosurgery
  - Balloon dilatation
  - Brachytherapy
  - Stenting
  - Endobronchial valve placement
  - Thermoplasty
  - Endobronchial ultrasound
  - Electromagnetic bronchoscopy
  - Needle aspiration

SUGGESTED READINGS

Carlos A, Mehta AC. Rigid versus flexible bronchoscopy in interventional pulmonology: perspective from the master clinicians. *Curr Opin Pulm Med*. 2025;31(1):1-10.

Facciolongo N, Patelli M, Gasparini S, et al. Incidence of complications in bronchoscopy: multicentre prospective study of 20,986 bronchoscopies. *Monaldi Arch Chest Dis*. 2009;71(1):8-14.

Islam S. Flexible bronchoscopy in adults: indications and contraindications. UpToDate. 2023.

Islam S. Flexible bronchoscopy in adults: overview. UpToDate. 2023.

Kavuru MS, Mehta AC, Turner JF, Jr. Applied anatomy of the airways. In: Wang K, ed. *Flexible Bronchoscopy*. 3rd ed. Blackwell Publishing Ltd; 2012:46-52.

Miller RJ, Casal RF, Lazarus DR, et al. Flexible bronchoscopy. *Clin Chest Med*. 2018;39(1):1-16.

Panda N, Auchincloss HG. Anatomy of the trachea. *Thorac Surg Clin*. 2025;35(1):1-10.

26.4

Tube Thoracostomy (Chest Tube)

Kristina Bermas

Introduction

- Tube thoracostomy is a procedure in which a flexible tube is inserted through the chest wall into the pleural space to evacuate air or liquid contents.
- There are two primary techniques for chest tube insertion: open surgical and Seldinger (described later).

Indications and Contraindications in the Intensive Care Unit (Table 26.4.1)

TABLE 26.4.1 Indications and Relative Contraindications for Tube Thoracostomy

Indications	Relative Contraindications
• Pneumothorax	• Coagulopathy
• Hemothorax	• Bleeding diathesis
• Pleural effusion	• Caution with pleural adhesions
• Pleurodesis	• Caution with rib fractures
• Chylothorax	• Extensive pulmonary blebs
• May be diagnostic (eg, patient with unstable trauma with signs of chest trauma)	

Complications

- Chest tube malpositioned location (most common)—intrafissure, intraparenchymal, subcutaneous
- Bleeding
  - Prehospital anticoagulation does not increase the mortality risk of chest tube placement.
- Infection—superficial (insertion site), deep (empyema, pneumonia)
  - Increased duration of chest tube and retained hemothoraces increase the risk for infection.
    - Early evacuation of retained hemothoraces decreases the risk of empyema.
- Organ injury—lung (most common), diaphragm, heart, liver, or spleen
- Reexpansion pulmonary edema
  - Occurs with rapid reexpansion of the lung after evacuation of a pneumothorax or rapid drainage of a large volume of fluid
  - Can be prevented by limiting drainage to $<$1,500 mL at a time

Considerations

- Chest tube size
  - Chest tubes range in sizes from 14F to 40F.
    - *Diameter in French/3 = Diameter in millimeter*
  - Recent studies have shown 14F pigtail catheters to be as effective as 28F to 32F chest tubes with no significant difference in complication rates and length of stay when used in nonemergent scenarios.
  - 14F catheters are better tolerated by patients compared to large-bore chest tubes.
  - There have been no studies on the use of 14F catheters in emergent trauma settings.
  - The 2020 EAST guidelines conditionally recommend the use of small-bore pigtail catheters over standard chest tubes in hemodynamically stable patients.
  - The Western Trauma Association guidelines recommend 28F or smaller chest tube for pneumothorax and stable patients with hemothorax. They recommend 28F chest tube in unstable patients with hemothorax.
- Technique
  - Percutaneous, Seldinger
    - Typically for smaller chest tubes
    - More comfortable for patients
    - Requires that the lung be collapsed at the point of insertion
  - Open/surgical
    - Typically for larger chest tubes
    - Allows dissection of intrapleural adhesions. Can be placed even when the lung is not fully collapsed
- Antibiotic prophylaxis
  - There is no clinical consensus regarding the use of prophylactic antibiotics for tube thoracostomies in the posttraumatic setting.
  - The American Association for the Surgery of Trauma Critical Care (AAST) Critical Care Committee did agree that if prophylactic antibiotics were used, one dose of cefazolin prior to the procedure is appropriate and does not need to be continued after tube placement.
- Insertion site
  - The insertion site depends on the indication and type of tube selected.
  - Image guidance, such as bedside ultrasound, should be considered to select the best insertion site for pleural effusions.
  - The 5th intercostal space in the midaxillary line is the best single all-purpose insertion site. The nipple or inframammary fold is the best landmark for the 5th intercostal space.
  - For pneumothoraces, tubes can be placed slightly higher or more anterior and directed apically and anteriorly.
  - For effusion of any sort, tubes can be placed slightly lower or more posterior and directed posteriorly.
  - When using the Seldinger technique, the operator should be sure, based on imaging (x-ray, computed tomography, or real-time ultrasound), that the lung is away from the chest wall at the site of insertion.

Procedure

- Open/surgical method
  - Patient should be placed in the supine position or the lateral position depending on what they can tolerate.
  - Full personal protective equipment and sterile prep and technique should be used.
  - Except in dire emergencies, a local anesthetic is used to provide pain control. The site of insertion is infiltrated all the way to the pleura.
  - Make a 1- to 2-cm incision parallel to the intercostal space.
  - A blunt clamp is used to bluntly dissect from the subcutaneous tissue to the rib.
  - Track up and over one rib space to help direct the chest tube cephalad and create a soft tissue flap upon the removal of the chest tube. This will help seal the site and prevent air from going back into the chest.
  - Once the rib is identified, the Kelly clamp is angled cephalad over the SUPERIOR EDGE OF THE RIB to avoid the nerve, artery, and vein bundle that runs just below each rib.
  - With the Kelly clamp in the closed position, force is used to punch the clamp into the pleural space.
  - Once the pleural space has been entered, the Kelly clamp is opened to widen the tract of the clamp as well as the entrance into the pleura.
  - A finger can be used to feel for proper position in the pleural space and clear any easily disrupted adhesions. Caution should be taken during this step if the patient has rib fractures or if the patient has significant pleural adhesions.
  - The Kelly clamp can be used to clamp the insertion end of the chest tube and can be used to guide the tube into the pleural space. It is typically guided toward the apex for pneumothorax or inferiorly/posteriorly for pleural effusions.
  - The tube should be advanced until the last drainage hole is inside the pleural space. Condensation/drainage from the tube should be observed to verify correct placement.
  - The chest tube should be sutured in place to avoid dislodgement and attached to the drainage system.
  - Chest radiograph should be obtained to verify position and assess lung expansion.
- Seldinger method
  - Position, prep, and anesthetize as earlier.
  - Advance a hollow-bore needle into the pleural space JUST SUPERIOR TO THE CHOSEN RIB. Air or fluid should be freely aspirated.
  - Introduce the guidewire into the pleural space.
  - Dilate the tract serially over the guidewire.
  - Introduce the tube into the pleural space over the guidewire.
  - Suture in place and attach to the drainage system as earlier.

Management

- Daily monitoring
  - Tidaling
    - Tidaling is when the fluid in the chamber or the tubing moves back and forth with respiration due to the negative pressure from the diaphragm. This is a sign that the chest tube is patent.
  - Air leak
    - Air leak should be assessed daily by noting the presence or absence of bubbling in the water chamber, and whether it is intermittent or continuous.

- Drainage
  - Drainage should be assessed after initial placement and regularly thereafter. Note volume and quality of the drainage.
  - For traumatic hemothorax, immediate drainage of 20 mL/kg or 1,500 mL or persistent drainage of >3 mL/kg or >200 mL/h for 4 hours indicates the need for emergent thoracotomy.
  - Rapid removal of large volumes may predispose the patient to reexpansion pulmonary edema.
- Removal
  - Chest tubes should be removed as soon as it is safe to do so.
  - A clamping trial of a few hours prior to removal has been shown to be safe.
    - Pneumothorax: remove once the lung is fully expanded and there is no visible air leak or accumulation of air with the chest tube off suction.
    - Effusion: remove once the lung is fully expanded and the daily output of fluid has decreased.

  The threshold for chest tube output prior to removal is individualized based on the indication for chest tube and other patient factors.

SUGGESTED READINGS

British Thoracic Society Pleural Disease Guideline Group. British Thoracic Society pleural disease guideline 2010. *Thorax*. 2010;65(suppl 2): ii1-ii76. Accessed December 2012. http://www.brit-thoracic.org.uk/guidelines/pleural-disease-guidelines-2010.aspx

Farrell MS, Agapian JV, Appelbaum RD, et al. Surgical and procedural antibiotic prophylaxis in the surgical ICU: an American Association for the Surgery of Trauma Critical Care Committee clinical consensus document. *Trauma Surg Acute Care Open*. 2024;9(1):e001305.

Lewis MR, Georgoff P. Minimally invasive management of thoracic trauma: current evidence and guidelines. *Trauma Surg Acute Care Open*. 2024;9(suppl 2):e001372.

Tarantino B, Wood M, Hancock D, Shah K. Does pre-injury anticoagulation make chest tubes any less safe? A nationwide retrospective analysis. *Am J Emerg Med*. 2024;82:47-51.

26.5

Thoracentesis, Paracentesis, and Pericardiocentesis

Spencer Lord

Thoracentesis

- A procedure that advances a needle through the chest wall to remove pleural fluid for therapeutic treatment and/or diagnostic purposes

Indications

- Diagnostic for patients with pleural effusion of unknown cause
- Diagnostic and therapeutic for patients with suspected parapneumonic effusions when the pleural fluid thickness is >1 cm on chest x-ray or >2 cm on computed tomography (CT)
- To confirm malignancy in patients with suspected malignant for cytological examination
- May be therapeutic for large effusions in patients with respiratory compromise
- To alleviate symptoms in refractory pleural effusions due to heart failure or hepatic hydrothorax
- Safe for diagnostic and treatment purposes in neutropenic patients with cancer or suspected infection
- Therapeutic for pleural effusions in veno-occlusive disease (VOD) that contribute to poor oxygenation and ventilation in the pediatric population

Contraindications

- Absolute contraindications
  - Lung adherent to the chest wall throughout the hemithorax: unable to safely access the pleural space
  - Uncontrollable cough: increases unnecessary procedural complications due to unsafe entry and movement of instruments
  - Severe respiratory distress or hypercapnic failure: Performing thoracentesis before securing airway can exacerbate their condition.
- Relative contraindications
  - Caution should be used in patients with coagulopathy, but thoracentesis can be performed with acceptable risk in patients where antiplatelet therapy cannot be interrupted and may have no higher risk of severe bleeding in coagulopathic patients.
  - Caution should be used in patients receiving mechanical ventilation, as positive pressure may increase the risk of pneumothorax.

Complications

- Pneumothorax occurs after 6% of thoracenteses, and is more likely if air was aspirated during the procedure; if chest pain, dyspnea, or hypoxemia develops; if multiple needle passes were required; or if the patient is critically ill or on mechanical ventilation.
- Only 2% of those who develop pneumothorax require chest tube placement.
- Reexpansion pulmonary edema occurs in 0.01% to 2.5% of patients.

- Reexpansion pulmonary edema is rare and can probably be avoided by limiting therapeutic aspirations to less than 1,500 mL or stopped sooner if pleural pressure drops below −20 cm H_2O. Prolonged collapse (>7 days) or large effusions (>3 L) increase reexpansion pulmonary edema.
- Hemothorax and significant bleeding only reported in 0.18% of cases.
- Other complications include localized infection, intraabdominal organ injury, and air embolism.

Procedure

- The patient should be sterilely prepped, draped, and positioned sitting upright, leaning over a table. Alternatively, the procedure may be performed in a supine or lateral decubitus position.
- The level of the effusion should be identified by ultrasound visualization to reduce complications.
- To avoid the peritoneal space, do not insert the needle below the ninth rib. Insert the needle one or two intercostal spaces below the level of the effusion.
- After anesthetizing the skin, insert a 22-gauge needle over the superior edge of the rib to anesthetize the tract and the parietal pleura.
- Attach an 18-gauge needle and catheter to a syringe and advance the needle along the superior surface of the rib. Once pleural fluid is obtained, advance the catheter over the needle and remove the needle. Attach a large syringe with a three-way stopcock to the catheter hub. Aspirate 50 mL of fluid for diagnostic thoracentesis.
- For a therapeutic thoracentesis, connect tubing to the stopcock and a large, evacuated container, never removing more than 1,500 mL at one time.
- When complete, remove the catheter during an end-expiratory breath hold and cover the site with an occlusive dressing.

Other Considerations

- Do not go through areas of prior scar or cellulitis.
- Avoid the inferior surface of the rib to prevent injury to the intercostal nerve and vessels.
- Complex and loculated pleural effusions require surgical consultation and intervention.

Postprocedure Management

- Patients should be monitored for development of a pneumothorax, hemothorax, and post expansion pulmonary edema.
- Fluid should be analyzed using Light's criteria to evaluate if it is a transudate or exudate. Fluid is an exudate if one or more of the following are present:
  - The pleural fluid protein to serum protein ratio is >0.5.
  - The pleural fluid lactic acid dehydrogenase (LDH) to serum LDH ratio is >0.6.
  - The pleural fluid LDH level is greater than two-thirds the upper normal limit for serum LDH.
- Common causes of *transudates* include congestive heart failure, cirrhosis, and other low-albumin states.
- Common causes of *exudates* include neoplastic diseases, infections, pancreatitis, and other inflammatory disorders.
- Fluid may also be sent for cell count, gram stain, culture, glucose, pH, triglyceride, adenosine deaminase, amylase measurements, and cytology.
- A parapneumonic effusion is an effusion associated with a pulmonary infection. An empyema is frank pus in the pleural space.
- Indications of an empyema include cloudy, milky, or thick fluid; a low fluid glucose; a low pH; an elevated white blood cells (WBC) >50,000; or an LDH >1.000.
- All patients with empyema should have a chest tube inserted and be treated with antibiotics. If drainage of the empyema is incomplete, thoracoscopy is required.

Paracentesis

- A procedure that advances a needle through the abdominal wall to remove ascites for therapeutic treatment and/or diagnostic purposes

Indications

- Diagnostic paracentesis should be considered in all patients with new onset ascites to determine if ascites is due to portal hypertension or other cause.
- Performed in patients with ascites if spontaneous bacterial peritonitis (SBP) is suspected
- Any clinical or biologic deterioration in patients with chronic ascites
- Hospitalized patients with cirrhosis and ascites: The American Association for the Study of Liver Diseases (AASLD) recommends diagnostic paracentesis, regardless of symptoms, to exclude SBP.
  - SBP should be considered in patients with ascites and any of the following: fever, abdominal pain, altered mental status, gastrointestinal (GI) bleed, sepsis, or shock.
- Should be considered in all patients being hospitalized with ascites
- Therapeutic paracentesis should be performed in hemodynamically stable patients with respiratory compromise, discomfort, or refractory ascites.
- Early (within 24 hours of hospitalization) paracentesis is associated with improved outcomes, reduced mortality, acute renal injury and infections.

Contraindications

- Disseminated intravascular coagulation and hyperfibrinolysis is a contraindication. Many patients have coagulopathy, but routine administration of fresh frozen plasma (FFP) or platelets is not recommended.
- There is no absolute platelet cutoff but thrombocytopenia less than 20,000/μL should warrant caution and consideration for correction.
- Severe coagulopathy: Although routine coagulation tests do not reliably predict bleeding risk in cirrhotic patients with an international normalized ratio (INR) >2.5 may necessitate correction before paracentesis.

- Caution should be taken in patients who are pregnant, have small bowel obstructions, or urinary retention.
- Therapeutic paracentesis may worsen hemodynamics and precipitate hypotension.

Complications

Major Complications

- Hemorrhage: Severe hemorrhage is rare occurring in 0.2% of cases, and is more common in patients with severe liver disease or renal dysfunction.
- Bowel perforation: rare (<0.001 events/cases); can lead to secondary bacterial peritonitis and abscess formation
- Infection
- Post-paracentesis circulatory dysfunction: hypovolemia and renal injury to rapid fluid removal; use of albumin infusion can mitigate this risk.
- Failure to visualize the inferior epigastric artery with ultrasound may lead to puncture and abdominal wall hematoma or hemoperitoneum).

Minor Complications

- Ascitic fluid leak: most common complication, occurring in 5% of procedures
- Abdominal wall hematoma: can be due to injury to abdominal wall vessels and may require angioembolization
- Transient hypotension: normally occurs in critically ill patients

Procedure

- The procedure may be performed at either a midline point 2 cm below the umbilicus or laterally in either lower quadrant, 2 to 4 cm medial and cephalad to the anterior superior iliac spine, lateral to the rectus sheath to avoid the inferior epigastric artery.
- Ultrasound should be used to identify the pocket of fluid, locate the inferior epigastric artery, and confirm lack of viscera immediately behind the marked site.
- After sterilely prepping and draping the patient, the skin and the planned tract are anesthetized with a 22-gauge needle.
- A nick is then made in the skin, and catheter-sheathed needle can be advanced either at a sharp angle through the skin or with a Z-technique to reduce leaking. Once ascites is obtained, the catheter is advanced over the needle and the needle removed. For a diagnostic procedure, a syringe should be connected to the catheter and 30 to 60 mL of fluid removed. If a therapeutic procedure is planned, the catheter may be connected to a container.

Other Considerations

- Do not insert the needle through areas of prior scar, abdominal wall hematoma, or cellulitis.

Postprocedure Management

- The fluid should be analyzed to evaluate for SBP.
  - Greater than 250 PMNs/mm^3 indicates SBP.
  - Patients should be treated with a third-generation cephalosporin.
- The fluid should be evaluated for the serum-ascites albumin gradient.
  - A ratio of >1.1 g/dL indicates portal hypertension.
  - A ratio of <1.1 g/dL indicates other causes, such as pancreatitis or cancer.
- Patients should be monitored for hemodynamic stability.
- Patients should be monitored for bleeding and leakage.
- Albumin should be transfused for large volume (>5 L) paracentesis to reduce the risk of hepatorenal syndrome. Treat with 6 to 8 g of albumin per liter of ascites fluid removed.

Pericardiocentesis

- A procedure that advances a needle through the chest or abdominal wall to remove pericardial fluid for therapeutic treatment and/or diagnostic purposes.
- Patients may develop pericardial effusions after cardiac catheterization, myocardial infarction, or cardiac surgery.
- Other common causes of pericardial effusions include neoplastic disease, uremia, idiopathic pericarditis, infectious, and tuberculosis.

Indications

- Pericardial drainage procedures are rarely diagnostic and should only be performed on patients with hemodynamic compromise or suspected bacterial or oncologic causes of pericardial effusion.
- Treatment of the underlying disorder should remain the therapeutic goal for patients with effusions that do not meet these criteria.
- Cardiac tamponade occurs along a spectrum. Clinical evidence of tamponade includes tachycardia, dyspnea, jugular venous distention, pulsus paradoxus, hypotension, and shock.
- Echocardiography is the preferred method of assessing for cardiac tamponade. Echo may demonstrate diastolic right atrial or right atrial and right ventricular collapse before clinical signs of tamponade develop.
- Emergent pericardiocentesis should only be performed at the bedside in cases of immediately life-threatening tamponade; otherwise, pericardiocentesis should be performed in the cardiac lab under echocardiographic or fluoroscopic guidance.
- Pericardiocentesis is rarely indicated in trauma patients, as patients with pericardial tamponade should undergo emergency thoracotomy.

Contraindications

- If the patient can wait to have the procedure performed in a controlled setting under direct visualization, bedside pericardiocentesis should not be performed.
- Blind or EKG-guided pericardiocentesis is no longer recommended.
- Aortic dissection: Pericardiocentesis is contraindicated in patients with aortic dissection-related hemopericardium due to recurrent pericardial bleeding and associated mortality.
- Uncorrected coagulopathy: Avoid procedure entirely unless emergent.
- Pulmonary hypertension (relative contraindication): associated with increased in-hospital mortality and higher rates of cardiovascular complications.

Complications

- When performed blindly, pericardiocentesis has a high complication rate.
- Dysrhythmias
- Coronary artery puncture/aneurysm
- Hemothorax/pneumothorax
- Pneumopericardium
- Hepatic injury
- Cardiac injury

Procedure

- As the patient with tamponade is being prepared for pericardiocentesis, continue to ensure adequate preload as to not precipitate hemodynamic collapse.
- Position the patient supine with the head of the bed to 30 to 45 degrees to bring the heart closer to the chest wall. Administer local anesthesia at the puncture site.
- Pericardiocentesis must be performed with adjunctive imaging, either ultrasound or fluoroscopy.
- Echocardiographic guidance of pericardiocentesis is available in most settings and allows the clinician to find the area where the most fluid is adjacent to the chest wall.
- The subxiphoid approach remains commonly used, although the intercostal approach may also be used under direct visualization as the provider should target the largest fluid pocket with the least intervening structures.
- Once the needle is in the pericardial space, introduce a guidewire through the needle followed by pigtail catheter placement to continue drainage.

Other Considerations

- Pericardiocentesis may be sufficient in idiopathic or viral pericarditis, however, in oncologic pericardial effusions or infectious purulent, the effusion may recur. These patients may require pericardial drainage catheters.
- Loculated effusion may require advanced imaging techniques such as CT-guided pericardiocentesis.
- Large pericardial effusions that have not previously caused tamponade may suddenly do so.

Postprocedure Management

- Monitoring and imaging: Echocardiogram and continuous hemodynamic monitoring should be used immediately after the procedure to detect any reaccumulation.
- Following cardiac tamponade from atrial fibrillation catheter ablation, the catheter can be removed if no ongoing bleeding after 30 minutes.
- Following malignant pericardial effusion, catheters should stay in for a minimum of 3 days due to recurrence.
- Catheter management: If a catheter is left in place, it is typically removed when there is less than 25 to 50 mL of fluid drainage over a 24-hour period and no evidence of reaccumulating.
- Anticoagulation can be safely restarted after 24-hour period of no further drainage or bleeding.
- The patient should be treated for the underlying condition that led to development of the pericardial effusion.
- Patients with inflammatory conditions or autoimmune pericardial effusions should be treated with aspirin or nonsteroidal anti-inflammatory (NSAID) medications and colchicine. Steroids are reserved for refractory cases.

SUGGESTED READINGS

American Thoracic Society. Management of malignant pleural effusions. *Am J Respir Crit Care Med*. 2000;162(5):1987-2001.

Biggins S, Angeli P, Garcia-Tsao G, et al. Diagnosis, evaluation, and management of ascites, spontaneous bacterial peritonitis and hepatorenal syndrome: 2021 practice guidance by the American Association for the Study of Liver Diseases. *Hepatology*. 2021;74(2):1014-1048.

Chetrit M, Lipes J, Mardigyan. A practical approach to pericardiocentesis with periprocedural use of ultrasound training initiative. *Can J Cardiol*. 2018;34(9):1229-1232.

Cho J, Jensen T, Reierson K. Recommendations on the use of ultrasound guidance for adult abdominal paracentesis: a position statement of the society of hospital medicine. *J Hosp Med*. 2019;14:E7-E15.

De Gottardi A, Thevenot T, Spahr L. Risk of complications after abdominal paracentesis in cirrhotic patients: a prospective study. *Clin Gastroenterol Hepatol*. 2009;7(8):906-909.

Desselle B, Bozeman P, Patrick C. Diagnostic utility of thoracentesis for neutropenic children with cancer. *Clin Infect Dis*. 1995;21(4):887-890.

Echevarria C, Twomey D, Dunning J, Chanda B. Does re-expansion pulmonary oedema exist? *Interact Cardiovasc Thorac Surg*. 2008;7(3):485-489.

Eryilmaz S, Emiroglu O, Eyileten Z, et al. Effect of posterior pericardial drainage on the incidence of pericardial effusion after ascending aortic surgery. *J Thorac Cardiovasc Surg*. 2006;132(1):27-31.

Fiorini F, Natali G, Battaglia Y. Ultrasound-guided paracentesis: technical, diagnostic and therapeutic aspects for the modern nefrologist. *G Ital Nefrol*. 2022;39(1):2022-vol1.

Fong C, Tan C, See K. Safety of thoracentesis and tube thoracostomy in patients with uncorrected coagulopathy: a systemic review and meta-analysis. *Chest*. 2021;160(5):1875-1889.

Glauser F, Barras A, Pache I, Monti M. Abdominal paracentesis. *Rev Med Suisse*. 2008;4(177):2324-2328.

Gordon CE, Feller-Kopman D, Balk EM, Smetana GW. Pneumothorax following thoracentesis: a systematic review and meta-analysis. *Arch Intern Med*. 2010;170(4):332-339.

Hiratzka L, Barkris G, Beckman J, et al. 2010 ACCF/AHA/AATS/ACR/ASA/SCA/SCAI/SIR/STS/SVM guidelines for the diagnosis and management of patients with thoracic aortic disease: a report of the American College of Cardiology Foundation/American Heart Association task force. *Circulation*. 2010;121(13):e266-e369.

Iliescu C, Grines C, Herrmann J, et al. SCAI expert consensus statement: evaluation, management, and special considerations of cardio-oncology patients in the cardiac catheterization laboratory. *Catheter Cardiovasc Interv*. 2016;87(5):E202-E223.

Light R. The light criteria: the beginning and why they are useful 40 years later. *Clin Chest Med*. 2013;34(1):21-26.

Luis S, Kane G, Luis C, Oh J, Sinak L. Overview of optimal techniques for pericardiocentesis in contemporary practice. *Curr Cardiol Rep*. 2020;22(8):60.

Mahadeo K, McArthur J, Adams, et al. Consensus report by the pediatric acute lung injury and sepsis investigators and pediatric blood and marrow transplant Consortium Joint Working Committees on supportive care guidelines for management of veno-occlusive disease in children and adolescents: part 2-focus on ascites, fluid and electrolytes, renal, and transfusion issues. *Biol Blood Marrow Transplant*. 2017;23(12):2023-2033.

Millington S, Koenig S. Better with ultrasound: paracentesis. *Chest*. 2018;154(1):177-184.

Mohammed A, Hochfeld U, Hong S, et al. Thoracentesis techniques: a literature review. *Medicine (Baltimore)*. 2024;103(1):e36850.

Pache I, Bilodeau M. Severe haemorrhage following abdominal paracentesis for ascites in patients with liver disease. *Aliment Pharmacol Ther*. 2005;21(5):525-529.

Patel I, Rahim S, Davidson J, et al. Society of Interventional Radiology consensus guidelines for the periprocedural management of thrombotic and bleeding risk in patients undergoing percutaneous image-guided interventions-Part II. *J Vasc Interv Radiol*. 2019;30(8):1168-1184.e1.

Patel N, Silvey S, O'Leary, et al. Early paracentesis is associated with better prognosis compared with late or no-paracentesis in hospitalized veterans with cirrhosis and ascites. *Liver Transpl*. 2023;29(9):919-927.

Philip V, Saugel B, Ernesti C. Effects of paracentesis on hemodynamic parameters and respiratory function in critically ill patients. *BMC Gastroenterol*. 2014;14:18.

Pinchot J, Kalva S, Majdalany B, et al. ACR Appropriateness Criteria® radiologic management of portal hypertension. *J Am Coll Radiol*. 2021;18 (5 suppl):S153-S173.

Porcel J. Nonmalignant pleural effusions. *Semin Respir Crit Care Med*. 2022;43(4):570-582.

Quiñones M, Douglas P, Foster E. American College of Cardiology/American Heart Association clinical competence statement on echocardiography: a report of the American College of Cardiology/American Heart Association/American College of Physicians—American Society of Internal Medicine task force on clinical competence. *Circulation*. 2003;107(7):1068-1089.

Rahman N, Ali N, Brown G, et al. Local anaesthetic thoracoscopy: British Thoracic Society pleural disease guideline 2010. *Thorax*. 2010;65 (suppl 2):54-60.

Runyon B. Management of adult patients with ascites due to cirrhosis. *Hepatology*. 2004;39(3):841-856.

Seferovic P, Ristic A, Makismovic R. Pericardial syndromes: an update after the ESC guidelines 2004. *Heart Fail Rev*. 2013;18(3):255-266.

Seo Y, Lim C, Lim J. Successful transcatheter arterial embolization of abdominal wall hematoma from the left deep circumflex iliac artery after abdominal paracentesis in a patient with liver cirrhosis: case report and literature. *Review*. 2024;83(4):167-171.

Shen K, Bribriesco A, Crabtree T, et al. The American Association for Thoracic Surgery consensus for the management of empyema. *J Thorac Cardiovasc Surg*. 2017;153(6):e129-e146.

Shen-Wagner J, Gamble C, MacGilvray P. Pleural effusion: diagnostic approach in adults. *Am Fam Physician*. 2023;108(5):464-475.

Sundaralingam A, Bedawi E, Harriss EK, Munavvar M, Rahman N. The frequency, risk factors, and management of complications from pleural procedures. *Chest*. 2022;161(5):1407-1425.

Vakamudi S, Ho N, Cremer P. Pericardial effusions: causes, diagnosis, and management. *Prog Cardiovasc Dis*. 2017;59(4):380-388.

Vasquez M, Iskander M, Mustafa M, et al. Pericardiocentesis outcomes in patients with pulmonary hypertension: a nationwide analysis from the United States. *Am J Cardiol*. 2024;210:232-240.

Wilcox M, Chong C, Stanbrook M, et al. Does this patient have an exudative pleural effusion? The rational clinical examination systematic review. *JAMA*. 2014;311(23):2422-2431.

Wong C, Holroyd-Leduc J, Thorpe K, et al. Does this patient have bacterial peritonitis or portal hypertension? How do I perform a paracentesis and analyze the results. *JAMA* 2008;299(10):1166-1178.

Zhao Q, Li L, Liu N, et al. Early vs delayed removal of the pericardial drain in patients with cardiac tamponade complicating radiofrequency ablation of atrial fibrillation. *J Cardiovasc Electrophysiol*. 2020;31(3): 597-603.

26.6

Feeding Tube Placement

Robert D. Sinyard and Casey M. Luckhurst

Indications

- Patients with functioning gastrointestinal (GI) tracts who cannot tolerate oral nutrition secondary to:
  - Impaired mental status
  - Foregut pathology (lack of coordinated peristalsis, weakness, obstruction, esophageal perforation, etc)
  - Prolonged mechanical ventilation
- Enteral nutrition is preferable to total parenteral nutrition (TPN) when GI function is intact (see Nutrition Support, Section 16.4).
- *Nasoenteric* access is appropriate for the short-term access in patients who are expected to recover the ability to eat and drink.
  - Examples:
    - Intubated patients expected to wean off the ventilator
    - Patients progressing with speech and language pathology treatment regimen to improve oropharyngeal coordination
- *Surgical* enteric access should be considered in cases of prolonged mental status impairment, ventilator dependence, or other barriers to oral intake.
  - Examples:
    - Patients with traumatic brain injury or stroke
    - Patients with chronic impairment of mentation or swallowing
    - Recurrent aspiration secondary to esophageal or oropharyngeal pathology
    - Ambulatory patients who suffer from chronic malnutrition

Modes of Access

- Nasogastric (NG) tubes
  - Salem sump
    - Large bore (14-18F)
    - Allows for aspiration of gastric contents, medication administration (crushed or liquid medications), and instillation of enteral tube feeding
    - Allows for monitoring of gastric residuals, though clinical evidence does not support the use of residuals, given the interruption in feeding and failure to prevent aspiration events
    - Attention required for nasal ala, given large-bore size and potential for pressure necrosis with prolonged use
  - Dobhoff
    - Small bore (8F)
    - Instillation only
    - Unable to aspirate
    - Better tolerated long term in terms of patient comfort and avoidance of pressure on nasal ala
- Postpyloric tubes
  - Indicated for patients with *gastroparesis*
  - No data to support routine placement in all intensive care unit (ICU) patients
    - No difference in incidence of pneumonia, ICU length of stay, or mortality, though some evidence for post-ligament of Treitz (ie, jejunal) access preventing aspiration events
    - Attempts to obtain postpyloric access can delay feeding.

- Bedside placement can be challenging; may require placement by fluoroscopy or endoscopy.
- Gastrostomy
  - Most common surgical feeding tube
  - Ideal for patients with normal gastric motility who require long-term enteral access
  - Allows for the measurement of residuals to monitor feeding tolerance
  - Open or laparoscopic surgical approach
    - Often required in patients with a history of prior upper abdominal surgery or for those unable to undergo upper endoscopy due to oropharyngeal or esophageal considerations
    - Anterior wall of the stomach is sutured to the anterior abdominal wall (Stamm approach).
  - Percutaneous approach
    - Endoscopically placed (percutaneous endoscopic gastrostomy or "PEG") and thus can be performed at bedside in ICU for mechanically ventilated patients
      - Inner tube bumper causes the anterior gastric wall to appose the anterior abdominal wall.
    - Fluoroscopic placement
      - Typically performed by interventional radiology under fluoroscopic guidance
      - Percutaneous access, typically using endogastric insufflation via NG tube, and radiographic confirmation
- Jejunostomy
  - Best option for patients requiring long-term access, who have gastric dysmotility, gastric outlet obstruction, or gastroesophageal (GE) junction pathology
  - Have higher long-term rate of complications (leak, luminal obstruction, adhesive small bowel obstruction) than gastrostomy tubes
  - Commonly placed after esophagectomy or total gastrectomy for temporary nutritional support
  - More complex operation, but can be performed open or laparoscopically
  - Some institutions place percutaneously under fluoroscopy by interventional radiology.

Procedure of Feeding Tube Placement

Nasogastric Tube

- Measure insertion length from nares, to ear, to just below left costal margin.
- Explain procedure to patient and consider anesthetization of nares and oropharynx with two sprays of aerosolized benzocaine or with topical lidocaine (urojet).
- Instruct patient to tuck chin. Pass NG tube through nostril until the tip abuts the hard palate.
- Provide cup of water and straw and instruct the patient to swallow. Loss of resistance should be appreciated with swallowing allowing for smooth and quick advancement of the tube into the gastric lumen.
- Immediately check placement with insufflation of air and auscultation of abdomen. Maintain a high index of suspicion for improper placement in patients unable vocalize or coughing during as well as after placement.
- Confirm placement in the stomach with abdominal x-ray. *Do not* instill feeds until placement confirmed.
  - In intubated, sedated patients who cannot cooperate, consider placement with laryngoscopy.
  - Alternatively, placing NG versus orogastric (OG) in intubated patient can be done based on tactile feedback.
  - For those patients with bronchial anastomoses or staple lines, consider initial placement to 30 cm, followed by chest x-ray to confirm correct placement in the esophagus

Postpyloric Nasoenteric Tube

- As earlier, but using a smaller bore, weighted tube with a stylet
- Use CO_2 detector to ensure the tube does not enter the airway.
  - In the presence of CO_2, color changes from purple (room air) to yellow (2%-5% CO_2).
  - Helps to differentiate between respiratory and GI placement in adult, mechanically ventilated patients
  - Cannot distinguish between esophageal, gastric, or duodenal placement
- Procedure
  - Give Reglan prior to placement.
  - Position right lateral decubitus.
  - Pass tube to ~30 cm, then insufflate the stomach with 300 to 600 mL of air.
  - Pass as far as possible. If resistance is met, the tip may be caught against the pylorus. Withdraw and attempt again.
  - Leave the stylet in place until placement is confirmed by x-ray.
  - Alternatively, leave in place with extra length to allow for peristalsis into a postpyloric position.

Percutaneous Endoscopic Gastrostomy

- Relative contraindications
  - Hepatosplenomegaly
  - Coagulopathy
  - Large volume of ascites
  - Prior upper GI surgery (specifically prior gastric resection)
  - Peritoneal dialysis
  - Portal hypertension with gastric varices
  - Ventral hernia
- Two operators: one to place tube, another to operate the endoscope
  - Insufflate the stomach with endoscope.
  - Choose a point two finger-breadths below the left costal margin, midaxillary line. Transilluminate the abdominal wall with the scope to confirm apposition to the stomach and make skin incision.
  - Pass needle and angiocatheter into the stomach, and confirm gastric entry with endoscope. Remove the needle and pass guidewire through angiocatheter.
  - Endoscopist grasps guidewire and pulls the guidewire out through the mouth.
  - Secure a lubricated PEG to the looped guidewire at the mouth. From the abdominal wall, withdraw the guidewire until the PEG exits the abdominal wall and the bumper is against the inner stomach wall.
  - Secure PEG to skin with Prolene or nylon suture and mark abdominal wall thickness as a reference for future tube position confirmation and adjustment.

- Can usually administer medications through the tube immediately, and begin feeding within 24 hours
- Wait 6 weeks before removing or replacing tube to ensure a mature tract.

Complications of Bedside Nasoenteric Tube Placement

- Misplacement
  - Occurs at a rate of 1% to 2.5% on review of > 2,000 insertions
  - Inadvertent airway intubation
    - Risk factors
      - Depressed sensorium
      - Depressed cough reflex
      - Mechanical ventilation
        - Occurs despite the presence of cuffed endotracheal tubes
    - More common with small-bore tubes
    - Usually enters the right mainstem bronchus
    - Can injure the lung
      - Lung abscess
      - Pneumothorax
      - Pneumonia
  - Side port(s) in the esophagus
    - Increases risk of aspiration
  - Coiling in the oropharynx
    - Increases risk of aspiration
  - **Radiography is the gold standard for placement confirmation.**
    - Auscultatory method *insufficient*
- Perforation
  - Cribriform plate
    - High risk in the setting of basilar skull fractures or transsphenoidal surgery
      - In these cases, place nasoenteric tubes with laryngoscopic or fluoroscopic guidance.
  - GI tract
    - Esophageal perforation is rare and occurs most commonly in preterm infants or those with altered esophageal anatomy.
- Aspiration
  - During placement, patients may gag and vomit.
    - Have suction at bedside
  - After placement, NG tube stents open the lower esophageal sphincter (LES), increasing the risk for reflux and aspiration.
    - Keep HOB >30 degrees
  - High risk for aspiration among patients with:
    - Gastroesophageal reflux disease (GERD)
    - Glasgow Coma Scale <9
    - Vomiting
- Sinusitis
  - Long-term complication
  - Remove tube as soon as feasible.
  - Consider oroenteric (rather than nasoenteric) tube placement in intubated patients.
- Epistaxis
  - Usually resolves spontaneously
  - May be significant in the setting of bleeding disorders
    - Consider nasal packing.
    - Embolization in severe cases refractory to packing

Complications of Percutaneous Endoscopic Gastrostomy Placement

- Misplacement
  - Colonic
    - Diarrhea that resembles tube feeds
    - Stool in the gravity bag
    - Confirm with tube study: inject undiluted Gastrografin into tube and obtain an abdominal film.
    - Requires surgical consultation
  - Transhepatic
    - Ensure no hemorrhage
    - If no bleeding, leave tube in place and allow the tract to mature.
- Dislodgement
  - If tract potentially *mature* (after 14 days), replace with Foley catheter. Inflate balloon, secure to the skin with a stitch, and obtain tube study for placement confirmation. Do not use until placement is confirmed radiographically.
  - If immediately *post-op*, evaluate for extravasation into the peritoneal cavity, via CT scan.
    - May need operative exploration
- Wound breakdown/site infection
  - Local wound care
- Bumper migration
  - Bumper can migrate (too loose) and cause gastric outlet obstruction. Corrected by securing PEG at the skin to the original tightness based on the time of initial operation.
  - Buried bumper syndrome—caused by overtightening of tube, causing bumper to migrate through the anterior gastric wall and into the abdominal wall. May correct with loosening to the original tightness but may also require surgical consultation

SUGGESTED READINGS

Baskin WN. Acute complications associated with bedside placement of feeding tubes. *Nutr Clin Pract*. 2006;21(1):40-55.

Chau JPC, Lo SHS, Fernandez R, Griffiths R. Use of end-tidal carbon dioxide detection to determine correct placement of nasogastric tube: a meta-analysis. *Int J Nurs Stud*. 2011;48(4):513-521.

Marik PE, Zaloga GP. Early enteral nutrition in acutely ill patients: a systematic review. *Crit Care Med*. 2001;29:2264-2270.

Marik PE, Zaloga GP. Gastric versus post-pyloric feeding: a systematic review. *Crit Care Med*. 2003;7(3):46-51.

Metheny NA, Meert KL, Clouse RE. Complications related to feeding tube placement. *Curr Opin Gastroenterol*. 2007;23:178-182.

Sorokin R, Gottlieb JE. Enhancing patient safety during feeding-tube insertion: a review of more than 2000 insertions. *JPEN J Parenter Enteral Nutr*. 2006;30(5):440-445.

SECTION 27

Intensive Care Unit Transport

Section Editor: Marvin G. Chang

27.1

Intensive Care Unit Transport

Ryan Dodge and Michael G. Fitzsimons

Definition

- Transport of the critically ill patient is a common activity that is fraught with significant challenges and potential risks.
- Often, patient transport occurs at a critical juncture of a patient's overall course, such as the requirement of escalation of care, the need for procedural intervention, or the requirement of advanced diagnostic testing. Therefore, this critical phase of the patient's care must not be overlooked.
- There are fundamental principles to safely and effectively transport critically ill patients, including adequate preparation, clear communication, vigilance during movement, appropriate recognition and intervention to physiologic changes, and comprehensive handoff at the receiving destination. These principles apply to both intrahospital and interhospital transport.

Types of Patient Transport

- Interhospital transport describes the movement of a patient from one medical facility to another facility. Reasons for interhospital transport include the need for specialized or higher level care, patient or family requests, or lack of capacity at the referring center.
- Intrahospital transport describes the movement of a patient from one location within a hospital to another location. Common destinations for travel from the intensive care unit (ICU) include the radiology suite for diagnostic and interventional procedures, the cardiac catheterization lab, the electrophysiology lab, and the operating room.
- Patients may also be transported back to the originating facility for further care or recovery. This is referred to as repatriation.

Preparation for Patient Transport Between Facilities

Appropriate patient and process preparation is critical to optimize outcomes associated with transport.

- The intent of the transport should be clear to all team members involved, as well as the patient and their family. Transport cannot be financially motivated according to the Emergency Medical Treatment and Active Labor Act (EMTALA) of 1986.
- The risks and benefits of transport must be considered.
- The patient must be stabilized to the best ability by the referring center, understanding that some conditions may only be stabilized with the expertise of the receiving facility.
- An agreement for the receiving facility to accept the patient must be established before patient movement.
- Communication between the referring and receiving facility is critical. Components of transport communication include patient identification, condition, treatment, reason for transport, and potential for deterioration during transport. Communication also includes sending appropriate records and studies to the accepting hospital.

Means to Transport Between Facilities

Patients may be transported between facilities by either ground or air.

- Ground transport occurs by ambulance. Benefits include immediate availability, low relative cost, minimal dependence on weather, and dependability. The downsides include speed and traffic delays.
- Air transport may include fixed-wing or rotor type (helicopter). Advantages of fixed wings include speed over longer distances, larger size, and the ability to transport more patients, providers, and equipment. Rotor aircraft can land in smaller areas and be mobilized quicker than fixed wings. Both methods pose risks of physiologic changes due to altitude, involve significant costs, and are weather dependent.

Preparation for Patient Transport Within a Facility

Transport within a single facility requires similar preparation to transport between facilities.

- The risks and benefits should be assessed, and other options should be considered. Many procedures previously performed in distant locations can now be performed at a patient's bedside (eg, endoscopy, ultrasound-guided procedures, computed tomography, tracheostomy).
- There must be appropriate personnel to accompany the patient, including a minimum of two individuals with expertise in airway management and the ability to administer medications. Providers with specialized skills may be necessary for the management of ventilators, extracorporeal membrane oxygenation (ECMO), intra-aortic balloon pumps (IABPs), or mechanical circulatory support (MCS).
- There must be clarification of responsibility for patient care and a plan for managing patient deterioration in the case of instability.

Equipment

Patient monitoring during transport should remain at the same level as before transport and should not be decreased. Transport is associated with acute hemodynamic instability; immediate recognition and management are critical.

- Maintain pretransport monitoring.
- Minimum continual monitoring should include blood pressure, pulse oximetry, and electrocardiography (ECG). Transport-associated noise may render alarms less effective; therefore, monitors should be continually visualized by transport care providers.
- The following additional pieces of equipment should be thoughtfully considered:
  - Portable defibrillators with the ability to perform defibrillation and cardioversion
  - Medications for pain management and resuscitation
  - Airway equipment, including intubation supplies, oxygen supply, artificial manual breathing unit (AMBU bag), and extra oxygen
  - Medication infusion pumps and infusion medications
  - Device to monitor end-tidal carbon dioxide ($EtCO_2$) to allow better assessment of ventilation than direct visualization or reliance on pulse oximetry
- Critical incidents are due to equipment issues nearly 40% of the time and are commonly due to poor protocols or training.

Physiologic Changes to Anticipate During Patient Transport

Airway

- Although the airway does not change during patient transport, accidental extubation is a risk that should be mitigated. Endotracheal tubes should be secured, and $EtCO_2$ should be monitored continually.
- Pretransport intubation and sedation should be considered for patients demonstrating a risk of deterioration during transport, especially those transported by ground or rotor wing.
- If a patient has a secure airway, there should be no tension on the breathing circuit, and the ventilator should be continually within the field of vision of the transporting providers.

Breathing

- Patients should be assessed for not only the adequacy of ventilation but also conditions likely to result in problems during transport, such as the requirement for high oxygen concentration (FiO_2) or positive end-expiratory pressure (PEEP), both of which are associated with deterioration. Simple pneumothorax may convert to tension pneumothorax at altitude during air transport. The dry air associated with elevation may impact secretions, causing mucus plugging. Pain with turbulence or rough roads may acutely worsen respiratory function. Patients who are stable while their head is elevated may experience decompensation when positioned supine.
- Those individuals skilled in manual ventilation may closely replicate that of a portable ventilator for short transport duration, but longer travel or transport with individuals less skilled in manual ventilation may benefit from a portable ventilator.
- Any period of transport while a patient is on supplemental oxygen runs the risk of inadequate oxygen supply. Oxygen, like any other medication administered, should be carefully checked for supply adequacy prior to patient transport.
- Ventilators or other life-sustaining devices that require battery power should be fully charged prior to transport. Backup breathing devices, such as an AMBU bag, can be temporarily used if there is power or equipment failure.

Circulation

- Hemodynamic changes, including hypertension, hypotension, and arrhythmias, occur in a high percentage of patients subject to transport. Factors associated with instability may include pretransport instability, the need for vasopressors or inotropic agents, preexisting arrhythmias, and cardiogenic shock.
- Patients requiring medications for hemodynamic status are likely to demonstrate more instability during transport. Contributing factors include movement itself, interruption of medication infusion, progression of the primary process, and the results of an intervention at the destination.
- Patients receiving advanced MCS often require transport to centers of specialty care. These devices are subject to dislodgement should tension inadvertently be applied during movement. IABP function may be reduced if pulled away from the proper position in the proximal descending aorta. The Impella device used for left ventricular support may be ineffective if pulled out of the ventricle. Dislodgement of cannulae for ECMO may result in life-threatening hemorrhage.

Neurologic Status

- Transport induces significant stress on the patient that may necessitate sedation and pain relief that requires careful monitoring to avoid additional instability.
- Intracranial injury can be exacerbated by changes encountered in transport, including hypoxemia, hypotension,

and intracranial hypertension. Intra-arterial blood pressure monitoring provides more immediate information and is less likely to be impacted by patient movement during transport. Direct monitoring of $EtCO_2$ for intubated patients may reveal detrimental hypotension or respiratory depression earlier than pulse oximetry or simple visual monitoring of respiratory rate. Invasive arterial lines and intracranial or spinal monitors must be appropriately leveled.

- Spinal injuries can be exacerbated by patient movement during transport. Stabilization devices should be checked before transport. Stabilization may reduce a patient's ability to protect their airway in the case of vomiting and may make it challenging to secure the airway should the patient require an advanced airway.

Environment and Other Factors

- The environment to consider when transporting includes temperature, humidity, atmospheric pressure (with flight), and physical movement.
- Transport moves patients from a temperature-controlled location, often with the ability to actively warm to a less controlled environment. Children, older patients, and patients suffering burn injuries are at the highest risk of hypothermia. Body temperature is easier to preserve than recover when reduced.
- Transport at elevation during air transport, cooler environments, and the use of supplemental oxygen risk dehydration and drying of secretions.
- Elevation associated with air transport exposes patients to lower atmospheric pressures, which may allow expansion of air in enclosed cavities such as the pleural space, abdomen, brain sinuses, and vasculature in the case of air embolization. The benefits of air transport must be balanced with the associated risks. Chest tube placement or orogastric tube placement before movement may be indicated.

Safety, Checklists, and Outcomes

- The majority of incidents associated with transport are patient or management issues and include communication failures, inadequate training, poor vigilance, inadequate preparation, and failure to follow established guidelines. Equipment-related incidents are somewhat less common but still make up nearly 40% of incidents.
- The use of a pretransport checklist is associated with improved safety, a lower incidence of critical events, improved compliance with protocols, and potential improvements in morbidity and mortality.
- The overall outcomes associated with interhospital patient transport are unclear, and additional study is needed.

SUGGESTED READINGS

Agizew TB, Ashagrie HE, Kassahun HG, Temesgen MM. Evidence-based guideline on critical patient transport and handover to ICU. *Anesthesiol Res Pract*. 2021;2021:6618709.

Beckmann U, Gillies DM, Berenholtz SM, Wu AW, Pronovost P. Incidents relating to the intra-hospital transfer of critically ill patients: an analysis of the reports submitted to the Australian Incident Monitoring Study in Intensive Care. *Intensive Care Med*. 2004;30(8):1579-1585.

Fan E, MacDonald RD, Adhikari NK, et al. Outcomes of interfacility critical care adult patient transport: a systematic review. *Crit Care*. 2006;10(1):R6.

Kikutani K, Shimatani T, Kawaguchi A, et al. Medical equipment that improve safety and outcomes of inter-facility transportation of critically ill patients: a systematic review. *Medicine (Baltimore)*. 2023;102(22):e33865.

Venn AM, Sotomayor CA, Godambe SA, et al. Implementation of an intrahospital transport checklist for emergency department admissions to intensive care. *Pediatr Qual Saf*. 2021;6(4):e426.

Warren J; Fromm RE, Orr RA, Rotello LC, Horst HM; American College of Critical Care Medicine. Guidelines for the inter- and intrahospital transport of critically ill patients. *Crit Care Med*. 2004;32(1):256-262.

SECTION 28

Epidemiology and Biostatistics

Section Editor: Edward A. Bittner

28.1

Epidemiology and Biostatistics

Edward A. Bittner and Marvin G. Chang

Overview

- Epidemiology is the study of the distribution and determinants of health-related states in populations, forming the foundation for evidence-based clinical practice.
- Biostatistics provides the analytic framework required to evaluate diagnostic tests, interpret measures of association, and judge the quality of clinical trials and predictive models.

Disease Burden

- Disease burden in a population is commonly quantified using prevalence and incidence.
- Summary metrics of population health include Disability-Adjusted Life Years (DALYs), which measure disease burden, and Quality-Adjusted Life Years (QALYs), which measure health gains from interventions.
- **Prevalence**: at a specific point in time
  - Number of people with disease/total number in population
- **Incidence**: over a time interval
  - Number newly diagnosed with disease/total number at risk of disease during that time
- DALY
  - Concept: measures health LOSS or BURDEN of disease. Used for public health/epidemiology (eg, "How big of a problem is sepsis compared to acute respiratory distress syndrome [ARDS]?")
  - Goal: TO MINIMIZE OR AVERT DALYs
  - Scale (disability weight): 0.0 (perfect health) to 1.0 (death)
    - Note this is the inverse scale of QALY.
  - Formula: YLL (years of life lost) + YLD (years lived with disability) = DALYs
    - Example 1 (mortality burden): a 45-year-old dies from sepsis (life expectancy 80). The YLL = 35 years. The total burden is 35 DALYs.
    - Example 2 (morbidity burden): the same 45-year-old from Example 1 survives sepsis but lives those 35 years with severe post–intensive care syndrome (PICS) (disability weight = 0.4). The YLD = 14 DALYs (35 years × 0.4). The total burden is 14 DALYs.
    - Example 3 (combined mortality + morbidity): the same 45-year-old from Example 1 develops sepsis and lives 10 years with severe PICS (disability weight = 0.4) before dying at age 55 (25 years before life expectancy). Total burden = 4 DALYs (YLD: 10 years × 0.4) + 25 DALYs (YLL) = 29 DALYs.
- QALY
  - Concept: measures health GAIN or BENEFIT. Used for cost-effectiveness (eg, "Is this new, expensive intervention worth the cost?")
  - Goal: To MAXIMIZE QALYs
  - Scale (utility value): 0.0 (death) to 1.0 (perfect health)
  - Formula: Years of life × Utility value = QALYs gained
    - Example (benefit of intervention): a new intensive care unit (ICU) protocol gives a survivor 10 extra years of life. Their post-ICU quality of life ("utility") is 0.7 (due to PICS). The intervention gained 7 QALYs (10 years × 0.7).

Diagnosis

- *Diagnostic tests* guide the physician's decision to determine if a patient has a disease or not (Table 28.1.1).
- Tests are typically evaluated in a diagnostic two-by-two table against a gold standard using the following metrics:
  - **Sensitivity**: proportion of individuals with disease who have a positive test result. Hint: Be sensitive to people with disease.
    - Sensitivity = TP/(TP + FN)

TABLE 28.1.1 Simple Classification System for Evaluating a Diagnostic Test

	Disease	
Test Result	**+**	**–**
+	True positive (TP)	False positive (FP)
–	False negative (FN)	True negative (TN)

- **Specificity**: proportion of individuals without the disease who have a negative test
  - Specificity = TN/(TN + FP)
- **Positive predictive value**: proportion of individuals with a positive test who have the disease
  - Positive predictive value = TP/(TP + FP)
- **Negative predictive value**: proportion of individuals with a negative test who do not have the disease
  - Negative predictive value = TN/(TN + FN)
- **Accuracy**: proportion of individuals correctly classified by the test
  - Accuracy = (TP + TN)/(TP + TN + FP + FN)
- **Negative likelihood ratio:** ratio of the probability of a negative test in patients with disease to the probability of a negative test in patients without disease
  - Negative likelihood ratio = [FN/(FN + TP)]/[TN/(TN + FP)]
  - Negative likelihood ratio = [1 − sensitivity]/specificity
- **Positive likelihood ratio:** ratio of the probability of a positive test in patients with disease to the probability of a positive test in patients without disease
  - Positive likelihood ratio = [TP/(TP + FN)]/[FP/(FP + TN)]
  - Positive likelihood ratio = sensitivity/(1 − specificity)

- **Limitations:**
  - These methods require binary classification of a test result using a cut-point.
  - Many tests lack meaningful cut-points.
  - These methods do not fully incorporate Bayesian methods such as pretest probabilities.

Measures of Association

- Describes the relationship between a risk factor and an outcome
- Reported measures of association must include the direction, magnitude, and statistical significance (Table 28.1.2).
  - *Direction* denotes whether the presence of a risk factor is associated with greater or lesser risk of disease.
  - *Magnitude* denotes the size of the association, which may be small, null, or large.
  - *Statistical significance* is a way to describe the certainty of an association.

TABLE 28.1.2 The Two-By-Two Table

	Disease	
Exposure	**+**	**–**
+	A	B
–	C	D

The Two-By-Two Table Is a Convention for Describing the Distribution of Disease by Exposure Status

- **Relative risk (risk ratio):** the risk of disease in the exposed group relative to the risk of disease in the unexposed group
  - In a cross-sectional study, this calculation is referred to as a prevalence ratio. The term *hazard ratio* is practically equivalent to relative risk.
    - Relative risk = risk of disease in exposed group/risk of disease in unexposed group
    - Relative risk = [A/(A + B)]/[C/(C + D)]
- **Odds ratio:** the odds of disease in the exposed group relative to the odds of disease in the unexposed group
  - The odds ratio approximates the relative risk when the prevalence of disease is low (<10%).
    - Odds ratio = (A/B)/(C/D)
    - Odds ratio = (A * D)/(C * B)
- ***Risk difference***, absolute risk reduction (or increase) is the difference in absolute risk between the exposed and unexposed groups.
  - Absolute risk reduction (ARR) = Risk in control group − Risk in treatment group = [C/(C + D)] − [A/(A + B)]
- *Number needed to treat* (NNT) is the number of patients who need to be treated to prevent one additional event.
  - This measure implies causality and should be calculated from a trial rather than observational study.
  - In this setting, a number needed to harm (NNH) may also be calculated using similar methods.
  - Number needed to treat = 1/ARR
  - When treatment increases risk (ARR <0), calculate NNH instead.
- *Kaplan-Meier curves* visually present survival experiences over time, usually in two or more groups.
  - To test for differences in survival experience, the *log-rank test* is commonly reported with a *P* value only.
- *Cox proportional hazards regression* allows adjustment for confounders while analyzing time-to-event data (eg, mortality, ventilator-free days).
- *Statistical significance* is determined by formal hypothesis testing. Common statistical terms are as follows:
  - The *P value* is NOT the probability that a research finding is false and NOT the probability that the null hypothesis is true.
  - The *P* value is the probability of obtaining a test statistic at least as extreme as the one observed in the study, assuming that the null hypothesis is true.
  - By convention, a *P* value < .05 is considered statistically significant.
  - The 95% confidence interval is the range of values calculated from sample data, such that if a study were repeated many times, 95% of the calculated intervals would contain the true population value.
  - *Type I error* occurs when the null hypothesis is rejected but is actually true (discovering something that is not true).
    - The probability of making a type I error is designated by α.
  - *Type II error* occurs when the null hypothesis is accepted but is actually false (failing to find something true) and is designated by β.
    - Power is 1 minus β

TABLE 28.1.3 Observational Studies

Design	Fundamental Feature	What Can Be Measured	Strengths	Limitations
Cross-sectional	Ascertain exposure and outcome at the same moment in time	• Prevalence of outcome • Prevalence of exposure • Prevalence ratio	• Very quick and inexpensive	• Preferentially describe survivors
Case-control	Select individuals based on disease status, subsequently determine exposure history	• Odds ratio	• Good for rare diseases, multiple exposures • Quick and inexpensive • Permits smaller sample sizes	• Susceptible to bias • Poor choice for rare exposures
Cohort (prospective or retrospective)	Select individuals based on exposure status, subsequently follow-up for disease occurrence	• Relative risk (risk ratio) • Prevalence of exposure • Incidence of disease	• Potentially less susceptible to bias • Good for rare exposures and evaluating multiple outcomes of a single exposure	• Require time and higher costs • Poor choice for rare diseases

  - *Sample size* may be calculated prior to a study to optimize efficiency.
    - Sample size calculations include many variables and always require an effect size of interest and the power desired.
  - Sample size and power are typically calculated before a study. After a study, confidence intervals are preferred to post hoc power calculations for interpreting null findings.
- *Receiver operating characteristic (ROC) curve* may be used to display the performance of a predictive model where the y-axis is the true positive rate (sensitivity) and the x-axis is the false positive rate (1 − specificity).
  - The area under an ROC curve is the c-statistic and lies between 0 and 1. Interpreting the c-statistic:
    - 1.0: perfect discrimination
    - 0.8 to 0.9: excellent discrimination
    - 0.7 to 0.8: acceptable discrimination
    - 0.5: discrimination no better than random chance
    - <0.5: discrimination worse than chance (the model is wrong more often than it is right)
- *Net reclassification improvement* is a technique used to quantify how successfully a new variable improves the predictive ability of a model.
  - Successful reclassification is a combination of decreasing risk estimates for patients without disease and increasing risk estimates for patients with disease.
- *t test* is used to compare means between two samples.
- *ANOVA (analysis of variance)* is used to compare the means among three or more samples.
- When normality assumptions of the data are not met, *nonparametric tests* (Mann-Whitney U, Wilcoxon) are used.
- *Chi-square tests* evaluate associations between categorical variables.
- *Regression analysis* (linear, logistic, and Cox) allows for adjusting for confounders, evaluating effect modification, and building predictive models, such as severity of illness scores.

Study Design

- An association between exposure (aka risk factor, marker) and disease (aka outcome, end point) may be causal or noncausal.
- Study design informs the strength of causal conclusions.
- *Descriptive studies* illustrate patterns, such as hospital readmission rates for congestive heart failure over a 5-year period.
- *Case report and case series* are descriptive and may provide clues to new patterns or rare conditions, such as a description of 14 patients who underwent hypothermia for severe ARDS.
- *Analytic studies* test hypotheses, such as testing the association between socioeconomic status and hospital readmission rate
  - Analytic studies may be observational (Table 28.1.3) or experimental.

Experimental Studies

- Referred to as *trials*
- Observational studies should NOT be called trials.
- Clinical trials are inherently prospective; terms like "retrospective randomized trial" are usually misnomers and would be better classified as observational cohort studies.

Strengths

- Trials are the current best method to determine causality.
- Randomization is required to avoid confounding.
- Optimal randomization includes concealed assignment to limit bias.
- Intention-to-treat analysis is needed to maintain the methodologic advantages of randomization.

Limitations

- Some exposures (parachute use when skydiving) may not be ethically tested for some outcomes (survival).
- Trial costs may be prohibitive due to recruitment, measurements, and follow-up.
- Findings from clinical trials are referred to as *efficacy* and may not persist in community settings that require *effectiveness*.
- Strict inclusion criteria may reduce external validity, a common issue in critical care trials.

Common Challenges to Study Validity

- *Bias* is systematic error and comes in many forms:
  - The fundamental issue is noncomparability, whether in how individuals are selected for a study (selection bias)

or how individuals' information is obtained (information bias).
  - Generally, bias cannot be corrected after a study is done.
- *Confounding* occurs when the association between an exposure and disease is distorted by a third variable (confounder).
  - Three criteria must ALL be met for a variable to be a confounder:
    - The confounder is associated with the exposure.
    - The confounder is an independent risk factor or cause of the disease.
    - The confounder is not in the causal pathway between exposure and disease (ie, not a mediator).
  - Confounding results in mixing of effects:
    - The observed association combines the true effect of the exposure with the effect of the confounder.
  - Detecting confounding in practice:
    - Confounding is suggested when the association between an exposure and disease changes after adjusting for a known risk factor.
  - Example: age confounds the relationship between ICU admission and mortality because:
    - Age is associated with ICU admission (older, sicker patients more likely admitted).
    - Age independently increases mortality risk.
    - Age is not caused by ICU admission (not a mediator).
  - Methods such as multivariable regression, propensity scoring, stratification, and inverse probability weighting are used to reduce confounding in observational studies.
  - Residual confounding occurs when statistical models cannot fully control for confounding. Common causes include unmeasured confounders, measurement error in measured confounders, and model misspecification.
- *Interaction*, or effect modification, occurs when the association between an exposure and disease varies by the presence of a third factor.
  - Confounding is made to disappear by adjustment.
  - Interaction is prominently displayed with stratification.
- *Internal validity* refers to the extent to which an association between an exposure and an outcome is true.
  - Confounding and bias are the major threats to internal validity.
- *External validity* refers to the extent to which an association between an exposure and an outcome may be applied to populations other than the one in a study:
  - Internal validity is a prerequisite for external validity.
  - Subsequently, patient selection/exclusion criteria are common threats to external validity.

Research Oversight and Ethics

- All research involving human subjects requires *Institutional Review Board* (IRB) review to ensure scientific validity, risk minimization, and protection of participant rights.
- In critical care, informed consent often relies on surrogate decision makers or may qualify for deferred or waived consent in emergency research.
- Ethical standards include fair subject selection, favorable risk-benefit balance, and transparency in reporting results.
- Conflicts of interest—particularly common in device and pharmaceutical research—must be disclosed and managed to preserve study integrity.

Value

- *Value* in health care may be defined using quality, safety, cost, and patient experience. Common concepts in health care improvement include the following:
  - *Outcome measures* are events that patients achieve, such as walking 12 weeks after knee replacement that are tracked for performance measurement.
    - Outcomes measures often require costly follow-up or are very rare (mortality).
  - *Process measures* are interventions made for patients, such as timely administration of antibiotics for patients who are septic that are tracked to improve quality.
    - Process measures may help to guide care but are often poor surrogates for outcome measures.
  - *Risk adjustment* is a statistical technique used to improve comparisons between or among care episodes by accounting for baseline differences in patient characteristics (eg, age, comorbidities, illness severity), enabling fair comparison of outcomes across different patient populations or institutions (eg, using Acute Physiology and Chronic Health Evaluation (APACHE) scores to compare ICU mortality rates).
    - Outcome measures may be risk adjusted.
    - Process measures are not risk adjusted.
- **Patient experience and patient-centered outcomes**
  - As health systems shift toward value-based care, assessments of communication quality, emotional support, shared decision-making, and care coordination have become core quality metrics.
  - ICU-specific experience instruments solicit feedback from patients, families and surrogate decision makers.
  - *Patient-centered outcomes* include functional recovery, cognitive health, psychological well-being, and caregiver burden—domains that reflect the long-term impact of critical illness and the prevalence of PICS.
  - Incorporating *patient experience* into quality frameworks broadens the definition of success from survival alone to achieving meaningful recovery aligned with patient values.

Quality Improvement

- *Quality improvement (QI)* efforts in critical care often use structured frameworks for reducing variation, enhancing reliability, and improving adherence to evidence-based practices
  - Frameworks such as Plan-Do-Study-Act cycles, Lean methodology, and Six Sigma emphasize iterative testing of changes, real-time feedback, and frontline engagement.
  - Successful QI depends on consistent definitions of measures (eg, ventilator-associated events, medication reconciliation accuracy), automated data capture when possible, and transparent reporting dashboards.
  - Embedding QI into daily workflows—using standardized rounding tools, daily goal sheets, and checklists—enhances both team communication and patient outcomes.

Prognostic Scoring Systems

- *Prognostic scoring systems* (eg, APACHE, Sequential Organ Failure Assessment [SOFA]) are used for risk stratification, benchmarking, and evaluation of outcomes in ICU populations.
- These systems quantify illness severity by integrating physiologic variables, laboratory values, and chronic health conditions into validated predictive models.
- Severity scores support clinical decision-making, allow for fair comparison of outcomes across institutions, and enable risk adjustment of mortality, length of stay, and resource use.
- The SOFA score provides a dynamic measure of evolving organ dysfunction and is commonly used as a primary or secondary end point in sepsis and critical care trials.
- Emerging data-driven models (eg, machine learning–based risk prediction) hold promise but must meet standards of calibration, discrimination, and external validation before routine clinical adoption.

Acknowledgments

We gratefully acknowledge the contributions of the previous edition author, Joseph Hyder, as portions of those chapters have been retained in this revision.

SUGGESTED READINGS

Curtis JR, Cook DJ, Wall RJ, et al. Intensive care unit quality improvement: a "how-to" guide for the interdisciplinary team. *Crit Care Med*. 2006; 34(1):211-218.

Desai N, Gross J. Scoring systems in the critically ill: uses, cautions, and future directions. *BJA Educ*. 2019;19(7):212-218.

Fletcher, GS (2021). *Clinical Epidemiology: The Essentials* (6th ed.). Lippincott Williams & Wilkins.

Nozari A, Stelfox HT, Bittner EA. Evidence-based practice and basic statistics in critical care. In: Bigatello LM, ed. *Critical Care Handbook of the Massachusetts General Hospital*. 5th ed. Lippincott Williams & Wilkins; 2010:225-235.

Sevransky JE, Checkley W, Martin GS. Critical care trial design and interpretation: a primer. *Crit Care Med*. 2010;38(9):1882-1889.

Teisberg E, Wallace S, O'Hara S. Defining and implementing value-based health care: a strategic framework. *Acad Med*. 2020;95(5):682-685.

SECTION 29

Hospital Infection Control and Isolation Techniques

Section Editor: Marvin G. Chang

29.1

Hospital Infection Control and Isolation Techniques

Bijan Safaee Fakhr and Lorenzo Berra

Isolation Techniques

- In the ICU, infection control programs focus on preventing device-related infections such as central line–associated bloodstream infection (CLABSI), catheter-associated urinary tract infection (CAUTI), and hospital- and ventilator-associated pneumonia (HAP/VAP).
- Infection control measures must be undertaken to decrease the risk of nosocomial infections and prevent transmission of blood-borne pathogens such as human immunodeficiency virus (HIV), hepatitis B virus (HBV), and hepatitis C virus (HCV); airborne pathogens such as SARS-CoV-2, *Mycobacterium tuberculosis*, influenza, and respiratory syncytial virus; and gastrointestinal pathogens such as *Clostridium difficile* between patients and intensive care unit (ICU) staff.
- Universal precautions apply to all patients and health care professionals, regardless of underlying diseases.
  - Barrier precautions and thorough handwashing are required when there is potential for contact with blood and other bodily secretions and fluids, as these may harbor infectious agents.
  - Barriers include face masks, gloves, protective eyewear or face shields, and gowns.
- Special precautions, including contact, airborne, and droplet precautions
  - They are used to limit the transmission of antibiotic-resistant bacteria from patients to health care workers and other patients, to limit the spread of viruses and bacteria present in respiratory secretions, and to protect immunocompromised hosts from infection (reverse isolation).
    - Reverse isolation, including neutropenic precautions, aims to reduce exposure to exogenous pathogens in profoundly immunocompromised patients such as hematopoietic stem cell transplant recipients and those receiving intensive induction chemotherapy for acute leukemia. Strategies include HEPA filtered positive pressure rooms when available, meticulous hand hygiene, visitor screening, and avoiding fresh flowers and plants.
- Contact precautions for multidrug-resistant organisms (MDROs)
  - General approach: Contact Precautions (gown and gloves for room entry and patient/environmental contact) are widely used to prevent transmission of MDROs in healthcare settings.
  - Methicillin-resistant Staphylococcus aureus (MRSA) and vancomycin-resistant Enterococcus (VRE)
    - Traditional: The Centers for Disease Control and Prevention (CDC) and the Healthcare Infection Control Practices Advisory Committee (HICPAC) recommend Contact Precautions for patients colonized or infected with MRSA or VRE.
    - Evolving evidence: In units with strong "horizontal" infection-prevention measures (high hand-hygiene adherence, daily chlorhexidine bathing, rigorous environmental cleaning, device-associated infection-prevention bundles), several hospitals have reported safely discontinuing routine Contact Precautions for endemic MRSA and VRE without clear increases in infection rates. Trials such as REDUCE MRSA and BUGG support the effectiveness of universal CHG-based strategies and suggest limited added benefit from further intensifying gown/glove use alone.
    - Current practice: Policies now vary by institution, but CDC/HICPAC still recommend Contact Precautions for MRSA and VRE, especially in

high-risk settings. For board exams, MRSA or VRE in the stem should still prompt Contact Precautions.

- High-consequence MDROs
  - Carbapenem-resistant Enterobacterales (CRE), carbapenemase-producing organisms (CPO), multidrug-resistant (MDR) Acinetobacter baumannii, and MDR Pseudomonas aeruginosa: Generally managed with Contact Precautions because of limited treatment options, high mortality, and transmission potential; many institutions add single rooms, dedicated equipment, and sometimes active surveillance of high-risk contacts.
  - Extended-spectrum beta-lactamase (ESBL)–producing organisms: Institutional policies vary; some hospitals use Contact Precautions routinely, while others rely mainly on horizontal measures and reserve Contact Precautions for higher-risk situations (e.g., uncontrolled diarrhea, draing wounds, or during outbreaks).

- Clostridioides difficile requires contact precautions plus enhanced measures::
  - Sporicidal environmental cleaning: Use an EPA-registered sporicidal disinfectant, such as a bleach-based product (≈1,000–5,000 ppm sodium hypochlorite), for daily and terminal cleaning of rooms housing patients with C. difficile infection (CDI).
  - Hand hygiene (evolving guidance): Historically, many guidelines and hospital policies emphasized soap and water after caring for CDI patients and often restricted alcohol-based hand rub (ABHR) because alcohol is not sporicidal. The 2022 SHEA/IDSA CDI prevention update acknowledges that the evidence for hand-hygiene method in CDI is low quality, suggests soap and water as the preferred method after caring for CDI patients, but also notes that facilities using ABHR have not seen higher CDI rates and that "soap-only" policies may reduce overall hand-hygiene compliance and increase other HAIs. Current CDC hand-hygiene guidance reflects this balance: ABHR remains the preferred method in most situations, including care of patients with CDI, with soap and water used when hands are visibly soiled and as an added step during CDI outbreaks, and access to ABHR should not be restricted.
  - Antimicrobial stewardship: Target high-risk agents (e.g., fluoroquinolones, clindamycin, broad-spectrum cephalosporins, carbapenems) and use the narrowest effective spectrum and shortest effective duration.
  - Diagnostic stewardship: Test only unformed (diarrheal) stool from patients with new-onset unexplained diarrhea (e.g., ≥3 unformed stools in 24 hours); avoid repeat testing within 7 days and do not perform "test-of-cure," as patients may remain colonized after successful treatment.
  - Airborne and droplet precautions limit the spread of pathogens in respiratory secretions.
    - Airborne precautions are used to limit the spread of SARS-CoV-2, *Mycobacterium tuberculosis*, varicella-zoster virus (VZV), rubeola, and multiple other viruses.
      - Airborne precautions necessitate the use of N95 respirators or powered air-purifying respirators (PAPRs) to protect health care providers and visitors against smaller particles (<5 μm) that remain suspended in the air for prolonged periods and can travel over greater distances.
      - A private negative pressure isolation room is preferred for patients with airborne precautions. If unavailable, alternative measures (eg, portable high-efficiency particulate arresting [HEPA] filters, enhanced ventilation) may be implemented depending on the clinical scenario and resource availability (eg, rural or resource-limited settings).
    - Droplet precautions are used to limit the spread of infectious agents such as *Neisseria meningitidis*, *Haemophilus influenzae*, *Mycoplasma pneumoniae*, adenovirus, and rubella virus.
      - Droplet precautions require surgical masks to protect against larger respiratory droplets (>5 μm) that travel short distances, typically <3 ft. In contrast, airborne precautions involve N95 respirators or PAPRs for smaller particles (<5 μm) that can remain suspended in the air over longer periods and distances.
      - Patients are placed in a private room if possible to minimize the risk of transmission.

- Ebola virus disease and other viral hemorrhagic fevers require high-level isolation:
  - Precautions: Standard plus Contact and Droplet Precautions with eye protection for all patient interactions.
  - Enhanced PPE: Fluid-resistant or impermeable gown or coverall, double gloves, full face shield or goggles, and a fit-tested N95 (or higher-level) respirator, especially for aerosol-generating procedures.
  - Designated facilities: Care should occur in designated high-level isolation or CDC-designated Ebola Treatment Centers when available.
  - Trained personnel only: Only staff specifically trained and fit-tested for this PPE should provide direct care, with supervised donning and doffing.
  - Minimize procedures: Limit aerosol-generating and nonessential invasive procedures whenever possible.
- To decrease transmission of blood-borne pathogens (HIV, HBV, HCV), it is recommended to immediately discard used needles without recapping them into special puncture-proof receptacles.
- Limiting the use of antibiotics
  - The frequent use of broad-spectrum antibiotics in the ICU has resulted in the emergence of microorganisms resistant to multiple antibiotics.
  - In 2019, 1.27 million deaths (95% uncertainty interval [UI] 0.911-1.71) were directly attributed to antimicrobial resistance.
  - Core principles of antimicrobial stewardship in the ICU include obtaining appropriate cultures before starting therapy, choosing empiric agents based on the likely source and local resistance patterns, rapidly narrowing or discontinuing therapy once culture data are available, avoiding treatment of colonization alone, and using the shortest effective duration of therapy.
  - The emergence of VRE was particularly concerning because it suggested that other more virulent Gram-positives, such as methicillin-resistant *Staphylococcus aureus* (MRSA), may also become resistant to vancomycin.

- To reduce the risk of promoting antibiotic-resistant organisms, clinicians should prioritize using the narrowest effective spectrum of antibiotics.
- When broad empiric antibiotic therapy is required, the regimen should be rapidly narrowed based on the results of cultures.
- Prophylactic perioperative antibiotics should not be routinely administered for all surgeries. When indicated, discontinue at surgical closure for most procedures; max duration <24 hours for high-risk cases (e.g., cardiac surgery, orthopedic procedures with implants).
- Many institutions have policies that limit the use of various antibiotics, require justification for the use of certain agents, and have guidelines for routine perioperative antibiotic prophylaxis.

General/Universal Precautions

- General infection control
  - Microorganisms are transmitted in hospitals by contact, droplets, airborne, and contaminated items.
- Contact
  - The spread of microorganisms can occur by direct and indirect contact.
  - Transmission by hand to the body surface is much more common than indirect contact with a contaminated surface.
  - For example, almost all cases of MRSA are transmitted by hand contamination of health care providers.
- Droplets: particles > 5 μm in diameter
  - Droplets can only be transmitted over a short distance—< 3 ft.
  - They are transmitted through coughing and sneezing.
  - Droplets transmit microorganisms, including *N. meningitidis*, *H. influenzae*, *M. pneumoniae*, adenovirus, rubella virus, and coronavirus
- Airborne particles are smaller (<5 μm) than droplets.
  - They can remain in the air for a long period of time.
  - Tuberculosis (TB), measles, varicella, disseminated VZV, and coronavirus are spread by airborne particles.
- Contaminated items
  - Infection from contaminated items is uncommon but well documented, particularly when devices are improperly cleaned or sterilized.
  - However, improper sterilization of bronchoscopes and endoscopes has led to infection with microorganisms such as Pseudomonas aeruginosa, Serratia marcescens, and Carbapenem-resistant Enterobacteriaceae (CRE).
  - Special attention should be made to regular cleaning and disinfection of high-touch surfaces, proper reprocessing of shared equipment (e.g., blood pressure cuffs, ultrasound probes, ventilator accessories), and attention to sinks and water sources to prevent biofilm-associated outbreaks.
  - Improper disinfection of stethoscopes can also lead to the transmission of nosocomial pathogens. The Centers for Disease Control and Prevention (CDC) recommends cleaning stethoscopes after examining each patient.
- Environmental cleaning
  - CDC emphasizes a multimodal, systems-based approach to environmental cleaning and disinfection to prevent healthcare-associated infection
  - Use U.S. Environmental Protection Agency (EPA)–registered hospital disinfectants and follow label contact time.
  - Standardize cleaning protocols that emphasize the physical removal of soil (e.g., friction and scrubbing) and use methods that minimize dispersing dust (e.g., wet mopping, wet vacuuming, and wet dusting).
  - Provide training and competency checks for environmental services staff.
  - Audit cleaning (e.g., direct observation, fluorescent markers, or adenosine triphosphate (ATP) bioluminescence) as part of a monitoring program.
  - Prioritize high-touch surfaces (bed rails, call buttons, IV poles, door handles).
  - Perform thorough terminal cleaning after discharge. For most multidrug-resistant organisms (MDROs) (e.g., MRSA, VRE, many gram-negative MDROs), standard EPA-registered hospital disinfectants are sufficient when used with proper technique and full contact time; specialized products (e.g., sporicidal agents or agents with specific label claims) are reserved for pathogens such as Clostridioides difficile, Norovirus, and Candida auris.

Needlestick Injuries

- Safe disposal of sharps in specially designed, safe containers is warranted.
- According to the Occupational Safety and Health Administration (OSHA), 385,000 needle injuries from needles and other sharps occur annually in hospitals throughout the United States.
- After a sharps injury, immediate wound cleansing, prompt reporting, baseline and follow-up testing, and time-sensitive HIV and hepatitis B post-exposure prophylaxis should be instituted according to institutional and CDC guidelines.
- The most important pathogens transmitted include HIV, HBV, and HCV.
- Pathogen-Specific Post-Exposure Prophylaxis (PEP) and management:
  - HIV: PEP is highly time-sensitive. A 28-day course of antiretroviral medication should be initiated as soon as possible, ideally within hours and not later than 72 hours of the exposure.
  - Hepatitis B (HBV): Management depends on the healthcare worker's vaccination and immunity status. If the worker is unvaccinated, incompletely vaccinated, or a known non-responder, they should receive both Hepatitis B immunoglobulin (HBIg) and the HBV vaccination series.
  - Hepatitis C (HCV): There is no vaccine or post-exposure prophylaxis available for HCV. Management is limited to baseline testing and follow-up serological monitoring to detect infection, with referral for antiviral treatment if infection develops.
  - Source patient testing (HIV, HBV, HCV) should be performed with informed consent per state law and institutional policy; when source testing is unavailable or refused, manage the exposed worker based on exposure severity and epidemiologic risk, often as if the source were potentially infected.
- OSHA requires all health care facilities to implement plans to decrease the transmission of blood-borne pathogens.

- These include the following measures:
  - Annual education for health care workers regarding the minimization of transmission of blood-borne pathogens
  - Standard precautions for working with all patients
  - Hepatitis B immunization as preexposure prophylaxis
  - Decreasing the use of sharps (eg, prefilled syringes, safety, and closed blood-collection systems) and engineering tools to reduce the risk of injury with sharps (self-containing needle systems, special containers, etc)

Prevention of Catheter-Related Sepsis

- Central venous catheters are a major source of device-related infection in the ICU, most commonly manifesting as central line–associated bloodstream infections (CLABSIs).
- The average intravascular central venous catheter (CVC)-related bloodstream infection rate in the United States is 2.7 to 0.8 per 1,000 catheter days.
- Despite a 46% decrease in catheter-associated bloodstream infections, there are still ~30,100 central line–associated bloodstream infections per year in ICUs and wards.
- The cost attributed to CVC-related bloodstream infections has been estimated at 46,000 US dollars per case.
- The most common way a patient develops a catheter-associated bloodstream infection is through the migration of skin organisms into the catheter and along the surface of the catheter at the insertion site or through direct contamination of the access ports.
- Hence, line infections have become a focal point of concern for hospital administrations and regulating agencies.
- Recent evidence demonstrated that using protocolized efforts, CVC-related infections could be largely eliminated.
- Measures recommended include:
  - The education of clinicians about best practices for controlling infection is pivotal to implementing a successful program to decrease CVC-related bloodstream infections.
  - A central line cart with all necessary supplies should be provided.
  - Catheter site selection
    - Guidelines versus recent evidence on insertion site and CLABSI
      - Traditional guidelines recommend avoiding femoral sites and prefer subclavian over internal jugular to minimize infection risk (Centers for Disease Control and Prevention (CDC); Society for Healthcare Epidemiology of America, Infectious Diseases Society of America, and Association for Professionals in Infection Control and Epidemiology (SHEA/IDSA/APIC); and Asia Pacific Society of Infection Control (APSIC))
      - 3SITES trial demonstrated subclavian had lowest infection/thrombosis rates compared to internal jugular and femoral sites, though ultrasound guidance was used relatively infrequently
      - Recent large ICU cohorts including the French REAREZO study with modern insertion bundles (ultrasound guidance, chlorhexidine antisepsis, maximal sterile barriers, chlorhexidine dressings) show minimal infection rate differences between sites, with all achieving very low CLABSI rates when bundles are rigorously applied
    - Individualize site selection by balancing infection and mechanical risks
      - Avoid subclavian: Hemodialysis patients or those with advanced kidney disease (stenosis risk); severe coagulopathy (non-compressible site); severe hypoxemia, ARDS, or COPD (pneumothorax risk); morbid obesity (technical difficulty)
      - Prefer compressible sites (femoral/IJ): Severe coagulopathy, high bleeding risk
      - Avoid femoral: Obesity (higher groin colonization rates); longer anticipated duration (higher DVT risk with femoral)
      - Avoid IJ: Presence of tracheostomy (contamination risk from secretions); prefer subclavian or consider femoral
      - Consider: Operator ultrasound experience, mechanical complication risk (pneumothorax, arterial injury); for anticipated duration >14-21 days, consider PICC or tunneled catheter
    - Bundle adherence is more important than site selection
      - Essential bundle components: Ultrasound guidance (especially with experienced operators; reduces infections 32%), chlorhexidine-based antisepsis, maximal sterile barriers, chlorhexidine-impregnated dressings, insertion checklists
  - Aseptic technique is recommended for the insertion of CVCs.
  - The importance of infection control practices should be included in the training of health care providers.
  - Operators should disinfect their hands with alcohol-based hand rub.
  - Sterile gloves, gowns, caps, surgical masks, and eye protection should be worn for insertion of central lines. Everyone in the room should wear a hat and mask when placing the catheter.
  - Complete sterile barrier drapes should be used.
- Skin preparation with an alcohol-based chlorhexidine solution (e.g., ≥0.5% chlorhexidine in 70% alcohol, commonly 2% chlorhexidine in 70% isopropyl alcohol) is the recommended standard and has been shown to be more effective than povidone–iodine or alcohol alone in reducing central line–associated infections.
- During the insertion of a line, one team member should run a checklist to ensure adherence to infection control practices and be empowered to hold the procedure (in nonemergency situations) if these practices are not followed.
- If a central line is placed in an emergent situation without complete adherence to the aseptic technique, the catheter should be replaced as soon as possible when it is considered safe for patient management.
- The need for central venous access should be reevaluated at daily rounds, and catheters should be removed as early as possible.

Other Strategies

- Selection of catheters
  - The material and coating of catheters influence the incidence of line infections.
    - Bacterial adherence is decreased in catheters made from polyurethane, Teflon, and silicone elastomers.

It is, therefore, recommended that catheters be made from one of these materials.

- Heparin sodium bonding decreases the incidence of catheter-related thrombosis. While some evidence suggests heparin-bonded catheters may reduce infection rates, the CDC/HICPAC and SHEA/IDSA do not recommend routine heparin bonding for CLABSI prevention; when used, it is mainly for thrombosis mitigation and must be weighed against the risk of heparin-induced thrombocytopenia (HIT).

- Chlorhexidine/silver sulfadiazine–impregnated catheters lead to a significant reduction in catheter colonization and catheter-related bacteremia.
- Minocycline/rifampin-impregnated catheters decrease the rate of line infections.
  - The impregnation does not cause changes in antibiotic resistance.
- Number of catheter lumens
  - Multilumen catheters have a higher number of infections.
  - When possible, it is recommended to insert catheters with a lower number of lumens.

- Feedback regarding the number and rates of catheter-related bloodstream infections should be provided to the care team regularly.
- These standardized insertion and maintenance bundles, checklists, and feedback of infection rates are central ICU quality-improvement initiatives and are required by many regulatory and accrediting bodies.
- Change of central lines
  - Routine changes of central lines, either by new stick or by guidewire change, do not decrease the incidence of line infection. Guidewire change should be avoided if the catheter is suspected or confirmed as a source of infection.
  - Instead of scheduled line changes, it is recommended that the patient be evaluated for line infection on a continuous basis.
- Percutaneously inserted central catheters (PICCs) are inserted centrally via peripheral arm veins, generally at the antecubital fossa.
  - Maintenance and follow-up are important since the line infection risk in the hospital setting is comparable to or even higher than that of central lines.
- Nonvascular transcutaneous devices (e.g., chest tubes, surgical drains, external ventricular drains, and enteral feeding tubes) can also serve as foci of infection; prevention principles include aseptic insertion, minimal manipulation, closed drainage systems when feasible, and prompt removal when no longer needed.
- Prevention of Ventilator-Associated Pneumonia (VAP) and Hospital-Acquired Pneumonia (HAP)
  - Hospital-Acquired Pneumonia (HAP):
    - Develops ≥ 48 hours after hospital admission
    - Occurs in patients who are NOT mechanically ventilated
    - This timing excludes infections present or incubating at admission
  - Ventilator-Associated Pneumonia (VAP):
    - Develops ≥ 48 hours after endotracheal intubation
    - Specifically occurs in mechanically ventilated patients
    - The 48-hour threshold helps distinguish it from pneumonia that was already developing before intubation
    - VAP affects 5–15% of ventilated patients with mortality rates of 20–50%, prolonging mechanical ventilation by 7–11.5 days.
  - Essential prevention practices (2022 SHEA/IDSA/APIC guidelines)
    - Avoidance of unnecessary intubation and reintubation and minimizing the duration of mechanical ventilation.; use noninvasive ventilation when appropriate
    - Minimize sedation with protocolized daily interruption and spontaneous breathing trials
    - Head of bed elevation 30–45 degrees (unless contraindicated)
    - Oral care with toothbrushing daily
    - Early mobilization and enteral nutrition
    - Use of endotracheal tubes with subglottic secretion drainage in patients expected to require prolonged mechanical ventilation.
  - Practices NOT recommended as VAP prevention strategies: chlorhexidine oral care, stress ulcer prophylaxis, probiotics
- Prevention of catheter-associated urinary tract infection is a key component of ICU infection prophylaxis, along with CLABSI and ventilator-associated pneumonia prevention bundles.
  - UTIs affect about 600,000 patients in acute care hospitals annually, comprising 1.8% of all annual hospitalizations, with 80% being non–catheter related.
  - The most common organisms include *Escherichia coli*, *Enterococcus*, *Klebsiella*, and *Pseudomonas*. In immunocompromised patients, *Candida* is another important organism involved.
  - About 1% of these patients develop severe Gram-negative sepsis with often multiresistant bacteria.
  - Similar to line infections, UTIs may be regarded as preventable complications that could have implications for future payments.
  - Catheter placement
    - Indwelling urinary catheters should be placed only in patients for whom frequent measurement of urinary output is beneficial.
    - Alternatives to indwelling devices, such as condom catheters or intermittent catheterization, should be considered.
    - Indwelling urinary catheters must be placed using a strict aseptic technique by trained personnel.
    - For most adult patients, a 14F–16F urinary catheter is appropriate; larger sizes may be used when clinically indicated (e.g., hematuria or high sediment load)
    - Smaller catheters are preferable in terms of infection prevention.
  - Catheter maintenance and removal
    - Clinicians should wash their hands and wear gloves prior to handling the indwelling catheter or drainage tubing.
    - Closed drainage systems should be utilized.
    - The incidence of UTI increases with breaks in the drainage system.
    - Catheters should be secured to the patient's leg to prevent movement or traction of the catheter.
    - Catheters should not be changed unless there is frequent occlusion of the catheter that requires repeated irrigation.

- Routine irrigation should be avoided.
- The most often cited strategies for avoiding catheter-associated UTIs are the following:
  - Daily reevaluation for prompt urinary catheter removal is crucial, as each day poses a 3–10% risk of bacteriuria, with 20–25% of those cases progressing to a symptomatic UTI.
  - Use of closed drainage systems.

Acknowledgments

We gratefully acknowledge the contributions of previous edition author(s), Sheri Berg Jessica Hines and Ulrich Schmidt, as portions of those chapters have been retained in this revision.

SUGGESTED READINGS

Asia Pacific Society of Infection Control (APSIC). Revised guidelines for prevention of central line-associated bloodstream infections (CLABSI) 2024. Published January 2025. Accessed 2026 Nov 16. https://apsic-apac.org/

Boulet B, Pereira B, Dupouy J, et al. Real-time ultrasound-guided versus landmark method for central venous catheterization: a systematic review and meta-analysis with trial sequential analysis. Crit Care. 2024; 28(1):378. doi:10.1186/s13054-024-05164-y

Buetti N, Marschall J, Drees M, et al. Strategies to prevent central line-associated bloodstream infections in acute-care hospitals: 2022 Update. Infect Control Hosp Epidemiol. 2022;43(5):553-569.

Centers for Disease Control and Prevention. Considerations for Reducing Risk: Surfaces in Healthcare Facilities. Published April 15, 2024. Accessed November 16, 2025. https://www.cdc.gov/healthcare-associated-infections/hcp/infection-control/index.html

Clinical Safety: Hand Hygiene for Healthcare Workers. Centers for Disease Control and Prevention. Published February 27, 2024. Accessed November 17, 2025. https://www.cdc.gov/clean-hands/hcp/clinical-safety/index.html

Clinical Guidance for C. diff Infection Prevention in Acute Care Facilities. Centers for Disease Control and Prevention. Published March 8, 2024. Accessed November 17, 2025. https://www.cdc.gov/c-diff/hcp/clinical-guidance/index.html

Cosme V, Massart N, Reizine F, et al; REAREZO Study Group. Central venous catheter-related infection: does insertion site still matter? A French multicentric cohort study. Intensive Care Med. 2024;50(11):1830-1840. doi:10.1007/s00134-024-07615-0

Centers for Disease Control and Prevention. Guidelines for environmental infection control in health-care facilities: recommendations of CDC and the Healthcare Infection Control Practices Advisory Committee (HICPAC). MMWR Recomm Rep. 2003;52(RR-10):1-48. Updated July 2019. Accessed November 16, 2025. https://www.cdc.gov/infection-control/media/pdfs/Guideline-Environmental-H.pdf

Centers for Disease Control and Prevention. *Bloodstream infection (BSI) events: central line-associated bloodstream infection (CLABSI) and non-central line-associated bloodstream infection*. 2024. Accessed June 30, 2024. https://www.cdc.gov/nhsn/psc/bsi/index.html

Centers for Disease Control and Prevention. *Paper presented at: Proceedings of the National Sharps Injury Prevention Meeting*. September 12, 2005; Crown Plaza Atlanta Airport Hotel, Atlanta, GA. https://www.cdc.gov/infection-control/media/pdfs/Sharps-Safety-Workbook-2008-P.pdf

Harris AD, Pineles L, Belton B, et al; Benefits of Universal Glove and Gown (BUGG) Investigators. Universal glove and gown use and acquisition of antibiotic-resistant bacteria in the ICU: a randomized trial. JAMA.

Huang SS, Septimus E, Kleinman K, et al; CDC Prevention Epicenters Program and the AHRQ DECIDE Network and Healthcare-Associated Infections Program. Targeted versus universal decolonization to prevent ICU infection. N Engl J Med. 2013;368(24):2255-22

Kalil AC, Metersky ML, Klompas M, et al. Management of adults with hospital-acquired and ventilator-associated pneumonia: 2016 clinical practice guidelines by the Infectious Diseases Society of America and the American Thoracic Society. Clin Infect Dis. 2016;63(5):e61-e111. doi:10.1093/cid/ciw353

Klompas M, Branson R, Cawcutt K, et al. Strategies to prevent ventilator-associated pneumonia, ventilator-associated events, and nonventilator hospital-acquired pneumonia in acute-care hospitals: 2022 Update. Infection Control & Hospital Epidemiology. 2022;43(6):687-713. doi:10.1017/ice.2022.88

Kociolek LK, Gerding DN, Carrico R, et al. Strategies to prevent Clostridioides difficile infections in acute-care hospitals: 2022 Update. Infect Control Hosp Epidemiol. 2023;44(4):527-549.

Kociolek LK, Gerding DN, Carrico R, Carling P, Donskey CJ, Dumyati G, Kuhar DT, Loo VG, Maragakis LL, Pogorzelska-Maziarz M, Sandora TJ, Weber DJ, Yokoe D, Dubberke ER. Strategies to prevent *Clostridioides difficile* infections in acute-care hospitals: 2022 Update. Infect Control Hosp Epidemiol. 2023 Apr;44(4):527-549.

Kollef M. SMART approaches for reducing nosocomial infections in the ICU. *Chest*. 2008;134(2):447-456.

McGlynn EA, Asch SM, Adams J, et al. The quality of health care delivered to adults in the United States. *N Engl J Med*. 2003;348(26):2635-2645.

O'Grady NP, Alexander M, Burns LA, et al; Healthcare Infection Control Practices Advisory Committee (HICPAC). Guidelines for the prevention of intravascular catheter-related infections. Clin Infect Dis. 2011; 52(9):e162-e193.

Parienti JJ, Mongardon N, Mégarbane B, et al; 3SITES Study Group. Intravascular complications of central venous catheterization by insertion site. N Engl J Med. 2015;373(13):1220-1229.

Pronovost PJ, Berenholtz SM, Goeschel CA. Improving the quality of measurement and evaluation in quality improvement efforts. *Am J Med Qual*. 2008;23(2):143-146.

Pronovost P, Needham D, Berenholtz S, et al. An intervention to decrease catheter-related bloodstream infections in the ICU. *N Engl J Med*. 2006;355:2725.

Rutala WA, Weber DJ, Healthcare Infection Control Practices Advisory Committee. Guideline for Disinfection and Sterilization in Healthcare Facilities, 2008. Centers for Disease Control and Prevention; 2008. Updated June 2024. Accessed November 16, 2025. https://www.cdc.gov/infection-control/media/pdfs/Guideline-Disinfection-H.pdf

SECTION 30

Emergent Airway Management

Section Editor: Edward A. Bittner

30.1

Emergent Airway Management

Omar Hyder

- Out-of-OR (operating room) emergent airway management (EAM) is typically performed in the emergency department (ED), the intensive care unit (ICU), or on hospital inpatient floors.
- EAM exists on a spectrum of urgency, from needing immediate securement of airway (eg, inability to protect airway against active aspiration) to situations where opportunity exists prior to intubation to quickly address severe physiologic abnormalities that may otherwise increase the risk of adverse outcomes (eg, severe hypovolemia).
- Rapid sequence intubation (RSI) is the most frequently used technique to secure the airway in EAM.
- RSI consists of several steps:
  - Preoxygenation with a tight-fitting face mask or bilevel positive airway pressure (BiPAP) +/− high-flow nasal cannula
  - Administration of induction agent and muscle relaxant (followed by 30-60 seconds delay)
  - Laryngoscopy and endotracheal intubation
  - Confirmation of endotracheal placement of tube with end-tidal carbon dioxide ($EtCO_2$) detection

Indications for Emergent Airway Management

- Respiratory failure (pulmonary edema, massive aspiration, pulmonary embolism, etc)
- Cardiac arrest/profound hemodynamic instability
- Severe metabolic acidosis (sepsis, cardiogenic shock)
- Altered mental status (stroke, intoxication, oversedation)
- Inability to protect airways (upper airway hemorrhage, copious secretions)
- Trauma

Complications of Emergent Airway Management

- Up to 45% patients may have complications with EAM, significantly higher than elective intubation.
- Physiologic complications: hypoxemia, hypercarbia, hypotension, hypertension, arrhythmias, or cardiac arrest
- Traumatic complications: dental injury, soft tissue injury, bleeding, tracheal injury, or arytenoid cartilage dislocation
- Procedure-related complications: aspiration of gastric contents, mainstem intubation, esophageal intubation, or bronchospasm
- Airway response team (ART)
  - Dedicated emergency ARTs improve patient outcomes.
  - ART team members have clearly assigned roles: team leader/event manager, airway proceduralist, airway assistant, and medication manager
  - ART team needs to have at least two practitioners with experience in EAM. This can be a combination of anesthesiologists, emergency medicine physicians, intensivists, and surgeons with experience in surgical airway management.

Procedure

- Evaluation of the patient
  - It is important to preempt difficulty in EAM and plan accordingly.
  - This can be anatomic (eg, difficult airway), physiologic (eg, severe heart failure), technical (eg, laryngoscopy during chest compressions), environmental (eg, intubation on cafeteria floor), or a combination of these.
  - Anesthesia/intubation records should be reviewed if available.

- Preparation for hemodynamic optimization
  - Hemodynamic instability during and after EAM is much more common than failed intubations. Preparations should be made to mitigate it.
  - Point-of-care transthoracic echocardiography can help with the assessment of gross cardiac function and hypovolemia.
  - Consider placement of an arterial line for beat-to-beat monitoring during induction in hemodynamically unstable patients.
- Vasopressors
  - Push-dose vasopressors should be available to use with induction agents to mitigate hypotension.
  - Use of an infusion of a vasopressor drug at a dosage suitable for the patient's preinduction hemodynamics and physiologic reserve may decrease periprocedural hypotension.
- Intravenous fluids
  - Administration of sedative medications to severely hypovolemic patients can drastically drop cardiac preload and result in cardiac arrest.
  - Every attempt should be made to resuscitate patients who are clinically hypovolemic prior to administration of induction medications.
  - Aggressive fluid loading with crystalloids or transfusion of blood products should be considered, as indicated by the clinical situation.
  - Fluid loading in patients without clinical signs of hypovolemia has not shown benefit.
- Predictors of difficult intubation
  - History of difficult intubation
  - Mallampati score III or IV
  - Limited neck range of motion
  - Short thyromental distance (<3 fingers)
  - Small mouth opening (<3 fingers)
- Preparation
  - Preoxygenation
    - In many critically ill patients requiring EAM, preoxygenation is not as effective as in elective circumstances in healthy patients.
    - Poor inspiratory effort, decreased functional residual capacity (FRC), increased metabolic demand, and intrapulmonary shunts contribute to quick desaturation.
    - Noninvasive ventilation (NIV/BiPAP) is a reasonable alternative to a conventional tight-fitting bag mask.
    - If a patient has been started on NIV for respiratory distress, then it should be continued until the very moment of laryngoscopy.
  - Aspiration precautions
    - All patients should be approached as having a full stomach.
    - Well-functioning suction with Yankauer should be present.
    - Nasogastric tube (NGT) (≥12F) should be placed on suction if patient already has one.
    - Gastrostomy tubes should be opened to gravity or placed on suction.
- Pharmacology
  - Induction agents
    - Dosing of induction agents needs to be tailored to each individual patient situation based on age, weight, physiologic reserve, and comorbidities.
  - Etomidate
    - Fast onset with increased cardiovascular stability
    - Compared to ketamine for unstable patients, etomidate produced more adrenal insufficiency, but no conclusive evidence that it increases mortality.
  - Ketamine
    - Preserves respiratory drive and produces sympathomimetic effect resulting in increases in heart rate, blood pressure, cardiac output, and myocardial oxygen demand
    - Maintains hemodynamics in hypovolemic and unstable patients
    - Dissociative effects allow agitated patients to preoxygenate with spontaneous breathing prior to administration of paralytic and apnea.
    - Rarely precipitates myocardial ischemia in the presence of severe coronary artery disease
  - Propofol
    - Should be used with caution in EAM; only in controlled conditions with vasopressor support in patients with robust physiologic reserve
    - Fast onset and dose-dependent intense suppression of consciousness and sympathetic drive, resulting in excellent intubating conditions at the cost of potentially severe hemodynamic instability
    - Negative inotropic effect and decreases systemic venous resistance (SVR) resulting in hypotension
    - Among critically ill patients, propofol is an independent predictor of postinduction hypotension and increased mortality.
  - Muscle relaxants
    - Use of neuromuscular blockers is standard of care for emergency intubation.
    - Rocuronium
      - Nondepolarizing muscle relaxant, has a relatively fast onset at appropriate dosing (1.2 mg/kg ideal body weight [IBW])
      - Onset: 45 to 60 seconds
      - Rapidly reversible with Sugammadex (16 mg/kg actual body weight)
    - Succinylcholine
      - Depolarizing muscle relaxant with very fast onset and produces superior conditions for intubation within 45 to 60 seconds
      - Due to depolarizing action, it briefly increases intraocular and intracranial pressures and can cause bradycardia.
      - Contraindicated in certain patient populations as it can cause hyperkalemia. The list is extensive and includes, but is not limited to, patients with recent trauma, recent burns, myopathies, prolonged immobilization, end-stage renal disease, and acetylcholine esterase deficiency.
- Airway equipment and techniques
  - Videolaryngoscopy
    - Videolaryngoscopy is the first-line technique for endotracheal intubation. It has demonstrated higher first-pass success (>90%), and multiple practitioners can view the airway status.
    - Several variations of videolaryngoscopes are available. Hyperangulated and nonhyperangulated blade types are available in both handheld and wheeled-tower form factors.

        - There are subtle differences in technique, ergonomics, and failure mechanisms with each type of device. The operator should choose based on their experience and availability.
        - Bougie introducer/Frova intubating stylet increases the success rate of intubation, especially in cases of poor glottic view (grade III-IV) when using direct laryngoscopy or videolaryngoscopy with Mac-type blades.
    - Laryngeal mask airway
        - Multiple sizes of laryngeal mask airways (LMAs) should be present in emergent airway kits.
        - Will augment ventilation when difficult intubation or ventilation is encountered
        - Can be used as an adjunct to fiberoptic intubation
    - Emergency cricothyroidotomy and percutaneous tracheostomy are the procedures of choice for establishing a surgical airway, depending on institutional practice and availability of skilled providers.
    - Awake fiberoptic intubation should be used in patients with a history of known difficult airway or a very high clinical suspicion. It is typically not a convenient procedure in EAM settings. Consider performing awake intubation in controlled settings in an OR with a surgeon on standby for percutaneous tracheal access.
- Post intubation care
    - After intubation, ensure adequate sedation as most patients will be paralyzed and/or uncomfortable.
    - Propofol, combination of benzodiazepines with opioids, or dexmedetomidine can be used for sedation.
    - Mechanical ventilation should be provided using lung-protective strategy: tidal volume of 6 to 8 mL/kg of IBW and positive end-expiratory pressure (PEEP) 5 to 10 cm H_2O.
    - Due to high incidence of hypotension after intubation, many patients frequently require volume resuscitation and administration of vasopressors.

SUGGESTED READINGS

Acquisto NM, Mosier JM, Bittner EA, et al. Society of Critical Care Medicine clinical practice guidelines for rapid sequence intubation in the critically ill adult patient. *Crit Care Med.* 2023;51(10):1411-1430.

Apfelbaum JL, Hagberg CA, Connis RT, et al. 2022 American Society of Anesthesiologists practice guidelines for management of the difficult airway. *Anesthesiology.* 2022;136(1):31-81.

Downing J, Yardi I, Ren C, et al. Prevalence of peri-intubation major adverse events among critically ill patients: a systematic review and meta analysis. *Am J Emerg Med.* 2023;71:200-216.

Frerk C, Mitchell VS, McNarry AF, et al. Difficult Airway Society 2015 guidelines for management of unanticipated difficult intubation in adults. *Br J Anaesth.* 2015;115(6):827-848.

Kornas RL, Owyang CG, Sakles JC, Foley LJ, Mosier JM. Evaluation and management of the physiologically difficult airway: consensus recommendations from Society for Airway Management. *Anesth Analg.* 2021;132(2):395-405.

Matchett G, Gasanova I, Riccio CA, et al. Etomidate versus ketamine for emergency endotracheal intubation: a randomized clinical trial. *Intensive Care Med.* 2022;48(1):78-91.

Pirotte A, Panchananam V, Finley M, Petz A, Herrmann T. Current considerations in emergency airway management. *Curr Emerg Hosp Med Rep.* 2022;10(4):73-86.

Prekker ME, Driver BE, Trent SA, et al. Video versus direct laryngoscopy for tracheal intubation of critically ill adults. *N Engl J Med.* 2023;389(5):418-429.

Russotto V, Myatra SN, Laffey JG, et al. Intubation practices and adverse peri-intubation events in critically ill patients from 29 countries. *JAMA.* 2021;325(12):1164-1172.

Tankard KA, Sharifpour M, Chang MG, Bittner EA. Design and implementation of airway response teams to improve the practice of emergency airway management. *J Clin Med.* 2022;11(21):6336.

30.2

Tracheostomy Complications

Christopher Piccuito and Lorenzo Berra

- Tracheostomy tubes are surgically placed using an open surgical or percutaneous technique.
- Immediate and late complications are similar between the two surgical techniques.

Immediate Complications

- Bleeding
    - A small amount of blood from the tracheostomy site is normal after placement.
    - Injury to anterior jugular vein
        - Hold pressure on the site of bleeding
        - May require ligation in severe cases
    - Frequent or improper tracheal suctioning
        - Avoid deep suctioning past the end of the tracheostomy tube.
        - Use safe suction pressure (maximum −200 mm Hg).
- Pneumothorax
    - Air collection in the pleural space
    - Signs and symptoms: early recognition is critical.
        - Chest crepitus
        - Increased heart rate
        - Decreased blood pressure
        - Decreased Spo_2
        - Asymmetrical chest rise
        - Diminished breath sounds
        - Jugular venous distention
    - Obtain chest x-ray.
    - Tension pneumothorax is an emergent situation.
    - Intervention to relieve pneumothorax
        - Needle decompression
        - Insert chest tube.
- Subcutaneous emphysema
    - Air or gas that has leaked into the tissues
    - Signs and symptoms
        - Chest or neck crepitus
        - Swelling around the neck

- Chest pain
- Ginkgo leaf sign on chest x-ray
- Could indicate pneumothorax

- Injury to recurrent lateral nerve
    - Recurrent lateral nerve is close to the tracheostomy surgical site.
    - Damage to the nerve may result in vocal cord paralysis.
    - Consider upper airway evaluation if the patient cannot tolerate a tracheostomy tube cap or speaking valve.
- Occluded tracheostomy tube
    - Can present as partial or total occlusion
    - Potential emergency
    - Signs and symptoms
        - Blood/tissue/phlegm visualized in the tracheostomy tube
        - Difficulty breathing or accessory muscle use
        - No exhaled air from the tracheostomy tube
        - Increased heart rate and respiratory rate
        - Decreased Spo_2
        - No chest rise with manual ventilation through the tracheostomy tube
        - Unable or difficult to pass a suction catheter through the tracheostomy tube
    - Assessing the tracheostomy tube in the following order:
        - Remove the tracheostomy cap or speaking valve.
        - Remove the inner cannula, if present.
        - Attempt to pass a suction catheter through the tracheostomy tube.
        - Deflate the tracheostomy tube cuff, if present.
        - Assess the airflow through the tracheostomy tube and the patient's mouth.
        - Assess the patient's vital signs.
        - If the patient is stable, may use bronchoscopy to assess the patency of the tracheostomy tube.
        - If there is no improvement, remove the tracheostomy tube and assess the patient's airway.
- Infection
    - Daily wound care is imperative.
    - Frequent tracheostomy tube changes to eliminate biofilm (every 30-60 days).
- Accidental displacement or dislodgement of tracheostomy tube
    - Dislodged: tracheostomy out of airway
    - Displaced into false passage: tracheostomy in the pretracheal space
    - Can occur at any point when a tracheostomy tube is present
    - Loss of the airway has a high mortality rate.
    - Patients with thick necks are at higher risk due to more pretracheal tissue.
    - Signs and symptoms
        - Difficulty breathing or accessory muscle use
        - No exhaled air from the tracheostomy tube
        - Increased heart rate and respiratory rate
        - Decreased Spo_2
        - No chest rise with manual ventilation through the tracheostomy tube
        - Unable or difficult to pass a suction catheter through the tracheostomy tube
        - Evidence of subcutaneous emphysema or pneumothorax
    - Assessing the tracheostomy tube in the following order:
        - Remove the tracheostomy cap or speaking valve.
        - Remove the inner cannula, if present.
        - Attempt to pass a suction catheter through the tracheostomy tube.
        - Deflate the tracheostomy tube cuff, if present.
        - Assess the airflow through the tracheostomy tube and the patient's mouth.
        - Assess the patient's vital signs.
        - If the patient is stable, may use bronchoscopy to assess the patency and the position of the tracheostomy tube.
        - If there is no improvement, remove the tracheostomy tube, assess the patient's airway, and provide appropriate support.
    - Prevention
        - Upon initial tracheostomy tube placement, secure the flange to the patient's skin with sutures.
        - Assess for proper tracheostomy tube securement.
            - Tracheostomy ties or securement devices should not be too tight or loose.
        - Initially, use sedation or paralytic for critical airways.
        - Use a flex-tube adapter to connect the tracheostomy tube to the mechanical ventilator.

Late Complications

- Tracheal stenosis
    - Abnormal narrowing of the trachea
    - May develop from prolonged endotracheal and/or tracheostomy tube placement
    - Tracheal scarring due to pressure injury
    - Signs and symptoms
        - Increased cough
        - Difficulty clearing secretions
        - High peak airway pressures with mechanical ventilation
        - Stridor
        - Inability to tolerate a tracheostomy cap or speaking valve
    - Diagnostics
        - Chest x-ray
        - Neck and chest computed tomography (CT) scan
        - Flexible bronchoscopy
    - Prevention
        - Monitor tracheostomy tube cuff pressure routinely.
        - Maintain between 20 and 30 cm H_2O.
        - Use an appropriately sized tracheostomy tube to limit pressure caused by the tube.
    - Treatment
        - Consider using an extra-long tracheostomy tube to bypass the point of stenosis.
- Tracheomalacia
    - Weakness in the airway wall, resulting in excessive airway narrowing during expiration
    - Tracheostomy or endotracheal intubation can damage the tracheal cartilage at the stoma or cuff site (friction/overinflation), respectively, weakening the tracheal wall.

- Signs and symptoms
  - Tracheostomy tube cuff leak
  - Need for overinflation of tracheostomy tube cuff
  - Difficulty breathing
- Diagnostics
  - Flexible bronchoscopy
  - Dynamic airway CT scan
- Prevention
  - Monitor tracheostomy tube cuff pressure routinely.
  - Maintain between 20 and 30 cm H_2O.
  - Use an appropriately sized tracheostomy tube to limit pressure caused by the tube.
- Treatment
  - Consider using an extra-long tracheostomy tube to bypass the point of malacia.
  - Airway stenting

- Tracheoesophageal fistula
  - Abnormal communication between the trachea or main bronchi and the esophagus
  - Caused by injury of the posterior tracheal wall from tracheostomy tube:
    - Insertion
    - Malposition
    - Movement/friction
    - Excessive cuff pressure >30 cm H_2O
  - Occurs in $<1\%$ of patients with a tracheostomy tube
  - Can be exacerbated by nasogastric tube placement
  - Signs and symptoms
    - Copious secretions
    - Aspiration
    - Ventilator-associated pneumonia (VAP)
    - Tube feedings suctioned from the tracheostomy tube or around the stoma
    - Increased dyspnea
    - Persistent cuff leak
    - Severe gastric distention due to excess air in the stomach
  - Diagnostics
    - CT scan
    - Endoscopy
    - Chest x-ray
      - Dilated esophagus
      - Overinflated tracheostomy tube cuff
  - Prevention
    - Use of high-volume, low-pressure endotracheal and tracheostomy tubes.
    - Monitor tracheostomy tube cuff pressure routinely.
    - Maintain between 20 and 30 cm H_2O.
    - Use an appropriately sized tracheostomy tube to limit pressure caused by the tube.
  - Treatment
    - Surgical repair
    - Stenting
- Tracheoarterial fistula
  - Rare but life-threatening airway emergency, typically involving the tracheoinnominate artery
  - Massive tracheal bleeding
  - Often within the first 3 weeks of tracheostomy tube placement
  - More common if tracheostomy is placed below the 3rd tracheal ring
  - Caused by:
    - Tissue necrosis from excessive movement of the distal tip of the tracheostomy tube
    - Excessive tracheostomy tube cuff pressure >30 cm H_2O
  - Signs and symptoms
    - Tracheal bleeding
    - Pulsation of the tracheostomy tube synchronous with heart rate
  - Diagnostics
    - Flexible bronchoscopy to determine the origin of bleeding
    - CT scan
    - Angiography
  - Prevention
    - Use of high-volume, low-pressure endotracheal and tracheostomy tubes.
    - Monitor tracheostomy tube cuff pressure routinely.
    - Maintain between 20 and 30 cm H_2O.
    - Use an appropriately sized tracheostomy tube to limit pressure caused by the tube.
  - Treatment
    - Occlusion of an artery by a digit or tracheostomy tube cuff
    - Immediate surgical repair
- Pneumonia
  - Increased aspiration risk
  - Higher risk for patients on mechanical ventilation (VAP)
  - Tracheostomy tube cuff inhibits swallowing
  - Secretion retention
  - Prevention
    - Swallow evaluation
    - Maintaining good airway clearance of secretions
    - Deflated cuff, when appropriate, to restore swallow
  - VAP prevention
    - Limit time on mechanical ventilation.
    - Perform routine oral care.
    - Use subglottic suction device.
    - Elevate the head of the bed to 30 degrees.
    - Promote early mobility.
    - Limit disconnections from the ventilator.

SUGGESTED READINGS

Bontempo LJ, Manning SL. Tracheostomy emergencies. *Emerg Med Clin North Am*. 2019;37(1):109-119.

Cipriano A, Mao ML, Hon HH, et al. An overview of complications associated with open and percutaneous tracheostomy procedures. *Int J Crit Illn Inj Sci*. 2015;5(3):179-188.

Fernandez-Bussy S, Mahajan B, Folch E, Caviedes I, Guerrero J, Majid A. Tracheostomy tube placement: early and late complications. *J Bronchology Interv Pulmonol*. 2015;22(4):357-364.

Hess DR, Altobelli NP. Tracheostomy tubes. *Respir Care*. 2014;59(6):956-973.

Iftikhar IH, Teng S, Schimmel M, Duran C, Sardi A, Islam S. A network comparative meta-analysis of percutaneous dilatational tracheostomies using anatomic landmarks, bronchoscopic, and ultrasound guidance versus open surgical tracheostomy. *Lung*. 2019;197(3):267-275.

Johnson-Obaseki S, Veljkovic A, Javidnia H. Complication rates of open surgical versus percutaneous tracheostomy in critically ill patients. *Laryngoscope*. 2016;126(11):2459-2467.

Klemm E, Nowak AK. Tracheotomy-related deaths. *Dtsch Arztebl Int*. 2017;114(16):273-279.

Klotz R, Probst P, Deininger M, et al. Percutaneous versus surgical strategy for tracheostomy: a systematic review and meta-analysis of perioperative and postoperative complications. *Langenbecks Arch Surg*. 2018; 403(2):137-149.

Meng X, Shao Y, Zhu W. Effect of open surgical and percutaneous dilatational tracheostomy on postoperative wound complications in patients: a meta-analysis. *Int Wound J*. 2024;21(1):e14368.

Roy CF, Silver JA, Turkdogan S, Siafa L, Correa JA, Kost K. Complication rate of percutaneous dilatational tracheostomy in critically ill adults with obesity: a systematic review and meta-analysis. *JAMA Otolaryngol Head Neck Surg*. 2023;149(4):334-343.

Waldron J, Padgham ND, Hurley SE. Complications of emergency and elective tracheostomy: a retrospective study of 150 consecutive cases. *Ann R Coll Surg Engl*. 1990;72(4):218-220.

Zouk AN, Batra H. Managing complications of percutaneous tracheostomy and gastrostomy. *J Thorac Dis*. 2021;13(8):5314-5330.

30.3

Neck Hematomas

Jay Saggu and Christoph G.S. Nabzdyk

Definitions

- Expanding neck hematomas are a potentially lethal complication of thyroid and parathyroid cancers, neck surgery, and trauma. Rare spontaneous cases have also been reported. In the postoperative patient, the incidence can be as high as 1% post-thyroid surgery, 1.4% after carotid endarterectomy (CEA), and up to 1.9% post-anterior cervical spine surgery, with most cases being diagnosed within 6 to 24 hours postoperatively.
- Anatomically, they may occur in the anterior neck or in the deeper cervical tissues. The anterior neck is often implicated in cases of thyroid or parathyroid surgeries, CEA, cervical spinal surgeries, neck dissections, central line placement, and nerve blocks. The retropharynx and prevertebral spaces can be implicated in spontaneous cases or cases of trauma or spine surgery. Risk factors include coagulopathy, preoperative antiplatelet agents, surgical technique and extent, high blood pressures, and increased venous pressures during coughing or vomiting.
- Neck hematomas can occur in blunt and penetrating neck trauma and may present with severe bleeding, audible bruits or palpable thrills, hemorrhagic shock, and airway compromise. Concomitant spinal cord injury or spinal fractures are not uncommon in high-energy impact injuries (eg, sports, motor vehicle collision, blast, hanging attempt).

Neck Anatomy

- Platysma is a thin muscle covering the anterior and lateral neck with fibers extending from the inferior mandibular border to the subcutaneous tissues of the superior pectoralis major. Deep cervical fascia is deep to the platysma and subdivides into the investing layer, the pretracheal layer, and the carotid sheath. These fascial layers are continuous with the cranial and thoracic fascia and communicate with the mediastinum and can help tamponade bleeding.
- The neck is also divided into zones craniocaudally, with the posterior border of the sternocleidomastoid muscle dividing the neck into anterior and posterior sections. These zones can aid in identifying potentially injured structures, particularly in penetrating neck trauma.
    - Zone 1 is the most caudal zone extending from the clavicle to the cricoid cartilage. Important structures include the proximal common carotid, subclavian and vertebral arteries, thyroid gland, trachea, esophagus, thoracic duct, jugular veins, lung apices, and spinal cord.
    - Zone 2 extends from the cricoid cartilage to the inferior mandibular border. Important structures in this zone include the laryngotracheal complex, pharynx, esophagus, jugular vein, carotid and vertebral arteries, spinal cord and vagus, recurrent laryngeal, and phrenic nerves.
    - Zone 3 is the most superior zone and extends from the mandibular border to the base of the skull. Important structures include the distal carotid and vertebral arteries, pharynx, spinal cord, cranial nerves (CNs) IX to XII, salivary glands, parotid glands with CN VII, and sympathetic chain.

Workup

- The severity and symptomatology of neck hematomas depend on their size, location, and effects on surrounding structures.
- Early on, patients may describe increasing neck pain, difficulty handling oral secretions, and voice changes. This may progress to respiratory distress, facial plethora, neck asymmetry, neck tightness and progressive neck, and submandibular swelling. Cyanosis, tracheal deviation, and respiratory failure are late findings and signs of imminent respiratory collapse. Initially, agitated patients may become somnolent and unresponsive in later stages. Hypertension and tachycardia are common, but bradycardia and hypotension may occur due to mechanical distortion of the carotid sinus and activation of the baroreceptor reflex.
- Cervicomediastinal hematomas, including prevertebral and retropharyngeal hematomas, may be more indolent on presentation. Classic symptoms such as dysphagia, hoarseness, dyspnea, and neck swelling may not be present early. Traditionally, these hematomas are associated with Capps triad: tracheal and esophageal compression, anterior tracheal displacement, and neck and chest bruising.
- Imaging studies can include ultrasound, plain film radiographs, computed tomography (CT), and magnetic resonance imaging (MRI) but may not be attainable in patients in distress. Thorough history and physical examination are vital for an early diagnosis.

- Neck hematomas should be included in the differential for neck swelling in post-neck surgery or trauma patients with careful assessment of patient's respiratory dynamics and airway patency.

Management

- It is essential to identify a neck hematoma early to avoid life-threatening complications.
- Airway compromise is the most feared complication as it can develop rapidly and precipitate cardiac arrest. Cephalad to the glottic opening, external compression can significantly displace, distort, and obscure the normal airway anatomy. Laryngeal and tracheal cartilage make the subglottic airways more resistant to external compression. Impaired venous and lymphatic drainage from the head results in significant swelling of supraglottic and glottic structures and tracheal mucosa. The combination of impaired drainage and direct compression can result in respiratory failure and make laryngoscopy and airway manipulation challenging. In postoperative neck hematomas in the anterior neck, reopening of skin and platysma incisions can facilitate laryngoscopy and may be required bedside.
- Airway management plans should be specific to the patient. Options for airway management include bag mask ventilation (use minimum amounts of positive pressure), and high-flow nasal cannula can be used to supplement oxygenation in the patient who is acutely hypoxic.
- Approaches to secure the airway include direct or video laryngoscopy, fiberoptic tracheal intubation, and laryngeal mask airway. However, prior to intubation, arrangements for emergent front-of-neck access with possible tracheostomy or cricothyroidotomy must be made. In general, anesthesia and head and neck or trauma surgery team involvement is recommended early due to the often-challenging airway anatomy and risk of inability to intubate or ventilate.
- Early recognition of impending airway obstruction, avoidance of positive pressure ventilation (can cause false track along injury and distort anatomy further), and placement of the endotracheal tube tip distal to the site of injury are vital in trauma cases. In-line cervical stabilization or immobilization is often necessary while the airway is secured in cases of blunt cervical injury.

Treatment

- Most postoperative hematomas require evacuation and reexploration of the wound in the operating room. Bleeding vessels often require ligation or cauterization, and hemostatic agents can be used as adjuncts to promote clot formation.
- In the absence of airway compromise or hemodynamic instability, treatment of cervical hematomas remains controversial. In cases of small hematomas, needle aspiration can be attempted. In other milder cases without ongoing expansion or significant volume accumulation, conservative management with fluid and steroids can be considered while keeping the patient in a highly monitored setting.
- In cases of both blunt and penetrating neck trauma, standard American Trauma and Life Support Guidelines should be followed with a stepwise evaluation and treatment of airway, breathing, circulation, and disability. Airway should be secured with any signs or symptoms of airway distress.
- Hard signs indicating immediate surgical consultation in penetrating neck injury include hemorrhagic shock, pulsatile bleeding or expanding hematoma, audible bruit or palpable thrill, neurologic deficits, and signs of airway compromise.
- Zone 1 and 3 penetrating injuries are often initially evaluated with angiography and triple endoscopy (laryngoscopy, bronchoscopy, esophagoscopy), in part, due to difficult surgical access. Zone 1 injuries may require cardiothoracic surgery in addition to trauma and head and neck surgery as sternotomy may be required. In the absence of the abovementioned signs, CT angiography and endoscopy can be considered depending on patient stability and symptomatology.
- Zone 2 is the most frequently affected zone in penetrating neck injuries. Signs of vascular injury include expanding hematoma, declining mental status, and bleeding from the aerodigestive tracts. Historically, surgical operative intervention was mandated for all penetrating injuries involving zone 2. With recent advancements in high-quality CT imaging, a modified "no-zone" approach is often recommended, with operative interventions offered based on the physiological status of the patient.
- In cases of blunt cervical injury, emergent vascular intervention may be necessary in high-grade blunt cerebrovascular injuries (BCVIs). Injuries that confer a high risk for BCVI include near hanging with cerebral anoxia, seatbelt sign of the anterior neck, basilar skull fracture involving the carotid canal, severe cervical hyperflexion/rotation/hyperextension, cervical vertebral body fracture or distraction, focal neurologic deficits, displaced facial fractures, and hard signs of vascular injury. Hard signs for vascular injury include pulsatile severe bleeding, expanding hematoma, audible bruit, palpable thrill, evidence of hemorrhagic shock, and absent brachial or radial artery pulses. Management for BCVI includes anticoagulation, antiplatelet therapy, and endovascular intervention. Surgical interventions are less common.

Conclusions

- Neck hematomas can occur spontaneously, postoperatively, or in cases of trauma.
- Airway distress can develop rapidly and result in complete obstruction, leading to acute respiratory failure and cardiac arrest. In emergent postoperative cases, relieving the skin and platysma incisions may aid in airway management.
- Management is dependent on the patient's signs and symptomatology and may require immediate operative exploration and intervention.
- Laryngoscopy can be difficult due to significant airway edema and distortion of the airway. Advanced airway equipment, experienced intubating personnel, and team members capable of obtaining emergent surgical airways should be immediately present prior to any induction of general anesthesia and surgical evacuation.

SUGGESTED READINGS

Argalious M. Airway management for an expanding neck hematoma. In: Doyle DJ, ed. *Clinical Airway Management*. Cambridge University Press; 2017.

Bittner EA. Silent pain in the neck. In *PSNet* [Internet]. Agency for Healthcare Research and Quality, U.S. Department of Health and Human Services; 2011. https://psnet.ahrq.gov/web-mm/silent-pain-neck

Gerasimov M, Lee B, Bittner EA. *Postoperative anterior neck hematoma (ANH): timely intervention is vital*. Anesthesia Patient Safety Foundation. 2021. https://www.apsf.org/article/postoperative-anterior-neck-hematoma-anh-timely-intervention-is-vital/

Iftikhar H, Awan MO, Abbas SA, et al. The risk factors for neck hematoma following thyroid surgery: an overview of systematic reviews. *Health Sci Rev*. 2022;3:100019.

Law JA. Management of the patient with a neck hematoma. In: Hung O, Murphy M, eds. *Management of the Difficult and Failed Airway*. McGraw-Hill; 2012.

Nowicki JL, Stew B, Ooi E. Penetrating neck injuries: a guide to evaluation and management. *Ann R Coll Surg Engl*. 2018;100:6-11.

Piaseczny M, La J, Chaplin T, Evans C. Protect that neck! Management of blunt and penetrating neck trauma. *Emerg Med Clin North Am*. 2023; 41:35-49.

Qureshi M, Patel K, Simon R. Neck level algorithmic approach to trauma. *Oper Tech Otolayngol Head Neck Surg*. 2020;31:289-294.

Shakespeare WA, Lanier WL, Perkins WJ, Pasternak JJ. Airway management in patients who develop neck hematomas after carotid endarterectomy. *Anesth Analg*. 2010;110:588-593.

Shilston J, Evans DL, Simons A, Evans DA. Initial management of blunt and penetrating neck trauma. *BJA Educ*. 2021;21:329-335.

Thakkar K, Nwangene NL, Maharjan R, et al. A comprehensive management of neck hematoma in post-thyroidectomy patient for papillary thyroid cancer: a case report. *Cureus*. 2023;15:e42689.

Thomas SA, Moideen SP, George SM, Ipe S, Menon DG. Management of spontaneous neck hematoma in patients on anticoagulant therapy: our experience from a tertiary care center. *Indian J Otolaryngol Head Neck Surg*. 2022;74:6362-6366.

30.4

Laryngectomy and Tracheal Reconstruction

Elisa C. Walsh

Anatomy of the Larynx and Trachea (Figure 30.4.1)

Larynx

- The larynx serves to maintain the patency of the upper airway, prevent aspiration into the tracheobronchial tree, and produce phonation.
- It is located in the anterior neck and spans roughly from the C3 to C6 level, with its superior border defined by the hyoid bone and its inferior border defined by the cricoid cartilage.
- It is a complex structure consisting of nine rigid cartilages (thyroid, cricoid, epiglottis; paired arytenoid, corniculate, and cuneiform) and several supporting muscles and ligaments.

Trachea

- The trachea serves as a conduit between the larynx and the bronchial tree, spanning roughly from the C6 to T4 to T5 level when it bifurcates into the mainstem bronchi at the carina.
- The anterior wall of the trachea is composed of 18 to 22 incomplete cartilaginous rings, while the posterior wall is composed of a fibromuscular membrane containing longitudinal smooth muscle known as the trachealis.

Laryngectomy

Indications

- Advanced laryngeal or hypopharyngeal malignancies with invasion of thyroid or cricoid cartilage and extralaryngeal soft tissue
- Failed response or predicted poor response (eg, specific histopathologic subtypes of tumors) to primary radiotherapy or chemoradiotherapy
- Severe laryngeal trauma prohibiting functional reconstruction
- Cranial nerve IX, X, or XI palsy leading to chronic aspiration and aphonia
- Recurrent laryngeal papillomatosis

Surgical Approach

- A traditional laryngectomy removes the entire larynx with attached prelaryngeal strap muscles, hyoid bone, thyroid lobe ipsilateral to the tumor, and any lymph nodes of concern with creation of a neopharynx.
- The proximal end of trachea is sutured to the anterior lower neck to create a stoma for ventilation.
- The procedure may include a percutaneous gastrostomy or sutured nasogastric tube.

Postoperative Care

- Speech Language Pathology (SLP) and Nutrition consults should be placed.
- A "obligate neck breather" or "postlaryngectomy" sign should be placed on the door to ensure no attempts at upper airway oxygenation or airway management in the event of emergency (Figure 30.4.2).
- Heat-moisture exchange (HME) applied over the stoma.
- Laryngectomy ("Lary") silicone tube often placed to maintain stoma patency
- Avoid any device exchange or reinstrumentation of the stoma within 7 to 10 days postoperatively to avoid creation of a false tract.

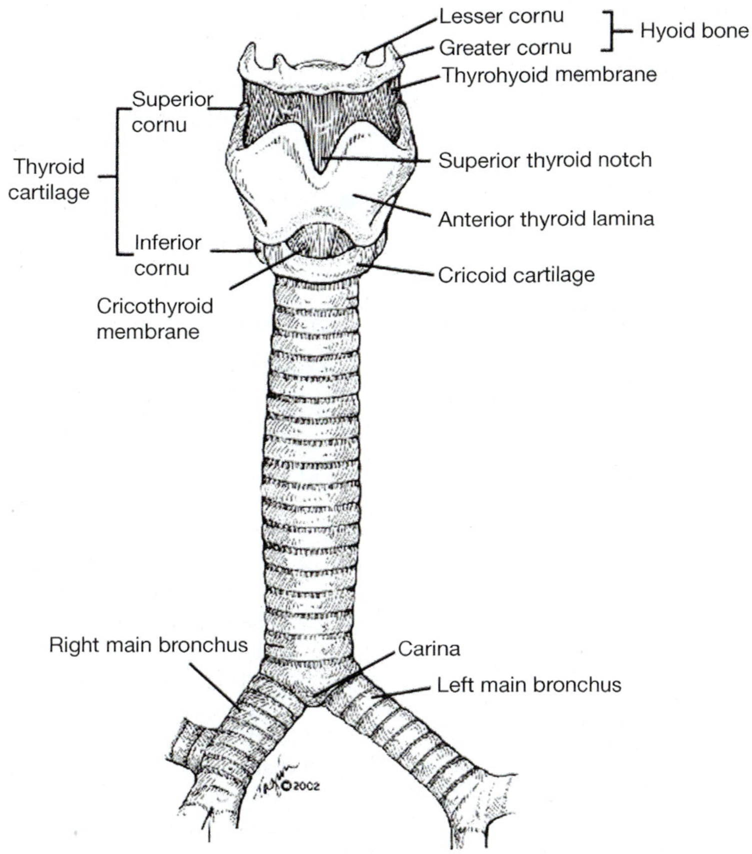

FIGURE 30.4.1 **Anatomy of the larynx and trachea.**

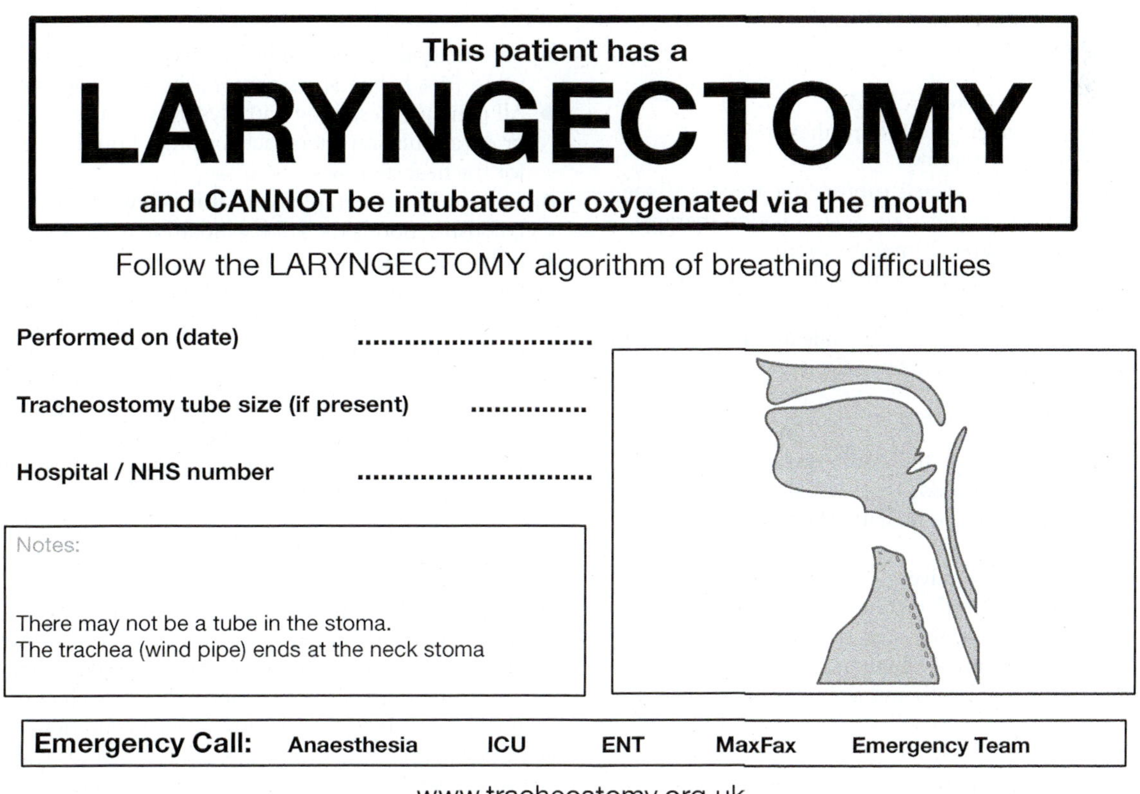

FIGURE 30.4.2 **An example bedhead sign for a postlaryngectomy patient.** ENT, ears, nose, and throat; ICU, intensive care unit. (© 2025 National Tracheostomy Safety Project.)

- Nutrition is initiated with tube feeds, with the goal of ultimately transitioning to per os intake.
- Antibiotics directed toward oropharyngeal flora are maintained until drain removal.
- Voice rehabilitation
  - Transesophageal puncture (TEP)
    - Prosthesis with a one-way valve inserted between the trachea and the esophagus
    - Airflow directed from lungs into esophagus (patient must occlude stoma externally) leads to vibration of the upper esophagus and neopharynx to reproduce voice.
  - Electrolarynx
    - Small electronic device that is applied directly to neck to produce vibrations of the trachea to reproduce voice
    - Esophageal voice

Complications

- Early
  - Airway compromise
    - Neck hematoma (see Chapter 30.3)
      - Usually within 24 hours postoperatively
    - Postoperative edema
  - Wound infection
  - Pharyngocutaneous fistula
    - Usually occurs within 7 to 10 days, but may occur later in postoperative course
    - Associated with prior and current smoking, prior radiotherapy, and poor nutritional status as indicated by serum hypoalbuminemia
    - Estimated overall postoperative rate of 14% to 30%
      - Hypocalcemia due to hypoparathyroidism
    - Late
      - Stomal or pharyngeal strictures
      - Hypothyroidism
      - Airway obstruction
        - Excessive secretion burden
        - Dislodgement of TEP prosthesis
  - Carotid blowout syndrome
    - Carotid or branch vessels rupture due to poor tissue integrity due to erosion (eg, post-radiation therapy, fistula leak) or direct tumor invasion.
    - Requires intubating the stoma with a cuffed airway device, external compression, and activating massive transfusion protocol while awaiting definitive surgical or interventional management

Emergency Airway Management

- Ventilate with 100% FIO_2 to the stoma via laryngeal mask airway or pediatric face mask. The Laerdal pediatric mask outperforms an Ambu pediatric mask in achieving peristomal seal.
- If >7 to 10 days postoperatively:
  - May intubate stoma with 6.0 cuffed endotracheal tube (ideally over fiberoptic scope or bougie)
  - In adjunct to fiberoptic evaluation, may remove any devices present (eg, HME) and attempt to pass suction catheter or use $etCO_2$ tracing to confirm and/or establish airway patency
    - If <7 to 10 days postoperatively:
      - Use fiberoptic scope for any stoma evaluation or device manipulation
      - Have primary surgical team at bedside if able

Future Directions

- Chemotherapy, immunotherapy, and radiation therapy regimens are constantly evolving and are often employed in lieu of surgical resection when possible.
- Partial laryngectomies allow preservation of a portion of the larynx when feasible.
- An artificial larynx has been described that allowed phonation, partial use of the upper airway, and largely prevented aspiration of saliva.

Tracheal Reconstruction

Indications

- Postintubation tracheal stenosis is by far the most common indication.
  - Risk factors include prolonged intubation, excessive cuff pressure (>20-25 mm Hg), and excessive motion of the endotracheal tube.
  - Incidence is estimated 10% to 22% postintubation and 1% to 2% posttracheotomy.
  - Historical endotracheal tubes had high-pressure, low-volume cuffs, which led to ischemia, circumferential scarring, and narrowing of the affected trachea. Modern endotracheal tubes have low-pressure, high-volume cuffs to help avoid ischemic injury.
- Primary or secondary malignancy
- Tracheoesophageal fistula
- Tracheoinnominate fistula
- Iatrogenic or traumatic injury to the trachea
- Other (eg, pregnancy related, rheumatologic)

Diagnosis

- Presentation can be insidious; the trachea can be narrowed up to 75% before any symptoms become apparent.
- All patients presenting with dyspnea after recent intubation or decannulation after tracheostomy should be evaluated for tracheal stenosis.
- Computed tomography with three-dimensional reconstruction is the gold standard for imaging.
- Pulmonary function testing shows airflow plateau on both the inspiratory and expiratory limbs of the flow volume loop due to fixed obstruction. Forced expiratory volume may also be reduced.
- Bronchoscopic evaluation to establish the proximal and distal extent of the stenosis may be performed outpatient or at the time of surgery. At the same time, gentle dilation may be performed to allow the trachea to accommodate a 5.5 endotracheal tube.

Management

- Patients with tracheal stenosis may be temporized with stents, dilations, and laser therapy to achieve airway patency.
- *Tracheal resection and reconstruction* is the definitive procedure to treat tracheal stenosis. As much as 50% of the trachea may be resected with optimal conditions.
- Total intravenous anesthetic is established to ensure anesthetic delivery despite interrupted ventilation and to increase the chance of smooth emergence.
- Right radial arterial access is often established to monitor for innominate artery compression.

- The most common incision is a low collar incision, sometimes extending inferiorly to divide the manubrium in distal stenoses; full sternotomy is rarely required.
- After dissection and exposure, cross-field ventilation with intermittent apnea is established via a reinforced endotracheal tube inserted into the distal airway to allow the surgeons to resect the portion of damaged trachea.
- Patients often receive a chin stitch to maintain neck flexion postoperatively and reduce tension on the new tracheal anastomosis. A suprahyoid laryngeal release may be performed as well.

Postoperative Care

- Patients are generally extubated and spontaneously breathing at the time of admission to the intensive care unit.
- Steroids are avoided to promote anastomotic healing.
- Continued neck flexion
- Bronchoscopy on postoperative day 7 to assess the integrity of the anastomosis and divide the chin stitch if placed

Complications

- Airway edema
- Anastomotic dehiscence
- Bleeding, including innominate artery erosion or damage

Emergency Airway Management

- Positive pressure ventilation and endotracheal intubation are avoided to prevent damage to the tracheal anastomosis.
- If intubation is required, the endotracheal tube must be placed past the anastomosis. Flexible bronchoscopy with the surgical team at bedside is recommended to confirm the site of the anastomosis.
- If necessary for airway management, the chin stitch may be severed. However, in the flex-flex position, direct laryngoscopy with a Miller blade often provides an excellent view of the vocal cords due to alignment of the orolaryngeal axes.

Outcomes

- Operative mortality is low (0.8%). However, the 30-day complication rate is almost 30%.
- Risk factors for worse outcomes include reoperation, diabetes mellitus, T tubes, tracheostomy present at resection, requirement for postoperative tracheostomy, and laryngeal involvement.
- Anastomotic complications occur in almost 25% of patients, with a 7% risk of major complication, including anastomotic necrosis and dehiscence.

SUGGESTED READINGS

Ceachir O, Hainarosie R, Zainea V. Total laryngectomy—past, present, future. *Maedica (Bucur)*. 2014;9(2):210-216.

Debry C, Vrana NE, Dupret-Bories A. Implantation of an artificial larynx after total laryngectomy. *N Engl J Med*. 2017;376(1):97-98.

Goepfert RP, Hutcheson KA, Lewin JS, et al. Complications, hospital length of stay, and readmission after total laryngectomy. *Cancer*. 2017; 123(10):1760-1767.

Goldenberg D, Ari EG, Golz A, Danino J, Netzer A, Joachims HZ. Tracheotomy complications: a retrospective study of 1130 cases. *Otolaryngol Head Neck Surg*. 2000;123(4):495-500.

Grillo, HC. *Surgery of the Trachea and Bronchi*. BC Decker; 2004.

Hasan Z, Dwivedi RC, Gunaratne DA, Virk SA, Palme CE, Riffat F. Systematic review and meta-analysis of the complications of salvage total laryngectomy. *Eur J Surg Oncol*. 2017;43(1):42-51.

Mathisen DJ. Tracheal resection and reconstruction: how I teach it. *Ann Thorac Surg*. 2017;103(4):1043-1048.

McGrath BA, Bates L, Atkinson D, Moore JA. Multidisciplinary guidelines for the management of tracheostomy and laryngectomy airway emergencies. *Anaesthesia*. 2012;67(9):1025-1041.

Powitzky R, Vasan N, Krempl G, Medina J. Carotid blowout in patients with head and neck cancer. *Ann Otol Rhinol Laryngol*. 2010;119(7):476-484.

Suárez C, Fernández-Alvarez V, Hamoir M, et al. Carotid blowout syndrome: modern trends in management. *Cancer Manag Res*. 2018;10:5617-5628.

Wright CD, Grillo HC, Wain JC, et al. Anastomotic complications after tracheal resection: prognostic factors and management. *J Thorac Cardiovasc Surg*. 2004;128(5):731-739.

Wright CD, Li S, Geller AD, et al. Postintubation tracheal stenosis: management and results 1993 to 2017. *Ann Thorac Surg*. 2019;108(5): 1471-1477.

SECTION 31

Preoperative Evaluation for Surgery

Section Editor: Marvin G. Chang

31.1

Preoperative Assessment

Amanda S. Xi

Preoperative History and Physical

- Assess functional status
  - Standard metabolic equivalent (MET): unit used to estimate the amount of oxygen used by the body during physical activity
    - 1 MET: energy used at rest
    - 4 METs (classically associated with readiness to undergo stress of surgery): ability to climb a flight of stairs, vacuum, and do light housework
- Identify areas for further testing (see later).
- Social history
  - Tobacco: associated with postoperative pulmonary complications and reactive airways
  - Marijuana: associated with increased anesthetic requirements, risk of withdrawal, increased postoperative pain/nausea
  - Alcohol: impaired liver function, risk of withdrawal
- Identify risk factors for perioperative complications (eg, frailty, delirium, organ failure).

Testing

- Driven by findings on history and physical and type of surgery
- Routine testing generally not indicated; indications for the following:
  - Labs
    - Hemoglobin/hematocrit: anemia; anticipated blood loss; premature infants
    - Platelets: personal/family history of bleeding diathesis; liver disease
    - Electrolytes: renal dysfunction, taking medications that affect Na^+/K^+ (antihypertensives/diuretics)
    - Coagulation factors: patient taking anticoagulants; liver disease
    - Transaminases: cirrhosis
    - Beta-human chorionic gonadotropin (β-hCG): controversial and institution specific—consider for all women of childbearing age
    - Arterial blood gas: patient mechanically ventilated prior to surgery
    - Type and screen/crossmatch: anticipated blood loss >500 mL
  - Electrocardiogram: age >60 years; major vascular surgery with at least one clinical risk factor (see American College of Cardiology/American Heart Association [ACC/AHA] guidelines later) of any age; intermediate-risk surgery with known coronary artery disease (CAD), peripheral vascular disease, or cerebrovascular disease; consider for patients undergoing major vascular disease with no risk factors
  - Chest x-ray: cardiopulmonary disease; age >50 years undergoing abdominal aortic aneurysm or upper abdominal/thoracic surgery
  - C-spine films: trisomy 21; rheumatoid arthritis with clinical signs; trauma
  - Pulmonary function tests (PFTs): see later
  - Echocardiography: age >50 years with new murmur (r/o aortic stenosis [AS]); new arrhythmia; assessment of known/suspected heart failure; known AS with prior echo >12 months; known moderate-to-severe valvular disease with prior echo >24 months, poor functional status

Evaluation of the Cardiac Patient for Noncardiac Surgery

- 2024 ACC/AHA perioperative cardiovascular evaluation for noncardiac surgery practice guidelines
  - High-risk surgery: major vascular
  - Intermediate-risk surgery: intraperitoneal and intrathoracic surgery, carotid endarterectomy, head and neck surgery, orthopedic surgery, prostate surgery
  - Low-risk surgery: endoscopic procedures, superficial procedure, cataract surgery, breast surgery, ambulatory surgery

TABLE 31.1.1 Lee Revised Cardiac Risk Index (RCRI)

Predictors	Derivation Cohort (%)	Validation Cohort (%)
None	0.5	0.4
1	1.3	0.9
2	3.6	6.6
≥3	9.1	11.0

- Active cardiac conditions typically take precedent over surgery: unstable coronary syndromes, decompensated heart failure, severe valvulopathy, and significant arrhythmia.
- Assessment of functional status to guide further cardiac testing
- Newest guideline includes risk modifiers that may benefit from further cardiac assessment.

- Lee Revised Cardiac Risk Index (RCRI)
  - Six independent risk factors for major postoperative complications
    - Risk factors are the same as those used for cardiac risk stratification (ie, high-risk surgical procedure, ischemic heart disease, congestive heart failure, history of cerebrovascular disease, insulin treatment, creatinine [Cr] >2 mg/dL).
    - Major complications: cardiac death, ventricular fibrillation, complete heart block, acute myocardial infarction (MI), pulmonary edema
    - *See Table 31.1.1 for additional details.*
- Other cardiac concerns
  - Pacemakers (PPM)/implantable cardioverter-defibrillator (ICD)/cardiac resynchronization therapy (CRT)
    - Determine device type, manufacturer.
    - Understand indication for implantation.
    - Last interrogation (PPM/CRT-P <6 months, ICD/CRT-D <3 months)
    - Understand function/programming
    - Understand magnet mode
    - *See Table 31.1.2 for additional details.*
  - Antiplatelet therapy
    - Primary prevention: aspirin 81 mg no longer recommended, given the second Perioperative Ischemic Evaluation trial (POISE 2), which found that in patients with or at risk for atherosclerotic disease, administering aspirin around the time of surgery did not lower the incidence of death or nonfatal MI, but it did increase the likelihood of major bleeding.
      - CAD risk factors include hypertension, hyperlipidemia, cigarette smoking, family history of premature death from MI, and age (men >55 years and women >65 years).
    - Secondary prevention
      - After MI: continue antiplatelet therapy if possible (aspirin alone at minimum) indefinitely.
      - After percutaneous coronary intervention (PCI)
        - Bare-metal stent (BMS): dual-antiplatelet therapy (DAPT): minimum 4 weeks
        - Drug-eluting stent (DES): DAPT: minimum 6 months (ideally 12 months)
      - Other indications: atrial fibrillation, stroke, noncardiac stents, diabetes mellitus (type 1 or 2), chronic kidney disease (Cr >2.0 mg/dL)
    - Management during the perioperative period
      - Discontinue aspirin for at least 4 days in patients taking the medication for PRIMARY prevention, given no significant clinical benefit and increased risk for bleeding (POISE 2 trial).
      - The decision to hold aspirin in patients taking the medication for SECONDARY prevention requires a multidisciplinary approach with input from surgeon, anesthesiologist, internist, and cardiologist.
      - If surgery necessitates stopping DAPT, prasugrel should be held for 7 days, clopidogrel for 5 days, and ticagrelor for 3 days prior to surgery.
        - The discussion and plan for postoperative resumption should be documented.
  - Anticoagulation therapy
    - Warfarin
      - Hold 5 days prior to procedure (6 days if international normalized ratio [INR] is >3.0).
      - Routine bridging with heparin is not routinely recommended for most patients.
      - Consider bridging only in patients at high thromboembolic risk.
        - Mechanical valve
          - Mechanical mitral valve
          - Caged ball or tilting-disk valve
          - Mechanical heart valve in any position with a recent stroke or transient ischemia attack (TIA) (within 3 months)
        - Atrial fibrillation
          - CHA_2DS_2-VASc score ≥7
          - CHA_2DS_2-VASc score of 5 to 6 with a recent stroke or TIA
          - Atrial fibrillation with rheumatic valvular heart disease
        - Venous thromboembolism (VTE)
          - Recent VTE (within 1-3 months)
        - Other conditions
          - Recent cardioembolic stroke (within 3 months)
          - Left ventricular (LV) thrombus (within 3 months)

TABLE 31.1.2 Pacemakers (PPM)/implantable Cardioverter-Defibrillator (ICD)/Cardiac Resynchronization Therapy (CRT)

Position I	Position II	Position III	Position IV	Position V
(Sensed)	(Paced)	(Response)	(Rate response)	(Multisite)
O = none	O = none	O = none		O = none
A = atrium	A = atrium	I = inhibited	O = none	A = atria
V = ventricle	V = ventricle	T = triggered	R = rate	V = ventricles
D = dual (A+V)	D = dual (A+V)	D = dual (T+I)	response	D = dual (A+V)

- Severe thrombophilia
- Antiphospholipid antibodies
- The BRIDGE trial showed no reduction in thromboembolism but a significant increase in major bleeding with bridging.
- Direct oral anticoagulants (DOACs)
  - No bridging not routinely recommended in majority of patients, given studies (RE-LY, ARISTOTLE, and ROCKET AF Trials) that showed bridging DOACs increased risk of bleeding without a reduction in thromboembolic risk.
  - Hold time before surgery depends on bleeding risk and renal function:
    - Low bleeding risk: hold 24 hours.
    - High risk: hold 48 hours.
    - Need for neuraxial: hold 3 to 5 days.
- Beta-blockade remains controversial, as it reduces the risk of perioperative MI but is associated with an increased rate of perioperative stroke.
  - Continue if patient currently taking.
  - Initiate in patients identified as having CAD or *high* cardiac risk undergoing vascular or intermediate-risk surgery.
  - May not be beneficial (possibly harmful) in lower risk patients
- Sodium-glucose cotransporter 2 (SGLT2) inhibitors
  - To reduce the risk for euglycemic diabetic ketoacidosis (DKA), hold 3 days before surgery for most (canagliflozin, dapagliflozin, empagliflozin); hold 4 days for ertugliflozin (longer half-life).
- Glucagon-like peptide-1 receptor agonist (GLP-1 RA) (2024 ASA Multisociety Guidance)
  - Initial concerns about aspiration risk from reduced gastric emptying led to conservative 2023 guidance. However, current evidence suggests that the actual incidence of aspiration is likely low, and in most cases, these agents can be continued perioperatively with appropriate precautions.
  - Most patients: continue GLP-1 agonists perioperatively (major reversal from 2023).
  - High-risk patients (escalation phase, gastrointestinal [GI] symptoms, weekly formulation, high dose):
    - 24-hour clear liquid diet before surgery
    - Consider point-of-care gastric ultrasound.
    - Shared decision-making about proceeding versus delaying
  - If holding is deemed necessary (uncommon):
    - Daily formulations: hold the day of surgery.
    - Weekly formulations: hold 7 days prior.
  - Follow institutional guidance as protocols are still being updated.
- Bacterial endocarditis prophylaxis
  - The AHA guidelines significantly limited the use of antimicrobial prophylaxis to include only patients with prosthetic valves, prior history of infectious endocarditis, unrepaired cyanotic congenital heart disease, repaired congenital heart disease within the first 6 months of repair with prosthetic material or those with residual defects preventing endothelialization, and recipients of cardiac transplantation who develop valvulopathy.

TABLE 31.1.3 Respiratory Failure Index

Preoperative Predictor	Point Value
Type of surgery	
Abdominal aortic aneurysm	27
Thoracic	21
Neurosurgery, upper abdominal, peripheral vascular	14
Neck	11
Emergency surgery	11
Albumin <3.0 g/dL	9
BUN >30 mg/dL	8
Partially or fully dependent functional status	7
History of chronic obstructive pulmonary disease	6
Age (years)	
>70	6
60-69	4

BUN, blood urea nitrogen.

  - Procedures for which prophylaxis is recommended include dental, respiratory tract, GI, or genitourinary (GU) procedures with active infection, surgery on infected soft tissue, and intracardiac surgery involving prosthetic materials.
  - Antimicrobial prophylaxis: amoxicillin/ampicillin first line
    - Dental and respiratory tract procedures: cefazolin, azithromycin, clarithromycin, clindamycin acceptable alternatives
    - GI/GU: vancomycin acceptable alternative
    - Skin/soft tissue: clindamycin or vancomycin second line

Pulmonary Evaluation

- Postoperative pulmonary complications are the most expensive of major postoperative medical complications and are associated with the longest length of stay.
- Risk factors for postoperative pulmonary complications:
  - Patient related: age >50 years, chronic pulmonary disease, tobacco, obesity, obstructive sleep apnea (OSA), pulmonary hypertension, heart failure, upper respiratory infection
  - Procedure related: surgical site (upper abdominal/thoracic), duration (>4 hours), emergency surgery
    - *See Tables 31.1.3 and 31.1.4 for additional details.*
- PFT: indications
  - All patients for proposed lung resection
  - Identifying medical optimization in patients with chronic obstructive pulmonary disease (COPD)/asthma

TABLE 31.1.4 Risk of Respiratory Failure

Class	Point Total	Percent Respiratory Failure
1	<10	0.5
2	11-19	1.8
3	20-27	4.2
4	28-40	10.1
5	>40	26.6

TABLE 31.1.5 Fasting Guidelines

Ingested Material	Minimum Fasting Period (h)
Clear liquids	2
Breast milk	4
Infant formula	6
Nonhuman milk	6
Light solid foods	6
Full meal	8

    - Differentiation from cardiac disease or deconditioning in patients with uncharacterized dyspnea/exercise intolerance

Preoperative Fasting Guidelines

- Recommendations to reduce the risk of pulmonary aspiration for healthy individuals undergoing elective procedures
- *See Table 31.1.5 for additional details.*

Other Perioperative Considerations

- Stress-dose steroids
    - Assume adrenal suppression for patients taking >20 mg prednisone/d.
    - Assume competent adrenal function for patients taking <5 mg prednisone/d.
    - Corticosteroid coverage for surgery in patients who are adrenally suppressed
        - Minor procedures: take usual morning steroid dose without supplementation.
        - Moderate surgical stress: usual morning dose
            - Additionally, hydrocortisone 50 mg intravenous (IV) prior to procedure and 25 mg IV every 8 hours for 24 hours, then resume usual dose
        - Major surgical stress: usual morning dose
            - Additionally, hydrocortisone 50 to 100 mg IV prior to procedure and 25 to 50 mg IV every 8 hours for 24 hours
            - Taper dose by half per day to maintenance

SUGGESTED READINGS

American Society of Anesthesiologists. *Multisociety Clinical Practice Guidance for the Safe Use of Glucagon-like Peptide-1 Receptor Agonists in the Perioperative Period.* 2024. https://www.asahq.org/about-asa/newsroom/news-releases/2024/10/new-multi-society-glp-1-guidance

American Society of Anesthesiologists. Practice advisory for the perioperative management of patients with cardiac implantable electronic devices: pacemakers and implantable cardioverter-defibrillators: an updated report by the American society of anesthesiologists task force on perioperative management of patients with cardiac implantable electronic devices. *Anesthesiology* 2011;114:247-261.

Arozullah AM, Daley J, Henderson WG, Khuri SF. Multifactorial risk index for predicting postoperative respiratory failure in men after major noncardiac surgery. *Ann Surg.* 2000;2:242-253.

Chang MG, Ripoll JG, Lopez E, et al. A scoping review of GLP-1 receptor agonists: are they associated with increased gastric contents, regurgitation, and aspiration events? *J Clin Med.* 2024;13(21):6336.

Committee on Standards and Practice Parameters; Apfelbaum JL, Connis RT, Nickinovich DG, et al. Practice advisory for preanesthesia evaluation. An updated report by the American Society of Anesthesiologists Task Force on Preanesthesia Evaluation. *Anesthesiology.* 2012;116:522-538.

Coursin DB, Wood KE. Corticosteroid supplementation for adrenal insufficiency. *Ann Intern Med.* 2003;139:194.

Fleischmann KE, Beckman JA, Buller CE, et al. 2009 ACCF/AHA focused update on perioperative beta blockade: A report of the American College of Cardiology Foundation/American Heart Association task force on practice guidelines. *Circulation.* 2009;120:2123-2151.

Fleisher LA, Beckman JA, Brown KA, et al. ACC/AHA 2007 guidelines on perioperative cardiovascular evaluation and care for noncardiac surgery: A report of the American College of Cardiology/American Heart Association Task Force on Practice Guidelines [published correction appears in *J Am Coll Cardiol.* 2008;52:794-797]. *J Am Coll Cardiol.* 2007;50:1707-1732.

Hepner DL. The role of testing in the preoperative evaluation. *CCJM.* 2009;76(suppl 4):S22-S27.

Lee TH, Marcantonio ER, Mangione CM, et al. Derivation and prospective validation of a simple index for prediction of cardiac risk of major noncardiac surgery. *Circulation.* 1999;100:1043-1049.

Levine GN, Bates ER, Bittl JA, et al. 2016 ACC/AHA guideline focused update on duration of dual antiplatelet therapy in patients with coronary artery disease: a report of the American College of Cardiology/American Heart Association Task Force on Clinical Practice Guidelines. *J Thorac Cardiovasc Surg.* 2016 Nov;152(5):1243-1275.

Parikh SS, Chung F. Postoperative delirium in the elderly. *Anesth Analg.* 1995;80:1223-1232.

Shah S, Schwenk ES, Sondekoppam RV, et al. ASRA pain medicine consensus guidelines on the management of the perioperative patient on cannabis and cannabinoids. *Reg Anesth Pain Med.* 2023;48(3):97-117.

Smetana GW, Lawrence VA, Cornell JE. Preoperative pulmonary risk stratification for noncardiac surgery: systematic review for the American College of Physicians. *Ann Intern Med.* 2006;144:581.

Thompson A, Fleischmann KE, Smilowitz NR, et al. 2024 AHA/ACC/ACS/ASNC/HRS/SCA/SCCT/SCMR/SVM Guideline for Perioperative Cardiovascular Management for Noncardiac Surgery: report of the American College of Cardiology/American Heart Association Joint Committee on Clinical Practice Guidelines. *Circulation.* 2024;150(19):e351-e442.

SECTION 32

Intensive Care Unit Administration and Practice Management

Section Editor: Edward A. Bittner

32.1

Intensive Care Unit Administration and Practice Management

Craig S. Jabaley

Definitions

- Administrative structures in critical care, including those within a given intensive care unit (ICU), play important roles in ensuring the delivery of, and access to, high-quality, value-based clinical care for critically ill patients.
- ICU administration can be broadly construed as including coordination of multidisciplinary teams, staffing oversight, ensuring access to services, and promoting the delivery of high-quality and value-based care.
- Successful ICU administration requires partnership between numerous stakeholders, including physicians, nurses, advanced practice providers, dietitians, respiratory therapists, and others.
- Critical care delivery has further evolved to better integrate technology, expand the number and scope of clinicians caring for patients, and incorporate family-centered care.

Organizational Structure of the Intensive Care Unit

- Critical care delivery has traditionally been confined to ICUs, and ICUs themselves have been historically conceptualized as physical brick and mortar spaces where critically ill patients are co-located to facilitate monitoring and take advantage of adjacencies. Contemporary critical care models also include the delivery of critical care beyond a given ICU.
- ICUs are often conceptualized as falling into one of three categories (Table 32.1.1):
  - Closed ICUs, wherein all aspects of patient care are managed by a dedicated critical care team with or without input from others, including those who may have admitted the patient to the ICU (where applicable)
  - Open ICUs, wherein those who admitted the patient to the ICU continue to manage the patient with the additional benefit of continuous monitoring, high-level nursing care, and other ICU resources with or without the consultative input of a critical care team
  - Hybrid ICUs that fall somewhere between these two ends of the spectrum but broadly include those where management responsibilities are shared between the admitting and critical care services
- ICUs can also be conceptualized in a complementary but slightly different manner:
  - ICUs may employ independent care models where a designated team is solely responsible for patient management (eg, admitting or critical care).
  - ICUs may employ collaborative care models wherein management is a shared responsibility between two or more teams. Collaborative care models are more common in specialized ICUs, such as those caring for surgical and/or transplant patients.
- Such designations, while sometimes conceptually helpful, rarely directly benefit patients served by a given ICU. Thus labeling ICUs in this manner is often less directly useful than ensuring care delivery models that best meet the needs of the patients served are designed and implemented.
- Regardless of a given ICU's organizational structure, all effective ICUs rely on multiprofessional collaboration to optimize clinical outcomes.

TABLE 32.1.1 Common Critical Care Organizational Structures and Their Characteristics

Critical Care Structure	Description	Advantages	Disadvantages	Patient Populations Typically Served
Closed ICU	All aspects of patient care are managed by a dedicated critical care team, typically with limited direct input from the admitting service	Improves adherence to best practices, reduces variability in care, ensures consistent intensivist involvement	Less autonomy for admitting services may be disenfranchising, potential challenges in building consensus, increased intensivist workload	Higher acuity medical and mixed medical and surgical patient populations
Open ICU	Admitting physicians retain full control of patient management with the benefit of ICU-level monitoring and resources	Greater autonomy for admitting service, preserves relationships between patients and admitting physicians	Increased variability in care, potential gaps in ICU-specific expertise, risks inconsistent or fragmented communication	Lower acuity patient populations (including monitoring only) or patients cared for by specialists very familiar with their needs
Hybrid ICU	A combination of open and closed models where management responsibilities are shared between teams with a focus on collaboration	Inherently promotes multispecialty input, recognizes specialist expertise, arguably helps promote comprehensive care for complex patients	Inherently increases complexity in decision-making, requiring strong communication and clearly defined roles to avoid delays or missteps in decision-making	Patients with highly specialized needs (such as transplant, cardiac surgery, and neurologic) who benefit from multispecialty input
Tele-ICU	Remote critical care specialists support on-site teams and patients through telemedicine technology offering monitoring, consultation, and/or direct management	Extends critical care expertise to otherwise underserved areas, supports on-staff clinicians, affords on-demand intensivist input	Relies on effective bidirectional communication and buy-in from bedside staff, requires infrastructure with associated financial barriers to entry	Patients in ICUs without 24/7 bedside intensivist coverage, including those in rural or resource-limited settings
Critical Care Consult Service	Critical care specialists support teams and patients at the bedside outside an ICU.	Can project critical care expertise outside of an ICU, improving the care of critically ill adults upstream or downstream from an ICU	Potential for delays in care if consultations are not timely, variability in adherence to recommendations, possible communication gaps	Patients with nascent or developing critical illness, such as in the emergency department or acute care floor

ICU, intensive care unit.

Aspirations and Attributes of an Intensive Care Unit

- Conceptualizing and/or defining the mission, vision, and values of a critical care delivery service can be a helpful exercise to inform goals and guide operations, particularly when developing new services or refining existing services.
  - The mission of an ICU should reflect its purpose, typically the provision of high-quality clinical care.
  - The vision of an ICU should define its future aspirations.
  - The values of an ICU are those that shape and guide both its daily and broader actions and decisions.
- These aspirations and the process by which they are developed with stakeholders can, in turn, help to delineate the attributes of an ICU or a critical care service that are important to stakeholders. Three key attributes important to an ICU typically emerge: quality, value, and access.
  - Whenever possible, these desired attributes should be aligned with those of the ICU's parent hospital and/or health care system.

Goals, Strategies, Execution, and Change Management in Intensive Care Unit Administration

- Having established an ICU's aspirations and desired attributes, the next task is to identify and set goals that, when achieved, further the ICU's desired attributes.
  - Ideal goals are specific, difficult but achievable, associated with concrete deadlines, and publicly known.
  - Goals should be aligned with desired attributes. For example:
    - A goal of reducing the time between deciding to admit a patient from the emergency department (ED) to the ICU and the patient's actual arrival time (ie, boarding) speaks to access as a desired attribute.
    - A goal of reducing central line–associated bloodstream infection speaks to quality as a desired attribute.
- A key component of effective ICU leadership is the development of strategies to achieve goals and the execution of those strategies.
  - Stakeholder engagement and consensus building are important aspects when developing strategy. When those responsible for execution are involved in planning, such efforts are more likely to be successful.
  - Consistent messaging, including a clear call to action, is a cornerstone of effective change management.
  - Barriers to change are often foreseeable, should be anticipated, and should be actively addressed or mitigated.
  - Effective leadership increases the likelihood of successful change management, which includes clear top-down communication about goals, strategies, and plans for execution.

Workforce and Staffing

- ICUs have both commonalities and sometimes marked differences in the composition of their workforce. For example, the provision of intensive nursing care to patients is common across ICUs around the world. However, the extent to which ICUs leverage other health care professionals in the care of critically ill patients is highly variable.

- Critical care delivery in the United States has, historically, been conceptualized as physician led and nurse driven. However, contemporary critical care has evolved to better reflect and acknowledge the value brought by myriad team members across professions and disciplines within those professions.
- From an administrative and organizational standpoint, it can be a helpful exercise to conceptualize elements of the ICU workforce as falling into one of three categories, as each has unique but important considerations (Table 32.1.2).
  - Constant workforce elements are those who are consistently present in the ICU. For example, nurses working in a given ICU are typically the most constant element of the workforce, dedicating all, or nearly all, of their professional effort to a given ICU.
    - Partially in response to increased turnover among nurses, a critically important constant workforce element, advanced practice providers have emerged as another key component of the constant workforce.
  - Cyclic workforce elements are those who work in the ICU on an intermittent but recurrently scheduled basis. For example, critical care physicians are typically cyclic in that they may devote professional effort to other endeavors, working in the ICU only intermittently.
  - Temporary workforce elements are those assigned to work in an ICU only transiently, such as physician trainees or contracted (ie, locum tenens or traveling) staff.
  - Furthermore, individuals within these workforce elements may work on a full-time, part-time, or contingent basis, adding further complexity.
- Staffing models must acknowledge and address the importance, role, and needs of all workforce elements.
- Achieving a stable and adequate workforce is essential to both providing consistent clinical care and reducing burnout, and meeting this goal is likely to require a mixture of different workforce elements. It is important to recognize that a workforce may be stable but inadequate, or adequate but unstable, and neither is a desirable state.
  - Staffing models that allow for flexibility in scheduling may not only better meet the needs of individuals but also allow more efficient allocation of personnel.
  - Strategies are necessary to promote the retention, development, and well-being of staff, and such strategies should acknowledge the unique priorities of individuals and the unique culture of a given ICU.

Team-Based Approaches to Operations and Effective Communication

- Teams are key not only to the delivery of clinical care within an ICU but also to championing and ensuring quality within the unit.
  - Trust, shared commitment and accountability, attention to (and visibility of) results, and productive conflict management are all foundational aspects of building a high-performing team.
- Operating plans can help teams bridge the gap between strategy and execution. Such plans should aim to detail how plans to meet goals are implemented, define the roles of team members, describe relevant workflows, and establish expectations (eg, timeliness).
  - A rudimentary operating plan may be as simple as codifying the time at which multidisciplinary rounds are to begin, which aims to align the activities and expectations of the workforce around a shared goal and activity.
  - In reality, minute-to-minute and hour-to-hour workflows between multidisciplinary team members are rarely perfectly aligned, and effective ICU administration includes identifying and addressing challenges in synchronizing different workflows within the ICU.
- The development, maintenance, and regular assessment of workforce competency are critical to developing and sustaining team performance.
  - Simulation training, skills checklists, and competency-based education are valuable tools to achieve these aims.

TABLE 32.1.2 Components of the ICU Workforce

Workforce Component	Description	Example Roles and Positions	Benefits to ICU Operations	Unique Challenges
Constant workforce	Staff consistently present in the ICU, dedicating nearly all their professional effort to the unit	Nurses, advanced practice providers, and often pharmacists	Create stability in clinical care delivery, in-depth knowledge of ICU processes and procedures forming the "memory" of the ICU	High risk of burnout due to high work intensity, instability in the constant workforce undermines ICU stability
Cyclic workforce	Staff who work in the ICU intermittently on a regularly scheduled basis, combining ICU work with responsibilities in other areas	Critical care physicians, and often respiratory therapists who may have shared roles	Flexibility in resource allocation, bring perspectives and knowledge from other areas, may be less prone to burnout	May be less familiar with ICU-specific operations, emphasizing the need for effective communication and transitions of care
Temporary workforce	Staff assigned to the ICU only transiently	Trainees and contract (ie, locum tenens or traveling) staff	Flexibility helps to address staffing shortages, including during surge demands.	Least familiar with ICU-specific operations with potential impacts on team cohesion, communication, and clinical care

ICU, intensive care unit.

  - Team training can help both to achieve coordinated, high-quality care and to build relationships. Approaches include standardized courses and curricula (eg, Advanced Cardiac Life Support) and in situ simulation training.
    - Team training also helps to develop shared mental models for common problems across members of the multidisciplinary workforce.
- The team-based, multiprofessional, and multidisciplinary nature of contemporary critical care both requires effective communication and simultaneously serves to complicate this laudable aim.
  - Real or imagined hierarchies between and within professions that constitute the ICU team are often meaningful barriers to effective communication.
    - These challenges are further potentiated by gradients in professional experience and the pervasive influences of stress and burnout in ICUs.
  - ICU leaders must aim to foster an environment where team members feel comfortable voicing concerns or clarifying ambiguous situations.
    - Productive conflict resolution skills are crucial for maintaining team cohesion. The absence of conflict, or conflict avoidance, is maladaptive and leaves important topics unaddressed.
    - Frameworks for clear communication (eg, SBAR or organ-system-based rounding) both enhance clarity and reduce the risk for lapses in communication completeness.
  - Regular meetings for clinical purposes (eg, rounds), quality purposes (eg, morbidity and mortality conferences), and administrative purposes help ICU leaders promote communication, orient and align the team toward important objectives, and address ongoing issues.
- Routine family involvement in decision-making has been shown to improve clinical and patient-centered outcomes and satisfaction. Creating processes and an environment that facilitates and welcomes family input, including open visiting hours and routine family meetings, is crucial.
  - Communication with families should aim to be honest, transparent, and clear, particularly during crises or when disclosing adverse events.
  - A consistent approach to family engagement and communication helps build trust and furnish emotional support.

Cost of Medical Care in the Intensive Care Unit

- Accurately accounting for the impact of critical illness on total U.S. health care expenditures is challenging. Critical care has been previously estimated to account for ~4% of national health care expenditures. For 2019, the Centers for Disease Control and Prevention (CDC) reported that such expenditures totaled 3.45 trillion dollars, in which case total ICU costs in the United States might be reasonably estimated to account for ~140 billion dollars annually.
- Questions about the cost of a day in the ICU often arise in clinical practice when trying to conceptualize the financial impact of extended critical care. Studies have demonstrated that first-day ICU costs are typically higher than costs on subsequent days and, to a greater extent, in surgical versus medical ICUs. Reasonable estimates of daily ICU costs are $4,500 on day 1 and $2,500 to $3,000 on subsequent days in medical ICUs, with higher costs in surgical and other specialized ICUs.
- Key contributors to ICU costs include:
  - Staffing, often found to represent the predominant driver of ICU costs
  - Medications
  - Diagnostic testing
  - Advanced therapies (eg, mechanical ventilation, renal replacement)
- Value in critical care can be conceptualized as the quality of outcomes relative to cost. Strategies to improve value include:
  - Reducing practice variability through standardized approaches (eg, protocols)
  - Implementation of decision support tools to reduce waste
  - Elimination or reduction of higher cost therapies, medications, and other approaches with unproven or unsupported benefit relative to cost
  - Clinically appropriate reduction of routine diagnostics that may not add value, such as daily laboratory testing and routine radiography.
- Given that ICUs are high-resource environments that typically entail substantial investment in staffing, physical plant, durable equipment, and other elements, collaborative financial management can also be used to help manage costs.
  - Successful ICU administration involves identifying what investments are required to meet the ICU's aspirations and goals and to further the development of its desired attributes. This may include staff, equipment, space or facilities, technology, and so forth.
  - Once needs have been identified, the next step is to develop a rationale for investment, which may be rooted in one or more of the following:
    - Supporting other services
    - Honoring or furthering desired attributes of the unit
    - Enhancing clinical care
    - Furthering staff well-being or satisfaction
    - Meeting regulatory requirements
    - Return on investment
  - ICU leaders should work closely with their multidisciplinary counterparts to control costs by exploring cost reduction initiatives and critically analyzing the impact of clinical care processes on both clinical outcomes and costs.

Population Health and the Intensive Care Unit

- The role of an ICU or critical care service in population health can be conceptualized as reducing preventable admissions through early intervention, reducing preventable readmissions, ensuring access to critical care services, improving care coordination, and addressing social determinants of health that might contribute to critical illness.
  - Coordination with outpatient, other inpatient, and post–acute care services may help prevent admissions

and readmissions by promoting a continuum of care in which the ICU is an important element.
  - Tele-ICU services are uniquely suited to extend the reach of critical care clinicians to underserved areas, which both improves access and remotely supports other clinicians at the bedside through monitoring, consultation, and/or direct management.
- Although population health principles are challenging to apply in an ICU setting, broader population health initiatives can reduce ICU admissions by improving chronic disease management and delivering preventive care.

Documentation, Billing, and Clinical Informatics in the Intensive Care Unit

- Accurate and timely clinical documentation is crucial to coordinate care delivery, preserve continuity of care, ensure compliance, and facilitate billing for services rendered.
- Clinical documentation and other interactions with the electronic health record are consistently identified as primary drivers of clinician dissatisfaction. As such, it is important that ICU leaders work to integrate the electronic health record as smoothly as is possible into clinical workflows in the ICU.
  - For structured data entry (eg, vital signs), approaches leveraging device integration and interoperability not only reduce the burden of documentation but may also promote greater accuracy and timeliness in creating a dynamic digital representation of a critically ill patient.
  - For unstructured data entry (eg, progress notes), approaches like templates, voice recognition, and ambient listening may all help reduce the burden of routine clinical documentation.
- Clinical documentation in the ICU should generally follow the established best practices for clinical documentation in other contexts, namely:
  - Clinical documentation should aim to both enhance care and record and validate the role of the author in that care.
  - Notes should delineate what the author personally saw and perceived, what the author thought or reasoned (ie, analysis and thought process), and what actions were recommended or taken by the author.
- Critical care billing in the United States is time based and uses two relevant Current Procedural Terminology (CPT) codes. Under recently revised guidance from the U.S. Centers for Medicare & Medicaid Services (CMS) related to critical care and split/shared billing, clinicians should approach billing for critical care services as follows:
  - CPT 99291 is used for the first 30 to 74 minutes of critical care, and only a single 99291 can be billed on a given calendar day.
  - CPT 99292 is used for additional 30-minute increments, and under revised CMS guidance from 2023, a 99292 should only be billed in addition to a 99291 when critical care services total 104 minutes (or more).
  - This revised CMS guidance also attributes aggregated critical care time to a single billing practitioner, which is the one who provides the "substantive portion" of services on a particular date.
- Note that billing and reimbursement approaches may differ between CMS and commercial payers, but over time, commercial payers tend to adopt CMS guidance.
- Given that billing for critical care is time based, professional charges for these services should be supported by recording additional elements in the clinical documentation, namely:
  - Why or how the patient is critically ill (eg, what organ failures were being addressed)
  - Relevant diagnoses
  - Documentation of the total time that was personally spent rendering services that did not overlap with other billing clinicians
    - This time does not need to be continuous.
    - Time spent can include direct patient management (that is not separately billed), time spent with the patient or family related to medical decision-making, and the time spent generating clinical documentation, all while proximate to the patient (eg, on the unit or floor).
- Robust clinical documentation also helps to ensure that the complexity and acuity of illness and associated clinical care are captured, which is important from both a quality and reimbursement standpoint.
- Clinical informatics can help to improve the timeliness and quality of care delivered in an ICU.
  - Clinical decision support tools may help facilitate earlier recognition of patient decompensation, ensure adherence to evidence-based best practices, and reduce variability.
  - Audit and feedback tools (eg, dashboards) can help track patient-centric and other performance metrics, such as compliance with the established best practices, which may reduce complications associated with critical illness.

Broader Administrative Models

- An organization can be broadly defined as an organized body with a purpose. Individual ICUs are, therefore, organizations in that they bring together a group of multiprofessional individuals (ie, an organized body) to care for critically ill patients (ie, a purpose).
- The ideal ICU would be a high-reliability organization with a focus on consistency in care delivery, standardization, and continuous learning.
- In pursuit of these goals on a larger scale, hospitals and health care systems are increasingly aiming to integrate multiple ICUs with the aim of improving oversight.
- Critical care organizations (CCOs) have arisen to meet these needs in organizing ICUs under a unified administrative structure, improving the quality of, value of, and access to critical care services at a larger scale.
  - CCOs often begin with horizontal integration by facilitating collaboration and standardization across ICUs.
  - CCOs may also aim to further vertical integration across the continuum of critical illness, which includes improving care before the ICU (eg, in the ED or on the floor) and after the ICU in championing ongoing care and follow-up of critical illness survivors.
- CCOs can often facilitate or accomplish goals that can be difficult or impossible for a single ICU, such as resource sharing, meeting surges in demand for critical care,

cross-training, promoting workforce stability across different ICUs, standardization of practice, and centralized quality and operational oversight.

- While CCOs offer myriad conceptual and practical benefits, their successful development and implementation is contingent on buy-in and support from key organizational leaders, investment in infrastructure (eg, technology and personnel), and support from staff.

Summary and Future Directions

- The key principles of ICU administration include defining aspirations, setting measurable goals, collaboratively developing strategies to achieve those goals, and ensuring effective execution. Consistent evaluation and adaptation are essential.
- Emerging trends in ICU administration include the use of telemedicine, integration of advanced analytics and machine learning, and an increased focus on effective team-based multiprofessional and multidisciplinary care.
- Moving forward, ICUs must focus on how to better organize critical care delivery to meet the needs of patients and stakeholders, surge planning for disasters, thoughtful ICU design that supports both patients and staff, and ethical considerations related to resource allocation and decision-making.

SUGGESTED READINGS

Centers for Disease Control and Prevention, National Center for Health Statistics. Health, United States, 2020–2021. Table HExpGDP. Gross domestic product, national health expenditures, per capita amounts, percent distribution, and average annual percent change: United States, selected years 1960–2019. Accessed July 1, 2024. https://www.cdc.gov/nchs/data/hus/2020-2021/HExpGDP.pdf

Davidson JE, Aslakson RA, Long AC, et al. Guidelines for family-centered care in the neonatal, pediatric, and adult ICU. *Crit Care Med*. 2017;45(1):103-128.

Gershengorn HB, Garland A, Gong MN. Patterns of daily costs differ for medical and surgical intensive care unit patients. *Ann Am Thorac Soc*. 2015;12(12):1831-1836.

Gershengorn HB, Kocher R, Factor P. Management strategies to effect change in intensive care units: lessons from the world of business. Part III. Effectively effecting and sustaining change. *Ann Am Thorac Soc*. 2014;11(3):454-457.

Halpern NA. Can the costs of critical care be controlled? *Curr Opin Crit Care*. 2009;15(6):591-596.

Halpern NA, Pastores SM. Critical care medicine beds, use, occupancy, and costs in the United States: a methodological review. *Crit Care Med*. 2015;43(11):2452-2459.

Kayser JB, Kaplan LJ. Conflict management in the ICU. *Crit Care Med*. 2020;48(9):1349-1357.

Kleinpell R, Grabenkort WR, Boyle WA, Vines DL, Olsen KM. The Society of Critical Care Medicine at 50 years: interprofessional practice in critical care: looking back and forging ahead. *Crit Care Med*. 2021;49(12):2017-2032.

Kreeftenberg HG, Pouwels S, Bindels AJGH, de Bie A, van der Voort PHJ. Impact of the advanced practice provider in adult critical care: a systematic review and meta-analysis. *Crit Care Med*. 2019;47(5):722-730.

Leung S, Gregg SR, Coopersmith CM, et al. Critical care organizations: business of critical care and value/performance building. *Crit Care Med*. 2018;46:1-11.

McCarthy C, O'Rourke NC, Madison JM. Integrating advanced practice providers into medical critical care teams. *Chest*. 2013;143(3):847-850.

Moitra VK. Critical care billing in 2023. *J Cardiothorac Anesth*. 2025;39(1):266-272.

Pastores SM, Halpern NA, Oropello JM, et al. Critical care organizations in academic medical centers in North America: a descriptive report. *Crit Care Med*. 2015;43:2239-2244.

Pastores SM, Kvetan V, Coopersmith CM, et al. Workforce, workload, and burnout among intensivists and advanced practice providers: a narrative review. *Crit Care Med*. 2019;47:550-557.

Sevransky JE, Agarwal A, Jabaley CS, et al. Standardized care is better than individualized care for the majority of critically ill patients. *Crit Care Med*. 2021;49:151-155.

Sikora A, Ayyala D, Rech MA, et al; for the MRC-ICU Investigator Team. Impact of pharmacists to improve patient care in the critically ill: a large multicenter analysis using meaningful metrics with the Medication Regimen Complexity-ICU (MRC-ICU) score. *Crit Care Med*. 2022;50(9):1318-1328.

Subramanian S, Pamplin JC, Hravnak M, et al. Tele-critical care: an update from the Society of Critical Care Medicine tele-ICU committee. *Crit Care Med*. 2020;48:553-561.

SECTION 33

Quality Improvement and Patient Safety

Section Editor: Edward A. Bittner

33.1

Quality Improvement and Patient Safety

Samer Shoshan and Jose L. Diaz-Gomez

Definitions

- Medical error: the Institute of Medicine (IOM) defined medical errors as a failure of a planned action to be completed as intended (errors of execution) or the use of a wrong plan to achieve an aim (errors of planning). Moreover, following patient's admission, errors can occur at any phase of care (diagnosis, treatment, or transition of care) that may results in harm to patient.
- Adverse event is a serious incident that cause harm to patients during their hospital stay by a medical intervention rather than the underlying disease itself. They have a wide range of complications from minor injuries to severe disabilities and death. Adverse events result into prolonged hospital stay and increased cost.
- Sentinel event is a severe form of adverse events and defined by The Joint Commission as a patient safety incident that reaches a patient and results in death, permanent harm, or severe temporary harm and intervention required to sustain life. For example, wrong site surgery, wrong procedure, suicide, or wrong medications result into major harm. These events always initiate an investigation and root cause analysis (RCA) seeking system failure and prevent future incidents.
- Misuse of medications and technology are errors that can be in medications prescribing, dispensing, administration, or monitoring. These errors are the most preventable known errors. Advanced technology plays a major role in mitigating such errors. Some examples include electronic prescription, order verification, barcoding systems, medication reconciliation, and smart pumps.

Medication Errors: Assessment and Prevention

- Medication reconciliation is the process by which a medical provider reviews the patient's home or active medications list and current prescribed medications. This is essential prior to patient's different care transition, including admission, transfer, and discharge. This can prevent medications duplications, missing medication, or wrong dosage. It is one of the effective ways to prevent medications errors and adverse drug events.
- Information technology to reduce medication errors has offered unquestionable help in preventing and mitigating medications errors. Computerized physician order entry (CPOE) within electronic health records (EHRs) assures handwritten prescription is no longer threat for errors. Now electronic prescription shows clear medication name, dose, and route with less confusion to the pharmacy team.
- *Automated pharmacy system:* currently with CPOE, a robotic system can pick and dispense the medications in a quick and efficient way minimizing human errors.
- *Clinical decision support system (CDSS):* electronic systems with pop-up messages and recommendations to help improve clinical decision for a patient's appropriate dosage, drug-drug interactions, risks for pregnancy or lactations, medication duplication, suggested alternatives, or antibiotic de-escalation. Barcoding system: patients now wear bracelets with barcodes to help in identification and medication verification so can prevent errors or wrong patient or wrong dose.

Crisis Management and Teamwork

- Simulation training in health care consists of practicing real clinical scenarios with persons acting like patients or smart mannequins to provide training for health care providers. Many health care facilitates have a simulation center or lab that care providers can access for training and practicing. Simulation training has been shown to be a very cost-effective method for elevating skills and improving patient safety. Cardiac arrest, trauma, difficult airways, and disaster medicine scenarios are common simulation examples. Simulation training helps with developing communication, leadership, and teamwork skills in a very safe and controlled environment. Debriefing is an important strategy after the scenario is completed. The instructor and candidates discuss together what went right and wrong and how to improve it next time.

- Crisis manuals and other cognitive aids in the health care industry are valuable as high reliability organizations are always expected to face unforeseen crisis and emergencies that can compromise patients' and providers' safety. During crisis and emergencies, quick and easily accessible resources or aids help in guiding health care providers to safely manage these challenging scenarios. Resources can be printed books, brochures, or online in the form of algorithms, checklist, or mnemonics. Training in the use of such manuals and aids can be provided via simulation or mandatory courses to be taken regularly. These materials should be revised and updated as new literature becomes available.
- Teamwork training is essential to crisis management. The Joint Commission has reported that communication and teamwork failures can contribute up to two-thirds of medical errors and adverse events. Currently, health care leaders have shown an increase in interest in teamwork collaboration and patient safety. A wide variety of strategies for teamwork training exist, including teaching contents (specific knowledge, skills, or attitude), tools, and delivery methods (dictations, demonstration, simulations, or role play).
    - TeamSTEPPS is an example of a well-established teamwork training program. Team building can also occur through leisure activities that can be done outside working hours. Such activities improve communications, identify leadership potential, build trust, and elevate a team's spirit.
- Handoff communication, also known as handover or care transition, occurs whenever responsibility for a patient's care is transferred to another provider or team. Breakdown in communication is common during this phase; hence, many methods have been adopted to ensure proper handoff and mitigate patient safety issues. As highlighted by the IOM, incrossing the quality chasm, 2001: "It is in inadequate handoffs that safety often fails first." Some of the most utilized for handoff communication tools include the SBAR (situation, background, assessment, recommendations) and the I-PASS (illness severity, patient information, action list, situational awareness and contingency plans, and synthesis by receiver) formats. These handoff tools provide a structured framework to deliver essential or information to the receiving team.
- Preoperative and procedural checklists are designed to reduce adverse events during and after surgery. The World Health Organization (WHO) developed the Surgical Safety Checklist approach after extensive research, aiming for improving safety, promoting teamwork, decreasing variances in practice, and applying best practices (Figure 33.1.1). This list is used before, during, and after surgery or procedure to ensure correct patient, correct procedure, correct site, available personals, tools, and equipment.

Quality Improvement Fundamentals

- Quality in health care has many definitions. The IOM in 1990 defined quality as "the degree to which healthcare services for individuals and populations increase the likelihood of desired health outcomes and are consistent with current professional knowledge." Another definition is doing the right thing at the right time in the right way for the right person and having the best results possible.
- The WHO in 2018 defined health care quality as "the degree to which health services for individuals and populations increase the likelihood of desired health outcomes." The provided care should be integrated, safe, timely, effective, efficient, equitable, and patient centered.

Design, Analysis, and Implementation of Quality Improvement Projects

- In order to improve quality, a framework is needed to assure all aspects have been addressed. One of most well-known frameworks used for quality improvement (QI) in health care was developed by Donabedian and consists of structure, process, and outcome measures.
- Measures of structure include intensive care unit (ICU) design and capacity, staffing, qualifications, technology, policies, procedures, and equipment. Process measures, sometime referred to as performance measures, include evidence-based practices to achieve the desired outcome.
- Examples of process measures include deep venous thrombosis (DVT) prophylaxis rate, stress ulcer prophylaxis rate, protective lung strategy for acute respiratory distress syndrome (ARDS), and aspirin initiation 24 hours post intravenous (IV) tissue plasminogen activator (tPA) for stroke. Outcome measures focus directly on the impact on care achieved for patients. Examples of outcome measures include mortality rate, readmission rate, satisfaction rate, and quality of life.
- By utilizing and analyzing the abovementioned measures, we can identify areas of underperformance.
- Another commonly used framework is the PDSA cycle or Plan-Do-Study-Act cycle. The cycle is a continuous, four-stage problem-solving technique used to enhance a process or implement change. It is one of the few QI frameworks that concentrates on the key component of change: "the conversion of thoughts and intentions into practices." It is a core aspect of numerous QI strategies, such as the model for improvement, lean, Six Sigma, and overall quality management. Data collection is essential for any QI project to identify underperformance, progress, and testing impact of interventions on care quality and patient's outcome. Data sources can be patient EHRs, patient surveys, wearable devices, and observations. Data must be relevant, accurate, reliable, and complying with regulatory needs also ensuring patient's confidentiality is protected.

Quality Improvement Metrics

- QI metrics represent indirect quantitative measurement of the quality of care provided. Quality metrics or indicators must be relevant, valid, accurate, reliable, actionable, meaningful, aligned with QI project goals, and feasible. Common QI metrics in the ICU setting include central line–associated bloodstream infections (CLABSIs), catheter-associated urinary tract infection (CAUTI), ventilator-associated events (VAEs), proportions of

Surgical Safety Checklist

World Health Organization | Patient Safety — A World Alliance for Safer Health Care

Before induction of anaesthesia → **Before skin incision** → **Before patient leaves operating room**

Before induction of anaesthesia

(with at least nurse and anaesthetist)

Has the patient confirmed his/her identity, site, procedure, and consent?
- ☐ Yes

Is the site marked?
- ☐ Yes
- ☐ Not applicable

Is the anaesthesia machine and medication check complete?
- ☐ Yes

Is the pulse oximeter on the patient and functioning?
- ☐ Yes

Does the patient have a:

Known allergy?
- ☐ No
- ☐ Yes

Difficult airway or aspiration risk?
- ☐ No
- ☐ Yes, and equipment/assistance available

Risk of >500ml blood loss (7ml/kg in children)?
- ☐ No
- ☐ Yes, and two IVs/central access and fluids planned

Before skin incision

(with nurse, anaesthetist and surgeon)

- ☐ **Confirm all team members have introduced themselves by name and role.**
- ☐ **Confirm the patient's name, procedure, and where the incision will be made.**

Has antibiotic prophylaxis been given within the last 60 minutes?
- ☐ Yes
- ☐ Not applicable

Anticipated Critical Events

To Surgeon:
- ☐ What are the critical or non-routine steps?
- ☐ How long will the case take?
- ☐ What is the anticipated blood loss?

To Anaesthetist:
- ☐ Are there any patient-specific concerns?

To Nursing Team:
- ☐ Has sterility (including indicator results) been confirmed?
- ☐ Are there equipment issues or any concerns?

Is essential imaging displayed?
- ☐ Yes
- ☐ Not applicable

Before patient leaves operating room

(with nurse, anaesthetist and surgeon)

Nurse Verbally Confirms:
- ☐ The name of the procedure
- ☐ Completion of instrument, sponge and needle counts
- ☐ Specimen labelling (read specimen labels aloud, including patient name)
- ☐ Whether there are any equipment problems to be addressed

To Surgeon, Anaesthetist and Nurse:
- ☐ What are the key concerns for recovery and management of this patient?

This checklist is not intended to be comprehensive. Additions and modifications to fit local practice are encouraged. Revised 1 / 2009 © WHO, 2009

FIGURE 33.1.1 The World Health Organization (WHO) surgical safety checklist. (© 2025 The World Health Organization.)

eligible patients received (stress ulcer prophylaxis, venous thromboembolism [VTE] prophylaxis, antibiotics in septic shock, protective lung ventilation in ARDS, and sedation interruption in mechanically ventilated patients), ICU length of stay, and mortality rate.

Patient Satisfaction Measurement

- Patient satisfaction is an indicator reflecting perception of the quality of care provided to them and their families. Involving patients and family members in decisions-making has a positive impact on increased satisfaction. Questionnaires and surveys obtained through phone calls, online, or direct with patient or family are commonly used methods for measuring the quality or satisfaction of care

Value-Based Care Incentives, Pay-for-Performance

- Methods to persuade medical providers to prioritize high-quality care and patient safety include linking payments, reimbursement, or rewarding based on preestablished targets for favorable patient outcome (readmission, complications, death). For example, the Centers for Medicare & Medicaid Services (CMS) has implemented the 2014 Hospital Value-Based Purchasing (Hospital VBP) Program, which adjusts hospitals' payments based on their performance on several safety and quality metrics, some of which are directly affected by the care patients receive in ICUs. Participating in such programs can provide an opportunity for QI.

Performance Assessment

- A performance assessment, in the context of hospitals, is a collection of aggregated, quantified, and analyzed data on specific health care measures that are considered to have the most significant positive impact on patient outcomes, allowing hospitals to track and demonstrate improvements in their quality of care when these measures show positive changes. The Joint Commission places more emphasis on accountability measures as follows:

1. Performing evidence-based care process improves health outcomes.
2. Performing the care process is closely connected to the patient outcome.
3. The measure accurately assesses whether or not the care process has actually been provided.
4. Implementing the measure has little or no chance of inducing unintended adverse consequences.

Dashboard and Individual Benchmarking

- Utilization of open-access online dashboards helps visualize performance assessment and safety measures in individual hospitals and comparison across other hospitals. A dashboard is a tool that facilitates the organization and interpretation of data at a macro level. Indeed, clinical dashboards have improved interconnectivity and patient care understanding between multidisciplinary teams and health care quality stakeholders. Moreover, continuous, concurrent tracking of performance measures in dashboards supports transparency, decision-making, dissemination of information, and transformative discussion that can guide innovative process management.

Group and Facilities Scorecards

- A scorecard is a strategic planning and performance measurement system that provides daily, weekly, or monthly information. It is considered a well-rounded set of quantifiable measures derived from an organization's strategy. The scorecards monitor organization performance against strategic goals while improving internal and external communication. Scorecards enforce accountability and provide actionable data; in contrast, dashboards provide drill-down capability and inform root cause. Despite their differences, evidence supports the best outcomes improvement when scorecards and dashboards are used together.

Public Reporting

- Federal quality payment program
  - The CMS Hospital VBP Program was designed to reward clinicians for providing high-value, high-quality patient-centered care. The program has two tracks. In the merit-based incentive payment system, the clinician earns performance-based payment adjustments for the services provided to Medicare patients. A second program, the advanced alternative payment model, is designed to provide tailored incentives to clinicians who are providing high-quality, high-value care, as it can focus on specific clinical conditions, care episodes, or populations.
- Anesthesia registries
  - The Anesthesia Quality institute launched the National Anesthesia Outcomes Registry (NACOR) to provide patient demographics reports and evidence-based rationale that inform treatment choices. Furthermore, the NACOR provides national and peer-group benchmarks that can lead to performance improvement. Additionally, the NACOR supports the quality and improvement activities components of the CMS merit-based incentive payment system through two quality reporting options (group practice reporting and individual).

Change Management Methods

- Peer-review and morbidity and mortality (M&M) conferences
- M&M conferences facilitate interprofessional and multidisciplinary discussions to learn from one's mistakes, providing a forum in which all personnel including institutional administrators can openly discuss errors while integrating system thinking and patient safety.
- Lean Six Sigma
  - Six Sigma is a disciplined, data-driven approach and methodology for eliminating defects.
  - Defects are defined as anything outside customer specifications. To achieve Six Sigma, a process must not produce >3.4 defects per million opportunities, which exemplifies a continuous journey toward perfection.
  - Six Sigma utilizes a framework for improvement—The DMAIC. This includes *Define* the problem to be addressed, *Measure* the baseline performance, *Analyze* processes and data to determine improvement needs, *Improve* the process by implementing solutions, and *Control* the process by establishing ongoing reviews of the performance. Additionally, each DMAIC component has tools to operationalize the framework as follows:
    - *Define*—stakeholder analysis & input, aim statement, project charter, small test of change
    - *Measure*—measurement plan, checking sheets, histograms, process observation, process capability, process mapping, value stream mapping, stratification, run charts, current state
    - *Analyze*—fishbone, Pareto diagram, RCA, cause-effect and scatter diagrams, correlation analysis, control charts, regression analysis
    - *Improve*—brainstorming, affinity analysis, future state mapping, PDSA cycles, visual control & andons, simulation, standardization, implementation plan
    - *Control*—control plan, transition plan, and project closure document, lessons learned, dashboard

Quality Improvement and the 5 S Processes

- The 5 S (sort, set in order, shine, standardize, and sustain) is a method for organizing, cleaning, developing, and sustaining a productive work environment.
  - *Sort:* needed items from the un-needed
  - *Set in order:* efficient access and identification
  - *Shine:* area is clean, and everything is maintained.
  - *Standardize:* consistent guidelines, visual indicators
  - *Sustain:* education, communication, and continual improvement so that behaviors become a habit
- The 5 S method has inherent benefits, such as eliminating wastes, improving team member flow, reducing search time, opening floor space, providing a foundation for visual management, reducing training time, and mitigating caregivers' stress.

Value Stream Mapping

- A value stream mapping (VSM) employs a flow diagram, which demonstrates all activities to process the patient, from start to finish. VSM as a tool to identify waste, reduce process cycle times, and implement process improvement. Its key features include process flow, information flow, process, wait & lead times, value analysis, and first-time quality (FTQ). The process time is the time to perform the work of the process step. It is the time from entering to exiting a process box—value-added time.
- Wait time (WT) is the amount of time between process steps when the product or service is not being worked on—non–value-added time. Total lead time (LT) is the time from when a service or product is requested until it is completed or delivered—process time + wait time. FTQ is the percentage of time a process step is completed accurately. Rolled FTQ is obtained multiplying the FTQ of each step in the process.

- The percentage of time the outcome of the entire product or service is completed accurately the first time—Value-added ratio = PT/LT × 100 (%). There are three versions of VSM, a current state (what is happening now), ideal state (what a perfect situation looks like), and future state (what is feasible in the near future).

Failure Mode and Effect Analysis

- Failure mode and effect analysis (FMEA) is a technique for capturing active and latent threats to safety. The likelihood that a specific process fails is combined with an estimate of the relative impact of that failure to produce a critically index. And this index facilitates a prioritization process as improvements targets. Furthermore, FMEA is advantageous because it combines the insights from both subject matter experts and frontline personnel to prioritize hazard and implement a timeline for QI. Indeed, the latter FMEA strength over other methods has been openly advocated by many health care organizations.

Root Cause Analysis

- Root Cause Analysis (RCA) is a structured facilitated team process to identify root causes of an event that resulted in an undesired outcome and develop corrective actions.
- The Joint Commission mandates an RCA following every sentinel event. The RCA requires complying with the following essential elements to be an effective investigation method:
  1. A skilled leader focused on key system defects and with an understanding of the entire range of contributing and causation factors
  2. An interprofessional and multidisciplinary approach, including institutional administrators and frontline caregivers
  3. An active participation of individuals involved in the case
  4. Identification of strong corrective action and prevention of future harm
  5. Implementation and sustainability of corrective actions including proper feedback and communication of lessons learned across the institution

Barriers to Quality Improvement

- Although organizational leadership support, data-driven practices, and active involvement of initiatives champions are QI facilitators, there are specific QI barriers that deserve further consideration. First, lack of caregivers' engagement in QI is identified as an important barrier. Second, a QI knowledge gap and poor motivation as barriers, especially in those institutions that lack consistent support or resources. Third, there is a need for genuine team building for QI success, and the lack of teamwork and organizational rigidity leads to inherent resistance to change. Lastly, there are practical examples of QI initiatives such as RCA investigations that have identifiable barriers (investigations of questionable quality or conducted under significant time pressure, poor design and implementation of risk controls, feedback without supportive learning, incidents investigated in isolation, and complex balance between individual and organizational responsibility). Therefore, all these factors should be optimized to make QI seamless, worthwhile, and rewarding.

Artificial Intelligence and Patient Safety

- Artificial intelligence (AI) tools can facilitate intelligent decision-making through learning from massive data flow. AI has been introduced into the health care setting with the aim of reducing workload on providers, facilitating better care delivery and increase patient flow.
- With proper use and aligned with local regulations, AI can be powerful tool to prevent medical errors and enhance quality of care through:
  - Early detection of clinical deterioration by analysis and continuous monitoring of patient's vital signs
  - Patient risk stratification
  - Clinical decision support
  - Reduction of medication errors

SUGGESTED READINGS

Agency for Healthcare Research and Quality. Quality in healthcare. *2019 National Healthcare Quality and Disparities Report* [Internet]. Agency for Healthcare Research and Quality (US); 2020. https://www.ncbi.nlm.nih.gov/books/NBK579353/

Aggarwal R, Mytton OT, Derbrew M, et al. Training and simulation for patient safety. *Qual Saf Health Care*. 2010;19:i34-i43.

Ahsani-Estahbanati E, Sergeevich Gordeev V, Doshmangir L. Interventions to reduce the incidence of medical error and its financial burden in health care systems: a systematic review of systematic reviews. *Front Med (Lausanne)*. 2022;9:875426.

Al-Elq AH. Simulation-based medical teaching and learning. *J Family Community Med*. 2010;17(1):35-40.

Bates DW, Levine D, Syrowatka A, et al. The potential of artificial intelligence to improve patient safety: a scoping review. *NPJ Digit Med*. 2021;4:54.

Blazin LJ, Sitthi-Amorn J, Hoffman JM, Burlison JD. Improving patient handoffs and transitions through adaptation and implementation of I-PASS across multiple handoff settings. *Pediatr Qual Saf*. 2020;5(4):e323.

Braun JP, Mende H, Bause H, et al. Quality indicators in intensive care medicine: why? Use or burden for the intensivist. *Ger Med Sci*. 2010;8:Doc22.

Chelluri LP. Quality and performance improvement in critical care. *Indian J Crit Care Med*. 2008;12(2):67-76.

Chhabra A, Singh A, Kuka PS, Kaur H, Kuka AS, Chahal H. Role of perioperative surgical safety checklist in reducing morbidity and mortality among patients: an observational study. *Niger J Surg*. 2019;25(2):192-197.

Choudhury A, Asan O. Role of artificial intelligence in patient safety outcomes: systematic literature review. *JMIR Med Inform*. 2020;8(7):e18599.

Cohen RI, Jaffrey F, Reitzner JB, Baumann MH. Quality improvement and pay for performance. *Chest*. 2013;143(6):1542-1547.

Costar DM, Hall KK. Improving team performance and patient safety on the job through team training and performance support tools: a systematic review. *J Patient Saf*. 2020;16(3S suppl 1):S48-S56.

Council of the Institute of Medicine. *America's Health in Transition: Protecting and Improving Quality*. National Academy Press; 1994.

de Vries EN, Ramrattan MA, Smorenburg SM, Gouma DJ, Boermeester MA. The incidence and nature of in-hospital adverse events: a systematic review. *Qual Saf Health Care*. 2008;17(3):216-223.

Delgado-Hito P, Alcalà-Jimenez I, Martinez-Momblan MA, et al. Satisfaction of intensive care unit patients linked to clinical and organisational factors: a cross-sectional multicentre study. *Aust Critical Care*. 2023;36(5):716-722.

Ellahham S, Ellahham N. Use of artificial intelligence for improving patient flow and healthcare delivery. *J Comput Sci Syst Biol*. 2019;12(3):1-6.

Greig PR, Zolger D, Onwochei DN, Thurley N, Higham H, Desai N. Cognitive aids in the management of clinical emergencies: a systematic review. *Anaesthesia*. 2023;78(3):343-355.

Institute of Medicine. *Preventing Medication Errors*. National Academies Press; 2006.

Institute of Medicine (US) Committee on Quality of Health Care in America; Kohn LT, Corrigan JM, Donaldson MS, eds. *To Err Is Human: Building a Safer Health System*. National Academies Press (US); 2000.

Institute of Medicine (US) Committee on Quality of Health Care in America. *Crossing the Quality Chasm: A New Health System for the 21st Century*. National Academies Press (US); 2001.

Jensen HI, Gerritsen RT, Koopmans M, et al. Satisfaction with quality of ICU care for patients and families: the EuroQ2 project. *Crit Care*. 2017; 21(1):239.

Joint Commission on Accreditation of Healthcare Organizations. Changes to definition of reviewable sentinel events. *Jt Comm Perspect*. 2005; 25(3):7.

Khanduja K, Scales DC, Adhikari NKJ. Pay for performance in the intensive care unit—Opportunity or threat? *Crit Care Med*. 2009;37(3):852-858.

Lindenauer PK, Remus D, Roman S, et al. Public reporting and pay for performance in hospital quality improvement. *N Engl J Med*. 2007;356(5): 486-496.

Lucian Leape Institute. *Patient safety and artificial intelligence: opportunities and challenges for care delivery*. Institute for Healthcare Improvement. 2024. Accessed January 1, 2026. https://www.ihi.org/initiatives/ihi-lucian-leape-institute/patient-safety-ai

Oyebode F. Clinical errors and medical negligence. *Med Princ Pract*. 2013; 22(4):323-333.

Patra KP, De Jesus O. Sentinel event. In: *StatPearls* [Internet]. StatPearls Publishing; 2024. Updated March 23, 2023. https://www.ncbi.nlm.nih.gov/books/NBK564388/

Ratwani RM, Bates DW, Classen DC. Patient safety and artificial intelligence in clinical care. *JAMA Health Forum*. 2024;5(2):e235514.

Sameera V, Bindra A, Rath GP. Human errors and their prevention in healthcare. *J Anaesthesiol Clin Pharmacol*. 2021;37(3):328-335.

Sharieff S, Sajjal A, Idrees A, Rafai W. Patient and family satisfaction in the intensive care unit of a quaternary care center. *Cureus*. 2023;15(9):e45795.

Skelly CL, Cassagnol M, Munakomi S. Adverse events. In: *StatPearls* [Internet]. StatPearls Publishing; 2024. Updated August 13, 2023. https://www.ncbi.nlm.nih.gov/books/NBK558963/

Tariq RA, Vashisht R, Sinha A, et al. Medication dispensing errors and prevention. In: *StatPearls* [Internet]. StatPearls Publishing; 2024. Updated February 12, 2024. https://www.ncbi.nlm.nih.gov/books/NBK519065/

Treadwell JR, Lucas S, Tsou AY. Surgical checklists: a systematic review of impacts and implementation. *BMJ Qual Saf*. 2014;23:299-318.

Weaver SJ, Dy SM, Rosen MA. Team-training in healthcare: a narrative synthesis of the literature. *BMJ Qual Saf*. 2014;23(5):359-372.

SECTION 34

Ethics and Medical Legal Issues

Section Editor: *Edward A. Bittner*

34.1

Ethics and Medical Legal Issues

Jun Soo Park and Matthew Sigakis

Medical Ethics

- When caring for critically ill patients, it is inevitable that ethical issues will arise.
  - Customs, laws, and ethical beliefs vary widely among societies and cultures, impacting moral and end-of-life issues in critical care settings.
  - This chapter explores a subset of ethical and legal topics that frequently arise in the intensive care unit.

Bioethical Principles

- Four key ethical tenets:
  - *Autonomy*: the right to self-govern without undue influence from a health care provider
  - *Beneficence*: the obligation to promote good and to prevent or remove harm
  - *Justice*: the goal to promote the greatest benefit to the largest number of individuals while inflicting the least amount of harm
  - *Nonmaleficence*: the need to refrain from inflicting harm
    - Nonmaleficence is considered the core of ethical and moral practice with decisions based on this tenet sometimes superseding even those based on beneficence and/or justice.
- *Patient autonomy* reflects an individual's right to make decisions about their medical care.
  - Autonomy is best preserved by obtaining informed consent and involving the patient in shared medical decision-making, whenever possible.
- Obtaining *informed consent* preserves patient autonomy, protects patients from harm, and is consequently an ethical responsibility of the treating clinician.
  - Informed consent ensures that patients understand their medical condition, the proposed treatment or procedure, potential risks and benefits, and any available alternatives.
  - Informed consent should be obtained for all procedures, therapies, and research.
  - Emergent situations may preclude the ability to obtain informed consent, and efforts should be made to explain care to the patient or surrogate decision maker at the earliest opportunity.

Decision-Making

- *Shared medical decision-making* recognizes patients as active participants in the decision-making process, affirming their autonomy by involving them in discussions and respecting their preferences and choices.
- *Competence* is a legal term; individuals over the age of 18 are presumed competent unless deemed incompetent through legal proceedings.
- In contrast, *decision-making capacity* is a medical term; individuals who can make their own informed health care decisions are deemed to have decision-making capacity.
  - If capacity is questioned, then a physician should evaluate the patient to determine if they can receive and understand medical information, discern various options presented, and choose a course based on the information offered.
  - In complicated situations where a patient's decision-making capacity is questioned, assessment by a consultant psychiatrist may be helpful.
- Many critically ill patients do not have decision-making capacity due to the gravity of their illness and/or because they are receiving sedative/analgesic medications to reduce suffering.
  - In these circumstances, an *advance directive* and/or a *surrogate* decision maker may be helpful.
- A *health care surrogate or durable power of attorney for health care* is a legal document prepared by the patient delineating

the person the patient would wish to make health care decisions under those circumstances.

- Using the principle of *substituted judgment*, a surrogate (typically a spouse, family member, or health care proxy) will make decisions for a patient when they cannot.
  - The surrogate is to make the decision that the *patient would make given the situation*; this decision may even differ from the surrogate's wishes.
  - If the surrogate does not know what the patient would decide, they should make the decision they feel is in the best interest of the patient and best reflects the patient's previously voiced beliefs and personality.
- An *advance directive* is a statement, in writing, specifying the patient's health care wishes should they become unable to make decisions.
  - The advanced directive is filled out by the patient themselves when they are in good health and of sound mind.
  - The directives ensure that patients' wishes are respected and followed when they are unable to express them, upholding the principle of patient autonomy.
  - <15% of the adult population have made advanced decisions regarding restrictions on life-supporting measures.
  - Increasingly, the US judicial system recognizes that advance directives may be verbal in nature and that what a patient has orally communicated to family, friends, or health care providers regarding treatment preferences may provide an acceptable framework for care decisions in the absence of written documentation.
- A *living will* is a type of advanced directive describing the medical treatments that a patient would wish to refuse or receive at the end of life.
  - These documents elucidate a patient's prior expressed wishes and should be considered in the decision-making process; however, US states vary as to whether living wills are legally binding.
  - The directives described in documents can vary from general principles to tremendously detailed requests.
  - Since it is impossible to predict exact circumstances surrounding severe illness, many living wills pertain only to the limited circumstances of brain death, persistent vegetative state, or a "terminal illness"; consequently, many living wills are only marginally helpful in a modern critical care environment.
  - Interpretation of the living will is best supplemented with formal goals of care discussions involving people closest to the patient.
- Family involvement in discussions involving treatment of a noncommunicative critically ill patient is vital to appropriate care and is best conducted in a quiet, private environment in an unhurried manner.
  - The patient should be included if they have capacity
  - When possible, a multidisciplinary team of social work, palliative care, and consultant providers can enhance the communication of the patient's clinical status to navigate medical decision-making.
  - The support of social work and palliative care can also assist the family's interpretation of the patient's wishes in the clinical context.
- *Palliative care* and *hospice care* are both approaches to care that focus on improving the quality of life for patients, but they have distinct differences in terms of their goals and eligibility criteria.
  - *Palliative care* aims to alleviate symptoms and reduce suffering alongside curative treatments, regardless of the stage of the disease.
  - *Hospice care* is specifically for patients nearing the end of life, who are no longer seeking curative interventions, focusing on emotional support and patient's comfort.
  - Hospice care requires a prognosis of ≤6 months.

End of Life, Withholding Therapies, and Withdrawing Care

- The goals of intensive care unit (ICU) therapy should always be confirmed with the patient and family.
  - For some patients, there are obvious goals such as preventing imminent death, curing acute disease, preventing /relieving pain and suffering, and eventually returning the patient to their premorbid level of function.
  - In some situations, patients may only hope to delay the disease process, and occasionally, ICU care is requested to prolong a patient's life long enough to allow for close relatives to arrive and pay last respects or to consent to organ donation prior to the patient's death.
- When discussing goals of therapy, the patient's values should be elicited and emphasized.
  - It is important for the health care team to discuss the patient's prognosis with the consultants involved and arrive at a consensus before meeting with the family.
  - The prognosis of the patient is very important in setting realistic therapeutic goals, but not always possible to provide early in the disease process.
  - If a definite prognosis cannot be determined, it is essential to describe the possible clinical trajectories and provide clear treatment options to the family.
- Once the prognosis has been discussed, the family or physician may propose a "*do not resuscitate*" (DNR) order.
  - The DNR status seeks to clarify which therapies will be offered to the patient in case of acute, life-threatening instability that requires immediate treatment to prevent death.
  - It must be emphasized to the family that an agreed-upon limitation of treatment, such as a DNR, does not signify that a patient's condition is "hopeless"; desired therapies will be continued unless further decisions, such as to withdraw life-sustaining treatments, are made.
  - DNR may be alternatively presented to family members using the term "allow natural death," which emphasizes the fact that death is natural and that the goals of care are for the patient to be comfortable rather than suffering unnecessarily.
  - A DNR order should be clearly documented in the medical record.
  - A DNR order can be reversed at any time by the patient if they have capacity, or by the health care decision maker.
  - Interventions to optimize the patient's quality of life can be continued throughout the ICU stay, even up to the moment of death, if needed.
  - When discussing a DNR order with patients and family, care providers may also describe this as "allowing natural death."

- In some situations, a decision to *withdraw* or *withhold* therapies may be made.
  - In this setting, most critically ill patients lack decision-making capacity, and a surrogate is involved in decision-making.
  - When a decision is made to withdraw or withhold therapy, critical care providers should support not only patients but also their family members throughout the dying process.
- If the patient's wishes regarding end-of-life care are unknown, the principle of *benefit versus burden* may be used.
  - In this process, the potentially helpful versus harmful effects of each therapy are weighed.
- Providers may also choose to initiate discussions regarding patient and family wishes after death, including organ donation and autopsy.
  - Although such discussions may be viewed as awkward while the patient still lives, most families appreciate honest attempts by the care team to prepare them for what lies ahead.
  - Studies evidence that for dying ICU patients, open, honest, and proactive communication decreases family member anxiety, distress, and posttraumatic stress disorder (PTSD) after patient death and is thought to decrease the incidence of complicated grief in family members.
- *Futility* refers to interventions that are unlikely to produce any significant benefit for the patient.
- If the team determines that ongoing care is *futile* (only serves to prolong the process of dying), the team may advise that therapies be withdrawn to reduce the suffering of the dying patient and move to a comfort focus.
  - While clinicians are ethically not required to provide futile care, only a few states have laws that enable a clinician team to withdraw life-sustaining treatments without the consent of family members.
  - Practical, proactive, compassionate, and clear communication between ICU clinicians and family members often prevents misunderstandings and averts the development of most situations where a family may compel a clinician to continue to provide futile care.
- If a clinician team is, due to futility, considering withdrawing life-sustaining treatments without the consent of the patient or family, the hospital ethics team should be proactively involved.
- Based on the principle of "double effect," clinicians provide medications to imminently dying patients with the *intent* to treat pain or suffering, even if these medications may have an unintended consequence of hastening death.
- For patients with intractable pain or suffering and when death is imminent, terminal sedation may be legally offered; however, terminal sedation should be directed by clinicians, such as palliative care providers, familiar with the process.
- Development of a withdrawal of life-sustaining treatment policy and procedure utilizing a standardized order set can improve care of the dying patient.

Institutional Ethics Committee

- Morally complex matters often arise in the ICU. If conflict arises, the input of the institutional ethics committee is advisable.
- The *institutional ethics committee* is generally composed of a group of health care professionals trained in medical ethics.
- The ethics committee offers an objective analysis of the patient's case and may draw on basic ethical principles to guide the patient, clinicians, and family to a consensus about the therapeutic course.
  - The role is one of an expert consultant, rather than an arbiter of dispute.
  - However, the committee may be involved with formulating and implementing an institutional *conflict resolution policy.*
- Ethics consultation is useful in rare circumstances of irreconcilable differences between the physician and patient and/or family and in which the usual mechanisms of decision-making, such as informal discussions, team meetings, assistance of social workers or clergy, prove ineffective.
- Hospital policy should describe a specific stepwise process toward achieving accord, or if none can be achieved, toward transferring the patient's care to another accepting physician, care team, or institution.
- Hospital or institutional policy may mandate input of the ethics committee in certain circumstances, such as withdrawal of life-sustaining treatments in traditionally "vulnerable" populations such as children or patients lacking a surrogate decision maker as well as in withdrawal of life-sustaining treatments in patients concurrently receiving neuromuscular blocking agents.
- Ethics consults focus on clinical dilemmas to discern morally and ethically acceptable treatment options, compared to palliative care consults, which help patients and families negotiate complex medical information, grapple with prognosis, and facilitate shared decision-making.

Special Populations

- The *pediatric patient* deserves special consideration regarding ethical considerations. Legally, such decisions are deferred to the parents.
  - Ethically, the child may participate in decisions depending on their developmental level and decision-making capacity.
  - Pediatric intensivists must be sensitive to individual family dynamics and parenting styles when approaching treatment decisions or end-of-life discussions with the pediatric ICU patient.
  - Even if not of legal age, some older children (such as teenagers) have been deemed to be able to provide consent for certain decisions and regardless, many children may provide *assent* for decisions.
- All adults have the right to refuse medical treatments. The fundamental right to refuse medical treatment is considered a *negative right*—the right to be free from unwanted medical interventions
  - Before honoring the patient's refusal, a physician must first assess the patient's competence and medical decision-making capacity.
  - This assessment involves evaluating whether the patient can understand the relevant information about the proposed treatment, appreciate the consequences of their decision, and communicate their choice in a consistent manner.
  - The physician should also ensure the patient is fully informed about the risks and benefits of the treatment and any available alternatives.

  - Once competence and decision-making capacity are established, the physician can respect the patient's autonomy by honoring their refusal of medical treatment, provided it is made voluntarily and without coercion.
- The Jehovah's Witness patient also deserves special consideration regarding ethical considerations.
  - Jehovah's Witnesses generally may refuse to receive blood or blood products based on their religious beliefs, even if such refusal may result in death.
  - Some patients may accept autotransfused or chest-tube salvaged blood, especially if it remains in contiguous circulation with their vasculature.
  - Special considerations may apply if the Jehovah's Witness patient is a minor, is incompetent, has responsibilities for dependents, and/or is in certain emergency circumstances.
  - Law and judicial practices vary from state to state, and health care practitioners must be familiar with their state's statutes or seek advice from hospital legal counsel.
  - Careful documentation of discussion and informed consent is mandatory.
  - Legal precedent generally supports patient autonomy regarding the acceptance of transfusion.
- The use of extracorporeal membrane oxygenation (ECMO) presents several ethical challenges for health care providers.
  - ECMO is a highly complex and foreign concept for patients and families. Explaining its intricacies, risks, benefits, and potential outcomes to patients or their family members can be difficult. Providers must convey medical information clearly, empathetically, and consistently.
  - The prognosis for patients on ECMO can be highly uncertain, and outcomes vary widely depending on the underlying condition and patient factors.
  - Deciding when to withdraw ECMO support is ethically challenging, particularly if the patient's condition is not improving, and there is little hope for recovery.
  - In this case, the principles of beneficence, nonmaleficence and equitable resource allocation are reconciled with patient autonomy and family's wishes.

Organ Donation, Neurologic Death, Circulatory Death

- *First-Person Authorization (FPA)*, also known as donor designation, is a law that allows adults to legally indicate their intent to donate organs or tissues.
  - This is usually done by signing a donor card, driver's license, or state identification card, or by enrolling in a donor registry.
  - The FPA cannot be overridden by family members.
- Donation after Neurologic Death (DND): patients who are declared brain dead and/or for whom, a surrogate consent may be considered for organ or tissue donation.
  - Due to a potential conflict of interest, conversations with the family regarding organ donation should not be conducted by the physician caring for the patient.
  - Federal regulations require these discussions be conducted by trained personnel for the regional organ procurement agency.
  - Early contact with the organ procurement agency (OPA) by ICU clinicians is critical as OPAs generally have specific guidelines regarding medications, ventilator settings, and blood work to be performed prior to organ donation.
- Brain death is a clinical syndrome defined as the irreversible loss of clinical function of the entire brain, including the brain stem. Prerequisites include the following:
  - The proximate cause of brain injury is known and irreversible.
  - Exclusion of complicating medical conditions that may confound clinical assessment
  - Absence of drug intoxication or poisoning
  - Absent evidence of neuromuscular blockade
  - Core temperature >36 °C
  - 24 hours of observation without clinical change is necessary for comas of unknown etiology.
- The three pivotal findings for brain death are coma, absent brainstem reflexes, and apnea.
- In the presence of confounding variables, brain death may be determined with the aid of ancillary testing.
  - Confirmatory ancillary tests may be used when uncertainty about the reliability of the neurologic examination exists, and apnea testing cannot be performed.
  - In clinical practice, electroencephalogram (EEG), cerebral angiography, nuclear scan, transcranial Doppler (TCD), computed tomographic angiography (CTA), and magnetic resonance imaging (MRI) are currently used as ancillary tests.
- Organ donation after cardiac death (DCD): critically ill patients who depend on life-sustaining treatments may be considered for organ DCD.
  - DCD patients must be expected to die imminently upon withdrawal of life-sustaining treatments.
  - DCD organ procurement is challenging and demands adherence to guiding ethical principles.
  - The institutional guidelines for DCD organ procurement should be followed.
- Care for the dying patient including analgesic and amnestic medications supersedes the goal of organ procurement.
- The institutional policy should clearly define the following:
  - The nonoverlapping of caregivers to the donor and the recipient to avoid conflict of interest
  - The physician responsible for pronouncing cardiac death
  - The time interval after asystole at which death is declared
  - The process for obtaining consent for and administering medications or procedures necessary for organ procurement, but not otherwise beneficial to the patient (ie, heparin administration, femoral arterial line placement, etc)
  - The process for allowing family presence at the time of death
  - The time interval after which organ procurement will not be attempted in the case of unexpected patient survival after the withdrawal of life-sustaining therapies

Research Ethics

- Ethical standards in research design are essential for ensuring the integrity and safety of research studies involving human subjects. Key research ethical principles include:

- *Scientific validity*: a study uses appropriate analyses while avoiding research misconduct, controlling biases, and ensuring transparency in reporting methods and results.
- *Fair subject selection*: a study does not unfairly exclude or disadvantage certain groups while avoiding exploitation, and the inclusion of underrepresented or vulnerable groups.
- *Favorable risk-benefit profile*: potential benefits of research outweigh the risks to participants. The risks may include physical harm, psychological distress, and loss of privacy.

- Conflicts of interest in medical research occur when organizations involved in the research have financial or personal interests that influence researchers' judgment, objectivity, or integrity.
- Financial disclosures refer to the formal declaration of financial relationships that researchers may have with external entities, such as pharmaceutical companies or medical device manufacturers.
- The Institutional Review Board (IRB) oversees the implementation of scientific trials to ensure the protection of human rights and to ensure the ethical conduct of research in accordance with established standards and regulations.

Professionalism, Impaired Providers, and Burnout

- Professionalism encompasses a set of core values and behaviors that health care professionals must adhere to provide high-quality, ethical care to patients.
  - Honesty involves providing truthful, accurate, and complete information to patients, colleagues, and the public.
  - Altruism is the selfless concern for the well-being of others, prioritizing the needs of the patient over the interests of the health care provider.
  - Integrity involves adhering to moral and medical ethical principles, maintaining consistency in actions.
  - Compassion is the empathetic recognition and understanding of patients' suffering.
  - Respect involves recognizing the inherent dignity, rights, and autonomy of patients.
- *Conflicts of interest* arise when personal or financial interests have the potential to influence a health care professional's judgment or actions.
  - Health care providers must disclose any conflicts of interest to patients and colleagues.
  - Professionals should avoid situations where conflicts of interest could compromise patient care.
- Professionals should maintain independence from commercial interests and marketing, ensuring that their recommendations are solely in the best interest of the patient.
- Physicians have an ethical responsibility to deliver competent, up-to-date medical care.
  - *Primary certification* is the recognition by a professional medical board that a physician has met the required standards of knowledge and clinical skills in a specialty. Certain specialty boards require recertification to ensure patients remain knowledgeable and competent.
  - Maintenance of certification requires physicians to engage in lifelong learning activities to maintain certification. This includes continuing medical education (CME), participating in quality improvement activities, and continuous self-assessment.
- Impairment of a health care professional is the inability or pending inability to practice according to accepted standards because of substance use, abuse, or dependency.
- It is estimated that ~10% to 15% of health care providers will misuse drugs or alcohol at least one time in their career.
- Though overall rates of drug abuse and dependence are similar to that in the general population, rates of benzodiazepine and opiate abuse are higher among health care professionals.
- Physicians have a moral obligation to protect patients against harm and a duty to report impaired providers to the medical board.
- Institutional, local, and statewide impaired clinician programs are available for treatment and rehabilitation; many of these programs help with reentry into practice.
  - Recovery rates are higher for health care professionals than for the general population.
  - Rarely is punitive action taken if the health care provider successfully undergoes treatment and follow-up.
- Burnout has been reported to be frequent among critical care clinicians and can impact clinicians quality of life and patient care.
  - Burnout is diagnosed by emotional exhaustion, depersonalization, and a sense of low personal accomplishment.
  - The Maslach Burnout Inventory–Human Services Survey (MBI–HSS) has become the definitive standard for evaluating burnout.
  - Studies have found burnout to be higher among residents, anesthesiologists, emergency medicine physicians, and oncologists.
  - Workplace determinants of burnout include workplace organization, duration of work hours, conflict, poor communication, and involvement in end-of-life care.
  - Improving overall health, increasing personal support, and improving work satisfaction may help decrease burnout.

Medical Errors in the Intensive Care Unit

- The rate of medical errors is higher in the ICU than in other areas of the hospital.
- Disclosure of an error should occur when harm has occurred; health care providers should recognize the decision made or action taken was incorrect.
- An empathetic, nondefensive demeanor is important.
- Open disclosure will help patients receive additional treatment required, facilitate financial adjustments, reduce concerns about an otherwise unexplained problem, reestablish trust, and strengthen the doctor-patient relationship.
- Failure to disclose has been linked to an increased desire to file an insurance claim; thus, compassionate and sensitive disclosure may reduce the risk of malpractice litigation.
- Medical errors (and identified near misses) should be reported through protected quality assurance processes, which often include a root cause analysis to identify the true sources of error and develop action plans for quality improvement and patient safety.

- Sleep deprivation is a critical issue that significantly impairs cognitive and physical abilities.
  - The risk of medical errors increases significantly with sleep deprived physicians.
  - Sleep deprivation can furthermore impair communication skills and decrease empathy, which can negatively affect patient outcomes.

Medical Legal

- Numerous legal considerations must be addressed when practicing in ICUs.
- Honest, open communication with patients and their families is the best way for the physician to resolve issues and avoid legal action.
- Federal rulings have outlined general principles regarding end-of-life care, but specific state statutes differ.
- The National Practitioner Data Bank (NPDB) is a database operated by the U.S. Department of Health and Human Services that contains medical malpractice claims and adverse action reports on health care professionals.

Medical Malpractice, Professionalism

- There are four elements of medical malpractice: duty, breach of duty, causation, and damages.
  - *Duty*: a health care provider has a duty to provide the same standard of reasonable care that another health care provider in a similar situation would deliver.
  - *Breach of duty*: a health care professional fails to meet the recognized standard of care when treating a patient.
    - Includes negligence, making errors in diagnosis or treatment, administering the wrong medication or dosage, failure to obtain informed consent, failure to adequately communicate with patients about their condition or treatment options
    - While a mistake can potentially lead to a breach of duty if it results in harm to the patient due to a departure from the standard of care, not all mistakes automatically constitute breaches of duty or negligence.
  - *Causation*: links the health care provider's breach of duty and the harm suffered by the patient
    - Establishing causation is crucial in medical malpractice cases because negligence alone is not sufficient to hold a health care provider liable.
  - *Damages*: actual harm resulting from the medical professional's negligence—can be physical, emotional, or financial

Patient Privacy

- Health care professionals have legal and ethical obligations to maintain patient confidentiality.
- Confidentiality in medicine is a fundamental principle that ensures patients' sensitive information is protected.
- Laws such as the Health Insurance Portability and Accountability Act (HIPAA) in the United States mandate strict protections for patient health information.
- There are certain circumstances where health care providers may breach confidentiality, such as when there is a risk of harm to the patient or others, or when required by law (eg, reporting certain infectious diseases).

Conclusion

- A few key principles are useful in aiding the clinician when confronted with ethical and end-of-life issues:
- Patient autonomy is primary in decision-making.
- Advance directives provide the best source of information for guidance in patients lacking capacity.
- The two types of advanced directives are *institutional directives* and *proxy directives*.
  - Institutional directives provide guidance for caregivers and health care agents when making decisions for patients by way of substituted judgment. Examples include living wills and The Five Wishes document.
  - Proxy directives name a patient's health care agent. Examples include the power of attorney.
- Oral communication can be utilized as advance directives, and the role of a surrogate in providing substitutive judgment has been supported.
- Individuals often have strong beliefs concerning desired ICU care, end-of-life care, and what is—to that person—a "meaningful quality of life."
- Moreover, patient, family, and surrogate beliefs may differ from those of the clinician team.
- Clear, compassionate, and proactive communication exploring the beliefs of all stakeholders can ensure that the level of care is appropriately aligned with a patient's wishes and beliefs.
- Involvement of social work and palliative care providers may be helpful in facilitating such goals of care discussions.
- Clinicians should be prepared to navigate through the various ethical challenges that special populations present in the ICU.
- Treatments, once rendered, may be withdrawn.
- There is no ethical difference between withdrawing and withholding a treatment; however, clinicians and family members often anecdotally report that withdrawing a treatment—as opposed to withholding it—is emotionally more difficult.
- End-of-life decisions are best addressed by the clinician and the patient/family, sometimes with help from institutional facilitators such as palliative care teams and/or ethics team consultants.
- Clinicians are not bound to provide care that they deem to be futile.
- It is advisable for a clinician to pursue every avenue of conflict resolution, including removing oneself from the care of the patient, before acting against the family's wishes.
- Clinicians should be aware of the principle of "double effect" and should treat pain and suffering, even if the medications have unintended consequences of hastening death.
- For unusual or questionable cases, it is appropriate to seek advice from an institutional ethics committee and legal counsel to assist with decision-making.
- Physicians have a moral obligation to protect patients against harm and a duty to report impaired providers to the medical board.
- Medical errors are bound to occur in the critical care setting—errors should be disclosed to the patient and family, reported to a quality assurance process, and analyzed through a root cause analysis.

- To avoid conflicts of interest, conversations regarding organ donation are not conducted by the physician taking care of the patient.
- Duty, breach of duty, causation, and damages make up the four elements of medical malpractice.

SUGGESTED READINGS

American medical association code of medical ethics' opinions on physicians' health and conduct. *Virtual Mentor.* 2011;13(10):700-702.

Baldisseri MR. Impaired healthcare professional. *Crit Care Med.* 2007;35(2 suppl):S106-S116.

Boyle D, O'Connell D, Platt FW, Albert RK. Disclosing errors and adverse events in the intensive care unit. *Crit Care Med.* 2006;34(5):1532-1537.

Embriaco N, Papazian L, Kentish-Barnes N, Pochard F, Azoulay E. Burnout syndrome among critical care healthcare workers. *Anesthesiology.* 2011;114(1):194-204.

Haberle TH, Shinkunas LA, Erekson ZD, Kaldjian LC. Goals of care among hospitalized patients: a validation study. *Am J Hosp Palliat Care.* 2011;28(5):335-341.

Hong CY, Goh LG, Lee HP. The advance directive—a review. *Singapore Med J.* 1996;37:411-418.

Hyman, SA, Michaels DR, Berry JM et al. Risk of burnout in perioperative clinicians: a survey study and literature review. *Curr Opin Crit Care.* 2007;13(5):482-488.

Kummer HB, Thompson DR. *Critical Care Ethics: A Practice Guide.* 2nd ed. Society of Critical Care Medicine; 2009.

Lo B, ed. *Disclosing Errors. Resolving Ethical Dilemmas: A Guide for Clinicians.* Lippincott Williams & Wilkins; 2013.

Mularskki RA, Puntillo K. Varkey B et al. Pain management within the palliative and end-of-life care experience in the ICU. *Chest.* 2009;135(5):1360-1369.

Norton SA, Hogan LA, Holloway RG, Temkin-Greener H, Buckley MJ, Quill TE. Proactive palliative care in the medical intensive care unit: effects on length of stay for selected high-risk patients. *Crit Care Med.* 2007;35(6):1530-1535.

Steinbrock R. Organ donation after cardiac death. *N Engl J Med.* 2007;357:209-213.

Varkey B. Principles of clinical ethics and their application to practice. *Med Princ Pract.* 2021;30(1):17-28.

Wijdicks EF, Varelas PN, Gronseth GS, Greer DM; American Academy of Neurology. Evidence-based guideline update: determining brain death in adults: report of the Quality Standards Subcommittee of the American Academy of Neurology. *Neurology.* 2010;74(23):1911-1918.

Wilmer A, Louie K, Dodek P, et al. Incidence of medication errors and adverse drug events in the ICU: a systematic review. *Qual Saf Health Care.* 2010;19:e7.

SECTION 35

Palliative Medicine and End-of-Life Care

Section Editor: Marvin G. Chang

35.1

Palliative Medicine and End-of-Life Care

Matthew Bartek

Background

- The complexities of critical illness, coupled with the emotional burden on patients and their families, create unique challenges in providing palliative and end-of-life care in this setting.
- Palliative care embodies a care philosophy that focuses on quality of life, relief of suffering, and family engagement.
- Palliative care includes end-of-life care, though it is not limited to care provided for the dying; palliative care can and should be administered in parallel with curative care.
- Three models of palliative care delivery include primary palliative care, consultative palliative care, and integrated palliative care.
- The iterative review of patient and family goals of care in the context of what is clinically and physiologically possible is important.
- Symptom management for critically ill patients should occur alongside the management of underlying illness.
- End-of-life care in the intensive care unit (ICU) should focus on symptom management, shared decision-making, clear communication, supporting family members' complex emotions and grieving; hospice agencies can often assist and even enroll patients who are dying in the ICU.

Principles of Palliative Care

- Address the family as the unit of care: while patient autonomy ultimately trumps conditions when there is disagreement, illness affects not only the patient but also the entire family, and posthospitalization care delivery often necessitates the engagement of families and friends. Palliative care teams work to provide support and resources to address the collective needs and concerns of patients and their families alike.
- Engage in multidisciplinary care: palliative care teams are by nature nonhierarchical and collaborative, drawing on expertise from physicians, nurses, social workers, chaplains, and others, who work together to address the complex needs of patients and their families.
- Assess prognostic awareness: sensitive exploration of a patient's understanding of their illness trajectory allows health care providers to tailor communication and care plans accordingly, ensuring patient autonomy and informed decision-making.
- Respond to emotion: acknowledging and validating the emotional experiences of patients and families fosters trust and allows for more efficient and effective navigation of complex decisions.
- Utilize effective communication techniques: employing effective communication skills, including active listening, empathy, and clear explanations, facilitates meaningful conversations about goals of care, treatment options, and end-of-life decisions.
- Aggressive symptom management: a proactive approach to identifying and treating distressing symptoms, such as pain, nausea, or anxiety, prioritizes patient comfort and enhances quality of life throughout the course of illness.
- Holistic care: suffering often stretches beyond the physiologic aspects of pain and so the relief of suffering must also extend to the physical, emotional, psychological, social, and spiritual needs of patients.
- Bereavement support: palliative care and hospice services include supporting families after the death of a loved one, providing resources and assistance during the grieving process.
- The conceptualization of palliative care has undergone a significant evolution over the past 15 years:
  - Historically associated primarily with end-of-life scenarios, current understanding emphasizes its role from the onset of serious illness and the delivery of critical care.
  - This timely integration is particularly salient in the ICU, where patients often face high symptom burdens and

significant functional impairments, irrespective of their ultimate survival.
  - This shift means critical care practitioners should not view palliative care as a consequence of treatment failure or a precursor to withdrawal of care. Instead, it is an essential, concurrent component of high-quality critical care, aimed at optimizing patient and family well-being from the moment of ICU admission for serious illness.

Care Models for Delivering Palliative Care in the Intensive Care Unit

- Primary palliative care: delivered by the ICU team without any specialty palliative care team involvement. This includes conducting family meetings, addressing the emotional needs of patients and families, and assessing the palliative care needs of patients early in their ICU stay.
- Specialty (secondary) palliative care: palliative care consults deliver services to patients in the ICU.
- Integrative or mixed palliative care delivery: close collaboration between critical care and palliative care teams to collaboratively identify patients with more complex palliative care needs and determine who should deliver this type of care; some models have automatically triggered palliative care consults based on prognostic mortality estimates.

Integrating Palliative Care Into Critical Care

- A palliative care assessment should be performed early in the ICU stay. This includes understanding: symptom burden (both physical and emotional), what is most important to the patient, their hopes and worries, and their own disease understanding.
  - Professional societies recommend performing a palliative care assessment within 24 hours of ICU admission if feasible and no later than 72 hours after admission; family meetings should be held within 72 hours of admission to the ICU.
  - Family meetings should be structured with multidisciplinary alignment about prognosis and care plans prior to family discussions.
    - Many frameworks exist for structuring complex discussions with patients and families. See Table 35.1.1 for components of complex discussions to consider.
- Prognosis should be iteratively reviewed and communicated to patients and their families, based on their expressed preferences on how to receive this type of information.
- Providers should be attentive and aware of the emotional burden of ICU stays, given the uncertainty combined with high risk/consequences of decisions.
- When to consult palliative care: criteria for early identification and referral:
  - Early integration of palliative care is strongly suggested for patients at high risk of mortality, those with end-stage disease, or those with a prolonged hospitalization.
  - There are no universally defined criteria to determine which patients are at the highest need of palliative care consultation.
    - Palliation should ideally begin at ICU admission and continuously adjust to evolving needs, mirroring curative care.
    - Standardized tools for symptom assessment, including psychosocial suffering and maladaptive coping, can aid in determining the need for specialty palliative care consultation.
- Continuous delivery of palliative care in the ICU
  - Partner with palliative care consulting teams, including social work, spiritual care consultants, and families, to iteratively assess and address sources of suffering and miscommunication.

TABLE 35.1.1 Evidence-Based Communication Strategies for Goals of Care Discussions

Communication Phase/Scenario	Key Strategy/Technique	Actionable Advice/Phrases	Rationale/Benefit
Setting Up the Conversation	Arrange for privacy; involve significant others; sit down; manage time constraints.	"I'd like to talk about (patient's condition) in a quiet place." "Who would you like to have present?"	Fosters a supportive environment, ensures focus, respects patient/family wishes
Assessing Patient/Family Perception	Determine what the patient/family knows or suspects; listen to their level of comprehension.	"What is your understanding of (patient's illness)?" "What have the doctors told you so far?"	Establishes baseline knowledge, identifies gaps, avoids overwhelming with unnecessary information
Delivering Difficult News	Give a "warning shot"; use simple, nontechnical language; be honest and direct; give information in small chunks; prepare and rehearse a "Headline Statement."	"I'm afraid I have some bad news." "The news is not good." "Your loved one has died." (avoid euphemisms)	Prepares for impact, ensures clarity, prevents shock, facilitates understanding
Responding to Emotion	Observe for emotion; identify the emotion; acknowledge and empathize; allow for silence.	"I can see this is very upsetting for you." "It's understandable to feel (sad/angry/scared)."	Fosters trust, validates feelings, creates space for processing, allows for more efficient conversations
Discussing Implications/Next Steps	Summarize information; discuss prognosis, treatment options, quality of life; offer resources.	"To summarize, we've discussed…" "Given this, our options are A, B, or C." "What questions do you have now?"	Ensures understanding, facilitates shared decision-making, provides a path forward
Interprofessional Communication	At least two team members present (eg, physician and social worker/chaplain); timely intrateam communication.	Physician shares medical info, social worker/chaplain support emotional and spiritual needs. "Let's align on the key messages before meeting the family."	Addresses medical, psychosocial, spiritual needs; ensures a united front; prevents misinformation

- Assess disease and prognostic understanding, patient and family hopes and worries, and overall sources of suffering.
  - Serious illness conversation scripts can aid in these conversations and should be reviewed progressively throughout a patients' stay to ensure goal-concordant care is being delivered.
- A detailed social history, including baseline functional status and posthospitalization expectations, is key to aligning visions of what is medically possible and what is likely.
  - Discussing best-case, worst-case, and most likely case scenarios can be a helpful tool to set expectations among patients and families.

- Family discussions should occur regularly and at inflection points in patients' care pathway; admission to the ICU may represent one of those inflection points.
  - Unique aspects of palliative care delivery in ICUs
- The palliative care needs of patients and their families in the ICU differ from those admitted to other inpatient units or who are managed as an outpatient.
- Prognostic uncertainty: the rapid and unpredictable nature of physiologic decline in critically ill patients often necessitates swift, high-stakes decisions by patients and families, frequently without a complete understanding of the long-term prognosis or the full spectrum of risks and benefits.
  - A major challenge is that a high percentage of ICU patients lack decision-making capacity, necessitating reliance on surrogates.
  - Clinicians must acknowledge the limitations of prognostication, especially in neurologic and terminal cases.
  - In cases of lacking capacity and absent surrogates, ad hoc decision-making is generally not recommended; legal or ethics consultation may be necessary.
- Unfamiliarity: many critically ill patients and their families have no prior experience with the ICU environment or its specialized care team, which can exacerbate feelings of vulnerability and confusion.
- High-stakes decisions: decisions made in the ICU are inherently life-altering or lifesaving, carrying immense emotional weight for all involved.

Evidence for Palliative Care in the Intensive Care Unit

- Aside from those patients with a cancer diagnosis, palliative care consultations are underutilized, as are the benefits of palliative care interventions.
- There is support for early palliative care consultations in the ICU to decrease ICU-related health care utilization, improve patient/family experience, and decrease unneeded procedures and time in the ICU, while not affecting overall mortality.
- Palliative care consultations in the ICU are associated with:
  - More goal-concordant care delivery
  - Increased rate of transition of code status to do-not-resuscitate/do-not-intubate (DNR/DNI)
  - Increased transfers from ICU to hospice
  - Reduction in unwanted and potentially inappropriate treatment
    - Goals of care, code status discussions, and limitations on lifesaving interventions
- Shared decision-making via a comprehensive assessment of patient and family values, goals, priorities, cultural context, and spiritual needs, is best practice care.
- For some patients, there are obvious goals, such as preventing imminent death, curing acute disease, preventing /relieving pain and suffering, and eventually returning the patient to their premorbid level of function.
  - In some situations, patients may only hope to delay the disease process, and occasionally, ICU care is requested to prolong a patient's life long enough to allow for close relatives to arrive and pay last respects or to consent to organ donation prior to the patient's death.
- When discussing goals of therapy, the patient's values should be elicited and emphasized.
  - It is important for the health care team to discuss the patient's prognosis and arrive at a consensus before meeting with the family.
  - The prognosis of the patient is very important in setting realistic therapeutic goals.
- All patients admitted to the ICU should have a discussion about code status preferences, in part to review wishes and communicate the increased likelihood of clinical decompensation that comes with ICU admission.
- The decision to permit or limit lifesaving interventions should not be phrased simply as a binary "life or death" choice but rather discussed in the context of what benefits and burdens would be offered by each choice, based on the likelihood of meaningful survival.
  - The GO-FAR (Good Outcome Following Attempted Resuscitation) Score can be used to help understand the chance of surviving an in-hospital cardiac arrest with good neurologic function.
  - Cardiopulmonary resuscitation (CPR) should be described in simple, realistic terms, emphasizing what it would entail, including the high likelihood of incurring injuries such as broken ribs, which may cause further suffering.
- Ideally, patients and families should be given time and space to consider limitations on interventions, including renal replacement therapy, mechanical ventilation, and CPR; the decision to withhold interventions can take hours or even some days to reach.
- If possible, engage in such decisions with patients alongside their families, serve a decision maker, and potentially nursing staff and social work.
- It must be emphasized to the family that an agreed-upon limitation of treatment, such as a DNR, does not signify that a patient's condition is "hopeless"; desired therapies will be continued unless further decisions, such as to withdraw life-sustaining treatments, are made.
- Interventions to optimize the patient's quality of life can be continued throughout the ICU stay, even up to the moment of death, if needed.
- Providers may also choose to initiate discussions regarding patient and family wishes after death, including organ donation and autopsy.
  - Although such discussions may be viewed as awkward while the patient still lives, most families appreciate honest attempts by the care team to prepare them for what lies ahead.

  - Moreover, studies evidence that for dying ICU patients, open, honest, and proactive communication decreases family member anxiety, distress, and posttraumatic stress disorder (PTSD) after patient death and is thought to decrease the incidence of complicated grief in family members.

Complex Symptom Management

Pain

- Assessment should include not only physical pain (visceral vs somatic, nociceptive vs neuropathic) but also spiritual, existential, and psychological pain; the concept of "total pain" emphasizes that the experience of pain is not only physical but also a complex multidimensional experience that includes psychological, social, and spiritual components.
- Opioids are the mainstay for treatment. Consider the route of administration, various pharmacologic interactions with a patient's underlying disease, kidney function, liver function, and tolerance to prior opioid medications.
- Adjuvant analgesics to manage neuropathic pain (anticonvulsants, antidepressants, topical agents) and/or inflammatory components of pain (nonsteroidal antiinflammatory drugs [NSAIDs], corticosteroids) may be helpful.

Dyspnea

- The sensation of breathlessness or "not getting enough air" can come from a complex interplay of physiologic and psychological factors.
- Treat underlying causes of hypoxia.
- Opioids can manage the sensation of air hunger via decreasing the central perception of dyspnea, the ventilatory drive to hypercapnia and hypoxia, and anxiety.
- Other adjuncts, such as benzodiazepines, nebulized furosemide (especially in chronic obstructive pulmonary disease [COPD]), and cool air being blown across the face, may provide relief as well.

Thirst and Xerostomia

- A majority of ICU patients, especially those on oxygen therapy and with high risk of dying, report the sensation of thirst, often to distressing levels.
- Topical agents, including artificial saliva, xylitol, and salivary flow stimulants, can be effective in managing xerostomia.
- Swabs of cold water, the use of a mouth and lip moisturizer, and sprays of cold water can decrease the sensation and discomfort of thirst, even in patients for whom oral intake is restricted (eg, those for whom diet is NPO).
- For patients who are not intubated, but are receiving oxygen therapy, consider the use of heated humidifiers to minimize the drying effect of oxygen.

End-of-Life Care

- Managing conflicts and addressing potentially inappropriate treatments
  - "Futile treatment" refers to interventions that cannot achieve their physiologic goal. "Potentially inappropriate" treatments may have some chance of effect but are ethically questionable to clinicians.
  - A multi-organization statement outlines a seven-step process for resolving disagreements concerning potentially inappropriate or futile treatments.
  - This process typically includes expert consultation, formal notice to surrogates, a second medical opinion, and interdisciplinary hospital committee review
  - Clinicians are not bound to provide care that they deem to be futile.
  - It is advisable for clinicians to pursue every avenue of conflict resolution, including removing oneself from the care of the patient, before acting against the family's wishes.

Palliative Sedation

- Palliative sedation is the monitored use of sedative medications to relieve refractory and intolerable suffering.
  - Based on the principle of "double effect," clinicians may and should provide imminently dying patients with medications with the intent to treat pain or suffering, even if these medications may have the unintended consequence of hastening death.
- It is considered a last resort when all other comfort-oriented interventions have failed to alleviate symptoms.
- Commonly used agents include midazolam, propofol, and benzodiazepines, titrated to effect.
- This intervention requires meticulous ethical consideration, shared decision-making with the patient or surrogate, and careful documentation.

Palliative Extubation

- The planned withdrawal of mechanical ventilation in a patient with a terminal illness or a poor prognosis
- This process represents a transition from life-sustaining treatment to a comfort-focused plan of care.
- A collaborative discussion among the clinical team, patient (if able), and family is essential to establish goals of care. It is important to review the likely clinical expectations following extubation with family members as well as an anticipated timeline leading to death.
- Immediately following extubation, a comfort care protocol with opioids and anxiolytics is initiated to manage dyspnea, anxiety, and pain.
- It is distinct from medical futility and is a withdrawal of treatment, not an act of euthanasia.

Hospice

- Hospice is a philosophy of care focused on comfort, quality of life, and support for patients with a terminal diagnosis and a prognosis of ≤6 months.
- The interdisciplinary hospice team includes physicians, nurses, social workers, chaplains, and volunteers.
- Care is provided in various settings, including the patient's home, assisted living facilities, or dedicated hospice inpatient units; many hospitals can also provide hospice care and transition patients to hospice agencies, even while a patient is still physically in the hospital.
- The primary goal of hospice is to maximize comfort and dignity, helping patients and families navigate the end-of-life process.

- Reviewing the option for hospice may be appropriate for patients, nearing the end of life, and may be a mechanism for honoring patient and family wishes.

Organ Donation

- Determination of death using brain criteria
- Brain death is a clinical syndrome defined as the irreversible loss of clinical function of the entire brain, including the brainstem. Prerequisites include the following:
  - Proximate cause of brain injury is known and irreversible
  - Exclusion of complicating medical conditions that may confound clinical assessment
  - Absence of drug intoxication or poisoning
  - Absent evidence of neuromuscular blockade
  - Core temperature >36.0 °C (96.8 °F)
  - A period of 24 hours of observation without clinical change is necessary for comas of unknown etiology.
  - In the presence of confounding variables, brain death may be determined with the aid of ancillary testing.
- The three pivotal findings for brain death are coma, absent brainstem reflexes, and apnea.
  - Confirmatory ancillary tests may be used when uncertainty about the reliability of the neurologic examination exists and apnea testing cannot be performed.
    - In clinical practice, electroencephalogram (EEG), cerebral angiography, nuclear scan, transcranial Doppler (TCD), computed tomography angiography (CTA), and magnetic resonance imaging/magnetic resonance angiography (MRI/MRA) are currently used in adults.
  - Organ donation after brain death: patients who are declared brain dead and/or for whom a surrogate consents may be considered for organ or tissue donation.
    - Due to a potential conflict of interest, conversations with the family regarding organ donation should not be conducted by the physician caring for the patient.
    - Federal regulations require these discussions be conducted by trained personnel for the regional organ procurement agency.
    - Early contact with the organ procurement agency (OPA) by ICU clinicians is critical as OPAs generally have specific guidelines regarding medications, ventilator settings, and blood work to be performed prior to organ donation.
  - Organ donation after cardiac death (DCD): critically ill patients who depend on life-sustaining treatments may be considered for organ DCD.
    - DCD patients must be expected to die imminently upon withdrawal of life-sustaining treatments.
    - DCD organ procurement is challenging and demands adherence to guiding ethical principles.
    - The institutional guidelines for DCD organ procurement should be followed.
  - Care for the dying patient, including analgesic and amnestic medications, supersedes the goal of organ procurement.
    - The institutional policy should clearly define the following:
      - The nonoverlapping of caregivers to the donor and the recipient to avoid conflict of interest
      - The physician responsible for pronouncing cardiac death
      - The time interval after asystole at which death is declared.
      - The process for obtaining consent for and administering medications or procedures that are necessary for organ procurement, but are not otherwise of benefit to the patient (ie, heparin administration, femoral arterial line placement, etc)
      - The process for allowing family presence at the time of death
      - The time interval after which organ procurement will not be attempted in the case of unexpected patient survival after the withdrawal of life-sustaining therapies

Concluding Considerations

- Patient autonomy is primary in decision-making. Advance directives provide the best source of information for guidance in patients lacking capacity.
  - Oral communication can be utilized as advance directives, and the role of a surrogate in providing substitutive judgment has been supported.
- Individuals often have strong beliefs concerning desired ICU care, end-of-life care, and what is—to that person—a "meaningful quality of life."
  - Moreover, patient, family, and surrogate beliefs may differ from those of the clinician team.
- Clear, compassionate, and proactive communication exploring the beliefs of all stakeholders can ensure that the intensity of care is appropriate to a patient's wishes and beliefs.
  - Involvement of palliative care providers may be helpful in facilitating such goals of care discussions.
- Treatments, once rendered, may be withdrawn.
  - There is no ethical difference between withdrawing and withholding a treatment.
  - However, clinicians and family members often anecdotally report that withdrawing a treatment—as opposed to withholding it—is emotionally more difficult.
- End-of-life decisions are best addressed by the clinician and the patient/family, sometimes with help from institutional facilitators such as palliative care teams and/or ethics team consultants.
- Clinicians are not bound to provide care that they deem to be futile.
  - However, it is advisable for a clinician to pursue every avenue of conflict resolution, including removing oneself from the care of the patient, before acting against the family's wishes.
- For patients with intractable pain or suffering and when death is imminent, terminal or palliative sedation may be legally offered; however, terminal sedation should be directed by clinicians, such as palliative care providers, familiar with the process.
- Physician-assisted death or medical aid in dying is currently legal in 11 states and the District of Washington; Euthanasia is currently not legal in the United States.

ACKNOWLEDGMENTS

We gratefully acknowledge the contributions of previous edition authors, Rebecca Kalman and Rebecca Aslakson, as portions of those chapters have been retained in this revision.

SUGGESTED READINGS

Center to Advance Palliative Care. *ICU: integrating palliative care—tools and resources—CAPC*. 2024. https://www.capc.org/toolkits/icu-integrating-palliative-care/

Comer A, Fettig L, Torke AM. Identifying goals of care. *Med Clin North Am*. 2020;104(5):767-775.

Curtis JR, Higginson IJ, White DB. Integrating palliative care into the ICU: a lasting and developing legacy. *Intensive Care Med*. 2022;48(7):939-942.

Kompanje EJO, Van Der Hoven B, Bakker J. Anticipation of distress after discontinuation of mechanical ventilation in the ICU at the end of life. *Intensive Care Med*. 2008;34:1593-1599.

Kon AA, Shepard EK, Sederstrom NO, et al. Defining futile and potentially inappropriate interventions: a policy statement from the Society of Critical Care Medicine Ethics Committee. *Crit Care Med*. 2016;44:1769-1774.

Long AC, Muni S, Treece PD, et al. Time to death after terminal withdrawal of mechanical ventilation: specific respiratory and physiologic parameters may inform physician predictions. *J Palliat Med*. 2015;18:1040-1047.

Ma J, Chi S, Buettner B, et al. Early palliative care consultation in the medical ICU: a cluster randomized crossover trial. *Crit Care Med*. 2019;47:1707-1715.

Rubins JB, Kinzie SD, Rubins DM. Predicting outcomes of in-hospital cardiac arrest: retrospective US validation of the good outcome following attempted resuscitation score. *J Gen Intern Med*. 2019;34(11):2530-2535.

SECTION 36

Health Care Disparities and Diversity, Equity, and Inclusion in Health Care

Section Editor: Casey M. Luckhurst

36.1

Health Care Disparities

Erika L. Rangel

Definitions

Social Determinants of Health

Definition: the conditions in which people are born, grow, work, live, and develop, as well as the broader set of forces, including economic policies, social norms, and political systems, which shape the conditions of daily life and impact health outcomes

Health Disparity

Definition: any differences in health status, health outcomes, and health care use that reflect a gap in the quality of care delivered, which may be caused by societal inequities

Considering Social Determinants of Health in Patient Management

Distinguishing Social Determinants of Health From Race or Ethnicity

- Social determinants of health (SDoH) should not be confused with race or ethnicity. Focusing on race as a result of health outcomes risks missing the true underlying drivers, leads to patient stigmatization, and can lead to inappropriate or ineffective interventions.
- Health disparities often attributed to race are actually mediated by SDoH, including:
  - Diabetes
  - Hypertension
  - Smoking: higher rates due to increased cultural exposure, predatory marketing, and maladaptive behavior to cope with stress
  - Asthma: drivers include exposure to pollutants and allergens due to poor-quality housing with dust, insects, rodents, or proximity to highways.

Impact of Residential Segregation on Minority Families

- Difficult to accumulate homeownership and generational wealth
- Poor access to healthy food and exercise spaces
- Exposure to environmental toxins (eg, lead)
- Increased exposure to community violence
- Decreased educational opportunities raise the risk of subsequent poor SDoH, such as underemployment and low income.

Interpersonal Trauma and Mental Health

- Disadvantaged access to resources is linked to depression, anxiety, posttraumatic stress disorder, substance use, and other mental health disorders.

Effects of Chronic Stress ("Weathering")

- Disadvantaged populations experience accelerated aging and deterioration of health from cumulative lifetime exposure to adverse socioeconomic conditions and discrimination.

Modification of Social Determinants of Health by Critical Illness

- *Financial:* changes to employment status due to critical illness–related disability and subsequent changes to insurance status
- *Adverse health impacts:* inability to access essential health care, increase in mental health problems

Improving Outcomes

- Use evidence-based care in all interactions.
- Explore unconscious biases and their potential impact on care.
- Use patient-friendly language and encourage patients and families to ask questions about care.
- Partner with community health to complete home safety assessments.

Maternal Health Care Disparities

Racial and Ethnic Disparities in Maternal Morbidity

- *Mortality*
  - Non-Hispanic Black women die at a rate 3 to 4 times greater than their White counterparts, regardless of socioeconomic factors.
  - Higher fatality rates for five specific pregnancy complications: preeclampsia, eclampsia, placental abruption, placenta previa, and hemorrhage
- *Maternal morbidity*
  - Pregnant Black, Hispanic, and Asian women have higher rates of acute respiratory distress syndrome, disseminated intravascular coagulation, heart failure, hemorrhage, and need for mechanical ventilation.
  - Black women have the highest rates of preterm birth, hemorrhage, and hypertensive disorders of pregnancy.
  - Hispanic women have the highest risk of gestational diabetes.

Influence of Social Determinants of Health on Maternal Health

- Poverty, lack of education, poor nutritional status, smoking, and neighborhood deprivation are associated with poor maternal and neonatal outcomes.

Disparities in Care

- Black and Hispanic women receive epidural analgesia for labor at lower rates than White women.
- Black women have a higher rate of cesarean delivery.
- Black women have limited access to doulas.
- Black women report higher pain scores compared to White women, are assessed less frequently for pain, and receive fewer opioids, including prescriptions for opioids at discharge.

Link Between Race and Health

- *Racism:* Black mothers are less often prescribed opioid pain relief.
- *Macrosocial factors:* minority individuals are underrepresented in medical research, given historical mistreatment and abuse, leading to distrust in medical researchers.
- *Biologic factors:* chronic stress experienced by minority women manifests in higher rates of chronic hypertension, diabetes, and other cardiovascular comorbidities.
- *Social status:* Black mothers are more likely to live in impoverished settings and lack insurance coverage.
- *Risk factors and resources:* Black mothers are more likely to deliver in hospitals with higher rates of severe maternal morbidity and mortality.

Hospital Factors and Provider Bias

- Hospital factors and provider bias contribute significantly to the morbidity and mortality of Black women.
- Systemic and institutional racism is the predominant cause of Black women's inequities in accessing care and their dramatic underrepresentation in research.

Improving Outcomes

- *Hospital quality:* improving hospital quality can reduce maternal deaths and near-misses.
- *Provider and system failures:* addressing provider and system failures through quality assurance processes tailored to seek out and address inequities in the delivery of care and outcomes
- *Provider bias training:* implementing system-wide provider bias training to raise awareness of structural competency
- *Incentivized team training:* team training programs, such as those conducted by large malpractice insurers, can improve patient outcomes.

Child and Adolescent Health Care Disparities

Relevance of Social Determinants of Health for Children and Adolescents

- SDoH are especially relevant for children and adolescents, particularly concerning mental health and respiratory disease.

Mortality Rates

- All minority children, particularly Black children, have higher death rates than White children across all age groups.

Illness Severity and Outcomes

- Multicenter pediatric intensive care unit (PICU) database studies show Hispanic, Black, publicly insured, and low-income children have higher illness severity, rates of PICU admission, rates of invasive mechanical ventilation, in-hospital mortality, readmission rates, and poorer functional outcomes.

Improving Outcomes

- Conduct universal social screening at admission in the PICU to allow risk stratification, tailoring of future community interventions, and placement of appropriate resource referrals (including reimbursement initiatives).
- Educate clinicians on the impact of SDoH.
- Employ a "strength-based approach" to recognize and celebrate unique family strengths that will allow families to build protective factors such as parental resilience and social support.
- Partner with pediatricians to provide integrated health services.

Intensive Care Unit Disparities and Outcomes

In studies, low socioeconomic status (SES) patients were usually defined as uninsured, underinsured, or treated in a safety net hospital, with a high proportion of uninsured/underinsured patients.

Racial, Ethnic, and Socioeconomic Disparities in Prevalence of Intensive Care Unit–Level Care Conditions (Compared to White and/or Privately Insured Individuals)

- Black patients
  - Higher prevalence of conditions requiring intensive care unit (ICU)-level care
  - More likely to have influenza-associated ICU admission
  - Higher incidence of sepsis, noncardiogenic acute respiratory failure, acute lung injury, acute respiratory distress syndrome (ARDS) after trauma, and cardiac arrest (both in and out of the hospital)
  - Women of childbearing age have a higher risk of venous thromboembolism (VTE).
- Minority patients
  - Indigenous people: more likely to require ICU admission for chronic obstructive pulmonary disease (COPD) exacerbations
- Low SES patients
  - More likely to develop ARDS after trauma
  - More likely to be hospitalized with COVID-19

Racial, Ethnic, and Socioeconomic Disparities in Presentation and Outcomes (Compared to White and/or Privately Insured Individuals)

- Black patients
  - Among men, sepsis develops at a younger age.
  - More likely to have Gram-positive infections, independent of the infection source
  - Higher proportion of invasive pneumococcal disease
  - Higher rates of influenza-associated mortality
  - More physiologic derangements and higher severity of illness at hospital and ICU admission
  - Lower survival to hospital discharge after cardiac arrest
- Minority patients
  - Black, Asian, Indigenous/Alaska Native: higher mortality after respiratory failure
  - Hispanic patients: higher adjusted odds of inpatient mortality after ICU admission for COVID-19
  - Indigenous people: longer length of stay and days on ventilator for COPD exacerbations
- Low SES patients
  - More severe clinical presentation (eg, organ failure)
  - Despite fewer comorbidities than insured patients, there is a higher likelihood of cirrhosis or HIV infection.
  - Higher mortality after trauma
  - Higher mortality after acute respiratory failure
  - Higher rates of mechanical ventilation and tracheostomy placement
  - Higher rates of sepsis-related mortality

Racial, Ethnic, and Socioeconomic Disparities in Intensive Care Unit Care (Compared to White and/or Privately Insured Individuals)

- Black patients
  - Black individuals with COVID-19 have higher rates of delayed treatment eligibility for dexamethasone or remdesivir.
- Minority patients
  - Pulse oximetry is less accurate in patients of color (Black, Asian, Hispanic), resulting in a higher incidence of occult hypoxemia.
  - End-of-life care and serious illness management
    - More often experience higher intensity or aggressive end-of-life care
    - Less likely to discontinue mechanical ventilation
    - Have higher symptom burden
    - Have poorer quality of life
    - Less likely to opt for palliative care
- Low SES patients
  - Socially disadvantaged populations have lower access to high-quality palliative care.
  - More likely not to receive appropriate low-tidal volume ventilation for ARDS
  - More likely to receive less interventions for sepsis
  - Less likely to be discharged to long-term care facilities
  - Less likely to have favorable functional status after traumatic injury

Factors Contributing to Disparities in Intensive Care Unit Care

- *Hospital factors*
  - Many racial/ethnic differences in critical care delivery and outcomes are attributable to between-hospital differences rather than between-patient differences.
  - Minority and uninsured patients tend to receive treatment at low-quality hospitals that fail to deliver guideline-adherent therapy.
  - Minority-serving hospitals have significant less improvement in ICU mortality rates than nonminority hospitals.
  - Urban hospitals that are more likely to serve Black and Hispanic populations are disproportionately challenged by funding models and the ability to recruit and retain health care workers.
- *Provider factors*
  - Differences in spirituality, religion, and language may impair communication between minority families and clinicians in the ICU.
  - Inconsistent use of a qualified interpreter may impact appropriateness of care and reduce trust with families.
  - Physician cognitive biases, age, experience, and gender affect clinical decision-making in the ICU.
- *Patient factors*
  - Communication with clinicians impaired by differences in spirituality and religion, language barriers, low health literacy, mistrust, values borne from surviving unjust conditions, and concern that clinicians will dismiss knowledge or beliefs.

Improving Outcomes

- *Community-based interventions*
  - Increase access to primary care in low SES neighborhoods
  - Uniform vaccination coverage among susceptible populations, such as minority nursing home residents
  - Further research to understand impact of implicit bias and racism among health care providers on processes of care for minority populations
- *Hospital-level interventions*
  - Reduce interhospital variation in clinical management, including analyzing physician adherence to treatment protocols and implementing clinical decision support.
  - Mitigate effects of insurance status as a source for disparities in management.
  - Establish uniform admission to post–acute care facilities.
  - Establish policies to assess health literacy to identify patients who may benefit from further education about discharge and follow-up instructions.
- *Provider-level interventions*
  - Racial and ethnic concordance between patients and physicians reduces language and cultural barriers and improves trust, use of preventive care, adherence, patient satisfaction, and health outcomes.
  - Aids to mitigating cognitive biases are being evaluated, including creating awareness among clinicians, decision-making training, and cognitive training.

SUGGESTED READINGS

Akande M, Paquette ET, Magee P, et al. Screening for social determinants of health in the pediatric intensive care unit: recommendations for clinicians. *Crit Care Clin*. 2023;39(2):341-355.

Barnato AE, Berhane Z, Weissfeld LA, et al; Robert Wood Johnson Foundation ICU End-of-Life Peer Group. Racial variation in end-of-life intensive care use: a race or hospital effect? *Health Serv Res*. 2006;41(6):2219-2237.

Beldhuis IE, Marapin RS, Jiang YY, et al. Cognitive biases, environmental, patient and personal factors associated with critical care decision making: a scoping review. *J Crit Care*. 2021;64:144-153.

Blank JA, Armstrong-Hough M, Valley TS. Disparities among patients with respiratory failure. *Curr Opin Crit Care*. 2023;29(5):493-504.

Breeding T, Ngatuvai M, Rosander A, et al. Trends in disparities research on trauma and acute care surgery outcomes: a 10-year systematic review of articles published in The Journal of Trauma and Acute Care Surgery. *J Trauma Acute Care Surg*. 2023;95(5):806-815.

Chatterjee P, Liao JM, Amagai K, Zhao Y, Shirk T, Navathe AS. Variation, Overlap, and Stability in Defining Safety Net Hospitals. JAMA Netw Open. 2025 Jul 1;8(7):e2523923. doi: 10.1001/jamanetworkopen.2025.23923. PMID: 40736736; PMCID: PMC12311695

Cotton NK, Shim RS. Social determinants of health, structural racism, and the impact on child and adolescent mental health. *J Am Acad Child Adolesc Psychiatry*. 2022;61(11):1385-1389.

DiMeglio M, Dubensky J, Schadt S, et al. Factors underlying racial disparities in sepsis management. *Healthcare (Basel)*. 2018;6(4):133.

Howell EA, Zeitlin J. Improving hospital quality to reduce disparities in severe maternal morbidity and mortality. *Semin Perinatol*. 2017;41(5):266-272.

Kasten MJ, Berman AC, Ebright AB, et al. Interpreters in health care: a concise review for clinicians. *Am J Med*. 2020;133(4):424-428.e2.

McGowan SK, Sarigiannis KA, Fox SC, et al. Racial disparities in ICU outcomes: a systematic review. *Crit Care Med*. 2022;50(1):1-20.

McPeake J, Boehm L, Hibbert E, et al. Modification of social determinants of health by critical illness and consequences of that modification for recovery: an international qualitative study. *BMJ Open*. 2022;12(9):e060454.

Minehart RD, Bryant AS, Jackson J, et al. Racial/ethnic inequities in pregnancy-related morbidity and mortality. *Obstet Gynecol Clin North Am*. 2021;48(1):31-51.

Najjar N, Opolka C, Fitzpatrick AM, et al. Geospatial analysis of social determinants of health identifies neighborhood hot spots associated with pediatric intensive care use for acute respiratory failure requiring mechanical ventilation. *Pediatr Crit Care Med*. 2022;23(8):606-617.

Soto GJ, Martin GS, Gong MN. Healthcare disparities in critical illness. *Crit Care Med*. 2013;41(12):2784-2793.

36.2

Diversity, Equity, and Inclusion in Health Care

Erika L. Rangel

Definitions

- *Underrepresented in medicine (URiM)*
  - *Definition*: racial and ethnic populations that are inadequately represented in the medical profession relative to their numbers in the general population. Includes Black, Hispanic/Latino, and Indigenous people
  - *Context in medicine*: underrepresented minorities in medicine often face systemic barriers to entry and advancement, resulting in a lack of diversity that can impact patient care and health outcomes.
  - *Approach*: addressing challenges requires targeted recruitment and retention efforts, mentorship programs, and institutional policies that promote diversity, equity, and inclusion at all levels of medical education and practice.
- *Diversity*
  - *Definition*: diversity refers to differences within a given setting, encompassing a range of attributes such as race, ethnicity, gender, age, sexual orientation, disability, and socioeconomic status.
  - *Context in medicine*: the medical workforce still lacks adequate representation of women and other groups historically URiM.
  - *Approach*: this can be pursued at the organizational level and with policies that actively promote the inclusion of diverse individuals.
- *Equity*
  - *Definition*: equity involves ensuring fair treatment, access, opportunity, and advancement for all individuals while striving to identify and eliminate barriers that have prevented the full participation of some groups.
  - *Context in medicine*: equity addresses disparities in health care access, outcomes, and representation within

the medical profession. It differs from diversity and is harder to achieve because it requires addressing systemic imbalances and biases.
  - *Approach*: implement targeted policies and practices that address systemic barriers to equity for health care workers, provide support tailored to the needs of underrepresented groups, and ensure equitable access to quality care for all patient populations.
- *Inclusion*
  - *Definition*: inclusion is the practice of creating environments in which any individual or group can feel welcomed, respected, supported, and valued. An inclusive climate embraces differences and offers respect in words and actions for all people.
  - *Context in medicine*: inclusion is less policy driven and more elusive than diversity, requiring ongoing individual and collective effort to foster a culture where all members feel they belong.
  - *Approach*: requires individual-level effort and commitment to actively engage with and value the contributions of all colleagues and patients

The Importance of Diversity, Equity, and Inclusion in the Workplace

- *Prioritized by the Institute of Medicine*
  - The landmark report, "In the Nation's Compelling Interest: Ensuring Diversity in the Health-Care Workforce," was published in 2004, urging increasing diversity in the health care workforce to represent shifting demographics.
  - Diverse health care was highlighted as critical to improving access to care, enhancing patient-provider communication, and delivering culturally competent health care services.
- *Diversity, equity, and inclusion (DEI) improves work performance*
  - Diversity fosters innovation, creativity, profitability, and better outcomes (including patient care and satisfaction).
  - DEI improves learning outcomes for trainees, including active thinking, empathy, intellectual engagement, and motivation.
  - Group performance across tasks is positively correlated with the proportion of females.
- *DEI in the research community benefits minority patient populations.*
  - Increasing diversity improves participation and benefits diverse groups previously underrepresented in clinical trials.
- *DEI in critical care*
  - Racial and ethnic concordance between patients and physicians reduces language and cultural barriers and improves trust, use of preventive care, adherence, patient satisfaction, and health outcomes.

Barriers to Diversity, Equity, and Inclusion in the Workplace and Academia

- *Systematic racism*
  - *Definition*: the institutional policies, practices, and cultural norms that perpetuate racial inequalities and discrimination within health care settings
  - *Context in medicine*: this form of racism is embedded in the structures and operations of health care institutions, leading to disparities in treatment, access, and opportunities for both patients and health care workers from marginalized racial groups.
- *Colorism/Shadeism*
  - *Definition*: the preferential treatment of individuals with lighter skin tones over those with darker skin tones within the medical system
  - *Context in medicine*: this bias can affect patients and health care workers, leading to disparities in medical treatment, diagnosis, and professional opportunities based on skin color rather than medical needs or professional merit.
- *Sexism*
  - *Definition*: discrimination or prejudice based on a person's sex or gender within the medical system
  - *Context in medicine*: this can manifest as unequal treatment of patients, with women and gender minorities potentially receiving less accurate diagnoses, fewer treatment options, and inadequate pain management. Additionally, sexism can impact health care workers, contributing to gender disparities in career advancement, salary, and leadership opportunities in the medical profession.
- *Discrimination against sexual orientation, gender identity, language, national origin, ethnicity, religion, immigration/citizenship status, age, familial status, and disability*
  - *Definition*: unjust or prejudicial treatment based on these characteristics
  - *Context in medicine*: this can manifest as unequal opportunities, harassment, or differential treatment in hiring, promotion, patient care, or workplace interactions, compromising both the well-being of health care workers and patient outcomes.
- *Implicit bias*
  - *Definition*: unconscious attitudes or stereotypes that affect understanding, actions, and behaviors toward individuals or groups
  - *Context in medicine*: this can impact medical decision-making, patient-clinician interactions, and results in disparities based on race, ethnicity, gender, or other characteristics.
- *Microaggressions*
  - *Definition*: minor yet damaging humiliations and indignities causing disrespect, devaluation, and exclusion
    - *Microassaults*: "old-fashioned" discriminatory statements that focus on the individual, not the group (eg, name-calling, "they are letting women be doctors now?")
    - *Microinsults*: subtle snubs or humiliations that may be unintentional to the perpetrator (eg, women or URiMs confused for nonmedical roles)
    - *Microinvalidations*: statements aimed to exclude, negate, or dismiss a person's thoughts, feelings, or experiential reality (eg, claiming color blindness to deny a minority group's experience)
    - *Environmental microaggressions*: when microassaults, microinsults, and microinvalidations are reflected in the workplace culture (eg, hallways decorated with pictures of white male surgeons)
  - *Context in medicine*: generates stresses equal to or worse than overt discrimination, associated with low self-esteem, depression, anxiety, and trauma responses

- *Stereotype threat*
  - *Definition*: apprehension or anxiety individuals experience when they fear confirming negative stereotypes about their social group
  - *Context in medicine*: individuals experiencing stereotype threat may perform below their actual abilities due to anxiety about conforming to negative stereotypes. This can undermine their confidence, hinder career advancement, reduce engagement and job satisfaction, and cause higher turnover.

Approaches to Improvement

- *Interventions in the workplace*
  - *Individual level*
    - Promote cultural and gender competency through education and training.
    - Encourage self-awareness and reflection on personal biases.
    - Be intentional in efforts to sponsor women and URiM trainees, who often lack representation in their departments, and advocate for them in their academic pursuits.
    - Teach allyship:
      - Bystanders are in an advantageous position to advocate because they are not the recipients of microaggressions. Understand that we all have privilege.
      - Be an active bystander by addressing microaggressions and discrimination, even when it may be uncomfortable. Shift the conversation back to the person who was interrupted, give credit or amplify someone who had the original idea, show support for those unfairly targeted
      - ACTION framework: Ask clarifying questions; Come from a place of curiosity, not judgment; Tell what you observed in a factual way; Impact exploration by discussing impact of the statement; Own your own thoughts about the situation; Next steps. (ie, "I am not sure I understood your comment. Can you explain that because I want to better understand. When I hear things like that it makes me feel like you think I have this position only because I am a minority, not because I am the most qualified to do the job." Follow with action items for those involved.)
      - Educate yourself: engage in discussions about race with the goal of learning and broadening your perspective. Acknowledge personal biases and be open to learning.
      - Refrain from gas-lighting techniques that delegitimize concerns.
  - *Interpersonal level*
    - Foster allyship versus performative action.
    - Promote upstander behavior over bystander passivity.
  - *Community level*
    - Encourage community engagement and support networks.
    - Create a caring environment that addresses family needs for both sexes (ie, inclusive parental leave policies, lactation facilities, assistance with childcare).
  - *Organizational level*
    - Develop and enforce DEI policies that ensure equal access to opportunities and resources.
    - Offices of Diversity and Inclusion can coordinate efforts to support URiM faculty, such as institution-wide seminars, workshops, and conferences focusing on diversity and inclusion; highlight the availability of resources for mentoring and career advancement; and promote work-life integration.
    - Create affinity groups that extend beyond a single discipline.
    - Promote representation over tokenism.
      - Instead of appointing a single representative from an underrepresented group to a leadership position for appearance's sake, ensure multiple leaders from diverse backgrounds are actively involved in decision-making processes.
      - Instead of hiring a few individuals from underrepresented groups sporadically, implement robust diversity recruitment and retention strategies.
    - Establish safe spaces for sharing concerns.
    - Make baseline assessments and elicit input from stakeholders regarding problems in institutional culture and practices, and obtain buy-in from leadership.
    - Develop concrete metrics for progress to drive accountability and commit to continuous self-assessment.
  - *Policy level*
    - Facilitate inclusivity by creating a "stop the line" policy to empower witnesses to bullying or sexual harassment to speak up or provide an explicit pathway for reporting concerns to leadership.
    - Advocate for inclusive policies that address assortativity versus homophily (the tendency of individuals to associate with similar others).

Interventions in Academia

- *Leadership*
  - Foster diverse leadership using diverse selection committees to build a culture of inclusivity at the top levels.
  - Improve the process of recruitment, including ensuring a diverse applicant pool, objective questions, and implicit bias training.
  - Ensure equal access to leadership development opportunities.
  - Leverage recruitment, mentoring, and networking opportunities by collaborating with organizations and allied societies
- *Scholarship*
  - Increase representation of diversity and race-related topics in research.
  - Emphasize the importance of inclusive language in academic reports.
  - Increase diversity in guideline panels, editorial boards, and manuscript authors.
  - Increase diversity among peer reviewers, as those with expertise face disproportionate demand for reviews, making appropriate expertise hard to find.

- *Promotion*
  - Consider faculty DEI efforts in promotion and tenure evaluation as these efforts are often initiated by URiM faculty and greatly benefit their institutions but are not traditionally considered to be "scholarly." This emphasizes an institution's commitment to DEI and encourages participation by all.
  - Define promotion criteria clearly and ensure transparent communication to all candidates. These should focus on merit, performance, and contributions aligned with organizational values rather than subjective factors.
  - Ensure diversity on promotion committees to bring multiple perspectives and reduce the likelihood of biases influencing decisions.
  - Provide mentorship, coaching, and professional development opportunities, particularly for those from URiM backgrounds.
  - Ensure equitable access to resources needed for promotion, such as research funding, administrative support, and opportunities for collaboration and networking.

SUGGESTED READINGS

Aguwa UT, Wang J, Woreta F, et al. Residency program diversity recruitment and education: survey of efforts and barriers to implementation. *J Surg Educ*. 2022;79(3):595-605.

Berman S, Brown T, Mizelle C, et al. Roadmap for trauma-informed medical education: introducing an essential competency set. *Acad Med*. 2023;98(8):882-888.

Brennan M. *Diversity metrics, measurement, and evaluation*. Accessed May 8, 2024.

Brown CE, Marshall AR, Snyder CR, et al. Perspectives about racism and patient-clinician communication among black adults with serious illness. *JAMA Netw Open*. 2023;6(7):e2321746.

Chatterjee P, Liao JM, Amagai K, Zhao Y, Shirk T, Navathe AS. Variation, Overlap, and Stability in Defining Safety Net Hospitals. JAMA Netw Open. 2025 Jul 1;8(7):e2523923.

Ehie O, Muse I, Hill L, Bastien A. Professionalism: microaggression in the healthcare setting. *Curr Opin Anaesthesiol*. 2021;34(2):131-136.

Flexman AM, Mehta S. Equity, diversity, and inclusion in anesthesiology and critical care: a time for reflection, acknowledgement, and change. *Can J Anaesth*. 2023;70(6):930-935.

Jagsi R, Griffith KA, Stewart A, et al. Gender differences in salary in a recent cohort of early-career physician-researchers. *Acad Med*. 2013;88:1689-1699.

Julien JS, Lang R, Brown TN, et al. Minority underrepresentation in academia: factors impacting careers of surgery residents. *J Racial Ethn Health Disparities*. 2014;1:238-246.

Nattinger AB. Promoting the career development of women in academic medicine. *Arch Intern Med*. 2007;167:323-324.

Person SD, Jordan CG, Allison JJ, et al. Measuring diversity and inclusion in academic medicine: the Diversity Engagement Survey. *Acad Med*. 2015;90:1675-1683.

Rock D, Grant H. *Why diverse teams are smarter*. Harvard Business Review. Accessed April 23, 2024. https://hbr.org/2016/11/why-diverse-teams-are-smarter

Sanfey H, Crandall M, Shaughnessy E, et al. Strategies for identifying and closing the gender salary gap in surgery. *J Am Coll Surg*. 2017;225:333-338.

Suraju MO, McElroy L, Moten A, et al. A framework to improve retention of Black surgical trainees: a Society of Black Academic Surgeons white paper. *Am J Surg*. 2023;226(4):438-446.

Torres MB, Salles A, Cochran A. Recognizing and reacting to microaggressions in medicine and surgery. *JAMA Surg*. 2019;154(9):868-872.

Underrepresented in Medicine Definition 2004. AAMC Unique Populations. Accessed November 21, 2025. https://www.aamc.org/learn-network/affinity-groups/gfa/unique-populations.

West MA, Hwang S, Maier RV, et al. Ensuring equity, diversity, and inclusion in academic surgery: an American Surgical Association White Paper. *Ann Surg*. 2018;268(3):403-407.

Zhuge Y, Kaufman J, Simeone DM, et al. Is there still a glass ceiling for women in academic surgery? *Ann Surg*. 2011;253(4):637-643.

SECTION 1 SHOCK

1.1 Distributive Shock

1. An 80-year-old female presents with fever, hypotension, and mental status changes. You suspect sepsis. Which of the following is NOT part of the sepsis bundle?
   A. Measure lactate.
   B. Obtain cultures.
   C. Start broad-spectrum antibiotics.
   D. All components of the sepsis bundle must be completed within an hour.

2. You are ordering cefazolin for a 35-year-old female with postoperative cellulitis. The electronic health record (EHR) alerts you that she is allergic to penicillin. You:
   A. Continue with the order for cefazolin.
   B. Change the order to vancomycin.
   C. Obtain more information about penicillin allergy.
   D. Hold off on antibiotics and observe.

1.2 Hypovolemic Shock

1. A 25-year-old male presents to the trauma bay after suffering a gunshot wound to his thigh during a hunting trip. His pants are soaked in blood, and he is in obvious pain. He appears pale and states he has no other past medical history. Which of the following hemodynamic parameter patterns would be expected for this patient?
   A. Mean arterial pressure (MAP), cardiac output (CO), pulmonary artery wedge pressure (PAWP), mixed venous oxygen saturation (Svo_2) will increase; systemic vascular resistance (SVR) will decrease.
   B. MAP, CO, PAWP, Svo_2 will decrease; SVR will increase.
   C. MAP will decrease; CO, PAWP, Svo_2, and SVR will increase.
   D. MAP and CO will decrease; PAWP, Svo_2, and SVR will increase.

2. A 69-year-old female is admitted to the intensive care unit (ICU) after undergoing emergent repair of a ruptured abdominal aortic aneurysm. She is intubated and sedated. Her blood pressure (BP) is 90/40 mm Hg, heart rate is 120 bpm, and central venous pressure (CVP) is 13. Which of the following statements is correct regarding the assessment of her volume status?
   A. CVP is the best indicator of volume status, and because this patient's CVP is normal, she should not receive volume.
   B. Pulse pressure variation will not be accurate because the patient is intubated.
   C. The patient should be given volume until her heart rate and BP are normalized.
   D. Multiple factors, including vitals, urine output, assessment with ultrasound or pulse pressure variation, as well as labs, including lactate and base excess, should be used to assess this patient's volume status.

1.3 Cardiogenic Shock

1. A 63-year-old man with a past medical history of hypertension, hyperlipidemia, and type II diabetes presents with chest pain for 3 days. Vital signs on presentation are: blood pressure (BP) 79/62 mm Hg, heart rate (HR) 103 bpm, respiratory rate (RR) 32 breaths/min, and O_2 saturation 88% on room air. Examination is notable for jugular venous distention, crackles on lung auscultation, and cool extremities. Salient laboratory results include N-terminal pro–brain natriuretic peptide (NT-proBNP) of 32,000 pg/mL (normal <125 pg/mL), high-sensitivity troponin of 1,000 ng/L (normal <14 ng/L), creatinine of 1.9 mg/dL, and lactate of 5.2 mmol/L. Electrocardiogram (ECG) demonstrates ST-segment elevations in leads V1 to V4 with associated Q waves and reciprocal depressions in leads II, III, and aVF. The MOST appropriate next step in treatment is:
   A. Initiate dobutamine therapy for cardiogenic shock.
   B. Load with dual antiplatelet therapy, start heparin, and transfer urgently to the cardiac catheterization laboratory.
   C. Place a pulmonary artery catheter to hemodynamically characterize the type of cardiogenic shock.
   D. Place an intra-aortic balloon pump at the bedside for stabilization.

2. A 33-year-old woman with World Health Organization (WHO) group I pulmonary hypertension presents with syncope at home. Her home medications are sildenafil 20 mg 3 times daily, which she has been taking regularly. Vital signs on presentation are BP 71/50 mmHg (MAP 61 mm Hg), HR 92 bpm, RR 28 breaths/min, and O_2 saturation 81% on room air. Examination is notable for jugular venous distention to the earlobe, clear lungs, and cool extremities. Laboratory studies are notable for an elevated alanine aminotransferase (ALT) of 1,240 U/L (normal <36 U/L), elevated aspartate aminotransferase (AST) of 1,400 U/L (normal <33 U/L), elevated creatinine (Cr) of 3.1 mg/dL (baseline 1.0 mg/dL), and lactate of 4.1 mmol/L. Limited ultrasound demonstrates a small and hyperdynamic left ventricular (LV) function, severely dilated and hypokinetic right ventricle, severe tricuspid regurgitation, and an estimated right ventricular systolic pressure of 90 mm Hg. Which of the following is the LEAST appropriate next step in management?
   A. Initiation of vasopressin for a goal MAP >65
   B. Initiation of milrinone
   C. Placement of a pulmonary artery catheter to monitor hemodynamics and target interventions
   D. Administration of fluids to increase left ventricular preload

1.4 Obstructive Shock

1. A 73-year-old male with a history of advanced chronic obstructive pulmonary disease and a metastatic pancreatic adenocarcinoma is brought by ambulance to the emergency department in acute distress. The examination is notable for

a heart rate of 116 beats per minute with a blood pressure of 70/45, and the oxygen saturation is 81% on 6 L/min on a nonrebreather facemask. He is severely tachypneic, and he has markedly diminished left-sided lung sounds, distant heart sounds, and hyperresonance to percussion of the left hemithorax. Which of the following is the best next step in managing this patient?
A. Intubation and mechanical ventilation
B. Needle pericardiocentesis
C. Needle thoracostomy
D. Stat chest radiography

2. A rapid response code is called for hypotension in a 37-year-old female who was admitted to the inpatient medicine service for workup of suspected antiphospholipid antibody syndrome. She is found to be tachycardic and mildly hypotensive, and she reports lightheadedness, dyspnea, and sharp chest pains worse on deep inspiration. While plans are made to obtain definitive imaging, which of the following bedside ultrasound findings would **MOST** support the likely diagnosis?
A. Diastolic collapse of the right ventricle
B. Failure to detect lung sliding
C. Inferior vena cava collapsibility
D. Interventricular septal flattening

SECTION 2 CARDIOVASCULAR

2.1 Coronary Artery Disease, Myocardial Ischemia, and Infarction

1. A 71-year-old woman is admitted to the medical intensive care unit after presenting with abdominal pain, nausea, and several episodes of large-volume coffee-ground emesis. Her medical history is notable for moderate coronary artery disease, type 2 diabetes, hypertension, and active tobacco use. Vital signs show heart rate (HR) 115, blood pressure (BP) 84/60 mm Hg, respiratory rate (RR) 12, and Spo$_2$ 99% on room air. Examination shows pallor but no other abnormalities. She begins to report chest discomfort. Electrocardiogram (ECG) shows submillimeter ST depressions in leads I and aVL. Laboratory testing shows acute anemia and an elevated high-sensitivity troponin value that continues to rise with serial testing. An echocardiogram is performed, which shows new hypokinesis of the anterolateral wall. What is the **MOST** likely diagnosis?
A. Distributive shock
B. Type 1 myocardial infarction
C. Type 2 myocardial infarction
D. Spontaneous coronary artery dissection

2. A 55-year-old male with prediabetes and active tobacco use experiences progressive nonradiating, central chest pain that culminates in a full day of symptoms at rest. He does not seek medical care, and his symptoms slowly resolve. Three days later, he suffers an out-of-hospital cardiac arrest and is brought to the emergency department for further evaluation. Initial ECG is notable for an inferior ST-segment elevation with prominent Q waves. He is taken urgently to the cardiac catheterization lab, which reveals a right dominant coronary system and organized thrombus in the mid-right coronary artery (RCA) extending into the posterior descending artery (PDA). A percutaneous left ventricular assist device and two drug-eluting stents are placed. Shortly following the procedure, he develops worsening hypoxemia and shock. A STAT echocardiogram is obtained (Q-Figure 2.1.1). Which of the following is the **MOST** likely diagnosis?
A. Papillary muscle rupture
B. Left ventricular apical aneurysm
C. Cardiac tamponade
D. Ventricular septal rupture

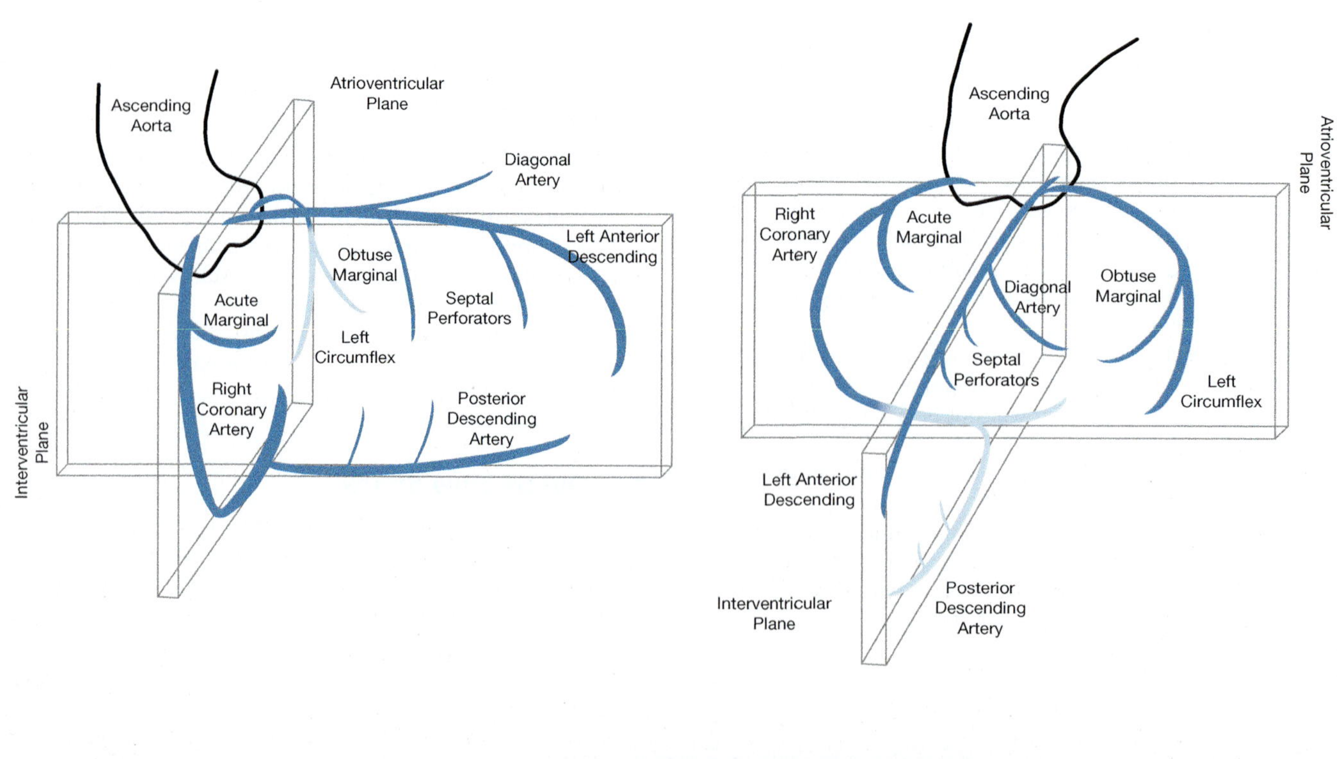

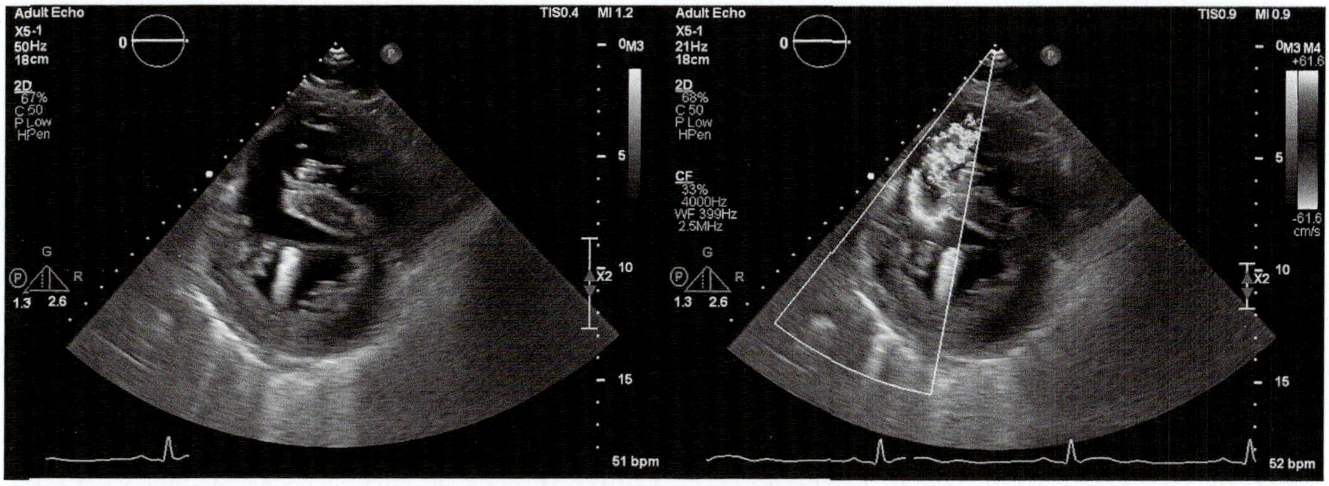

Q-Figure 2.1.1 **Transthoracic echocardiogram demonstrating postinfarction ventricular septal rupture.** Left panel shows two-dimensional echocardiography with an inferoseptal defect. Right panel shows color Doppler imaging, revealing systolic left-to-right shunt flow across the interventricular septum as indicated by the direction of color flow. This mechanical complication typically occurs 3 to 14 days following transmural myocardial infarction.

2.2 Heart Failure

1. A 59-year-old male was admitted with acute on chronic decompensated heart failure due to heart failure with preserved ejection fraction (HFpEF) in the setting of chronic hypertension with thickened left ventricular (LV) walls, and now will be approaching discharge. Which of the following medications may be less effective?
   A. Mineralocorticoid receptor antagonist (MRA)
   B. Loop diuretic
   C. Beta-blocker
   D. Sodium-glucose cotransporter-2 inhibitor (SGLT2i)

2. A 59-year-old male was diagnosed with end-stage restrictive heart disease and has undergone a successful donation after brain death (DBD) heart transplant and returns to the intensive care unit (ICU) with an initial cardiac index of 1.7 L/min/m^2. Intraoperative transesophageal echocardiography showed hyperdynamic LV and mildly reduced right ventricular (RV) function while receiving milrinone infusion. The pulmonary capillary wedge pressure is 12 mm Hg, the central venous pressure is 9 mm Hg, and the pulmonary artery pulsatility index is 1.8. What steps would not likely help guide the ICU clinician to optimize cardiac output in the immediate postoperative state?
   A. Adding inhaled nitric oxide to the ventilator circuit
   B. Titrating inotropic agents, including adding a second agent
   C. Reducing heart rate to avoid increased myocardial oxygen demand
   D. Considering trial of additional preload to assess optimal systemic filling pressure

2.3 Rhythm Disturbances

1. A 63-year-old female with a history of hypertension (HTN), heart failure with reduced ejection fraction (HFrEF) (EF 20%), paroxysmal atrial fibrillation (on apixaban), and coronary artery disease (CAD) presents with progressive dyspnea and peripheral edema. A pulmonary artery catheter was placed, and the patient was admitted to the intensive care unit (ICU) due to her low EF, but blood pressure was normal. Her electrocardiogram (ECG) is shown in Q-Figure 2.3.1.

   What is the best course of treatment?
   A. Intravenous (IV) metoprolol 10 mg
   B. IV diltiazem 5 mg
   C. IV amiodarone 150 mg bolus
   D. Synchronized cardioversion
   E. Defibrillation

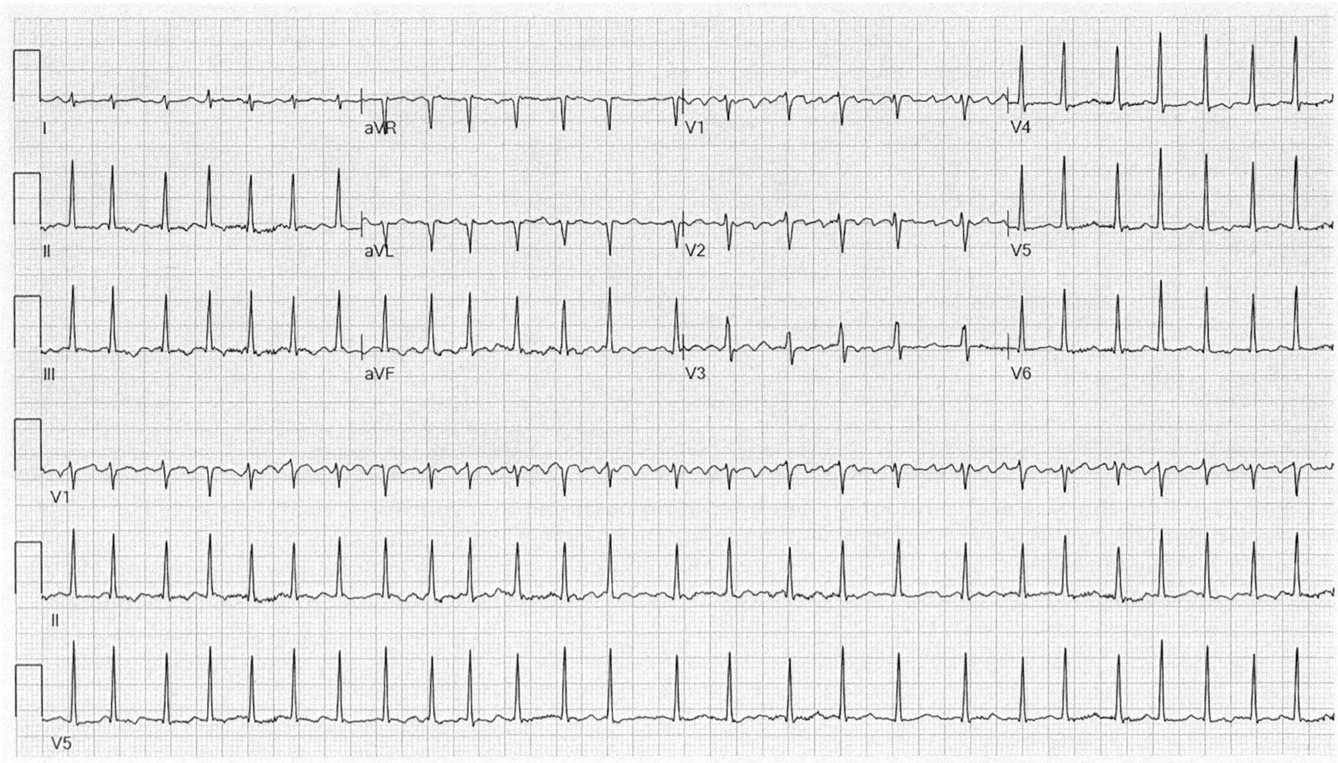

2. A 54-year-old man with a history of chronic obstructive pulmonary disease (COPD) and HTN presented with a witnessed loss of consciousness after several days of reported chest pain. Emergency medical services (EMS) found him in ventricular fibrillation/ventricular tachycardia (VT/VF), and cardiopulmonary resuscitation (CPR) was performed with return of spontaneous circulation (ROSC). He was brought to the hospital. Cardiac catheterization showed 95% proximal left anterior descending (LAD) occlusion and left ventricular ejection fraction (LVEF) ~20% with anterior wall akinesis. He received a drug-eluting stent and was admitted. On day 2 of hospitalization, the patient reported chest discomfort to his nurse. His pulse is rapid. Arterial line showed a blood pressure of 90/50. His ECG (Q-Figure 2.3.2.) is shown.

What is the best next step in management?
A. Defibrillation
B. Synchronized cardioversion
C. IV amiodarone 300 mg bolus
D. IV lidocaine 1 mg/kg bolus

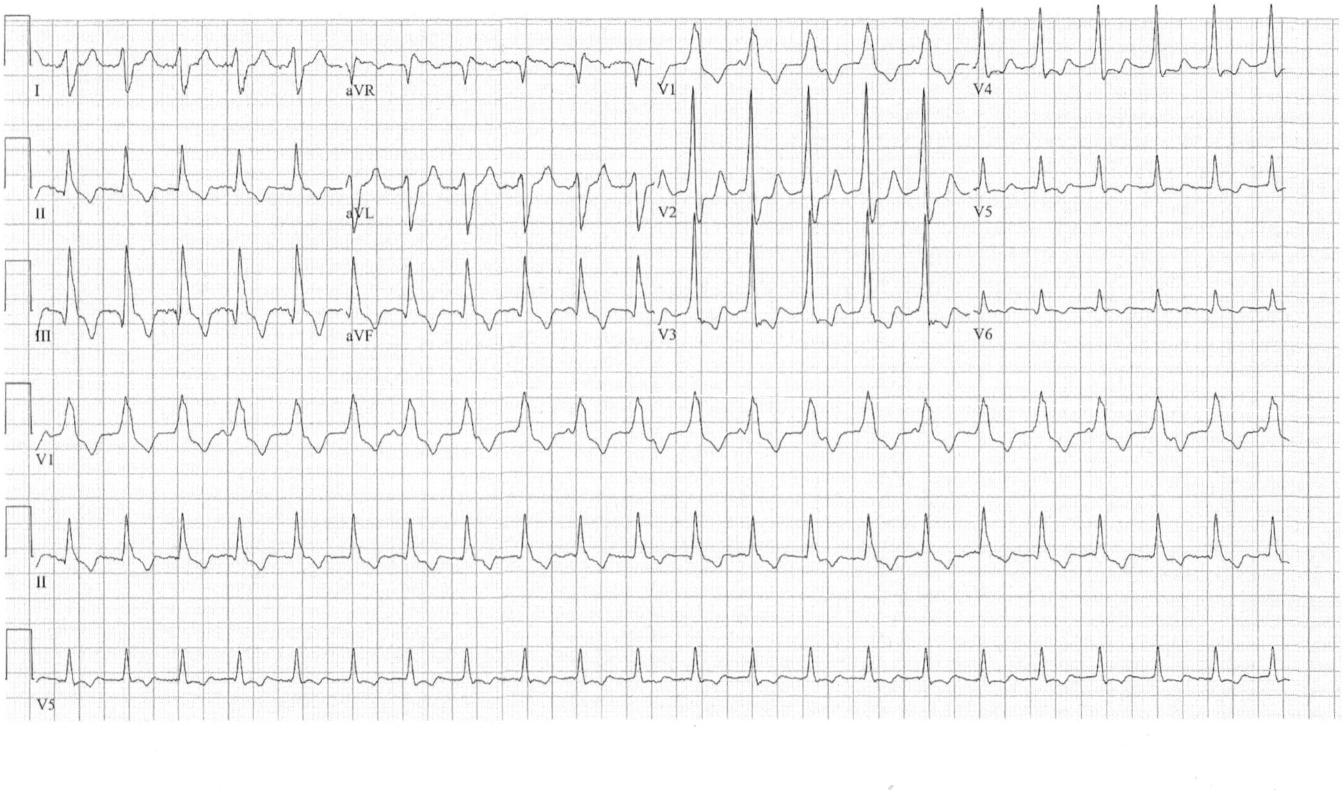

2.4 Valvular Disorders

1. A 74-year-old woman who presented to the emergency department 3 days prior with an uncomplicated ST-segment elevation myocardial infarction (STEMI) s/p percutaneous coronary intervention of the left circumflex artery develops acute shortness of breath. Her vitals are notable for blood pressure 84/52 mm Hg, respiratory rate 36 breaths per minute, heart rate 116 beats per minute, and pulse oximetry of 84% on room air. On bedside ultrasound, there is hyperdynamic left ventricular function, eccentric anteriorly directed jet of mitral regurgitation, and no pericardial effusion. What is the likely mechanism of her acute decompensation, and what intervention would help temporarily stabilize the patient?
   A. Cardiac tamponade; pericardiocentesis
   B. In-stent thrombosis; repeat coronary angiography ± percutaneous coronary intervention
   C. Pulmonary embolism; catheter-directed lysis
   D. Papillary muscle rupture; intra-aortic balloon pump
   E. Pneumonia; antibiotics

2. A 62-year-old man with a history of severe bicuspid aortic stenosis s/p bioprosthetic aortic valve replacement 20 years prior presents to the emergency department with an acute onset of shortness of breath. Emergency medical service (EMS) is called, and on arrival, his vitals are notable for blood pressure 74/48 mm Hg, respiratory rate 24 breaths per minute, heart rate 142 beats per minute, and pulse oximetry of 96% on room air. Electrocardiogram (ECG) shows atrial fibrillation with rapid ventricular response. In the emergency department, he quickly requires maximum dose phenylephrine and high-dose norepinephrine to maintain a mean arterial pressure of 65 mm Hg. His labs are notable for creatinine (Cr) 2.1 (baseline 1.1), lactate 6.2, high-sensitivity troponin T 82, aspartate aminotransferase (AST) 897, and alanine aminotransferase (ALT) 1,200. An echocardiogram is completed and shows a flail prosthetic leaflet with resultant severe aortic regurgitation. What is the most appropriate next step?
   A. Continue with medical management of cardiogenic shock.
   B. Urgent transcatheter aortic valve replacement.
   C. Place an intra-aortic balloon pump for hemodynamic support.
   D. Activate the coronary catheterization lab for emergency coronary angiography ± percutaneous coronary intervention.

2.5 Pericardial Disease

1. A 54-year-old man with a past medical history of hypertension and hyperlipidemia presents to the emergency department with significant dyspnea on exertion in the setting of nonspecific viral symptoms × 1 week. Vital signs are notable for T 99.1° F, heart rate (HR) 111 beats/minute, blood pressure (BP) 104/76 mm Hg, and respiratory rate 22 breaths/minute. Physical examination is notable for normal mentation, distant heart sounds without new murmurs, elevated jugular venous pressure (JVP), clear lungs, and lukewarm extremities. Electrocardiogram (ECG) demonstrates diffuse ST elevations and low voltage; bedside transthoracic echocardiogram (TTE) demonstrates a large pericardial effusion with right ventricular (RV) diastolic collapse. Prior to urgent pericardiocentesis, what is the next best step in management?
   A. Dobutamine 2 μg/min
   B. 1 L normal saline
   C. Furosemide 40 mg IV
   D. Norepinephrine 5 μg/min

2. Which of the following hemodynamic findings would confirm a diagnosis of effusive-constrictive pericarditis:
   A. Diastolic pressure equalization of all four cardiac chambers
   B. Prominent X- and Y-descents
   C. Blunted Y-descent
   D. Failure of right atrial pressures to decrease by >50% following pericardiocentesis

2.6 Myocardial Disorders

1. Hypertrophic cardiomyopathy (HCM) is the most common cause of sudden cardiac death (SCD) in young individuals and is most often due to genetic mutations in MYH7 and MYBPC3. For secondary prevention, implantable cardioverter-defibrillator (ICD) placement is a Class I recommendation in patients with prior cardiac arrest or sustained ventricular arrhythmias. In patients with HCM, which of the following clinical features are considered major risk factors warranting primary prevention ICD placement (Class IIa)?
   A. Unexplained syncope
   B. HCM-related SCD in relative
   C. Left ventricular (LV) apical aneurysm
   D. LV ejection fraction (LVEF) ≤50%
   E. All of the above

2. Restrictive cardiomyopathy (RCM) is associated with reduced ventricular compliance. Which of the following best explains why vasodilators and negative chronotropic agents should be used with caution in patients with RCM?
   A. They reduce arrhythmias by reducing myocardial demand and ischemia.
   B. They reduce preload and heart rate, compromising cardiac output.
   C. They improve lusitropy and diastolic filling time.
   D. They improve systemic vascular resistance and augment cardiac output.
   E. None of the above is true.

2.7 Congenital Heart Disease in Adults

1. Which of the following interventions is least likely to worsen right-to-left shunting and hypoxemia in a patient with a ventricular septal defect (VSD)?
   A. Permissive hypercapnia
   B. Increasing positive end-expiratory pressure (PEEP) on the ventilator
   C. An intravenous infusion of vasopressin
   D. Therapeutic hypothermia

2. An 18-year-old man with right aortic arch, infundibular, and valvar pulmonic stenosis presented for surgical correction. Postoperatively, following infundibular resection and pulmonic valve replacement, he developed severe acute heart failure. Which of the following was the most likely etiology?
   A. Perioperative myocardial infarction
   B. Sudden pulmonary embolism
   C. Left-to-right shunt through an associated VSD once right ventricular (RV) pressure declined
   D. Overaggressive fluid resuscitation intraoperatively

2.8 Cardiogenic Pulmonary Edema versus Noncardiogenic Pulmonary Edema

1. A 65-year-old male presents to the emergency department with shortness of breath and orthopnea. His physical examination reveals bilateral crackles on lung auscultation and jugular venous distension. Chest x-ray shows bilateral perihilar opacities. Which of the following is the most appropriate initial treatment for this patient?
   A. Antibiotics
   B. Intravenous furosemide
   C. Nitroglycerin
   D. Intravenous fluids
   E. Noninvasive positive pressure

2. A 45-year-old male is admitted to the intensive care unit (ICU) after a near-drowning incident. He is hypoxemic and has diffuse crackles on lung auscultation. Chest x-ray shows bilateral infiltrates. Pulmonary capillary wedge pressure (PCWP) <18 mmHg. Which of the following is the most appropriate next step in management?
   A. Start diuretics.
   B. Administer intravenous fluids.
   C. Initiate mechanical ventilation with low tidal volume.
   D. Administer vasodilators.
   E. Perform a thoracentesis.

2.9 Systemic Hypertension

1. A 57-year-old woman is admitted to the cardiac intensive care unit (ICU) after undergoing a percutaneous coronary intervention to the right coronary artery for non–ST-segment myocardial infarction. 90 minutes after admission, the patient notes the abrupt onset of sharp stabbing chest pain and upper back pain. The patient's medical history includes hypercholesterolemia, a 25 pack-year history of smoking cigarettes, chronic hypertension, and asthma. Her home medications include atorvastatin, lisinopril, and as-needed albuterol inhaler. On physical examination in the ICU, blood pressure is 210/110 mm Hg in the right arm and 190/110 mm Hg in the left arm, pulse is 120 beats per minute, respiratory rate 22 per minute, and oxygenation saturation of 94% on 2 L of nasal cannula. Physical examination reveals a postprocedural awake patient in visible discomfort, tachycardia, a 3/6 diastolic murmur at the upper left sternal boarder, and clear lungs on auscultation

   Which is the **MOST** appropriate initial treatment for this patient's blood pressure?
   A. Nicardipine
   B. Nitroprusside
   C. Captopril
   D. Esmolol
   E. Hydralazine

2. A 28-year-old woman at 36 weeks of pregnancy is admitted to the obstetric service in the surgical ICU for severe headache and blurred vision for 4 hours. Her past history is notable for one prior pregnancy complicated by preeclampsia and gestational diabetes in this pregnancy. Her home medications include a multivitamin and baby aspirin. On examination, she has a blood pressure of 220/110 mm Hg, heart rate of 90 per minute, respiration rate of 22 per minute, and oxygen saturation of 99% on room air. Her examination is unremarkable. Labs demonstrate hemoglobin of 12 g/dL, platelet count of 120,000/μL, and a urine protein:creatinine ratio of 600 mg/g. Upon presentation, she is treated with intravenous (IV), labetalol which is continued as an infusion when she is admitted to the surgical ICU.

   What is the next **MOST** appropriate management of her condition?
   A. IV enalapril
   B. IV nitroprusside
   C. Delivery of the fetus
   D. IV betamethasone
   E. None of the above

2.10 Pulmonary Hypertension

1. In a patient with pulmonary hypertension (PH), which of the following does **NOT** worsen right ventricular (RV) function?
   A. Hypercarbia
   B. Acidemia
   C. Hyperoxia
   D. High positive end-expiratory pressure (PEEP)

2. Which of the following clinical scenarios is **MOST** likely to be associated with a mean pulmonary arterial pressure (mPAP) = 28 mm Hg, pulmonary capillary wedge pressure (PCWP) of 10 mm Hg, and pulmonary vascular resistance (PVR) of 1 WU?
   A. Pulmonary arterial hypertension (PAH)
   B. Recurrent pulmonary embolisms
   C. Severe mitral regurgitation
   D. Septic shock

2.11 Aneurysms and Dissections

1. A 64-year-old male patient presents to the emergency department with 1 hour of abrupt onset chest pain. Computed tomography demonstrates 8 mm eccentric thickening of the aorta distal to the left subclavian artery. The aortic wall appears hyperdense on noncontrast imaging, and there is intimal calcium displacement. On contrast imaging, there is no evidence of a false lumen. The patient has a heart rate of 104 bpm and a blood pressure of 125/85 and reports that his chest pain is improving. Which of the following is the **MOST** appropriate next step in management?
   A. Urgent transesophageal echocardiography
   B. Open surgical repair
   C. Thoracic endovascular aortic repair (TEVAR)
   D. Metoprolol
   E. Vitamin K

2. A 32-year-old woman presents after an episode of chest pain followed by syncope. On evaluation in the emergency department, she is awake and alert with a heart rate of 69 and a blood pressure of 115/75. Physical examination discloses a tall, slender woman with pectus excavatum. No murmurs are auscultated on cardiac examination. A computed tomography angiogram is ordered and demonstrates an enlarged aortic root with an intimal tear that extends from the right sinotubular junction into the innominate artery. On repeat evaluation, the patient reports that her chest pain has substantially improved. Which of the following is the **MOST** appropriate next step in management?

A. Urgent transesophageal echocardiography
B. Urgent magnetic resonance imaging
C. Intravenous esmolol
D. Urgent surgical consultation for open surgical repair
E. Urgent surgical consultation for endovascular repair

2.12 Cardiovascular Infections

1. Which of the following is a major criterion for the diagnosis of *infective endocarditis (IE)* by the Modified Duke Criteria?
   A. Fever
   B. Embolic phenomena
   C. New murmur
   D. Blood cultures positive for a typical organism
   E. Immunologic phenomena

2. A 45-year-old with a history of injection drug use (IDU) presents to the emergency department (ED) with fever to 38.3 °C and chills and is found to have positive blood cultures (2/4 sets grow *Staphylococcus aureus*). Transthoracic echocardiogram (TTE) is of fair quality and shows no obvious valvular vegetation. What is the next best step in management?
   A. No further imaging; IE has been ruled out
   B. Cardiac computed tomography (CT)
   C. Transthoracic echocardiogram (TEE)
   D. Fluorodeoxyglucose (18F) ^{18}F-FDG positron emission tomography (PET)/CT
   E. All of the above

2.13 Implantable Cardiac Devices

1. A 70-year-old male with a history of myocardial infarctions and heart failure with reduced ejection fraction (HFrEF) was evaluated 2 weeks after he underwent primary prevention dual-chamber implantable cardiac defibrillator (ICD) and had been discharged following chest radiography and device interrogation. He now presents with sudden pleuritic chest pain at rest with dyspnea and diaphoresis. Laboratory evaluation showed new mild anemia and a leukocytosis, but undetectable troponin. Chest radiography showed a new pleural effusion. Electrocardiography (ECG) showed new ST-segment elevation in inferior and precordial leads. Bedside ultrasonography showed pericardial effusion. Thirty minutes after arrival, the patient's blood pressure dropped to 77/44 mm Hg with a pulse of 60 bpm. What is the next best step?
   A. Emergency coronary angiography
   B. Imaging to exclude aortic dissection
   C. ICD interrogation
   D. Rheumatology and Infectious Diseases consultation

2. What would the expected QRS complex in a patient with 100% biventricular pacing (cardiac resynchronization therapy [CRT]) be expected to look like?
   A. Right bundle branch block; QRS negative in leads I and aVL
   B. Right bundle branch block; QRS positive in leads I and aVL
   C. Left bundle branch block; QRS negative in leads I and aVL
   D. Left bundle branch block; QRS positive in leads I and aVL

3. A 65-year-old man with ischemic cardiomyopathy is admitted to the hospital with decompensated heart failure for intravenous (IV) diuresis. He has been consistently taking maximally tolerated doses of guideline-directed medical therapy and is followed closely by a heart failure team. A transthoracic echocardiogram reveals an ejection fraction of 30%, similar to 6 months prior. An ECG shows sinus bradycardia with a heart rate of 55 bpm, PR interval of 260 millisecond, and QRS interval of 110 millisecond, unchanged from prior. Which of the following implantable cardiac devices is *MOST* appropriate at this time?
   A. Dual-chamber permanent pacemaker (PPM)
   B. Leadless PPM
   C. ICD
   D. Cardiac resynchronization therapy defibrillator (CRT-D)

4. A 76-year-old woman undergoes dual-chamber PPM placement for symptomatic sick sinus syndrome. The procedure is uneventful, and she returns to the ward. One hour later, she notes lightheadedness. She is afebrile, with a blood pressure of 70/40 and a heart rate of 120 bpm. ECG shows sinus tachycardia. Her extremities are cool, and she has distended neck veins. Which of the following is least helpful during the initial evaluation and stabilization?
   A. Chest x-ray
   B. Limited transthoracic echocardiogram
   C. Complete blood count
   D. Device interrogation

2.14 Hemodynamic Monitoring and Bioengineering

1. An 82-year-old female is status post bioprosthetic mitral valve replacement for calcific mitral stenosis. Her preoperative echocardiogram demonstrated a small left ventricular (LV) cavity with mild left ventricular hypertrophy (LVH) and normal biventricular systolic function. No hemodynamically significant valvular disease other than the known mitral stenosis. During the postoperative period, she was started on dobutamine for a low cardiac index but but subsequently developed worsening hypotension. What is the **MOST** likely explanation for the hypotension in this case?
   A. Failure of mitral valve surgery
   B. Left ventricular outflow tract (LVOT) obstruction
   C. Acute heart failure due to myocardial ischemia
   D. Increased preload from fluid overload

2. A 65-year-old man presented to the emergency department with new-onset dyspnea on exertion that started several weeks earlier. The shortness of breath has progressively worsened to the point that he is now breathless at rest. He also notes worsening lower extremity edema and orthopnea. He has no prior medical history and is on no medication. His physical examination demonstrates a man with obesity and a thick neck. Jugular venous pulsations are difficult to visualize. Heart sounds are regular but distant. There is 1+ lower extremity edema bilaterally. His initial laboratory studies are normal, except for an elevated brain natriuretic peptide. Bedside echocardiography reveals a normal ejection fraction without significant valvular abnormalities. Upon admission to the intensive care unit (ICU), which one of the following clinical developments would prompt you to pursue pulmonary artery (PA) catheter placement for this patient?
   A. New atrial fibrillation
   B. Worsening renal function on intravenous furosemide
   C. Fevers and hypotension requiring vasopressor support
   D. Initiation of bilevel positive airway pressure

3. An 80-year-old woman with a history of atrial fibrillation in the ICU is being monitored for acute respiratory failure secondary to septic shock. The team is using the ClearSight system to obtain continuous noninvasive blood pressure measurements and cardiac output readings. What is a potential limitation of using the ClearSight device in this patient?
   A. Inaccurate measurements in patients with peripheral vascular disease
   B. Dependence on arterial waveforms for accuracy
   C. Inability to measure cardiac output continuously
   D. Requirement for invasive monitoring

2.15 Cardiac Imaging

1. In a patient with severe pulmonary hypertension, what sign are you **MOST** likely to see in tamponade on echocardiogram?
   A. Right atrial collapse
   B. Right ventricular collapse
   C. Left atrial collapse
   D. Inferior vena cava dilation/reduced collapse
   E. Both C and D

2. For a patient undergoing a transesophageal echocardiogram, which of the following are absolute contraindications?
   A. Esophageal varices
   B. Active upper gastrointestinal (GI) bleeding
   C. Esophageal stricture
   D. Restricted neck mobility
   E. Both B and C

2.16 Pharmacologic Therapies for Cardiac Disorders

1. Which of the following drugs *MOST* likely cause an elevation in plasma triglycerides?
   A. Nicardipine
   B. Clevidipine
   C. Nitroprusside
   D. Procainamide

2. A 52-year-old man is admitted to the intensive care unit (ICU) after cardiac surgery. His examination is notable for agitation, tremors, and hyperthermia (39.5 °C). His preoperative medications include citalopram, quetiapine, and buspirone for anxiety and major depressive disorder. Based on his examination and home medications, you suspect he may be experiencing serotonin syndrome. Which of the following intraoperative medications *MOST* likely contributed to this diagnosis?
   A. Hydroxocobalamin
   B. Milrinone
   C. Methylene blue
   D. Epinephrine

2.17 Cardiac Arrest and Resuscitation

1. A high-quality team is performing cardiopulmonary resuscitation in the intensive care unit (ICU). An advanced airway is placed and connected to waveform capnography. During the resuscitation, there is a sudden increase in the end-tidal carbon dioxide from 10 to 30 mm Hg. What does this most likely signify?
   A. Esophageal intubation
   B. Return of spontaneous circulation
   C. Resuscitative efforts are unlikely to succeed
   D. Pneumothorax

2. A 54-year-old female transported by emergency medical service (EMS) presents to the emergency department after an out-of-hospital cardiac arrest. Initial rhythm with EMS was pulseless electrical activity (PEA). Return of spontaneous circulation is achieved in the emergency ward with an estimated total downtime of 25 minutes. She is subsequently intubated and has a central line placed to infuse norepinephrine to maintain a mean arterial pressure (MAP) >65 mm Hg. Targeted temperature management at 36 °C is started. Initial head computed tomography (CT) prior to transport to the ICU is unremarkable. She remains comatose in the ICU. What is the next best step in management?
   A. Start broad-spectrum antibiotics.
   B. Actively warm the patient to normothermia.
   C. Begin renal replacement therapy.
   D. Initiate electroencephalogram (EEG) monitoring.

2.18 Hemodynamic and Mechanical Circulatory Support

1. A patient is supported by femoral-femoral venoarterial extracorporeal membrane oxygenation (ECMO) with parameters blood flow rate: 4 L/min, sweep gas flow rate: 3 L/min, and fraction of delivered oxygen 100%. Mechanical ventilator settings: V_t: 450, respiratory rate (RR): 12, positive end-expiratory pressure (PEEP): 8, and FIO_2: 90%. Right radial artery blood gas: pH: 7.42, $PaCO_2$: 38 mm Hg, PaO_2: 64 mm Hg. Hemodynamic measures: central venous pressure (CVP): 15, pulmonary artery pressure 45/30, and pulmonary capillary wedge pressure 28. Heart rate: 100, arterial blood pressure: 105/80, pulsatile with each electrical beat. Dobutamine is at 7.5 µg/kg/min. What is the **MOST** logical next step?
   A. Diuresis, increase PEEP, decrease afterload, decrease ECMO blood flow.
   B. Convert to venovenous eECMO.
   C. Place a left-sided transvalvular microaxial flow pump.
   D. Decrease dobutamine dose to 5 µg/kg/min.

2. A patient is receiving mechanical circulatory support for acute left ventricular failure after myocardial infarction with a left-sided transvalvular microaxial flow pump. Despite attempts at volume removal with diuresis, reducing afterload, and increasing pump settings, the patient is short of breath. Pump flow reads 4.5 L/min. Placement signals appear normal. A right heart catheter shows CVP: 14, pulmonary artery pressure: 50/30, pulmonary capillary wedge pressure: 27, and Fick-derived cardiac output: 3.2 L/min. Mean arterial pressure is 65 mm Hg. What is the **MOST** logical next step?
   A. Start inotropic support with milrinone.
   B. Initiate venovenous ECMO to supplement total body blood flow.
   C. Obtain a chest radiograph to assess device placement.
   D. Obtain a transthoracic echocardiogram for cardiac valve assessment.

2.19 Cardiac and Vascular Surgery Postoperative Management and Perioperative Complications

1. A 65-year-old female undergoes three-vessel coronary artery bypass grafting (CABG) and is taken to the intensive care unit (ICU). Shortly after arrival, the patient's chest tubes are noted to have zero output for an hour. Approximately an

hour later, the patient develops pulseless ventricular tachycardia. What is the best next step in management?
A. Start chest compressions
B. Defibrillate
C. Transthoracic or transesophageal echo
D. Pericardiocentesis

2. A 57-year-old male undergoes an open thoracoabdominal aneurysm repair with preoperative spinal drain placement. Several hours after the patient arrives to the ICU, the bedside nurse notices reduced strength in the bilateral lower extremities. What is the best next step in management?
A. STAT magnetic resonance imaging (MRI)
B. Observation
C. Decrease spinal drain output
D. Increase the mean arterial pressure (MAP)

SECTION 3 PULMONARY

3.1 Pulmonary Mechanics

1. A mechanically ventilated patient is placed on assist-control ventilation. The peak inspiratory pressure (PIP) is measured at 30 cm H_2O, and the plateau pressure (P_{plat}) is 22 cm H_2O. The set tidal volume is 500 mL, and the PEEP is 10 cm H_2O. What is the patient's *respiratory system compliance (CRS)?*
A. 25 mL/cm H_2O
B. 41.7 mL/cm H_2O
C. 50 mL/cm H_2O
D. 62.5 mL/cm H_2O

2. Which of the following clinical situations would most likely result in a widened difference between PIP and P_{plat}?
A. Pulmonary fibrosis
B. Emphysema
C. Bronchospasm
D. Flail chest

3.2 Respiratory Failure, Mechanical Ventilation, and Weaning

1. Which of the following is not a typical physiologic cause of hypoxemic respiratory failure?
A. Diffusion defect
B. Alveolar hypoventilation
C. Pulmonary shunt
D. Increased CO_2 production

2. Which of the following is true regarding the spontaneous breathing trial (SBT)?
A. A duration of 2 hours is preferred to 30 minutes to ensure success.
B. SBT is typically performed using a set respiratory rate and tidal volume.
C. A positive cuff leak test indicates significant airway edema.
D. The most common cause of failed SBT is persistence of underlying disease.

3.3 Acute Respiratory Distress Syndrome

1. A 68-year-old man presents to the hospital with 3 days of fevers, chills, shortness of breath, and productive cough. A chest radiograph obtained in the emergency department reveals multifocal infiltrates bilaterally. He is admitted to the medical ward but has progressive hypoxemia, ultimately requiring intubation and transfer to the medical intensive care unit. His ventilator settings are respiratory rate set to 28, tidal volume set to 420 mL (6 mL/kg ideal body weight), positive end-expiratory pressure (PEEP) of 8, and an FIO_2 set to 1. Her PaO_2 on these settings is 90. Which of the following has been shown to reduce mortality in this patient?
A. Maintaining a negative fluid balance
B. Initiation of inhaled pulmonary vasodilator therapy
C. Titrating PEEP to achieve a driving pressure <15 cm H_2O
D. Prone positioning

2. A 48-year-old woman presents to the hospital with fever, cough, and progressive dyspnea. Four days prior to presentation, she was diagnosed with influenza A and has been receiving oseltamivir. A chest radiograph reveals multifocal pneumonia bilaterally, and she requires initiation of high-flow nasal oxygen in the emergency department. Three days after admission to the medical intensive care unit, she is intubated, and her ventilator settings are optimized. Over the ensuing 48 hours, she is ultimately administered continuous neuromuscular blockade, placed in the prone position, and initiated on inhaled pulmonary vasodilators. Despite these interventions, her PaO_2-to-FIO_2 ratio is 60 on FIO_2=1 or 100%. Which of the following statements regarding the role of venovenous extracorporeal membrane oxygenation (VV-ECMO) is most correct?
A. Transfer to a center capable of providing VV-ECMO is associated with a mortality benefit even if VV-ECMO is not ultimately initiated.
B. The duration of her illness precludes the initiation of VV-ECMO.
C. The duration of her time on mechanical ventilation precludes the initiation of VV-ECMO.
D. VV-ECMO should be considered only after a trial of inverse ratio ventilation as a salvage maneuver.

3.4 Ventilator-Induced Lung Injury and Ventilator-Associated Lung Injury

1. Mechanical ventilation that induces an inflammatory response resulting in lung injury is referred to as what?
A. Barotrauma
B. Biotrauma
C. Volutrauma
D. Atelectrauma

2. Which of the following strategies is least likely to minimize the risk of ventilator-induced lung injury (VILI) in patients receiving mechanical ventilation?
A. Low tidal volumes
B. Driving pressure <15 cm H_2O
C. Optimizing positive end-expiratory pressure (PEEP)
D. Maintaining normocapnia

3.5 Pulmonary Embolic Disorders

1. A 56-year-old woman presents with sudden-onset shortness of breath, pleuritic chest pain, and tachycardia. She recently underwent knee replacement surgery. Her Wells score is 7.5. What is the **MOST** appropriate next step in diagnosis?
A. Obtain a D-dimer level.
B. Perform a lower extremity ultrasound.

C. Proceed directly to pulmonary computed tomographic angiography (CTA).
D. Order a ventilation-perfusion scan.

2. Which of the following patients with confirmed pulmonary embolism is at high-intermediate risk and should be considered for closer monitoring but not immediate thrombolysis?
A. A 48-year-old woman with stable vitals and elevated B-type natriuretic peptide (BNP) but normal right ventricle (RV) size on CTA
B. A 65-year-old man with stable vitals, RV hypokinesis on transthoracic echocardiogram (TTE), and elevated troponin
C. A 71-year-old woman in shock with systolic blood pressure (SBP) 78 mm Hg and large saddle embolus
D. A 55-year-old man with no RV strain, no biomarker elevation, and no symptoms of hypotension

3.6 Severe and Life-Threatening Asthma Exacerbation

1. A 28-year-old female with past medical history of migraines, asthma, and allergic rhinitis with nasal polyps presents to the hospital with dyspnea at rest. She states that her symptoms started some hours before coming to the emergency department, and they got progressively worse over time. She also complains of wheezing, chest tightness, and rhinorrhea. Her asthma and her migraines are usually well controlled since she started maintenance therapy with inhaled steroids and amitriptyline, respectively. However, she developed a migraine the day before presentation for which she took diclofenac with improvement. She is hemodynamically stable, with a normal abdomen, cardiovascular, and skin examination. Her pulmonary examination is notable for diffuse inspiratory and expiratory wheezes. The patient was found to have a severe asthma exacerbation and was started on albuterol and ipratropium via a nebulizer, intravenous magnesium, and methylprednisolone. What further therapy would **MOST** likely be most beneficial to this patient?
A. Intravenous theophylline
B. Intravenous montelukast
C. Bilevel noninvasive ventilation
D. Helium-oxygen gas

2. The patient in Question 3.6.1 does not respond to initial therapy and requires intubation and mechanical ventilation. She has been started on epinephrine continuous infusion, is sedated, and paralyzed. Chest x-ray shows hyperinflation. Blood pressure is 90/60 mm Hg. Initial mechanical ventilation settings are in volume control with a tidal volume of 540 mL (ideal body weight of 60 kg), respiratory rate 20, positive end-expiratory pressure (PEEP) 5 cm H_2O, Fio_2 0.5, and flow 60 L/min (descending ramp). On these settings, the patient has a peak inspiratory pressure of 50 cm H_2O, plateau pressure of 28 cm H_2O, pressure on expiratory pause of 18 cm H_2O, and her arterial blood gases show: pH 7.31, $paco_2$ 52, bicarbonate 24, Pao_2 90, and Spo_2 98%. Which ventilator change would not improve the patient's hyperinflation and respiratory status?
A. An increase in inspiratory flow
B. A decrease in the respiratory rate
C. An increase in PEEP
D. A change in the flow pattern to a square waveform

3.7 Chronic Obstructive Pulmonary Disease

1. A 68-year-old man with a 45-pack-year smoking history presents with progressive dyspnea on exertion and chronic productive cough. He has experienced two exacerbations in the past year. Physical examination reveals prolonged expiration and diminished breath sounds. Pulmonary function testing shows:

Forced expiratory volume in 1 second (FEV_1): 55% predicted
Forced vital capacity (FVC): 82% predicted
FEV_1/FVC: 0.59 (postbronchodilator)
Total lung capacity (TLC), forced residual capacity (FRC), and residual volume (RV): increased
Diffusion lung capacity for carbon monoxide (DLCO): normal

Which of the following **BEST** describes the interpretation of these findings?
A. Restrictive lung disease due to interstitial lung pathology
B. Moderate airflow obstruction consistent with chronic obstructive pulmonary disease (COPD)
C. Severe asthma with reversible obstruction
D. Upper airway obstruction from a central mass
E. Normal spirometry in an older patient

2. A 72-year-old woman with known COPD presents to the emergency department with 3 days of worsening dyspnea, increased cough, and purulent sputum. She is afebrile, with respiratory rate (RR) 28, heart rate (HR) 102, Spo_2 89% on room air. Arterial blood gas (ABG) shows:

pH: 7.29
$Paco_2$: 58 mm Hg
Pao_2: 59 mm Hg
Complete blood count (CBC) reveals an eosinophil count of 420/μL. Chest radiograph is negative for consolidation.

Which of the following is the **MOST** appropriate next step in her management?
A. High-dose systemic corticosteroids without bronchodilators
B. Empiric cefepime for potential *Pseudomonas* infection
C. Initiate noninvasive ventilation and systemic steroids.
D. Immediate intubation and mechanical ventilation
E. Begin pulmonary rehabilitation and long-term oxygen therapy.

3.8 Restrictive Lung Diseases

1. A 26-year-old female presents to the hospital with fever, dyspnea, and cough for 1 week. She is a graduate student who has never been hospitalized, and her medication list is only notable for fluoxetine and cetirizine. She denies tobacco use and endorses almost daily inhalational marijuana use. Physical examination is notable for inspiratory crackles bilaterally without wheezing, and Spo_2 is 87% on room air. Chest x-ray (CXR) shows bilateral patchy infiltrates, and high-resolution computed tomography (HRCT) shows diffuse ground-glass opacities (GGOs) and centrilobular nodules. She is admitted and is started on broad-spectrum antibiotics and supplemental oxygen. Her infectious workup (respiratory viral panel and sputum culture) is negative, and she continues to have respiratory symptoms and worsening hypoxemia despite completing a course of antibiotics. A repeat CXR shows worsening pulmonary infiltrates, and she is transferred to the intensive care unit (ICU) and intubated. On examination, the lung fields are notable for crackles

and no wheezing. She is afebrile. Complete blood count (CBC) is notable for normal white blood cell (WBC) and mild peripheral eosinophilia. What is the **MOST** appropriate next step?

A. Treat empirically for asthma exacerbation with prednisone 40 mg for 5 days.
B. Broaden antibiotics to cover multidrug-resistant (MDR) organisms.
C. Perform a diagnostic bronchoscopy with bronchoalveolar lavage (BAL).
D. Thoracic surgical consultation for lung biopsy.

2. A 48-year-old man with no past medical history presents to the hospital with 1 week of progressive dyspnea, myalgias, and cough. Initial examination reveals hypoxemia requiring nasal cannula oxygen supplementation, and chest radiograph reveals bilateral airspace opacities. Initial laboratory studies reveal leukocytosis, normal metabolic panel, normal amylase, normal lipase, normal troponin, and modestly elevated C-reactive protein and creatine kinase. Sputum cultures are unrevealing, and he is initiated on broad-spectrum antibiotics. Over the course of 5 days, his clinical status worsens, and he is intubated and transferred to the ICU where he requires 80% of F_{IO_2} to maintain an arterial Pa_{O_2} >60 mm Hg. BAL is performed and reveals inflammation without viral or bacterial pathogens detected by polymerase chain reaction (PCR) or culture. A chest CT scan is performed and reveals widespread, bilateral GGOs and regions of organizing pneumonia with subpleural sparing. Laboratory studies are repeated and notable for an elevated serum aldolase. What is the **MOST** appropriate next step?

   A. Broaden antibiotics to cover MDR organisms.
   B. Thoracic surgical consultation for lung biopsy.
   C. Administer high-dose immunosuppression.
   D. Send autoimmune serologic studies.

3.9 Aspiration Syndromes

1. Which of the following is a risk factor for aspiration?
   A. Presence of protective airway reflexes
   B. Effective cough mechanism
   C. Dysphagia and compromised airway defenses
   D. Absence of gastroesophageal reflux

2. A 75-year-old woman with a history of stroke presents with a sudden onset dyspnea and low-grade fever. A chest x-ray shows infiltrates in the lower lobes. What is the **MOST** probable cause of her condition?
   A. Viral pneumonia
   B. Aspiration pneumonitis
   C. Pulmonary embolism
   D. Tuberculosis

3.10 Pneumonia

1. A 76-year-old man with no health care contacts and a history of bronchiectasis presented to the emergency department with 3 days of worsening cough, mucous production, and fevers. His family became concerned when he seemed to be more confused and disoriented on the day of admission. He can state his name and that he is in a hospital but does not know the day or month. Laboratory studies show a negative rapid viral swab, white blood cell (WBC) of 11 × 10³/μL, creatinine 1.3 mg/dL, and blood urea nitrogen (BUN) 24 mg/dL. He has a 3-L oxygen requirement by nasal cannula but is breathing comfortably with a systolic blood pressure of 140 mm Hg. A rapid viral swab is negative. What is the **MOST** appropriate course of action?
   A. Discharge home with supplemental oxygen and azithromycin.
   B. Admit to the general medical service and treat with ceftriaxone and azithromycin.
   C. Admit to the intensive care unit (ICU), start hydrocortisone 200 mg intravenously (IV), cefepime, and ciprofloxacin.
   D. Admit to the general medical service and treat with cefepime and ciprofloxacin.

2. A 56-year-old woman with a history of alcohol misuse was admitted to the ICU 4 days ago after being found unresponsive in her home by emergency medical service (EMS). She was intubated shortly after presentation to the hospital due to hypoxemia, hypotension, and her altered mental status. She was started on broad-spectrum antibiotics, including ceftriaxone and IV ciprofloxacin immediately on admission to the hospital and has been receiving appropriate low tidal volume ventilation, IV hydrocortisone, and a ventilator-associated pneumonia prevention bundle. Her respiratory cultures have since grown. *Streptococcus pneumoniae* and her antibiotics tailored appropriately. Despite appropriate antibiotics and an improvement in her oxygen requirement since arrival, she continues to have vasopressor dependence, fevers to 39.4 °C, and rising leukocytosis without eosinophilia. A chest x-ray was obtained (Q-Figure 3.10.1).

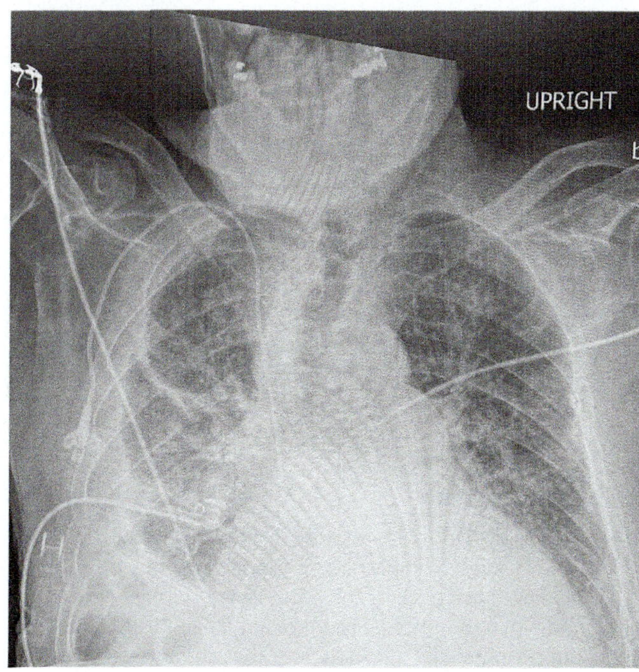

   What is the **MOST** likely cause of her ongoing critical illness?
   A. She has a new ventilator-associated pneumonia.
   B. She is suffering from a noninfectious fever secondary to exposure to antibiotics.
   C. She has developed an empyema.
   D. She has worsening acute respiratory distress syndrome (ARDS) and needs advanced ventilator management.

3.11 COVID-19

1. A 68-year-old man with a history of diabetes mellitus and coronary artery disease presents to the hospital after a positive polymerase reaction chain (PCR) test for COVID-19. He is febrile and reports a cough, chest pain, and sore throat but is on room air. Which medication is **NOT** indicated in this patient?
   A. Remdesivir
   B. Dexamethasone
   C. Enalapril
   D. Enoxaparin

2. A 74-year-old woman with a history of hypertension and chronic obstructive pulmonary disease (COPD) is positive for COVID-19 and is admitted to the intensive care unit (ICU) for worsening hypoxemia and respiratory distress from the medicine floor. She has been treated with 5 days of dexamethasone 6 mg/kg, remdesivir, treatment dose enoxaparin, and supported with bilevel positive airway pressure (BiPAP) while on the floor. Which are the next **BEST** steps to treat this patient upon arrival in the ICU?
   A. Continue current medications with the addition of tocilizumab and change oxygen support to high-flow nasal cannula (HFNC).
   B. Trial of prone positioning before intubation. Continue dexamethasone and add baricitinib or tocilizumab.
   C. Continue current medical therapy with closer monitoring and hold home captopril.
   D. Consider early intubation. Continue dexamethasone and add baricitinib or tocilizumab. Stop remdesivir and change treatment dose enoxaparin to prophylactic dosing.

3.12 Pleural Disease

1. Which pleural fluid characteristic **MOST** strongly predicts the need for chest-tube drainage in parapneumonic effusion?
   A. Lactate dehydrogenase (LDH) >500 U/L
   B. pH <7.20
   C. Glucose >60 mg/dL
   D. Protein >3.0 g/dL

2. When should recurrence prevention (pleurodesis or surgery) be offered for spontaneous pneumothorax?
   A. After any first episode
   B. After the second primary or first secondary episode
   C. Only if bilateral
   D. After three recurrences

3.13 Hemoptysis

1. A 68-year-old woman with a medical history of atrial fibrillation and stage IV breast adenocarcinoma with pulmonary metastases presents to the emergency department with 12 hours of hemoptysis. She takes apixaban for thromboembolism prophylaxis. She estimates that she has coughed up 1 cup of blood (~230 mL) in total. Her respiratory rate is 24, and her oxygen saturation is 91% on ambient air. Which of the following is the **MOST** appropriate next step?
   A. Perform computed tomography (CT) scan of the chest with intravenous contrast.
   B. Administer andexanet alfa (factor Xa inhibitor reversal agent).
   C. Consult pulmonology for flexible bronchoscopy.
   D. Consult interventional radiology for bronchial artery angiography.

2. A 38-year-old woman with a medical history of frequent rhinosinusitis presents with 3 days of fatigue, rhinorrhea, sore throat, and cough productive of specks of blood. Initial laboratory workup is notable for an elevated creatinine, elevated blood urea nitrogen, and urinalysis with microscopic hematuria. On hospital day 3, the patient develops worsened hemoptysis now productive of ~10 to 20 mL of blood every 10 minutes, and her oxygen saturation has now dropped to 88% on ambient air. She has started on supplemental oxygen and transferred to the intensive care unit (ICU). A computed tomography angiography (CTA) of the chest reveals patchy ground-glass opacities throughout the bilateral lungs without an obvious focal source of bleeding. Which of the following medications will **MOST** effectively treat the source of her hemoptysis?
   A. Nebulized tranexamic acid
   B. Intravenous tranexamic acid
   C. Topical epinephrine
   D. Intravenous corticosteroids

3.14 Upper Airway Diseases and Disorders

1. A 64-year-old female underwent an uneventful hemithyroidectomy. On POD#1, she has acute neck swelling and requires return to the operating room (OR) for emergency open hematoma evaluation and cauterization of bleeding vessels within the thyroid bed. Upon awakening from general anesthesia, she has a weak, breathy voice and complains of coughing while drinking thin liquids. What is the most likely diagnosis?
   A. Laryngeal hematoma from emergency intubation
   B. Unilateral vocal fold paralysis
   C. Cricoarytenoid joint dislocation
   D. Laryngeal cancer

2. A 21-year-old female admitted for tonsillitis starts to complain of difficulty swallowing and voice changes. Her voice sounds muffled. Examination shows good mouth opening and a fluctuant, unilateral swelling around the left tonsil and soft palate. What is the next step in management?
   A. Obtain a neck computed tomography (CT) scan.
   B. Perform an incision and drainage intraorally.
   C. Start intravenous (IV) antibiotics.
   D. Prepare to intubate or secure a surgical airway.

3.15 Pulmonary Vasculitic and Autoinflammatory Disorders

1. Which of the following is **MOST** characteristic of eosinophilic granulomatosis with polyangiitis (EGPA)?
   A. PR3-ANCA positivity in >80% of patients
   B. Adult-onset asthma and marked eosinophilia

C. Linear immunoglobulin G (IgG) deposition on alveolar basement membrane
D. Pulmonary artery aneurysms on computed tomographic angiogram (CTA)

2. What is first-line induction therapy for severe granulomatosis with polyangiitis (GPA) with diffuse alveolar hemorrhage (DAH)?
A. High-dose steroids alone
B. Cyclophosphamide + plasmapheresis
C. Rituximab + glucocorticoids
D. Mepolizumab

3.16 Inhalational Injuries and Tracheobronchitis in the Intensive Care Unit

1. A 45-year-old man is rescued from a house fire and presents with facial burns, singed nasal hairs, and a hoarse voice. On arrival, he is alert and speaking in full sentences, but you note progressive stridor and accessory muscle use. What is the **MOST** appropriate next step in management?
A. Administer racemic epinephrine.
B. Observe closely in the intensive care unit (ICU) with serial examinations.
C. Intubate the patient immediately.
D. Administer corticosteroids.
E. Obtain a chest computed tomography (CT) scan.

2. A 60-year-old man is admitted after exposure to chlorine gas during an industrial accident. He develops dyspnea, wheezing, and a nonproductive cough. Chest x-ray (CXR) is initially unremarkable. What is the **MOST** appropriate next step in his management?
A. Start systemic corticosteroids.
B. Perform urgent bronchoscopy.
C. Begin empiric antibiotics.
D. Provide humidified oxygen and bronchodilators.
E. Administer nebulized sodium bicarbonate routinely.

3.17 Pulmonary Contusion

1. Which of the following factors most strongly influences the clinical impact of pulmonary contusions?
A. The radiodensity of the contusions as measured by Hounsfield units
B. The radiologic volume of the contused lung
C. The mechanism of injury
D. The presence or absence of hemoptysis

2. Which of the following is the most useful in diagnosing pulmonary contusions?
A. X-ray
B. Ultrasound
C. Computed tomography
D. Bronchoscopy

3.18 Flail Chest and Surgical Stabilization of Rib Fractures

1. Current evidence of the benefit of surgical stabilization of rib fractures is strongest for which of the following scenarios?
A. An intubated patient with two fractures in each of ribs 4 to 7
B. A patient with mild chronic obstructive pulmonary disease (COPD) with nondisplaced single fractures of ribs 3 to 8
C. A patient with three rib fractures each displaced by half a shaft-width
D. A patient with nondisplaced single fractures of ribs 2 to 9 with poor pain control

2. When should surgical stabilization of rib fractures (SSRF) be performed?
A. 3 to 4 days after initial trauma to allow for resolution of pulmonary contusions
B. 1 to 3 days after initial trauma to allow for serial assessment of clinical trajectory prior to operative intervention
C. >4 days after initial trauma, if the patient remains ventilator dependent
D. Immediately after trauma, or as soon as it is safe to do so.

3.19 Sleep-Related Breathing Disorders

1. Which of the following is true regarding the apnea-hypopnea index (AHI) and diagnosis of obstructive sleep apnea (OSA)?
A. AHI >5 is sufficient to diagnose OSA in all patients, regardless of symptoms.
B. AHI includes apneas, hypopneas, and respiratory effort–related arousals (RERAs) per hour of sleep.
C. Respiratory disturbance index (RDI) is used to assess OSA severity in asymptomatic patients.
D. AHI >15 is diagnostic of OSA in asymptomatic individuals.

2. Which of the following is a recognized perioperative complication in patients with untreated OSA?
A. Increased risk of pulmonary embolism due to impaired venous return
B. Reduced intraoperative blood loss due to airway collapse
C. Postoperative arrhythmias due to sedative-induced loss of upper airway tone
D. Increased risk of anaphylaxis due to continuous positive airway pressure (CPAP) use

3.20 Pulmonary Imaging

1. A 57-year-old female with a past medical history of hypertension (HTN), type 2 diabetes mellitus (DM2), morbid obesity, congestive heart failure (CHF), obstructive sleep apnea (OSA), tobacco use disorder (TUD), and metastatic ovarian cancer was transferred to the intensive care unit (ICU) for observation following an uneventful hyperthermic intraperitoneal chemotherapy (HIPEC) procedure. In the ICU, the patient was initially on 2 L nasal cannula (NC), hemodynamically stable, and comfortably resting in the bed. During the ICU stay the next morning, she started having shortness of breath and increased work of breathing along with high O_2 requirements. Now she is receiving 10 L of O_2 through a nonrebreather mask; vitals: Sao_2 88%, blood pressure (BP) 85/45, heart rate (HR) 115, temperature 36.9 °C, and respiratory rate (RR) 29. The ICU team ordered a STAT chest radiography (CXR) and performed a bedside lung ultrasound (LUS). What is the correct

combination of the findings on the LUS and the necessary clinical intervention given the Q-Figure 3.20.1?

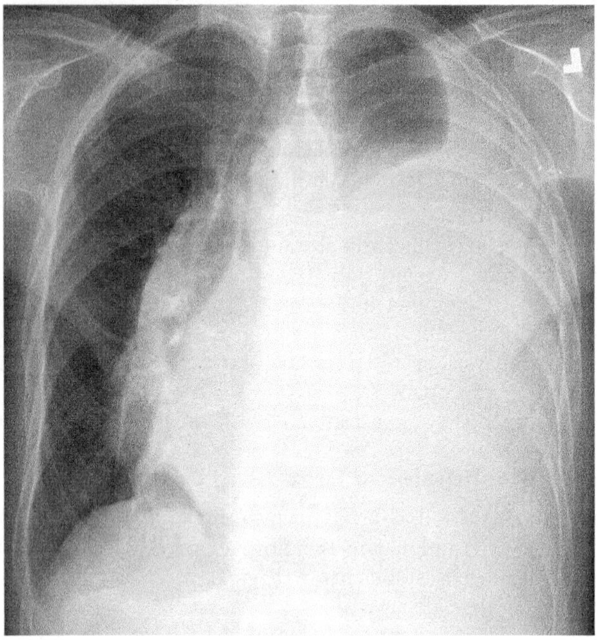

A. Static air bronchograms and lung pulse—perform bronchoscopy.
B. B′-profile and "Shred sign"—start antibiotics and vasopressors.
C. *Positive "spine sign"—perform L thoracentesis.*
D. Diffuse B-profile and normal pleural sliding—start diuretics.

2. A previously healthy 37-year-old male was transported to the ICU following Motor Vehicle Accident (MVA). The patient sustained third-degree burns of over 30% of the body surface area. He was intubated at the scene. Given the ongoing resuscitation efforts, the ICU team decides to obtain central venous access in the left subclavian vein. After unsuccessful attempts, the procedure was aborted, and central venous catheter (CVC) was placed in the right femoral vein instead. Shortly after the procedure, the respiratory therapist (RT) notified the team that the end-tidal CO_2 ($EtCO_2$) on capnography increased to 60s, and increasing the minute ventilation did not correct the $EtCO_2$. A STAT CXR was ordered. The bedside LUS revealed Q-Figure 3.20.2.

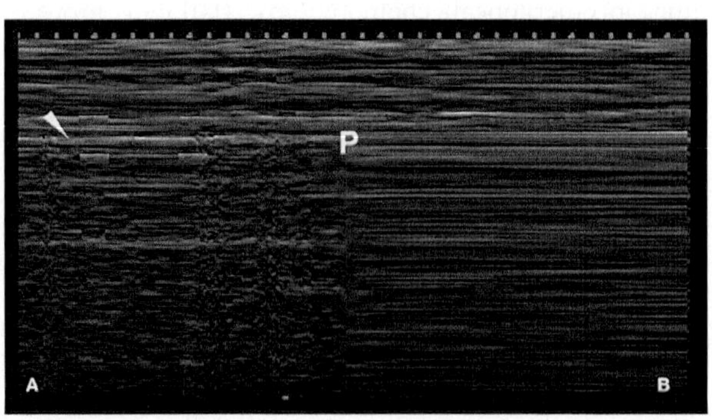

Which of the following CXRs would confirm the suspected diagnosis?

A. **Q-Figure 3.20.3A**

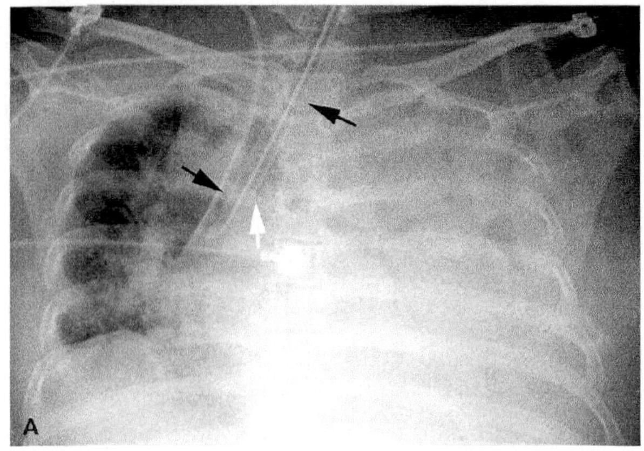

B. **Q-Figure 3.20.3B**

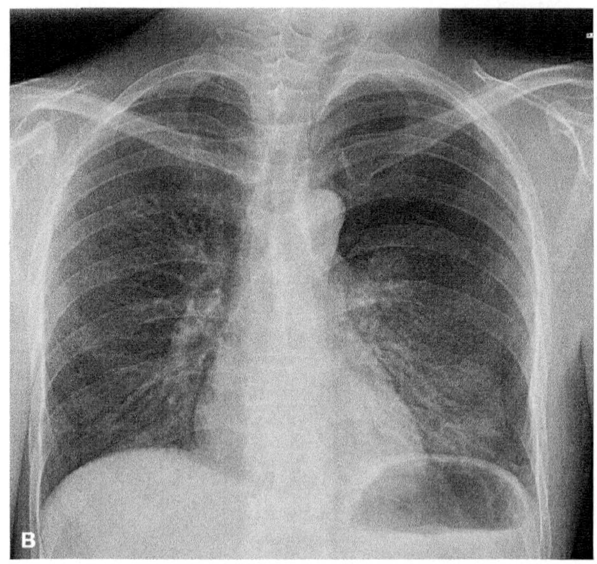

C. **Q-Figure 3.20.3C**

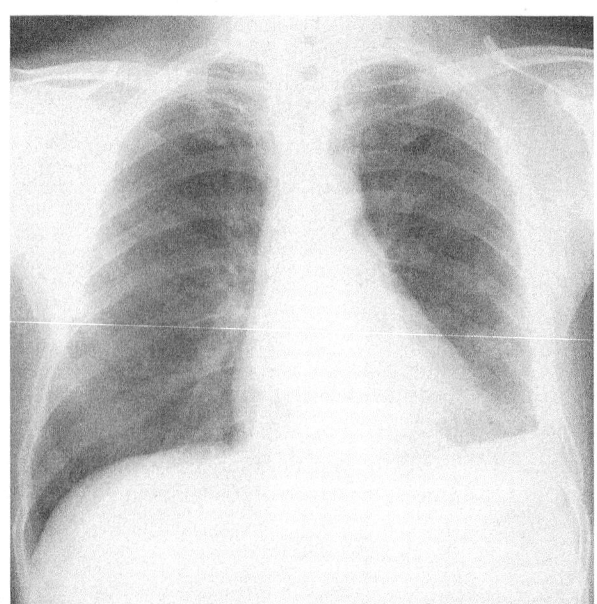

D. Q-Figure 3.20.3D

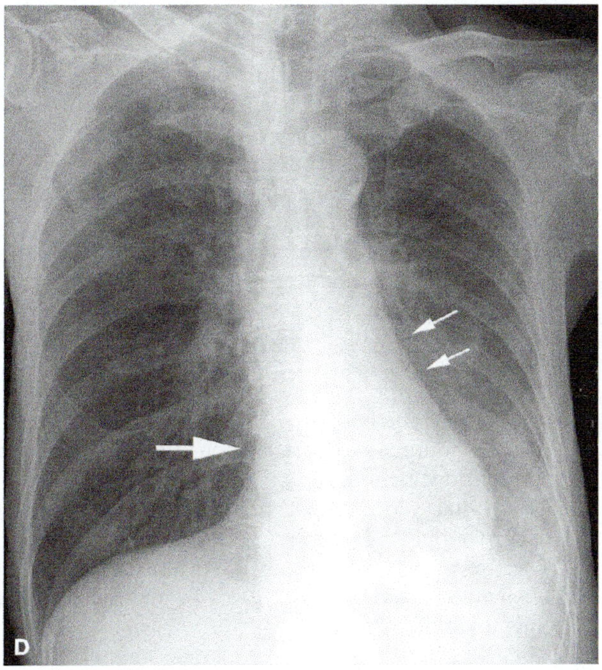

3.21 Pharmacologic Therapies for Pulmonary Disorders

1. A 68-year-old female with a past medical history of chronic obstructive pulmonary disease (COPD), diabetes, hypertension, and atrial fibrillation presents to the emergency department (ED) with profound dyspnea, which has been progressing over the last 24 hours. Baseline COPD medications include aclidinium 400 μg/formoterol 12 μg (1 inhalation) twice daily and rescue albuterol inhaler, which she reports using every 4 hours for the last week. This is her second hospitalization in the past 6 months for severe COPD exacerbations. Which one of the following is the best recommendation regarding initial bronchodilator therapy?
   A. Double the dose of maintenance inhaler therapy, aclidinium 400 μg/formoterol 12 μg (2 inhalations) twice daily.
   B. Continue Ipratropium and albuterol, followed by 0.5 mg ipratropium bromide/2.5 mg albuterol nebulized every 6 hours, with as-needed doses every 1 to 4 hours.
   C. Initiate theophylline loading dose 5 to 7 mg/kg followed by a continuous infusion of 0.4 to 0.6 mg/kg/h to maintain a serum concentration of 10 to 15 mg/L.
   D. Add budesonide 2 mg nebulized every 6 hours to aclidinium/formoterol.

2. A 53-year-old female with COPD is brought into the ED with complaints of severe shortness of breath, fatigue, and chest pain on exertion. She reports the use of methamphetamine for weight loss in the last couple of years. Echocardiogram reveals normal left ventricular ejection fraction (LVEF), no evidence of left atrial (LA) enlargement or diastolic dysfunction. A right heart catheterization reveals mean pulmonary artery pressures of 60 mm Hg and a normal pulmonary capillary wedge pressure. She does not have a positive vasodilator challenge. Cardiac index is 1.8, and the patient is short of breath at rest and admitted to the intensive care unit (ICU). You have tadalafil, macitentan, and intravenous (IV) epoprostenol available to you. What is the best initial therapy?
   A. Start a trial of tadalafil.
   B. Start a trial of macitentan.
   C. Start tadalafil and macitentan.
   D. Consider expert consultation if available and start IV epoprostenol.

3.22 Thoracic Surgery Postoperative Management and Perioperative Complications

1. A 55-year-old man undergoes a right pneumonectomy for pulmonary mucormycosis. On postoperative day 2, she becomes hypoxemic and requires reintubation. Chest radiograph demonstrates extensive airspace opacities in the left lung, concerning for postpneumonectomy pulmonary edema and acute respiratory distress syndrome (ARDS). What is the risk of mortality associated with postpneumonectomy pulmonary edema?
   A. 1%
   B. 2%
   C. 20%
   D. >50%

2. A 65-year-old woman undergoes left upper lobectomy for non–small cell lung cancer. Her chest tube output remains high at 400 mL/24 hours despite diuresis. A chyle leak is suspected, and triglycerides are checked in the pleural fluid. What level of triglycerides is diagnostic of chyle?
   A. >20 mg/dL
   B. >50 mg/dL
   C. >110 mg/dL
   D. >200 mg/dL

3.23 Veno-Venous Extracorporeal Membrane Oxygenation

1. A 65-year-old man develops acute respiratory distress syndrome (ARDS) with refractory hypoxemia despite conventional management and is cannulated to venovenous extracorporeal membrane oxygen (VV ECMO). On day 4 of his ECMO run, his circuit is set to a flow of 5 LPM, Fdo_2 0.7, sweep 3 LPM. There have been no issues with flow, and the pressure difference across the membrane lung has not changed over the past 4 days. An arterial blood gas is drawn from the patient's left radial artery with the following results: pH 7.38, $Paco_2$ 42, Pao_2 58. The patient's flow rate is increased to 6 LPM and Fdo_2 is increased to 1.0, and the patient's Pao_2 increases to only 62 mm Hg. Pre- and post-membrane blood gases are obtained: $PpreO_2$ is 194, while $PpostO_2$ is 260. Which of the following is the most likely cause of this patient's hypoxemia?
   A. Chugging
   B. Membrane lung malfunction
   C. Pump malfunction
   D. Recirculation

2. A 32-year-old woman presents in status asthmaticus and is cannulated to VV ECMO for refractory hypercapnic respiratory failure. Prior to ECMO cannulation, an arterial blood gas is obtained with the following results: pH 6.88, $Paco_2$ 112, Pao_2 71. Her initial circuit is set to flow of 6 LPM, Fdo_2 1.0, sweep 8 LPM. Thirty minutes after cannulation, an arterial blood gas is obtained with the following results: pH 7.44,

$Paco_2$ 46, Pao_2 302. The patient's rapid reduction in $Paco_2$ puts her at risk for which of the following?
A. Limb ischemia
B. Intracerebral hemorrhage
C. Prolonged asthma exacerbation
D. ECMO pump failure

SECTION 4 GASTROINTESTINAL AND HEPATOBILIARY

4.1 Abdominal Compartment Syndrome

1. A 30-year-old male is admitted to the intensive care unit (ICU) with severe pancreatitis. On the third hospital day, the patient is noted to have a tense, distended abdomen with worsening hypotension despite increasing vasopressors, anuria, and rapidly worsening oxygenation with elevated peak pressures on the ventilator. Which of the following is the **MOST** important next step?
   A. Obtain computed tomography (CT) scan of the abdomen and pelvis
   B. Urgent surgical consultation for possible abdominal compartment syndrome
   C. Measurement of bladder pressure
   D. Continue current care as this is the expected evolution of severe pancreatitis

2. A 27-year-old male is shot in the abdomen and undergoes an exploratory laparotomy with massive transfusion. Postoperatively, he is admitted to the ICU for further resuscitation. Which of the following would not be consistent with a developing abdominal compartment syndrome?
   A. Increasing peak airway pressures
   B. Worsening hypotension and oliguria
   C. Improving compliance on the ventilator
   D. Elevated bladder pressure

4.2 Acute Pancreatitis

1. Which of the following are definitive indications for procedural intervention in acute pancreatitis?
   A. Acute interstitial pancreatitis
   B. Inability to tolerate oral intake
   C. Infected pancreatic or peripancreatic necrosis
   D. Severe acute pancreatitis requiring intensive care unit (ICU) admission

2. Fluid resuscitation in acute pancreatitis should be guided by which of the following?
   A. End-organ perfusion parameters
   B. Use of normal saline over lactated Ringer
   C. 250 to 500 mL/h of normal saline during the first 24 to 48 hours
   D. Continued aggressive fluid resuscitation after 48 hours

4.3 Hepatic Dysfunction and Hyperbilirubinemia

1. A patient is recovering from sepsis-induced hepatic dysfunction in the intensive care unit (ICU). Although the majority of his liver function tests have reverted to normal, he still has a significant direct hyperbilirubinemia. During rounds, a medical student points out that conjugated bilirubin has a half-life of about 4 hours; therefore, the patient's hyperbilirubinemia should have subsided by now. Your response is:
   A. Given the worrying persistence of hyperbilirubinemia, the patient should be worked up for recurrence of sepsis or other causes of liver dysfunction.
   B. The patient has elevated levels of delta bilirubin, and an extensive workup is unnecessary at this point.
   C. Bilirubin binds covalently to scleral elastin, and thus, patients appear jaundiced for longer than they actually have hepatic dysfunction.
   D. Patients with conjugated hyperbilirubinemia will invariably also have bilirubinuria.

2. Which of the following statements regarding hepatic blood flow is false?
   A. The liver has the highest oxygen extraction capacity of any organ in the body.
   B. If cardiac output and portal venous flow fall, the hepatic arterial flow increases.
   C. The portal venous flow provides 80% of the liver's oxygen supply.
   D. The oxygen consumption of the liver can remain unchanged, even with decreases in total hepatic blood flow up to 50%.

3. Which of the following statements regarding new-onset hepatic dysfunction in the ICU is true?
   A. The most common cause of new jaundice in the ICU is viral hepatitis.
   B. Hepatic dysfunction is very rarely seen in ICUs.
   C. Hepatic dysfunction does not have a significant impact on prognosis.
   D. In the ICU, liver dysfunction is relatively common.

4.4 Hepatic Encephalopathy

Clinical Case 4.4.1

A 67-year-old male with a history of alcoholic cirrhosis and esophageal varices presents to the emergency department (ED) with massive hematemesis and shock. He is intubated for airway protection and emergently transferred to the endoscopy suite for control of his variceal bleeding. Due to his hemodynamic instability, the anesthesiologist chooses a fentanyl- and midazolam-based anesthetic. He is appropriately resuscitated, and his variceal bleeding is controlled, but he does not regain consciousness at the end of the case. He is transferred to the intensive care unit (ICU) for further management. At this point, it is unclear whether the patient has any prior history suggestive of encephalopathy. An ammonia level in the ICU is reported as 70 μmol/L (normal range 10-60 μmol/L).

1. In Case 4.4.1, all of the following are true regarding the diagnosis and initial management of hepatic encephalopathy (HE), except:
   A. The combination gastrointestinal (GI) bleeding and benzodiazepines was likely responsible for precipitating the encephalopathy.
   B. The patient's serum ammonia level is diagnostic of HE.
   C. It is reasonable to start lactulose via nasogastric tube (NGT) as part of his initial management.
   D. A thorough evaluation should be undertaken to identify other precipitating causes of HE.
   E. A computed tomography (CT) scan of the patient's head is a reasonable part of the diagnostic workup.

2. Which of the following statements regarding the management of the patient in Case 4.4.1 in the ICU is correct?
   A. Flumazenil 1 mg intravenous (IV) should be part of the standard of care in this patient.
   B. His feeding regimen should not include >0.6 g protein/kg to reduce the risk of recurrence.
   C. Although frequently used, lactulose has never been definitively shown to be more effective than placebo.
   D. Propofol should not be used to sedate these patients since they are at an elevated risk of propofol infusion syndrome (PRIS).
   E. Transmigration of lipopolysaccharide (endotoxin) from intestinal gram-negative flora plays a key role in the pathogenesis of HE, and hemoperfusion over polymyxin B columns improves recovery from HE.

3. Lactulose is thought to exert its effects in HE through which of the following mechanisms?
   A. Acidifying the colonic contents and converting NH_3 to NH_4^+, which does not effectively enter the circulation
   B. Inhibition of NH_3 synthesis by colonic bacteria
   C. Reduction of fecal transit time, leading to decreased ammonia release
   D. Inhibition of ammonia synthesis by colonic bacteria
   E. All of the above

4.5 Hepatorenal Syndrome

1. A 59-year-old female with difficult-to-control type II diabetes, atrial fibrillation, and known cirrhosis secondary to alcohol use disorder decompensated by ascites is admitted to the hospital with 3 days of worsening diffuse abdominal pain. Her creatinine on admission is 3.1 mg/dL, up from a baseline of 1.5 mg/dL. She is treated empirically for spontaneous bacterial peritonitis, but despite appropriate antimicrobial therapy and gentle volume expansion, her creatinine continues to rise daily. She is euvolemic on examination and continues to make urine. Which of the following tests is **MOST** helpful in determining the cause of her AKI?
   A. Paracentesis for Gram stain, culture, and sensitivity
   B. Computed tomography (CT) scan of the abdomen and pelvis to rule out obstructive kidney disease
   C. Emergent kidney biopsy
   D. Urine sodium levels

2. A 65-year-old man presents to the emergency department with worsening dyspnea and lower extremity edema. He has a history of heart failure with reduced ejection fraction as well as cirrhosis secondary to chronic hepatitis B infection. His chest x-ray demonstrates pulmonary edema, and he is admitted to the medical service for diuresis. After 2 days of diuresis with high-dose intravenous furosemide, his dyspnea improves, but his estimated glomerular filtration rate (eGFR) begins to decline rapidly. The resident overnight suspects hepatorenal syndrome-acute kidney injury (HRS-AKI) and begins treatment with terlipressin and 25% albumin therapy after reviewing the treatment guidelines. Shortly after beginning treatment, the patient develops profound respiratory distress and is intubated emergently for hypoxemia. Which of the following would have prevented this complication of treatment?
   A. Using a thiazide diuretic instead of furosemide
   B. Using midodrine instead of terlipressin
   C. Obtaining an echocardiogram on admission
   D. Focused clinical examination to assess intravascular volume status

4.6 Bowel Ischemia and Perforation

1. A 55-year-old male presents to the emergency department with new-onset atrial fibrillation and acute abdominal pain. A computed tomography (CT) scan is performed that shows proximal occlusion of the superior mesenteric artery with diffuse hypo-enhancement of the small bowel. Which of the following is the least important next step in the care of this patient?
   A. General surgery consultation
   B. Vascular surgery consultation
   C. Initiation of heparin for anticoagulation
   D. Initiation of intravenous (IV) antibiotics
   E. Arterial line placement for hemodynamic monitoring

2. A 47-year-old patient is admitted to the intensive care unit (ICU) 1 week after a total knee replacement. She was recovering well after the operation until the day of admission when she developed acute abdominal pain in her mid-epigastrium. On further questioning, she reports taking daily narcotics since the operation, as well as ibuprofen 3 to 4 times a day. She is tachycardic, normotensive, and has diffuse abdominal tenderness. What is the best imaging study?
   A. Plain x-ray
   B. CT without contrast
   C. CT with oral contrast only
   D. CT with oral and IV contrast

4.7 Acute Mesenteric Ischemia

1. A 74-year-old female with peripheral arterial disease, carotid artery disease, and coronary artery disease with prior stents is admitted to the medical intensive care unit (ICU) with pyelonephritis. She is treated with antibiotics and eventually meets the criteria to leave the unit. She suddenly starts complaining of severe abdominal pain. On further questioning, she mentions that she has been suffering from some abdominal pain after eating for the past 2 months with a 15-lb weight loss. What is the **MOST** likely etiology of the patient's current symptoms?
   A. Mesenteric arterial embolism
   B. Mesenteric arterial thrombosis
   C. Mesenteric venous thrombosis
   D. Nonocclusive mesenteric ischemia

2. A 32-year-old female with a history of deep venous thrombosis (DVT), previously on anticoagulation, and recent initiation of oral contraceptive use presents with generalized abdominal pain that has progressively worsened over the past week. She notes that her pain is most pronounced after a meal. Her electrocardiogram (ECG) shows normal sinus rhythm. She has diffuse tenderness without rigidity or rebound. There is concern for mesenteric ischemia. What would be the **MOST** likely etiology of this patient's ischemia?
   A. Mesenteric arterial embolism
   B. Mesenteric arterial thrombosis
   C. Mesenteric venous thrombosis
   D. Nonocclusive mesenteric ischemia

3. A 70-year-old woman undergoes percutaneous coronary intervention (PCI) for ST-elevation myocardial infarction (STEMI) and develops severe abdominal pain. Computed tomographic angiography (CTA) shows diffuse severe narrowing of the superior mesenteric artery (SMA) and its branches without evidence of bowel infarction. Aggressive supportive care is initiated, and the patient is weaned off all pressors with little improvement. What is the next **BEST** step in treatment?
   A. Balloon angioplasty of the SMA and its branches
   B. Retrograde open mesenteric stenting
   C. Aorto-SMA bypass
   D. Direct intra-arterial infusion of papaverine

4.8 Gastrointestinal Bleeding

1. Which condition is characterized by tears in the mucosa and submucosa at the gastroesophageal junction, typically caused by severe retching or vomiting?
   A. Esophageal varices
   B. Mallory-Weiss tear
   C. Gastritis
   D. Dieulafoy lesion

2. Which imaging study can detect bleeding at a rate of 0.1 to 0.35 mL/min but has a low spatial resolution with an accuracy of 40% to 60%?
   A. Computed tomographic (CT) angiography
   B. Tagged red blood cell (RBC) scan
   C. Angiography
   D. Push enteroscopy

4.9 Malabsorption in the Critically Ill Patient

1. A 68-year-old male admitted to the surgical intensive care unit following damage control surgery for severe intra-abdominal sepsis develops significant diarrhea, abdominal distension, and feeding intolerance after initiation of enteral nutrition. He has a history of chronic pancreatitis. Stool analysis shows numerous fat globules on Sudan stain. Which of the following is the **MOST** likely underlying cause of malabsorption and the best initial diagnostic test to evaluate it in this critically ill patient?
   A. Small intestinal bacterial overgrowth (SIBO); hydrogen breath test
   B. Pancreatic exocrine insufficiency (PEI); fecal elastase-1
   C. Intestinal ischemia; serum lactate
   D. *Clostridium difficile* infection; stool polymerase chain reaction (PCR) for *C. difficile* toxin gene

2. A 45-year-old female in the surgical intensive care unit suffered massive bowel loss requiring extensive small intestine resection due to acute mesenteric ischemia. She has < 100 cm of residual small bowel and requires nutritional support. Attempts to advance continuous nasojejunal feeds with a standard polymeric formula have resulted in high-volume watery diarrhea and significant electrolyte losses. What is the **MOST** appropriate adjustment to the nutritional management strategy in this patient with suspected severe short-bowel syndrome malabsorption?
   A. Transition to bolus feeding of the current polymeric formula to stimulate adaptation.
   B. Stop enteral feeding completely and rely solely on total parenteral nutrition (TPN).
   C. Change to a low-fat, semi-elemental or elemental enteral formula delivered continuously.
   D. Increase the caloric density of the current polymeric formula to compensate for malabsorption.

4.10 Ileus And Acute Colonic Pseudoobstruction (Ogilvie Syndrome)

1. A 58-year-old male is on postoperative day 3 following an uncomplicated open colectomy. He complains of significant abdominal distension and nausea and has not passed flatus or stool. On physical examination, his abdomen is distended and tympanitic with absent bowel sounds. A plain abdominal radiograph shows diffusely dilated small and large bowel loops with multiple air-fluid levels. He is receiving intravenous (IV) opioids for pain control. Which of the following findings on subsequent imaging would best help distinguish prolonged postoperative ileus from a mechanical small bowel obstruction?
   A. Presence of gas in the rectum
   B. Identification of a distinct transition point where dilated bowel abruptly narrows
   C. Visualization of a normal caliber colon
   D. Detection of mild ascites

2. An 85-year-old hospitalized patient developed acute, significant abdominal distension 2 days after hip fracture repair. He has a history of multiple medical problems and is on several medications, including oxycodone for pain. Abdominal computed tomography (CT) scan confirms massive dilation of the colon (cecal diameter 14 cm) without evidence of mechanical obstruction, consistent with acute colonic pseudo-obstruction (Ogilvie syndrome). Initial conservative management (cessation of opioids, IV fluids, NPO) over 24 hours has not improved the dilation. The patient's heart rate is 75 bpm, blood pressure 130/70 mm Hg, and creatinine is within normal limits. What is the **MOST** appropriate next step in management?
   A. Urgent colonoscopic decompression.
   B. Administer IV neostigmine.
   C. Continue conservative management for another 24 hours.
   D. Initiate IV metoclopramide.
   E. Prepare for emergent surgical cecostomy.

4.11 *Clostridium difficile* and Toxic Megacolon

1. A 58-year-old male without significant past medical history was admitted to the hospital with severe *Clostridioides difficile* colitis (first episode). He has been receiving treatment with oral vancomycin 500 mg every 6 hours and intravenous (IV) metronidazole 500 mg every 8 hours for the past 2 days. You get notified that the patient is now reporting worsening abdominal pain. On assessment, his blood pressure is 80/50 and heart rate is 120 beats/min despite resuscitation with IV fluid boluses. His abdomen is distended and tender to palpation diffusely. Which of the following would be the most appropriate next step?
   A. Fecal microbiota transplantation
   B. Proceed to the operating room for a subtotal colectomy with end ileostomy
   C. Addition of bezlotoxumab to the treatment regimen
   D. Proceed with a computed tomography (CT) scan of the abdomen/pelvis

2. A 71-year-old male with Crohn disease on maintenance with adalimumab presents to the hospital with the initial episode of *C. difficile* colitis. He is hemodynamically normal. His abdomen is tender to palpation, but there are no peritoneal signs. His white blood cell (WBC) is 16,000/mm and creatinine is 1.6 mg/dL. Treatment is initiated with oral vancomycin 125 mg every 6 hours. What is another treatment option that can be considered for this patient?
   A. Probiotics
   B. Fecal microbiota transplantation
   C. Bezlotoxumab
   D. Subtotal colectomy with end ileostomy

4.12 Gastrointestinal and Intra-Abdominal Infections

1. A 65-year-old man presents to the emergency department (ED) with severe abdominal pain. He appears unwell but is awake and talking, and his vitals include heart rate (HR) 120, blood pressure (BP) 80/40, respiratory rate (RR) 24, and O_2 sat 97% on room air. He has large-bore intravenous (IV) access. On abdominal examination, he has peritonitis. Which of the following management steps should be initiated **FIRST**?
   A. Fluid resuscitation with 30 mL/kg crystalloid
   B. Computed tomography (CT) of the abdomen/pelvis with IV contrast
   C. Broad-spectrum antibiotic therapy with vancomycin, cefepime, and flagyl
   D. Direct to operating room (OR) for an emergent laparotomy

2. A 70-year-old woman presents to the ED with an acute onset, severe abdominal pain she developed while recovering from a knee replacement she underwent 2 weeks prior. She has been taking ibuprofen around the clock since the surgery. On arrival to the ED, she is overall well appearing but appears to be in pain. Her vitals include HR 105, BP 110/70, RR 18, and O_2 sat 98% on room air. IV access is obtained, and crystalloid resuscitation is initiated. Which of the following are **NOT** part of the initial management of her suspected disease process while in the ED?
   A. Blood cultures followed by broad-spectrum antibiotics, including antifungals
   B. Proton pump inhibitors
   C. Empiric treatment for *H. pylori*
   D. CT of the abdomen/pelvis with IV and oral contrast

4.13 Inflammatory Bowel Disease

1. A 25-year-old man was admitted with an ulcerative colitis flare, with 15 bloody bowel movements each day, three bloody bowel movements overnight, abdominal cramping, and tenesmus. Computed tomography (CT) scan demonstrates inflammation of the entire colon and rectum, with no perforation. Flexible sigmoidoscopy demonstrates friable, edematous mucosa extending from the rectum up through at least the descending colon. He was started on intravenous (IV) methylprednisolone 60 mg/d; however, he did not clinically improve over the following 4 days. What is the next best step?
   A. Start infliximab.
   B. Test for *Clostridioides difficile* and cytomegalovirus (CMV) infections.
   C. Consult colorectal surgery.
   D. All of the above are the best steps.

2. A 28-year-old woman with ulcerative colitis was admitted with worsening bloody bowel movements and abdominal pain despite escalation of outpatient medical therapy. She has been on high-dose oral steroids for the past 2 months and has been unable to tolerate weaning off steroids. In the hospital, she clinically worsened despite IV steroids and infliximab. She developed a colonic perforation and underwent emergent total abdominal colectomy with end ileostomy 2 days ago. Steroids were weaned off. She has continued to have abdominal pain and tenderness on examination and has continued to be hypotensive. What is on your differential diagnosis for her continued hypotension?
   A. Abdominal sepsis from rectal stump dehiscence
   B. Adrenal insufficiency
   C. Postoperative bleeding
   D. All of the above

4.14 Vascular Diseases of the Small Bowel

1. A 42-year-old man who is obese presents to the emergency department (ED) with progressively worsening abdominal pain over the past 10 days. He reports a family history of deep venous thrombosis (DVT). His labs are normal. What would be most useful to diagnose his condition?
   A. Abdominal x-ray
   B. Computed tomography (CT) scan with oral (PO) and intravenous (IV) contrast
   C. Diagnostic laparoscopy
   D. Duplex ultrasound (US)
   E. CT angiography with arterial and venous phases

2. A 27-year-old female is admitted to the intensive care unit after presenting with gastrointestinal (GI) bleeding and was found to have a duodenal arteriovenous malformation. She has undergone multiple endoscopic attempts to stop the bleeding with no success. What would be the next best step in management?
   A. Laparotomy and bowel resection
   B. Conservative management and resuscitation
   C. Angiographic intervention with embolization
   D. Transfer to another hospital

4.15 Obesity

1. According to the American Society for Parenteral and Enteral Nutrition (ASPEN) guidelines, which of the following is recommended for the nutritional management of patients who are critically ill obese?
   A. High-protein, low-calorie feeding to promote weight loss
   B. Standard enteral feeding formulas with no adjustments for protein content
   C. Hypocaloric, high-protein feeding to maintain lean body mass
   D. Aggressive calorie restriction to achieve rapid weight loss

2. In the context of critical care for patients who are obese, which of the following pathophysiologic changes primarily contribute to hypoxemia?
   A. Increased ventilation-perfusion ($\dot{V}/\dot{Q}$) mismatch due to atelectasis
   B. Decreased pulmonary artery pressure leading to reduced perfusion
   C. Enhanced alveolar-capillary membrane diffusion capacity
   D. Increased tidal volume and minute ventilation improving oxygenation

4.16 Gastrointestinal Diagnostic Modalities

1. For a patient who underwent liver transplant 4 days ago and is now suspected to have hepatic synthetic dysfunction as well as encephalopathy, what modality is best for assessing liver structure and portal vein patency?
   A. Liver biopsy
   B. Abdominal ultrasound with Doppler
   C. Computed tomography (CT) of the abdomen
   D. Esophagogastroscopy

2. An intubated patient in your intensive care unit (ICU) after polytrauma develops marked abdominal distension and has not had a bowel movement or passed gas in at least 5 days. What is the best initial test?
   A. Colonoscopy
   B. CT of the abdomen and pelvis
   C. Barium enema
   D. Sigmoidoscopy

4.17 Pharmacologic Therapies for Gastrointestinal Disorders

1. A 55-year-old female patient in the intensive care unit (ICU) is experiencing enteral feeding intolerance with high gastric residual volumes. She was started on metoclopramide 10 mg 2 times daily(bid) 48 hours ago with initial improvement, but her intolerance has now returned. What is the **MOST** effective next step to manage her dysmotility?
   A. Increase the dose of metoclopramide
   B. Place a post-pyloric feeding tube and discontinue all prokinetic agents
   C. Add erythromycin to the current metoclopramide regimen
   D. Discontinue metoclopramide and switch to erythromycin monotherapy

2. A patient is being treated for a severe upper gastrointestinal (GI) bleed. After initial resuscitation and endoscopic therapy, which pharmacologic strategy is recommended for the subsequent 72 hours to reduce the risk of rebleeding?
   A. High-dose intravenous proton pump inhibitor (PPI) therapy
   B. Scheduled intravenous H2-receptor antagonist (H2RA) administration
   C. A single dose of intravenous tranexamic acid (TXA)
   D. Continuous infusion of octreotide

4.18 Gastrointestinal and Abdominal Postoperative Management and Perioperative Complications

1. A 56-year-old male presents a week after an open inguinal hernia repair. He reports mild swelling at the incision site. There is a small area of fluctuance but no overlying erythema, induration, or drainage. His vitals and labs are within normal limits, and he is otherwise healthy. An ultrasound shows a 3-cm simple fluid collection. What is the **MOST** appropriate next step in management?
   A. Observation
   B. Ultrasound-guided aspiration
   C. Ultrasound-guided drain placement
   D. Incision and drainage

2. A 65-year-old female becomes febrile and tachycardic on postoperative day 5 after a partial colectomy for cancer. She has lower abdominal tenderness and has not had a bowel movement in 3 days. She has a leukocytosis to 20. This is **MOST** concerning for the development of what postoperative complication?
   A. Bowel obstruction
   B. Pulmonary embolism
   C. Anastomotic leak
   D. Intra-abdominal hematoma

SECTION 5 RENAL

5.1 Acute Kidney Injury

1. A patient with a history of scleroderma is admitted to the intensive care unit (ICU) with severe hypertension, rising creatinine (Cr), and anuria. Proteinuria and hematuria are noted. Which of the following medications should be started?
   A. Captopril
   B. Mannitol
   C. Intravenous immune globulin
   D. Hydrocortisone

2. What is the benefit of the AKIN criteria compared to the RIFLE criteria to define acute kidney injury (AKI)?
   A. AKIN criteria focus on urine output as opposed to serum Cr.
   B. AKIN criteria do not require a timeline for definition.
   C. AKIN criteria do not require a baseline Cr.
   D. AKIN criteria have better correlation with morbidity and mortality.

5.2 Infections of the Urinary Tract

1. A 50-year-old male has had an indwelling urinary catheter for 3 days while being admitted to the intensive care unit (ICU) with COVID-19 acute respiratory distress syndrome (ARDS). He begins having a fever of 38.5 °C and endorses suprapubic tenderness. Vital signs are otherwise unremarkable. After ruling out other sources of fever, a catheter-associated urinary tract infection (UTI) is suspected. Of the following, what is the **MOST** appropriate next step in diagnosis and management?
   A. Replace the urinary catheter
   B. Culture urine from the current catheter
   C. Initiate antibiotics
   D. Microanalysis only

2. A 36-year-old female presents with 7 days of painful, frequent, and hesitant urination. She also endorses fevers and flank pain that does not radiate to the groin. Costovertebral angle tenderness is present on examination. Her vitals include temperature (T) 38.3 °C, heart rate (HR) 105, blood pressure (BP) 126/64, and respiratory rate (RR) 20. Urine analysis findings include large leukocyte esterase, positive nitrites, leukocyte casts, and no crystals. Serum creatinine is within normal limits. Of the following, what is the **MOST** appropriate next step in evaluation?
   A. Computed tomography (CT) of the abdomen/pelvis without intravenous (IV) contrast
   B. CT of the abdomen/pelvis with IV contrast
   C. No imaging
   D. Ultrasound of the abdomen

5.3 Acid-Base Physiology and Disorders

1. A 42-year-old female with an unknown past medical history is admitted to the intensive care unit with altered mental status, agitation, and abdominal pain. She is intubated for airway protection, and the patient remains sedated and synchronous on controlled mechanical ventilation. Initial chemistries are notable for values including Na^+ 151 mEq/L, K^+ 3.9 mEq/L, Cl^- 117 mEq/L, and HCO_3^- 11 mEq/L. An arterial blood gas returns with pH 7.18, $Paco_2$ 30 mm Hg, and Pao_2 90 mm Hg on a delivered Fio_2 of 40%. Which of the following primary acid-base disorders is **MOST** likely present?
   A. Anion gap metabolic acidosis
   B. Metabolic alkalosis
   C. Non–anion gap metabolic acidosis
   D. Respiratory alkalosis

2. A 25-year-old male with no significant medical history presents to the emergency department with weakness and lethargy after 3 days of unremitting gastrointestinal distress. Laboratory studies are notable for Na^+ 136 mEq/L, K^+ 3.1 mEq/L, Cl^- 85 mEq/L, and HCO_3^- 36 mEq/L. An arterial blood gas returns with pH 7.52, $Paco_2$ 50 mm Hg, and Pao_2 98 mm Hg on room air. Which of the following would be **MOST** useful in pinpointing the etiology of the patient's primary acid-base disorder?
   A. Serum albumin
   B. Serum anion gap
   C. Urine anion gap
   D. Urine chloride

5.4 Renal Replacement Therapy

1. A 56-year-old woman is admitted to the intensive care unit (ICU) with acute liver failure. She has developed an oliguric acute kidney injury (AKI) with persistent hyperkalemia despite medical management. She is encephalopathic, with a serum ammonia level of 400 μg/dL. She is hemodynamically stable. What is the **MOST** appropriate modality of renal replacement therapy (RRT) for this patient?
   A. Intermittent hemodialysis (IHD)
   B. Continuous venovenous hemofiltration (CVVH)
   C. Slow continuous ultrafiltration (SCUF)
   D. Accelerated venovenous hemofiltration (AVVH)

2. You are about to initiate CVVH for a patient in the ICU. Which of the following is the **MOST** appropriate initial dose for therapy?
   A. 15 mL/kg/h
   B. 25 mL/kg/h
   C. 35 mL/kg/h
   D. 45 mL/kg/h

3. A patient is admitted to the ICU with septic shock. He is intubated for respiratory distress. He develops an oliguric AKI thought to be secondary to acute tubular necrosis (ATN). After 24 hours, his urine output remains minimal. Blood urea nitrogen (BUN) has increased to 80 mg/dL, but all other electrolytes remain within normal limits. His fluid balance is 3 L positive on admission. Oxygenation is stable on minimal ventilator settings. He remains on low-dose norepinephrine infusion. What is the **MOST** appropriate course of action for his AKI?
   A. Initiate continuous renal replacement therapy (CRRT) promptly
   B. Initiate IHD
   C. Aggressive fluid challenge
   D. Expectant management

5.5 Renal Imaging and Other Diagnostic Modalities

1. A 69-year-old man with new-onset renal failure is being evaluated in the intensive care unit (ICU), and after consultation with nephrology, the ICU team decides to acquire imaging of the kidneys and measure glomerular filtration rate (GFR). What form of imaging will provide the **MOST** functional information and quantitative data?
   A. Magnetic resonance imaging (MRI) urography
   B. Intravenous (IV) urography
   C. Renal scintigraphy
   D. None of the above

2. A 52-year-old woman with chronic kidney disease presents to the emergency department with severe abdominal pain and an acute rise in her baseline creatinine. The fellow on call would like to obtain imaging, but the patient reports a history of anaphylaxis with the administration of contrast dye. What type of contrast would be safest to administer in this patient?
   A. Microbubble contrast
   B. Iodinated contrast
   C. Gadolinium-based contrast
   D. None of the above

5.6 Pharmacologic Therapies for Renal Disorders

1. A 64-year-old man is recovering in the intensive care unit (ICU) after a type A aortic dissection repair. He is volume overloaded and is being actively diuresed with furosemide. He has baseline chronic obstructive pulmonary disease (COPD) and is a known CO_2 retainer. He has developed a profound metabolic alkalosis leading to further CO_2 retention, complicating his ventilator weaning. The addition of which agent would help correct the alkalosis while allowing continued diuresis?
   A. Albumin
   B. Acetazolamide
   C. Torsemide
   D. Mannitol

2. A 77-year-old woman with an ischemic cardiomyopathy has been admitted to the ICU in decompensated heart failure. She is responding well to loop diuretics but is becoming progressively hypernatremic. The addition of which agent would help correct the hypernatremia while allowing continued diuresis?
   A. Acetazolamide
   B. Torsemide
   C. Mannitol
   D. Chlorothiazide

5.7 Pharmacologic Implications of Altered Renal Clearance

1. A 67-year-old woman with acute renal failure is receiving intravenous vancomycin treatment. Her estimated glomerular

filtration rate (GFR) has declined from 80 mL/min/1.73 m^2 to 30 mL/min/1.73 m^2. Which of the following is true regarding vancomycin administration?
A. Dosing frequency may require reduction, but dosage strength is never changed.
B. Dosage strength may require reduction, but frequency is never changed.
C. Both dosing frequency and dosage strength may require reduction.
D. Dosing changes are not required since vancomycin is not renally cleared.

2. A 53-year-old female being treated for septic shock develops acute tubular necrosis of the kidneys. Changes in what mechanisms may alter the clearance of medications that primarily undergo elimination by the kidneys?
A. Glomerular filtration
B. Tubular secretion
C. Tubular reabsorption
D. All of the above

5.8 Genitourinary Emergencies

1. A 40-year-old man presents to the emergency department with fever, chills, and hypotension. He remains hypotensive after fluid resuscitation with 2 L crystalloid solution and is started on norepinephrine and vasopressin infusions. Broad-spectrum antibiotics are administered. Physical examination is notable for erythema and purple discoloration of the perineum with palpable crepitus. Vasopressor requirements continue to rise precipitously, and serum lactate is now 5.0 mmol/L. What is the best next step?
A. Continue medical management only
B. Urgent surgical exploration
C. Computed tomography (CT) of the abdomen/pelvis with intravenous (IV) contrast
D. Start continuous venovenous hemofiltration

2. A 48-year-old man is admitted to the hospital with acute decompensated heart failure. A Foley catheter is placed to measure hourly urine output. Several hours later, the patient reports severe penile pain. On examination, the foreskin appears retracted and edematous and is tender to palpation. The Foley catheter is draining clear urine. What is the **MOST** likely diagnosis?
A. Penile fracture
B. Traumatic urethral injury
C. Urinary tract infection
D. Paraphimosis

3. A 50-year-old woman is admitted to the intensive care unit after falling off a ladder. Her trauma burden is notable for right distal radius fracture, right-sided posterior rib fractures, and an American Association for the Surgery of Trauma (AAST) grade III traumatic renal injury on the right side. CT of the abdomen/pelvis demonstrated a 2-cm renal parenchymal laceration with adjacent perirenal hematoma. Admission hemoglobin was 6.9 g/dL. She does not take anticoagulant medications. One unit of packed red blood cells was transfused with an appropriate increase in hemoglobin. She remains hemodynamically stable. What is the best next step in management?
A. Close monitoring with nonoperative management
B. Urgent surgical exploration
C. Percutaneous nephrostomy tube placement
D. Administration of prothrombin complex concentrate

SECTION 6 HEMATOLOGY/ONCOLOGY

6.1 Anemia

1. A 40-year-old patient with newly diagnosed Burkitt lymphoma, whose initial treatment course is complicated by tumor lysis syndrome requiring rasburicase, is transferred to the intensive care unit (ICU) with severe anemia (hemoglobin [Hb] = 5.5), dyspnea, and cyanosis requiring escalation in supplemental oxygenation therapy. Arterial blood gas (ABG) is notable for the brown appearance of blood. What is the **MOST** likely cause?
A. Gastrointestinal bleeding
B. Microangiopathic hemolytic anemia
C. Iron deficiency
D. G6PD deficiency

2. Which of the following is NOT a common cause of isolated anemia in the ICU?
A. Renal insufficiency
B. Inflammation of acute illness
C. Hemoglobinopathy
D. Phlebotomy

6.2 Thrombocytopenia

1. An 86-year-old man with well-controlled HIV and a history of immune-mediated thrombotic thrombocytopenic purpura (TTP) for which he received plasma exchange, prednisone, and rituximab 1 year ago, is admitted to the intensive care unit (ICU) with respiratory failure from aspiration pneumonia and a left-sided pulmonary embolus. He is started on amoxicillin-sulbactam and unfractionated heparin. After 5 days, his respiratory status improves and he is transferred to the floor. On hospital day 7, blood work shows worsening thrombocytopenia with a platelet count that dropped from 200,000 on admission to 60,000 that day. Examination reveals new swelling in the left leg.

Which of the following studies is **MOST** likely to lead to diagnosis of his thrombocytopenia?
A. Drug-dependent platelet antibodies
B. Peripheral blood smear
C. Heparin-platelet factor 4 (PF4) antibody testing with reflex to serotonin release assay
D. HIV viral load
E. ADAMTS13 activity

2. A 35-year-old woman presents to the emergency department with gum bleeding and bruising. She has a history of depression and has been taking sertraline for 3 years. She drinks one alcoholic beverage weekly. Physical examination reveals a well-appearing young woman with a few petechiae in the mouth and scattered bruises over the arms and legs. There is no lymphadenopathy or organomegaly. A complete blood

count (CBC) shows a normal white blood cell (WBC) and hemoglobin and a platelet count of 6,000. There are no priors for comparison. A peripheral blood smear confirms true thrombocytopenia.

Which of the following approaches is **MOST** likely to treat her underlying disease?
A. Glucocorticoids
B. Therapeutic plasma exchange
C. Platelet transfusion
D. Stop sertraline
E. Alcohol cessation

6.3 Thrombocytosis

1. A 48-year-old man with a history of Crohn disease presents to the hospital with norovirus gastroenteritis. On admission, his complete blood count (CBC) shows a normal white blood cell (WBC), a hemoglobin of 10 g/dL with a low mean corpuscular value (MCV) of 75 fL and an elevated red cell distribution width (RDW) at 15%, and a platelet count of 550,000. A prior CBC from 1 year ago was normal. Physical examination shows a slightly tired man who has mild conjunctival pallor and mild generalized abdominal discomfort on palpation.

   What is the **MOST** appropriate next step for addressing his thrombocytosis?
   A. Initiate therapeutic anticoagulation with unfractionated heparin.
   B. Start aspirin 81 mg daily.
   C. Send iron studies and replete if deficient.
   D. Send JAK2 testing.

2. A 60-year-old woman presents to the hospital with abdominal pain. Computed tomography (CT) scan reveals an acute portal vein thrombus. CBC shows a WBC of 10 with neutrophil predominance, hemoglobin of 12 g/dL (MCV 92 fL), and a platelet count of 700,000. No previous CBCs are recorded in the system. Therapeutic anticoagulation is started.

   What is the next best diagnostic test?
   A. Iron studies
   B. JAK2 mutation testing
   C. von Willebrand panel
   D. Erythrocyte sedimentation rate (ESR), C-reactive protein (CRP)

6.4 Neutropenia

1. A 55-year-old with newly diagnosed acute myeloid leukemia (AML) is transferred to the intensive care unit with septic shock. The patient is on day 23 of induction chemotherapy and has been neutropenic for 11 days and persistently febrile for 72 hours. On examination, he has right lower quadrant abdominal tenderness. His current antimicrobial regimen is intravenous cefepime monotherapy. Which of the following etiologies is LEAST likely to represent the etiology of febrile neutropenia?
   A. Enteric Gram-negative rods
   B. Influenza A
   C. Anaerobic bacteria
   D. Fungal pathogens

2. The patient in Q1 is placed on vancomycin, meropenem, and micafungin, and his shock slowly improves. One week later, he appears well, has started to have hematologic recovery (platelet count now 75k and transfusion independent), and is ready for transfer to the leukemia unit. Peripheral blood flow cytometry reveals decreased blast fraction. However, he remains neutropenic. Which of the following represents the most likely etiology?
   A. Carbapenem-resistant infection
   B. Drug toxicity
   C. Relapsed leukemia
   D. Vitamin B12 deficiency

6.5 Hemoglobinopathies

1. A 28-year-old male with known hemoglobin (Hb) SS sickle cell disease presents to the emergency department reporting severe pain in his low back and lower leg joints. He took oral oxycodone 10 mg every 4 hours over the past 24 hours without much pain relief. Vitals show temperature of 98.5 °F, blood pressure of 112/72 mm Hg, heart rate of 88 beats per minute, and SpO_2 of 98% on room air. Labs are obtained. Which is the best indicator that this is a vaso-occlusive pain episode?
   A. Hb level
   B. Reticulocyte count
   C. Patient's report
   D. Lactate dehydrogenase (LDH)

2. A 25-year-old female with Hb SC disease admitted for a vaso-occlusive pain episode 3 days ago develops a new oxygen requirement of 4 L nasal cannula with SpO_2 of 94%. Heart rate is 110 beats per minute, blood pressure 136/80 mm Hg, and temperature of 100.5 °F. Chest x-ray reveals a new infiltrate in the left lower lobe that was not present on the admission chest x-ray. Labs obtained since development of oxygen requirement shows a Hb of 8.2 g/dL (9.8 g/dL on admission), reticulocyte of 16% (8% on admission), total bilirubin 5 mg/dL (2 mg/dL on admission), direct bilirubin 1.2 mg/dL (0.5 mg/dL on admission), and LDH 510 U/L (325 U/L on admission). She continues to have an increasing oxygen requirement, now up to 15 L nonrebreather. What is the most appropriate management?
   A. Simple transfusion
   B. Exchange transfusion
   C. No transfusion
   D. Intravenous fluids

6.6 Hematopoietic Cell Transplantation

1. A 55-year-old with central nervous system (CNS) lymphoma is on day 12 after a thiotepa-, busulfan-, and cyclophosphamide-based autologous hematopoietic cell transplant (HCT). His white blood cell count recently normalized. He is admitted to the intensive care unit (ICU) with hypoxemic respiratory failure. On examination, he has a faint rash and bilateral leg swelling. His chest imaging shows bilateral interstitial opacification without effusions. His pre-HCT ejection fraction was normal. Which of the following is the MOST likely diagnosis?
   A. Pulmonary embolism
   B. Chemotherapy-associated cardiomyopathy
   C. Engraftment syndrome
   D. Aspiration pneumonitis

2. A 44-year-old who is 45 days out from recent haploidentical allogeneic transplant for high-risk acute myeloid lymphoma (AML) is admitted to the hospital with severe diarrhea and found to have grade 4 gastrointestinal (GI) graft-versus-host disease (GVHD). He is treated with high-dose steroids and improves; however, on hospital day 13, he develops shock requiring transfer to the ICU. Which of the following is the most appropriate next steps in management?
   A. Increase corticosteroid dose
   B. Start empiric broad spectrum antibiotics
   C. Obtain chest CT scan
   D. Obtain a trans-thoracic echocardiogram

6.7 Tumor Lysis Syndrome

1. A 46-year-old male presents with fatigue, epistaxis, and exertional dyspnea. He is found to have severe anemia, thrombocytopenia, and a white cell count of 51.2 K/μL with 85% circulating myeloblasts. He is diagnosed with acute myeloid leukemia and commenced on treatment with daunorubicin and cytarabine. He is given allopurinol 300 mg daily, rasburicase 3 mg once, and normal saline infusion at 125 mL/h. On day 2 of chemotherapy, he develops altered mental status and oliguria and is found to have the following laboratory results:

	Day 1	Day 2	Units	Normal Range
Sodium	139	138	mmol/L	(135-145)
Potassium	4.8	5.4	mmol/L	(3.4-5.0)
Creatinine	0.77	1.43	mg/dL	(0.50-1.00)
Calcium	8.2	7.1	mg/dL	(8.5-10.5)
Phosphorus	4.8	10.2	mg/dL	(2.6-4.5)
Uric acid	9.8	2.0	mg/dL	(2.3-6.6)
Lactate dehydrogenase (LDH)	838	2,135	U/L	(110-210)

   What is the **MOST** important next step in the management of this patient?
   A. Add furosemide to augment diuresis and potassium excretion.
   B. Increase the dose of allopurinol to 600 mg daily.
   C. Repeat dose of rasburicase 3 mg.
   D. Initiate dialysis.
   E. Calcium gluconate infusion.

2. A 36-year-old female presents with abdominal pain, unexpected weight loss, and night sweats. Computed tomography (CT) imaging of the chest, abdomen, and pelvis reveals widespread lymphadenopathy and a 10-cm ileal mass. Cervical lymph node biopsy demonstrates a diagnosis of Burkitt lymphoma, and the patient will be treated with immunochemotherapy. Baseline labs reveal LDH 5,000 U/L, uric acid level of 10.3 mg/dL, and acute kidney injury with creatinine 1.2 mg/dL.

   Which intervention will most reduce the risk of worsening urate nephropathy in this patient after initiating chemotherapy?
   A. Urinary alkalinization
   B. Normal saline infusion
   C. Allopurinol
   D. Rasburicase
   E. 7-Day course of prednisone prior to starting intensive chemotherapy

6.8 Solid Tumors

1. A Do Not Resuscitate/Do Not Intubate (DNR/DNI) 45-year-old woman with triple-negative breast cancer metastatic to the brain, liver, and bone presents with fatigue and dry cough and is admitted to the intensive care unit (ICU) with hypoxemic respiratory failure requiring high-flow nasal cannula 60% FIO_2 at 60 L/min. She received palliative outpatient chemotherapy with pembrolizumab and paclitaxel 7 days prior to admission. Home medications include dexamethasone 4 mg 2 times daily (bid) as part of a prolonged taper after being diagnosed with brain metastases 6 weeks ago. Computed tomographic (CT) pulmonary angiogram shows bilateral ground-glass opacities with patchy superimposed consolidations without evidence of pulmonary emboli. White blood cell (WBC) count is 3,800/μL, with 80% neutrophils and 10% lymphocytes. She was started on vancomycin, cefepime, and azithromycin in the emergency department (ED). Broadening antimicrobial coverage with the addition of which of the following medications is **LEAST** appropriate?
   A. Trimethoprim-sulfamethoxazole (TMP-SMX)
   B. Letermovir
   C. Ganciclovir
   D. Voriconazole

2. A 55-year-old man presents to the ED with hematemesis, is intubated for airway protection, started on high-dose proton pump inhibitor therapy, and admitted to the ICU. He has a history of metastatic pancreatic cancer on palliative chemotherapy and was discharged from the hospital 4 weeks ago after an episode of acute pancreatitis related to gemcitabine, managed conservatively. CT scan shows splenomegaly and splenic vein thrombosis with gastric varices. Octreotide is administered by infusion. Esophagogastroduodenoscopy shows large gastric varices with adherent clot without active bleeding, not amenable to endoscopic intervention. What is the **MOST** appropriate next step?
   A. Systemic anticoagulation
   B. Gastrectomy
   C. Splenic artery embolization
   D. Transjugular intrahepatic portosystemic shunt (TIPS)

6.9 Critical Care Management of Severe Immune-Related Adverse Events

1. What is the incidence of intestinal perforation in immune-related colitis?
   A. ~ 1%
   B. 5%
   C. 50%
   D. 90%

2. Which grade of intensive care unit (ICI) pneumonitis involves life-threatening respiratory compromise and usually requires ICU admission?
   A. Grade 1
   B. Grade 2
   C. Grades 3 and 4
   D. Grade 5

6.10 Coagulopathy

1. A 79-year-old with a history of atrial fibrillation on apixaban presents to the emergency department with acute left-sided weakness, NIHSS 15. Computed tomography (CT) head

shows subarachnoid hemorrhage (SAH). Which of the following is an appropriate next treatment?
A. Observe in the intensive care unit (ICU) and repeat CT of the head in 4 hours.
B. Administer andexanet alpha.
C. Administer tissue plasminogen activator (tPA).
D. Administer prothrombin complex concentrate (PCC) 50 U/kg.
E. Emergent craniotomy.

2. A 33-year-old man with no medical history is involved in a motor vehicle collision. In the emergency department, he is found to have a positive FAST examination and is taken to the operating room for an exploratory laparotomy. In the ICU post-op, he is found to have increased bloody drain output. What is likely contributing to his coagulopathy?
A. Hypothermia
B. Consumption and/or dilution of coagulation factors
C. Acidemia
D. All of the above
E. None of the above

6.11 Hematology Diagnostic Modalities

1. A 62-year-old man in the intensive care unit (ICU) develops a sudden drop in hemoglobin from 10 to 7 g/dL over 24 hours, with jaundice and dark urine. His labs show lactate dehydrogenase (LDH) = 900 U/L (↑), haptoglobin = 10 mg/dL (↓), and a peripheral smear with schistocytes. Which test will **MOST** directly distinguish immune-mediated hemolysis from a nonimmune microangiopathic process?
A. Reticulocyte count
B. LDH level
C. Direct antiglobulin (Coombs) test
D. D-dimer

2. A 40-year-old patient with trauma with massive hemorrhage is being resuscitated. A point-of-care thromboelastography (TEG) shows: R = 12 minutes (normal 5-10), K = 1.0 minutes (normal 1-3), α-angle = 65 degree angle (normal 53-72), MA = 55 mm (normal 50-70), and LY30 = 2% (normal 0-8). Which blood product should you administer first?
A. Platelets
B. Cryoprecipitate
C. Fresh frozen plasma (FFP)
D. Tranexamic acid

6.12 Disseminated Intravascular Coagulopathy

1. Which of the following patients with suspected disseminated intravascular coagulopathy (DIC) should receive a platelet transfusion?
A. A 57-year-old man with an intracranial bleed and a platelet count of 105,000/μL
B. An 81-year-old woman with urosepsis and a platelet count of 7,000/μL
C. A 63-year-old man with decompensated liver failure and a platelet count of 21,000/μL
D. A 41-year-old woman who is oozing from intravenous (IV) sites with a platelet count of 34,000/μL

6.13 Hypercoagulable States

1. A 67-year-old male with cirrhosis is involved in a severe motor vehicle accident. His primary injury is a traumatic chest wall deformity. He has required venovenous extracorporeal membrane oxygenation (VV-ECMO) for the last 15 days due to acute respiratory distress syndrome (ARDS). He has been on a heparin drip for the last 8 days for a right lower extremity deep vein thrombosis that was found on day 7 of his hospitalization. His activated partial thromboplastin time (aPTT) and anti-factor Xa assay levels have been within therapeutic range. His platelet count has dropped from 125,000 to 55,000/μL since admission. Which of the following is the **MOST** likely cause of his thrombocytopenia?
A. Polytrauma
B. VV-ECMO
C. Heparin-induced thrombocytopenia (HIT)
D. Antibiotics
E. Cirrhosis

2. Which of the following patients should undergo thrombophilia screening?
A. A 65-year-old male with a newly diagnosed venous thromboembolism (VTE) 2 days following a left hemicolectomy
B. A 62-year-old female with idiopathic VTE
C. A 49-year-old male with active intravenous drug use (IVDU) diagnosed with popliteal deep venous thrombosis (DVT)
D. A 22-year-old male with osteosarcoma found to have a femoral DVT
E. None of the above

6.14 Coagulation Management Strategies

1. A 19-year-old male arrives at the trauma bay with pronounced bleeding from a gunshot wound to the proximal left lower extremity. He is hypotensive with a blood pressure of 80/40. A massive transfusion protocol is activated. Which of the following is the earliest laboratory abnormality that you would expect to find in this patient?
A. Hypocitricemia
B. Decreased R-time on thromboelastometry (TEG)
C. Hypofibrinogenemia
D. Hypokalemia
E. Hypernatremia

2. A 64-year-old female on warfarin for paroxysmal atrial fibrillation is admitted to the intensive care unit (ICU). She is obtunded in the setting of a large subdural hematoma. A computed tomography (CT) scan of the head demonstrates a pronounced midline shift. Which of the following is the correct management of the patient's warfarin anticoagulation?
A. Hold warfarin.
B. Administer a 4-factor prothrombin complex concentrate (PCC).
C. Administer intravenous (IV) vitamin K.
D. Recheck prothrombin time/international normalized ratio (PT/INR) every 4 to 6 hours to ensure that INR becomes normal (<1.4 in most laboratories).
E. All of the above are correct.

6.15 Complications of Immunosuppressive Drugs

1. A 45-year-old man with past medical history (PMH) of nonalcoholic steatohepatitis (NASH) cirrhosis, hypertension, and hyperlipidemia underwent liver transplantation 4 weeks ago and is maintained on triple immunosuppressive therapy with tacrolimus, mycophenolate mofetil, and prednisone.

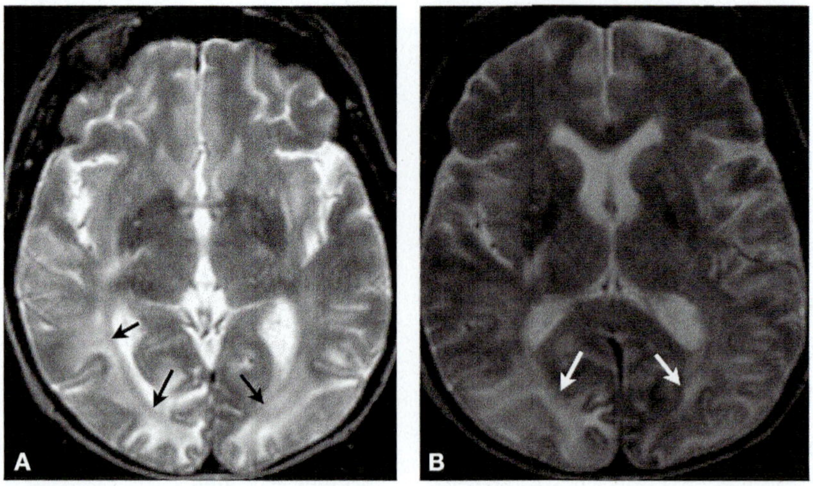

QFIGURE 6.15.1 (From Klein J, Vinson EN, Brant WE, Helms CA. *Brant and Helms' Fundamentals of Diagnostic Radiology*. 4th ed. Wolters Kluwer; 2019. Figure 7.16.)

The patient developed progressively worsening altered mental status, and now he is admitted to the intensive care unit (ICU) with new-onset generalized tonic-clonic seizures. On examination, the patient has bilateral visual field deficits. Vitals: blood pressure (BP) 182/106 mm Hg, heart rate (HR) 92, and Spo_2 94% on room air, T 36.8 °C. Laboratory studies show normal electrolytes and renal function. Trough levels of tacrolimus are within goal range. Stat computed tomographic (CT) of the head was negative, and the ICU team ordered a brain magnetic resonance imaging (MRI) (QFigure 6.15.1).

Which of the following is the **MOST** likely diagnosis and appropriate next step?
A. Hypertensive crisis with intracerebral hemorrhage; initiate nicardipine and continue tacrolimus.
B. Posterior reversible encephalopathy syndrome (PRES); reduce or discontinue tacrolimus.
C. Calcineurin inhibitor–induced thrombotic microangiopathy; initiate plasma exchange.
D. Ischemic stroke; administer aspirin and initiate permissive hypertension.

2. A 49-year-old man underwent orthotopic liver transplantation for hepatitis C–related cirrhosis. He is maintained on tacrolimus, mycophenolate mofetil, and prednisone. He received standard perioperative antimicrobial prophylaxis and remains on trimethoprim-sulfamethoxazole for *Pneumocystis jirovecii* prevention. At his 3-month posttransplant visit, he reports a 1-week history of fever, malaise, and nonproductive cough. Examination reveals oral thrush and scattered rhonchi on lung auscultation. Chest radiograph shows patchy right upper lobe consolidation. Laboratory studies are notable for leukopenia. Which of the following pathogens is **MOST** likely responsible for his presentation?
A. *Pseudomonas aeruginosa*
B. Cytomegalovirus
C. *Streptococcus pneumoniae*
D. JC polyomavirus

6.16 Complications of Chemotherapy

1. A 62-year-old man with metastatic gastric cancer is receiving high-dose methotrexate therapy. Two days after initiation, he develops confusion, slurred speech, and right-sided weakness. Magnetic resonance imaging (MRI) shows bilateral symmetric restricted diffusion in cerebral white matter beyond vascular territories. Which of the following best describes the mechanism and appropriate management of this complication?
A. Acute subcortical hemorrhage from methotrexate-induced platelet dysfunction; treat with platelet transfusion.
B. Acute/subacute leukoencephalopathy from methotrexate-induced disruption of metabolism; treat with high-dose folinic acid.
C. Aseptic meningitis from intrathecal methotrexate; treat with corticosteroids.
D. Posterior reversible encephalopathy syndrome from methotrexate-induced hypertension; treat with blood pressure control.
E. Ischemic stroke from methotrexate-induced carotid artery thrombosis; treat with anticoagulation.

2. A 55-year-old woman with breast cancer develops acute dyspnea, chest discomfort, and hypotension while receiving continuous 5-fluorouracil (5-FU) infusion. Electrocardiogram (ECG) shows diffuse ST-segment depression. Which of the following statements regarding this complication is most accurate?
A. It is mediated by immune complex deposition in the coronary arteries; management is aspirin and corticosteroids.
B. It represents type I (irreversible) cardiotoxicity; dexrazoxane is indicated.
C. It represents type II (reversible) cardiotoxicity due to coronary microvascular vasoconstriction; infusion should be stopped immediately.
D. It is caused by dose-dependent oxidative stress and mitochondrial injury; beta-blockers are preventive.
E. It typically resolves with diuretic therapy and high-flow oxygen without altering chemotherapy administration.

SECTION 7 ENDOCRINE

7.1 General Neuroendocrine Axis

1. A patient is admitted to the intensive care unit (ICU) with a traumatic brain injury after a high-speed motor vehicle collision. He is hemodynamically stable but develops polyuria. What is the **MOST** likely injury?
   A. Damage to the neurohypophysis with reduced antidiuretic hormone (ADH) release
   B. Injury to the adenohypophysis with reduced adrenocorticotropic hormone (ACTH) release
   C. Injury to the adenohypophysis with reduced vasopressin release
   D. Damage to the hypothalamus with reduced corticotropin stimulation release

2. A 45-year-old female is admitted to the ICU with a sudden-onset severe headache, visual disturbances, and altered mental status. Imaging reveals a sellar mass with suprasellar extension compressing the optic chiasm. What is the **MOST** likely associated symptom?
   A. Hypertension
   B. Irregular or no menstrual periods
   C. Tachycardia
   D. Acromegaly

7.2 Diabetes Mellitus

1. A 60-year-old female with a history of hypertension, heart failure, and type 2 diabetes mellitus on empagliflozin, losartan, and carvedilol presents to the operating room (OR) for a laparoscopic cholecystectomy for acute cholecystitis. She is tachycardic and hypotensive during the case and shows improvement with vasopressor and multiple fluid boluses. Urine output has been marginal. Her emergence from anesthesia is delayed, and she exhibits an erratic breathing pattern. She is transported to the intensive care unit (ICU) intubated, where labs are significant for pH 7.0, Pco_2 32, LA 1.8, Na 142, K 3.4, Cl 110, HCO_3 16, serum glucose 196 mg/dL, creatinine is 1.8 mg/dL, and urinalysis demonstrates large urine ketones.

   Which of the following interventions prior to surgery is **MOST** likely to have prevented this complication?
   A. Delay the case 24 hours to avoid medication complications.
   B. Initiate continuous vasopressor infusion prior to induction of anesthesia.
   C. Delay surgery for 24 hours while treating cholecystitis with antibiotics.
   D. Initiate insulin and dextrose infusions and monitor blood gas.

2. A patient in the neurologic ICU for the management of severe traumatic brain injury. In addition to standard therapies and precautions for elevated intracranial pressure, which of the following strategies is **MOST** appropriate for the management of blood glucose to prevent further neurologic injury?
   A. Permissive hyperglycemia due to the expected response to steroid therapy
   B. Initiate insulin drip at blood glucose 140 mg/dL and titrate to 80 to 110 mg/dL.
   C. Initiate insulin drip at blood glucose 180 mg/dL and titrate to 140 to 180 mg/dL.

7.3 Adrenal Gland

1. Potential causes of primary hypoaldosteronism are all of the following, except:
   A. Propofol
   B. Infection
   C. Adrenal hemorrhage
   D. Etomidate
   E. Ketoconazole

2. What are the electrolyte perturbations and presenting symptoms characteristic of primary adrenal insufficiency (mineralocorticoid deficiency)?
   A. Hyponatremia, hyperpigmentation, hyperkalemia
   B. Hyponatremia, hypopigmentation, hyperkalemia
   C. Hyponatremia, hypopigmentation, hypokalemia
   D. Hypernatremia, hyperpigmentation, hypokalemia

7.4 Pituitary Hormone Disorders

1. An 80-year-old man is admitted to the hospital after being found down at home. He was last seen normal yesterday and is functional at baseline. He is a longtime smoker with chronic obstructive pulmonary disease (COPD) and was recently diagnosed with lung cancer. On physical examination, he is lethargic and confused. Laboratory evaluations are notable for serum sodium 120 mEq/L, urine osmolarity 275 mOsm/kg, urine sodium 45 mEq/L, and serum osmolarity 265 mOsm. Which of the following is the **MOST** appropriate next step in management?
   A. Start fluid restriction of 1,000 mL/d.
   B. Desmopressin
   C. 0.9% isotonic saline infusion
   D. 3% hypertonic saline infusion

2. A 48-year-old woman with a history of headaches is admitted for elective pituitary adenoma resection. Following an otherwise uncomplicated procedure, she is admitted to the intensive care unit (ICU) for observation. ~12 hours postoperatively, urine output has increased to 1,000 mL over the last 3 hours while the serum sodium increased from 140 to 146 mEq/L. What are the next steps in management to prevent worsening hypernatremia?
   A. Start maintenance intravenous (IV) fluids with 0.9% normal saline.
   B. Start maintenance fluids with dextrose 5% in water until the sodium level returns to baseline.
   C. Ask to measure the urine osmolarity, and if <300 mOsm/kg, administer a dose of desmopressin and allow the patient to drink to thirst.
   D. Start fluid restriction of 1.5 L/d and recheck sodium in another 12 hours.
   E. Ask the surgical team if 3% hypertonic saline was given intraoperatively.

7.5 Thyroid Disorders

1. A 65-year-old male developed an acute onset of lower extremity weakness a few hours after having dinner. Prior to the event, he had been experiencing palpitations for weeks but denied any other symptoms. He was brought to the emergency department (ED), where a head computed tomography (CT) was obtained and was negative for intracranial

abnormalities. His symptoms resolved completely within 72 hours without any deficits. What was the etiology of his clinical presentation?
A. Transient ischemic attack
B. Thyrotoxic periodic paralysis
C. Guillain-Barré syndrome
D. Disk herniation

2. Which of the following is the **MOST** common precipitating factor for myxedema coma?
A. Overexposure to heat
B. Infection
C. Excessive exercise
D. Overconsumption of iodine-rich foods

7.6 Pharmacologic Therapies for Endocrine Disorders

1. Which of the following medications has the highest risk of euglycemic diabetic ketoacidosis (DKA) if not held within the perioperative period?
A. Metformin
B. Empagliflozin
C. Insulin glargine
D. Glimepiride

2. Which beta-blocker would be most appropriate for use in thyroid storm?
A. Propranolol
B. Metoprolol
C. Carvedilol
D. Labetalol

SECTION 8 NEUROLOGY

8.1 Coma, Encephalopathy, Delirium, and Other Altered States of Consciousness

1. A 48-year-old man is admitted to the intensive care unit for severe traumatic brain injury after he was struck by a motor vehicle while crossing the street. Intracranial trauma burden was notable for scattered, sulcal subarachnoid hemorrhage, bifrontal contusions, and grade 2 diffuse axonal injury. He is status post placement of tracheostomy and gastrostomy tube, and his hospital course was complicated by acute kidney injury and ventilator-associated pneumonia. On hospital day 35, as he is approaching readiness for discharge, his neurologic examination is notable for spontaneous eye opening but no tracking or regarding of the examiner. Pupillary, corneal, cough, and gag reflexes are intact. His arms and legs withdraw when stimulated. He does not follow commands. Which of the following is the best descriptor of the patient's disorder of consciousness?
A. Coma
B. Unresponsive wakefulness state
C. Minimally conscious state
D. No disorder of consciousness

2. A 77-year-old man with a past medical history of Parkinson disease and atrial fibrillation on apixaban is admitted to the intensive care unit after a fall from a ladder resulting in a 5mm right cerebral convexity subdural hemorrhage. Examination on admission is notable for a heart rate of 44, blood pressure 91/58, disorientation to year, and pronator drift in the left arm. He receives four-factor prothrombin complex concentrate and is evaluated by the neurosurgical team, who recommend nonsurgical management. The following evening, he is oriented to himself only, inattentive, and agitated. Repeat computed tomography (CT) scan of the head is stable. The following morning, his agitation has improved, but he is less alert. Which of the following medications should be considered if the patient develops recurrent agitation?
A. Haloperidol
B. Quetiapine
C. Valproic acid
D. Dexmedetomidine

8.2 Status Epilepticus

1. A 59-year-old male with little known past medical history presents to the emergency department via emergency medical services (EMS) after being found down on the street with witnessed generalized convulsive activity for 6 minutes. He received 4 mg intravenous (IV) lorazepam prior to arrival and is no longer convulsing. On examination, he remains altered and confused and unable to appropriately follow commands, Glasgow Coma Scale (GCS) 10. His vital signs include a heart rate of 98 bpm, blood pressure of 110/70, and oxygen saturation of 98% on 2 L nasal cannula. What is the next best step in this patient's management?
A. Continue supportive care and monitor for clinical improvement.
B. Load with 60 mg/kg levetiracetam (maximum dose of 4 g, pending normal renal function), obtain computed tomography (CT) of the head, and admit for observation.
C. Load with 60 mg/kg levetiracetam (maximum dose of 4 g, pending normal renal function), obtain urgent CT of the head and electroencephalography (EEG).
D. Prepare for intubation and start IV sedation with propofol.

2. In accordance with the most recent definition of status epilepticus per the International League Against Epilepsy (ILAE), what defines t_2 in convulsive status epilepticus?
A. t_2 denotes the time point at which there is failure of intrinsic mechanisms responsible for the termination of seizures and occurs at 5 minutes for convulsive status epilepticus.
B. t_2 denotes the critical time point beyond which there is long-term neurologic injury or neuronal cell death and occurs at 5 minutes for convulsive status epilepticus.
C. t_2 denotes the time point at which there is failure of intrinsic mechanisms responsible for termination of seizures and occurs at 10 minutes for convulsive status epilepticus.
D. t_2 denotes the critical time point beyond which there is long-term neurologic injury or neuronal cell death and occurs at 30 minutes for convulsive status epilepticus.

8.3 Depressive Disorders

1. A 35-year-old woman with a history of diabetes mellitus and major depressive disorder is admitted to the intensive care unit (ICU) in diabetic ketoacidosis. She is started on an insulin drip and is medically stabilized. However, she is noted to be tearful at times and is somewhat withdrawn. Upon interview, she complains of depressed mood, anhedonia,

poor energy, low interest, hypersomnia, increased appetite, and poor concentration. She denies suicidal thoughts. She informs you that she has tried fluoxetine and sertraline (two selective serotonin reuptake inhibitors [SSRIs]) in the past (at adequate doses and for adequate duration) with little effect. She has significant peripheral neuropathy as a result of her diabetes mellitus. What medication would be the **MOST** appropriate next step treatment for this patient's depression?
A. Fluvoxamine
B. Duloxetine
C. Mirtazapine
D. Dextroamphetamine

2. A 56-year-old man with a history of cocaine and alcohol dependence is admitted to the ICU for severe alcohol withdrawal. The patient suffers from significant autonomic hyperactivity (with blood pressure [BP] as high as 200/140 and pulse in 160s), visual and tactile hallucinations, diaphoresis, and tremor. He is treated with intravenous diazepam with improvement in his symptoms. Once the benzodiazepine is tapered, the patient complains of significantly depressed mood and neurovegetative symptoms of depression. He has a history of similar symptoms while withdrawing from alcohol and cocaine but has not had depressive episodes when abstinent for prolonged periods of time. What is the appropriate treatment for his depressive symptoms?
A. Citalopram
B. Methylphenidate
C. Mirtazapine
D. None of the above

3. Which of the following would not be considered first-line treatment for newly diagnosed major depressive disorder?
A. Sertraline
B. Bupropion
C. Nortriptyline
D. Venlafaxine

8.4 Central Nervous System Infections

1. A 30-year-old man with no pertinent medical history presents for evaluation after experiencing a generalized tonic-clonic seizure at home. Per family, he was complaining of headache and neck stiffness for 2 days. He was febrile, but otherwise his vital signs were stable. Basic labs and blood cultures were collected. Which of the following would be the **MOST** appropriate antimicrobial regimen to initiate?
A. Ceftriaxone, vancomycin, steroids
B. Ceftazidime, vancomycin, ampicillin, acyclovir
C. Ceftriaxone, vancomycin, ampicillin, steroids
D. Ceftriaxone, vancomycin, acyclovir, steroids

2. A 79-year-old woman with a history of hypertension is brought by her family for evaluation of fever and altered mental status. The patient was slightly confused the day prior and was experiencing a mild headache. In the emergency department, she developed status epilepticus and required endotracheal intubation for airway protection due to ongoing seizure activity. Computed tomography (CT) of the head was unremarkable. Blood cultures were collected, and a lumbar puncture was performed. She was started on empiric antimicrobial therapy and admitted to the intensive care unit. Brain magnetic resonance imaging (MRI) the following day showed patchy areas of T2 hyperintensity in the left temporal lobe. Which of the following CSF profile patterns is **MOST** consistent with her presentation?
A. Normal cell count, high protein, normal glucose
B. High cell count, high protein, normal glucose
C. Normal cell count, normal protein, low glucose
D. High cell count, low protein, high glucose

8.5 Acute Traumatic Brain Injury and Intracranial Hypertension

1. A 35-year-old male is involved in a high-speed motor vehicle collision. He is intubated and sedated in the intensive care unit (ICU) on hospital day 1 and has an invasive multimodality neuromonitor in place due to a presenting Glasgow Coma Score (GCS) of 6. His intracranial pressure (ICP) is 17 mm Hg and $Pbto_2$ is 35 mm Hg. Three hours later, his ICP is 25 mm Hg and his $Pbto_2$ is 30 mm Hg. His mean arterial pressure (MAP) is 90 mm Hg and $Paco_2$ is 35 mm Hg. What is the Next best step in management?
A. Increase MAP
B. Neurosurgical consultation for immediate decompressive craniectomy
C. Intermittent boluses of hyperosmolar therapy
D. Continuous infusion of hyperosmolar therapy

2. An 18-year-old female is admitted after a suicide attempt where she jumped out a third-story window. Her admission GCS was 7 and her Marshall classification was III, with evidence of mild brain swelling. The remainder of her trauma computed tomography (CT) scans showed femur and calcaneal fractures, and a pelvic fracture without active bleeding. An ICP monitor was placed, and her femur fractures were externally fixated. Soon after admission to the ICU, her ICP rises from 20 to 30 mm Hg, her $Pbto_2$ drops from 30 to 5 mm Hg, she develops new anisocoria, and she develops hypotension (MAP 50) and tachycardia (heart rate [HR] 150) associated with a bedside FAST showing new intraabdominal free fluid. What is the Next best step in management?
A. Immediate CT scans of the head, chest, abdomen, and pelvis
B. Emergent surgical evaluation of intraabdominal free fluid
C. Emergent neurosurgical evaluation of suspected herniation syndrome
D. Increase Fio_2 to 100% and transfuse blood to a hemoglobin (Hb) >9 g/dL to improve cerebral oxygenation

8.6 Spinal Cord Injury

1. Which of the following statements about blunt cerebrovascular injury (BCVI) is **TRUE**?
A. BCVI rarely occurs in the setting of cervical spine fractures.
B. Neurologic symptoms are required to consider BCVI diagnosis.
C. Computed tomographic (CT) angiography is used to screen for BCVI in high-risk patients.
D. Antiplatelet therapy is contraindicated due to the risk of bleeding in patients with trauma.

2. Which of the following is the preferred vasopressor in managing neurogenic hypotension following spinal cord injury due to its combined alpha- and beta-adrenergic activity?
A. Phenylephrine
B. Dopamine
C. Epinephrine
D. Norepinephrine

8.7 Ischemic Stroke

1. A 76-year-old man with a history of hypertension and diabetes mellitus presents to the emergency department (ED) with sudden-onset, left-sided weakness and dysarthria. His symptom onset was witnessed by his family 60 minutes before arrival. His blood pressure in the ED was 145/70. His National Institutes of Health Stroke Scale (NIHSS) is 5. The noncontrast computed tomography (CT) of the head revealed no evidence of hypodensity or hemorrhage. Computed tomographic angiography (CTA) of the head and neck revealed no large vessel occlusion. Which of the following is the **MOST** appropriate next step in this setting?
   A. Aspirin
   B. Intravenous thrombolysis
   C. Mechanical thrombectomy
   D. Clopidogrel

2. A 68-year-old woman with a past medical history of atrial fibrillation on apixaban is brought to the ED with right-sided weakness and expressive aphasia. She was last known normal 3 hours before presentation in the ED. Her NIHSS is 12. Her blood pressure is 135/70. The CT of the head is negative for hemorrhage. CTA of the head and neck revealed a proximal left middle cerebral artery (MCA) occlusion. Which of the following next step is **MOST** appropriate?
   A. Intravenous thrombolysis
   B. Mechanical thrombectomy
   C. Magnetic resonance imaging (MRI) of the brain
   D. Normal saline bolus

8.8 Intracerebral Hemorrhage

1. A 62-year-old man not on any medications is brought into the emergency department an hour after collapsing to the ground while walking home from work. On examination, he is awake but appears agitated and confused with incomprehensible speech. His left arm and leg are moving spontaneously, but his right arm only slightly withdraws to noxious stimuli in the plane of the bed. Blood pressure is 192/115. A noncontrast head computed tomography (CT) shows a 52-mL left frontal lobe hemorrhage. CT angiogram does not show any vascular abnormality. Complete blood count is within normal limits, partial thromboplastin time (PTT) is 26, and international normalized ratio (INR) is 1.3. Which of the following is the **MOST** appropriate treatment strategy for this patient?
   A. Initiate nicardipine to target a systolic blood pressure of 140 and admit to the intensive care unit for close monitoring.
   B. Initiate nicardipine to target a systolic blood pressure of 140 and administer prothrombin complex concentrate.
   C. Initiate nicardipine to target a systolic blood pressure of 140 and consult neurosurgery for minimally invasive hemorrhage evacuation.
   D. Initiate nicardipine to target a systolic blood pressure of 140 and consult neurosurgery for a decompressive hemicraniectomy.

2. A 58-year-old woman with past medical history of hypertension, atrial fibrillation on apixaban, and coronary artery disease on aspirin 81 mg presents with inability to move her left arm and leg. Her blood pressure is 210/120. A noncontrast head CT shows a 22-mL right basal ganglia hemorrhage. She has a platelet count of 230, PTT 22, INR 1.3, and fibrinogen 250. Which of the following treatments should be administered at this time?
   A. Platelet transfusion
   B. Idarucizumab
   C. Cryoprecipitate + tranexamic acid
   D. Andexanet alfa

8.9 Subarachnoid Hemorrhage and Vascular Malformations

1. Which scale is used as a predictor of risk for vasospasm and delayed cerebral ischemia (DCI) following aneurysmal subarachnoid hemorrhage?
   A. Modified Fisher Scale
   B. Hunt-Hess Scale
   C. Spetzler-Martin Grading System
   D. Raymond-Roy Occlusion Classification

2. Cavernous malformations are often associated with which other vascular malformation?
   A. Aneurysm
   B. Arteriovenous malformation
   C. Developmental venous anomaly
   D. Telangiectasia

8.10 Cerebral Venous Thrombosis

1. What is the most common symptom of cerebral venous thrombosis (CVT)?
   A. Seizures
   B. Headache
   C. Visual disturbances
   D. Nausea

2. Which of the following is a transient risk factor for CVT?
   A. Genetic thrombophilia
   B. Antiphospholipid syndrome
   C. Pregnancy/postpartum
   D. Malignancy

3. What imaging modality is considered optimal for confirming a diagnosis of CVT?
   A. Noncontrast computed tomography (CT)
   B. Magnetic resonance imaging (MRI)
   C. CT venography
   D. Ultrasound

4. What is the recommended initial treatment for CVT?
   A. Oral vitamin K antagonists
   B. Direct oral anticoagulants
   C. Parenteral heparin
   D. Decompressive hemicraniectomy

5. Which statement regarding the use of direct oral anticoagulants (DOACs) in CVT is true?
   A. They are not recommended.
   B. They have been shown to significantly increase recurrence rates.
   C. They are considered a safe and effective alternative to vitamin K antagonists.
   D. They should only be used in patients without any risk factors.

6. When is endovascular treatment (EVT) considered in patients with CVT?
   A. When the patient has a headache
   B. In cases of clinical or radiographic progression despite medical management
   C. As the first-line treatment for all patients with CVT
   D. Only in patients with no identifiable risk factors

8.11 Autoimmune Encephalitis and Demyelinating Disease

1. A 23-year-old female with a recent diagnosis of anxiety developed progressive cognitive decline marked by memory loss, as well as decreased level of arousal and dysautonomia over the course of 4 to 6 weeks. On review of history with her family, she had additionally begun to demonstrate abnormal behavior and involuntary movements that raise a question of epileptic seizures. Brain magnetic resonance imaging (MRI) is normal; however, an electroencephalogram (EEG) reveals epileptic discharges. Metabolic, infectious, and toxicology studies have been unrevealing. In addition to initiating antiseizure medications, what should you consider?
   A. Activated charcoal because substance intoxication is suspected
   B. Empiric immunosuppression with high-dose steroids (ie, intravenous [IV] methylprednisolone 1 g daily for 3-5 days) with potential additions of intravenous immunoglobulin (IVIg) or therapeutic plasma exchange pending steroid response
   C. No other treatment, an antiseizure medication start will be sufficient
   D. Empiric broad-coverage antibiotics

2. A 40-year-old female with no formal medical history presents for evaluation of severe, bilateral vision loss (visual acuity [VA] 20/200 OU) associated with pain with eye movements. MRI of the orbits demonstrates T2 FLAIR (Fluid Attenuated Inversion Recovery) hyperintensities and gadolinium-contrast enhancement of both optic nerves and the optic chiasm. She reports that in the past 1 to 2 weeks, she has also noted a band-like tightness around her lower torso and has had difficulty with urinary incontinence. MRI of her cervical and thoracic spine is obtained and displays both a longitudinally extensive lesion involving T6-T10 with patchy enhancement and two short segment lesions in the cervical spine without clear enhancement. Which of the following management is **MOST** likely for this patient?
   A. Start high-dose IV steroids (IV methylprednisolone 1 g daily for 3-5 days) only.
   B. Start high-dose IV steroids (IV methylprednisolone 1 g daily for 3-5 days) and then discharge with an oral prednisone taper thereafter.
   C. Start high-dose IV steroids (IV methylprednisolone 1 g daily for 3-5 days) with a plan to closely assess steroid response, as a lack of timely vision improvement will prompt a need for therapeutic plasma exchange.
   D. Start empiric IV ceftriaxone.

8.12 Neuromuscular Disorders

1. A 58-year-old woman with a history of acetylcholine receptor antibody–positive myasthenia gravis was hospitalized for small bowel obstruction. She underwent surgery for lysis of peritoneal adhesions. Prior to surgery, she was "*nil per os*" and with nasogastric tube to low wall intermittent suction. After surgery, she immediately failed extubation and required urgent reintubation. Which of the following medications is **MOST** likely to have caused an exacerbation of her myasthenia gravis?
   A. Fentanyl 50 μg/kg intravenously (IV), as part intubation procedure
   B. Magnesium sulfate 4 g (IV), as part of an order set for electrolyte replacement
   C. Nicardipine drip at 5 mg/h to reduce blood pressure during surgery
   D. Metronidazole 500 mg within 60 minutes prior to surgery as antibiotic prophylaxis

2. A 68-year-old man is admitted to the intensive care unit (ICU) for respiratory distress. History is significant for a self-limited gastrointestinal illness 5 days prior to presentation. He reports dysesthesia of the feet and weakness of his legs that started around 2 days prior and that have worsened. Examination is notable for dysphoria and poor compliance. His heart rate is 64 beats/min, and respiratory rate is 35 breaths/min. Deep tendon reflexes are absent. Arterial blood gas showed a pH of 7.38, $Paco_2$ of 42 mm Hg, and Pao_2 of 91 mm Hg. Given the most likely diagnosis, what is the **MOST** appropriate treatment?
   A. Obtain vital capacity and negative inspiratory pressure to assess respiratory muscle strength.
   B. Perform cerebrospinal fluid (CSF) analysis with cell and protein count.
   C. Start treatment with intravenous immune globulin (IVIG) (2 g/kg over 2-5 days).
   D. Induce pharmacologically and perform endotracheal intubation.

8.13 Brain Death/Death by Neurologic Criteria

1. A 65-year-old man is admitted with a large left thalamic hemorrhage and herniation. On hospital day 4, he is still comatose, has no brainstem reflexes, and is not spontaneously breathing on the ventilator despite being off sedation since admission. His temperature is 34.5 °C, and blood pressure is 106/70 mm Hg. Complete blood count (CBC), basic metabolic panel (BMP), liver panel, and thyroid-stimulating hormone (TSH) were unremarkable. Blood and urine toxicology screens are negative. An evaluation for brain death/death by neurologic criteria (BD/DNC) is considered. Which of the following prerequisites would preclude this patient from clinical examination for BD/DNC determination?
   A. Etiology for presentation
   B. Core body temperature
   C. Toxicology screen
   D. Systolic blood pressure reading

2. Ancillary testing is required in which of the following patients to determine BD/DNC?
   A. Patient with thoracic cord injury
   B. Patient with core body temperature of 33 °C
   C. Patient with blood pressure of 105/68 mm Hg on low-dose vasopressors
   D. Patient with suspected chronic hypercarbia and unknown baseline $PaCO_2$

8.14 Anoxic Brain Injury, Temperature Control, and Neuroprognostication

1. A 65-year-old man is brought to the emergency department after an out-of-hospital ventricular fibrillation arrest. Return of spontaneous circulation was achieved after 16 minutes of resuscitation. He is currently hemodynamically stable but unresponsive and not following commands on examination. He is found to be hypothermic at 34 °C. What is the next best step in postcardiac arrest management?
   A. Initiate therapeutic hypothermia to 31 °C.
   B. Allow slow rewarming (≤0.5 °C per hour) and continue to monitor temperature, initiating temperature control only if temperature exceeds 38 °C.
   C. Allow slow rewarming (≤0.5 °C per hour) with active fever prevention for goal temperature ≤37.5 °C.
   D. Initiate active rewarming to 37 °C at a rate of 1 °C per hour with active fever prevention for a goal temperature ≤37.5 °C.

2. Five days after his arrest, the above patient remains unresponsive with preserved pupillary reflexes and demonstrates no motor response to noxious stimuli in any extremity. Electroencephalogram (EEG) performed on days 0 to 3 off sedation shows diffuse voltage suppression. Magnetic resonance imaging (MRI) of the brain was unable to be performed as the patient has a non–MRI-compatible permanent pacemaker. Noncontrast head computed tomography (CT) performed on day 3 shows hypodensity of the bilateral basal ganglia. Somatosensory evoked potentials (SSEPs) performed on day 4 show a bilateral absent N20 response. Which of the following combination of results is most concerning for a high likelihood of poor neurologic outcome at 90 days?
   A. Bilateral basal ganglia hypodensity on CT and absent motor response to noxious stimuli in all four extremities
   B. Absent N20 on SSEPs and EEG with diffuse voltage suppression
   C. EEG with diffuse voltage suppression and bilateral basal ganglia hypodensity on CT
   D. Absent motor response to noxious stimuli in all four extremities and absent N20 on SSEPs

8.15 Neurooncology

1. A 55-year-old woman with no past medical history presents with 2 weeks of progressive blurry vision, nausea, and difficulty walking. She takes no medications and denies any recent trauma or substance abuse. Her vital signs are within normal limits, and she is alert and oriented without evidence of aphasia or dysarthria. She has evidence of direction-changing nystagmus and ataxia on finger-nose-finger testing bilaterally. The remainder of her physical examination is reassuring, and a noncontrast head computed tomography (CT) does not show evidence of hydrocephalus, large territorial hypodensity, or hemorrhage and is read as normal. Which of the following is the **MOST** likely diagnosis?
   A. Myasthenia gravis
   B. Toxic-metabolic encephalopathy
   C. Paraneoplastic syndrome
   D. Small ischemic stroke
   E. Benign paroxysmal positional vertigo

2. A 60-year-old woman with widely metastatic breast cancer, including leptomeningeal carcinomatosis, is admitted to the hospital for worsening headaches, nausea, and vomiting. In the emergency department, she is sleepy but interactive, providing her own history and oriented to time, place, and situation. Her neurologic examination is otherwise nonfocal, and she is admitted to the hospital for workup. On hospital day 1, she is repositioned in bed for a turn and suddenly becomes unresponsive, with no verbal responsiveness, pupils 4 mm bilaterally and weakly responsive to light, and no response to painful stimuli in any limb. Her blood pressure is 110/70, heart rate is 75, oxygen saturation is 97% on room air, and fingerstick glucose is 110. She receives Narcan twice without improvement but slowly regains awareness over the course of minutes and is again following commands in all four limbs. A CT scan of her head does not show a large territorial infarct, hemorrhage, or overt hydrocephalus. She receives 60 mg/kg of levetiracetam and is begun on continuous electroencephalography (EEG) monitoring. In the intensive care unit (ICU), she is helped onto a bedpan and has another episode of altered awareness, which lacks an epileptiform correlate on EEG. Which of the following is the **MOST** likely diagnosis?
   A. EEG-negative seizure
   B. Ischemic stroke of the basilar artery
   C. Intracranial pressure crisis/plateau wave
   D. Paraneoplastic syndrome
   E. Immune checkpoint inhibitor encephalitis

8.16 Analgesia, Sedation, Neuromuscular Blockade, and Other Pharmacologic Therapies for Neurologic Disorders

1. A 70-year-old man with influenza pneumonia has been mechanically ventilated for 7 days with volume-controlled mode. He has received intermittent boluses of midazolam for sedation over the past 3 days due to hypertriglyceridemia, and his pain appears well controlled with hydromorphone boluses. During the spontaneous awakening trial (SAT), he is found to be delirious and restless, necessitating early termination of the trial. However, his Spo_2 remains adequate on pressure support ventilation and 40% Fio_2. What is the **MOST** appropriate next step in the management of his sedation and delirium?
   A. Continue current sedation regimen with intermittent midazolam.
   B. Discontinue midazolam and initiate a low-dose dexmedetomidine infusion to target lighter levels of sedation.
   C. Limit frequency of awakening trials to prevent agitation and dyspnea.
   D. Start continuous hydromorphone infusion to improve tolerability of future SATs/SBTs (spontaneous breathing trials).

2. A 62-year-old woman has been receiving mechanical ventilation for 3 days due to moderate-to-severe acute respiratory distress syndrome (ARDS). On examination, she is deeply sedated (RASS-4) with propofol and hydromorphone infusions but continues to exhibit frequent dyssynchrony (double triggering) accompanied by large tidal volumes. She has not tolerated SATs because of significant desaturations and increased work of breathing. What is the **MOST** appropriate next step in the management of her sedation and ventilation?
   A. Increase the rates of propofol and hydromorphone infusions to improve ventilator synchrony.

B. Switch from propofol to dexmedetomidine infusion.
C. Initiate cisatracurium infusion and reassess the need for neuromuscular blockade daily.
D. Continue current management awaiting resolution of dyssynchrony over time.

8.17 Neurosurgical Management and Perioperative Complications

1. A 65-year-old woman is postoperative day 2 from a left-sided craniotomy for Falcine meningioma resection. Her post-op course has been uncomplicated, but she is now complaining of headache and has profound right-sided weakness. A noncontrast computed tomography (CT) demonstrates a left frontal hemorrhage with extensive perihematomal edema. What is the **MOST** likely etiology of her hemorrhage?
   A. Uncontrolled hypertension
   B. Venous infarction
   C. Residual tumor hemorrhage
   D. Hemorrhagic conversion of ischemic stroke

2. A 50-year-old man undergoes lumbar drain placement for refractory high intracranial pressure in the setting of cryptococcal meningitis. Two days afterward, he undergoes a routine CT scan, and upon transport back to the unit, he becomes progressively obtunded. It is noted that his lumbar drain was not clamped for transport, and 60 mL of cerebrospinal fluid (CSF) was inadvertently drained. STAT repeat CT demonstrates thin bilateral subdural hematomas and descent of the brainstem. What is the **BEST** next step in management?
   A. Emergent bilateral craniotomy for subdural hematoma evacuation
   B. Hyperosmolar therapy with mannitol
   C. Clamping of the lumbar drain and expectant management
   D. Rapid infusion of 60 mL normal saline via the lumbar drain

SECTION 9 INFECTIOUS DISEASE

9.1 Infectious Disease and Virulence Factors

1. A 39-year-old female with gastrointestinal dysmotility and a tunneled central venous catheter (CVC) for total parenteral nutrition (TPN) is admitted to the intensive care unit (ICU) with septic shock from *Escherichia coli* bacteremia. Intravenous (IV) ceftriaxone is started on admission, and by hospital day 2, she has defervesced, repeat blood cultures are negative, and she is clinically improving. Your attending asks if her CVC needs to be removed because of the bacteremia. Based on your review of the IDSA central line–associated bloodstream infection (CLABSI) guidelines, what is your suggestion about this infection?
   A. This is a complicated infection in a patient with a long-term CVC; remove the catheter and treat with systemic antibiotics.
   B. This is a complicated infection in a patient with a long-term CVC; you can try to leave the line in and do systemic antibiotics and lock therapy.
   C. This is an uncomplicated infection in a patient with a long-term CVC; you must remove the catheter and treat with systemic antibiotics.
   D. This is an uncomplicated infection in a patient with a long-term CVC, with no indication for removal, systemic antibiotics only.
   E. This is an uncomplicated infection in a patient with a long-term CVC; options for treatment include removal and systemic antibiotics or a trial of catheter salvage with systemic and lock therapy.

2. Routine fever workup in the ICU includes all of the following except:
   A. Blood cultures
   B. Thorough physical examination
   C. Chest x-ray
   D. C-reactive protein (CRP)
   E. Advanced imaging (ie, computed tomography [CT] of the chest/abdomen/pelvis) if localizing symptoms or recent surgery

9.2 Antibiotic Therapy and Resistance

1. A 43-year-old female is admitted to the intensive care unit (ICU) with *Enterobacter cloacae* bacteremia from a urinary source. In vitro testing demonstrates susceptibility to ceftriaxone, piperacillin/tazobactam, cefepime, and meropenem. Which antibiotic would be the best treatment?
   A. Ceftriaxone
   B. Piperacillin/tazobactam
   C. Meropenem
   D. Cefepime

2. A 75-year-old female has been intubated in the ICU for 4 days for the treatment of alcohol withdrawal. On day 5, she develops a fever to 38.5 °C, new leukocytosis to 13,000, and thick secretions from the endotracheal tube. The ICU team is concerned about pneumonia. Tracheal aspirates are sent for culture. Which empiric regimen would be the *MOST* appropriate while awaiting culture results?
   A. Ceftriaxone + azithromycin
   B. Vancomycin + ceftriaxone
   C. Vancomycin + cefepime
   D. Vancomycin + cefepime + azithromycin
   E. Daptomycin + cefepime
   F. Daptomycin + cefepime + azithromycin

SECTION 10 IMMUNOLOGY

10.1 The Immune System and Immunologic Disorders

1. A 50-year-old man presents to the emergency department with 1 week of progressive shortness of breath and reports scant hemoptysis. A chest x-ray shows diffuse patchy opacities, and he is intubated for acute hypoxemic respiratory failure. He undergoes bronchoscopy with bronchoalveolar lavage that is notable for sequentially bloodier aliquots. For the month leading up to this, he has had recurrent fevers, migratory joint pain (involving primarily the knees and wrists), and sinus pain with dark brown, crusty nasal discharge. Workup is notable for hemoglobin of 8 g/dL, creatinine of 2.3 mg/dL (baseline 0.9), and erythrocyte sedimentation rate (ESR) 90 mm/h, and C-reactive protein (CRP) 130 mg/dL. Urinalysis shows hematuria with occasional red

blood cell (RBC) casts. Which serologic test would be **MOST** likely to suggest the underlying diagnosis?

A. Antinuclear antibody (ANA)
B. Antineutrophil cytoplasmic antibody (ANCA)
C. Rheumatoid factor (RF)
D. Ribonucleoprotein (RNP)

2. A 23-year-old woman with a recent diagnosis of systemic lupus erythematosus with lupus nephritis 4 months ago (currently on prednisone 10 mg daily, hydroxychloroquine 200 mg daily, mycophenolate 1500 mg twice daily, belimumab 200 mg subcutaneous weekly) presents to urgent care with 2 days of fevers and cough. She denies other symptoms, including joint pains, rashes, and oral ulcers. Her oxygen saturation is 90% on room air, heart rate is 110 beats per minute, and blood pressure is 110/70 mm Hg. Physical examination is notable for decreased breath sounds and rhonchi over the right middle lobe without other focal abnormalities. She has not had any recent antibiotic exposure or hospitalizations. In addition to appropriate laboratory evaluation and imaging, what would be the **MOST** appropriate medication regimen at this time?

A. Increase prednisone to 40 mg daily; continue hydroxychloroquine, mycophenolate, and belimumab.
B. Start intravenous (IV) ceftriaxone and azithromycin; hold the prednisone, hydroxychloroquine, mycophenolate, and belimumab.
C. Start IV ceftriaxone and azithromycin; continue prednisone 10 mg daily and hydroxychloroquine, and hold mycophenolate and belimumab.
D. Start IV ceftriaxone and azithromycin; continue prednisone 10 mg daily, hydroxychloroquine, mycophenolate, and belimumab.

SECTION 11 Dermatology

11.1 Dermatologic Conditions

1. After an extensive resection of a necrotizing infection of the scrotum (Fournier gangrene), the patient with a medical history of intravenous (IV) substance abuse is admitted to the intensive care unit (ICU). Culture results of the resected tissue are pending. Which of the following antibiotics should be empirically prescribed with clindamycin until the culture results are finalized?

A. Cefazolin
B. Ceftriaxone
C. Vancomycin
D. Meropenem

2. A 42-year-old woman is admitted to the ICU following a fall that resulted in a subdural hematoma. With increasing neurologic symptoms and agitation, a follow-up computed tomography was planned. She was intubated after propofol and rocuronium. Within 5 minutes after intubation, her lips became swollen and she developed multiple raised rashes. What is the best initial treatment?

A. Diphenhydramine 50 mg IV
B. Epinephrine 0.3 mg IV
C. Hydrocortisone 100 mg IV
D. Sugammadex 200 mg IV

SECTION 12 THERMOREGULATION

12.1 Fever

1. Which statement regarding fever management in the intensive care unit (ICU) is **MOST** correct?

A. Routine use of antipyretics is recommended to prevent fever-related complications, assuming normal liver and renal functions.
B. Arterial catheters do not need to be removed during a line holiday as they are lower risk for infection than central venous catheters.
C. Fever can result from dexmedetomidine infusion.
D. Fever can result from thyroid storm or serotonin syndrome, and acetaminophen should be scheduled for these syndromes.

2. A 65-year-old patient was admitted to the ICU 3 days post-chemotherapy for the management of pain control and hyperglycemia, which are now well controlled, and he is awaiting a floor bed. On rounds, he presents with a temperature of 38.5 °C sustained over 2 hours. Pertinent vitals include a blood pressure of 85/50 mm Hg, heart rate of 110 beats/min, and a respiratory rate of 28 breaths per minute. Pertinent labs include an absolute neutrophil count of 354 cells/μL of blood. Which of the following sequences of actions is most appropriate?

A. Perform a thorough physical examination, volume resuscitate, initiate broad-spectrum antibiotics, and monitor closely.
B. Perform a thorough physical examination, volume resuscitate, obtain cultures, and initiate empirical antibiotic therapy.
C. Administer acetaminophen, wait for the temperature to stabilize, and then assess for other signs of infection.
D. Investigate for noninfectious causes, consult infectious disease specialist, and perform a chest x-ray.

12.2 Malignant Hyperthermia

1. Which of the following anesthetic agents is not a reported trigger for malignant hyperthermia?

A. Desflurane
B. Nitrous oxide
C. Succinylcholine
D. None of the above

2. Which of the following signs of malignant hyperthermia is most likely to occur *after* the others?

A. Increase in end-tidal CO_2 ($EtCO_2$)
B. Sinus tachycardia
C. Hyperthermia
D. Muscle rigidity

12.3 Neuroleptic Malignant Syndrome

1. Which of the following characteristics differentiates neuroleptic malignant syndrome (NMS) from serotonin syndrome?

A. Hyperreflexia
B. Lead-pipe rigidity
C. Hyperthermia
D. Myoclonus

2. Which of the following statements about hyperthermia in NMS is **MOST** correct?

A. Hyperthermia occurs early in the course of the syndrome.
B. Hypothermia is more typical of NMS.
C. Hyperthermia occurs late in the course and is secondary to sustained muscle contraction.
D. Hyperthermia is an uncommon feature.

12.4 Serotonin Syndrome

1. A 50-year-old woman with a history of depression presents to the emergency department with a recent onset of confusion, tremors, and involuntary movements. He reports that these symptoms began shortly after a change in her medications. Which is the **MOST** appropriate first step in management?
   A. Review her medications to check for serotonergic agents.
   B. Administer cyproheptadine immediately.
   C. Initiate physical cooling measures, intubation, and neuromuscular blockade.
   D. Discontinue all medications.

2. A 65-year-old man hospitalized for a week develops worsening delirium, requiring escalating doses of multiple medications to manage agitation. Over the last few hours, he has developed hyperreflexia, clonus, and hyperthermia. Which intervention is **MOST** effective for controlling his elevated temperature?
   A. Acetaminophen
   B. Physical cooling measures
   C. Antihistamines
   D. Haloperidol

12.5 Heat Stroke

1. A 25-year-old woman complains of dizziness and nausea after running a marathon on a hot day. She is conscious but confused, and her skin is hot and dry to the touch. What is the *MOST* likely cause of her symptoms?
   A. Dehydration
   B. Heat stroke
   C. Sunburn
   D. Muscle strain

2. A 70-year-old man is brought to the emergency department after collapsing outside on a hot, humid day. He is disorientated and has a core body temperature of 41 °C (105.8 °F). What is the *MOST* important initial treatment for this patient?
   A. Administering acetaminophen to reduce his temperature
   B. Placing him in a cool environment and applying cold compresses
   C. Giving him a large amount of fluids to drink orally
   D. Prescribing antibiotics to treat a possible infection

12.6 Hypothermia

1. A 28-year-old female with a history of depression and substance abuse is found obtunded on a ski slope in the winter. In the hospital examination, she is found to have fixed dilated pupils with blood pressure (BP) of 98/40 mm Hg and heart rate (HR) of 37/min. After securing her airway, her measured core temperature is 27 °C. What step would be *MOST* helpful to further guide management?
   A. Rewarming patient
   B. Perform an apnea test
   C. Initiate extracorporeal membranous oxygenation (ECMO)
   D. Start transcutaneous pacing

2. A 32-year-old homeless male with a history of intravenous drug use (IVDU) was found outside lethargic with a temperature of 30 °C, HR 51/min, BP 100/60, and oxygen saturation of 94% on room air. Despite forced warm air and resuscitation with warm intravenous fluids, the patient's temperature only increases by 0.5 °C over the next 4 hours. What is the *MOST* appropriate next step?
   A. Initiate ECMO
   B. Discontinue warming efforts
   C. Consider an alternative etiology of hypothermia while continuing warming efforts
   D. Start transcutaneous pacing

SECTION 13 OBSTETRICS

13.1 Preeclampsia/Eclampsia and HELLP Syndrome

1. A 28-year-old female at 36 weeks of gestation presents with new-onset hypertension (160/100 mm Hg) and severe right upper quadrant pain. Laboratory results reveal platelet count 85,000/µL, aspartate aminotransferase (AST) 150 IU/L, alanine aminotransferase (ALT) 160 IU/L, and lactate dehydrogenase (LDH) 700 IU/L. Which of the following is the **MOST** appropriate initial management?
   A. Immediate delivery without stabilization
   B. Magnesium sulfate for seizure prophylaxis and blood pressure control before delivery
   C. Watchful waiting with close fetal monitoring
   D. Immediate administration of corticosteroids

2. A 32-year-old female presents at 34 weeks of gestation with new-onset blurred vision and a persistent headache that does not improve with acetaminophen. Her blood pressure is 165/110 mm Hg. Additional findings include urine protein 400 mg/24 hours, platelet count 120,000/µL, and creatinine 1.3 mg/dL. Which of the following complications poses the **MOST** immediate risk to this patient?
   A. Placental abruption
   B. Cerebral hemorrhage
   C. Disseminated intravascular coagulation (DIC)
   D. Fetal growth restriction

13.2 Acute Fatty Liver of Pregnancy

1. A 34-year-old female at 36 weeks of gestation presents with confusion, nausea, severe hypoglycemia (glucose 35 mg/dL), coagulopathy (international normalized ratio [INR] 2.5), hyperbilirubinemia (total bilirubin 5.8 mg/dL), and abdominal pain. Laboratory studies reveal elevated transaminases and acute kidney injury. Ultrasound demonstrates ascites and increased liver echogenicity. What is the **MOST** appropriate next step in her management?
   A. Administer corticosteroids
   B. Immediate delivery of the fetus
   C. Plasma exchange
   D. Liver biopsy to confirm diagnosis

2. A 32-year-old female at 37 weeks of gestation presents with nausea, vomiting, and severe fatigue. On examination, she appears jaundiced and confused. Laboratory results are as follows: blood glucose 40 mg/dL, total bilirubin 5.6 mg/dL,

alanine aminotransferase (ALT) 300 IU/L, creatinine 2.5 mg/dL, prothrombin time (PT) 20 seconds, and platelet count 65,000/μL. Which of the patient's findings is **MOST** helpful for distinguishing acute fatty liver of pregnancy (AFLP) from hemolysis, elevated liver enzymes, and low platelets (HELLP) syndrome?

A. Severe hypoglycemia
B. Abdominal pain
C. Encephalopathy
D. Coagulopathy

13.3 Amniotic Fluid Embolism

1. A 35-year-old woman undergoing labor develops sudden respiratory failure, hypotension, and coagulopathy. Which of the following is the **MOST** appropriate treatment of this patient's condition?
   A. Broad-spectrum antibiotics
   B. Corticosteroid therapy
   C. Supportive care focused on hemodynamic stabilization and correction of coagulopathy
   D. Emergent cesarean delivery regardless of fetal status

2. A 36-year-old woman undergoing labor develops sudden dyspnea, hypotension, and a sense of impending doom. She rapidly progresses to cardiac arrest. Advanced Cardiac Life Support (ACLS) is initiated, including manual left uterine displacement and chest compressions. Amniotic fluid embolism (AFE) is suspected. Despite ongoing resuscitation efforts, return of spontaneous circulation (ROSC) is not achieved after 4 minutes. What is the **MOST** appropriate next step in this patient's management?
   A. Continue chest compressions and administer additional doses of epinephrine.
   B. Perform a resuscitative hysterotomy.
   C. Administer corticosteroids.
   D. Insert an arterial line and pulmonary artery catheter to monitor hemodynamic status.

13.4 Postpartum Hemorrhage

1. A 32-year-old woman develops significant postpartum hemorrhage (PPH) 2 hours after a vaginal delivery. According to the World Health Organization (WHO) recommendations, which of the following is the appropriate management regarding tranexamic acid administration?
   A. Administer 1 g of tranexamic acid intravenously within 3 hours of delivery; a second dose may be given if bleeding continues after 30 minutes or restarts within 24 hours.
   B. Administer 1 g of tranexamic acid intravenously within 6 hours of delivery; a second dose may be given if bleeding continues after 60 minutes or restarts within 12 hours.
   C. Administer 2 g of tranexamic acid intravenously within 3 hours of delivery; a second dose may be given if bleeding continues after 30 minutes or restarts within 24 hours.
   D. Administer 1 g of tranexamic acid intravenously within 3 hours of delivery; a second dose may be given if bleeding continues after 60 minutes or restarts within 12 hours.

2. A 32-year-old woman experiences severe PPH unresponsive to medical management and conservative surgical interventions. Which surgical procedure is considered definitive when all other measures have failed to control life-threatening hemorrhage?
   A. Uterine artery ligation
   B. B-Lynch uterine compression sutures
   C. Hysterectomy
   D. Intrauterine tamponade balloon

13.5 Peripartum Cardiomyopathy

1. A 36-year-old G2P1001 African American female presents at 39 weeks 6 days estimated gestation with symptoms of orthopnea, shortness of breath on exertion, and peripheral edema. A transthoracic echocardiogram shows a left ventricular ejection fraction (LVEF) of 40% and normal right ventricular function. Her pregnancy has been otherwise uncomplicated. She is diagnosed with presumed peripartum cardiomyopathy. Which of the following is a poor prognostic indicator?
   A. LVEF 40%
   B. Lack of other pregnancy-related complications
   C. African American race
   D. Single gestation pregnancy

2. A 41-year-old G3P3003 female at 22 days postpartum presents with heart failure symptoms and is diagnosed with peripartum cardiomyopathy. Her LVEF is 30%, and she has mild right ventricular systolic dysfunction on a transthoracic echocardiogram. She is breastfeeding. Which of the following medications is most likely indicated?
   A. Sacubitril-valsartan
   B. Therapeutic enoxaparin
   C. Bromocriptine
   D. Lisinopril

13.6 Peripartum Infections

1. A 36-year-old G2P1001 female who is 29 weeks pregnant ruptured her membranes 1 week ago and developed a fever, uterine tenderness, and vaginal leukorrhea. She has already received betamethasone for fetal maturation and was started on antibiotics, given fluids, and is in the intensive care unit (ICU) for vasopressors. What is the next best step in therapy?
   A. Immediate delivery
   B. Magnetic resonance imaging (MRI) of the abdomen and pelvis
   C. Amniocentesis to confirm diagnosis
   D. Intraamniotic lavage with normal saline

2. A 23-year-old G1P0 at 25 weeks gestation arrives with a 1-week history of dysuria and a 2-day history of back pain, fever, and dizziness. She is started on empiric antibiotic therapy, given 30 mL/kg of fluids for hypotension, and has a lactic acid of 4.6 mmol/L. What is the next best step in therapy for her if she remains hypotensive?
   A. Change antibiotics from ceftriaxone to cefepime.
   B. Give an additional 2 L bolus of crystalloid.
   C. Immediate delivery.
   D. Start norepinephrine.

13.7 Posterior Reversible Encephalopathy Syndrome

1. A 20-year-old woman presented thunderclap headache 2 weeks after an uncomplicated vagubak delivery. A brain computed tomography (CT) scan did not reveal any

intracranial bleeding. In addition, a cerebral angiogram showed strings and beads appearance in medium-sized arteries. Which of the following is the **MOST** likely diagnosis?
   A. Posterior reversible encephalopathy syndrome (PRES)
   B. Subarachnoid hemorrhage
   C. Reversible cerebral vasoconstriction syndrome (RCVS)
   D. Cluster headache

2. Which of the following factors is associated with poor outcomes after PRES?
   A. Acute respiratory insufficiency
   B. Recurrent seizures
   C. Postpartum
   D. Bilateral posterior white matter edema

13.8 Other Obstetric Emergencies

1. When performing Advanced Cardiac Life Support (ACLS) on a pregnant person, which of the following should be considered?
   A. Defibrillation should be withheld in shockable rhythms due to concern for fetal harm.
   B. Medications should be given in increased doses compared to the nonpregnant patient.
   C. Fetal assessment should not be performed during resuscitation.
   D. Resuscitative hysterotomy/perimortem cesarean section should be considered after 20 minutes of cardiac arrest.

2. A 32-year-old pregnant woman who is at 20 weeks of gestation presents with right lower quadrant abdominal pain, mild tachycardia, a low-grade fever of 38.1 °C, and a white blood cell count of 13,200 cells/μL. Concern is for acute appendicitis. The most recent meal was 3 hours prior. Which of the following is **MOST** likely to be true?
   A. Fetal heart rate (FHR) monitoring should take place throughout a surgical procedure.
   B. General anesthesia has not been definitively shown to affect fetal neurocognitive outcomes.
   C. The patient should be treated nonoperatively, given the fetal risk incurred by anesthetic exposure.
   D. Rapid sequence induction with succinylcholine is contraindicated.

13.9 Obstetric Imaging Modalities

1. A 38-year-old female presents to the emergency department with an acute-onset, left-sided weakness and slurred speech that started 45 minutes prior to arrival. The patient's partner notifies you that she is ~6 weeks pregnant with a desired pregnancy. Which of the following imaging modalities is the **BEST** initial imaging to obtain?
   A. Obtain Stat ultrasound to confirm pregnancy viability.
   B. Magnetic resonance imaging (MRI) of the brain without contrast
   C. Computed tomography (CT) scan with and without contrast
   D. Defer CT scan to reduce radiation exposure to the fetus.

2. A 42-year-old female with a known 16-week pregnancy arrives to her clinical appointment 1 hour late, stating, "I am so sorry, I was stuck in terrible commute traffic for 3 hours." During the evaluation, she becomes acutely short of breath, and vital signs are checked, revealing temp 98.9 °F, pulse 128, blood pressure 114/67, O_2 sat 83%, and respiratory rate 26/min. You suspect she may have a pulmonary embolism and are considering obtaining a CT angiography to make the diagnosis. At this time, your colleague reminds you that she is 16 weeks pregnant and cannot have a CT scan due to the radiation. Which of the following responses is **MOST** correct?
   A. Thank you for catching that—let's obtain a $\dot{V}/\dot{Q}$ scan to avoid radiation!
   B. In that case, we can forego imaging and start treatment for a presumed pulmonary embolism.
   C. While there is a risk to the pregnancy with radiation, this risk is far outweighed by the benefit of early diagnosis.
   D. Despite the pregnancy status, a CT angiography is appropriate after performing a pregnancy viability ultrasound and obtaining consent.

SECTION 14 FLUID MANAGEMENT

14.1 Fluid Management

1. An 83-year-old male presents to the emergency department with a 1-day history of worsening flank pain, intermittent gross hematuria, confusion, and shaking chills. Vitals are notable for a temperature of 39.1 °C, heart rate of 113 beats per minute, and mean arterial pressure of 57 mm Hg. His extremities are warm, and he is diaphoretic. The total body weight is 80 kg. Which of the following would be the **MOST** appropriate for initial fluid resuscitation in this patient?
   A. 1 L of 5% human albumin
   B. 2.5 L of lactated Ringer solution
   C. 2.5 L of normal saline
   D. 3 units of packed red blood cells

2. A 69-year-old female with a known history of ischemic cardiomyopathy and a depressed ejection fraction presents with several days of fevers, progressive shortness of breath, and severe emesis. Her blood pressure is 93/49 mm Hg, and the examination is notable for faint bibasilar crackles and 1+ pitting edema of the lower extremities. Oxygen saturation is measured at 97% on 2 L/min supplemental oxygen by nasal cannula. Which of the following would be **MOST** reliable in guiding fluid resuscitation for this patient?
   A. Central venous pressure
   B. Chest radiography
   C. Lactate concentration
   D. Passive leg raising

14.2 Sodium and Chloride Balance

1. Which of the following is **MOST** accurate regarding sodium disorders?
   A. Patients with hypotonic hyponatremia always present with orthostatic symptoms.
   B. Syndrome of inappropriate antidiuretic hormone (SIADH) is most commonly associated with hypervolemic hypotonic hyponatremia than with euvolemic hypotonic hyponatremia.
   C. Urine osmolality is a useful tool in the differential diagnosis of hypotonic hyponatremia.
   D. Urine osmolality is a useful tool in the differential diagnosis of hypertonic hyponatremia.

2. A 35-year-old man was admitted to the emergency department after a major polytrauma. After the resuscitation phase, the arterial blood gas analysis showed hyperchloremia and metabolic acidosis. What is the **MOST** probable cause of the hyperchloremia?
   A. Diabetes insipidus
   B. Chloride-rich intravenous fluid therapy
   C. Posthypocapnia state
   D. Diuretics

14.3 Potassium Balance

1. A 40-year-old male with stage IV acute kidney injury was transferred to the intensive care unit (ICU) for monitoring after telemetry changes were noticed. On arrival, he was alert and oriented, but his potassium was found to be 6.7 mmol/L. Which electrocardiographic change is **MOST** likely to be seen in this patient?
   A. Increased P-wave amplitude
   B. Peaked T waves
   C. Ventricular fibrillation
   D. Prominent U waves

2. If you were taking care of the abovementioned patient, what would be the fastest-acting treatment you could administer to avoid further cardiac compromise?
   A. Loop diuretics
   B. Kayexalate
   C. Digoxin
   D. Calcium

14.4 Calcium, Magnesium, and Phosphorous Balance

1. A 58-year-old man with chronic alcoholism presents to the intensive care unit (ICU) in septic shock and atrial fibrillation with rapid ventricular rate. Initial serum potassium is 2.8 mEq/L. Following two separate 20 mEq infusions of potassium chloride, his serum potassium is still 2.9 mEq/L. Which of the following is the **MOST** appropriate next step to correct this patient's hypokalemia?
   A. Administer intravenous insulin and dextrose.
   B. Check a serum magnesium level.
   C. Switch to a potassium phosphate infusion.
   D. Give an additional 40 mEq of potassium chloride.

2. A 45-year-old woman with Crohn is recovering well after her colectomy and ileostomy following an ICU admission for toxic megacolon. Vasopressor support has been discontinued, and she is awaiting transfer to the surgical inpatient ward. Due to profound malnutrition, total parenteral nutrition (TPN) is initiated. The next day, she develops progressive weakness and tachypnea. Her serum phosphorus is 0.8 mg/dL, ionized calcium is 1.2 mmol/L, and magnesium is 2.0 mg/dL. This patient's symptoms are **MOST** likely due to which of the following?
   A. Diaphragmatic weakness
   B. Impaired oxygen delivery
   C. Acute metabolic acidosis
   D. Symptomatic hypocalcemia

SECTION 15 NUTRITION

15.1 Basal and Stress Energy Requirements

1. What is an accurate marker of adequate nutrition in the intensive care unit (ICU) patient?
   A. Albumin
   B. Prealbumin
   C. Retinol-binding protein
   D. None of the above

2. For which of the following patient populations is enteral nutrition not indicated?
   A. Intubated healthy patient who has been without nutrition for 72 hours
   B. Older patient with chronic wasting from an ongoing malignancy
   C. Patient with body mass index (BMI) 45 and pancreatitis admitted to the ICU
   D. None of the above
   E. All of the above

15.2 Stress Hormone Response

1. A 38-year-old female is admitted to the surgical intensive care unit (ICU) after a motor vehicle collision and sustaining multiple orthopedic injuries and a 30% total body surface area burn to her chest, abdomen, and lower extremities. After 48 hours of intensive care, the intensivist would like to start a medication to attenuate the catabolic process seen in this hypermetabolic patient. Which medication should she implement?
   A. Rectal acetaminophen
   B. Seroquel
   C. Propranolol
   D. Dilaudid

2. A 59-year-old female with a history of insulin-dependent diabetes insipidus, chronic obstructive pulmonary disease (COPD), coronary artery disease, and hyperlipidemia is admitted to the ICU with a COPD exacerbation. The patient's respiratory status deteriorates and is intubated on hospital day 2. On hospital day 4, the patient has marked hyperglycemia that requires initiation of an insulin drip for glucose control. Which of the following is contributing to her hyperglycemia?
   A. Increased availability of blood cortisol
   B. Lipolysis
   C. Hepatic gluconeogenesis
   D. All of the above

15.3 Nutritional Deficiency States

1. A 65-year-old male with a history of hypertension, obesity, diabetes, and peripheral arterial disease is admitted to the burn intensive care unit (ICU) after sustaining a 50% total body surface area burn to his chest, abdomen, and upper and lower extremities. A nasogastric tube is placed. When should enteral tube feeding be initiated?
   A. After the first bowel movement
   B. As soon as possible, ideally within the first 6 hours

C. Only if patient cannot take voluntary oral (PO) nutrition
D. No enteral nutrition should be given. Start parenteral nutrition.

2. A 79-year-old female with a history of diabetes, hypertension, and dementia is admitted to the ICU after concerns of failure to thrive at her skilled nursing facility. The patient is found to be hypotensive and is given 30 mL/kg of crystalloid for resuscitation, followed by initiation of norepinephrine, given signs of sepsis. On examination, she has a sacral ulcer with surrounding cellulitis. Which of these is not associated with malnutrition?
   A. Poor wound healing
   B. Reduced risk of infection
   C. Peripheral muscle weakness
   D. Altered mental status

15.4 Nutrition Support

1. How often should gastric residuals be checked in the intensive care unit (ICU)?
   A. Hourly
   B. Every 4 hours
   C. Every 8 hours
   D. They should not be checked regularly.

2. Which of the following is false regarding enteral nutrition?
   A. Protective effect on gut mucosa
   B. Improves wound healing
   C. Contraindicated when on low-dose vasopressors
   D. Contributes to immune function

15.5 Refeeding Syndrome

1. A 44-year-old male has remained in the hospital for the past 8 days following traumatic pancreatitis with poor oral (PO) intake. Improved pain management has improved his symptoms, and he no longer feels nauseous and is requesting to eat. You start him on a full liquid diet at 10 kcal/kg/d and increase to 30 kcal/kg/d after 3 days. This is adequate for his needs. On day 3, you notice a significant drop in the patient's phosphate from 3.2 mEq/L → 1.1 mEq/L and potassium from 4.2 mEq/L → 2.6 mEq/L despite daily labs and replacement. Over the next day, the patient's electrolytes remain difficult to replete. What would be the best management strategy for this patient?
   A. Continue aggressive electrolyte repletion, increase lab frequency from twice daily to at least 4 times a day and maintain patient at his current caloric intake.
   B. Continue aggressive electrolyte repletion, increase lab frequency from twice daily to at least 4 times a day, reduce caloric intake by 50%, and advance by roughly 1/3rd of the patient's goal every 1 to 2 days.
   C. Continue aggressive electrolyte repletion, maintain lab frequency, and switch to total parenteral nutrition. Stop all enteral nutrition.
   D. Continue aggressive electrolyte repletion, increase lab frequency and increase daily lab frequency from twice a day to 4 times a day, and increase daily caloric intake to 40 kcal/kg/d.

2. A 56-year-old woman with a history of homelessness, chronic alcohol use, type 2 diabetes, chronic obstructive pulmonary disease (COPD), body mass index (BMI) of 15, and bowel resection following traumatic enterotomies due to penetrating trauma recently found a stable living situation with state aid for groceries and job training. The patient arrives confused, with acute hypercarbic respiratory failure, and labs significant for a phosphate below assay, sodium 126 mEq/L, chloride 88 mEq/L, bicarbonate 6 mEq/L, potassium 3.0 mEq/L, glucose 45 mEq/L, and lactic acid of 18 mmol/L. The patient uses an inhaler, otherwise is on no other medication. After airway and hemodynamic management, what is the next recommended step?
   A. Give glucose.
   B. Give phosphate.
   C. Give thiamine.
   D. Start dialysis.
   E. Infuse sodium bicarbonate.

SECTION 16 PHARMACOLOGY AND TOXICOLOGY

16.1 Basic Pharmacokinetics and Pharmacodynamics

1. Which of the following changes is most likely to increase the required loading dose of a medication?
   A. Converting to an administration route with greater bioavailability
   B. Resolution of an acute kidney injury
   C. Development of pancreatitis
   D. Coadministration of a medication known to inhibit cytochrome P450 3A4

2. Two drugs (A and B) are both able to increase a patient's mean arterial blood pressure when administered intravenously. Drug A produces its effect significantly faster than drug B but must be administered at a higher dose to achieve the same increase in blood pressure. Which of the descriptions of these medications is most likely true?
   A. Drug A—higher Emax, drug B—more likely has a reversible effect
   B. Drug A—more likely has a reversible effect, drug B—more likely has a direct effect
   C. Drug A—more likely has a direct effect, drug B—more potent
   D. Drug A—more potent, drug B—higher *E*max

16.2 Drug-Drug Interactions

1. A 78-year-old female with a past medical history of epilepsy, maintained on valproic acid, is admitted for urosepsis with increasing vasopressor requirements. Which of the following broad-spectrum antibiotics is *MOST* likely to interact with her valproic acid and increase the risk of seizures?
   A. Levofloxacin
   B. Tobramycin
   C. Meropenem
   D. Linezolid

2. A 54-year-old man with a past medical history of atrial fibrillation on warfarin is admitted for a skin and soft tissue infection. Which antimicrobial is *MOST* likely to interact with his warfarin?
   A. Ceftriaxone
   B. Doxycycline
   C. Sulfamethoxazole-trimethoprim
   D. Clindamycin

16.3 Toxicology, Drug Overdose, and Poisoning

1. A 46-year-old undomiciled man with a history of alcohol use disorder presents to the emergency department (ED) via emergency medical services (EMS) after being found unresponsive. His vital signs are significant for heart rate (HR) 120, respiratory rate (RR) 30, blood pressure (BP) 89/55, and T 37.9 °C. On examination, he is unresponsive; there is dried blood around his mouth; he is tachypneic and has crackles on lung auscultation, tachycardic with no murmurs, capillary refill is delayed; and he appears malnourished. You appreciate a fruity odor on his breath. Labs are significant for sodium of 125, chloride 98, bicarbonate 22, blood urea nitrogen (BUN) 24, creatinine 1.2, glucose 72, ethanol <1 mg/dL, and measured serum osmolarity 300 mOsm/kg. After intubating the patient for airway protection, which of the following therapies is the most appropriate?
   A. Fomepizole
   B. Hemodialysis
   C. Multidose-activated charcoal
   D. Supportive care

2. A 23-year-old woman with a history of G6PD deficiency presents after being rescued from a house fire. She reports having a headache, feeling lightheaded, and is nauseated. On examination, HR is 130, RR 32, BP 146/82, T 37.7 °C, and Spo_2 87% on room air. She has no obvious burns and no soot in her oropharynx, but she does seem confused. She has crackles on lung auscultation. Labs are drawn, and your nurse reports they may have inadvertently obtained arterial blood instead of venous blood. Urine qualitative pregnancy test is positive. In addition to supplemental oxygen, which of the following medications is the best option?
   A. Sodium nitrite and sodium thiosulfate
   B. Hydroxocobalamin
   C. Hyperbaric oxygen
   D. Methylene blue

16.4 Toxicology, Drug Overdose, and Poisoning

1. A 46-year-old undomiciled man with a history of alcohol use disorder presents to the emergency department (ED) via emergency medical services (EMS) after being found unresponsive. His vital signs are significant for heart rate (HR) 120, respiratory rate (RR) 30, blood pressure (BP) 89/55, and T 37.9 °C. On examination, he is unresponsive; there is dried blood around his mouth; he is tachypneic and has crackles on lung auscultation, tachycardic with no murmurs, capillary refill is delayed; and he appears malnourished. You appreciate a fruity odor on his breath. Labs are significant for sodium of 125, chloride 98, bicarbonate 22, blood urea nitrogen (BUN) 24, creatinine 1.2, glucose 72, ethanol <1 mg/dL, and measured serum osmolarity 300 mOsm/kg. After intubating the patient for airway protection, which of the following therapies is the most appropriate?
   A. Fomepizole
   B. Hemodialysis
   C. Multidose-activated charcoal
   D. Supportive care

2. A 23-year-old woman with a history of G6PD deficiency presents after being rescued from a house fire. She reports having a headache, feeling lightheaded, and is nauseated. On examination, HR is 130, RR 32, BP 146/82, T 37.7 °C, and Spo_2 87% on room air. She has no obvious burns and no soot in her oropharynx, but she does seem confused. She has crackles on lung auscultation. Labs are drawn, and your nurse reports they may have inadvertently obtained arterial blood instead of venous blood. Urine qualitative pregnancy test is positive. In addition to supplemental oxygen, which of the following medications is the best option?
   A. Sodium nitrite and sodium thiosulfate
   B. Hydroxocobalamin
   C. Hyperbaric oxygen
   D. Methylene blue

SECTION 17 TRANSFUSION THERAPY

17.1 Transfusion Medicine

1. Which donor is **MOST** suitable for the potential manufacture of whole blood (WB) that will be stocked in an emergency department for trauma resuscitation?
   A. Type AB, RhD negative, 33 yo G2P2 female, regular prior blood donor
   B. Type O, RhD negative, 26 yo G1P1 female, first-time blood donor
   C. Type O, RhD positive, 25 yo male, regular prior blood donor
   D. Type AB, RhD negative, 25 yo male, first-time blood donor

2. What is the **MOST** common cause of transfusion-associated mortality in the United States?
   A. ABO-incompatible red blood cell (RBC) transfusion
   B. RhD-incompatible RBC transfusion
   C. Transfusion-associated circulatory overload (TACO)
   D. Transfusion-associated graft-versus-host disease (TA-GVHD)

SECTION 18 TRANSPLANTS

18.1 Transplants: Lung, Heart, Liver, and Other Organs

1. A 45-year-old male patient underwent a liver transplant 48 hours ago. Postoperatively, the patient shows signs of worsening liver function, including rising liver enzymes, coagulopathy, and encephalopathy. Despite adequate blood flow to the graft as confirmed by Doppler ultrasound, the patient continues to deteriorate. Which of the following is the **MOST** likely diagnosis?
   A. Acute rejection
   B. Hepatic artery thrombosis
   C. Primary nonfunction of the graft

D. Chronic rejection
E. Biliary stricture

2. A 48-year-old male patient is in the intensive care unit (ICU) after undergoing a heart transplant 3 days ago. He is on tacrolimus as part of his immunosuppressive regimen. The patient suddenly develops altered mental status, generalized tonic-clonic seizures, and has no prior history of epilepsy. Laboratory tests show normal electrolytes and renal function. Which of the following is the **MOST** likely cause of his seizures?
   A. Electrolyte imbalance
   B. Central nervous system infection
   C. Tacrolimus-induced neurotoxicity
   D. Acute ischemic stroke
   E. Hypoglycemia

18.2 Organ Donation

1. Which of the following best explains the primary cardiovascular consequence of brain death and its effect on donor organ quality?
   A. Persistent hypotension due to adrenal insufficiency
   B. Systemic inflammation from gut bacterial translocation
   C. A biphasic cardiovascular response initiated by a catecholamine surge followed by vasodilation and hypoperfusion
   D. Chronic myocardial ischemia due to coronary artery occlusion
   E. Increased coronary blood flow resulting in improved myocardial oxygenation

2. Which of the following statements regarding controlled donation after circulatory death (cDCD) is most accurate?
   A. DCD kidneys are not used due to high rates of delayed graft function.
   B. Functional warm ischemia time (fWIT) has little impact on liver graft outcomes.
   C. The withdrawal of life support and declaration of death must be performed independently of the transplant team.
   D. Thoracoabdominal normothermic regional perfusion (ta-NRP) is only used for uncontrolled DCD cases.
   E. A mandatory 10-minute waiting period must be observed after cardiac arrest before procurement begins.

SECTION 19 TRAUMA MANAGEMENT

19.1 Fluid Resuscitation/Transfusion Guidelines

1. A 30-year-old male presents after a high-speed motor vehicle collision. On initial survey, he is hypotensive, tachycardic, and has an unstable pelvic fracture. What is the best systolic blood pressure to target when resuscitating the patient while he awaits angioembolization?
   A. 70 mm Hg
   B. 90 mm Hg
   C. 110 mm Hg
   D. 130 mm Hg

2. A 25-year-old male presents after a stab wound to the upper extremity. A tourniquet was placed by emergency medical services (EMS) due to pulsatile bleeding. On arrival, he is hypotensive and tachycardic. What is the best initial fluid to use for resuscitation?
   A. Lactated Ringer
   B. Normal saline
   C. Albumin
   D. Blood

19.2 Basic Management

1. A 56-year-old male telephone line worker presents after falling an estimated 30 ft while working on a telephone pole. On arrival to the emergency department, his heart rate (HR) is 110, blood pressure (BP) 103/78, respiratory rate 10, with an oxygen saturation of 98%. His Glasgow Coma Scale (GCS) is 15. He is able to speak in full sentences and is complaining of left hip and left leg pain. He has a scalp laceration to the level of bone as well as a left elbow laceration that does not appear to extend into the joint. Focused assessment with sonography for trauma (FAST) examination is negative, chest x-ray demonstrates no pneumothorax or hemothorax, though he appears to have at least two left-sided rib fractures. Pelvic x-ray demonstrates a widening of the pubic symphysis as well as a fracture through the left sacral ala, and left superior and inferior pubic rami. What is the best next step in the management of this patient?
   A. Transfuse 1 unit of packed red blood cells (pRBCs) for tachycardia and low systolic BP.
   B. Transport to computed tomography (CT) scan for head, cervical spine, chest, abdomen, and pelvis imaging.
   C. Place a pelvic binder.
   D. Establish femoral central venous access.
   E. Transport to the intensive care unit (ICU), consult orthopedic surgery for bony injuries, and perform serial hemoglobin checks.

2. A 46-year-old male presents with a right distal thigh impaled by an arrow shot by a compound bow. The arrow is still present in the leg, and a tourniquet was placed proximally due to excessive bleeding in the field. He is pale, diaphoretic, with an HR of 124 and BP of 80/43. He is awake and alert. He has no other injuries. He is given 2 units of whole blood, and his BP improves to 110/84, HR 97. He is able to move his right foot and toes and has full sensation. When the tourniquet is taken down a large amount of bright red blood pours out around the arrow, with no return of dorsalis pedis (DP) or posterior tibial (PT) pulses on examination. What is the next best step for this patient?
   A. Put up a tourniquet, perform a computed tomographic angiogram (CTA) with runoff to the right leg.
   B. Proceed directly to the operating room for exploration.
   C. Remove the arrow and explore the wound in the trauma bay with the tourniquet up.
   D. Continue resuscitation and perform lateral x-rays of leg to evaluate for bony injury.
   E. Administer tranexamic acid (TXA), remove the arrow, and maintain pressure after taking down the tourniquet.

19.3 FAST: Focused Assessment With Sonography

1. An 89-year-old female is presenting after mistakenly pressing the gas instead of the brake pedal and suffering a motor vehicle accident (MVA) as a single-restrained driver versus

a tree at an estimated 60 mph. She had prolonged extrication and was confused at the scene, though responsive. On arrival to the trauma bay, she was noted to have a blood pressure (BP) of 82/45 with a heart rate of 76. She is given a unit of blood, and her BP improves to 112/78. FAST examination is positive in the right upper quadrant. She has a small nonbleeding laceration to her forehead. Chest x-ray demonstrates multiple left-sided rib fractures without hemothorax or pneumothorax. Pelvis x-ray is negative. She is saturating at 100% on a nasal cannula. While completing the secondary survey, she is again noted to dropped her BP to 78/43. What would be the best next steps in management?
   A. Transfuse an additional 1 unit of packed red blood cells (pRBCs) and proceed to a computed tomography (CT) scan to evaluate all injuries.
   B. Establish central intravenous (IV) access for massive transfusion protocol (MTP) and transfuse to achieve a mean arterial pressure (MAP) >65.
   C. Transfuse blood product as needed and proceed directly to the operating room (OR) for exploration.
   D. Establish an arterial line for accurate BP monitoring to determine if the patient's initial cuff pressures are accurate.
   E. Administer tranexamic acid (TXA), transfuse blood product to maintain MAP >65, and perform a diagnostic peritoneal lavage (DPL) to confirm FAST examination results.

2. A 58-year-old male presents to the trauma bay with a self-inflicted butcher knife wound to the anterior left chest after an argument with his spouse. His pericardial FAST examination is positive for a pericardial effusion. He is intoxicated but able to communicate in full sentences. Chest x-ray demonstrates a widened mediastinum with a small hemothorax, with lung fields up and bilateral breath sounds. His BP is 98/55, and he is tachycardic to 137. He is saturating at 96% on room air. He has no other injuries. What is the appropriate next step in management?
   A. Left chest tube placement
   B. Pericardiocentesis
   C. Central venous access
   D. Proceed directly to the OR for pericardial window
   E. Emergency department (ED) thoracotomy for chest exploration

19.4 Complications

1. Which of the following injuries is most commonly associated with a 10% incidence of avascular necrosis of the femoral head?
   A. Anterior dislocations
   B. Posterior fracture dislocations
   C. Subcapital femoral fractures
   D. Intertrochanteric fractures

2. Which of the following correctly describes the presentation and management of syndrome of inappropriate antidiuretic hormone secretion (SIADH) following traumatic brain injury?
   A. Presents with hypernatremia and hypovolemia; treated with aggressive hydration
   B. Presents with hyponatremia and euvolemia or hypervolemia; treated with fluid restriction and/or hypertonic saline
   C. Presents with hypernatremia and hypervolemia; treated with diuretics and sodium restriction
   D. Presents with hyponatremia and hypovolemia; treated with fluid restriction and desmopressin

3. Which of the following treatments has been shown to decrease complications and shorten hospital stays in patients with retained hemothorax despite tube thoracostomy placement?
   A. Second chest tube
   B. Antibiotics
   C. Use of fibrinolytic agents (eg, tissue plasminogen activator [tPA]) combined with DNase and/or early thoracoscopy
   D. Repeated thoracentesis

SECTION 20 PEDIATRIC EMERGENCIES

20.1 Airway and Pulmonary Emergencies

1. A 3-year-old child presents to the emergency department with fever, stridor, tachypnea, and wheezing, which have been worsening gradually over the course of 4 days. Neck x-ray demonstrates subglottic narrowing and an irregular tracheal contour. What pathogen is **MOST** likely causing this child's illness?
   A. *Haemophilus influenzae* B (HIB)
   B. Respiratory syncytial virus (RSV)
   C. *Staphylococcus aureus*
   D. Parainfluenza virus

2. An 8-year-old boy is brought to the emergency department with an asthma exacerbation. Albuterol and ipratropium were administered; however, his symptoms have continued to progress, and he now appears somnolent and bradypneic with poor air movement on chest auscultation. He is receiving 4 L of supplemental oxygen by nasal cannula, and his Spo_2 is 88%. Which of the following options is the least reasonable next step in management?
   A. Intramuscular epinephrine
   B. Intravenous dexamethasone
   C. High-flow nasal cannula
   D. Heliox

20.2 Surgical Emergencies

1. The pediatric resuscitation team is called to the operating room immediately following the birth of a 39 4/7 weeks of gestation infant with limited prenatal care. Upon arrival, the team finds an alert and vigorous infant with a notable abdominal wall defect and evisceration of bowel. Which of the following is an important first step in the stabilization of this neonate?
   A. Immediate endotracheal intubation
   B. Wrapping the bowel with sterile saline dressings covered with plastic wrap
   C. Providing positive pressure bag-mask ventilation
   D. Attempting to manually reduce the hernia

2. An outside hospital calls for a potential transfer of a 16-month-old patient to your tertiary care pediatric hospital who presented to their emergency department with

intermittent abdominal pain and lethargy. An abdominal film was taken, which revealed massively distended loops of bowel and two concentric radiolucent circles superimposed on the right kidney. In this scenario, what is the **MOST** important factor in deciding to accept this patient to your institution?

A. The lack of a pediatric surgical team readily available at the referring hospital
B. The radiographic findings indicating the need for specialty surgical expertise
C. The mental status of the patient
D. The preference of the parents

20.3 Cardiovascular Emergencies

1. A 2-year-old male is rushed to the emergency department by his parents after being found unresponsive at home. He has a patent airway, and successful bag-valve ventilations are started. He has a weak pulse and is still unresponsive. Intravenous (IV) access is being obtained. The cardiac monitor shows a narrow complex tachycardia at a rate of 220 bpm and no discernible p waves. What is the next step in management?
   A. Shock the patient with 200 J.
   B. Shock the patient with 0.5 J/kg.
   C. Shock the patient with 2 J/kg.
   D. Administer epinephrine 0.01 mg/kg IV.

2. A 1-week-old ex-full-term female presents with fast breathing at home and pallor. Family reports the infant has been interested in feeding but is taking over an hour to finish a bottle. Chart review shows limited access to prenatal care but a normal delivery. Vitals on arrival are temperature 37.4 °C, heart rate (HR) 190, blood pressure (BP) 50/30, and 80% on room air. Examination reveals a pale, lethargic appearing infant, weak but palpable pulses, with capillary refill of 5 seconds, mottled extremities, fine crackles on auscultation without an obvious murmur, and palpable liver edge with slightly rounded abdomen. Chest radiograph shows an enlarged cardiac silhouette with pulmonary edema. Which empiric intervention should you consider based on the above clinical features?
   A. 20 mL/kg fluid bolus
   B. Prostaglandin infusion initiation
   C. Acetaminophen for fever prevention
   D. Milrinone infusion initiation

SECTION 21 ADVANCED CARDIAC LIFE SUPPORT (ACLS) AND ADVANCED TRAUMA LIFE SUPPORT (ATLS)

21.1 Advanced Cardiovascular Life Support and Advanced Trauma Life Support Guidelines

1. A 60-year-old man with a history of hypertension and type 2 diabetes mellitus is brought to the emergency room in cardiac arrest. He achieves return of spontaneous circulation (ROSC) after cardiac compressions, two defibrillations, and a dose of epinephrine. Which of the following is NOT appropriate postresuscitation care?
   A. Immediate cardiac catheterization
   B. Maintaining oxygen saturation of 100%
   C. Crystalloid and vasopressor administration to maintain systolic blood pressure >90 mm Hg and mean arterial pressure >65 mm Hg
   D. Electroencephalogram (EEG) to detect seizures

2. A 20-year-old pedestrian is brought to the emergency department after being hit by a motor vehicle. Trauma evaluation reveals multiple rib fractures, pelvic radiograph shows pelvic fracture, and right leg deformity suggestive for femur fracture. His blood pressure is 80/60, heart rate 125 bpm, respiratory rate 22 breaths per minute. He is agitated and confused, and his extremities are cool. What is his approximate blood loss?
   A. <15% blood volume
   B. 15%-30% blood volume
   C. 31%-40% blood volume
   D. >40% blood volume

SECTION 22 POINT-OF-CARE ULTRASOUND IN THE ICU

22.1 Point-of-Care Ultrasound in the ICU

1. During a focused transthoracic echocardiography (TTE) exam, which view is MOST appropriate for assessing pericardial effusion?
   A. Parasternal long-axis view
   B. Apical four-chamber view
   C. Subcostal four-chamber view
   D. Suprasternal notch view

2. In the evaluation of a patient with suspected deep venous thrombosis (DVT), which of the following is the primary diagnostic ultrasound finding?
   A. Lack of venous compressibility
   B. Presence of B-lines
   C. Increased gain artifacts
   D. Collapsed venous lumen

SECTION 23 BURNS AND THERMAL INJURIES

23.1 Burns and Thermal Injuries

1. A 30-year-old woman sustains severe burns to her face, neck, and upper chest from a kitchen accident. She has singed nasal hairs, carbonaceous sputum, and mild stridor. What is the next best step in management?
   A. High-flow oxygen via a nonrebreather mask
   B. Nebulized epinephrine
   C. Immediate endotracheal intubation
   D. Bronchoscopy to assess airway injury

2. A 50-year-old male with full-thickness burns covering 40% of his total body surface area (TBSA) is being evaluated for surgical management. Which of the following is the best approach to optimize wound healing and reduce mortality?

A. Early excision and autografting within 48 to 72 hours
B. Delayed excision and grafting after 2 weeks to allow for eschar demarcation
C. Enzymatic debridement followed by secondary intention healing
D. Use of topical antimicrobials alone with delayed reconstruction

SECTION 24 DISASTER MANAGEMENT, EXPOSURES, AND OTHER ENVIRONMENTAL INJURIES

24.1 Mass Casualty, Triage, and Epidemic/Pandemic Response

1. Which of the following is the primary goal in the initial response to a mass casualty incident (MCI)?
   A. Transporting all victims to the hospital as quickly as possible
   B. Providing advanced medical care on-site
   C. Ensuring the safety of responders and preventing further casualties
   D. Completing detailed medical histories for each victim

2. During a pandemic, what is the primary purpose of implementing a triage system in health care facilities?
   A. To isolate all infected patients from the general population
   B. To prioritize medical care based on the severity of patients' conditions
   C. To reduce the overall number of patients seeking medical care
   D. To ensure all patients receive equal attention and resources

24.2 Chemical, Biological, Radiological, and Nuclear Exposures

1. A first responder develops acute respiratory distress after recently being exposed to chlorine gas. Despite receiving oxygen therapy, the patient's condition deteriorates. What is the next best step in management?
   A. Administration of corticosteroids
   B. Endotracheal intubation and mechanical ventilation
   C. Nebulized albuterol therapy
   D. Chest computed tomography (CT) to evaluate for pulmonary edema

2. A patient presents to the emergency department after handling an unknown substance at an industrial site. He reports drooling, muscle twitching, and difficulty breathing. After decontamination, atropine is administered. What additional treatment is critical to address the suspected agent's mechanism of toxicity?
   A. Diazepam for seizure prophylaxis
   B. Sodium bicarbonate to correct acidosis
   C. Pralidoxime to regenerate acetylcholinesterase
   D. High-dose steroids to reduce inflammation

24.3 Drowning

1. A 12-year old boy is found unconsciousness in a swimming pool. What is the **MOST** likely cause of cardiac arrest?
   A. Arrhythmia
   B. Myocardial infarction
   C. Hypoxemia
   D. Aspiration

2. While out on a boat trip in a community lake, you notice your friend is thrashing in the water and starting to gurgle and spit out water. After calling for your help on the boat radio, what is the next step in the Drowning Chain of Survival?
   A. Jump in the water and swim to rescue your friend.
   B. Provide flotation to prevent submersion.
   C. Drive boat to the shore to obtain extra help.
   D. Provide basic life support.

24.4 Hanging and Strangulation

1. What is the most common injury that occurs in long-drop hanging?
   A. Asphyxiation
   B. Cerebral edema from acute compression of the neck vasculature
   C. Cervical spine injury
   D. Decapitation

2. Which of the following is NOT an injury typically observed from hanging?
   A. Cerebral edema
   B. Pneumothorax
   C. Vertebral artery dissection
   D. High cervical spine injury
   E. Subarachnoid hemorrhage

24.5 Altitude Injury

1. Two hours after ascending to 3,000 m, a 50-year-old climber develops a headache, fatigue, and nausea. Which of the following pharmacotherapies would have **MOST** likely prevented these symptoms?
   A. Nimodipine
   B. Acetazolamide
   C. Acetaminophen
   D. Ginkgo biloba

2. After ascending to 4,000 m, a mountain climber begins to feel irritable. As he continues to climb, he passes out and becomes unresponsive. What is the **MOST** likely life-threatening diagnosis?
   A. Acute mountain sickness
   B. Carbon monoxide poisoning
   C. High altitude cerebral edema
   D. Meningitis

SECTION 25 INTENSIVE CARE UNIT PROPHYLAXIS

25.1 Prophylaxes and Harm Reduction in the Intensive Care Unit

1. A 62-year-old man with hypertension presents to the emergency department with shortness of breath and is found to be hypoxemic and hypotensive with systolic readings consistently <90 mm Hg despite appropriate volume resuscitation.

He is initiated on antibiotics and vasopressors and is admitted to the intensive care unit (ICU). Lab data are notable for a creatinine of 1.6 mg/dL (baseline creatinine [Cr] several months ago was 0.8 mg/dL), an international normalized ratio (INR) of 1.9, a hemoglobin of 12.9 g/dL, and platelets of 72,000 per microliter. He is requiring 3 L supplemental oxygen via nasal cannula to maintain oxygen saturation in the mid-90s. He does not have a history of chronic liver disease or malignancy, he does not take anticoagulation, his only home medication is lisinopril, and he does not have any known drug allergies. What is the **MOST** appropriate stress ulcer prophylaxis for this patient?

A. Stress ulcer prophylaxis not indicated
B. Proton pump inhibitor as needed for heartburn symptoms
C. Standing daily histamine-2 receptor antagonist
D. Standing daily proton pump inhibitor

2. A 77-year-old woman with a history of chronic obstructive pulmonary disease and chronic low back pain has been admitted to the ICU for 3 days. She initially presented with hypoxemic respiratory failure and septic shock secondary to community-acquired pneumonia. She received intravenous fluids, empiric antibiotics, norepinephrine, and vasopressin. She has been sedated with propofol alone and mechanically ventilated since her initial presentation. Today, she is beginning to show signs of improvement, is requiring less ventilatory support, and is using lower doses of vasopressors to maintain goal physiologic parameters. Her hospital unit uses a daily checklist using the ABCDEF ICU liberation bundle. The purpose of the ABCDEF bundle is to ensure which of the following?

A. Vasopressor doses target the correct blood pressure goal.
B. The patient's pain is appropriately treated.
C. Broad-spectrum antibiotics are used appropriately.
D. Sufficient intravenous fluid resuscitation

SECTION 26 PROCEDURES

26.1 Tracheostomy

1. A 65-year-old female underwent a bedside percutaneous tracheostomy procedure 4 days ago for prolonged intubation. The initial postprocedural course was uncomplicated with successful weaning of her sedation and ventilatory settings. Overnight, she becomes acutely delirious and inadvertently decannulates herself. Prior to decannulation, she was requiring pressure support ventilation with minimal supplemental oxygen. After decannulation, her oxygen saturation is 90% on 15 L non-rebreather mask and remains delirious. What is the next best next step in management?

A. Trial of high-flow nasal cannula therapy
B. Careful replacement of the tracheostomy tube
C. Orotracheal intubation
D. Cricothyroidotomy

2. A 70-year-old male suffered a large right middle cerebral artery (MCA) stroke requiring intubation and urgent thrombectomy 7 days ago. He remained intubated in the intensive care unit during this time due to ventilator-associated pneumonia and poor mental status. After a week of antibiotic therapy, his condition improved, and he was extubated to nasal cannula. Over the course of the next day, he became increasingly somnolent with a weak cough requiring deep suctioning and required reintubation. Bronchoscopy demonstrated no evidence of ongoing infection but a significant burden of clear, thin secretions. Postintubation, the patient remains on minimal ventilatory settings. What is the best next step in management?

A. Complete a course of broad-spectrum antibiotics prior to reattempting extubation
B. Bedside percutaneous tracheostomy in the next 24 to 48 hours
C. Delayed tracheostomy after a course of broad-spectrum antibiotics
D. Extubation after aggressive mucolytic therapy and adequate inline suctioning

26.2 Cricothyroidotomy

1. In which of the following scenarios would an emergent cricothyroidotomy *MOST* likely be indicated?

A. A 45-year-old male with facial fractures after being ejected off a scooter. Heart rate 105, blood pressure 98/65, respiratory rate 22, Spo_2 93% on nonrebreather mask
B. A 24-year-old female unable to move any of her extremities after a motor vehicle collision. Heart rate 53, blood pressure 91/54, respiratory rate 18, Spo_2 96% by nonrebreather mask
C. A 75-year-old male with advanced oropharyngeal cancer who presented with pneumonia. Heart rate 123, blood pressure 95/58, respiratory rate 32, Spo_2 80% on nonrebreather mask
D. A 25-year-old male with significant ligature marks from a hanging injury. Heart rate 109, blood pressure 114/75, respiratory rate 10 and agonal, Spo_2 88% on nonrebreather mask

2. You are called for an emergent surgical airway on a 45-year-old obese male who presented to the emergency department with angioedema whom they could not intubate and could not oxygenate. Which surgical airway technique would *MOST* likely be best in this case?

A. Percutaneous cricothyroidotomy with Seldinger technique
B. Percutaneous tracheostomy
C. Scalpel-Finger-Bougie cricothyroidotomy technique
D. Standard open tracheostomy

26.3 Bronchoscopy

1. A 67-year-old male smoker is found to have a central right upper lobe pulmonary nodule on lung cancer screening computed tomography (CT). He undergoes flexible bronchoscopy with transbronchial lung biopsy. In the recovery unit, he requires a 3-L nasal cannula to maintain saturations >90%. He complains of shortness of breath and pleuritic chest pain. What is the best next step in his workup?

A. Increase supplemental oxygen
B. Administer a nebulizer
C. Obtain a chest x-ray
D. Return to the operating room for repeat bronchoscopy

2. A 59-year-old male undergoes tracheostomy tube exchange. Due to a positional cuff leak, a longer tracheostomy tube is selected. Following insertion of the new tube, end-tidal CO_2 is confirmed. A flexible bronchoscope is inserted through

the tracheostomy tube to confirm the appropriate position. Upon entering the airway, several small lumens are seen straight ahead as well as a branch to the right of the screen. What is the best next step in management?

A. Nothing, as the tracheostomy tube is in the appropriate position
B. Remove the tracheostomy tube and proceed with endotracheal intubation
C. Obtain a chest x-ray
D. Insert a shorter tracheostomy tube

26.4 Tube Thoracostomy (Chest Tube)

1. A 56-year-old male presents to the emergency department with progressive chest pain and shortness of breath since he fell 1 week ago. Chest x-ray shows near-complete obliteration of the left lung. You place a 28F chest tube that immediately drains 2,100 mL of thin old blood. The patient's symptoms resolved, but after a few minutes, the patient again complains of shortness of breath and is now diaphoretic and hypoxic. What is the **MOST** likely diagnosis?
   A. Lung injury
   B. Cardiac injury
   C. Reexpansion pulmonary edema
   D. Chest tube malposition

2. An 85-lb 70-year-old female presented to the emergency department with subcutaneous emphysema of the left chest and up to the neck. A chest x-ray shows a small left hemopneumothorax. She is dyspneic and mildly hypoxic but otherwise hemodynamically stable. You decide that she needs a chest tube. What type of chest tube would be **MOST** appropriate?
   A. 28F straight chest tube
   B. 14F pigtail catheter
   C. 30F angled chest tube
   D. 7F straight catheter

26.5 Thoracentesis, Paracentesis, and Pericardiocentesis

1. A 55-year-old male with a history of alcohol-induced cirrhosis presents with 10 L of ascites removed from his abdomen via ultrasound guided paracentesis in the left lower quadrant. Two hours after the procedure, he becomes hypotensive. His laboratory results show an international normalized ratio (INR) of 1.4, hemoglobin 7.5, a platelet count of 110,000. What is the most appropriate next step in management?
   A. Give 2 L of lactated ringer.
   B. Give 25 g of albumin.
   C. Give 75 g of albumin.
   D. Give 2 units of fresh frozen plasma (FFP).
   E. Give 2 units of packed red blood cells (pRBCs).

2. You have been consulted regarding a 66-year-old female patient with a progressively worsening right-sided pleural effusion in the setting of acute on chronic heart failure. Patient is currently on 4 L nasal cannula. The effusion has been drained before without complication and with significant symptomatic improvement. She has had this current effusion for over 2 weeks and has not improved with medical optimization. INR is 1.5, platelets 180,000. Patient consents to the procedure. You access the pleural space via ultrasound guidance, identify placement of your wire and pass the catheter into the pleural space without complication. You drain roughly 1 L of fluid without complication before the patient reports mild chest pain. You pause briefly, the patient assures you she is okay, and the pain is manageable. You continue to remove another liter, but the patient becomes more dyspneic, and hypotensive requiring you to abort the procedure and place your patient on noninvasive positive pressure ventilation. How could you have reduced the likelihood of this event?
   A. Using a pleural pressure monitor
   B. Prophylactic noninvasive positive pressure support
   C. Placing the patient in left lateral decubitus position
   D. Prophylactic low dose vasopressor

26.6 Feeding Tube Placement

1. Which of the following is an absolute contraindication to percutaneous endoscopic gastrostomy (PEG) tube placement?
   A. Ascites
   B. No clear window for placement on computed tomography (CT)
   C. Coagulopathy
   D. Inability to endoscopically transilluminate
   E. Ventral hernia

2. What is the minimum amount of time a PEG tube should remain in place prior to safe removal with spontaneous closure of the tract?
   A. 3 to 5 days
   B. 2 weeks
   C. 4 to 6 weeks
   D. 12 weeks

SECTION 27 INTENSIVE CARE UNIT TRANSPORT

27.1 Intensive Care Unit Transport

1. Which of the following monitors/devices should be considered when transporting a critically ill patient from one unit to another within a hospital?
   A. Defibrillator
   B. Electrocardiogram (ECG) and pulse oximeter
   C. End-tidal carbon dioxide
   D. All of the above

2. A critically ill patient with a pneumothorax needs to be transported from a community hospital to a tertiary care center 30 miles away. Which of the following modes of transportation is safest for transporting?
   A. Helicopter
   B. Fixed-wing propeller aircraft
   C. Ambulance
   D. Charter jet

SECTION 28 EPIDEMIOLOGY AND BIOSTATISTICS

28.1 Epidemiology and Biostatistics

1. Which study design is **MOST** appropriate for studying a rare disease?

A. Cross-sectional
B. Case-control
C. Prospective cohort
D. Randomized trial

2. A 52-year-old woman is admitted to the intensive care unit (ICU) with septic shock. Her Sequential Organ Failure Assessment (SOFA) score increases from 6 on admission to 10 on hospital day 2. Which of the following statements regarding the change on SOFA is **MOST** correct?
   A. The patient's mortality risk is decreasing due to a rising score.
   B. The SOFA score is static and should not change over time.
   C. Worsening organ dysfunction is occurring, indicating a higher mortality risk.
   D. SOFA cannot be used to monitor dynamic changes in organ failure.

3. A machine learning model is developed to predict extubation failure in ICU patients. The area under the receiver operating characteristic (ROC) curve (c-statistic) for the model is 0.82 when tested on an external population. Which of the following interpretations of the c-statistic for this model is **MOST** correct?
   A. Poor discrimination
   B. Good discrimination
   C. Perfect discrimination
   D. No better than chance

SECTION 29 INFECTION CONTROL

29.1 Infection Control

1. Which central access carries the lowest risk of infection?
   A. Femoral
   B. Jugular
   C. Subclavian
   D. All of the above

2. Airborne precautions are required for the following infection?
   A. SARS-CoV-2
   B. *Neisseria meningitidis*
   C. Rubella virus
   D. *Haemophilus influenzae*

SECTION 30 EMERGENT AIRWAY MANAGEMENT

30.1 Emergent Airway Management

1. A 74-year-old male adult patient with an acutely altered mental status requires a rapid-sequence intubation in the intensive care unit (ICU). After induction of anesthesia, two attempts to intubate the patient with direct and video laryngoscopy by experienced physicians fail. You have called for additional help. Bag mask ventilation with an appropriately sized oral airway is inadequate. Which of the following is the **MOST** appropriate next airway intervention?
   A. Surgical cricothyrotomy
   B. Repeat laryngoscopy attempt
   C. Placement of supraglottic airway
   D. Extracorporeal membrane oxygenation (ECMO) cannulation

2. A 59-year-old female with a history of chronic obstructive pulmonary disease (COPD) is admitted to the ICU with influenza pneumonia, causing moderate acute respiratory distress syndrome (ARDS). She has failed a trial of noninvasive ventilation and needs endotracheal intubation for initiation of mechanical ventilation. Which of the following is the **MOST** likely adverse event observed after induction of anesthesia for emergent airway management (EAM)?
   A. Aspiration of gastric contents
   B. Cardiovascular instability
   C. Cardiac arrest
   D. Severe hypoxia

30.2 Tracheostomy Complications

1. A 60-year-old man with a recent history of acute respiratory failure due to COVID-19 has been mechanically ventilated for the last 14 days. The team has decided to move forward with tracheostomy tube placement to help facilitate ventilator weaning. Two hours after the procedure, the patient develops swelling around the neck and chest and neck crepitus. What is the **MOST** likely tracheostomy tube complication?
   A. Tracheal stenosis
   B. Bleeding
   C. Injury to recurrent lateral nerve
   D. Subcutaneous emphysema

2. A 70-year-old female had a tracheostomy tube placed 3 weeks ago. During mechanical ventilation, the tracheostomy tube cuff requires 10 mL of air to prevent a leak around the cuff. The cuff pressure is measured at 50 cm H_2O. Which of the following complications could develop if the cuff pressure remains greater than the recommended safe range of 30 cm H_2O?
   A. Bleeding
   B. Tracheomalacia
   C. Pneumothorax
   D. Subcutaneous emphysema

30.3 Neck Hematomas

1. Which of the following is NOT considered a risk factor for developing expanding neck hematomas?
   A. Preoperative antiplatelet agents
   B. High blood pressures
   C. Low venous pressures during coughing or vomiting
   D. Coagulopathy

2. You are called to see a 65-year-old female with coronary artery disease, hypertension, hyperlipidemia, asthma, and chronic obstructive pulmonary disease who presents with acute-onset shortness of breath and dysphagia about 1 hour postoperatively from a total thyroidectomy. Her vitals are Spo_2 98% on room air, blood pressure 138/82 mm Hg, pulse 115 beats per minute, and temperature of 37.2 °C. On examination, you notice an asymmetric neck and appreciate a stridor, but no wheezes. Which of the following is the **MOST** appropriate next step in management?
   A. Inform the surgical team and obtain a STAT computed tomography examination of the neck to evaluate for bleeding and hematoma formation.

B. Inform the surgical team and perform a nasopharyngoscopy to evaluate for acute postoperative recurrent laryngeal nerve palsy.
C. Obtain STAT surgical and anesthesia consults and prepare to secure the airway.
D. Inform the surgical team and obtain and place the patient on telemetry and continuous pulse oximeter monitoring and monitor the patient closely in the intensive care unit.

30.4 Laryngectomy and Tracheal Reconstruction

1. You are called to evaluate a 67-year-old male patient who is postoperative day 3 status post laryngectomy for squamous cell carcinoma. He is in respiratory distress with a peripheral oxygen saturation of 88%. Which of the following is the best approach to initially addressing this patient's airway management?
   A. Intubate the stoma with a 6.0 endotracheal tube.
   B. Use a mask to ventilate the stoma.
   C. Use a mask to ventilate the oropharynx.
   D. Intubate the stoma using a Lary tube.

2. A 74-year-old male patient with a history of chronic obstructive pulmonary disease, type 2 diabetes mellitus, and squamous cell carcinoma of the larynx status post total laryngectomy with bilateral neck dissection and adjuvant radiotherapy complicated by pharyngocutaneous fistula s/p partial pharyngectomy and creation of a neopharynx presents to the emergency department with large-volume bleeding from his oral cavity. According to emergency medical services, the patient was found unresponsive in his apartment by a neighbor with a trail of blood around him. He was intubated in the emergency department with a 7.0 cuffed Portex tracheostomy tube, confirmed via tracheoscopy. After stabilization, what is the next best study to confirm the diagnosis?
   A. Computed tomography
   B. Magnetic resonance imaging
   C. Upper endoscopy
   D. Bronchoscopy

SECTION 31 PREOPERATIVE EVALUATION FOR SURGERY

31.1 Preoperative Assessment

1. A 60-year-old patient with a history of hypertension, congestive heart disease with preserved ejection fraction, type 2 diabetes mellitus on insulin, and expanding aortic aneurysm is presenting for open aortic aneurysm repair. Which risk factor is not part of the Lee Revised Cardiac Risk Index (RCRI)?
   A. Hypertension
   B. Congestive heart disease
   C. Type 2 diabetes mellitus on insulin
   D. Surgical procedure type

2. An 84-year-old patient is scheduled for an elective transjugular intrahepatic portosystemic shunt (TIPS). Based on the preoperative fasting guidelines, what is the minimum fasting period for this patient if the patient consumed toast and the procedure is not urgent or emergent?
   A. 2 hours
   B. 4 hours
   C. 6 hours
   D. 8 hours

SECTION 32 ICU ADMINISTRATION AND PRACTICE MANAGEMENT

32.1 Intensive Care Unit Administration and Practice Management

1. An attending physician in the intensive care unit (ICU) works for a week at a time and staffs the unit 10 weeks a year. Which of the following workforce categories **BEST** describes this physician?
   A. Constant
   B. Cyclic
   C. Temporary
   D. None of the above

2. An ICU medical director is working to develop strategies to reduce central line–associated bloodstream infection. Which of the following approaches has been **MOST** clearly associated with increased odds of change management success?
   A. Team member engagement in planning
   B. Implementing a zero-tolerance policy
   C. Mandating extended training for all staff
   D. None of the above

SECTION 33 QUALITY IMPROVEMENT AND PATIENT SAFETY

33.1 Quality Improvement and Patient Safety

1. A community hospital leadership aspires to enhance its patient safety after recognizing an increase in perioperative adverse events. Some of these adverse events include adverse drug events in postanesthesia care unit (PACU) that have concerned the patient safety and quality improvement committee within the Department of Anesthesiology. Which of the following medication safety strategies in addition to technology-related solutions can mitigate the risk of medication administration errors?
   A. Applying the principle of the "Five Rights"
   B. Checklist for medication administration
   C. Allowing simultaneous use of mobile phones by all providers for medication verification
   D. An interdependent check process

2. The Department of Anesthesiology Quality Improvement team is genially invested in ensuring eliminating defects related to the administration of tidal volumes over 8 mL/kg (predicted body weight) to all patients receiving mechanical ventilatory support during general anesthesia. Which of the following framework should be employed?
   A. PDSA cycle—Plan-Do-Study-Act cycle
   B. DMAIC—define, measure, analyze, improve, control
   C. The 5 S—sort, set in order, shine, standardize, sustain
   D. FMEA—failure mode and effect analysis

SECTION 34 ETHICS AND MEDICAL LEGAL ISSUES

34.1 Ethics and Medical Legal Issues

1. Which of the following best describes the principle of beneficence in medical ethics?
   A. The right to self-govern without undue influence from a health care provider
   B. The obligation to promote good and to prevent or remove harm
   C. The goal to promote the greatest benefit to the largest number of individuals while inflicting the least amount of harm
   D. The need to refrain from inflicting harm

2. In the context of critically ill patients, what is the primary purpose of obtaining informed consent?
   A. To ensure the physician has legal protection
   B. To preserve patient autonomy and involve them in shared medical decision-making
   C. To comply with hospital policies and regulations
   D. To document the patient's medical history accurately

SECTION 35 PALLIATIVE MEDICINE AND END-OF-LIFE CARE

35.1 Palliative Medicine and End-of-Life Care

1. Which statement regarding palliative sedation is most accurate?
   A. It is used for any patient experiencing anxiety in the intensive care unit (ICU).
   B. It is initiated when all other comfort-oriented interventions have failed to relieve intolerable suffering in a dying patient.
   C. It is equivalent to euthanasia if death is hastened.
   D. It should be implemented without shared decision-making to avoid burdening the family.

2. Which of the following best describes *primary palliative care* in the ICU?
   A. Palliative care delivered exclusively by a specialty-trained palliative care team.
   B. Palliative care initiated at the end of life after all disease-directed treatments have failed.
   C. Palliative care provided by the ICU team without specialty palliative care involvement.
   D. Automatic palliative care consultation triggered by prognostic mortality estimates.

SECTION 36 HEALTH CARE DISPARITIES AND DIVERSITY, EQUITY, AND INCLUSION IN HEALTH CARE

36.1 Health Care Disparities

1. Ashley, a 28-year-old Black woman, is pregnant with her second child. During her first pregnancy, she experienced preeclampsia and had a traumatic birth experience. Despite expressing severe pain during labor, her pain was underassessed and undertreated. Ashley's current pregnancy is complicated by chronic hypertension. She is concerned about the quality of care she will receive due to her previous experience and has limited access to prenatal care. What factor is **MOST** likely contributing to Ashley's concern about the quality of care she will receive?
   A. Cultural beliefs about pregnancy
   B. History of preeclampsia
   C. Racial and ethnic disparities in health care
   D. Limited access to prenatal care

2. Mrs Rodriguez, a 70-year-old Spanish-speaking woman from a low socioeconomic background, is admitted to the intensive care unit (ICU) with advanced heart failure. Despite her critical condition, her family wishes to pursue all possible life-sustaining treatments. However, they express concerns about the quality of care she will receive, citing past experiences of perceived bias due to their socioeconomic status and language barriers. What is the **MOST** likely reason for Mrs Rodriguez's family expressing concerns about the quality of end-of-life care?
   A. Lack of understanding of Mrs Rodriguez's medical condition
   B. Previous negative experiences with health care due to socioeconomic and language barriers
   C. Cultural differences in end-of-life care preferences
   D. Limited access to advanced medical facilities

36.2 Diversity, Equity, and Inclusion in Health Care

1. Dr Patel, a department chair at a large teaching hospital, realizes that their residency program has a very low representation of underrepresented minorities. Despite their efforts to recruit diverse candidates, the application pool remains predominantly homogeneous. Dr Patel wants to implement an effective strategy to improve the diversity of their residency program. Which of the following actions would be the **MOST** effective initial step to address this issue?
   A. Increase advertising efforts to promote the residency program in diverse medical schools and communities.
   B. Implement a mentorship program for current underrepresented in medicine (URiM) medical students to encourage them to apply.
   C. Review and revise the selection criteria and processes to ensure they do not unintentionally disadvantage URiM applicants.
   D. Host diversity and inclusion workshops for current faculty and staff to create a more welcoming environment.

2. Dr Lee, a senior resident, notices that her colleague, Dr Johnson, often dismisses the concerns of female and URiM trainees during team discussions. This behavior seems to be affecting their confidence and participation. Dr Lee decides to address this issue with Dr Johnson to foster a more inclusive environment. What would be the **MOST** effective way for Dr Lee to address Dr Johnson's behavior?
   A. Publicly call out Dr Johnson during a team meeting to set an example.
   B. Have a private conversation with Dr Johnson, using the ACTION framework to discuss the impact of his behavior.
   C. Report Dr Johnson's behavior to the hospital's HR department without addressing him directly.
   D. Encourage the affected trainees to speak up more during discussions.

SECTION 1 SHOCK

1.1 Distributive Shock

1. **Answer: D.** Sepsis is a medical emergency and physicians must act quickly. This is emphasized by the 1-hour sepsis bundle, which consists of:
   - Measure lactate (remeasure if initial lactate >2).
   - Obtain blood cultures.
   - Start broad-spectrum antibiotics.
   - Administer 30 mL/kg of fluid if hypotension or lactate >4.
   - Start vasopressors to maintain mean arterial pressure (MAP) ≥65.

However, there is the recognition that not all components can be completed within an hour (especially in resource-poor areas).

2. **Answer: C.** Historically, the cross-reactivity between penicillin and cephalosporins was reported to be around 10%. However, the true cross-reactivity is likely less than 2%. Furthermore, cross-reactivity is primarily determined by the R1 side chain and limited primarily to first- and second-generation cephalosporins. Of note, the R1 side chain of cefazolin has a very low cross-reactivity with penicillin. Management of this patient should include a detailed history of their penicillin allergy, including type of reaction (rash, pruritus, bronchospasm, severe cutaneous adverse reactions), time course of reaction (immediate [within an hour] vs delayed [usually >6 hours, although can be weeks to months]), how many years ago was the reaction, how was the reaction treated (hospitalization? epinephrine?), and whether the patient had tolerated other similar medications (eg, ampicillin, other cephalosporins). Patients with mild reactions (rash, lack of mucosal and/or organ involvement, no severe skin reactions) should be able to receive cephalosporins with dissimilar side chains (including cefazolin). Patients who have had immunoglobulin E (IgE)-mediated reactions (anaphylaxis, angioedema, bronchospasm) -or other hypersensitivity reactions

1.2 Hypovolemic Shock

1. **Answer: B.** Rationale: This patient is experiencing acute hemorrhagic (hypovolemic) shock from significant blood loss due to a gunshot wound. Loss of intravascular volume leads to reduced venous return and preload, resulting in a decrease in pulmonary artery wedge pressure (PAWP) and cardiac output (CO). The fall in CO contributes to a decreased mean arterial pressure (MAP). In response, the sympathetic nervous system is activated, causing peripheral vasoconstriction to preserve perfusion to vital organs, which leads to an increase in systemic vascular resistance (SVR). Tissue hypoxia and reduced oxygen delivery increase oxygen extraction at the tissue level, resulting in a decreased mixed venous oxygen saturation (SvO_2).

   Thus, the expected hemodynamic pattern is decreased MAP, CO, PAWP, and SvO_2, with a compensatory increase in SVR, consistent with answer B.

2. **Answer: D.** Assessment of intravascular volume status in critically ill patients is complex and cannot rely on a single parameter. Although this patient has a "normal" CVP, CVP alone is a poor predictor of fluid responsiveness and does not reliably reflect true preload or circulating volume, particularly in postoperative, mechanically ventilated, or vasoplegic patients.

   Dynamic indices (e.g., pulse pressure variation), vital signs, urine output, bedside ultrasound (cardiac and venous assessments), and laboratory markers (e.g., lactate, hemoglobin trends) each provide complementary information, but all have important limitations when interpreted in isolation. Therefore, an integrated, multimodal approach is required to accurately assess volume status and guide resuscitation. This makes answer D correct.

1.3 Cardiogenic Shock

1. **Answer: B.** The patient's clinical syndrome and electrocardiogram indicate cardiogenic shock due to acute myocardial infarction (AMI-CS). The definitive treatment for AMI-CS is coronary revascularization. A pulmonary artery catheter will likely be placed to assist management, but not necessarily to characterize the type of shock; dobutamine may be indicated based on the hemodynamic profile, but it does not represent the most immediate appropriate step. While mechanical circulatory support (MCS) may be indicated, the IABP-SHOCK II trial showed no overall benefit of intraaortic balloon pump (IABP) in AMI-CS.

2. **Answer: D.** The patient's clinical syndrome and data indicate right ventricular (RV) failure as the cause of cardiogenic shock. Optimization of this shock will require a pulmonary artery catheter to guide therapies, including maintenance of MAP (ideally with an agent that does not raise pulmonary vascular resistance [PVR], such as vasopressin), RV inotropic support (milrinone), and perhaps RV unloading (eg, nitric oxide). While an increase in LV preload is needed, judging by the ultrasonographic appearance of a small and hyperdynamic LV, administration of intravenous (IV) fluids (especially without knowing central venous pressure [CVP] and pulmonary capillary wedge pressure [PCWP]) can further dilate and tax the RV without directly increasing LV preload. Augmentation of LV preload will be accomplished best by other measures to improve RV function. The intensivist should also consider indications for right-sided MCS early in a patient with RV failure, such as this.

1.4 Obstructive Shock

1. **Answer: C.** This patient exhibits classic hallmarks of a tension pneumothorax, including tachycardia, hypotension, hypoxia, and evidence of lung collapse with likely mediastinal shift on examination. The diagnostic suspicion is further heightened by the patient's history of severe obstructive lung disease, which may predispose him to a secondary spontaneous pneumothorax from the rupture of a bleb or bulla. The immediate next step is needle decompression (ie, needle thoracostomy), which should relieve the positive pressure within

the left hemithorax to restore cardiac preload while also improving ventilation. A chest tube should then be placed to avoid reexpansion of the pneumothorax. While this patient exhibits severe hypoxia and respiratory distress in the setting of advanced lung disease, the temptation to proceed directly to tracheal intubation (A) should be avoided in the setting of suspected tension pneumothorax. This is because the initiation of positive pressure ventilation could force additional air into the pleural space and accelerate the patient's hemodynamic deterioration. Needle pericardiocentesis (B) would be the appropriate lifesaving intervention for cardiac tamponade. However, this case is significantly more concerning for tension pneumothorax, which may also produce distant heart sounds through shift of the mediastinal contents or movement of the heart away from the left chest wall as intrapleural air accumulates. Lastly, though a stat chest radiograph (D) would certainly support a diagnosis of tension pneumothorax, the patient requires an emergent intervention to avert cardiovascular collapse. Tension pneumothorax is chiefly a clinical diagnosis, and prompt needle thoracostomy should not be delayed for confirmatory imaging.

2. **Answer: D.** The leading concern in this case is for acute pulmonary embolism (PE), a diagnosis that would be supported by the patient's pleuritic chest pain, tachycardia, dyspnea, and history of a likely hypercoagulable state with hospitalization. The first-line modality to confirm the diagnosis of PE in most patients is a computed tomography (CT) pulmonary angiogram, which can be obtained in tandem with initiation of resuscitative measures, PE response team activation, and systemic anticoagulation depending on the patient's presentation. However, bedside ultrasonography can provide valuable information to immediately guide hemodynamic resuscitation and may support the diagnosis. Point-of-care echocardiography in a patient with an intermediate- or high-risk PE may show right ventricular enlargement, flattening or bowing of the interventricular septum (a "D-sign"), right ventricular free wall hypokinesis with apical sparing (the McConnell sign), an underfilled and hyperkinetic left ventricle, and/or a thrombus appearing as a density within the right heart or pulmonary arteries. In some cases, severe tricuspid regurgitation may also be evident, and right ventricular systolic function may be visibly reduced. By contrast, diastolic right ventricular collapse (A) is a specific sign of increased pericardial pressure in the setting of cardiac tamponade and would be unlikely to occur in PE. A lack of lung sliding (B), which is highly sensitive but nonspecific for pneumothorax, would not be a classic finding in the setting of PE. Finally, an increase in respirophasic collapsibility of the inferior vena cava (C) would suggest a decreased right atrial pressure in a spontaneously breathing patient. In the setting of acute right ventricular strain and decreased systolic performance, the opposite—namely, decreased caval collapse in the setting of increased central venous and right atrial pressures—would be more likely, though this finding would still be nonspecific for high-risk PE.

SECTION 2 CARDIOVASCULAR

2.1 Coronary Artery Disease, Myocardial Ischemia, and Infarction

1. **Answer: C.** The diagnosis of acute myocardial infarction (MI) can be made due to the presence of acute myocardial injury (elevated and dynamic troponin levels) with clinical evidence of ischemia (chest discomfort, electrocardiogram [ECG], new wall motion abnormality). The distinction between type 1 and type 2 MI depends on the presence or absence of coronary atherothrombosis, and clinical context is the key. In this case, the patient's presentation is consistent with an acute upper gastrointestinal bleed, which results in anemia, hypotension, and tachycardia. All of these can lead to myocardial oxygen supply-demand mismatch. Type 2 MI can be seen in patients with existing coronary artery disease (CAD) who experience an acute stressor and is a common mechanism for MI in the intensive care unit (ICU) settings. Type 1 MI certainly remains a possibility in this setting; evaluating this possibility would be vital since type 1 MI would require treatment with antiplatelet and anticoagulant agents, which would be relatively contraindicated in acute upper gastrointestinal bleed.

2. **Answer: D.** The image from transthoracic echocardiography demonstrates the presence of a ventricular septal defect as an inferoseptal defect on two-dimensional (2D) echo with color flow from the left ventricle to the right ventricle during systole. The patient's history is worrisome for possible missed MI. Though patients will stop experiencing pain once the infarcted territory is no longer viable, they remain at risk for electrical and mechanical complications of MI as a result of an untreated transmural infarction. In this case, the patient experienced a large inferior wall infarct (right coronary artery [RCA] and posterior descending artery [PDA] territory) and subsequently suffered a cardiac arrest due to presumed ventricular arrhythmia, as well as ventricular septal rupture across the inferior portion of the interventricular septum. Complications from myocardial necrosis are most common 3 to 14 days after MI and are a medical emergency once recognized.

2.2 Heart Failure

1. **Answer: C.** Contemporary "four pillar" of chronic heart failure with reduced ejection fraction (HFrEF) treatment consists of beta-blocker, renin-angiotensin-aldosterone system inhibitor (RAASi) ± neprilysin inhibitor, mineralocorticoid receptor antagonist (MRA), and sodium-glucose cotransporter-2 inhibitor (SGLT2i). The success of these agents in heart failure with preserved ejection fraction (HFpEF) has been suboptimal. Diuretics have a class I indication as needed for symptom relief. SGLT2i has a class 2a recommendation (reducing heart failure hospitalization). The mainstay of HFpEF therapy is in risk factor modification, including management of hypertension and diabetes. Guidelines confer class 2a recommendations for both MRA and angiotensin receptor blocker/angiotensin receptor-neprilysin inhibitor (ARB/ARNi) in HFpEF. Beta-blockers may reduce contractility but contribute to chronotropic incompetence, especially in a ventricle that has impaired relaxation and inability to augment stroke volume (SV). Beta-blockers in some studies have been associated with a higher risk of HF hospitalizations in HFpEF, especially with EF >60%.

2. **Answer: C.** This patient has posttransplant right ventricular (RV) dysfunction. Multiple strategies are used to assist the RV in this state, including: preload optimization, RV afterload reduction, inotropy, and chronotropy. The patient is receiving inotropes, and additional inotropes may be considered (answer B). RV afterload is being addressed with milrinone as well as adding inhaled nitric oxide, both of which will

lower pulmonary vascular resistance (PVR) and help the RV to eject (answer A). In the posttransplant state, the myocardium may be ischemic and the walls edematous; the ventricles may require higher filling pressures for optimization. A central venous pressure (CVP) of 9 mm Hg is mildly elevated for a normal heart, but not necessarily for this immediate posttransplant state; additionally, the ratio of CVP to pulmonary capillary wedge pressure (PCWP) pressure of 0.75 is elevated and corroborates RV dysfunction. Careful trial of crystalloid (answer D), guided by invasive hemodynamic measurements, could improve overall cardiac output (CO). In posttransplant patients, higher pacing rates are often used to augment overall CO when the SV is relatively constrained by a dysfunctional ventricle. Many patients are atrially paced via surgical epicardial wires, at rates >100 bpm; therefore, answer C is incorrect.

2.3 Rhythm Disturbances

1. **Answer: C.** Calcium channel blockers and beta-blockers should be used cautiously in patients with severely impaired left ventricular (LV) dysfunction, as they can precipitate cardiogenic shock through negative inotropic impacts, as well as reduction of heart rate needed to maintain cardiac output. Synchronized cardioversion could be performed if the atrial fibrillation (AF) was causing hypotension; however, the paroxysmal nature suggests that cardioversion may not be successful; and the cardioversion has the potential of stunning the heart. Amiodarone may facilitate rhythm control with the least acute adverse effects.

2. **Answer: B.** This is a regular wide-complex tachycardia, but with evidence of atrioventricular dissociation as shown by discordance of the P waves and QRS complexes (best visualized in the V1 rhythm strip). Given acute hypotension and symptoms, cardioversion would be the next best step according to the Advanced Cardiovascular Life Support (ACLS) algorithm. Of course, the intensivist would also be evaluating multiple causes of hypotension in this patient, which could include in-stent thrombosis, retroperitoneal hemorrhage, and tamponade.

2.4 Valvular Disorders

1. **Answer: D.** This patient has suffered ischemic injury to the posteromedial papillary muscle, which typically has a single coronary blood supply. The result is acute severe mitral regurgitation (MR), which requires diuresis, inotrope, and mechanical circulatory support as a bridge to repair. While all of the other choices are possible and should be evaluated by an intensivist, answers A and B are less likely based on the ultrasonographic result.

2. **Answer: B.** Acute severe aortic regurgitation (AR) is an emergency, and requires definitive intervention; medical management (answer A) is insufficient "and coronary intervention (D) does not directly address the underlying problem." Intra-aortic balloon pump (answer C) is contraindicated in severe AR.

2.5 Pericardial Disease

1. **Answer: B.** Support of preload, with crystalloid, is the first immediate step in the treatment of pericardial tamponade; diuresis would be incorrect. If hypotension develops, then vasoactive agents may be needed for support as a next step, prior to definitive pericardiocentesis.

2. **Answer: D.** Effusive-constrictive pericarditis is a syndrome with concurrent pericardial effusion and pericardial constriction, defined by the failure of the right atrial (RA) pressure to decrease >50% or to <10 mm Hg following pericardiocentesis. In tamponade, diastolic pressure equalization in all four chambers and a blunted Y-descent may be observed, but these do not confirm effusive-constrictive pericarditis. In constrictive pericarditis, the X- and Y-descents are prominent, but without the pericardial effusion and failure of RA pressure to decrease, effusive-constrictive pericarditis is not confirmed.

2.6 Myocardial Disorders

1. **Answer: E.** Presence of at least one of the aforementioned risk factors should prompt implantable cardioverter-defibrillator (ICD) placement for primary prevention (Class IIa).

2. **Answer: B.** Due to impaired lusitropy, reduced ventricular compliance, fixed stroke volume, and rate-dependent cardiac output (CO), vasodilators and negative chronotropic agents should be used with caution in RCM. Excessive preload reduction in restrictive cardiomyopathy (RCM) compromise left ventricular (LV) filling and result in decreased CO. Afterload reducing agents (angiotensin-converting enzyme inhibitor [ACEi], angiotensin receptor blocker [ARB], angiotensin receptor-neprilysin inhibitor [ARNI], nitrates) should be titrated carefully to avoid hypotension and low CO. Similarly, CO in RCM is dependent on higher heart rate (HR) due to relatively fixed and reduced stroke volume. Prolonged diastole at low HR may exacerbate pulmonary congestion. Consequently, calcium channel blockers and beta-blockade should also be administered with caution.

2.7 Congenital Heart Disease in Adults

1. **Answer: C.** The right-to-left shunt fraction is impacted by relative intrachamber pressures and the relative pulmonic versus systemic resistance. The intensivist should recall factors that may increase pulmonary valve resistance (PVR), which, in this case, will render it more difficult for the right ventricle (RV) to eject into the pulmonary artery (PA), thus favoring right-to-left shunt flow. Factors that increase PVR include hypercapnia, positive pressure ventilation, and hypothermia, as well as hypoxemia, acidosis, and others.

2. **Answer: C.** The patient had infundibular and valvar pulmonic stenosis, with chronically elevated RV pressures. If an associated VSD was present, it would have been predominantly right-to-left prior to surgery due to high RV pressure. Following resection and valve replacement, RV pressure drops rapidly, reversing the shunt to left-to-right. This would result in acute pulmonary overcirculation, left-sided volume overload, and clinical heart failure. Perioperative MI or PE are possible but less likely in this setting, and the timing is more consistent with a hemodynamic shift.

2.8 Cardiogenic Pulmonary Edema versus Noncardiogenic Pulmonary Edema

1. **Answer: B.** This patient is presenting with signs and symptoms of acute cardiogenic pulmonary edema (shortness of breath, bilateral crackles, and orthopnea), likely due to heart failure. The most appropriate initial treatment is intravenous furosemide (a loop diuretic), which will help reduce fluid overload. Noninvasive positive pressure, continuous (CPAP)

or Bilevel (BiPAP), may also be useful in this scenario, but diuretics should be prioritized to decrease pulmonary congestion.

A. Intravenous antibiotics would be used if there was evidence of infection, which is not indicated here.
B. Nitroglycerin can be added to the diuretic therapy to reduce preload and improve symptoms. It lowers the venous tone and is useful in patients with persistent symptoms or an inadequate response to diuretics.
C. Intravenous fluids would worsen pulmonary edema by increasing fluid overload.
D. Noninvasive positive pressure can help with oxygenation and decrease the work of breathing but does not directly address fluid overload.

2. **Answer: C.** The patient's presentation is consistent with noncardiogenic pulmonary edema due to a near-drowning event. This form of acute lung injury causes fluid accumulation in the alveoli without an elevation in pulmonary capillary wedge pressure (PCWP). The most appropriate treatment is supportive care, including mechanical ventilation with low tidal volume to prevent ventilator-induced lung injury.
   A. Diuretics may not be as helpful in noncardiogenic pulmonary edema, where fluid overload is not the primary issue.
   B. Intravenous fluids could exacerbate pulmonary edema by increasing fluid in the lungs.
   C. Vasodilators are not indicated in this setting.
   D. Thoracentesis is typically used to remove pleural effusions, not to treat alveolar edema.

2.9 Systemic Hypertension

1. **Answer D.** The patient has evidence of hypertensive emergency with a type A aortic dissection and requires emergent surgery. The most appropriate initial medical treatment is to administer intravenous esmolol (D). Dissection occurred after coronary angiography and percutaneous coronary intervention. Aortic dissection is a rare complication of coronary angiography, but when it occurs, it is most frequently associated with catheter trauma following percutaneous coronary intervention (PCI) to the right coronary artery (RCA). Esmolol is a beta-1 selective adrenergic receptor blocker that is extremely rapid in onset (1-2 minutes after administration). Esmolol can rapidly reduce heart rate and blood pressure (BP), reducing aortic shear wall stress and limiting dissection propagation. Based on the 2025 American College of Cardiology/American Heart Association (ACC/AHA) BP guidelines, patients with a hypertensive emergency with evidence of end-organ malperfusion should be treated to reduce systolic blood pressure (SBP) to <140 mm Hg during the first hour and <120 mm Hg specifically for aortic dissection.

   Treatment with a rapidly acting calcium channel blocker such as nicardipine (A) or vasodilator such as nitroprusside (B) should not be initiated before beta-adrenergic receptor blockade. In the absence of beta-blockade, vasodilator treatment can induce reflex activation of the sympathetic nervous system, resulting in tachycardia and increased ventricular contraction. Other afterload reducing agents such as hydralazine (E) and captopril (C) should not be initiated before esmolol. Hydralazine may promote ventricular contractility (or cause reflex tachycardia) and thus is additionally not recommended.

2. **Answer C.** The most appropriate next step for this patient with preeclampsia with severe features is delivery. Preeclampsia is a gestational hypertensive condition characterized by hypertension (HTN) occurring after 20 weeks of gestation and evidence of end-organ dysfunction. In this patient's case, she demonstrates headache and blurred vision along with an elevation of proteinuria. Other possible features of preeclampsia include elevated liver transaminases in the serum greater than 2 times the upper limit of normal, thrombocytopenia with platelets <100,000/ µL, or kidney injury as evidenced by an elevation in serum creatinine >1.1 mg/dL. Definitive treatment of preeclampsia beyond 34 weeks of gestation is delivery of the fetus after initial immediate stabilization of severe hypertension.

   Delivery should not be delayed administering glucocorticoids such as betamethasone (D), which may promote fetal lung maturity before 34 weeks of gestation in patients with gestational hypertensive disorders. Angiotensin-converting enzyme inhibitors such as enalapril (A) are teratogenic and should be avoided in pregnancy. Recommended first-line antihypertensives to control BP in pregnancy include intravenous labetalol, hydralazine, and immediate-release nifedipine. Intravenous nitroprusside (B) is only recommended for hypertensive emergencies resistant to first-line therapy and the presence of end-organ malperfusion. It carries with it the risk of cyanide and thiocyanate toxicity and can increase intracranial pressure in some patients.

2.10 Pulmonary Hypertension

1. **Answer: C.** The right ventricle (RV) is sensitive to acute increases in pulmonary vascular resistance (PVR). Hypoxia, NOT hyperoxia, is responsible for hypoxic pulmonary vasoconstriction, which can acutely lead to an increase in PVR. Both hypercarbia and acidemia independently lead to increases in pulmonary vascular constriction. High levels of positive end-expiratory pressure (PEEP) may overdistend lungs above functional residual capacity and may lead to increased pulmonary vasculature constriction. However, if optimized, PEEP may decrease pulmonary vascular constriction by maintaining lung volumes near functional residual capacity and its potential to improve oxygenation.

2. **Answer: D.** Pulmonary arterial hypertension (PAH) and recurrent pulmonary embolisms would be associated with >2 WU or elevated PVR. Severe mitral regurgitation would be a cause of left heart–associated pulmonary hypertension (PH) and would be consistent with a pulmonary capillary wedge pressure (PCWP) of >15. In the case of septic shock, PH may be secondary to a high cardiac output state. In high-output PH, PCWP is typically <15 mm Hg, reflecting normal or low left atrial pressures, while the PVR of 1 WU is consistent with low PVR, characteristic of this condition where PVR ≤2 WU.

2.11 Aneurysms and Dissections

1. **Answer: D.** This patient presents with acute onset chest pain and has findings consistent with an uncomplicated type B intramural hematoma (IMH). IMH results from spontaneous rupture of the vasa vasorum, leading to medial hemorrhage. Classic findings on computed tomography include focal, crescentic thickening of the aortic wall, which appears hyperattenuating on noncontrast imaging. The presence of inward intimal calcium displacement can distinguish IMH from mural thrombus. In the absence of complicated IMH

(malperfusion, tamponade, periaortic hematoma, rupture, refractory chest pain) or high-risk imaging features (large or increasing aortic diameter, large or increasing hematoma thickness, progression to aortic dissection), medical management of type B IMH is appropriate. Thus, beta-blockade for impulse control would be the most reasonable next step in this scenario (answer option D). Transesophageal echocardiography (answer option A) is not appropriate as the diagnosis has already been made by computed tomography. Open surgical repair (answer option B) or thoracic endovascular aortic repair (TEVAR) (answer option C) could be considered if the patient develops complicated IMH or high-risk imaging features on a subsequent scan. Vitamin K (answer option E) is not an appropriate therapy for IMH.

2. **Answer: D.** This patient presents after an episode of chest pain and syncope and is noted to have findings consistent with a Stanford type A/DeBakey type II aortic dissection on computed tomography. The involvement of the innominate artery suggests that her syncopal episode may have been related to transient carotid artery occlusion. The patient's young age coupled with her physical examination findings are suggestive of a connective tissue disorder, such as Marfan syndrome. Regardless of the patient's hemodynamic status, the management of all acute type A aortic dissections involves urgent surgical consultation for open surgical repair (answer option D). Transesophageal echocardiography (answer option A) is an appropriate study to characterize ventricular and valvular function after the patient arrives in the operating room (OR); however, surgical consultation should not be delayed for this exam. Intravenous esmolol (C) is a reasonable answer option for impulse control in patients with elevated heart rate; however, surgical consultation is the priority in this case. Magnetic resonance imaging (answer option B) and endovascular repair (answer option E) are not appropriate in this scenario.

2.12 Cardiovascular Infections

1. **Answer: D.** Based on the Modified Duke Criteria, major criteria include positive blood cultures for typical microorganisms, positive laboratory tests, echocardiographic evidence of a vegetation, or direct intraoperative evidence of infective endocarditis (IE). Duke Criteria require two major criteria, or a combination of major and minor criteria, for the diagnosis of IE.

2. **Answer: C.** Transesophageal echocardiogram (TEE) is recommended as the next best imaging modality if suspicion remains for IE despite a negative transthoracic echocardiogram (TTE). Here *Staphylococcal* bacteremia is a higher risk situation for which the sensitivity of TTE alone is insufficient. TEE has a higher sensitivity and specificity than both cardiac computed tomography (CT) and fluorodeoxyglucose (18F) ^{18}F-FDG positron emission tomography (PET)/CT for native valve endocarditis. If the patient is unable to undergo TEE or if TEE (which requires sedation) is not within the goals of care, cardiac CT (choice B) may be the next best option.

2.13 Implantable Cardiac Devices

1. **Answer: C.** This patient's presentation is concerning for device migration and lead perforation, which requires a high index of suspicion to diagnose. Inferior ST-segment elevations may indicate myocardial injury from the lead perforating the right ventricular (RV) free wall, which would cause hemopericardium and, depending on the extent of the migration, could also cause hemothorax; hypotension could result from tamponade and/or blood losses. In this patient, device interrogation showed the inability of the lead to "capture" the RV and abnormal impedance. Migration was confirmed on computed tomography, with the lead tip perforating the pericardium and epicardial fat, and into the pleural space, and with imaging consistent with hemothorax. Prompt surgical repair was performed.

2. **Answer: A.** In biventricular pacing, the ventricular impulse arises from the RV septum (RV lead) and the left ventricular (LV) lateral wall (coronary sinus lead), in order to optimize mechanical ventricular synchrony. In single-lead ventricular pacing, the complex arising from the RV septum will typically have a left bundle branch block morphology and a positive QRS in lateral leads I and aVL as the impulse propagates from the RV to the LV. In biventricular pacing, the impulse from the LV lead would generate a right bundle branch block complex, and because the impulse propagates from LV to RV, the QRS would be negative in leads I and aVL. Ideally, biventricular pacing will reduce the width of the QRS compared to the native complex. Biventricular pacing spikes may be able to be identified as well. These are general rules, and depending on the specific insertion sites and electrical properties of the myocardium, other patterns can be seen (eg, about 10% of patients will exhibit a right bundle morphology from single-RV lead ventricular pacing), but these general rules are useful for the intensivist to understand.

3. **Answer: C.** This patient has symptomatic heart failure with reduced ejection fraction (HFrEF). Despite >3 months of guideline-directed medical therapy, his ejection fraction (EF) remains <35%. He is at risk of ventricular arrhythmias and sudden cardiac death and thus would benefit from implantation of an implantable cardiac defibrillator (ICD) for primary prevention. Cardiac resynchronization therapy defibrillator (CRT-D) is most strongly indicated in patients with HFrEF with EF <35% who have a QRS >150 millisecond and left bundle branch block. For this patient with a mildly prolonged QRS and no bundle branch block, cardiac resynchronization is not indicated (D). Although the patient is bradycardic, it is sinus with a first-degree atrioventricular (AV) block and unlikely to be contributing to his symptoms. Moreover, his bradycardia and AV block are likely the result of his guideline-directed medical therapy (eg, beta-blocker). A pacemaker of any type is, therefore, unnecessary (A, B).

Key Point: ICD placement is indicated for primary prevention of sudden cardiac death in patients with HFrEF <35% for >3 months despite maximally tolerated guideline-directed medical therapy.

4. **Answer: D.** This patient is experiencing an acute, early postimplant complication after receiving a permanent pacemaker (PPM). A patient with hypotension, tachycardia, and distended neck veins is concerning for cardiac tamponade or tension physiology. A chest x-ray (A) to evaluate for pneumothorax and limited echocardiogram (B) to evaluate for new or enlarging pericardial effusion and signs of tamponade should be performed emergently. Bleeding, usually in the form of device pocket hematoma, can also cause tachycardia and hypotension, though unlikely to explain the patient's distended neck veins. A complete blood count (C) is still

useful during the initial evaluation to investigate potential bleeding and in case the patient requires additional procedures (eg, pericardial drain, chest tube). Lead dislodgement and loss of capture or other device dysfunction can happen in the early postimplant period, but it is unlikely to explain this tachycardic patient's deterioration. A device interrogation (D) is, therefore, not helpful in the immediate workup and stabilization.

Key Point: Pneumothorax, cardiac perforation with tamponade, and hematoma are differential diagnoses to consider when evaluating a patient with acute hypotension in the early postimplant period.

2.14 Hemodynamic Monitoring and Bioengineering

1. **Answer: B.** This patient developed left ventricular outflow tract (LVOT) obstruction following the initiation of dobutamine. This can occur if the mitral-aortic angle is narrowed post-mitral valve repair (MVR), particularly in patients with a small left ventricular cavity, a thickened interventricular septum, or systolic anterior motion of the anterior mitral leaflet. In some cases, fixed LVOT obstruction may result from the protrusion of a high-profile prosthetic valve into the outflow tract or due to abnormal subvalvular positioning of the valve, but this is not the case in this question.
2. **Answer: B.** The only clinical scenario that warrants invasive monitoring and assessment is worsening renal function despite intravenous furosemide. In this scenario, a pulmonary artery (PA) catheter can help determine the cause and/or therapeutic intervention required to improve symptoms and renal function in a patient who is failing medical therapy.
3. **Answer: B.** The ClearSight system relies on the analysis of finger arterial pressure waveforms, which can be affected by factors such as peripheral circulation, patient movement, and cuff placement. In patients with atrial fibrillation, where the waveforms are irregular, leading to inaccuracies.

2.15 Cardiac Imaging

1. **Answer: E.** Inferior vena cava (IVC) dilation and reduced collapse are sensitive signs for tamponade in general. In pulmonary hypertension, with elevated right-sided pressures, the right-sided chamber pressures are less likely to collapse due to higher pericardial pressure. The left atrium collapse is a more common sign of tamponade in these patients. In most patients without high right-sided pressures, right atrial collapse is usually quite sensitive and right ventricular collapse is more specific (as it requires higher pericardial pressures).
2. **Answer: E.** Active upper gastrointestinal (GI) bleeding and esophageal strictures are absolute contraindications to transesophageal echocardiogram (TEE). Varices and restricted neck mobility are relative contraindications, and risk-benefit assessment should be performed by the operating providers.

2.16 Pharmacologic Therapies for Cardiac Disorders

1. **Answer: B.** Clevidipine is supplied in a 20% lipid emulsion (0.2 g/mL), which leads to elevated plasma triglycerides with high doses or prolonged use. Triglyceride monitoring is recommended when use extends >24 hours or with concurrent use of agents like propofol, which also provide exogenous lipids. Use clevidipine with caution in patients with egg/soy allergy.
2. **Answer: C.** Methylene blue is a vasopressor used to treat refractory vasodilatory shock, such as sepsis or vasoplegia after cardiopulmonary bypass. Methylene blue's therapeutic effect comes from interfering with the nitric oxide pathway by inhibiting nitric oxide synthase, but it also acts as a monoamine oxidase inhibitor (MAOI). Use of methylene blue in patients receiving serotonergic agents can lead to serotonin syndrome via monoamine oxidase inhibition.

2.17 Cardiac Arrest and Resuscitation

1. **Answer: B.** Waveform capnography is a useful measure to monitor the quality of cardiopulmonary resuscitation (CPR) as end-tidal CO_2 ($ETCO_2$) directly correlates with cardiac output. $ETCO_2$ can be utilized with both bag-mask valve ventilation and an advanced airway during CPR. Patients with an advanced airway who have an initial $ETCO_2$ >20 mm Hg at 20-minutes into a resuscitation are strongly predictive of achieving return of spontaneous circulation (ROSC). A sudden increase in $ETCO_2$ during CPR suggests ROSC has occurred. An $ETCO_2$ <10 mm Hg in intubated patients suggests return of spontaneous circulation is unlikely. An esophageal intubation would demonstrate flat tracing of zero or near zero, while tracheal intubation during cardiac arrest will still have a rectangular waveform during ventilation, and high-quality CPR can generate $ETCO_2$ >20 mm Hg. A pneumothorax will not increase $ETCO_2$ and may cause a decrease in $ETCO_2$ if obstructive shock develops.
2. **Answer: D.** Seizures occur in 5% to 20% of postarrest patients. The incidence may be even higher as the diagnosis of seizures by clinical examination is challenging in patients due to sedation and neuromuscular blockade. Seizure identification and treatment in the postarrest phase of care are important as seizures may lead to a second neurologic insult in a vulnerable patient. Electroencephalogram (EEG) monitoring should be initiated in the postarrest patient who remains comatose. Nonconvulsive status epilepticus may not be clinically apparent and requires EEG for diagnosis. Seizure needs to be ruled out as a cause of the continued comatose state postarrest to accurately neuroprognosticate the patient's clinical course and likelihood of recovery. Prophylactic antibiotics are of unclear benefit in postarrest care and would not promptly address a mental status change. Targeted temperature management should be maintained for at least 24 hours before rewarming. Renal replacement therapy may be useful in certain toxidromes or if severe uremia is present with oliguric or anuric renal failure.

2.18 Hemodynamic and Mechanical Circulatory Support

1. **Answer: A.** Despite F_{DO_2} 100% and F_{IO_2} 90%, the right radial arterial line Pa_{O_2} is only 64 mm Hg. North-south syndrome is a phenomenon that occurs when deoxygenated blood is ejected from the heart due to poor lung function or inadequate ventilator settings. Poor lung function can be due to a variety of reasons, including parenchymal disease such as pneumonia or pulmonary edema, airway disease such as mucus plugging or bronchospasm, or inappropriately low ventilator settings. In this case, the patient has evidence of significant cardiac congestion (due to pulmonary edema) by

right heart catheter-derived hemodynamics. Additionally, the patient has evidence of high afterload based on the arterial line blood pressure of 105/80. Given that the patient has pulsatile arterial pressure with every heartbeat, the most appropriate next step is bedside noninvasive maneuvers to reduce cardiac filling pressures, such as diuresis, increasing positive end-expiratory pressure (PEEP), decreasing afterload with intravenous vasodilators, and reducing extracorporeal membrane oxygenation (ECMO) flows. Diuresis decreases filling pressures by reducing preload. Increasing PEEP decreases left atrial pressure and reduces left ventricular afterload. Decreasing afterload with intravenous vasodilators augments forward flow from the heart, increasing stroke volume and decreasing filling pressures. Decreasing ECMO flows reduces afterload and potentially increases stroke volume. Venovenous ECMO to address hypoxemia would be deleterious, given that cardiac decompensation is the most likely reason for pulmonary edema and north-south syndrome in this case. Although placement of a transvalvular microaxial flow pump may be required, initiating less invasive bedside maneuvers is lower risk and can be performed in more rapid manner, or while in parallel with considering a mechanical unloading strategy. Reducing the dobutamine dose would worsen cardiac contractility and further increase cardiac congestion.

2. **Answer: D.** Valvular insufficiency in patients undergoing support with transvalvular heart pumps can occur for multiple reasons, including entanglement in the mitral valve apparatus, aortic valve insufficiency due to the transvalvular nature of the device, and, rarely, damage to aortic valve leaflets. This patient is exhibiting signs of significant aortic insufficiency, given the combination of elevated pulmonary artery catheter-derived filling pressures, a significant mismatch in flow between the pulmonary artery catheter-derived cardiac output and pump-derived flows, and clinical signs of congestion. Given the possibility of a mechanical cause of valvular insufficiency, initiating pharmacologic inotropic support would be unlikely to address the underlying issue. Initiating venoarterial ECMO before assessing valvular function could result in worsening of aortic insufficiency and pulmonary congestion. While a chest radiograph can assess pulmonary congestion, it is not the ideal mechanism of assessing for valvulopathy or proper device placement. A transthoracic echocardiogram can simultaneously assess for mitral valve regurgitation, aortic valve regurgitation, and device positioning with respect to the mitral valve apparatus. Additionally, transthoracic echocardiography is simple, risk free, and can be performed expeditiously without the need for transportation or sedation.

2.19 Cardiac and Vascular Surgery Postoperative Management and Perioperative Complications

1. **Answer: B.** In an intensive care unit (ICU) with continuous monitoring, a patient who develops pulseless ventricular tachycardia or ventricular fibrillation should be defibrillated up to three times within the first minute. Subsequently, if the patient has not converted, chest compressions should be initiated. There is a much higher risk of chest compressions in patients who have a fresh sternotomy, as the sharp sternal edges may cause laceration of the myocardium. Thus, deviation from standard Advanced Cardiac Life Support (ACLS) is warranted. The best next step is to determine why the patient has developed a malignant arrhythmia; in this case, it is likely due to cardiac tamponade, heralded by the decreased chest tube output, and which will require immediate drainage.

2. **Answer: D.** When reduced motor capabilities are noticed on physical examination after a thoracoabdominal aneurysm repair, there should be significant concern for spinal cord perfusion. The best next step is to increase mean arterial pressure (MAP) and decrease the cerebrospinal fluid (CSF) pressure, which can be done by increasing the spinal drain output. This can be conceptualized by the equation: spinal cord perfusion pressure = MAP − CSF pressure (or central venous pressure [CVP]). While imaging may be warranted at some point, the best first step is to optimize spinal cord perfusion.

SECTION 3 PULMONARY

3.1 Pulmonary Mechanics

1. **Answer: B.** $C_{RS} = V_T/(P_{plat} - \text{PEEP}) = 500/(22 - 10) = 500/12 = 41.7$ mL/cm H_2O. Note that this value is at the lower end of normal (50-100 mL/cm H_2O), suggesting decreased respiratory system compliance.

2. **Answer: C.** *Inspiratory resistance* is the respiratory parameter most reflected in the (PIP–P_{plat}) difference, where PIP is peak inspiratory pressure. Thus, the correct answer is that which causes an increase in airways resistance: C. Bronchospasm increases airway resistance by constricting airways, increasing PIP without changing P_{plat} significantly. This is the classic cause of an increased resistive component in mechanical ventilation. Answer A, pulmonary fibrosis: decreases lung compliance, raising P_{plat}, not the PIP−P_{plat} difference. Answer B, emphysema: increases lung compliance, often with dynamic hyperinflation, but not typically an isolated increase in resistance unless accompanied by bronchospasm. Answer D, flail chest: increases chest wall compliance (paradoxical movement), which may affect total compliance but not specifically airway resistance.

3.2 Respiratory Failure, Mechanical Ventilation, and Weaning

1. **Answer: D.** D is correct because increased CO_2 production is a cause of hypercapnic, not hypoxemic, respiratory failure. While CO_2 retention may accompany some forms of respiratory failure, it is not a primary cause of hypoxemia. A is incorrect as diffusion defect is a classic cause of hypoxemic respiratory failure due to impaired oxygen transfer across the alveolar-capillary membrane. B is incorrect as hypoventilation (reduced minute ventilation) can lead to both hypercapnia and hypoxemia and is listed as a cause of hypoxemic failure. C is incorrect as shunt physiology (perfusion without ventilation) is a major cause of refractory hypoxemia.

2. **Answer: D.** D is correct as explained in the chapter as it emphasizes that failure of a spontaneous breathing trial (SBT) is most often due to incomplete resolution of the original cause of respiratory failure. A is incorrect as SBTs

lasting >30 minutes have not been shown to improve predictive value and are, therefore, not routinely recommended. B is incorrect as SBTs are typically performed with minimal ventilator settings (pressure support [PS] 0-5 cm H_2O, positive end-expiratory pressure [PEEP] 0-5 cm H_2O), not with set rate/volume-controlled modes. C is incorrect as a positive cuff leak test indicates the absence of significant airway edema, not its presence.

3.3 Acute Respiratory Distress Syndrome

1. **Answer: D.** Maintaining a negative fluid balance (A) has been shown to reduce time on the ventilator and in the intensive care unit, but has not been associated with mortality. Similarly, initiation of inhaled pulmonary vasodilators (B) has been shown to improve oxygenation but has not been shown to improve mortality. No study has yet shown how to appropriately select positive end-expiratory pressure (PEEP) (C). Finally prone position (D) was shown in the PROSEVA study to reduce mortality in patients meeting the inclusion criteria defined as: Pao_2:Fio_2 ratio <150 mm Hg on an Fio_2 ≥60% and a PEEP ≥5 cm H_2O.

2. **Answer: A.** Duration of illness (B) and duration of mechanical ventilation (C) can be relative contraindications, and although no specific guidelines exist, many centers err on a duration of illness <14 days and a duration of mechanical ventilation <7 days, as there is concern about a lack of ability to recover and exacerbation of lung injury from a protracted period of injurious ventilation. (D) Inverse ratio ventilation can increase the Pao_2 in patients with severely reduced Pao_2 but can be injurious to the lungs; it should not preclude consideration of venovenous extracorporeal membrane oxygenation (VV-ECMO). Transfer to a center capable of providing VV-ECMO (D) was shown in the CESAR trial to improve outcomes in patients who did not ultimately go on ECMO, and in light of the aforementioned considerations regarding duration of illness, early consideration of transfer in patients with severe acute respiratory distress syndrome (ARDS) is crucial.

3.4 Ventilator-Induced Lung Injury and Ventilator-Associated Lung Injury

1. **Answer: B.** The complexity of ventilator-induced lung injury (VILI) pathophysiology highlights the importance of individualized ventilation strategies. Each mechanism (barotrauma, volutrauma, atelectrauma, and biotrauma) contributes uniquely to lung injury, but they often occur simultaneously, in that one mechanism may affect another. For example, while increasing positive end-inspiratory pressure (PEEP) can prevent atelectasis and atelectrauma, it must be balanced carefully to avoid barotrauma. Additionally, the inflammatory cascade initiated by biotrauma not only damages the lungs but can also lead to multiorgan dysfunction, emphasizing the systemic impact of VILI. Understanding these mechanisms is crucial for developing more effective ventilation strategies, which can improve patient outcomes and reduce the incidence of VILI.

2. **Answer: D.** Low tidal volume ventilation and optimal PEEP levels are foundational elements of lung-protective strategies that reduce the risk of overdistension and alveolar collapse. Limiting driving pressure <*15 cm H_2O* can also help reduce barotrauma. Permissive hypercapnia, although counterintuitive, mitigates further lung injury by avoiding high pressures and volumes. Integrating these strategies requires a nuanced approach, tailored to the patient's dynamic respiratory mechanics and clinical condition. Continuous monitoring and adjustments are essential to ensure these interventions are effective without compromising respiratory function. By prioritizing lung protection, clinicians can significantly decrease the incidence of VILI, leading to better short- and long-term outcomes for patients.

3.5 Pulmonary Embolic Disorders

1. **Answer: C.** This patient has a high pretest probability of pulmonary embolism (PE) based on the Wells score >6, and recent surgery is a significant risk factor. In this setting, the correct next step is pulmonary computed tomographic angiography (CTA), which is highly specific and sensitive when matched to clinical suspicion. A D-dimer is not helpful in high-probability cases as its utility lies in ruling out PE in low-risk patients. A lower extremity ultrasound can be useful, but in this context, it is not definitive and should not delay definitive imaging. A ventilation-perfusion ($\dot{V}/\dot{Q}$) scan may be appropriate if CTA is contraindicated (eg, contrast allergy or renal failure), but CTA is preferred when available. A is incorrect: D-dimer is best used when pretest probability is low; it would not rule out PE here. B is incorrect: While positive deep venous thrombosis (DVT) on ultrasound may support a PE diagnosis, it cannot rule out PE if negative and is not sufficient alone in a high-risk case. D is incorrect: $\dot{V}/\dot{Q}$ scan is second line; CTA is preferred unless contraindicated.

2. **Answer: B.** This patient meets high-intermediate risk criteria: hemodynamically stable with evidence of right ventricular (RV) strain on imaging and biomarker elevation. This group benefits from close monitoring and possibly catheter-directed therapy if deterioration occurs, but systemic thrombolysis is not standard unless they decompensate. A is incorrect: only one criterion (biomarker elevation) is met; this is low-intermediate risk. C is incorrect: This patient is in shock, consistent with high risk, and thrombolysis should be strongly considered unless contraindicated. D is incorrect: no RV strain or biomarker elevation and stable vitals indicate low risk.

3.6 Severe and Life-Threatening Asthma Exacerbation

1. **Answer: B.** This patient presents with a severe asthma exacerbation most likely related to the use of a nonsteroidal antiinflammatory drug. She does have asthma and allergic rhinitis with nasal polyps, and the fact that she took diclofenac the day before supports the possibility of aspirin-exacerbated respiratory disease (AERD). Although usually seen with aspirin, any nonsteroidal antiinflammatory can cause an exacerbation in these patients. Intravenous montelukast may be effective in this patient. Although there are no randomized clinical trials to strongly support its use, the leukotriene receptor antagonist blocks the leukotriene pathway, which is usually overactivated in those patients.

2. **Answer: C.** On the current settings, the patient has significant hyperinflation, which is leading to increased dead space and hypotension. Any maneuver that increases expiratory time and/or decreases minute ventilation should reduce the

hyperinflation. A decrease in respiratory rate or tidal volume will decrease minute ventilation. However, these maneuvers could cause worsening respiratory acidosis (depending on the effects on dead space). In patients with asthma, tolerating a low pH is recommended as long as it does not affect the patient's hemodynamics. Increasing the flow rate or switching to a square waveform will reduce inspiratory time and increase the time for expiration, although peak inspiratory pressures will increase. An increase in positive end-expiratory pressure (PEEP) will not reduce minute ventilation or increase the time for expiration. In fact, increased PEEP could worsen hyperinflation by decreasing the driving pressure during expiration.

3.7 Chronic Obstructive Pulmonary Disease

1. **Answer: B.** The forced expiratory volume in 1 second/forced vital capacity (FEV_1/FVC) <0.70 postbronchodilator is diagnostic for airflow obstruction under GOLD criteria. An FEV_1 of 55% predicted places this patient in the moderate category. Increased total lung capacity (TLC), forced residual capacity (FRC), and residual volume (RV) are consistent with air trapping. A normal diffusion lung capacity for carbon monoxide (DLCO) is common in nonemphysematous chronic obstructive pulmonary disease (COPD) (bronchitis-predominant).

   Why the other answers are incorrect:
   A. Restrictive lung disease: This would show reduced TLC and FVC and a normal or high FEV_1/FVC, which are not seen here.
   C. Severe asthma: Asthma typically has reversible obstruction; this case shows persistent airflow limitation postbronchodilator.
   D. Upper airway obstruction: This would present with flattened flow-volume loops and not the pattern seen here.
   E. Normal spirometry: An FEV_1/FVC <0.70 is not normal, even in older adults. The ATS/ERS would use the lower limit of normal, which would likely also be abnormal in this case.

2. **Answer: C.** This patient meets criteria for acute exacerbation of COPD (AECOPD) with respiratory acidosis and hypoxemia. Her elevated eosinophil count supports use of systemic glucocorticoids. Noninvasive ventilation (NIV) improves outcomes and can reduce the need for intubation. *Why the other answers are incorrect?* Option A: Steroids alone without bronchodilators: incomplete. Bronchodilators are first-line symptomatic treatment for AECOPD. Option B: Cefepime: broad-spectrum and unnecessary unless risk factors for *Pseudomonas* are present (eg, recent hospitalization, bronchiectasis). Doxycycline or azithromycin would be preferred here. Option D: Intubation: not indicated initially. NIV is preferred unless the patient fails or is obtunded. Option E: Pulmonary rehabilitation and long-term oxygen are part of outpatient management, not the acute setting.

3.8 Restrictive Lung Diseases

1. **Answer: C.** The diagnosis is acute eosinophilic pneumonia (risk factors in this patient include selective serotonin reuptake inhibitor (SSRI) and inhalational marijuana use). The correct answer is (C). A bronchoalveolar lavage (BAL) with cell count demonstrating >25% eosinophils would confirm the diagnosis and guide appropriate management (at least several weeks of steroids). Asthma is unlikely in the absence of wheezing and presence of hypoxemia and parenchymal abnormalities. She would likely clinically respond to steroids, though would require a longer course for AEP (A), she does not have risk factors for multidrug-resistant (MDR) organisms and does not appear to be acutely infected (B), and additional less invasive workup should be completed before entertaining a surgical lung biopsy (D).

2. **Answer: C.** The likely diagnosis is myositis-related interstitial lung disease (ILD). Although a rare diagnosis, the constellation of mixed nonspecific interstitial pneumonia (NSIP) and organizing pneumonia (OP) on chest imaging, biochemical evidence of muscle injury (creatine kinase, aldolase elevation), and rapidly progressive hypoxemic respiratory failure should together raise concern for this extremely aggressive form of autoimmune ILD. The correct answer is (C), and empiric therapy (typically in consultation with Rheumatology) should be initiated without delay, given the high mortality associated with myositis ILD. Broadening antibiotics (A) might be reasonable, but there is little evidence of any bacterial infection in the available history and data. Surgical lung biopsy (B) in a critically ill intubated patient would be morbid and delay therapy. Autoimmune serological studies (D) should certainly be sent, but as they can take days to weeks to result, they should not delay immunosuppressive therapy in the interim.

3.9 Aspiration Syndromes

1. **Answer: C.** Aspiration is facilitated by conditions that compromise the protection of the lower airways, such as dysphagia and impaired cough reflex. These factors allow substances to enter the lower airways more easily, leading to aspiration syndromes.

2. **Answer: B.** Aspiration pneumonitis is common in patients with predisposing conditions like a history of stroke, which can lead to impaired swallowing and a weak cough reflex, allowing oropharyngeal or gastric contents to enter the lungs. This results in symptoms such as dyspnea and fever, with characteristic infiltrates on the chest x-ray.

3.10 Pneumonia

1. **Answer: D.** It is important to identify risk factors for pseudomonal infection as well as disease severity when selecting antibiotic therapy and the most appropriate setting for management. This patient has an elevated CURB-65 score of 3 (patient's age, blood urea nitrogen [BUN] ≥19 mg/dL, and confusion), raising his 30-day risk of mortality to 14%. While not all the elements of the CURB-65 score are provided, these three findings confirm that outpatient management is inappropriate, *Answer A*. His history of bronchiectasis is a risk factor for pseudomonal infection, and antibiotic selection must include coverage for this pathogen, *Answer B*. This patient needs to be treated in the hospital; however; his oxygen requirement is small, and he is normotensive; therefore, intensive care unit (ICU) admission is not essential, *Answer C*. Further, since the patient is only on 3 L/min nasal cannula, hydrocortisone for severe community-acquired pneumonia (CAP) is not indicated, *Answer C*. This patient can be reasonably managed in the general hospital ward with appropriate antipseudomonal coverage.

2. **Answer: C.** There are several important parts of this patient's history to take note of first, she is under age 60, she has a history of alcohol misuse, and she was unconscious at the

time of presentation, all of which are strong risk factors for empyema. Empyema is further suggested by the culture of *Streptococcus pneumoniae* on respiratory specimens, *Answer C*. While many of her risk factors for empyema are shared with the development of a ventilator-associated pneumonia (VAP), the time course, appropriate antibiotic selection, and the chest imaging are all more consistent with an empyema, *Answer A*. Over the course of the hospital stay, she has had an improvement in her oxygen requirement, making worsening acute respiratory distress syndrome (ARDS) incorrect, *Answer D*. Antibiotics, especially penicillin-derived agents, are amongst the most common causes of drug fever in the ICU. It is rare for a drug fever to cause shock, and there is often a development of eosinophilia and examination findings such as rash or blistering of the skin, *Answer B*.

3.11 COVID-19

1. **Answer: B.** Steroid therapy is not indicated in COVID-19–positive patients without hypoxemia and may cause harm.

2. **Answer: D.** Early intubation upon arrival in the intensive care unit (ICU) is associated with better outcomes. Baricitinib or tocilizumab should be added for patients with severe hypoxemic respiratory failure, and there is no indication for remdesivir in immunocompetent ICU patients. Given the bleeding risks, treatment dose enoxaparin should be changed to prophylactic dosing for patients in the ICU.

3.12 Pleural Disease

1. **Answer: B.** pH <7.20 indicates a complicated effusion requiring drainage.

2. **Answer: B.** The American College of Clinical Pharmacy (ACCP) guidelines recommend recurrence prevention after the second primary spontaneous pneumothorax (PSP) or first secondary spontaneous pneumothorax (SSP).

3.13 Hemoptysis

1. **Answer: B.** This is a patient presenting with massive hemoptysis as defined by both volume and physiologic consequences. The priority is, therefore, to stabilize and rapidly intervene on any reversible underlying etiologies. A computed tomography (CT) scan (A) would be a reasonable method to localize the source(s) of bleeding but should not be performed before reversal of anticoagulation. Bronchoscopy (C) and invasive angiography (D) might be appropriate diagnostic and therapeutic interventions but also should occur only after reversal of coagulopathy.

2. **Answer: D.** The patient has a pulmonary-renal syndrome, most consistent with vasculitis. Corticosteroids represent the only presented choice that intervenes on the underlying source of hemoptysis.

3.14 Upper Airway Diseases and Disorders

1. **Answer: B.** The most common complication after thyroidectomy is vocal fold paralysis. The recurrent laryngeal nerve is prone to injury in this scenario because of the proximity of the thyroid gland to the nerve as it enters the larynx. The rates of injury increase with emergency cases, and the nerve would be difficult to identify in the wound in cases of hematoma evacuation.

2. **Answer: B.** The clinical scenario describes an acute tonsillitis evolving into a peritonsillar abscess. The scenario does not suggest impeding airway distress. A computed tomography (CT) scan is unlikely to be necessary given the clear physical examination findings, and intravenous antibiotics alone are not sufficient to treat the abscess. For a stable patient with fluctuant swelling around the tonsil, an incision and drainage is most appropriate. This can be performed bedside or in the operating room.

3.15 Pulmonary Vasculitic and Autoinflammatory Disorders

1. **Answer: B.** Eosinophilic granulomatosis with polyangiitis (EGPA) is highly associated with antecedent atopic disease and characteristically exhibits MPO-ANCA (rather than PR3-ANCA positivity, B). Linear immunoglobulin G (IgG) deposition (C) would be more consistent with Goodpasture syndrome while pulmonary artery (PA) aneurysms are classic in Behçet syndrome.

2. **Answer: C.** For patients critically ill with complications of GPA, current guidelines recommend high-dose steroids and rituximab as induction therapy. Steroids alone (A) are unlikely to provide adequate disease control at doses tolerable for long-term use, and B-cell depleting agents require weeks for maximal effect. Cyclophosphamide (B) is comparably effective to rituximab but has a more severe side-effect profile, and there is no role for plasmapheresis in antineutrophil cytoplasmic antibody (ANCA)-associated vasculitis. Mepolizumab (D) would be an appropriate therapy for EGPA but has no role in the treatment of GPA.

3.16 Inhalational Injuries and Tracheobronchitis in the Intensive Care Unit

1. **Answer: C.** This patient shows signs of impending airway obstruction from thermal injury to the upper airway. Delaying intubation risks complete obstruction due to edema. Chest imaging (E) and corticosteroids (D) will not prevent obstruction. Racemic epinephrine (A) is useful for laryngotracheitis, but not for thermal injury.

2. **Answer: D.** Supportive care is first line for chemical inhalation injuries. Humidified air and bronchodilators help mitigate airway inflammation and bronchospasm. Corticosteroids (A) and antibiotics (C) are not routinely indicated. Bronchoscopy (B) is not urgent unless there is diagnostic uncertainty or airway obstruction. Nebulized bicarbonate (E) has anecdotal use, but is not standard of care.

3.17 Pulmonary Contusion

1. **Answer: B.** The volume of contused lung, or more specifically the ratio of contused and total lung volume, predicts the severity of respiratory failure and progression to acute respiratory distress syndrome (ARDS) or pneumonia.

2. **Answer: C.** X-ray and ultrasound are easily accessible and quick to perform and can reveal the presence of airspace disease. However, computed tomography (CT) offers significant advantages over each: It can further characterize airspace disease, quantify and delineate the anatomy of the involved lung, and provide additional information about concomitant bony thoracic trauma. Nevertheless, the other imaging

modalities do have a role in serial assessment to inform ongoing management. Bronchoscopy can be a useful diagnostic and therapeutic tool when bronchial occlusion due to secretions, blood, or aspirated foreign bodies is suspected.

3.18 Flail Chest and Surgical Stabilization of Rib Fractures

1. **Answer: A.** Recent clinical trial evidence (Dehghan et al 2022) demonstrated that operative management of rib fractures improved outcomes for the subset of patients who were intubated and ventilated at the time of randomization. Operative management similarly improves outcomes for individuals with flail chest (Marasco et al 2013). Surgical stabilization of rib fractures (SSRF) may be appropriate in any of the other scenarios, but the evidence base is not as strong.

2. **Answer: D.** A substantial body of retrospective clinical evidence has shown that time-to-surgery directly affects outcomes in patients undergoing SSRF. While ongoing hemodynamic instability, or higher priority injuries requiring operative intervention may cause necessary delays, SSRF should be performed as soon as possible after the decision to operate is made.

3.19 Sleep-Related Breathing Disorders

1. **Answer: D.** According to the criteria, an apnea-hypopnea index (AHI) or respiratory disturbance index (RDI) >15 events/hour can diagnose obstructive sleep apnea (OSA), even in the absence of symptoms. A is incorrect as AHI >5 requires symptoms (eg, fatigue, sleepiness, snoring) to diagnose OSA. B is incorrect as AHI includes only apneas and hypopneas—respiratory effort–related arousals (RERAs) are not included; those are part of the RDI. C is incorrect as AHI is the primary index used to assess OSA severity and make the diagnosis. RDI includes RERAs and may identify upper airway resistance syndrome, but is not used alone for severity grading.

2. **Answer: C.** Patients with OSA are at risk for postoperative arrhythmias due to sedation-related decreases in upper airway dilator muscle tone and blunted central respiratory drive, which exacerbate sleep-disordered breathing during recovery. A is incorrect because while OSA is associated with cardiovascular disease, pulmonary embolism is not a recognized direct consequence of impaired venous return in this context. B is incorrect as airway collapse increases perioperative airway resistance, but is not associated with reduced blood loss. D is incorrect as continuous positive airway pressure (CPAP) use is generally safe, including during pregnancy, and not associated with anaphylaxis.

3.20 Pulmonary Imaging

1. **Answer: C.** The chest radiography (CXR) demonstrates a large left pleural effusion, left lung atelectasis, and contralateral mediastinal shift (tension hydrothorax). Note the widened intercostal space on the left. The pleural effusion creates an acoustic window, which helps visualize the thoracic spine above the diaphragm (spine sign). Soft blood pressure (BP) is likely due to the decreased preload.

   Choice A describes the findings in atelectasis, which could be due to the mucous plug. In atelectasis, there is an ipsilateral mediastinal shift and a narrowed intercostal space.
   Choice B describes pneumonia.
   Choice D describes cardiogenic pulmonary edema, which usually has bilateral manifestation.

2. **Answer B.** The bedside lung ultrasound (LUS) shows a pathognomonic sign of pneumothorax called the lung point. M mode shows the transition from the seashore to the stratosphere sign and indicates the separation of the visceral pleura from the chest wall at the margin of pneumothorax (PTX). Choice B demonstrates the left PTX. Note the separation of visceral pleura.

   Choice A shows endotracheal tube (ETT) migration into the right main bronchus, resulting in complete left lung collapse.
   Choice C shows the left costophrenic angle obliterated due to the pleural effusion.
   Choice D demonstrates left lower lobe atelectasis due to mucous plugging.

3.21 Pharmacologic Therapies for Pulmonary Disorders

1. **Answer: B.** Short-acting beta-2 agonist, with or without a short-acting anticholinergic, is the preferred initial treatment for acute chronic obstructive pulmonary disease (COPD) exacerbations (B is correct). Currently, there are no clinical studies that have demonstrated a benefit from the use of long-acting bronchodilators (either beta-2 agonist or anticholinergic) with or without inhaled corticosteroid during the acute exacerbation. Although these medications can be continued during an acute exacerbation, there is no evidence increasing the dosage of maintenance inhalers for severe COPD exacerbation (A is incorrect). Intravenous methylxanthines (theophylline or aminophylline) are not recommended to use due to the significant side effects, including atrial and ventricular arrhythmias and seizures (C is incorrect). Escalation to triple therapy with long-acting beta-2 agonist, long-acting antimuscarinic, and inhaled corticosteroid is warranted at the time of discharge due to ongoing exacerbations; there is no role in acute exacerbation management (D is incorrect).

2. **Answer: D.** Advanced symptomatic heart failure with decreased cardiac output has to be treated acutely, and IV epoprostenol can be initiated for acute management in the intensive care unit (ICU); the short half-life allows rapid dose adjustments. If available, expert consultation with pulmonary hypertension specialist familiar with medications and side effects is useful but should not delay treatment (D is correct). While drugs such as tadalafil and macitentan can be used in the long-term management of pulmonary arterial hypertension (PAH), prostacyclin analogs such as epoprostenol and treprostinil are considered first-line medications in acute/severe decompensated PAH. In the setting in which a PDE5 was initiated, sildenafil would be preferred due to its shorter half-life compared to tadalafil (A, B, C are incorrect).

3.22 Thoracic Surgery Postoperative Management and Perioperative Complications

1. **Answer: D.** Development of postpneumonectomy pulmonary edema is a potentially devastating complication that can quickly lead to acute respiratory distress syndrome (ARDS), with a high associated mortality of >50%. The risk is higher after right pneumonectomy, and the causes

are multifactorial including barotrauma or high delivered oxygen concentration during single-lung ventilation in the operating room, perioperative fluid overload, and reperfusion injury to the remaining lung. Treatment is supportive starting with supplemental oxygen and diuresis. If mechanical ventilation is required, lung-protective ventilation strategies should be employed using low-tidal volumes of 6 mL/kg of predicted body weight and ensuring plateau pressures are <30 cm H_2O.

2. **Answer: C.** Chylothorax can usually be diagnosed clinically by the identification of milky chest tube output after the patient has started eating fat-containing food. However, about 30% of chylothoraces present without the classic milky appearance. If the patient is unable to eat or if the chest tube output remains high despite diuresis, the fluid can be tested for triglycerides, lymphocytes, and chylomicrons. Triglyceride level >110 mg/dL, lymphocyte count >90%, or any detection of chylomicrons in the fluid is diagnostic of chyle.

3.23 Veno-Venous Extracorporeal Membrane Oxygenation

1. **Answer: D.** The most likely cause of this patient's hypoxemia is recirculation. Recirculation is a common phenomenon in venovenous extracorporeal membrane oxygen (VV ECMO) and is characterized by the drainage of oxygenated, postmembrane blood through the drainage limb before it reaches systemic circulation. All patients will have some degree of recirculation, and its clinical relevance increases as the percentage of recirculated ECMO flow increases. To confirm the presence of recirculation, pre- and postmembrane oxygen saturation (or blood gases) can be checked, in addition to Svo_2. An elevated premembrane oxygen saturation (or Po_2) suggests that the drainage limb is draining oxygenated blood and confirms the presence of recirculation, while if the premembrane oxygen saturation is equal to Svo_2, there is no recirculation. A chest x-ray should be performed to evaluate cannula positioning. Recirculation can be mitigated by reducing flow rates, ensuring proper cannula positioning (~10 cm apart), or adding an additional limb, in certain cases.

2. **Answer: B.** The rapid reduction in this patient's $Paco_2$ puts her at risk for intracerebral hemorrhage. In patients with severe respiratory acidosis, rapid reductions in $Paco_2$ have been associated with an increased risk of intracerebral hemorrhage and an increased risk of neurologic injury. The optimal rate of reduction in $Paco_2$ has not been defined; however, a gradual reduction in the first 24 hours with close monitoring of blood gases is recommended to reduce this risk.

SECTION 4 GASTROINTESTINAL AND HEPATOBILIARY

4.1 Abdominal Compartment Syndrome

1. **Answer: B.** Abdominal compartment syndrome (ACS) is a clinical diagnosis that requires urgent surgical evaluation. Signs of compartment syndrome include oliguria/anuria, rising creatinine, tense abdominal distention, and difficulty with ventilation. Objective measures can include bladder pressure or proton pump inhibitors (PIPs), but these should not delay clinical decision-making. There is no definitive radiographic finding that diagnoses compartment syndrome. Definitive treatment includes laparotomy to relieve the pressure. Adjuncts include muscle relaxation and diuresis as able.

2. **Answer: C.** The high intra-abdominal pressures of ACS cause upward displacement of the diaphragm, resulting in decreased thoracic volumes and pulmonary compliance, which lead to an increase in peak airway pressures, ventilation and perfusion mismatch, hypoxia, hypercapnia, and acidosis. This can be measured with bladder pressure, as the abdominal pressures are directly translated to the bladder. Additionally, this abdominal pressure compresses the kidneys and obstructs venous outflow, resulting in decreased glomerular filtration rate (GFR) and urine output.

4.2 Acute Pancreatitis

1. **Answer: C.** There are multiple types of pancreatic fluid collections, but sticking to strict indications for intervention helps avoid unnecessary procedures and concomitant complications. Acute interstitial pancreatitis requires no acute intervention, though patients may progress to develop collections ultimately requiring procedural involvement. The inability to tolerate oral intake can often be managed with enteral access or parenteral support. Severe acute pancreatitis warranting intensive care unit (ICU) admission may require multiple critical care adjuncts, but the pancreatitis itself does not necessarily demand immediate intervention. Infected pancreatic collections almost always require intervention following the step-up approach.

2. **Answer: A.** The severe inflammatory response associated with acute pancreatitis frequently leads to capillary leak and intravascular hypovolemia. Consequently, crystalloid resuscitation has become a key principle for management. However, recognizing the complications of volume overload should cause providers to be judicious with their use of fluid. Doing so involves a clear focus on end-organ function as opposed to set rates without consistent reevaluation of an ongoing need for volume. Balanced crystalloid solutions have demonstrated improved outcomes as compared to normal saline.

4.3 Hepatic Dysfunction and Hyperbilirubinemia

1. **Answer: B.** Part of direct bilirubin includes conjugated bilirubin that is covalently linked to albumin. This fraction is called delta bilirubin. Delta bilirubin makes up a significant portion of total bilirubin in patients with hepatobiliary disease or cholestatic jaundice. Because it is bound to albumin, delta bilirubin's half-life is >12 to 14 days compared with about 4 hours for conjugated bilirubin. It, therefore, remains even after other markers of liver dysfunction have gone. And because it is bound to albumin, it is not excreted in urine. In the abovementioned scenario if there is no other evidence of ongoing liver damage and no bilirubinuria, an extensive workup is unnecessary.

2. **Answer: C.** The portal vein provides 80% of the liver's blood flow, not its oxygen supply. Because the portal vein contains much less oxygen than the blood in the hepatic artery, both contribute approximately equally to the liver's oxygen supply.

The liver does have the highest oxygen extraction capacity of any organ in the body, which is why it can maintain its oxygenation even when hepatic blood flow is significantly reduced. If cardiac output drops and portal venous flow decreases, the *hepatic artery buffer response* causes a compensatory increase in hepatic blood flow. This is thought to be due to the vasodilating properties of local metabolites, such as adenosine.

3. **Answer: D.** Liver dysfunction is relatively common in intensive care units (ICUs), being seen in 10% to 30% of patients. It has also been associated with worse overall outcomes in some studies. Most hepatic dysfunction in the ICU is multifactorial in nature, with sepsis being the most common cause. De novo viral hepatitis is quite unusual in the ICU.

4.4 Hepatic Encephalopathy

1. **Answer: B.** Although it is reasonable to measure a serum ammonia level in this setting, this mildly increased ammonia level is of no clinical importance, since similar levels may be seen in patients with cirrhosis but without overt hepatic encephalopathy (HE). A computed tomography (CT) of the head, while not a critical part of a workup for HE (unless looking for evidence of increased intracranial pressures in fulminant hepatic failure), is useful to rule out a massive stroke, given the patient's presentation in shock.

2. **Answer: C.** While lactulose is the de facto gold standard modality in the treatment of HE, no randomized controlled trials exist that have demonstrated its efficacy—at this point, it would probably be considered unethical to compare lactulose with a placebo. A few small studies support the use of flumazenil in HE, but it is not considered a standard of care. Protein in the diet is a source of nitrogenous compounds, including ammonia. However, a low-protein diet is no longer recommended in these patients since they tend to be malnourished at baseline. HE is not a risk factor for propofol infusion syndrome (PRIS)—propofol is an excellent choice for sedation in these patients. The use of polymyxin B hemoperfusion is common in some countries (such as Japan) to treat sepsis; they have no role in the treatment of HE.

3. **Answer: E.** All the choices reflect potential mechanisms for the beneficial effect of lactulose.

4.5 Hepatorenal Syndrome

1. **Answer: D.** Hepatorenal syndrome-acute kidney injury (HRS-AKI) is often precipitated by an acute event. It is a diagnosis of exclusion, but a high index of suspicion must be maintained in patients with cirrhosis. It is characterized by a rise in serum creatinine by $\geq$0.3 mg/dL ($\geq$26.5 μmol/L) within 48 hours, or an increase in serum creatinine to $\geq$1.5 times baseline in the prior 7 days that does not respond to volume expansion. Prerenal AKI often occurs secondary to infection, but after adequate treatment with antibiotics for spontaneous bacterial peritonitis, and with appropriate volume resuscitation, one would expect that AKI related to this would plateau or resolve with standard therapy. When investigating the cause of an AKI in a patient at risk for HRS-AKI, urine sodium levels are helpful as ongoing intense sodium avidity in the absence of other causes of prerenal physiology increases the diagnostic likelihood of HRS-AKI.

Key Point: HRS-AKI is a diagnosis of exclusion. AKI is a common diagnosis in hospitalized patients, so the index of suspicion for HRS-AKI should be high in hospitalized patients with cirrhosis. Urine sodium is an affordable, noninvasive, and useful test in this scenario.

2. **Answer: D.** An increase in splanchnic vascular tone, coupled with volume expansion, is the current therapeutic paradigm for HRS-AKI. The use of terlipressin and 25% albumin is considered first-line therapy. Terlipressin increases vascular tone and, therefore, hydrostatic pressure in the pulmonary circulation. Albumin increases colloid oncotic pressure. The resultant change in Starling forces at the pulmonary capillary-alveolar interface because of therapy may cause pulmonary edema and resultant hypoxia. In patients who already have intravascular volume overload from heart failure, treatment for HRS-AKI may precipitate hypoxic respiratory failure. Clinical examination with a focus on intravascular volume status should be performed before therapy is initiated to mitigate against adverse respiratory events.

Key Point: In patients with HRS-AKI, intravascular volume status should be assessed before starting treatment due to the high risk of pulmonary edema associated with volume expansion therapy.

4.6 Bowel Ischemia and Perforation

1. **Answer: E.** This patient is presenting with acute mesenteric ischemia, likely from an embolus secondary to atrial fibrillation. His computed tomography (CT) scan shows an occlusion of the superior mesenteric artery (SMA) and poor perfusion of his small bowel. Time is of the essence. Prompt surgical evaluation by both general and vascular surgeries, with simultaneous initiation of anticoagulation is key. Initiation of broad-spectrum antibiotics is also important in this patient who may already have bowel ischemia. While the patient may become ill and ultimately benefit from arterial line placement for hemodynamic monitoring, this is not a top priority at this time, and efforts should be focused on fixing the problem at hand.

2. **Answer: D.** Given that this patient is hemodynamically stable, obtaining a CT scan with intravenous (IV) and oral contrast will be the highest diagnostic yield. Specifically, with concerns for a perforated ulcer, the addition of oral contrast is helpful. IV contrast allows for better definition of the organs and for assessment of ischemia. A plain film may be helpful, specifically in the patient who may be in undifferentiated shock and is too unstable to obtain a CT, but that is not this patient.

4.7 Acute Mesenteric Ischemia

1. **Answer: B.** The patient has a history of significant vascular disease, which likely puts the patient at high risk of atherosclerotic disease of the mesenteric vasculature. This is further supported by her history of postprandial abdominal pain and weight loss over the prior several months. Although she is admitted to the hospital with another issue, it is not uncommon for patients with significant vascular disease to develop acute thrombosis of chronic atherosclerotic lesions. As such, the most likely etiology of this patient's mesenteric ischemia is mesenteric arterial thrombosis.

2. **Answer: C.** This relatively young patient with a history of deep venous thrombosis (DVT) and recent oral contraceptive pill (OCP) use with no other vascular risk factors is likely presenting with mesenteric venous thrombosis. Her history should be suspicious for a baseline hypercoagulable state, especially when she is not on anticoagulation. Her electrocardiogram (ECG) is normal, which also decreases the likelihood that she has an embolic phenomenon.

3. **Answer: D.** The patient has concern for mesenteric ischemia after being admitted with an ST-elevation myocardial infarction (STEMI). Computed tomographic angiography (CTA) does not demonstrate any evidence of embolic or thrombotic disease of the superior mesenteric artery (SMA), but rather diffuse narrowing, involving the branches as well. The history and imaging findings are specifically concerning for nonocclusive mesenteric ischemia. Aggressive supportive care is the initial treatment of choice with reversal of the underlying condition and optimization of cardiac output and elimination of vasopressors. If this fails to resolve the ischemia, then local intra-arterial papaverine can be attempted.

4.8 Gastrointestinal Bleeding

1. **Answer: B.** Mallory-Weiss tears are longitudinal mucosal lacerations found at the gastroesophageal junction or in the gastric cardia. They are most commonly caused by severe vomiting or retching, often after excessive alcohol intake. These tears lead to upper gastrointestinal bleeding and typically present with hematemesis. The other options are not characterized by mucosal lacerations.

2. **Answer: B.** A tagged red blood cell (RBC) scan, also known as a nuclear medicine bleeding scan, uses radiolabeled RBCs to detect active gastrointestinal (GI) bleeding. It can identify bleeding at low rates (0.1-0.35 mL/min), making it sensitive for intermittent or slow bleeds. However, its spatial resolution is poor, and it often cannot precisely localize the bleeding site, leading to accuracy rates of only 40% to 60%. Computed tomographic (CT) angiography detects bleeding at a higher rate of 0.3 to 0.5 mL/min but has lower spatial resolution. Angiography requires faster bleeding (≥0.5-1.0 mL/min) and offers the ability to both diagnose and treat (embolization). Push enteroscopy is a diagnostic endoscopic technique used to evaluate the small intestine, not to detect bleeding rates.

4.9 Malabsorption in the Critically Ill Patient

1. **Answer: B.** The patient's history of chronic pancreatitis, coupled with symptoms of diarrhea, feeding intolerance, and particularly the finding of fat globules in the stool (steatorrhea), strongly suggests pancreatic exocrine insufficiency (PEI). Severe critical illness and abdominal surgery can acutely worsen preexisting PEI. Fecal elastase-1 is a noninvasive and relatively easy-to-perform stool test that has fair sensitivity and specificity for diagnosing PEI, especially severe cases, making it the best initial diagnostic step in this context. While small intestinal bacterial overgrowth (SIBO) (A) can cause similar symptoms, PEI is more directly suggested by the history and steatorrhea; breath tests for SIBO are often unreliable in critically ill patients with dysmotility. Intestinal ischemia (C) is a critical concern in sepsis and surgery, but while it can cause malabsorption, the prominent steatorrhea points away from primary ischemia as the *most likely* initial cause, and serum lactate is a marker of global hypoperfusion/anaerobic metabolism, not a direct test for the cause of malabsorption. *Clostridium difficile* infection (D) is common in critically ill patients, especially after antibiotic exposure, and causes diarrhea, but it does not typically cause significant steatorrhea as the primary malabsorptive feature; stool testing for *C. difficile* is appropriate to rule out coinfection or alternative cause of diarrhea, but PEI remains the more likely explanation for the constellation of symptoms including steatorrhea in this patient.

2. **Answer: C.** In a critically ill patient with severe short-bowel syndrome following extensive resection, significant malabsorption and high-volume output are expected. While total parenteral nutrition (TPN) is necessary for primary nutritional support, attempting to provide some enteral nutrition is crucial for promoting intestinal adaptation and maintaining gut integrity. Continuous feeding (as opposed to bolus, A) is generally better tolerated in patients with limited bowel length. Using a low-fat, semi-elemental, or elemental formula (C) bypasses the need for significant digestion (particularly fat, which is often poorly absorbed) and presents nutrients in a more readily absorbable form, potentially reducing osmotic load and diarrhea compared to a standard polymeric formula. Stopping enteral feeding completely (B) would prevent any chance of intestinal adaptation. Increasing the caloric density of the current polymeric formula (D) without addressing the malabsorption and osmotic load is likely to worsen diarrhea and feeding intolerance.

4.10 Ileus And Acute Colonic Pseudoobstruction (Ogilvie Syndrome)

1. **Answer: B.** Prolonged postoperative ileus is a functional impairment resulting in diffuse bowel dilation, typically without a clear transition point. Mechanical small bowel obstruction (SBO), conversely, is caused by a physical blockage and is characterized by dilation of bowel loops proximal to the obstruction and collapse of bowel distally. The hallmark radiographic finding of a mechanical obstruction is a distinct transition zone where the caliber of the bowel changes abruptly. Gas in the rectum (A) can be seen in both conditions or be absent. A normal caliber colon (C) might suggest SBO, but colonic dilation can also occur in ileus or with a competent ileocecal valve in SBO, making it less definitive than identifying a transition point. Mild ascites (D) is a nonspecific finding that can be associated with surgery, inflammation, or other medical conditions but does not directly differentiate functional from mechanical obstruction.

2. **Answer: B.** Acute colonic pseudo-obstruction with a cecal diameter >12 cm carries a high risk of ischemia and perforation, necessitating prompt intervention after failure of initial conservative measures. Intravenous neostigmine (B) is the recommended first-line pharmacologic treatment for Ogilvie syndrome in patients without contraindications (such as mechanical obstruction, bradycardia, bronchospasm, or severe renal insufficiency). The patient's vital signs and renal function are permissible for neostigmine use. Urgent colonoscopic decompression (A) is the next step if neostigmine is contraindicated or fails. Continuing conservative management

(C) with a cecal diameter of 14 cm poses an unacceptable risk of perforation. Intravenous metoclopramide (D) is generally ineffective for colonic pseudo-obstruction. Emergent surgical cecostomy (E) is reserved for cases refractory to medical and endoscopic management or those presenting with complications like perforation or ischemia.

4.11 *Clostridium difficile* and Toxic Megacolon

1. **Answer: B.** ~1% of all patients with *Clostridioides difficile* infection and about 30% of those with severe-complicated or fulminant disease may eventually require surgery. Typically, the recommended procedure is a subtotal colectomy with end ileostomy. In this scenario, the patient has been receiving appropriate medical treatment and suddenly becomes hemodynamically unstable with a concerning abdominal examination. These patients warrant immediate attention and resuscitation as the first step. Transfer to the intensive care unit (ICU) should be initiated if the patient is not already there. If there is no response or only partial response to resuscitation and there is ongoing hemodynamic instability, surgery should be the next step for source control. Computed tomography (CT) scan is not necessary in this context as it will only delay definitive treatment. Fecal microbiota transplantation does not have a role in the treatment of the initial episode of *C. difficile* infection. In addition, it should not be considered in the presence of hemodynamic instability and/or peritonitis. Similarly, bezlotoxumab can be considered as an adjunct treatment in high-risk patients but has no role in an acutely decompensating patient.

Key point: In patients with severe-complicated or fulminant disease who become hemodynamically unstable and develop signs of peritonitis, urgent operative intervention with a subtotal colectomy and end ileostomy is recommended.

2. **Answer: C.** Bezlotoxumab is a monoclonal antibody that binds exotoxin B and has been approved by the U.S. Food and Drug Administration (FDA) for the treatment of *C. difficile* infection. It should be considered as an adjunct treatment to decrease the risk of recurrence in high-risk patients, such as those of advanced age, patients who are immunosuppressed, patients with inflammatory bowel disease, or other significant comorbidities. A single intravenous dose of 10 mg/kg has led to a 40% relative risk reduction for recurrent infection and has been associated with decreased hospital length of stay. Fecal microbiota transplantation should be considered in recurrent cases of *C. difficile* infection. Surgery should typically be reserved for patients with colonic perforation or severe or fulminant colitis who do not improve with medical management. There is some evidence that probiotics may be useful in the prevention of recurrent infections but do not have a role in the treatment of *C. difficile* infection.

Key point: Bezlotoxumab should be considered as an adjunct treatment to decrease the risk of recurrence in high-risk patients, such as those of advanced age, patients who are immunosuppressed, patients with inflammatory bowel disease, or other significant comorbidities.

4.12 Gastrointestinal and Intra-Abdominal Infections

1. **Answer: A.** Ultimately, this patient may need all of these interventions while he is in the emergency department (ED), but the question asks which to initiate first. The initial approach to an ill, hemodynamically unstable patient in the ED should be the ABCs (airway, breathing, circulation). In this patient, airway and breathing are intact (albeit with some tachypnea), but he is hypotensive and tachycardic. Fluid resuscitation must be initiated first. Following this, labs can be drawn, including blood cultures, and broad-spectrum antibiotics can be initiated empirically. Once the patient has stabilized, a computed tomography (CT) scan can be obtained to work up the etiology of his severe abdominal pain.

2. **Answer: C.** Empiric treatment for *Helicobacter pylori* is *not* part of the initial management of a patient with suspected peptic ulcer disease. This patient, with her recent history of significant nonsteroidal antiinflammatory drug (NSAID) use following her knee replacement, is at risk for peptic ulcer disease. While we do not yet know that a perforated peptic ulcer is responsible for her symptoms, initiating treatment with broad-spectrum antibiotics after blood cultures are drawn, starting a proton pump inhibitor (PPI), and planning for a CT scan are all very reasonable steps while she is in the ED. An *H. pylori* stool antigen test should be sent while she is in the hospital, but not necessarily in the ED. Empiric treatment for *H. pylori* can be considered upon discharge in patients who are at risk for poor follow-up postoperatively. In general, treatment is only initiated in those patients who test positive for *H. pylori*.

4.13 Inflammatory Bowel Disease

1. **Answer: D.** Patients with acute severe ulcerative colitis (UC) flares are often require hospitalization. Medical management is the mainstay of therapy, with intravenous (IV) steroids and the addition of infliximab or cyclosporine if not responsive to steroids by 3 to 5 days. Flexible sigmoidoscopy should be performed to confirm the diagnosis and take biopsies to assess for cytomegalovirus (CMV) infection. *Clostridioides difficile* is often concurrent with UC flares and is associated with worse prognosis and should be ruled out. There is no evidence for the routine use of antibiotics. Critically ill patients with UC should be on deep venous thrombosis (DVT) prophylaxis due to increased risk of venous thromboembolism. Repeat imaging should be considered, as high-dose steroids can sometimes mask peritonitis associated with colonic perforation. Colorectal surgery should be consulted early to begin discussions with the patient on surgical options and stoma teaching, in case the patient requires urgent surgery. ~20% of patients with UC require surgery, which, in the urgent setting, is usually a total abdominal colectomy with end ileostomy.

Key point: Patients with acute severe UC flares who fail to improve after 3 to 5 days of IV steroids should be started on rescue therapy with infliximab or cyclosporine, tested for concomitant *C. difficile* and CMV infections, reimaged to rule out colonic perforation, and should have an early surgical consult.

2. **Answer: D.** UC can oftentimes be managed medically as an outpatient, with 5-aminosalicylic acid (5-ASA) enemas, oral 5-ASA, and budesonide. Oral systemic corticosteroids and/or anti-tumor necrosis factor (TNF) agents can be added to induce remission. Patients who clinically worsen are often admitted for escalation in therapy. Patients who develop colonic perforations require urgent total abdominal colectomy

with end ileostomy. Possible complications include bleeding, intra-abdominal abscesses, rectal stump dehiscence, and missed enterotomies. Because the rectum is often extremely inflamed and friable, surgeons take measures to decrease the risk of a rectal stump dehiscence, including placement of a transanal rectal tube for decompression, creation of a mucus fistula, or implanting the rectal stump in the subcutaneous tissues above the fascia (so that a rectal stump leak causes a superficial surgical site infection, not abdominopelvic sepsis). It is important to keep adrenal insufficiency on the differential diagnosis for these patients, as they have often been on high-dose steroids for several months. Fast steroid tapers after surgery can lead to adrenal insufficiency, which often presents with hypotension, but can also be associated with more vague symptoms, such as abdominal pain, nausea, vomiting, fatigue, and lethargy.

Key point: The differential diagnosis for abdominal pain and hypotension after urgent total abdominal colectomy with end ileostomy for UC flare includes bleeding, rectal stump leak, missed enterotomy, and adrenal insufficiency (for patients who have been on high-dose steroids).

4.14 Vascular Diseases of the Small Bowel

1. **Answer: E.** Given the patient's young age with risk factors for hypercoagulability (ie, obesity, family history of deep venous thrombosis [DVT]), mesenteric venous thrombosis should be in the differential for this patient. An abdominal x-ray would not provide a definitive diagnosis. While duplex ultrasound (US) may be utilized, bowel gas and obesity make it very difficult to properly visualize the intra-abdominal structures. It would be improper to take this patient to the operating room without any evidence of an acute abdomen to perform a diagnostic laparoscopy. While a computed tomography (CT) scan with oral (PO) and intravenous (IV) contrast would likely give you some information, venous thromboses may be missed and/or difficult to visualize without the thin cuts of a CT angiography (CTA) with venous delays.

2. **Answer: C.** If endoscopic attempts to stop arteriovenous malformation bleeding are unsuccessful, the next step would be to attempt angiographic embolization. Bowel resection is reserved for patients who have refractory bleeding with failure of both endoscopic attempts and angiographic embolization. Conservative management with resuscitation would be incorrect in this patient who has bleeding despite endoscopic attempts at stopping the bleeding. Transfer to another hospital should only be performed in relatively stable patients when angiographic embolization capabilities do not exist at the current hospital.

4.15 Obesity

1. **Answer : C.** According to the American Society for Parenteral and Enteral Nutrition (ASPEN) guidelines, the nutritional management of patients who are critically ill obese should focus on providing adequate protein to preserve lean body mass while avoiding overfeeding. This approach is known as hypocaloric, high-protein feeding. The goal is to meet the protein needs of the patient, which are higher due to critical illness, while avoiding the complications associated with overfeeding, such as hyperglycemia, fatty liver, and increased carbon dioxide production.

   High-protein, low-calorie feeding (option A) is partially correct while not using high-caloric input and also the rationale is not to lose weight. Standard enteral feeding formulas (option B) may not provide sufficient protein or appropriate caloric restriction. Aggressive calorie restriction (option D) is not recommended, as it can lead to malnutrition and poor outcomes in critically ill patients.

2. **Answers: A.** In patients who are obese, several pathophysiologic changes contribute to hypoxemia, a condition characterized by low levels of oxygen in the blood. One of the primary mechanisms is the increased ventilation-perfusion ($\dot{V}/\dot{Q}$) mismatch. Obesity can lead to atelectasis particularly in the dependent lung regions. These changes result in areas of the lung that are perfused, but not ventilated, consequently causing hypoxemia.

   Decreased pulmonary artery pressure (option B) is incorrect; patients who are obese are more likely to have increased pulmonary artery pressure due to hypoxemia Enhanced alveolar-capillary membrane diffusion capacity (option C) is incorrect; in fact, the diffusion capacity is often impaired due to interstitial edema not necessarily related to obesity. Increased tidal volume and minute ventilation (option D) is incorrect because obesity often leads to restricted lung expansion, reducing tidal volume and minute ventilation.

4.16 Gastrointestinal Diagnostic Modalities

1. **Answer: B.** Doppler ultrasound is noninvasive and evaluates for active flow in the setting of vascular etiologies for the patient's worsening liver function (eg, portal vein thrombosis, hepatic vein thrombosis, hepatic artery thrombosis).

2. **Answer: B.** This patient likely has acute colonic pseudo-obstruction (Ogilvie syndrome). A computed tomography (CT) scan with intravenous (IV) contrast of the abdomen and pelvis rules out true mechanical obstruction or perforation before considering pharmaceutical or mechanical decompression.

4.17 Pharmacologic Therapies for Gastrointestinal Disorders

1. **Answer: C.** Combination therapy with metoclopramide and erythromycin has superior efficacy and delays tachyphylaxis, making it the preferred strategy in this scenario. Increasing the dose of metoclopramide is unlikely to overcome tachyphylaxis and may increase the risk of side effects. Switching to another single agent will likely also lead to tachyphylaxis within a few days. While a postpyloric tube is an option for feeding intolerance, addressing the underlying dysmotility pharmacologically is a primary step.

2. **Answer: A.** High-dose proton pump inhibitor (PPI) therapy is the standard of care postendoscopy for nonvariceal upper gastrointestinal bleed (UGIB) to maintain a high gastric pH, which promotes clot stability and reduces rebleeding risk. H2RAs are less potent acid suppressors than PPIs and are not the first-line recommendation for preventing rebleeding after an acute UGIB. Octreotide is primarily used for variceal bleeding by reducing splanchnic blood flow, not as the primary agent for preventing rebleeding in nonvariceal cases. Large trials like HALT-IT did not show a benefit for routine tranexamic acid (TXA) use in UGIB, and it is not the standard of care for postendoscopy rebleeding prophylaxis.

4.18 Gastrointestinal and Abdominal Postoperative Management and Perioperative Complications

1. **Answer: A.** A small seroma can be observed since there is no sign of infection or other wound complications.

2. **Answer: C.** This presentation is consistent with an intra-abdominal infection, given her fever, tachycardia, leukocytosis, and new post-op ileus. The most likely reason for this would be due to an anastomotic leak at the resection site.

SECTION 5 RENAL

5.1 Acute Kidney Injury

1. **Answer: A.** Captopril is used to treat scleroderma renal crisis. Titrate to systolic body pressure (SBP).

2. **Answer: C.** With the RIFLE classification baseline serum creatinine (SCr) is necessary to define and classify AKI; however this baseline value is frequently unknown in clinical practice. Baseline SCr is not necessary in the AKIN classification, instead it requires at least two values of SCr be obtained within a period of 48 h.

5.2 Infections of the Urinary Tract

1. **Answer: A.** Most urinary catheters will become colonized with bacteria within the first few days of placement. A quarter of colonized catheters will progress to a pathologic infection. It is estimated that <1% of catheter-associated urinary tract infections (CAUTIs) will advance to bacteremia. The initial management includes removing the urinary catheter and culturing either midstream clean catch if capable or from a newly placed catheter. The presence of a catheter alone may cause bladder irritation without infection. There are many reasons for a fever in the critically ill, so starting antibiotics in an otherwise compensated patient is not advised pending urinary culture data. Microscopic analysis will only confirm the presence of bacteriuria and pyuria as both are nondiagnostic for CAUTI; it may be useful in subsequent steps to evaluate for pyelonephritis, where leukocyte casts may be noted.

2. **Answer: C.** In a patient with suspected pyelonephritis without features of critical illness, nephrolithiasis, and obstructive uropathy, it is recommended to defer imaging until determining initial response to appropriate antibiotics. If the fever persists >48 to 72 hours after antibiotics, a computed tomography (CT) of the abdomen/pelvis with intravenous (IV) contrast is usually appropriate. If crystalline nephropathy is suspected after initial labs, then a CT of the abdomen/pelvis without IV contrast would be appropriate. In patients with evidence of renal dysfunction and concerns for radiation exposure, ultrasound of the abdomen may be reasonable.

5.3 Acid-Base Physiology and Disorders

1. **Answer: A.** The patient's laboratory studies indicate a primary metabolic acidosis. This is evident based on the patient's acidemia (pH 7.18) with a low serum bicarbonate (11 mEq/L). Next, the presence of adequate respiratory compensation may be assessed using the Winters formula: $(1.5 \cdot 11) + 8 \pm 2$ = expected $Paco_2$ ~22.5 to 26.5 mm Hg. Since the $Paco_2$ of 30 mm Hg is higher than this value, respiratory compensation is inadequate, and a concomitant respiratory acidosis is present. There is, therefore, also no evidence of a primary respiratory alkalosis (D). Finally, the patient's anion gap (AG) is calculated based on the formula $AG = Na^+ - Cl^- - HCO_3^-$, which gives $AG = 151 - 117 - 11 = 23$ mEq/L. This elevated value indicates that the patient has a primary AG metabolic acidosis, which could be further related to acid-forming processes such as toxic ingestions, lactate or ketone accumulation, or severe uremia. Of note, the corrected bicarbonate could additionally be calculated based on the formula corrected $HCO_3^- = (AG - 12) +$ measured $[HCO_3^-]$, which here gives corrected $[HCO_3^-] = (23 - 12) + 11 = 22$ mEq/L. Since the corrected bicarbonate lies between 22 and 26 mEq/L, there is no compelling evidence of a concurrent metabolic alkalosis (B) or non-AG metabolic acidosis (C).

2. **Answer: D.** The patient's laboratory studies indicate a primary metabolic alkalosis. This is evident based on the patient's alkalemia (pH 7.52) with an elevated serum bicarbonate (36 mEq/L). In the setting of a primary metabolic alkalosis, the urine chloride concentration—in conjunction with assessments of volume status and blood pressure—may be used to narrow the differential diagnosis to saline-responsive or saline-unresponsive etiologies. In the case of gastroenteritis with possible recurrent vomiting, the patient's low blood pressure, hypochloremia, and likely hypovolemia may be accompanied by a low urine chloride concentration (<20 mEq/L), and volume resuscitation with normal saline may aid in the resolution of the alkalosis while restoring the circulating plasma volume. The serum albumin value (A) is primarily useful in clarifying expected serum electrolyte values, allowing for estimation of ionized calcium and correction of the AG. The serum AG itself (B) allows the clinician to differentiate between metabolic acidosis with an elevated AG, which is usually caused by accumulation of abnormal acids in the serum, and non-AG metabolic acidosis, which is generally caused by a sustained depletion of serum bicarbonate. Lastly, the urine AG (C) may be used in determining the likely site of bicarbonate wasting in a patient with a non-AG metabolic acidosis, with a positive urine AG suggesting renal losses and a negative urine AG indicating extrarenal losses of bicarbonate.

5.4 Renal Replacement Therapy

1. **Answer: B.** This patient should be started on renal replacement therapy (RRT) for refractory hyperkalemia. Even though she is hemodynamically stable, a continuous renal replacement therapy (CRRT) modality, such as continuous venovenous hemofiltration (CVVH), is still the most appropriate choice due to the high serum ammonia level. The danger of initiating intermittent hemodialysis in this scenario would be rapid clearance of ammonia, leading to a rapid drop in serum osmolarity, which could precipitate fluid shifting into the brain and cause cerebral edema. Slow continuous ultrafiltration (SCUF) is a CRRT modality that is used solely for slow volume removal; hence, it would not be effective in clearing hyperkalemia in this scenario. Accelerated venovenous hemofiltration (AVVH) is a hybrid therapy that would not be

preferred in this scenario, since it can also lead to overly rapid clearance of ammonia compared to CRRT.

2. **Answer: B.** Kidney Disease: Improving Global Outcomes (KDIGO) recommends an effluent flow rate of 20 to 25 mL/kg/h. In practice, the prescription can be written for 25 to 30 mL/kg/h to account for treatment interruptions due to filter clotting or circuit disconnections for patient transport or procedures. These dosage recommendations come from randomized controlled trial (RCT) data, including the RENAL trial, which found that there was no difference between intensive (40 mL/kg/h) and less-intensive (25 mL/kg/h) doses in terms of mortality or renal recovery. Higher doses may be associated with the risk of hypophosphatemia.

3. **Answer: D.** Though this patient has been oliguric for 24 hours, he does not have an urgent indication for initiation of RRT. The AKIKI, IDEAL-ICU, and STARRT-AKI trials found no difference in mortality between early and delayed initiation of RRT in patients with severe acute kidney injury (AKI) who did not have an urgent indication for dialysis. Furthermore, a significant percentage of patients in the delayed cohorts did not even require RRT, suggesting that expectant management may spare patients from unnecessary RRT. An aggressive fluid challenge is not recommended in this situation, since the patient is already 3 L positive for the admission, hemodynamically stable on low-dose vasopressor, and at risk for volume overload, given prolonged oliguria.

5.5 Renal Imaging and Other Diagnostic Modalities

1. **Answer: C.** Renal scintigraphy allows for assessment of renal function, anatomy, and perfusion. Here, a labeled radiotracer is administered to the patient, and a series of images are collected at timed intervals relative to the passage of the tracer itself. In dynamic imaging, the radiotracer technetium-99m diethylene triamine pentaacetic acid (Tc-99m DTPA) allows for concurrent glomerular filtration rate (GFR) measurement.

2. **Answer: A.** The patient has had a previous anaphylactic reaction to iodinated contrast dye. She has not been premedicated, and it would likely trigger the same reaction if administered in the emergency department (ED) for imaging. Gadolinium-based contrast is not without complications in chronic kidney disease (nephrogenic systemic fibrosis), but the risk is quite low. However, microbubble contrast would be the safest option for this patient. Microbubbles are phospholipid shells that contain inert gases, which can be eliminated through exhalation.

5.6 Pharmacologic Therapies for Renal Disorders

1. **Answer: B.** Acetazolamide is a carbonic anhydrase inhibitor. It acts to prevent bicarbonate reabsorption in the proximal convoluted tubule, increasing sodium excretion. When combined with a loop diuretic, it can help counteract the induced contraction alkalosis from the diuresis while continuing to facilitate active diuresis in volume overloaded patients.

2. **Answer: D.** Chlorothiazide is a thiazide diuretic. It acts to inhibit sodium reabsorption in the distal convoluted tubule. Loop diuretics lead to the excretion of dilute hypotonic urine. Patients being treated with loop diuretics can reabsorb sodium in the distal convoluted tubule, so the addition of a thiazide diuretic promotes natriuresis, leading to correction of the hypernatremia.

5.7 Pharmacologic Implications of Altered Renal Clearance

1. **Answer: C.** Medications that are subject to renal clearance may require dose modifications in states of altered renal clearance. Vancomycin is primarily eliminated from the body by renal excretion. Specifically, it undergoes renal filtration and tubular secretion. In patients with significantly impaired renal function, both the dose of vancomycin and its administration frequency may need adjustment to avoid toxic serum concentrations.

2. **Answer: D.** Acute tubular necrosis is a type of kidney injury that affects the renal tubules. Injury to the renal tubules causes disruption in tubular secretion and reabsorption and can also decrease glomerular filtration. These changes affecting glomerular filtration, tubular secretion, and/or tubular reabsorption can alter renal clearance.

5.8 Genitourinary Emergencies

1. **Answer: B.** This patient is presenting with septic shock and is hemodynamically unstable despite appropriate medical management. Physical examination is highly concerning for Fournier gangrene. Given the patient's hemodynamic instability, the most appropriate next step is urgent surgical exploration and debridement of necrotic tissue to contain the infection. Although computed tomography (CT) of the abdomen/pelvis with intravenous (IV) contrast would ideally be obtained to solidify the diagnosis and delineate the extent of tissue involvement, operative intervention should not be delayed to acquire imaging if the patient is clinically worsening and requires expeditious source control. Although the patient has lactic acidosis, likely from septic shock, continuous venovenous hemofiltration should not be started for the sole purpose of clearing lactic acid in the absence of urgent indications for dialysis; rather, treating the underlying cause remains paramount.

2. **Answer: D.** This patient presents after Foley catheter placement with painful, retracted, and edematous foreskin, which is most consistent with paraphimosis. This scenario may occur when the foreskin is retracted for Foley catheter placement but is not reduced after successful catheterization. The retracted foreskin forms a tight band that can lead to swelling and ischemia of the tissues. Penile fracture, in contrast, presents with "eggplant deformity" and rapid detumescence with a history of sexual intercourse. Traumatic urethral injury is possible after Foley catheter placement, but this is less likely due to the lack of hematuria and the presence of foreskin edema, which would be more consistent with paraphimosis. Urinary tract infection is a known complication of urethral catheterization that can present with dysuria, but ascending infection of the bladder is unlikely to occur so soon after initial placement of a urethral catheter.

3. **Answer: A.** This patient is presenting with an American Association for the Surgery of Trauma (AAST) grade III traumatic renal injury (laceration >1 cm, active bleeding).

It appears that the bleeding may have slowed down or stopped altogether, as evidenced by the appropriate bump in hemoglobin after a packed red blood cell transfusion. Reassuringly, she remains hemodynamically stable. In this scenario, the best next step is close monitoring with nonoperative management. If the patient becomes hemodynamically unstable with brisk bleeding, urgent surgical intervention would be indicated. Alternatively, if the patient remains hemodynamically stable but has evidence of continued, slow bleed, it may be reasonable to proceed with angiography and embolization. There is no role for percutaneous nephrostomy in this scenario, as there is no evidence of urinary extravasation or distal genitourinary injury requiring renal pelvis decompression. There is no role for prothrombin complex concentrate administration in this scenario, as the patient is not taking any anticoagulant medications that need to be reversed.

SECTION 6 HEMATOLOGY/ONCOLOGY

6.1 Anemia

1. **Answer: D.** G6PD deficiency is the most common inherited red blood cell disorder and predisposes to hemolytic anemia in response to oxidative stress. Triggers include medications, foods, and illness (especially infection). In this case, rasburicase triggered a severe hemolytic crisis and methemoglobinemia. Management is supportive with transfusions and respiratory/ventilatory support. Due to suspicion of G6PD deficiency, methylene blue (MB) should be avoided in the management of methemoglobinemia as MB can also trigger G6PD crises. Gastrointestinal bleeding (A) and iron deficiency (C) are common causes of ICU anemia but is not associated with brown appearance of blood or rasburicase administration. Microangiopathic hemolytic anemia (MAHA) is associated with schistocyte formation and mechanical shearing of RBCs. It is less likely to occur in the context of rasburicase administration.

2. **Answer: C.** Phlebotomy, inflammation of acute illness, and acute kidney injury are the most common causes of anemia in the intensive care unit. Patients with hemodynamic compromise and worsening anemia should be evaluated for sources of blood loss. Hemoglobinopathies, such as sickle cell disease (SCD) and thalassemias are uncommon causes of anemia in the ICU.

6.2 Thrombocytopenia

1. **Answer: C.** The most likely diagnosis is heparin-induced thrombocytopenia (HIT). He has a high probability of HIT with a 4T score of 6: 2 points for degree of thrombocytopenia, 2 points for timing of platelet fall, 1 point for a suspected thrombosis based on new leg swelling, and 1 point for possible other causes of thrombocytopenia. Evidence of hospital-acquired thrombocytopenia and new venous thrombosis in a patient receiving heparin should immediately raise concern for HIT. Drug-induced immune thrombocytopenia (ITP) from amoxicillin is possible but does not present with thrombosis. Drug-dependent platelet antibodies can be tested to support a putative diagnosis of drug-induced ITP (DITP), but the diagnosis is ultimately clinical based on the improvement in platelet count after withdrawing the offending agent. Schistocytes on peripheral smear and a low ADAMTS13 activity support a diagnosis of immune-mediated thrombotic thrombocytopenic purpura (TTP). Without new anemia or evidence of microvascular thrombosis, TTP is less likely. Active, poorly controlled HIV is associated with thrombocytopenia and ITP.

2. **Answer: A.** ITP is the most likely diagnosis in an otherwise well-appearing individual who presents with isolated thrombocytopenia in the absence of obvious causes. Glucocorticoids are used as first-line treatment to reduce aberrant autoantibody production and platelet destruction. TTP presents with a microangiopathic hemolytic anemia and thrombocytopenia. Prompt initiation of therapeutic plasma exchange temporizes immune-mediated TTP by removing pathologic ADAMTS13 autoantibodies and replenishing ADAMTS13 levels. Treatment of the underlying disease commonly involves both glucocorticoids and rituximab for immune suppression. A platelet transfusion is indicated in patients with clinically relevant bleeding or those with a platelet count <10,000 at risk of spontaneous bleeding. Patients with ITP with only mild mucocutaneous bleeding do not require platelet transfusion, even among those with counts <10,000. These patients classically have poor response to platelet transfusion due to accelerated autoantibody-mediated clearance. Rates of spontaneous bleeding are lower than in other thrombocytopenic diseases due to the presence of young, reactive platelets that are generated in the face of rapid turnover. Sertraline-induced ITP is unlikely, given the chronicity of use. Alcohol-mediated thrombocytopenia is unlikely with infrequent use.

6.3 Thrombocytosis

1. **Answer: C.** This patient presents with thrombocytosis that is likely multifactorial. He has a probable reactive component from inflammatory bowel disease (IBD) and acute gastroenteritis. In addition, complete blood count (CBC) shows a microcytic anemia with elevated red cell distribution width, suspicious for iron deficiency. Treatment of his underlying issues with immune modulation for IBD, supportive care for acute gastroenteritis, and correction of iron deficiency are the appropriate next steps for addressing his thrombocytosis. Therapeutic anticoagulation and antiplatelet therapy are not indicated for reactive thrombocytosis, which, unlike autonomous thrombocytosis, is rarely symptomatic and does not typically lead to clotting. JAK2 testing for a myeloproliferative disorder is recommended when thrombocytosis is persistent despite addressing underlying reactive causes.

2. **Answer: B.** JAK2 testing is indicated to evaluate for a myeloproliferative neoplasm in this patient, who presents with thrombocytosis and a new thrombosis. In particular, portal vein thrombosis that occurs in the absence of a clear underlying predisposition, such as cirrhosis or liver cancer, raises suspicion for an acquired thrombophilia, especially a JAK2 mutation. Her normal hemoglobin and mean corpuscular value (MCV) are not consistent with thrombocytosis in the setting of an underlying iron deficiency. Extremely elevated platelet counts (typically >1,000,000) may lead to acquired von Willebrand disease. Routine testing is not indicated for patients with moderate thrombocytosis in the absence of bleeding symptoms. Erythrocyte sedimentation rate (ESR)

and C-reactive protein (CRP) are helpful to support a diagnosis of reactive thrombocytosis.

6.4 Neutropenia

1. **Answer: B.** Neutropenic fever is a common complication in the treatment of aggressive hematologic malignancies, such as acute myeloid leukemia (AML). While the most common cause of neutropenic fever is thought to be enteric Gram-negative rods, other infectious pathogens to consider are Gram-positive bacteria (indwelling lines), anaerobic bacteria (especially in a patient with right lower quadrant pain concerning for typhlitis), and fungal (prolonged neutropenic fever). In a patient who is neutropenic with septic shock and persistent fever, broadening antimicrobial coverage to include Gram-positive and anaerobic bacteria and fungi (yeast/mold) is prudent while obtaining additional information and infectious disease consultation. Influenza infection is a less likely cause in a hospitalized patient under appropriate neutropenic precautions.

2. **Answer: B.** Cytopenias in a patient with AML are always potentially concerning for relapsed or refractory disease. However, in this case, the isolated nature of the neutropenia implicates medical causes. In the intensive care unit (ICU), it is important to remember that antibiotics (in this case, vancomycin and meropenem) are important causes of neutropenia. Running the medication list is an important first step in the evaluation of neutropenia. Resistant infection and B12 deficiency are less likely.

6.5 Hemoglobinopathies

1. **Answer: C.** There is no established objective laboratory marker of an acute vaso-occlusive pain episode; thus, patient report of pain is the gold standard and should be taken seriously.

2. **Answer: B.** This patient has acute chest syndrome (ACS) based on fever, respiratory symptoms (oxygen requirement), and a new infiltrate on chest x-ray and is considered severe, given rapidly increasing oxygen requirement, dropping hemoglobin, and worsening hemolytic markers. Guidelines recommend red cell exchange transfusion over simple transfusions in patients with sickle cell disease (SCD) and severe ACS. This patient in particular also has a relatively higher hemoglobin due to having SC, and an exchange transfusion allows for lowering the S percent without increasing the hemoglobin level significantly, which can also cause issues with hyperviscosity.

6.6 Hematopoietic Cell Transplantation

1. **Answer: C.** Hypoxemic respiratory failure is one of the most common indications for intensive care unit (ICU) transfer in patients who have recently received a stem cell transplant. The differential diagnosis is broad, including infectious pneumonia (bacterial, viral, fungal), diffuse alveolar hemorrhage, inflammatory syndromes, and toxic drug injury. The clinical situation here is most consistent with engraftment syndrome, given recent neutrophil engraftment, volume overload, and rash. The diagnostic process often requires bronchoscopy with bronchioalveolar lavage to rule out infection and hemorrhage. Treatment of engraftment syndrome is a short course of intravenous (IV) corticosteroids.

2. **Answer: B.** The treatment of severe graft-versus-host disease (GVHD) typically hinges on augmented immunosuppression, and corticosteroids remain first-line treatment for gastrointestinal (GI) GVHD. Infections are common complications in the treatment of GVHD, and maintaining a broad infectious differential for immunosuppressed patients in the first 100 days after allogeneic transplant is essential for patients transferred to the ICU with septic shock. Considerations include enteric bacterial translocation, line infection (bacterial or yeast), invasive fungal infection, and viral infection, including cytomegalovirus (CMV) disease. Increased steroid dosing (A) would not be expected to treat shock in the setting of ongoing corticosteroid administration. Chest imaging and/or TTE could evaluate for infection, new cardiac dysfunction, and endocarditis but should not delay timely empiric antibiotics.

6.7 Tumor Lysis Syndrome

1. **Answer: D.** This patient has developed severe tumor lysis syndrome (TLS) with marked hyperphosphatemia and hypocalcemia. The phosphate-calcium product ($Ca \times PO_4$) is calculated to be 72.42 mg²/dL² (7.1 mg/dL × 10.2 mg/dL), and the patient has become oliguric with acute kidney injury. Generally, for severe hyperphosphatemia and a calcium-phosphate product >70 mg²/dL², dialysis should be considered, and this patient with evolving kidney injury, altered mental status, and oliguria is likely to require dialysis. Of note, the patient had a high white cell count, elevated phosphorus, and increased uric acid prior to starting treatment, indicating a baseline level of spontaneous TLS and a high risk for progression to severe TLS after starting chemotherapy.

2. **Answer: D.** *Several randomized trials and meta-analyses* have shown that rasburicase reduces serum uric acid levels *faster and more effectively* than allopurinol. Rasburicase use is associated with a *lower incidence of acute kidney injury* and dialysis requirement in patients with high-risk TLS, as compared with allopurinol. Normal saline infusion is important in reducing the risk of kidney injury and maintaining urate excretion but does not immediately lower urate levels. Urinary alkalinization is no longer recommended to prevent urate nephropathy because it has low efficacy and carries the potential for adverse effects, including increased renal precipitation of xanthine and hypoxanthine. Prephase treatment with prednisone may reduce the degree of tumor lysis at the time of chemotherapy initiation but will have a minimal impact on uric acid levels.

6.8 Solid Tumors

1. **Answer: B.** This patient with cancer is significantly immunosuppressed due to corticosteroids (>20 prednisone equivalents daily) and recent lymphodepleting chemotherapy. There are nonspecific chest computed tomographic (CT) findings. The most likely diagnosis is pneumonia, though the differential diagnosis includes drug toxicity (eg, pembrolizumab or paclitaxel-induced pneumonitis), cancer progression (less likely based on CT imaging), and pulmonary embolism (ruled out by CT). There is appropriate empiric coverage for community- and hospital-acquired pneumonias. However, this patient is at risk for opportunistic infections, including *Pneumocystis jirovecii* pneumonia (PJP), most significantly (steroids, lack of prophylaxis despite indication, lymphopenia) but also cytomegalovirus (CMV) (lymphopenia)

and aspergillus (steroids). Trimethoprim-sulfamethoxazole (TMP-SMX) (option A) is the first-line therapy for PJP. In this Do Not Intubate (DNI) patient on high-flow nasal cannula (HFNC), it is reasonable to treat empirically for PJP as diagnosis relies on obtaining a bronchoalveolar lavage (BAL) sample, which is not feasible in this clinical context. Ganciclovir (option C) is first-line therapy for severe CMV pneumonitis. Empiric treatment of CMV is reasonable given risk factors and that confirming the presence of CMV viremia might take excessively long in this critically ill patient. Voriconazole (option D) has a wide spectrum of antifungal activity and is the recommended initial therapy for invasive aspergillosis. In this patient with risk factors, empiric treatment is reasonable. Letermovir (option B) is approved for CMV prophylaxis in immunocompromised populations and is not indicated for empiric antimicrobial therapy.

2. **Answer: C.** This is a patient with cancer who developed splenic vein thrombosis as a sequela of chemotherapy-related acute pancreatitis. Splenic vein thrombosis causes left-sided portal hypertension, with dilation of the short gastric veins resulting in gastric varices that cannot be decompressed with right-sided interventions such as transjugular intrahepatic portosystemic shunt (TIPS) (option D). However, these gastric varices can be definitively managed with splenic artery embolization (option C) or splenectomy. In this patient with life-threatening bleeding, systemic anticoagulation (option A) is excessively risky. Gastrectomy (option B) is overly invasive in this poor surgical candidate and fails to address the underlying venous hypertension.

6.9 Critical Care Management of Severe Immune-Related Adverse Events

1. **Answer: A.** Intestinal perforation occurs in ~1% of cases of immune-related colitis. This is uncommon but is a potential severe complication of immune-related colitis. Patients at risk of intestinal perforation may present with sudden, severe abdominal pain, distension, fever, and signs of peritonitis (inflammation of the abdominal lining). Important to note that this can be difficult to recognize in patients on high-dose steroids.

2. **Answer: C.** Immune-related pneumonitis is typically assessed through clinical evaluation, symptoms, and signs on imaging (namely, chest computed tomography [CT] scans). All immune-related adverse events are graded with the Common Terminology Criteria for Adverse Events (CTCAE) grading criteria, which is free and available online Common Terminology Criteria for Adverse Events (CTCAE) (cancer.gov). For pneumonitis, the grading is as follows:

   Grade 1: asymptomatic pneumonitis that may affect one lobe or <25% of lung parenchyma
   Grade 2: symptomatic pneumonitis involving multiple lobes or 25% to 50% of lung parenchyma
   Grade 3: severe pneumonitis with symptoms that significantly limit self-care activities. It involves all lobes or >50% of lung parenchyma. Patients are generally hospitalized.
   Grade 4: life-threatening pneumonitis causing respiratory compromise. This grade indicates severe hypoxemia that requires intensive care unit (ICU) admission and potentially mechanical ventilation to manage respiratory failure.
   Grade 5: death related to pneumonitis

6.10 Coagulopathy

1. **Answer: B.** For a patient with an intracranial bleed, rapid reversal of apixaban or rivaroxaban anticoagulation should be achieved with andexanet alpha. However, the recently published ANNEXA-I study showed that while better hemostasis was achieved for patients receiving andexanet alpha, there was also an increase in thrombotic events.

2. **Answer: D.** Patients with trauma are at high risk for coagulopathy secondary to a variety of factors, including those stated. Maintaining balanced transfusion, normothermia, and correcting pH abnormalities are critical to the care of these patients.

6.11 Hematology Diagnostic Modalities

1. **Answer: C.** The direct antiglobulin test (DAT) detects antibodies or complement bound to red blood cells (RBCs) and is the definitive test for immune-mediated hemolysis. A positive DAT confirms that red cells are being destroyed by an antibody-mediated process. Reticulocyte count (A) reflects bone marrow response but does not distinguish immune from nonimmune hemolysis. Both will raise retics. Lactate dehydrogenase (LDH) (B) is elevated in hemolysis but is nonspecific—levels rise in any cell injury. D-dimer (C) indicates fibrin turnover, useful in thrombosis/disseminated intravascular coagulation (DIC), but does not diagnose hemolysis or its mechanism.

2. **Answer: C.** The prolonged R-time indicates delayed clot initiation due to clotting factor deficiency; fresh frozen plasma (FFP) replenishes these factors, shortening R. MA (clot strength) is normal, so platelet function/number (A) is adequate. K-time and α-angle are normal, indicating sufficient fibrinogen (B). Cryoglobulin transfusion primarily targets low fibrinogen. LY30 is within normal range, so fibrinolysis is not excessive; antifibrinolytics (D) are not indicated.

6.12 Disseminated Intravascular Coagulopathy

1. **Answer: B.** While these decisions can be made on a case-by-case basis, platelet transfusions should typically be reserved for patients with a platelet count <10,000 to 20,000/μL, <50,000/μL with significant bleeding or who are undergoing major surgery, or <100,000/μL with intracranial bleeding.

6.13 Hypercoagulable States

1. **Answer: C.** The cause of this patient's thrombocytopenia is concerning for a diagnosis of heparin-induced thrombocytopenia (HIT). The timing is consistent with HIT (~7 days after initiation of heparin) as is the degree of thrombocytopenia (>50% from baseline). An antiplatelet PF4 antibody test should be sent immediately, and the patient transitioned to a nonheparin anticoagulant. The other answers could all be contributing to his thrombocytopenia as well, making these cases particularly challenging.

2. **Answer: E.** Routine testing for thrombophilia is expensive and is not currently supported, particularly in patients with critical illness.

6.14 Coagulation Management Strategies

1. **Answer: C.** In major trauma, early depletion of fibrinogen can be due to hemodilution from resuscitation, blood loss, consumption in clot formation, hypothermia, fibrinogenolysis, and acidosis. Low levels of fibrinogen are associated with mortality. With hemorrhagic shock, one would expect hypercitricemia (citrate is an anticoagulant used in blood products), increased R-time (due to coagulopathy), and hyperkalemia (due to hemolysis of stored packed red blood cells [pRBCs]).

2. **Answer: E.** Rapid reversal agents should be considered in severe, life-threatening acute intracranial hemorrhage where urgent need for anticoagulant reversal outweighs the risk of thrombosis. Intravenous (IV) vitamin K has a slower onset (4-12 hours) and works by promoting the synthesis of factors II, VII, IX, and X in the liver. The onset of prothrombin complex concentrate (PCC) is fast (5-15 minutes) and has a duration of up to 24 hours when given in combination with IV vitamin K. Of note, fresh frozen plasma (FFP) can also be given to reverse warfarin; however, FFP can take up to 30 minutes to thaw, blood banks may not have an adequate supply of universal (type AB) FFP and thus additional time must be considered for type and screen, and the onset of action is longer (1-4 hours).

6.15 Complications of Immunosuppressive Drugs

1. **Answer: B.** The patient presents with acute neurologic symptoms (visual disturbances and acute Mountain sickness [AMS]), severe hypertension (HTN), and magnetic resonance imaging (MRI) findings (T2 signal abnormality within the parieto-occipital lobes) consistent with posterior reversible encephalopathy syndrome (PRES), a known complication of calcineurin inhibitors such as tacrolimus. PRES is often reversible with prompt blood pressure control and reduction or discontinuation of the offending agent (in this case, tacrolimus). Therapeutic trough levels do not preclude PRES. Answer A is incorrect as computed tomographic (CT) imaging shows no hemorrhage, and continuing tacrolimus would worsen PRES. Answer C describes thrombotic microangiopathy (TMA), which presents hemolysis, thrombocytopenia, and renal failure, not seizures and imaging changes. Answer D is unlikely, given the radiographic distribution, clinical findings, and acute presentation.

2. **Answer: B.** This patient is in the intermediate posttransplant period (1-6 months after solid organ transplantation), when immunosuppression is at its peak and the risk for opportunistic infections and latent viral reactivation is highest. Cytomegalovirus (CMV) is a classic pathogen in this window, particularly in seronegative recipients from seropositive donors. Pulmonary involvement may include interstitial pneumonia, and other manifestations include fever, malaise, cytopenias, and mucosal involvement (eg, thrush). Answer A: *Pseudomonas aeruginosa* is more commonly seen in the early perioperative phase (<1 month) when nosocomial pathogens and surgical complications dominate. Answer C: *Streptococcus pneumoniae* is a typical late-phase (>6 months), community-acquired infection, when immunosuppression has tapered and risk is similar to the general population. Answer D: JC polyomavirus causes progressive multifocal leukoencephalopathy, a late-phase complication (>6 months) in patients with profound or prolonged immunosuppression, not acute pulmonary disease.

6.16 Complications of Chemotherapy

1. **Answer: B.** Methotrexate, especially in high intravenous (IV) doses, can cause acute/subacute leukoencephalopathy characterized by stroke-like symptoms and symmetric restricted diffusion on magnetic resonance imaging (MRI). It is associated with folate deficiency, elevated homocysteine, and altered methionine metabolism. High-dose folinic acid (leucovorin) can be beneficial. The following answer options are incorrect because:
   - *A:* Methotrexate does not cause acute subcortical hemorrhage via platelet dysfunction; myelosuppression may occur but is not the primary mechanism here.
   - *C:* Aseptic meningitis is seen after *intrathecal* methotrexate, not IV high-dose therapy, and presents with headache, fever, nuchal rigidity.
   - *D:* Posterior reversible encephalopathy syndrome (PRES) is not a typical methotrexate complication; it is more often seen with calcineurin inhibitors or hypertensive crises.
   - *E:* Methotrexate does not directly cause carotid artery thrombosis; ischemic stroke in this setting would be rare and unrelated to the described MRI findings.

2. **Answer: C.** Continuous infusion 5-fluorouracil (5-FU) can cause type II cardiotoxicity via profound coronary microvascular vasoconstriction, leading to ischemia. Management includes immediate discontinuation and treatment as for acute coronary syndrome. The following answer options are incorrect because:
   - *A:* There is no evidence for immune complex–mediated vasculitis in 5-FU cardiotoxicity.
   - *B:* Type I cardiotoxicity (irreversible) is seen with anthracyclines, not 5-FU; dexrazoxane is used for anthracycline cardiotoxicity prevention.
   - *D:* Oxidative stress and mitochondrial injury describe anthracycline toxicity, not 5-FU–induced vasospasm.
   - *E:* Supportive care alone is inadequate without stopping the causative drug; oxygen/diuretics are not primary therapy here.

SECTION 7 ENDOCRINE

7.1 General Neuroendocrine Axis

1. **Answer: A.** The polyuria is likely secondary to a deceleration injury causing diffuse axonal injury (DAI) of the neurohypophysis. The decreased vasopressin secretion will cause central diabetes insipidus.

2. **Answer: B.** Prolactinomas are the most common pituitary tumor. Symptoms include increased lactation, infertility, loss of libido, and lethargy. In this case, the sudden-onset headache, visual disturbances, and altered mental status suggest pituitary apoplexy—a rare but critical emergency where the tumor bleeds or loses blood supply. The headache is typically severe because the swelling stretches the dura, while visual changes arise from pressure on the optic chiasm,

leading to characteristic visual field deficits. This condition requires immediate intensive care unit (ICU) care for stabilization and hormone replacement therapy, along with surgical evaluation.

7.2 Diabetes Mellitus

1. **Answer D.** The patient is demonstrating a metabolic acidosis with mild hyperglycemia, a presumed acute kidney disease (AKI), and ketonuria. These sequelae, combined with the sodium-glucose cotransporter-2 (SGLT-2) inhibitor empagliflozin, are concerning for euglycemic diabetic ketoacidosis (EDKA). EDKA is a state of carbohydrate deficit in the setting of decreased serum insulin and increased counterregulatory hormones, including glucagon. Increased glucagon/insulin ratio leads to increased lipolysis, free fatty acids, and ketoacidosis. Anion gap metabolic acidosis can cause nausea, anorexia, and vomiting, which can exacerbate volume depletion and exacerbate glucagon effects, worsening lipolysis, and ketogenesis.

   SGLT-2 inhibitors' mechanism of action is enhanced excretion and blocked reabsorption of glucose in the proximal convoluted tubule. Urinary loss of glucose creates carbohydrate depletion and osmotic diuresis, which can result in hypovolemia and dehydration. Carbohydrate depletion leads to an increased glucagon/insulin ratio. SGLT-2 inhibitors have half-lives of 11 to 16 hours, so they are recommended to be discontinued 3 to 4 days prior to surgery. Replacement of carbohydrate loss with dextrose infusion and decreasing the glucagon/insulin ratio with an exogenous insulin infusion can decrease lipolysis, generation of free fatty acids, and ketoacidosis.

   Continuous vasopressor infusion may increase blood pressure but may not improve perfusion in the setting of dehydration and hypovolemia and will not prevent ketoacidosis. Likewise, while infection may exacerbate ketoacidosis, it is unlikely to prevent ketoacidosis in the setting of decreased intake with acute cholecystitis and active use of SGLT-2 inhibitors.

2. **Answer C.** While admission hyperglycemia is related to the increased mortality rate in patients with a head injury, multiple trials since NICE Sugar have demonstrated significantly increased episodes of severe hypoglycemia and mortality among patients with intensive blood glucose goals. Subgroup analysis of patients in the neuro intensive care unit (ICU) and with traumatic brain injury (TBI) likewise found no difference in mortality but significantly greater episodes of moderate and severe hypoglycemia. Steroid therapy is ineffective at improving outcomes and is associated with increased complications and mortality. Blood glucose goals in patients with TBI should be the same as those of other critically ill patients.

7.3 Adrenal Gland

1. **Answer: A.** Propofol does not precipitate hypoaldosteronism.

2. **Answer: A.** Primary adrenal insufficiency (mineralocorticoid deficiency or Addison disease) is characterized by hyponatremia, hyperkalemia, and hyperpigmentation of skin.

7.4 Pituitary Hormone Disorders

1. **Answer: D.** The patient's history and laboratory studies are consistent with severe hyponatremia. Based on the presentation, the most likely cause is syndrome of inappropriate antidiuretic hormone (SIADH). SIADH is caused by excess secretion of antidiuretic hormone (ADH) from the posterior pituitary gland or unregulated production from an ectopic source (ie, tumor cells in lung cancer). Elevated ADH leads to hyponatremia and hypo-osmolarity by decreasing renal free water excretion. For this patient presenting with acute-onset, severe, symptomatic hyponatremia, correction of the serum sodium is needed. Three percent hypertonic saline infusion will begin correcting the sodium fastest. Recall that sodium should not be corrected no >9 mEq/L in 24 hours to avoid osmotic demyelination syndrome. Ultimately, the underlying cause of SIADH (likely lung cancer in this case) will need to be treated.

   Fluid restriction would be appropriate for mild hyponatremia for SIADH, but this patient is a more severe case. Desmopressin (DDAVP) acts similarly to ADH and would worsen the effects of SIADH by further increasing free water retention and hyponatremia. Isotonic saline infusion would not be expected to correct the hypernatremia sufficiently.

2. **Answer: C.** The constellation of polyuria, dilute urine, and a rise in serum sodium point to a diagnosis of diabetes insipidus (DI). This patient, status post neurosurgery, is most likely experiencing central DI. A decrease in ADH leads to polyuria. Additional tests that help confirm the diagnosis include urine osmolarity and serum sodium. In DI, urine is dilute, as evidenced by <300 mOsm. With the loss of dilute urine, serum sodium will rise. The hypernatremia may cause patients significant thirst and resultant polydipsia.

   DDAVP is a synthetic vasopressin analog, acting on the V2 receptor. Administering DDAVP in central DI will replace the lack of ADH and reverse the effects of free water loss. Monitor urine output and serum sodium closely after initiating DDAVP to titrate the dose effectively and prevent hyponatremia from overcorrection.

   Answer A is incorrect because starting normal saline with hypotonic fluid loss in urine may further increase serum sodium. Answer B is incorrect because the mild hypernatremia is not causing symptoms at this time. Fluid restriction, as in answer D, would likely cause hypovolemia (from continued polyuria) while raising the serum sodium.

7.5 Thyroid Disorders

1. **Answer: B.** Thyrotoxic periodic paralysis is a rare but severe and reversible complication of hyperthyroidism, more common in men (30:1) and people of Asian origin. It presents with acute attacks of muscle weakness or paralysis, typically occurring at night or early morning after heavy meals, alcohol, or exercise, with recovery within 72 hours. The lower limbs are affected first, followed by the girdle and upper limbs, rarely involving respiratory muscles. It is critical to distinguish thyrotoxic periodic paralysis from other causes of acute paralysis, such as Guillain-Barré syndrome or electrolyte disturbances, through clinical history and laboratory findings, including serum potassium and thyroid function tests. Most patients are undiagnosed with hyperthyroidism before the attacks, which are characterized by hypokalemia due to thyroid hormone–induced Na^+ K^+-ATPase activity, increasing K^+ transport into cells and reducing K^+ output. The degree of hypokalemia varies, and normal potassium levels do not rule out the condition. Acute treatment includes

potassium to prevent life-threatening arrhythmias and respiratory issues, and nonselective beta-blockers such as propranolol, not only manage acute episodes but also help prevent recurrences by inhibiting adrenergic stimulation of the Na^+/K^+-ATPase. Prompt and stable restoration of euthyroidism is essential. Ablative treatment of the thyroid gland is recommended for all patients, but prophylactic potassium supplementation is unnecessary when euthyroid.

2. **Answer: B.** Infection is the most common precipitating factor for myxedema coma. This severe form of hypothyroidism can also be triggered by other stressors such as cold exposure, surgery, administration of sedative drugs, especially opioids, or trauma, but infections are the primary catalyst. Proper management of hypothyroidism, along with prompt identification and treatment of infections or other precipitating factors, is crucial to stabilize the patient and improve outcomes in myxedema coma. Options A, C, and D are less commonly associated with triggering myxedema coma. Proper management of hypothyroidism and prompt treatment of infections are crucial to prevent this life-threatening condition.

7.6 Pharmacologic Therapies for Endocrine Disorders

1. **Answer: B.** Sodium-glucose cotransporter 2 (SGLT-2) inhibitors have an increased risk of euglycemic diabetic ketoacidosis (DKA), especially if not held in the perioperative setting. Metformin has a risk of lactic acidosis, not euglycemic DKA. Insulin and glimepiride would have a risk of hypoglycemia if not held, not euglycemic DKA.

Key Point: SGLT-2 inhibitors should be held in the perioperative setting to minimize the risk of euglycemic DKA.

2. **Answer: A.** Propranolol is considered the beta-blocker of choice for the management of thyroid storm, due to not only its effects on the hyperadrenergic disease state but also its ability to inhibit peripheral conversion of T4 to T3. The other beta-blockers do not possess this inhibitory effect on peripheral conversion, making them less ideal.

Key Point: Propranolol is considered part of the standard of care treatment for thyroid storm. In addition to targeting the hyperadrenergic response, it uniquely inhibits peripheral conversion of T4 to T3.

SECTION 8 NEUROLOGY

8.1 Coma, Encephalopathy, Delirium, and Other Altered States of Consciousness

1. **Answer: B.** Patients with spontaneous eye opening and sleep-wake cycles without awareness of self or the environment are described as having unresponsive wakefulness syndrome. This is in contrast with coma, in which patients are neither awake nor alert and cannot interact with the environment, and the minimally conscious state, in which purposeful behaviors, such as command following, visual fixation or tracking of gaze (typically to a mirror), reaching for objects, localization to pain (not flexion alone) and object recognition (appropriate use, for example, of a comb or ball), intelligible verbalization, or attempts at communication, are present and reproducible. The difference between flexion response to pain and localization to pain is typically considered either reproducibly crossing midline to a painful response or taking a clearly avoidant response from pain that is not stereotyped or merely consistent with a reflexive movement. Differentiating between these disorders of consciousness is important in that patients who progress to the minimally conscious state are more likely to recover consciousness.

2. **Answer: B.** The patient's fluctuating mental status with inattention on examination and stable brain imaging are most consistent with delirium. The mainstay of treatment of delirium is identifying and reversing the underlying medical cause. The goal of pharmacologic therapy in patients with delirium with agitation is to ensure the safety of the patient and staff after verbal de-escalation has failed. In this patient, use of a first-generation antipsychotic could worsen the motor symptoms of Parkinson disease. When used as a prophylactic treatment for seizures after traumatic brain injury, valproic acid was associated with increased mortality. Dexmedetomidine should be avoided in patients with bradycardia and is not a first-line therapy for agitation. Atypical antipsychotics, such as quetiapine, are less likely to exacerbate motor symptoms when used sparingly and at low dose and are the treatment of choice for agitation in patients with Parkinson disease.

8.2 Status Epilepticus

1. **Answer: C.** A patient with convulsive seizure activity lasting >5 minutes without return to baseline meets criteria for status epilepticus (SE), which is a neurologic emergency. First-line treatment in SE with convulsive motor activity is the administration of a benzodiazepine as this patient received. Given that the patient has not returned to baseline and remains altered, there is substantial concern for ongoing nonconvulsive seizure activity. Loading with an appropriate antiseizure medication, such as levetiracetam, is the appropriate next step in addition to promptly assessing for any acute intracranial findings on head imaging. Urgent placement of an electroencephalography is important in this patient to assess for appropriate treatment of seizure activity and to assess for any nonconvulsive subclinical seizure activity that may require escalation of antiseizure medications. In situations where SE presents with hemodynamic and respiratory instability, securing the airway with urgent intubation and intravenous sedation with appropriate.

2. **Answer: D.** In accordance with the International League Against Epilepsy's (ILAE) definition of SE, two critical time points (t_1) and (t_2) are characterized. t_1 is the time point at which intrinsic mechanisms responsible for seizure termination fail, and t_2 is the time point beyond which there is concern for long-term neurologic injury and cell death. For convulsive SE, t_1 is defined as 5 minutes and t_2 at 30 minutes. For nonconvulsive SE, t_1 is defined as 10 minutes, and t_2 is less poorly defined but speculated to be ~60 minutes.

8.3 Depressive Disorders

1. **Answer: B.** Duloxetine would be the most appropriate next step treatment for this patient. Not only does duloxetine work by a different mechanism than selective serotonin reuptake inhibitor (SSRI) medications, but it is also helpful for peripheral neuropathy, a prominent symptom in this patient

with diabetic neuropathy. Fluvoxamine, another SSRI, could be chosen; however, given that it does not ameliorate peripheral neuropathy, it is not the *most appropriate* choice. Mirtazapine is another option that does not help with peripheral neuropathy. Furthermore, its side-effect profile of sedation and appetite stimulation makes it less appropriate for this woman who already suffers from elevated appetite and hypersomnia. Finally, dextroamphetamine and other stimulants are not typically used as first- or second-line medications for major depressive disorders. It also does not treat peripheral neuropathy.

2. **Answer: D.** The patient does not suffer from major depressive disorder but instead suffers from alcohol-induced mood disorder. As the patient's depressive symptoms have always resolved after a period of abstinence, supportive and substance abuse treatment would be most effective at this time. Some patients can have residual depressive symptoms, even weeks after the cessation of substance use.

3. **Answer: C.** The American Psychiatric Association practice guidelines for the treatment of major depressive disorder state that SSRIs, serotonin-norepinephrine reuptake inhibitors (SNRIs), bupropion, and mirtazapine can be considered first line for the treatment of major depressive disorder. Electroconvulsive therapy (ECT) can also be used first line in patients with severe psychosis, catatonia, or severe suicidal ideation who require improvement as quickly as possible. However, nortriptyline, a tricyclic antidepressant, would be considered second or third line, given the possibility of arrhythmias, especially in overdose.

8.4 Central Nervous System Infections

1. **Answer: D.** Acute meningitis represents a neurologic emergency, and early recognition and initiation of appropriate treatment are key to successful management. Patients present with headache, neck stiffness, fever, altered mental status, seizures, and focal neurologic deficits. The latter two imply brain parenchymal involvement and are suggestive of meningoencephalitis, rather than isolated meningitis. Initial management involves the assessment of airway, breathing, and circulation, as with any emergency. Given the high morbidity and mortality, empiric antimicrobial therapy is initiated prior to testing and confirmation of the diagnosis. Blood cultures should be immediately collected as many patients have bacteremia. Lumbar puncture (LP) must never delay treatment. Careful review of indications for imaging prior to LP and attention to whether a patient is coagulopathic remain essential. Patients with community-acquired meningitis are treated with a third-generation cephalosporin (ceftriaxone) to cover *Streptococcus pneumoniae* and *Neisseria meningitidis* and vancomycin to cover potentially ceftriaxone-resistant *S. pneumoniae* species. In patients who are immunocompromised or older than 50 years, ampicillin is added for *Listeria monocytogenes* coverage. If meningoencephalitis is suspected, as in this case, the regimen must include acyclovir until herpes encephalitis is ruled out due to high morbidity and mortality. Steroids should be administered before or with the first dose of antibiotics, as they are associated with mortality benefits in adults with *S. pneumoniae* meningitis.

Key point: In patients with suspected meningoencephalitis, empiric antimicrobial therapy includes ceftriaxone, vancomycin, and acyclovir, with the addition of ampicillin for those who are immunocompromised or older than 50 years, and steroids.

2. **Answer: B.** Herpes simplex encephalitis is the most common cause of viral encephalitis and is associated with high morbidity and mortality. Patients present with fever, altered mental status, seizures, and focal neurologic deficits. Cerebrospinal fluid (CSF) most commonly shows a viral pattern of inflammation with lymphocytic pleocytosis, mildly elevated protein, and normal CSF glucose. Brain magnetic resonance imaging (MRI) is abnormal in nearly all patients and shows patchy areas of inflammation with a predilection for temporal lobe involvement. Electroencephalography may show focal slowing, epileptiform discharges, or seizures. Diagnosis is made by detecting herpes simplex virus via polymerase chain reaction in the CSF. Treatment with acyclovir for 14 to 21 days.

Key point: Herpes simplex encephalitis shows a viral pattern of inflammation in the CSF with lymphocytic pleocytosis, mildly elevated protein, and normal CSF glucose.

8.5 Acute Traumatic Brain Injury and Intracranial Hypertension

1. **Answer: C.** Intracranial hypertension can occur after traumatic brain injury (TBI), and patients presenting with a Glasgow Coma Score (GCS) <8 should be considered for intracranial pressure (ICP) and/or invasive multimodal neuromonitoring. A central principle of TBI management is to prevent secondary injury, which requires close monitoring to correct hemodynamics, blood gases, electrolyte abnormalities, and ICP. If the patient displays signs of sustained intracranial hypertension (ICP >22 mm Hg) with normal brain tissue oxygenation (Pbto$_2$ >20 mm Hg), first-line immediate therapies include ensuring appropriate sedation/analgesia, maintaining cerebral perfusion pressure (CPP) >60 mm Hg, maintaining Paco$_2$ at low normal, draining cerebrospinal fluid (CSF) if an intraventricular drain is in place, and administering hyperosmolar therapy.

In this patient, the CPP (MAP—ICP) is 65 mm Hg and is appropriate, and thus increasing the MAP is less likely to benefit the patient. A salvage decompressive craniectomy may eventually become indicated, but this is a third-line therapy with generally poor long-term outcomes. Continuous infusion of hyperosmolar therapy is unlikely to be effective in this rapidly changing situation because a continuous infusion takes hours to appreciably increase the serum osmolarity. Intermittent boluses of hyperosmolar therapy are the most appropriate next step in this situation, given its ability to rapidly change serum osmolarity and draw water from the intracranial compartment. The intermittent hyperosmolar boluses should be discontinued once the ICP normalizes.

Key Point: Hyperosmolar therapy for acute elevations in ICP should be dosed in a bolus manner.

2. **Answer: B.** Patients with TBI frequently present with concomitant traumatic injuries, all of which need to be considered as sources of morbidity and mortality. This patient with polytrauma demonstrated signs of hemorrhagic shock related to new intraabdominal bleeding concurrent with neurologic deterioration soon after admission. While she indeed had a documented TBI and her new intracranial

hypertension could be due to a neurosurgically correctable lesion, her neurologic deterioration was more likely due to hypotension from hemorrhagic shock. This patient is now actively bleeding, and thus, immediate operative intervention is required for hemorrhage control.

Because this patient is unstable and actively bleeding, a computed tomography (CT) scan will delay hemorrhage control. Furthermore, the CT scanner is not a safe place for an unstable patient. Neurosurgical intervention may eventually be indicated, but first, the patient's hemodynamics need to be stabilized. The patient's low cerebral oxygenation is likely due to her hypotension, and increasing the FIO_2 will not help. Certainly, one would transfuse blood in this situation, but not to a target of 9 g/dL for the purposes of improving cerebral oxygenation.

Key Point: Hypotension will lead to secondary brain injury in patients with TBI. The cause of any life-threatening hypotension must be addressed immediately.

8.6 Spinal Cord Injury

1. **Answer: C.** Blunt cerebrovascular injury (BCVI) has a strong association with cervical spine fractures, even in the absence of neurologic symptoms. Computed tomographic (CT) angiography is the recommended screening tool, and early initiation of antiplatelet or anticoagulation therapy significantly reduces the risk of stroke, especially within the first 24 hours.

2. **Answer: D.** Norepinephrine is the first-line agent for managing hypotension in spinal cord injury due to its effective vasoconstriction (alpha activity) and ability to increase heart rate and cardiac output (beta activity), making it ideal in treating both hypotension and bradycardia.

8.7 Ischemic Stroke

1. **Answer: B.** The patient presents with disabling symptoms and is within the therapeutic window for intravenous thrombolysis of 4.5 hours from his last known normal. His scan also did not reveal any evidence of hemorrhage or an established large acute infarct. (B) Intravenous thrombolysis is, therefore, the correct answer. He would not be a candidate for mechanical thrombectomy (C) as there is no evidence of large vessel occlusion on the computed tomographic angiography (CTA) of the head and neck. Aspirin and/or clopidogrel (A, D) can be considered if a patient presents with nondisabling symptoms, is outside the therapeutic window of 4.5 hours, or has another relative/absolute contraindication for intravenous thrombolysis.

2. **Answer: B.** The patient was last known normal 3 hours before presentation. Although she is within the therapeutic window for intravenous thrombolysis (ie, <4.5 hours from last known normal), she is not a candidate as she is on apixaban (A). She is a candidate for mechanical thrombectomy (B) as she presents with disabling symptoms with National Institutes of Health Stroke Scale (NIHSS) >6 and has evidence of a proximal occlusion of her left middle cerebral artery (MCA). Magnetic resonance imaging (MRI) of the brain (C) is usually obtained as part of the stroke workup but would not be the next best step in this case. Normal saline bolus (D) is not indicated in this case.

8.8 Intracerebral Hemorrhage

1. **Answer: C.** In patients with spontaneous lobar intraparenchymal hemorrhage (IPH), volume 30 to 80 mL, Glasgow Coma Scale (GCS) 5 to 14, National Institutes of Health Stroke Scale (NIHSS) >5, baseline modified Rankin Scale (mRS) <2, last known well <24 hours, and absence of culprit vascular abnormality, treatment with minimally invasive trans-sulcal parafascicular surgery plus medical management was associated with better functional outcomes than with medical management alone (Pradilla et al, 2024). Prothrombin complex concentrate (PCC) (choice B) is not indicated, given that the patient is not on anticoagulation and does not have an elevated international normalized ratio (INR) (>1.4). Decompressive hemicraniectomy (choice D) has no clear effect on functional outcome and is reserved as a lifesaving measure in patients with supratentorial ICH who are in a coma, have significant mass effect, or have elevated intracranial pressure (ICP) refractory to medical management.

2. **Answer: D.** Andexanet alfa is the reversal agent for direct oral anticoagulants, such as apixaban, and should be administered to patients who suffer acute intracerebral hemorrhage (ICH) while taking these medications. PCC can be used as an alternative to Andexanet alfa in patients with ICH while taking a direct oral anticoagulant (regardless of INR) if andexanet alfa is unavailable or if felt to be more clinically appropriate for a given patient. (Andexanet alfa is associated with less hematoma expansion, but higher thrombotic risk than PCC.) In patients with normal platelet counts on antiplatelet medications, platelet transfusions should only be considered if there is a plan for emergent neurosurgery. Platelet transfusions are otherwise potentially harmful in ICH. Idarucizumab is the reversal agent for dabigatran. Cryoprecipitate + tranexamic acid can be used for tissue plasminogen activator (tPA) reversal.

8.9 Subarachnoid Hemorrhage and Vascular Malformations

1. **Answer: A.** Modified fisher scale. The modified Fisher scale classifies the severity of aneurysmal subarachnoid hemorrhage (aSAH) based on the thickness and distribution of blood on CT with its associated risk of vasospasm (Table 8.9.2). Reported rates of symptomatic vasospasm are approximately 0% for grade 0, 6–24% for grade 1, 15–33% for grade 2, 33–35% for grade 3, and 34–40% for grade 4.

2. **Answer: C.** Developmental Venous anomaly. Cavernous malformations are reported to be associated with developmental venous anomalies (DVA) in approximately 2–33% of cases. One explanation for the association is that DVAs increase local venous pressure which can promote microhemorrhages that stimulate cavernoma formation.

8.10 Cerebral Venous Thrombosis

1. **Answer: B.** Headache is the most frequent presenting symptom of CVT, reported in up to 80–90% of cases. It results from increased intracranial pressure due to impaired venous drainage and secondary cerebral edema. While seizures and focal deficits are common, headache remains the most consistent and earliest symptom.

2. **Answer: C.** Pregnancy and the puerperium are well-established transient risk factors due to hypercoagulability, vascular changes, and dehydration. In contrast, genetic thrombophilias and antiphospholipid syndrome are chronic prothrombotic states, while malignancy provides a persistent systemic risk.

3. **Answer: C.** CT venography (CTV) is considered a fast, widely available, and reliable modality for confirming CVT, showing direct evidence of sinus occlusion and venous filling defects. MRI with MR venography can also be diagnostic, but CTV has superior accessibility and accuracy in acute settings compared to noncontrast CT or ultrasound.

4. **Answer: C.** Anticoagulation with low-molecular-weight or unfractionated heparin is the first-line treatment, even in the presence of hemorrhagic venous infarcts, as it prevents thrombus propagation and promotes recanalization. Oral vitamin K antagonists or DOACs are reserved for maintenance, and surgery (e.g., hemicraniectomy) is reserved for severe refractory cases.

5. **Answer: C.** Randomized and observational studies (e.g., RE-SPECT CVT, SECRET, ACTION-CVT) show similar efficacy to warfarin with low recurrence rates and a favorable or comparable bleeding profile, so DOACs (dabigatran, rivaroxaban, apixaban) are now considered safe alternatives for long-term management after initial heparin therapy.

6. **Answer: B.** Endovascular therapy (mechanical thrombectomy, thrombolysis) is not first-line, but it may be considered in patients who deteriorate clinically or radiographically despite adequate anticoagulation. EVT is generally reserved for severe, refractory CVT with impending herniation or rapid progression. Overall, high quality data are still limited, and efficacy and safety are not yet firmly established.

8.11 Autoimmune Encephalitis and Demyelinating Disease

1. **Answer: B.** The clinical vignette of a young woman with subacute neuropsychiatric decline with associated new-onset epileptic seizures and dysautonomia should raise a strong suspicion for an autoimmune/paraneoplastic limbic encephalitis. It is critical to exclude alternative etiologies and initiate empiric immunosuppression for the treatment of limbic encephalitis in a timely manner, once infectious etiologies are reasonably excluded.. It is not appropriate to await autoantibody results to then initiate empiric first-line immunosuppression, as delayed treatment portends poor outcomes. This has particularly been noted in anti-NMDAR autoimmune encephalitis, which more commonly affects young women who subacutely develop neuropsychiatric decline, seizures, and dysautonomia and may have an associated ovarian teratoma that requires resection as a component of their treatment plan. The NEOS score is a prognostic prediction tool for anti-NMDAR autoimmune encephalitis.

2. **Answer: C.** This clinical vignette describes a 40-year-old woman who presents with severe optic neuritis that is bilaterally and radiographically involved in the optic chiasm. Severe, bilaterally optic neuritis or optic chiasm involvement should provoke testing for MOG-IgG (myelin oligodendrocyte glycoprotein antibody disease [MOGAD]) and AQP4-IgG (neuromyelitis optica spectrum disorder [NMOSD]), as these features are more commonly seen with these conditions rather than multiple sclerosis. Given that MOGAD and NMOSD are more likely the underlying etiologies of this patient's presentation, immediate initiation of glucocorticoids is essential, with close surveillance for appropriate treatment response. MOGAD tends to be more steroid responsive of the two, but severe cases may warrant second-line approaches, such as therapeutic plasma exchange. In NMOSD, therapeutic plasma exchange for severe optic neuritis is most certainly warranted. It is best practice to institute intravenous steroids followed by a taper, while also concurrently evaluating for the need of a second-line approach in patients with an undifferentiated, incident demyelinating event, as MOGAD and NMOSD, unlike multiple sclerosis (MS), do require prompt and prolonged treatment for clinical recovery.

8.12 Neuromuscular Disorders

1. **Answer: B.** Magnesium intravenous (IV) can exacerbate myasthenia gravis (MG) symptoms. Oral magnesium is less associated with MG exacerbation and can be used with caution. Opioid medications such as fentanyl, morphine, or oxycodone are generally well tolerated in patients with MG, although high doses can suppress respiratory function. Metronidazole is less frequently linked to MG exacerbation as compared to other antibiotics, such as ciprofloxacin or gentamycin. Current literature reviews do not associate calcium channel blockers, such as nicardipine, with MG exacerbations.

2. **Answer: D.** The most likely diagnosis of this clinical vignette is Guillain-Barré syndrome (GBS). The absence of hypocarbia and normal pH in the setting of tachypnea suggests respiratory muscle exhaustion and should warrant an early intubation. Respiratory mechanics, such as vital capacity and negative inspiratory pressure, are helpful to assess expiratory muscle strength but can be unreliable in a noncompliant patient. In the early phases of the disease, the cerebrospinal fluid (CSF) analysis can be unrevealing, and in the described vignette, lumbar puncture should be postponed until after achieving clinical stability. Immunomodulatory therapies, such as intravenous immune globulin (IVIG), can help the prognosis of GBS, but the time to benefit onset can be up to a week.

8.13 Brain Death/Death by Neurologic Criteria

1. **Answer: B.** brain death/death by neurologic criteria (BD/DNC) should only be considered in patients who are comatose, have absent brainstem reflexes, and are not breathing spontaneously, as in this case. There are several prerequisites required prior to initiating a BD/DNC evaluation. An etiology (such as intracranial hemorrhage in this case) should be identified, and its course and severity should be known to cause irreversible neurologic injury (presence of brain herniation). Patients should be assessed for the presence of certain BD/DNC mimics (eg, fulminant Guillain-Barré syndrome or high cervical cord injuries) or confounders (severe electrolyte derangements, metabolic abnormalities, or positive toxicology), all of which are absent in our patient. Clinicians must ensure that the patient is not hypotensive before performing BD/DNC evaluation. Systolic and mean arterial blood pressure readings should be maintained $\geq$100 and $\geq$75 mm Hg, respectively. Finally, hypothermia can

lead to reversible brainstem areflexia and coma; therefore, a core body temperature ≥36 °C must be achieved prior to BD/DNC evaluation.

Key Point: Hypothermia can affect the neurologic examination. Achieving a core body temperature ≥36 °C is a required prerequisite prior to the initiation of BD/DNC evaluation.

2. **Answer: D.** Ancillary testing is pursued when the clinical evaluation for BD/DNC determination is incomplete or inconclusive. Patients with BD/DNC mimics should be considered for ancillary testing. For example, a high cervical (not thoracic) cord injury warrants ancillary testing. Patients who are hypothermic should rewarmed, and clinicians should wait a minimum of 24 hours after rewarming to ≥36 °C before clinical examination and apnea testing. Hypothermia in itself is not an indication for ancillary testing. Systolic blood pressure readings should be maintained ≥100 mm Hg prior to and during BD/DNC evaluation. This can be achieved using fluids or vasopressors/inotropes. Ancillary testing should only be pursued if there are risks of cardiopulmonary decompensation, significant vasopressor support, or unstable cardiac arrhythmias. Ancillary testing is not required in patients without a known history of chronic hypercarbia or those with a known history of hypercarbia and known baseline $PaCO_2$ levels. However, in patients with suspected chronic hypercarbia and unknown baseline $Paco_2$ level, ancillary testing must be performed.

Key Point: Ancillary tests are supportive of BD/DNC diagnosis under certain circumstances and should never be used alone. For patients with suspected chronic hypercarbia and unknown baseline $PaCO_2$ level, ancillary testing must be performed in addition to the clinical examination and apnea test.

8.14 Anoxic Brain Injury, Temperature Control, and Neuroprognostication

1. **Answer: C.** This patient is comatose after return of spontaneous circulation (ROSC), and temperature control should be initiated, which can be performed with active fever prevention (goal ≤37.5 °C) or targeted temperature management with mild hypothermia (33-36 °C) depending on the context and institutional practice. Aggressive treatment should be initiated as soon as possible, and treatment should not be withheld awaiting fever of 38 °C. For patients with mild hypothermia, rapid rewarming >0.5 °C per hour should be avoided.

2. **Answer: B.** Of the described diagnostic results, somatosensory evoked potentials (SSEPs) with bilateral absent N20 responses and electroencephalogram (EEG) with diffuse voltage suppression are most concerning for poor neurologic prognosis. Per the 2023 Neurocritical Care Society guidelines, SSEP with bilateral absent N20 responses in the absence of confounding factors is considered a reliable predictor of poor functional outcome at 3 months (weak recommendation, moderate quality evidence) and EEG with diffuse voltage suppression factors is considered a moderately reliable predictor of poor functional outcome at 3 months (weak recommendation, low-quality evidence). Bilateral basal ganglia hypodensity on computed tomography (CT) and absent motor response to noxious stimuli in the extremities are not reliable predictors of poor functional outcome at 3 months.

8.15 Neurooncology

1. **Answer: C.** The patient's progressive symptoms over 2 weeks suggest a subacute process (which would not be consistent with a small ischemic stroke). The direction-changing nystagmus suggests localization to the cerebellum, whereas untreated benign paroxysmal positional vertigo would not be expected to cause direction-changing nystagmus (and the time course is typically acute onset and severe with head turns). Her being alert and oriented (and presenting in the emergency department [ED]) is not congruent with toxic-metabolic encephalopathy, where there is a global change in the level of arousal, typically in the set of medications or prolonged illness. Breast and ovarian cancers are associated with anti-Yo (PCA-1) antibodies that can cause a subacute cerebellar syndrome such as the one presented here, although a broader workup for new-onset ataxia should also be conducted (including nutritional screening, autoimmune causes, magnetic resonance imaging [MRI] of the brain with and without contrast, and lumbar puncture). Paraneoplastic syndromes often cause symptoms prior to the malignancy itself, and the presence of symptoms of a paraneoplastic syndrome should prompt an aggressive workup for malignancy.

2. **Answer: C.** This patient has known leptomeningeal disease and presents to the hospital with headaches, nausea, and vomiting, suggesting elevated intracranial pressure (ICP). Positional changes often provoke ICP crises as the mean arterial pressure drops or the ICP rises, causing a drop in cerebral perfusion pressure. This is a challenging diagnosis to make, and emergent head computed tomography (CT) and electroencephalography (EEG) should be performed to ensure other treatable pathologies are not missed. EEG is always indicated because patients with intracranial metastases are at high risk of seizure. However, after a levetiracetam load, the episode recurred, which makes this less likely. EEG can be insensitive for rare, deep seizures, with atypical semiologies, but given that this patient was completely unresponsive (invoking the entire cortex bilaterally), we would expect some epileptiform activity to be detected if seizure were the mechanism. Ischemic stroke would be a reasonable concern initially, especially given that CT is insensitive to acute ischemic strokes, especially in the posterior fossa (and a large brainstem infarct could plausibly mimic this presentation). However, the stereotyped nature of the episodes, return to baseline after the initial event, and the provocation of these episodes, which change in position, would be highly atypical for acute ischemic stroke. Paraneoplastic syndromes most often occur early in a patient's course, and it would be unusual to develop a paraneoplastic syndrome after the malignancy has metastasized so widely. Moreover, paraneoplastic syndromes most often cause altered awareness via seizure or encephalitis, and the patient's return to baseline over minutes without an epileptiform correlate on EEG would not be consistent with encephalitis (where the altered awareness would be expected to be progressive with time). Immune checkpoint inhibitor encephalitis is unlikely for the same reasons. Note that although an ICP crisis may resolve initially, any drop in cerebral perfusion pressure can lead to ischemic injury to the brain (which itself causes edema, swelling, and further increases in ICP). Without rapid cerebrospinal fluid (CSF) diversion via a ventriculoperitoneal (VP) shunt or lumbar drain, patients experiencing plateau waves will progress quickly to death.

8.16 Analgesia, Sedation, Neuromuscular Blockade, and Other Pharmacologic Therapies for Neurologic Disorders

1. **Answer: B.** Delirium and agitation are the major barriers to ventilator weaning and extubation in this patient. Discontinuing midazolam and initiating a low-dose dexmedetomidine infusion (B) is the most appropriate intervention, as benzodiazepines are strongly associated with increased risk of delirium and identified as a modifiable risk factor in the 2018 Society of Critical Care Medicine (SCCM) Prevention and Management of Pain, Agitation/Sedation, Delirium, Immobility, and Sleep Disruption (PADIS) guidelines. Dexmedetomidine facilitates lighter sedation and has been associated with lower delirium risk and faster liberation from mechanical ventilation compared to benzodiazepines, with the 2025 SCCM PADIS Focused Update providing conditional recommendation favoring dexmedetomidine over propofol when delirium reduction is a priority. Continuing intermittent midazolam (A) maintains benzodiazepine exposure and ongoing delirium risk. Limiting awakening trials (C) contradicts evidence-based practice, as daily spontaneous awakening trials reduce the duration of mechanical ventilation, and the patient's adequate oxygenation on pressure support indicates readiness for continued weaning attempts. Starting continuous hydromorphone (D) does not address benzodiazepine-associated delirium and may lead to excessive opioid exposure without improving sedation quality.

2. **Answer: C.** This patient is experiencing persistent ventilator dyssynchrony despite deep sedation, resulting in large tidal volumes that prevent lung-protective ventilation in acute respiratory distress syndrome (ARDS). While dexmedetomidine is often preferred to propofol for light sedation and may reduce delirium risk, switching sedatives (B) would not address the fundamental problem of refractory dyssynchrony with injurious tidal volumes. The patient requires deep sedation (RASS -4) and cannot tolerate spontaneous awakening trials, indicating she is not a candidate for lighter sedation strategies at this time. Further escalation of current sedative dosing (A) is unlikely to resolve dyssynchrony and increases the risk of complications. Continuing current management (D) allows ongoing potentially injurious ventilation. Initiating a neuromuscular blocking agent such as cisatracurium (C) is appropriate when persistent ventilator dyssynchrony cannot be managed with optimized sedation and lung-protective ventilation strategies. When neuromuscular blockade is used, it should be reassessed daily and discontinued as soon as possible. The ROSE trial showed that routine early continuous neuromuscular blockade in moderate-to-severe ARDS did not improve mortality, but current guidelines support selective use for refractory hypoxemia or persistent ventilator dyssynchrony despite optimized sedation.

8.17 Neurosurgical Management and Perioperative Complications

1. **Answer: B.** The delayed onset of hemorrhage and edema out of proportion to hemorrhage size are consistent with venous infarction. Falcine meningioma resection necessitates exposure of the superior sagittal sinus, and often the vein of Trolard. Occlusion of either of these from surgical sacrifice or thrombosis could predispose to venous infarction. A computed tomographic venography (CTV) would be a reasonable next step.

2. **Answer: D.** This patient is suffering from severe intracranial hypotension as a result of cerebrospinal fluid (CSF) overdrainage. His altered mental status and CT findings are concerning for impending herniation. The only fast-acting intervention in this case is reinfusion of saline to replace the CSF overdrainage. His head of bed could also be laid flat to mitigate the effects of gravity.

SECTION 9 INFECTIOUS DISEASE

9.1 Infectious Disease and Virulence Factors

1. **Answer: E.** This patient has a long-term central venous catheter (CVC), which she uses for total parenteral nutrition (TPN) outside the hospital setting. In the setting of a long-term CVC infection with Gram-negative bacilli, options include removal of the CVC and systemic antibiotics for 7 to 14 days, or catheter salvage with systemic and antibiotic lock therapy for 10 to 14 days, with the removal of CVC if the clinical response is inadequate. Response to antimicrobial and lock therapy and discussion with your patient about their options will help guide decision-making.

2. **Answer: D.** C-reactive protein (CRP) is an acute-phase reactant and can be high in many inflammatory states. CRP measurement has a low specificity for sepsis, and routine use in the workup of fever/sepsis is not recommended.

9.2 Antibiotic Therapy and Resistance

1. **Answer: D.** *Enterobacter cloacae* commonly harbor inducible chromosomal genes coding for the AmpC beta-lactamase enzyme that can hydrolyze many penicillins and cephalosporins. These organisms often display ceftriaxone or ceftazidime sensitivity in vitro but may become nonsusceptible to these agents during treatment (especially for treatment courses longer than a few days). The treatment of choice for AmpC organisms is cefepime. Fluoroquinolones may also be used if susceptibility is documented.

2. **Answer: C.** The patient's clinical syndrome is consistent with a ventilator-associated pneumonia (VAP). Because this is a nosocomial (hospital-acquired) infection, broad empiric coverage for both methicillin-resistant *Staphylococcus aureus* (MRSA) and *Pseudomonas aeruginosa* (PsA) should be initiated while workup is ongoing. Vancomycin treats MRSA appropriately, and cefepime treats PsA. If the patient had a recent negative MRSA nasal swab and local MRSA pneumonia prevalence is low, then it would also be reasonable to consider cefepime monotherapy, depending on the patient's clinical condition. Choice B is not correct because PsA is a common organism causing VAP—depending on the patient's other risk factors and clinical condition, double coverage for PsA may be warranted. Azithromycin (choices D, F) is typically not needed for VAP treatment unless *Legionella* infection is strongly suspected. Ceftriaxone and azithromycin (choice A) is appropriate community-acquired pneumonia coverage. Daptomycin (choices E, F) treats MRSA but is inactivated by pulmonary surfactant and is not used for pneumonia.

SECTION 10 IMMUNOLOGY

10.1 The Immune System and Immunologic Disorders

1. **Answer: B.** Antineutrophil cytoplasmic antibody (ANCA)-associated vasculitis (AAV) can present with diffuse alveolar hemorrhage (DAH) and glomerulonephritis. Other manifestations of AAV can include sinonasal involvement (including sinusitis, epistaxis, nasal crusting, saddle nose deformity), fever and constitutional symptoms, ocular manifestations (including scleritis, conjunctivitis, lacrimal gland involvement), arthritis (classically migratory arthritis), and palpable purpura indicative of cutaneous vasculitis. Laboratory testing for ANCA consists of detection by immunofluorescence assays, which have lower specificity; more specific autoantibodies can be confirmed by ELISA assays for PR3 or MPO, which have higher specificity. Antinuclear antibody (ANA) is a nonspecific test. It may be positive in this patient but would not help to support a diagnosis of AAV. Rheumatoid factor (RF) can be positive in rheumatoid arthritis and other diseases (eg, cryoglobulinemic vasculitis, Sjögren syndrome); these diseases are less consistent with the patient's presentation. Ribonucleoprotein (RNP) can be positive with systemic lupus erythematosus (SLE) or mixed connective tissue disease (MCTD). While patients with SLE can present with DAH and glomerulonephritis, the sinus pain and dark brown, crusty nasal discharge are typical symptoms of AAV and are not typical of SLE or MCTD.

Key Point: AAV commonly presents with pulmonary (eg, diffuse alveolar hemorrhage) and renal (eg, glomerulonephritis) manifestations.

REFERENCES

Boyle N, O'Callaghan M, Ataya A, et al. Pulmonary renal syndrome: a clinical review. *Breathe (Sheff)*. 2022;18(4):220208.

Kitching AR, Anders HJ, Basu N, et al. ANCA-associated vasculitis. *Nat Rev Dis Primers*. 2020;6(1):71.

2. **Answer: C.** It is important to have a high level of concern for infection in patients who are on multiple immunosuppressive medications as infection remains a leading cause of mortality for individuals on glucocorticoids and other forms of immunosuppression. While flares of lupus can present with fevers, this patient has other localizing symptoms concerning for pneumonia. Given the high risk for infection, starting antibiotics while awaiting infectious evaluation is often necessary. Most immunosuppressive medications should be held temporarily when there is concern for acute infection. Hydroxychloroquine is not immunosuppressive and can be safely continued in patients with infections. While prednisone exposure should be limited in patients with infection, it should not be stopped abruptly, given the risk of adrenal insufficiency with chronic use. Multidisciplinary discussion could involve a further dose reduction in prednisone in the setting of treating infection, though, as earlier, it should not be stopped altogether. As she had recent lupus nephritis, her immunosuppressive regimen can likely be restarted shortly after improvement on antibiotics.

Key Point: Infection is a leading cause of morbidity and mortality in individuals with systemic rheumatic diseases receiving glucocorticoids and/or other forms of immunosuppression.

REFERENCES

Dixon-Zegeye M, Rutherford A. Infections in systemic autoimmune diseases. In: Atzeni F, Galli M, Juan J. Reino G, Galloway J, eds. *Infections in Systemic Autoimmune Diseases: Risk Factors and Management. Handbook of Systemic Autoimmune Diseases*. Elsevier; 2020:143-166.

Pego-Reigosa JM, Nicholson L, Pooley N, et al. The risk of infections in adult patients with systemic lupus erythematosus: systematic review and meta-analysis. *Rheumatology (Oxford)*. 2021;60(1):60-72.

SECTION 11 DERMATOLOGY

11.1 Dermatologic Conditions

1. **Answer: D.** Polymicrobial infections constitute up to 75% of necrotizing infections. Treatment until definitive cultures are required to cover Gram-positive, Gram-negative, and anaerobic microbes. Clindamycin inhibits bacterial protein synthesis, exerts a prolonged postantibiotic effect, decreases toxin production, and increases microbial opsonization and phagocytosis. Of the choices, meropenem will provide the broadest coverage of Gram-positive, including methicillin-resistant *Staphylococcus aureus* (MRSA) and methicillin-resistant *Staphylococcus epidermidis* (MRSE), and anaerobic pathogens.

2. **Answer: B.** The swollen lips and raised lesions are compatible with the diagnosis of anaphylaxis. Of the neuromuscular blockers, succinylcholine and rocuronium have been reported as triggers for anaphylaxis. Sugammadex, the reversal again for steroidal neuromuscular blockers, has been proposed as a treatment for rocuronium-induced anaphylaxis, but sugammadex itself has been reported to cause anaphylaxis. Diphenhydramine and steroids are treatments of anaphylaxis; however, epinephrine in the face of multiple life-threatening symptoms is the preferred drug of choice.

SECTION 12 THERMOREGULATION

12.1 Fever

1. **Answer: C.** Dexmedetomidine, a commonly used sedative agent in the intensive care unit ICU, can sometimes lead to fever as a side effect. This occurs through its action on alpha-2 adrenergic receptors in the hypothalamus, altering the body's thermoregulation. It is important for clinicians to recognize this potential cause of fever in ICU patients receiving dexmedetomidine. Routine use of antipyretics in the ICU is not recommended solely to prevent fever-related complications unless the fever is causing significant distress or contributing to other complications. Arterial catheters, like central venous catheters, carry a risk of infection and should be managed according to infection control protocols during line holidays. Treatment of hyperthermia syndromes such as serotonin syndrome and thyroid storm is to address the underlying cause and provide supportive care. In case of serotonin syndrome, benzodiazepine and cyproheptadine may be beneficial. Thyroid storm has a complex treatment algorithm involving steroids, beta-blockers, and antithyroid medications.

2. **Answer: B.** Given the patient's recent chemotherapy, neutropenia, and hypotension, there is a heightened suspicion for an infectious cause of fever, possibly sepsis. Immediate volume resuscitation, administration of broad-spectrum antibiotics, and obtaining cultures are crucial initial steps. Delaying antibiotic therapy or relying solely on symptomatic relief with acetaminophen, as suggested in other options, risks allowing the infection to progress unchecked and worsen the patient's condition. While consulting an infectious disease specialist or performing a chest x-ray may be part of the comprehensive diagnostic approach, they should not delay the urgent initiation of antibiotic treatment.

12.2 Malignant Hyperthermia

1. **Answer: B.** All volatile anesthetics (eg, sevoflurane, isoflurane, desflurane) have been shown to trigger malignant hyperthermia in susceptible individuals. Succinylcholine is also a trigger for hyperthermia. Nitrous oxide, an inhalational but not volatile anesthetic, has not been shown to trigger malignant hyperthermia.

2. **Answer: C.** Early signs of malignant hyperthermia most commonly include an increase in CO_2 production, sinus tachycardia, muscle rigidity (especially masseter muscle), and myoglobinuria. Late signs of malignant hyperthermia most commonly include tachypnea, rhabdomyolysis, hyperthermia, metabolic acidosis, and cardiac arrhythmias.

12.3 Neuroleptic Malignant Syndrome

1. **Answer: B.** Lead-pipe rigidity is characteristic of neuroleptic malignant syndrome (NMS), whereas hyperreflexia and myoclonus are more commonly associated with serotonin syndrome. Both conditions can present with hyperthermia and altered mental status, but the presence of lead-pipe rigidity is a key distinguishing feature in NMS.

2. **Answer: C.** Hyperthermia in NMS occurs later in the course of the syndrome and is due to sustained muscle contractions and rigidity.

12.4 Serotonin Syndrome

1. **Answer: A.** Serotonin syndrome can develop following the introduction or dose escalation of serotonergic agents, most commonly with monoamine oxidase inhibitor (MAOi) or selective serotonin reuptake inhibitors (SSRIs). Special caution should be given to patients on polypharmacy. Treatment depends on the severity of symptoms.

2. **Answer: B.** Physical cooling measures are necessary, as hyperthermia in this context results from increased muscular activity and does not respond to antipyretics. Temperature control is crucial in preventing complications.

12.5 Heat Stroke

1. **Answer: B.** This woman is conscious but confused. In severe heat stroke, a person might not become unconscious or experience seizures. However, her symptoms do point toward a heat-related illness, and heat exhaustion is a possibility on the spectrum leading to heat stroke. It is best to err on the side of caution and consider heat stroke a possibility. She needs immediate medical attention to assess her core body temperature and receive proper treatment.

   Dehydration can definitely cause dizziness and nausea, especially after exercise on a hot day. However, the hot and dry skin, combined with confusion, suggests a more severe issue than just dehydration.

   Sunburn can cause discomfort and even nausea, but it would not explain the other symptoms like confusion and hot, dry skin. Muscle strain can cause pain and weakness, but it would not typically cause dizziness, nausea, or confusion.

2. **Answer: B.** Because heat stroke is suspected. Rapid cooling is essential to prevent organ damage and death. While reducing temperature is crucial, acetaminophen is not effective for heat stroke. Rehydration is important, but in cases of severe heat stroke with disorientation, the person might not be able to swallow safely. Oral fluids are not the most effective way to cool the body down initially.

   While infection is a possibility, it is not the most likely cause of his symptoms in this scenario. Heat stroke is the primary concern, and treating the high body temperature is the most critical initial step.

12.6 Hypothermia

1. **Answer: A.** The next step after Basic Life Support for this patient is initiating rewarming. Findings that might appear ominous in patients who are normothermic, such as comatose, loss of brainstem reflexes, and dilated pupils, will reverse with rewarming. Therefore, doing an apnea test as a part of brain death evaluation is not warranted unless the findings persist after the patient is warmed. Bradycardia is a physiologic response to hypothermia and will improve once warm; therefore, in the absence of refractory shock, pacing or extracorporeal membranous oxygenation (ECMO) is not indicated.

2. **Answer: C.** The expected rate of temperature change during rewarming is about 0.5 °C to 2 °C per hour. If, despite active rewarming, the patient's temperature is <0.5 °C per hour, consider other etiologies of hypothermia while continuing rewarming efforts. Although ECMO is an effective rewarming method for patients who suffer from severe accidental hypothermia and cardiac arrest, this patient is still hemodynamically stable. Other causes of hypothermia include endocrine disorders, drug intoxication, and sepsis.

SECTION 13 OBSTETRICS

13.1 Preeclampsia/Eclampsia and HELLP Syndrome

1. **Answer: B.** This patient meets the diagnostic criteria for HELLP (hemolysis, elevated liver enzymes, and low platelets) syndrome, as evidenced by hemolysis (elevated lactate dehydrogenase [LDH]), elevated liver enzymes, and low platelet count. Initial management includes maternal stabilization with seizure prophylaxis (magnesium sulfate) and blood pressure control (eg, labetalol, hydralazine, or nifedipine) prior to delivery. Delivery is the definitive treatment, but stabilization reduces the risk of maternal complications, such as stroke or seizure. Corticosteroids are not indicated in this case because the pregnancy has reached

36 weeks of gestation, beyond the period (<34 weeks) when corticosteroids are used to promote fetal lung maturity prior to preterm delivery.

2. **Answer: B.** This patient has severe preeclampsia, as evidenced by blood pressure ≥160/110 mm Hg, proteinuria, persistent headache, and end-organ dysfunction (elevated creatinine). Cerebral hemorrhage is the leading cause of maternal mortality in preeclampsia and occurs secondary to hypertensive crisis and endothelial dysfunction. While placental abruption and disseminated intravascular coagulation (DIC) are potential complications, the immediate risk of hypertensive encephalopathy and intracranial hemorrhage is greater.

13.2 Acute Fatty Liver of Pregnancy

1. **Answer: B.** This patient's clinical presentation is highly suggestive of acute fatty liver of pregnancy (AFLP), given that the patient meets the Swansea criteria, exhibiting six or more clinical features, including nausea/vomiting, abdominal pain, severe hypoglycemia, hyperbilirubinemia, transaminitis, coagulopathy, acute renal failure, ascites, and echogenic liver on ultrasound imaging. The definitive treatment for AFLP is prompt delivery of the fetus, as this removes the source of hepatotoxic fatty acids contributed by the fetus, resolving the maternal condition. Supportive therapies, such as plasma exchange, continuous renal replacement therapy (CRRT), or molecular adsorbent recirculating system (MARS), may be considered in cases of severe liver failure but are not the primary treatment. Corticosteroids are not a standard treatment for AFLP. A liver biopsy is rarely necessary when clinical and laboratory findings meet Swansea criteria.

2. **Answer: A.** Severe hypoglycemia is a hallmark of AFLP and rarely occurs in hemolysis, elevated liver enzymes, and low platelets (HELLP) syndrome, making it the most helpful feature for distinguishing between the two conditions. Abdominal pain is common in both AFLP and HELLP, so it is not specific. Encephalopathy and coagulopathy are more typical of AFLP but can also occur in HELLP, making them less reliable for differentiation.

13.3 Amniotic Fluid Embolism

1. **Answer: C.** This patient is exhibiting the classic presentation of amniotic fluid embolism (AFE), which includes sudden hypoxia, hypotension, and coagulopathy. Management focuses on supportive care, prioritizing stabilization of blood pressure, respiratory function, and correction of coagulopathy through transfusion protocols as necessary. Antibiotics are not routinely required unless there is a specific concern for infection. Corticosteroids are not standard treatment for AFE. In cases where fetal distress is evident, emergent cesarean delivery may be warranted; however, it is not performed in all cases.

2. **Answer: B.** AFE is a rare but catastrophic condition that can result in sudden cardiovascular collapse. In cases of maternal cardiac arrest where return of spontaneous circulation (ROSC) is not achieved within 4 minutes, a resuscitative hysterotomy (perimortem cesarean delivery) should be performed. This intervention improves maternal hemodynamics by relieving aortocaval compression, enhances oxygen delivery, and may improve the likelihood of neonatal survival if the fetus is viable. While continuing Advanced Cardiac Life Support (ACLS), measures such as chest compressions and epinephrine administration are essential, resuscitative hysterotomy is the definitive next step. Corticosteroids are not indicated in AFE. A resuscitative hysterotomy should be prioritized over invasive monitoring when ROSC has not been achieved within 4 minutes of a cardiac arrest.

13.4 Postpartum Hemorrhage

1. **Answer: A.** The World Health Organization (WHO) recommends the early use of intravenous tranexamic acid (TXA 1 g IV) as soon as possible after the onset of postpartum hemorrhage and within 3 hours of delivery for women with postpartum hemorrhage. This recommendation is based on evidence from the WOMAN trial, which demonstrated that early administration of TA reduces mortality due to bleeding in women with postpartum hemorrhage. If bleeding continues after 30 minutes or restarts within 24 hours of the initial dose, a second dose of 1 g IV may be administered. TXA should be slowly administered over 10 minutes to reduce the risk of transient hypotension.

2. **Answer: C.** In the management of life-threatening postpartum hemorrhage, initial interventions include medical therapies (eg, uterotonic agents) and conservative surgical procedures such as uterine artery ligation, B-Lynch compression sutures, and intrauterine tamponade using devices like the Bakri balloon. These measures aim to control bleeding while preserving the uterus. However, when these interventions fail to achieve hemostasis, hysterectomy is considered the definitive surgical procedure to control life-threatening hemorrhage.

13.5 Peripartum Cardiomyopathy

1. **Answer: D.** African American race is a predictor of poor outcomes in peripartum cardiomyopathy (PPCM). Other poor prognostic indicators include left ventricular ejection fraction (LVEF) <30%, right ventricular (RV) dysfunction, and multiple gestation pregnancy.

2. **Answer: B.** Therapeutic anticoagulation should be strongly considered in all cases of PPCM with LVEF <35%, as this increases the risk of LV thrombus formation. There are little data on newer guideline-directed medical therapy (GDMT) medications, such as sacubitril-valsartan, in lactating patients. Bromocriptine may provide benefit, but the data are varied at this time. Enalapril and captopril are both safe in breastfeeding patients; lisinopril should be avoided.

13.6 Peripartum Infections

1. **Answer: A.** This patient likely has an intraamniotic infection (chorioamnionitis) requiring immediate that should be treated with antibiotics, supportive care, and removal of the infected source—in this case, the fetus and placenta. Antibiotics and supportive care are important but insufficient alone, as they do not eliminate the infected source. Chorioamnionitis is always an indication for delivery, regardless of gestational age, to prevent severe maternal complications, such as sepsis and multiorgan dysfunction, and to reduce the risk of neonatal sepsis and long-term neurologic injury.

2. **Answer: D.** The patient requires acute resuscitation, and the surviving sepsis campaign recommends starting norepinephrine as first-line treatment due to its efficacy in increasing systemic vascular resistance without compromising uteroplacental perfusion. Fetal heart rate monitoring should also be initiated to ensure adequate uteroplacental oxygenation and assess for signs of fetal distress during maternal resuscitation. Dopamine, if she were bradycardic can be considered but is not suggested in the question's stem. The stem does not provide data for hypovolemia; therefore, additional fluids are not recommended. More fluids may induce pulmonary edema. Ceftriaxone is an appropriate first-line medication for pyelonephritis. Delivery of a 25-week fetus may be considered, but there are other measures that can be considered prior to delivery.

13.7 Posterior Reversible Encephalopathy Syndrome

1. **Answer: C.** Reversible cerebral vasoconstriction syndrome (RCVS) is characterized by sudden, severe headaches due to reversible spasm of cerebral arteries. Its hallmark is the sudden onset of a severe, "thunderclap" headache, often described as the worst headache the patient has ever experienced. Thus, it shares similarities with subarachnoid hemorrhage. However, a characteristic vasoconstriction (focal or diffuse) in the proximal and medium-sized cerebral arteries facilitates the diagnosis in this case, especially in the absence of intracranial hemorrhage in brain computed tomography (CT) imaging. Although some patients with RCVS have a history of migraine and some authors have described possible association, cluster headaches occur in cyclical patterns lasting weeks to months at a time, with pain-free periods in between. Brain CT imaging and angiogram are normal in cluster headaches. Posterior reversible encephalopathy syndrome (PRES) does not typically present as a thunderclap headache, and the neuroimaging findings instead reveals cerebral edema predominantly in the posterior regions (occipital and parietal lobes).

Key Point: RCVS has a distinctive headache pattern of severe, "thunderclap" headache with signs of cerebral vasoconstriction (proximal and medium-sized arteries) on neuroimaging without permanent damage. Risk factors include medications (vasoconstrictors), postpartum state, hypertension, physical exertion, and autoimmune disease.

2. **Answer: B.** PRES typically presents with acute headache, seizures, visual disturbances, or altered mental status, resulting from vasogenic edema predominantly in the posterior regions (occipital and parietal lobes). The following are recognized risk factors: hypertension, eclampsia, acute or chronic renal failure, and immunosuppressive treatments. PRES is typically reversible with timely recognition and treatment. However, several factors are associated with poor outcomes, including late recognition, malignant hypertension, eclampsia, renal failure, immunosuppressive therapy, older age, altered level of consciousness, and recurrent seizures. Recurrent seizures must prompt aggressive management as prolonged and recurrent seizures can worsen neurologic outcomes in an otherwise potentially reversible condition. Acute respiratory insufficiency is not prevalent in PRES unless the patient has a decreased level of consciousness (more specifically, Glasgow Coma Scale [GCS] <8) or preexisting advanced lung disease. In pregnancy-associated PRES, delivery often facilitates recovery by removing a major inciting trigger (eclampsia). However, the postpartum period remains a recognized risk window for PRES due to ongoing hemodynamic and endothelial changes. Although expected neuroimaging findings include cerebral edema, hemorrhagic transformation of cerebral edema in usual PRES regions is an adverse prognostic factor, cerebral edema is the hallmark of PRES. Yet, early recognition is desirable to establish proper intervention and measures.

Key Point: Early recognition and aggressive seizure management are crucial in PRES to prevent deterioration from prolonged or recurrent seizures.

13.8 Other Obstetric Emergencies

1. **Answer: C.** During Advanced Cardiac Life Support (ACLS) for the pregnant patient, focus should remain on high-quality cardiopulmonary resuscitation (CPR), defibrillation when indicated (ventricular fibrillation or pulseless ventricular tachycardia), and medication administration. Fetal monitoring is not indicated, as any signs of fetal distress are going to be addressed with the same continued management of the arrested pregnant patient. In fact, fetal monitoring may be deleterious, not only as a distracting task but also as one that may impair the ability to do other recommended measures, including manual left uterine displacement, resuscitative hysterotomy/perimortem cesarean section, or extracorporeal membrane oxygenation (ECMO) cannulation.

Defibrillation should not be withheld for a shockable rhythm with concern for fetal harm (option A), and electrical restoration of a perfusing rhythm should not be delayed. Medications should be given in standard doses (option B) during ACLS and should preferably be given via access above the diaphragm so that the gravid uterus does not obstruct venous return of the administered medications. Perimortem cesarean section/resuscitative hysterotomy should be performed within 4 minutes of cardiac arrest (option D), with the goal to get the fetus delivered within 5 minutes of arrest; if maternal viability is unlikely or not possible, perimortem cesarean delivery should commence immediately.

2. **Answer: B.** Nonobstetric surgery during pregnancy for urgent/emergent indications occurs in 0.5% to 2% of pregnancies. Acute appendicitis necessitating appendectomy can be safely accomplished in the pregnant patient. General anesthesia has not been shown to affect behavioral or cognitive outcomes in the fetus with antenatal anesthetic exposure (option B).

For previable pregnancies (usually assumed to be <22 weeks of gestation), fetal heart tones should be assessed before and after surgery, but generally do not require continuous fetal heart rate (FHR) monitoring during the procedure (option A). For viable pregnancies (>22 weeks of gestation), continuous FHR and uterine monitoring should be considered, as operative delivery can be done in cases of severe fetal distress. Though regional/neuraxial techniques may be considered or even preferred, pregnant patients with an operative urgency or emergency should not be withheld general anesthesia for fear of fetal risk (option C). Both succinylcholine and rocuronium are appropriate medications for rapid sequence induction in the pregnant patient, as uteroplacental transfer of these agents is low and has not demonstrated fetal risk (option D).

13.9 Obstetric Imaging Modalities

1. **Answer: C.** CT scan with and without contrast is the best initial imaging modality because early detection of ischemic or hemorrhagic stroke is critical for maternal and fetal survival. The benefits of imaging and early intervention outweigh the minimal risks associated with radiation exposure at this stage of pregnancy.

2. **Answer: C.** While radiation exposure carries a theoretical risk, the benefits of accurately diagnosing pulmonary embolism (PE), which poses a significant risk to both mother and fetus, far outweigh this risk. CT angiography provides superior diagnostic accuracy for PE and lower radiation exposure compared to a V/Q scan in most cases.

SECTION 14 FLUIDS AND ELECTROLYTES

14.1 Fluid Management

1. **Answer: B.** This patient's presentation is concerning for sepsis arising from a urinary source, likely obstructive pyelonephritis. Guidelines put forth by the Society of Critical Care Medicine's Surviving Sepsis Campaign recommend fluid resuscitation with 30 mL/kg isotonic crystalloid within 3 hours of presentation for patients with suspected sepsis. A balanced isotonic crystalloid, such as lactated Ringer solution, is the most reasonable choice per current guidelines. While albumin solutions (A) may reduce the time to discontinuation of pressors in patients with low serum albumin and sepsis, there is insufficient clinical evidence of benefit to its use over crystalloids, especially for initial resuscitation, in most patients. However, albumin may eventually aid in the avoidance of over-resuscitation in patients who have already received large volumes of crystalloid solution. Balanced crystalloids are often preferred over 0.9% saline (C) for many critically ill and non-critically ill hospitalized patients due to lower chloride content and associations with fewer major adverse kidney events (composite of death, dialysis, or persistent renal dysfunction) in some studies (SMART and SALT-ED trials); however, large randomized trials in ICU patients showed no clear difference in 90-day mortality or AKI (PLUS and BaSICS trials), and a hospital-wide crossover trial found no difference in the composite of death or readmission (FLUID trial). Finally, blood products (D) are not indicated for volume resuscitation in sepsis in the absence of hemorrhage or anemia. While this patient has hematuria, his clinical picture is far more consistent with sepsis and developing distributive shock rather than significant blood loss.

2. **Answer: D.** Dynamic indices of volume responsiveness—those which demonstrate changes in cardiac output in response to varying preload conditions—have been repeatedly shown to be superior in guiding fluid administration compared to static metrics. Of all the options, only a passive leg raise (PLR) maneuver serves as a dynamic assessment of volume responsiveness. PLR transiently increases preload by mobilizing venous blood from the lower extremities to the right heart, effectively serving as a reversible autotransfusion. If this maneuver results in a significant increase, typically ≥10% to 12%, in stroke volume or cardiac output, it indicates the heart is preload responsive, and the patient may benefit from fluid administration. To perform an ideal PLR, the patient is first placed in a sitting or semi-recumbent position while stroke volume or cardiac output is monitored (eg, via pulse contour analysis or bedside echocardiography). The patient is then placed supine with the legs elevated to 45 degrees, which results in the return of ~200 to 300 mL of blood from the lower extremities to the right atrium. A meaningful increase in stroke volume or cardiac output confirms volume responsiveness. While central venous pressure (A) remains a useful metric of volume tolerance and systemic perfusion pressure in specific circumstances, it is a static measure with demonstrated low accuracy in identifying volume-responsive patients. Chest radiographs (B) similarly may be useful in supporting a diagnosis of volume overload, but they provide static information that is insufficient to determine whether a patient may respond to additional fluid. The serum lactate (C) may be trended as a marker of tissue perfusion and may guide resuscitation over time, but it does not provide a reliable index of responsiveness to volume.

14.2 Sodium and Chloride Balance

1. **Answer: C.** Hyponatremia may coexist with different volume statuses, and syndrome of inappropriate antidiuretic hormone (SIADH) is commonly associated with euvolemic hypotonic hyponatremia because excess water distributes throughout the total body water space. Measuring urine osmolality is a critical diagnostic tool for hypotonic hyponatremia, as it helps determine whether the kidney's ability to dilute urine is impaired (eg, in SIADH, where urine osmolality is high) or intact (eg, psychogenic polydipsia, where urine osmolality is low).

2. **Answer: B.** Chloride-rich intravenous fluids (eg, 0.9% saline), when administered in large volume, can cause hyperchloremia. In this case, hyperchloremia is associated with a metabolic acidosis due to a decrease in the strong ion difference (SID).

14.3 Potassium Balance

1. **Answer: B.** The most likely electrocardiogram (ECG) finding associated with high potassium levels (hyperkalemia) is peaked T waves. Ventricular fibrillation would be a late finding on an unstable/unresponsive patient. Increased P-wave amplitude and prominent U waves are seen in severe hypokalemia.

2. **Answer: D.** Calcium is the fastest-acting treatment for stabilizing the cardiomyocyte membrane and preventing further rhythm degeneration into malignant arrhythmias, particularly if there are ECG changes. Of note, calcium treatment does not lower serum potassium levels and should be combined with other therapies to lower serum potassium. Loop diuretics and Kayexalate will work to eliminate potassium from the body, but they have a delayed onset of action. Digoxin should be avoided in hyperkalemia.

14.4 Calcium, Magnesium, and Phosphorous Balance

1. **Answer: B.** This patient has refractory hypokalemia, which is a classic presentation for coexisting hypomagnesemia. Hypomagnesemia prevents the correction of hypokalemia, in

part by causing a loss of potassium channel inhibition, which leads to renal potassium wasting. Therefore, the magnesium level should be checked and repleted before the potassium can normalize. Administering insulin (A) would worsen the hypokalemia by causing an intracellular shift. Administering potassium phosphate (C) is indicated for concurrent hypophosphatemia, for which there is no evidence. Giving more potassium chloride (D) will likely remain ineffective until the underlying magnesium deficiency is corrected.

2. **Answer: A.** This patient is experiencing refeeding syndrome, a life-threatening condition characterized by severe hypophosphatemia (<1.0 mg/dL) resulting from a transcellular phosphate shift after nutrition is initiated. A primary complication of severe hypophosphatemia is profound muscle weakness, which affects the diaphragm and leads to respiratory failure. While impaired oxygen delivery (due to decreased 2,3-DPG) also occurs with severe hypophosphatemia, it is the diaphragmatic weakness that is the direct cause of respiratory muscle failure and the patient's shallow breathing. Symptomatic hypocalcemia (D) can be caused by hyperphosphatemia, not hypophosphatemia.

SECTION 15 NUTRITION

15.1 Basal and Stress Energy Requirements

1. **Answer: D.** There is no accurate laboratory marker that can reliably indicate nutritional status in critically ill patients. Serum albumin is a good surrogate measure of outpatient nutritional status but albumin takes 21 days to turnover in the body, and serum levels may be affected (lowered) by acute inflammation. Prealbumin has a shorter turnover in the body (4-7 days), but serum levels are also lowered by acute inflammation. Retinol-binding protein is a biomarker that can more quickly reflect response to nutritional therapy (half-life is ~12 hours), either alone or in conjunction with prealbumin; however, it is likewise affected by inflammation and infection.

2. **Answer: D.** All of these patients should have the initiation of enteral nutrition. While healthy patients can go without nutrition for 1 to 2 weeks, enteral nutrition should be initiated early in an intensive care unit (ICU) admission if intubation is anticipated to be prolonged to minimize muscle wasting and malnutrition. The older patient with ongoing malignancy and the patient with pancreatitis are both in pro-inflammatory states and should thus get early initiation of nutrition. Lastly, body mass index (BMI) is a poor predictor of nutrition, and an elevated BMI does not suggest an over-nourished state; in fact, patients with elevated BMI typically have inadequate micronutrient consumption.

15.2 Stress Hormone Response

1. **Answer: C.** Beta-blockade, specifically propranolol, has shown to decrease energy expenditure and reverse the catabolic effects of severe burns. Randomized trials in adults and children have shown the benefit of reducing the metabolic demands to promote wound healing and increase net muscle protein compared to controls. Propranolol should be started after the resuscitation period and adjusted to a 20% reduction in heart rate.

2. **Answer: D.** Hyperglycemia is a common stress response. Increased cortisol levels lead to hyperglycemia via increased release of glucagon from the pancreas, reduced glucose uptake in muscle cells, and gluconeogenesis in the liver. Lipolysis results in free fatty acids and glycerol, with the latter being the substrate used in gluconeogenesis within the liver. Hepatic gluconeogenesis converts glycerol, lactate, and amino acids into glucose.

15.3 Nutritional Deficiency States

1. **Answer: B.** Severe burn injuries result in a hypermetabolic response that leads to a net catabolic state. Wound healing is largely dependent on adequate nutrition. Generally, total caloric intake should be 25 kcal/kg/d plus 30 kcal per % total body surface area burn. Protein intake should be 1 g/kg/d plus 3 g/d per % total body surface area burn. Nutrition should start as early as possible.

2. **Answer: B.** Malnutrition is the deficiency of essential nutrients needed for sustaining homeostasis. Deficiencies in essential nutrients lead to poor wound healing, muscle loss, altered metabolic pathways, and an increased risk of infection via impairment of the immune system.

15.4 Nutrition Support

1. **Answer: D.** Gastric residuals should not be routinely checked. However, some nursing protocols call for routine monitoring of gastric residuals, and in this case, current guidelines recommend to hold feeds for volumes >500 mL.

2. **Answer: C.** Enteral nutrition should be avoided only in the case of uncontrolled shock and high-dose vasopressors.

15.5 Refeeding Syndrome

1. **Answer: B.** The gentleman in this vignette has developed refeeding syndrome. Due to the severity of his electrolyte disturbances, adequate replacement can be difficult without increasing the frequency of laboratory draws. The safest way to reach the patient's nutritional goals is to decrease daily caloric intake by 50% and slowly increase the calorie count by one-third every 1 to 2 days. While total parental nutrition can be used to meet caloric needs in patients without enteral nutrition, patients still have the risk for developing.

2. **Answer: C.** This patient has a concerning differential that includes refeeding syndrome and thiamine deficiency, as well as a severe metabolic acidosis. Further, the patient presents hypoglycemic. While there is not enough information, thiamine deficiency should be treated first as glucose administration prior to thiamine could exacerbate thiamine deficiency since thiamine is required for glucose metabolism. Critical deficiency in thiamine can lead to poor end-organ function, including neurocognitive function, leading to Wernicke encephalopathy. The patient still needs phosphate repletion, but this should not take priority over thiamine than glucose repletion. There is not enough information to determine whether the patient will need bicarbonate administration or dialysis.

SECTION 16 PHARMACOLOGY AND TOXICOLOGY

16.1 Basic Pharmacokinetics and Pharmacodynamics

1. **Answer: C.** The loading dose of a medication increases proportionally with the desired blood concentration and the volume of distribution and decreases with increasing bioavailability. Converting to a route of administration with greater bioavailability (option A) will, therefore, decrease the required loading dose. Medications that are administered orally and absorbed through the intestines undergo first-pass elimination by the liver, which decreases bioavailability, before reaching systemic circulation. Therefore, inhibition of hepatic cytochrome P450 enzymes (option D) would increase the bioavailability and decrease the required loading dose for oral medications and have no impact on routes that do not undergo first-pass elimination. Other forms of metabolism and elimination (such as increased renal clearance, option B) impact the required maintenance dose of a medication, but not its loading dose. The development of pancreatitis (option C) is associated with increased vascular permeability, accumulation of extravascular fluid, and a resulting increase in the volume of distribution and an increase in the required loading dose.

2. **Answer: C.** The *E*max of a drug determines the strongest effect that it can have, regardless of the dose that is given. The amount of drug required to achieve half of that maximum effect is called EC50, and medications with smaller EC50 are said to be more potent. Drugs with direct effects have fewer intermediate steps between binding to their target and the creation of the desired effect, so they tend to act faster than drugs with indirect effects. The reversibility of a drug effect determines whether its effect goes away when the medication is removed from the body or persists until the binding target is replaced, so irreversible medications tend to have longer lasting effects. In this example, drug A acts faster than drug B, so it is more likely to have a direct effect. Additionally, drug B requires a lower dose to achieve its effect than drug A, so it is more potent. Option C pairs these two descriptions. No information is given about the strongest possible effect of either drug or the duration of their action, so descriptions of *E*max and reversibility of effect (options A, B, and D) cannot be accurately predicted.

16.2 Drug-Drug Interactions

1. **Answer: C.** Carbapenems are known to clinically significantly reduce concentrations of valproic acid. Since the patient is on valproic acid for a seizure disorder, administration of a carbapenem will reduce concentrations of valproic acid immediately, and persist for up to weeks of discontinuation, leading to an increased risk of seizures given that she has a history of epilepsy requiring an antiepileptic. An alternative antiepileptic plan should be prepared if a carbapenem is clinically necessary. This interaction does not exist with the other three broad-spectrum antibiotics.

Key Point: Avoid using carbapenems in patients on valproic acid for seizure disorders, given the rapid clearance of valproic acid and increased risk of seizures with subtherapeutic antiepileptics. If broad-spectrum antibiotics must be used, consider another antibiotic class or utilizing an alternative antiepileptic plan to replace valproic acid if a carbapenem is clinically necessary.

2. **Answer: C.** Sulfamethoxazole-trimethoprim is an inhibitor of CYP2C9, and warfarin is a substrate of CYP2C9. The inhibition of this enzyme leads to increased concentrations of warfarin, thus increasing the international normalized ratio (INR) and potential bleeding risk. Warfarin doses often require reduction when initiating CYP2C9 inhibitors and may be reduced by as much as 50%.

Key Point: In patients taking warfarin, it is important to always assess for drug interactions that may impact the metabolism of warfarin and may require subsequent dose adjustments to maintain therapeutic anticoagulation and mitigate the risk of bleeding or thrombosis.

16.3 Toxicology, Drug Overdose, and Poisoning

1. **Answer: B.** Massive ingestions of isopropyl alcohol can result in coma and shock. Isopropyl alcohol is metabolized to acetone via alcohol dehydrogenase, yielding a fruity odor. These patients will develop an elevated serum osmolar gap but may not have a high anion gap metabolic acidosis as patients who consume ethylene glycol or methanol (ie, ketosis without acidosis). The serum osmolality is calculated via the following equation:

   Serum osmolality =

   $$(2 \times [\text{Na}]) + \left(\frac{[\text{Glucose}]}{18}\right) + \left(\frac{[\text{BUN}]}{2.8}\right) + \left(\frac{[\text{ETOH}]}{2.8}\right)$$

   Therefore,

   $$(2 \times [125]) + \left(\frac{[72]}{18}\right) + \left(\frac{[24]}{2.8}\right) + \left(\frac{[0]}{4.6}\right) = 263 \text{ mOsm/kg.}$$

   The serum osmolality gap is 37 (300 − 263), which denotes a significant gap. The constellation of symptoms in a patient with an elevated osmolar gap without an elevated anion gap metabolic acidosis is suggestive of isopropyl toxicity. While patients with isopropyl alcohol toxicity generally have favorable outcomes, isopropyl alcohol is readily dialyzable and can be considered in massive ingestions.

2. **Answer: B.** Cyanide is a rapidly acting toxin that forms during combustion, and cyanide toxicity is likely to occur in patients presenting from house fires. Cyanide inhibits cytochrome oxidase to disrupt oxidative phosphorylation, leading to anaerobic metabolism. Anaerobic metabolism relies on glucose to produce adenosine triphosphate (ATP) as opposed to oxygen. Peripheral tissue no longer extracts oxygen, which leads to venous blood with a higher oxygen content, thus appearing bright red like arterial blood. Cyanide toxicity causes headaches, confusion, pulmonary edema, and tachypnea, among other symptoms. Early in toxicity, patients may be hypertensive, but eventually may progress to cardiovascular collapse. The treatment of choice for patients with cyanide toxicity is hydroxocobalamin. While sodium

nitrite and sodium thiosulfate also treat cyanide toxicity, sodium nitrite induces methemoglobinemia and may induce a hemolytic crisis in patients with G6PD deficiency and may also cause fetal hypoxia in pregnancy.

16.4 Toxicology, Drug Overdose, and Poisoning

1. **Answer: B.** Massive ingestions of isopropyl alcohol can result in coma and shock. Isopropyl alcohol is metabolized to acetone via alcohol dehydrogenase, yielding a fruity odor. These patients will develop an elevated serum osmolar gap but may not have a high anion gap metabolic acidosis as patients who consume ethylene glycol or methanol (ie, ketosis without acidosis). The serum osmolality is calculated via the following equation:

$$\text{Serum osmolality} = (2 \times [\text{Na}]) + \left(\frac{[\text{Glucose}]}{18}\right) + \left(\frac{[\text{BUN}]}{2.8}\right) + \left(\frac{[\text{ETOH}]}{2.8}\right)$$

Therefore,

$$(2 \times [125]) + \left(\frac{[72]}{18}\right) + \left(\frac{[24]}{2.8}\right) + \left(\frac{[0]}{4.6}\right) = 263 \text{ mOsm/kg.}$$

The serum osmolality gap is 37 (300 − 263), which denotes a significant gap. The constellation of symptoms in a patient with an elevated osmolar gap without an elevated anion gap metabolic acidosis is suggestive of isopropyl toxicity. While patients with isopropyl alcohol toxicity generally have favorable outcomes, isopropyl alcohol is readily dialyzable and can be considered in massive ingestions.

2. **Answer: B.** Cyanide is a rapidly acting toxin that forms during combustion, and cyanide toxicity is likely to occur in patients presenting from house fires. Cyanide inhibits cytochrome oxidase to disrupt oxidative phosphorylation, leading to anaerobic metabolism. Anaerobic metabolism relies on glucose to produce adenosine triphosphate (ATP) as opposed to oxygen. Peripheral tissue no longer extracts oxygen, which leads to venous blood with a higher oxygen content, thus appearing bright red like arterial blood. Cyanide toxicity causes headaches, confusion, pulmonary edema, and tachypnea, among other symptoms. Early in toxicity, patients may be hypertensive, but eventually may progress to cardiovascular collapse. The treatment of choice for patients with cyanide toxicity is hydroxocobalamin. While sodium nitrite and sodium thiosulfate also treat cyanide toxicity, sodium nitrite induces methemoglobinemia and may induce a hemolytic crisis in patients with G6PD deficiency and may also cause fetal hypoxia in pregnancy.

SECTION 17 TRANSFUSION THERAPY

17.1 Transfusion Medicine

1. **Answer: C.** Allogeneic blood products can be collected as whole blood by phlebotomy, or using apheresis technologies to directly collect a specific blood fraction. After whole blood is collected by phlebotomy, it can be manufactured into components, such as packed red blood cells (RBCs) or plasma, or it can be labeled for patient use as "whole blood." For emergency use, whole blood should be type O (A and D are not). Due to the plasma in whole blood, it should be sourced from a donor that is "transfusion-related acute lung injury (TRALI) mitigated"; that is, from a donor who is unlikely to have anti-HLA (human leukocyte antigen) antibodies in their plasma. The most common source of anti-HLA antibodies is through pregnancy; therefore, whole-blood donors must either be male, women who have never been pregnant, or women who have been pregnant but who have been tested and found not to have anti-HLA antibodies (B is not TRALI mitigated). Because there are both RBCs and plasma in whole blood, a plasma ABO incompatibility will arise with non-type O individuals (ie, patients who are type A, B, or AB), so blood services typically select donors who have low isohemagglutinin titers to minimize the potential for passive hemolysis of the patient's native RBCs from anti-A, anti-B, or anti-A,B in the plasma from a type O donor. Such a product is called "low-titer O whole blood" (LTOWB). Repeated donors have typically had isohemagglutinin titers measured on at least one prior occasion, and although titers can change over time, an ideal donor for LTOWB would be choice C. Choices A and D are not type O. Choice B is not TRALI mitigated. Although donor B is O, RhD negative, blood stocked for emergency resuscitation may be O RhD positive due to the limited availability of O RhD-negative blood donors.

Key Point: When used in emergency resuscitation, whole blood (that has not been made into components) should be type O and from a TRALI-mitigated donor. Routine stocking of RhD-positive whole blood is an acceptable strategy for emergency release due to the difficulty procuring RhD-negative units.

2. **Answer: C.** The only mandated hemovigilance system in the United States is the reporting of fatalities suspected to be due to transfusion or in blood donors. 32% of transfusion-associated fatalities in the United States annually are due to transfusion-associated circulatory overload (TACO). Laboratory practices and standards in the United States have focused on preventing transfusion reactions that can be mitigated using pretransfusion testing protocols, such as the requirement for two distinct specimens for patient ABO and RhD typing, rigid requirements for product labeling, and strict rules regarding donor and recipient identification. Moreover, patient factors are important in the natural history of an ABO-incompatible mistransfusion; that is, some patients can tolerate a large volume of incompatible blood transfusion, but others may experience serious effects with as little as 5 mL. Although ABO-incompatible transfusions can be fatal due to preformed isohemagglutinins, pretransfusion testing and transfusion administration protocols have substantially reduced acute hemolytic events and the delayed-type hemolytic reactions that can occur with RhD-incompatible transfusions are rarely fatal (A and B). Transfusion-associated graft-versus-host disease (TA-GVHD) is a rare complication of transfusion due to widespread protocols, including irradiation for at-risk patients. Leukoreduction and pathogen reduction techniques reduce TA-GVHD risks even further. The per-unit risk of TACO is ~1% for platelet and plasma components and ~2.7% for RBC transfusions. Patients with congestive heart failure, renal disease, atrial fibrillation, or

low total blood volumes are at particular risk of TACO. TACO can be prevented by transfusing at rates of about 2 to 4 mL/min in routine transfusion situations when the patient is not hemorrhaging. Once recognized, the transfusion should be stopped, oxygen support should be started, and interventions to remove volume, such as diuresis or even therapeutic phlebotomy may be necessary. TACO is largely underrecognized, and bedside providers performing transfusions are critical stakeholders in both reporting and reducing this transfusion complication.

Key Point: TACO is an underrecognized but serious complication of transfusion that is much more common than hemolytic reactions. In a patient with risk factors for circulatory overload, slow transfusion is preferred in the appropriate clinical context.

SECTION 18 TRANSPLANTS

18.1 Transplants: Lung, Heart, Liver, and Other Organs

1. **Answer: C.** Primary nonfunction (PNF) is a rare but serious complication following liver transplantation, characterized by the immediate failure of the transplanted liver to function. It typically presents within the first few days posttransplant with signs of worsening liver function, including elevated liver enzymes, coagulopathy, and encephalopathy, despite adequate blood flow to the graft. This condition necessitates urgent retransplantation.

2. **Answer: C.** Tacrolimus, a calcineurin inhibitor commonly used for immunosuppression after organ transplantation, can cause neurotoxic effects, including seizures. This is particularly relevant in the intensive care unit (ICU) setting, where patients may be receiving high doses or have fluctuating levels of the drug. The absence of other common causes of seizures (eg, electrolyte imbalance, infection, or stroke) and the recent initiation of tacrolimus make tacrolimus-induced neurotoxicity the most likely diagnosis. Seizures may occur due to elevated tacrolimus levels or increased sensitivity to the drug. Monitoring drug levels and adjusting the dosage are critical to managing this complication.

18.2 Organ Donation

1. **Answer: C.** Brain death results in a catecholamine storm caused by massive sympathetic discharge due to increased intracranial pressure and medullary herniation. This initially produces hypertension and tachycardia but is quickly followed by vasodilation, hypotension, and hypoperfusion, secondary to sympathetic depletion, spinal ischemia, and loss of vascular tone. This biphasic response contributes to global ischemia, especially in the myocardium, kidneys, and lungs, and requires aggressive hemodynamic management (fluids, inotropes, hormone replacement) to preserve organ viability.
   A. Option A and B represent secondary mechanisms.
   B. Option D is incorrect because coronary occlusion is not the primary mechanism.
   C. Option E misinterprets the nature of the catecholamine surge. While coronary blood flow may increase transiently, oxygen delivery to the myocardium is impaired, not improved.

2. **Answer: C.** In controlled donation after circulatory death (DCD), ethical integrity requires that decisions regarding withdrawal of care and declaration of death are made independently of the transplant team to avoid conflicts of interest. This is a cornerstone of maintaining public trust in the DCD process.
   A. Option A is incorrect: DCD kidneys are widely used, and although they carry a higher risk of delayed graft function, long-term outcomes are comparable to those from brain-dead donors.
   B. Option B is incorrect: functional warm ischemia time (fWIT) is a major determinant of liver viability, particularly regarding ischemic cholangiopathy and graft function.
   C. Option D is incorrect: thoracoabdominal normothermic regional perfusion (ta-NRP) is typically used in controlled DCD to improve organ perfusion and reduce ischemic injury.
   D. Option E is misleading: while some centers use a 5-minute waiting period, there is no mandatory 10-minute interval, and 2 to 5 minutes is the most commonly adopted duration based on ethical and physiologic considerations.

SECTION 19 TRAUMA MANAGEMENT

19.1 Fluid Resuscitation/Transfusion Guidelines

1. **Answer: B.** As long as the patient is able to maintain adequate mentation, targeting a systolic blood pressure around 90 mm Hg has been shown to decrease transfusion requirements and improve mortality. This is in keeping with the tenets of permissive hypotension in the trauma setting.

2. **Answer: D.** Blood product should be used when available to resuscitate a patient in hemorrhagic shock in order to correct the oxygen-carrying capacity deficit and coagulation deficit, which was lost due to hemorrhage, and to avoid further dilutional coagulopathy associated with crystalloids.

19.2 Basic Management

1. **Answer: C.** This patient with polytrauma is presenting with an open-book pelvic fracture in addition to multiple other injuries. He is not hypotensive as his mean arterial pressure (MAP) is 85, and though his tachycardia could be explained by hemorrhagic shock, pain from multiple bony fractures may also cause tachycardia. He should get a pan scan to evaluate the extent of his injuries prior to transport to an intensive care unit (ICU); however, *the presence of an open book pelvic fracture should result in a binder being placed as a reflexive initial step.* Central access in the groin should be avoided if possible due to the need for multiple interventions for pelvic fixation and possible hemorrhage control.

2. **Answer: B.** This patient is presenting with a penetrating injury to the right thigh and hard signs of vascular injury. Even if his blood pressure normalizes, he should be taken directly to the operating room for vascular exploration and repair of his arterial injury. X-rays may be useful in penetrating gunshot wounds to evaluate for bony fracture, but these can be performed in the operating room and are unlikely

with an arrow, given the relatively lower velocity. The arrow should not be removed until vascular control proximally and distally is obtained. A computed tomographic angiogram (CTA) is unnecessary if hard signs of vascular injury (pulselessness, pulsatile bleeding, loss of sensation/motor function, expanding hematoma).

19.3 FAST: Focused Assessment With Sonography

1. **Answer: C.** This patient is presenting with blunt trauma, hypotension, and a positive FAST examination. Any positive FAST in the setting of hypotension is hemorrhagic shock until proven otherwise. A computed tomography (CT) scan is not needed nor is any other confirmatory imaging. Additionally, a patient with trauma does not need central access to be adequately resuscitated; two large-bore peripheral intravenous (IV) are sufficient. The patient should be resuscitated with blood product and taken directly to the operating room (OR) for exploration to achieve hemorrhage control.

2. **Answer: D.** This patient is presenting with a penetrating injury concerning for heart or great vessel injury. FAST examination confirms this possibility. He is saturating well, and there may be some decompression of his pericardium into his left chest, but he does have signs of tension physiology. As he is not profoundly hypotensive, he should be transported directly to the OR for a pericardial window and likely sternotomy. A pericardiocentesis should be avoided as it does not address the underlying issue, and if there is a heart laceration, the patient may simply exsanguinate through a pericardial drain.

   A chest tube would not be beneficial as the hemothorax is small and the patient is saturating well. A central line is not needed. The patient should not be induced with anesthesia until his chest is prepped and draped, as the loss of sympathetic drive may result in cardiovascular collapse and death on induction. An Emergency department (ED) thoracotomy would not be indicated unless the patient lost vital signs.

19.4 Complications

1. **Answer: B.** Avascular necrosis (AVN) of the femoral head is a condition where the blood supply to the femoral head is interrupted, leading to bone cell death and subsequent collapse of the bone structure. Posterior fracture dislocations are commonly associated with a 10% incidence of AVN due to the higher likelihood of disrupting the blood vessels that supply the femoral head during the dislocation and fracture event.

2. **Answer: B.** Syndrome of inappropriate antidiuretic hormone secretion (SIADH) following traumatic brain injury typically presents with hyponatremia and concentrated urine (usually UOsm >300 mOsm) in the context of euvolemia or hypervolemia. It usually resolves spontaneously. The treatment involves fluid restriction and, if symptomatic, hypertonic saline; demeclocycline may be used in refractory cases.

3. **Answer: C.** In patients with retained hemothorax despite tube thoracostomy placement, the use of fibrinolytic agents such as tissue plasminogen activator (tPA) combined with DNase and/or early thoracoscopy within 7 days postinjury has been shown to decrease complications and shorten hospital stays.

SECTION 20 PEDIATRIC EMERGENCIES

20.1 Airway and Pulmonary Emergencies

1. **Answer: C.** The most likely diagnosis in this toxic-appearing child with tracheal irregularity on x-ray is bacterial tracheitis, which is commonly caused by *Staphylococcus aureus* and *Staphylococcus pneumoniae*. *Haemophilus influenzae* B (HIB), prior to the vaccine advent in 1985, commonly caused epiglottitis ("thumbprint sign"). Respiratory syncytial virus (RSV) and parainfluenza are normally associated with diagnoses of bronchiolitis and croup, respectively.

Key Point: *S. aureus* is a common pathogen identified in bacterial tracheitis. Typical x-ray findings in bacterial tracheitis include subglottic and tracheal narrowing and an irregular tracheal contour.

2. **Answer: D.** This child is demonstrating signs of impending respiratory failure with somnolence, bradypnea, and hypoxia. Intravenous dexamethasone and intramuscular epinephrine are mainstays of treatment of severe/refractory asthma exacerbations. High-flow nasal cannula is reasonable to trial in this patient with hypoxia as a temporizing method prior to intubation. Evidence for heliox in asthma is mixed, and it is not a good choice in patients who are hypoxic as it reduces the amount of supplemental oxygen able to be delivered.

Key Point: Heliox has theoretical utility in asthma, but evidence is mixed. It should be avoided in patients who are hypoxemic as it limits the deliverable amount of supplemental oxygen.

20.2 Surgical Emergencies

1. **Answer: B.** The neonate presenting in this vignette has physical examination findings consistent with gastroschisis, a full-thickness paraumbilical abdominal wall defect usually associated with evisceration of bowel and sometimes other organs. Neonates with gastroschisis can have profound fluid losses and are at risk for insensible fluid losses from exposure of the bowel and third spacing from sequestration of intestinal fluid. One of the first immediate steps in the delivery room is thermal and fluid regulation, including wrapping the bowel in sterile saline dressings covered with plastic wrap to preserve heat and minimize ongoing fluid losses. Surgical repair is typically performed in the first few hours of life. While checking for patency of the airway is an important first step, immediate intubation and/or use of positive pressure is not routinely necessary.

2. **Answer: A.** The child in this vignette has clinical and radiographic signs of intussusception, including the "target" sign on abdominal plain film. Intussusception refers to the telescoping of a part of the intestine into itself. It is the most common abdominal emergency in early childhood, particularly in children younger than 2 years of age. The diagnosis of intussusception is typically made by ultrasound by experienced technologists. The treatment of choice is typically nonoperative reduction using hydrostatic or pneumatic pressure by enema. This treatment relies on a patient who is clinically stable and appropriate radiologic facilities and personnel. While nonoperative reduction is typically successful, there is a risk of perforation and tension pneumoperitoneum during the procedure, necessitating the notification and availability of a pediatric surgeon. Surgical intervention also may be necessary if nonoperative reduction fails to reduce the

intussusception. Lethargy is a common presenting sign of intussusception and does not correlate with the severity of illness. While the radiographs in this film heighten concern for obstruction, given the dilated loops of bowel, the patient should be transferred to a center with pediatric surgical expertise regardless of whether obstruction is present or not.

20.3 Cardiovascular Emergencies

1. **Answer: B.** Given this pediatric patient has a narrow complex tachycardia with a rate of >180 and no visualized p waves on the cardiac monitor, the rhythm is concerning for supraventricular tachycardia (SVT). The patient is unresponsive and has weak pulses, which are evidence of cardiopulmonary compromise. These findings signify the patient is in an unstable SVT. Based on the Pediatric Advanced Life Support (PALS) algorithm, the treatment for unstable SVT involves synchronized cardioversion with an initial dose of 0.5 to 1 J/kg. If not effective, the next dose can be increased to 2 J/kg. Of note, vagal maneuvers and adenosine can be administered but should not delay synchronized cardioversion in the setting of unstable SVT. A dose of 200 J is common in the adult population but would be an inappropriate dose for a 2-year-old patient. Epinephrine would be a medication that is administered if the patient were to progress to cardiac arrest or shock necessitating vasoactive support.

2. **Answer: B.** The patients presenting clinical features of tachypnea, feeding difficulty, cyanosis, signs of poor perfusion (weak pulses, mottled extremities), hepatomegaly, and radiologic evidence of cardiomegaly with pulmonary edema are concerning for congestive heart failure (CHF). Given the patient's age, his CHF would most commonly be the result of a ductal-dependent congenital heart lesion, likely transposition of the great arteries (TGA). Congenital heart defects can be missed if there is limited access to prenatal care, and newborn infants can tolerate some cyanosis/hypoxia as they transition from fetal physiology. This infant's current presentation is likely in the setting of impending patent ductus arteriosus (PDA) closure and thus necessitates a prostaglandin infusion to maintain ductal patency. The administration of a 20 mL/kg fluid bolus could exacerbate respiratory distress by causing further pulmonary edema. Given the lack of fever, acetaminophen would not be indicated for this patient. Milrinone is a vasodilator medication that provides cardiac contractility and relaxation to help improve cardiac output but does have potential harmful side effects, including hypotension, kidney injury, and tachyarrhythmias. For stabilization, the infant above requires adequate oxygenation, which, at minimum, would require patency across the ductus arteriosus through a prostaglandin infusion and would not be achieved with an infusion of milrinone.

SECTION 21 ADVANCED CARDIAC LIFE SUPPORT (ACLS) AND ADVANCED TRAUMA LIFE SUPPORT (ATLS)

21.1 Advanced Cardiovascular Life Support and Advanced Trauma Life Support Guidelines

1. **Answer: A.** Postarrest patients are critically ill requiring support of multiple organ systems. Respiratory support includes intubation and lung protective ventilation. Hemodynamic goals include maintaining a systolic blood pressure >90 mm Hg and a mean arterial pressure >65 mm Hg with fluids and vasopressors. Evaluation for neurologic injury should receive as high a priority as evaluation for cardiac intervention. Neurologic injury is a frequent cause of death and disability postcardiac arrest and thus care should be focused on reducing injury to the brain by optimizing cerebral perfusion pressure, maintaining normocarbia, maintaining oxygenation with goal oxygen saturation of 92% to 98% (avoid hyperoxia), detecting and preventing seizures, and targeted temperature measurement (32-36 °C for 24 hours using a cooling device with a feedback loop) if the patient does not follow commands. Cardiac arrest due to shockable rhythms is associated with a high rate of severe coronary artery disease. Evaluation for cardiac intervention should start with a 12-lead electrocardiogram (ECG). While some studies have shown an association of improved outcomes with PCI, a large study that randomized over 500 patients successfully resuscitated from out-of-hospital cardiac arrest with no evidence of ST elevation to either immediate coronary angiography or coronary angiography after neurologic recovery found no difference in survival or neurologic outcomes. Emergent cardiac intervention is indicated in patients with ST-elevation myocardial infarction (STEMI) if the patient has unstable cardiogenic shock or requires mechanical circulatory support.

2. **Answer: C.** This patient has signs of inadequate perfusion including a narrow pulse pressure, tachycardia, tachypnea, vasoconstriction, and mental status changes. Patients with <30% blood volume loss usually do not have hypotension, tachycardia, and mental status changes (though tachycardia and decreased pulse pressure may occur with higher range blood loss). Other signs of higher blood volume loss (>31% blood volume) include base deficit >−6 mEq/L and decreased urine output. Some studies have questioned the validity of clinical signs used in the ATLS classification. There is some evidence that the Shock Index (heart rate/systolic blood pressure) and base deficit may better reflect blood loss in the trauma patient.

SECTION 22 POINT-OF-CARE ULTRASOUND IN THE ICU

22.1 Point-of-Care Ultrasound in the ICU

1. **Answer: C.** The subcostal four-chamber view is considered the best view for assessing pericardial effusion, because it provides a clear, unobstructed visualization of the pericardial space, particularly in critically ill patients where other views may be limited by lung interference or patient positioning. While this view is ideal, findings should be confirmed in other views, such as the parasternal or apical four-chamber views, to rule out artifacts and ensure diagnostic accuracy. The suprasternal notch view is primarily used to evaluate great vessels, such as the aortic arch, and is not suitable for pericardial assessment.

2. **Answer: A.** The lack of full compressibility of the vein when gentle pressure is applied with the ultrasound transducer is the primary diagnostic finding for deep vein thrombosis (DVT), with high sensitivity and specificity for thrombus.

A collapsed lumen typically results from external compression or normal physiology and suggests no thrombus at the imaging site. B-lines are vertical artifacts typically seen on lung ultrasound, originating from the pleural line, and are not typically associated with venous imaging. Gain artifacts are technical adjustments and not diagnostic findings.

SECTION 23 BURNS AND THERMAL INJURIES

23.1 Burns and Thermal Injuries

1. **Answer: C.** Inhalation injuries affecting the upper airway can rapidly progress to *airway edema and obstruction* due to thermal injury and inflammation. *Early intubation is critical* because airway swelling can make securing the airway increasingly difficult.
    - *High-flow oxygen* (option A) is useful but does not prevent worsening airway obstruction.
    - *Nebulized epinephrine* (option B) may help with mild airway edema but is not sufficient for impending obstruction.
    - *Bronchoscopy* (option D) is useful for diagnosing *lower airway injuries*, but it should not delay *airway protection*.

2. **Answer: A.** Early excision and grafting (within 48-72 hours) is the standard of care for deep partial-thickness and full-thickness burns covering a significant total body surface area (TBSA). This approach has been shown to reduce mortality, decrease infection risk, and shorten hospital stay by removing necrotic tissue and preventing systemic inflammatory complications.
    - Delayed excision (option B) increases the risk of sepsis and multiorgan failure due to prolonged exposure to necrotic tissue.
    - Enzymatic debridement (option C) can be helpful for smaller burns but is not a substitute for surgical excision in large burns.
    - Topical antimicrobials alone (option D) may help prevent infection but do not promote timely wound closure, leading to increased morbidity and mortality.

SECTION 24 DISASTER MANAGEMENT, EXPOSURES, AND OTHER ENVIRONMENTAL INJURIES

24.1 Mass Casualty, Triage, and Epidemic/Pandemic Response

1. **Answer: C.** In the initial response to a mass casualty incident (MCI), the foremost priority is scene safety. Ensuring the safety of responders and controlling ongoing hazards (e.g., fire, structural instability, active violence, hazardous materials) prevents additional injuries and preserves the ability to provide care. Without a safe scene, effective triage, treatment, and transport cannot occur. Rapid transport (A) and advanced on-site care (B) are secondary priorities that follow stabilization of the scene, while completing detailed medical histories (D) is inappropriate in the acute MCI phase, where rapid triage and life-saving interventions take precedence.

2. **Answer: B.** During a pandemic, triage systems are implemented to allocate limited health care resources effectively by prioritizing patients according to the severity of illness and likelihood of benefit from medical intervention. This approach aims to maximize overall outcomes when demand exceeds capacity. While isolation of infected patients (A) is an important infection control strategy, it is not the primary purpose of triage. Reducing the number of patients seeking care (C) is not a goal of triage, and ensuring equal attention and resources for all patients (D) is neither feasible nor appropriate during resource-constrained pandemic conditions, where care must be guided by clinical urgency and potential benefit.

24.2 Chemical, Biological, Radiological, and Nuclear Exposures

1. **Answer: B.** Chlorine gas exposure can cause acute lung injury and airway obstruction. Intubation and mechanical ventilation are critical to maintain oxygenation and prevent respiratory failure when oxygen therapy alone is insufficient. Corticosteroids and nebulized albuterol may be considered adjuncts, but definitive airway management is the priority. Imaging is secondary in acutely deteriorating patients.

2. **Answer: C.** The symptoms are consistent with organophosphate poisoning, which inhibits acetylcholinesterase, leading to an accumulation of acetylcholine. While atropine addresses muscarinic effects, pralidoxime reactivates acetylcholinesterase, targeting the root cause of toxicity. Diazepam is used for seizures, which may occur, but it does not address the enzymatic inhibition.

24.3 Drowning

1. **Answer: C.** Hypoxemia is the most common cause of cardiac arrest from drowning. Resuscitation should focus on rescue breaths in addition to chest compressions. Arrhythmias can occur from cold water exposure yet infrequently lead to cardiac arrest. Myocardial infarction may precipitate drowning in adults with coronary artery disease. Aspiration is common during drowning and may accelerate hypoxemia.

2. **Answer: B.** According to the Drowning Chain of Survival, a flotation device should be provided to a drowning victim after recognizing distress and calling for help. Jumping in the water to rescue the victim should occur only if conditions are safe and the rescuer has appropriate training.

24.4 Hanging and Strangulation

1. **Answer: C.** Long-drop hanging is still a method used for execution in parts of the world. The drop distance is at least the height of the subject, and the intended outcome is a cervical spine injury. In cases when this is not achieved, asphyxiation may occur. If the drop distance is exceedingly high, decapitation can occur.

2. **Answer: B.** Direct compression of and traction on the jugular veins and neck arterial vessels from hanging can result in cerebral edema and vertebral artery dissection. Although the mechanism is not firmly established, vertebral artery dissection is one suspected etiology behind the presence of subarachnoid hemorrhages seen in victims of hanging. High

cervical spine injuries, such as Hangman fractures, are commonly seen in longer drop distances.

24.5 Altitude Injury

1. **Answer: B.** Acetazolamide helps prevent and treat altitude sickness by inhibiting an enzyme called carbonic anhydrase in the kidneys, leading to bicarbonate excretion and a mild metabolic acidosis that stimulates breathing and enhances oxygenation, thereby speeding up acclimatization. Acetazolamide is more commonly used and better validated for use as prophylaxis. Dexamethasone is more effective than acetazolamide at rapidly relieving the symptoms of moderate-to-severe altitude sickness.

2. **Answer: C.** High altitude cerebral edema (HACE) is a severe and potentially fatal condition associated with high altitude illness that is often thought of as a late or end-stage acute mountain sickness (AMS). It is often characterized by ataxia, fatigue, and altered mental status.

SECTION 25 INTENSIVE CARE UNIT PROPHYLAXIS

25.1 Prophylaxes and Harm Reduction in the Intensive Care Unit

1. **Answer: D.** Stress ulcer prophylaxis is recommended for intensive care unit (ICU) patients at high (4%-8%) and highest (8%-10%) risk of gastrointestinal (GI) bleed. This patient is at high risk of GI bleed based on the presence of coagulopathy with an international normalized ratio (INR) >1.7 not on anticoagulation as well as shock with acute kidney injury. Other key risk factors—which are not present in this patient—include mechanical ventilation with and without enteral nutrition as well as chronic liver disease. All stress ulcer prophylaxes should be ordered on a standing basis. Once-daily proton pump inhibitors (PPIs) are the agent of choice for gastric acid suppression for critically ill patients at sufficient risk. Histamine-2 receptor antagonists (H2RAs) comprise a second-line option that can be used when the patient has an allergy to PPIs or is receiving other medications whose metabolism may be affected by PPI (eg, certain antiretrovirals). H2RAs are typically dosed at least twice per day for stress ulcer prophylaxis.

Key Point: A standing PPI is the agent of choice for stress ulcer prophylaxis in patients at high risk of GI bleed.

2. **Answer: B.** The ICU Liberation or ABCDEF Bundle is an evidence-based, society-recommended collection of assessments and interventions intended to be reviewed daily for each ICU patient to lower the risk of a variety of avoidable outcomes—including mortality, ICU readmission, delirium, and the use of physical restraints—using evidence-based interventions. The acronym stands for Assess, prevent, and manage pain; Both spontaneous awakening and breathing trials daily; Choice of sedation and analgesia should be individualized; Delirium assessment, management, and prevention; Early mobility and exercise; and Family engagement and empowerment at the bedside. This older patient has a history of chronic low back pain, which, if not evaluated and addressed, could increase her risk of delirium and subsequent complications. The other management decisions, while important, are not part of the ABCDEF bundle.

Key Point: The ABCDEF ICU liberation bundle of evidence-based interventions prompts clinicians to address some of the risks inherent to ICU care that can be easily overlooked.

SECTION 26 PROCEDURES

26.1 Tracheostomy

1. **Answer: C.** Option A is incorrect because high-flow nasal cannula is not a durable airway. While the patient may be currently maintaining her oxygen saturations, she was requiring positive pressure ventilatory support prior to inadvertent decannulation and still requires significant amounts of supplemental oxygen. Option B is incorrect as replacement of the tracheostomy tube through an immature tract (<7 days) is a dangerous maneuver that should not be attempted. There is high potential for creation of a false passage in the subcutaneous and pretracheal spaces. Ventilatory support in the extratracheal space has the potential to cause subcutaneous emphysema, pneumomediastinum, and tension pneumothorax exacerbating the respiratory decline. Option C is correct because in the setting of impending respiratory failure, orotracheal intubation is the safe and correct maneuver. Option D is incorrect because cricothyroidotomy should not be performed if transoral endotracheal intubation is feasible.

2. **Answer: B.** Option A is incorrect because although the patient may benefit from additional antibiotics, his primary issue is secretion management and poor mental status, which would be better addressed with a tracheostomy. Patients who have suffered a significant neurologic event, such as a significant stroke, are at high risk of prolonged intubation and ventilator-associated complications, making tracheostomy a preferable option. Option B is correct because the patient has multiple indications for a tracheostomy, including neurologic injury and difficulty managing secretions. A tracheostomy would provide easier secretion management and a more stable airway as the patient recovers from the stroke and reduces the risk of further ventilator-associated complications. Option C is incorrect because while additional antibiotics may be beneficial, delaying the tracheostomy in a patient who has already failed extubation after a prolonged intubation would increase the risk of ventilator-associated complications. Option D is incorrect because the patient is at high risk of failing extubation again after a major neurologic event, ventilator-associated pneumonia, and reintubation. Mucolytic therapy may be useful for conditions like cystic fibrosis or chronic obstructive pulmonary disease (COPD), where mucous trapping is a significant issue. However, this patient's overwhelming secretions are more likely due to deconditioning and neurologic impairment, which requires durable access for effective secretion management, making a tracheostomy the best solution.

26.2 Cricothyroidotomy

1. **Answer: C.** The patients in each of these options have potential indications for cricothyroidotomy. However, unlike in the other scenarios, this patient in "C" is not able to be oxygenated.

2. **Answer: C.** This is a "Cannot Intubate, Cannot Oxygenate" (CICO) scenario. The patient requires an emergent cricothyroidotomy, which eliminates options "B" and "D." The Difficult Airway Society deems that the open cricothyroidotomy technique is faster and more reliable than the percutaneous technique.

26.3 Bronchoscopy

1. **Answer: C.** Option A is incorrect; while increasing supplemental oxygen may temporize this patient's shortness of breath and hypoxia, it does not address the underlying cause of his symptoms. Option B is incorrect, as a nebulizer would appropriately treat bronchospasm, which is common after bronchoscopy. While bronchospasm may be associated with shortness of breath and hypoxia, pleuritic chest pain is atypical and raises concern for pneumothorax in this patient who underwent transbronchial lung biopsy. This should be further investigated with a portable chest x-ray. Option C is correct, as the constellation of shortness of breath, pleuritic chest pain, and hypoxia after transbronchial lung biopsy is concerning for postprocedural pneumothorax. The most appropriate next step is to obtain a chest x-ray. This can be performed at the bedside. Transbronchial lung biopsy entails violation of the visceral pleura during specimen collection, posing a risk of air leak and consequent pneumothorax. Risk factors for pneumothorax include the type of biopsy forceps, use of mechanical ventilation, presence of emphysema, lesion location, and number of samples taken. Option D is incorrect, as repeat bronchoscopy is unlikely to diagnose or treat the underlying cause of this patient's symptoms.

2. **Answer: D.** Option A is incorrect, as the multiple small lumens represent segmental bronchi, indicating that the tracheostomy tube is within the right mainstem bronchus and is too long for the patient. Option B is incorrect, as both end-tidal CO_2 and bronchoscopy have confirmed placement of the tracheostomy tube within the tracheobronchial tree and suggest adequate ventilation. Endotracheal intubation is, therefore, unnecessary, and a shorter tracheostomy tube may be inserted through the same tract. Option C is incorrect, as chest x-ray is unnecessary as flexible bronchoscopy clearly demonstrates placement of the tracheostomy tube within the right mainstem bronchus. Detailed knowledge of airway anatomy is critical for all bronchoscopists to identify complications such as those presented in the vignette. Option D is correct, as the bronchoscopist is currently visualizing the division of the right upper lobe bronchus and bronchus intermedius. This indicates that the tracheostomy tube is in the right mainstem bronchus and is too long for the patient. The most appropriate next step is to insert a shorter tracheostomy tube. Flexible bronchoscopy should be repeated thereafter to confirm visualization of the carina and hence appropriate positioning of the tracheostomy tube in the trachea.

26.4 Tube Thoracostomy (Chest Tube)

1. **Answer: C.** Reexpansion pulmonary edema is a common complication after quick drainage of a large amount of pleural fluid due to rapid reexpansion of the lung.

2. **Answer: A.** Percutaneous technique required in the insertion of small-bore catheters is not recommended when the lung is not collapsed, eliminating choices "B" and "D." A 30F catheter is not superior to a 28F catheter, and there is no indication in this case for an angled chest tube.

26.5 Thoracentesis, Paracentesis, and Pericardiocentesis

1. **Answer: C.** This patient underwent a large volume paracentesis and has developed paracentesis-induced circulatory dysfunction (PICD), typically seen when greater than 5 L of ascites fluid is removed at one time. Albumin replacement should be between 6 and 8 g/L removed; therefore, 75 g should be sufficient for this patient. The mechanism of this hypotension is due to a combination of arteriole vasodilation, compensatory reaction of the renin-angiotensin-aldosterone system (RAAS) following abrupt changes in intrabdominal pressure, and proinflammatory response. Often patients with cirrhosis are dependent on their systemic vascular resistance to maintain their mean adequate pressure (MAP) due to poor cardiac compensation. Albumin mitigates PICD by exerting a higher oncotic pressure to maintain intravascular volume and suppress RAAS and maintaining blood volume. Twenty-five grams of albumin would not be sufficient for the volume removed. Fresh frozen plasma (FFP) and blood products will improve oncotic pressure but are not indicated in this patient. Crystalloids, such as lactated ringers, do not exert the same oncotic pressure as albumin.

2. **Answer: A.** Using a pleural pressure monitor. The patient is experiencing reexpansion pulmonary edema. Pleural pressure monitoring reduces the incidence of reexpansion pulmonary edema (RPE). It is critical to avoid a pleural pressure drop below −20 mm H_2O or a decline of more than 10 cm H_2O between two measurements to a value less than or equal to −10 mm H_2O. This threshold indicates cessation of fluid removal to avoid RPE. Manometry should be performed at the beginning of the procedure and after every 250 mL of fluid withdrawn. There are some studies that show prophylactic continuous positive airway pressure (CPAP) reduces the risk of RPE, but more studies are needed to standardize this care. There is no data supporting a particular patient position to reduce the risk of RPE. Vasopressors do not reduce the risk of RPE.

26.6 Feeding Tube Placement

1. **Answer: D.** Abdominal ascites, coagulopathy, and a ventral hernia pose relative contraindications to percutaneous endoscopic gastrostomy (PEG) placement but can typically be managed appropriately to allow for safe PEG placement. While a lack of an obvious window on computed tomography (CT) should raise concerns about a safe tract for PEG placement, the inability to endoscopically access the stomach or clear transillumination of the abdominal wall after gastric insufflation should result in abandonment of the procedure.

2. **Answer: D.** Tract maturation occurs between 4 and 6 weeks, thus enabling safe removal with minimal risk for peritonitis. Removal of a tube without surgical closure of the gastrocutaneous fistula prior to this 4- to 6-week period may result in free leakage of gastric contents into the peritoneum. It is important to consider nutrition and patient-specific wound healing factors, as these may influence your timeline for PEG removal.

SECTION 27 INTENSIVE CARE UNIT TRANSPORT

27.1 Intensive Care Unit Transport

1. **Answer: D.** Patient monitoring during transport should remain at the same level as before transport and should not be decreased. Transport is associated with acute hemodynamic instability; immediate recognition and management are critical.

2. **Answer: C.** Simple pneumothorax may convert to tension pneumothorax at altitude during air transport. Ground transportation is the safest option for relatively short distances and to avoid altitude changes associated with aircraft.

SECTION 28 EPIDEMIOLOGY AND BIOSTATISTICS

28.1 Epidemiology and Biostatistics

1. **Answer: B.** Case-control studies start with diseased individuals, making them efficient for *rare diseases* and allowing the evaluation of multiple exposures. Cross-sectional and cohort designs are inefficient for rare outcomes.

2. **Answer: C.** The Sequential Organ Failure Assessment (SOFA) score is dynamic, with increasing values indicating worsening organ dysfunction and a higher risk of death.

3. **Answer: B.** The c-statistic (also known as the *concordance statistic*), provides a measure of how good a model is at correctly classifying outcomes. It has the following interpretations:
   - A value below 0.5 indicates a poor model.
   - A value of 0.5 indicates that the model is no better at classifying outcomes than random chance.
   - The closer the value is to 1, the better the model is at correctly classifying outcomes.
   - A value of 1 means that the model is perfect at classifying outcomes.

Thus, the c-statistic of 0.82 means that the model has good discrimination to differentiate patients who will fail extubation from those who will succeed.

SECTION 29 INFECTION CONTROL

29.1 Infection Control

1. **Answer: C.** Although the subclavian central line is thought to carry the lowest risk of infection, followed by the jugular access and then the femoral, its placement should also take into account the risk of developing other complications, such as bleeding or pneumothorax.

2. **Answer: A.** SARS-CoV-2 requires airborne precautions. *Neisseria meningitidis*, rubella virus, and *Haemophilus influenzae* all require droplet precautions.

SECTION 30 EMERGENT AIRWAY MANAGEMENT

30.1 Emergent Airway Management

1. **Answer: C.** Supraglottic airway (SGA) devices provide a rapid, effective means of adequate ventilation when traditional intubation methods and bag mask ventilation are unsuccessful. Use of SGAs as the next step in unanticipated cannot ventilation-cannot intubate emergent airway management (EAM) scenarios may allow more time for difficult airway equipment and personnel to be available and review how to proceed. Use of SGA device after failed intubation is recommended by the American Society of Anesthesiologists and the Difficult Airway Society.

   Cricothyrotomy provides rapid, temporary access to the airway, allowing for immediate ventilation, and is typically used in emergency situations. In unanticipated difficult airway management, surgical airway techniques like cricothyrotomy and tracheostomy serve as critical, last-resort options when noninvasive methods, including SGAs and endotracheal intubation, fail.

   After initial unsuccessful laryngoscopy attempts by experienced personnel using appropriate equipment, continued laryngoscopy attempts are often a manifestation of task fixation. This should be avoided unless there is reasonable evidence that a change of personnel, equipment, or technique will lead to success.

   Extracorporeal membrane oxygenation (ECMO) is a crucial adjunct in extreme cases where conventional airway management techniques fail and/or rapid deterioration occurs, offering a bridge to definitive airway management. It is not a first-line intervention due to its complexity and resource requirements.

2. **Answer: B.** Hemodynamic instability during the induction of anesthesia for emergency airway management is common, potentially complicating an already high-risk scenario. Ideally, potentially modifiable risk factors for hemodynamic instability, including hypovolemia and acute blood loss anemia, should be corrected prior to the induction of anesthesia. However, many EAM situations do not afford time for such correction. Availability of appropriate venous access, vasopressors, and intravenous (IV) fluids should be ensured for EAM. Preparation and aggressive management of hemodynamic instability may decrease the risk of progression to life-threatening hemodynamic compromise and cardiac arrest.

   Severe hypoxia may occur in 9% to 15% of patients during EAM. Patients with severe lung disease are at higher risk.

   Aspiration of gastric contents, causing aspiration pneumonia or pneumonitis, is less frequent than hemodynamic instability. Rapid sequence intubation, deep level of muscle relaxation prior to laryngoscopy, and suctioning out stomach contents if an appropriate gastric tube is already in place can potentially reduce the risk of aspiration of gastric contents.

   The INTUBE study, an international, prospective, observational study of emergency, out-of-OR (operation room) intubation practices, found that 43% patients had cardiovascular instability, 9% patients had severe hypoxia, and 3% patients suffered cardiac arrest.

30.2 Tracheostomy Complications

1. **Answer: D.** Subcutaneous emphysema and/or pneumomediastinum can occur if the tracheostomy tube is placed into a false passage anterior to the trachea rather than the lumen of the trachea itself. It can also occur if the guidewire punctures the posterior or lateral wall of the trachea during placement of a percutaneous tracheostomy. If suspected, a chest radiograph should be obtained and a chest tube placed for pneumothorax, if indicated. If confirmed, the tracheostomy tube should be removed, and ventilation continued via placement of an endotracheal tube.

2. **Answer: B.** Tracheostomy can damage the tracheal cartilage at the stoma or cuff site, respectively, which weakens the tracheal wall, leading to tracheomalacia. Management of cuff pressures is important to prevent tracheomalacia. Factors that can affect cuff pressure include tracheal size, tracheostomy tube size, ventilatory pressures, and patient position. Maintaining a cuff pressure range between 20 and 30 cm H_2O is recommended in adult patients to prevent tracheal injury. When tracheomalacia occurs due to an overinflated cuff, the walls protrude at the level of the cuff and become weakened. If the patient is on mechanical ventilation, there may be a persistent leak. If more air is placed into the cuff to achieve a seal, this can then further damage the tracheal wall. If the diagnosis is confirmed for tracheomalacia, the tracheostomy may be changed to a longer tracheostomy tube to bypass the level of tracheal wall damage and create an optimal seal.

30.3 Neck Hematomas

1. **Answer: C.** High venous pressure that occurs during the Valsalva response during coughing or vomiting is associated with neck hematoma formation. Preoperative risk factors for the development of neck hematoma include high blood pressures, preoperative antiplatelet agents, coagulopathy, high venous pressures during coughing and vomiting, and certain surgical techniques.

2. **Answer: C.** This postthyroidectomy patient with asymmetric neck is at a high risk for a postoperative neck hematoma formation. Her symptomatology of dyspnea and dysphagia and her physical examination findings of stridor and asymmetric neck swelling support this diagnosis. These patients are at risk for imminent airway collapse, and securing the airway is essential. The airway is often difficult due to soft tissue edema from venous and lymphatic drainage obstruction and direct distortion. Surgical airway may be necessary; therefore, STAT surgical airway consultation is recommended. A computed tomography (CT) of the neck may be appropriate; however, airway must take priority. A recurrent laryngeal nerve palsy may cause similar symptoms but is not typically associated with an asymmetric neck.

30.4 Laryngectomy and Tracheal Reconstruction

1. **Answer: B.** If a patient is less than 7 postoperative days from a laryngectomy, there is a risk of creating a false tract with any device manipulation in the stoma. If any intervention is done, it should be performed with a fiberoptic bronchoscope and ideally with the primary surgical team at bedside. Initial management should thus focus on establishing mask ventilation over the stoma. After 7 to 10 postoperative days, the patient may be intubated with a 6.0 cuffed endotracheal tube in the stoma (ideally over the fiberoptic scope or bougie).

2. **Answer: A.** Carotid blowout syndrome (CBS) occurs when carotid or branch vessels rupture due to poor tissue integrity due to erosion or direct tumor invasion. It most frequently occurs in patients with advanced or recurrent tumors that have required aggressive treatment. The most important risk factor for CBS after surgery is previous irradiation of the neck. Patients may present with a sentinel bleed or a catastrophic hemorrhage from either the neopharynx or the stoma. Computed tomographic (CT) angiography of the head and neck is the next best study to confirm the diagnosis once the patient has been stabilized. Management may entail intubating the stoma with a cuffed airway device, providing external compression, and activating massive transfusion protocol while awaiting definitive surgical or interventional management.

SECTION 31 PREOPERATIVE EVALUATION FOR SURGERY

31.1 Preoperative Assessment

1. **Answer: A.** The six independent risk factors for major postoperative complications of the Lee Revised Cardiac Risk Index (RCRI) are as follows:
   - High-risk surgical procedure
   - Ischemic heart disease
   - Congestive heart failure
   - History of cerebrovascular disease
   - Insulin treatment
   - Creatinine >2 mg/dL

This patient has three risk factors: high-risk surgical procedure, congestive heart failure, and type 2 diabetes mellitus on insulin. Hypertension is not a risk factor cited in the RCRI.

2. **Answer: C.** This patient consumed toast, which is considered a light solid food. See the following table for the minimum fasting periods for the types of ingested material.

Ingested Material	Minimum Fasting Period (h)
Clear liquids	2
Breast milk	4
Infant formula	6
Nonhuman milk	6
Light solid foods	6
Full meal	8

SECTION 32 ICU ADMINISTRATION AND PRACTICE MANAGEMENT

32.1 Intensive Care Unit Administration and Practice Management

1. **Answer: B.** In conceptualizing an intensive care unit (ICU) workforce, it can be helpful to categorize constituents into

constant, cyclic, or temporary groups as each has unique considerations and needs. In this example, the attending physician works cyclically in the ICU, which is to say that their professional time is likely divided between multiple commitments. Cyclic team members, especially those who are new, may not have a collective memory of the unit equal to that of more constant workforce elements and may lack familiarity with routine processes and procedures, especially those that are dynamic. In contrast, more constant workforce elements (eg, nurses) typically have the best longitudinal knowledge of an ICU's workflows, while temporary workforce elements (eg, trainees) lack such insights to the greatest extent.

2. **Answer: A.** Setting goals and developing strategies to meet them is a key element of ICU administration. Best practices in this process include the engagement of those responsible for executing strategies during the planning process. This helps to increase buy-in and also increases the likelihood that the agreed-upon processes will account for unit-level practice and cultural nuances. Approaches that subvert team member buy-in, such as zero-tolerance policies and lengthy education, have not been associated with success. Furthermore, education has been demonstrated to be less effective in promoting change as compared to architecting process improvement, such as standardization.

SECTION 33 QUALITY IMPROVEMENT AND PATIENT SAFETY

33.1 Quality Improvement and Patient Safety

1. **Answer: A.** With the ever-increasing growth in available medications, administration medication occurs at any point in the medication prescription or administration, the latter is more often recognized in the anesthesiology practice. Furthermore, in this specific setting in the postanesthesia care unit (PACU), the nursing staff is administering medications prescribed by anesthesiologists. A long-standing nursing principle is known as the "Five Rights" (right patient, right route, right dose, right time, right drug). Thus, it is expected that the nurse make the "Five Rights" before administering medication to a patient. Interestingly, some others have argued to have additional checks right action, right response, or even right of patient to refuse a medication). Indeed, the additions to the "Five Rights" illustrate the limitations of human vigilance as a safety bulwark. Although checklist is considered a method to ensure adherence to key care processes, their most application and impact has been in supporting teamwork and improving surgical safety. Preventing unnecessary distractions and interruptions at the time of medication administration is utmost important. Therefore, simultaneous use of mobile devices by multiple providers even for purposes of getting medication-related information is inappropriate. Double-check is a well-known method utilized in other high-risk industries (aviation, navy) to ensure that critical processes are executed correctly. Whenever double-check is required by policy, it is critical to ensure that they are independent.

Key Point: In addition to computerized physician order entry (CPOE) and computerized decision support, other important medication safety strategies include standardization, checking "Five Rights," double-checks, preventing unnecessary distractions and interruptions, and performing medication reconciliation at the time of care transitions.

2. **Answer: B.** The Joint Commission emphasizes accountability and performance of evidence-based processes that lead to improved health outcomes. Therefore, best practices such as delivering lung-protective mechanical ventilation in the perioperative period have been proposed as another quality metric. A PDSA is a systematic, iterative approach used to drive continuous improvement in processes and implement change. It is particularly useful in small-scale testing and iterative learning through quick experimentation. Indeed, it is often used for refining processes over time, with an emphasis on rapid cycles of improvement and flexibility. The DMAIC is a framework utilized under the Six Sigma data–driven approach for improving existing processes. The DMAIC uses statistical tools to analyze data in the *Analyze* phase. Additionally, it is a more rigorous approach to process improvement. Given its strong emphasis on statistical analysis and focus on reducing variation and achieving process control, it is the best methodology to reduce defects. In this case, it will be a specific decrease in cases receiving tidal volume over 8 mL/kg (predicted body weight). The 5 S method is more focused on eliminating waste, teamwork, productivity, and enhance efficiency. It was popularized by Toyota as it demonstrated the lean manufacturing principles. The FMEA is a systematic approach utilized to identify potential failures, assess their impact, and prioritize actions to mitigate risks. It is more helpful in the early design or process stages to improve the quality, reliability, and safety of health care organization services.

Key Point: The DMAIC process is mostly used in the Six Sigma frameworks, and it is typically used for solving specific, significant problems in processes with a focus on defining measurable improvements.

SECTION 34 ETHICS AND MEDICAL LEGAL ISSUES

34.1 Ethics and Medical Legal Issues

1. **Answer: B. Beneficence** refers to the duty of health care providers to act in the best interest of the patient—promoting well-being, preventing harm, and removing existing harm when possible. The right to self-govern without undue influence from a health care provider describes autonomy (A is incorrect). The goal to promote the greatest benefit to the largest number of individuals while inflicting the least amount of harm reflects is incorrect as beneficence is focused on the individual patient's welfare, not the collective good (C is incorrect). The need to refrain from inflicting harm describes the principle of non-maleficence (D is incorrect).

2. **Answer: B.** Obtaining informed consent allows patients (or their surrogates, in the critically ill setting) to understand their diagnosis, the risks/benefits of proposed interventions, alternatives, and the potential outcomes, thereby protecting the patient's autonomy. While documentation of informed consent can provide some medicolegal protection, this is not its primary purpose (A is incorrect). Hospitals require

consent for certain procedures, but this is a procedural requirement, not the core ethical reason (C is incorrect). Medical history is collected separately during history taking, not through the consent process (D is incorrect).

SECTION 35 PALLIATIVE MEDICINE AND END-OF-LIFE CARE

35.1 Palliative Medicine and End-of-Life Care

1. **Answer: B.** The chapter defines palliative sedation as a last-resort, ethically justified intervention based on the principle of double effect, used when symptoms are otherwise unmanageable. The following answer options are incorrect because:
    - C. *Incorrect.* Palliative sedation is not euthanasia—the intent is to relieve suffering, not to cause death.
    - A. *Incorrect.* Palliative sedation is not a routine treatment for anxiety; it is reserved for *refractory* symptoms in imminently dying patients.
    - D. *Incorrect.* Shared decision-making and clear documentation are essential; families and/or surrogates should be part of the process.

2. **Answer: C.** Primary palliative care in the intensive care unit (ICU) is performed by the existing ICU team—this includes conducting family meetings, addressing emotional needs, and early assessment of symptom burden. The following answers are incorrect because:
    - A. *Incorrect.* This describes specialty (secondary) palliative care, not primary palliative care.
    - B. *Incorrect.* Modern palliative care is not restricted to the terminal phase; it should be integrated early and alongside curative treatments.
    - D. *Incorrect.* This is a feature of integrative/mixed palliative care models, where prognostic triggers may automatically initiate a specialty consult.

SECTION 36 HEALTH CARE DISPARITIES AND DIVERSITY, EQUITY, AND INCLUSION IN HEALTH CARE

36.1 Health Care Disparities

1. **Answer: C.** This vignette highlights the significant impact of racial and ethnic disparities on maternal health care outcomes. Ashley's experience underscores a broader systemic issue where Black women face higher risks of maternal morbidity and mortality, often due to inadequate pain management and biased clinical decision-making. This vignette illustrates how these disparities can lead to increased anxiety and concern among Black pregnant women about their care quality, potentially impacting their overall health and pregnancy outcomes.

Key Point: Racial and ethnic disparities in health care significantly affect the quality of care and health outcomes for minority patients. Addressing these disparities requires systemic changes, including bias training for health care providers and ensuring equitable access to quality care for all patients, especially in critical areas like maternal health.

2. **Answer: B.** This vignette highlights how previous negative experiences with bias due to socioeconomic status and language barriers can lead to distrust and concerns about the quality of care at the end of life. Mrs Rodriguez's family's apprehensions reflect broader systemic issues where patients from low socioeconomic backgrounds and minority groups often face disparities in the management and quality of end-of-life care. These disparities can lead to more aggressive treatments and a lack of alignment with patient and family preferences for palliative care.

Key Point: Socioeconomic and language barriers significantly impact the quality and decision-making of end-of-life care. These disparities can result in mistrust and a preference for more aggressive treatments among patients and their families. Addressing these issues requires improving cultural competence, reducing provider biases, and ensuring that patient and family preferences are respected and integrated into care plans.

36.2 Diversity, Equity, and Inclusion in Health Care

1. **Answer: C.** Reviewing and revising the selection criteria and processes is a critical first step because it directly addresses potential systemic barriers that may be preventing underrepresented in medicine (URiM) candidates from being selected. While increasing advertising, implementing mentorship programs, and hosting workshops are all beneficial actions, they do not address potential biases in the selection process itself, which is essential for creating a truly inclusive program.

Key Point: Ensuring that selection criteria and processes are fair and unbiased is essential for improving diversity in residency programs.

2. **Answer: B.** The ACTION framework provides a structured and respectful way to address sensitive issues. By having a private conversation and using this framework, Dr Lee can help Dr Johnson understand the impact of his behavior without causing public embarrassment or defensiveness. This approach is more likely to result in a positive change in behavior. Options A and C might escalate the situation without resolving the underlying issue, and option D puts undue pressure on the trainees rather than addressing the root cause.

Key Point: Using structured frameworks like ACTION for private, respectful conversations can effectively address and change problematic behaviors in the workplace.

Index

Note: Page numbers followed by "f" indicate figure; those followed by "t" indicate table.

B

J

K

L

Q

R